D0531827

American
Medical
Association

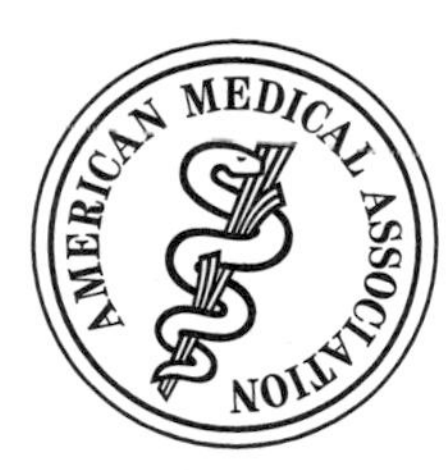

Complete Guide to Women's Health

Other books by the American Medical Association

American Medical Association Family Medical Guide

American Medical Association Encyclopedia of Medicine

American Medical Association Guide to Your Family's Symptoms

American Medical Association Seven Weeks to Better Sex

American Medical Association Handbook of First Aid and Emergency Care

American Medical Association Pocket Guide to Emergency First Aid

American Medical Association Pocket Guide to Sports First Aid

American Medical Association Pocket Guide to Calcium

American Medical Association Pocket Guide to Back Pain

American Medical Association

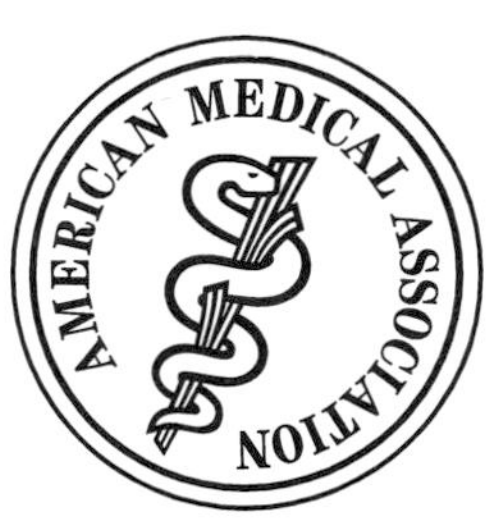

Complete Guide to Women's Health

Ramona I. Slupik, MD
Medical Editor

Written by
Kathleen Cahill Allison

Produced by
Alison Brown Cerier Book Development, Inc.

Random House New York

The recommendations and information in this book are appropriate in most cases; however, they are not a substitute for medical diagnosis. For specific information concerning your personal medical condition, the AMA suggests that you consult a physician. The names of organizations, products, or alternative therapies appearing in the book are given for informational purposes only. Their inclusion does not imply AMA endorsement, nor does the omission of any organization, product, or alternative therapy indicate AMA disapproval.

Photographs of healthy bone and bone with osteoporosis on page 34, copyright SPL/Custom Medical Stock Photo

Photographs of muscle tissue, coronary angiogram, and healthy artery and narrowed (atherosclerotic) artery on pages 35, 36, and 37, copyright Custom Medical Stock Photo

Photograph of fibroid on page 38, copyright Binor/Custom Medical Stock Photo

Photograph of mammogram on page 39, copyright Moore/Custom Medical Stock Photo

Photograph of conception on page 40, copyright Rawlins/Custom Medical Stock Photo

Chart, "Body mass index," on page 97, reprinted by permission of *Western Journal of Medicine* (George A. Bray and David S. Gray, "Obesity," 1988, volume 149: 429.41)

Table, "Healthy weights for women," on page 99, reprinted Courtesy of Metropolitan Life Insurance Company

Photographs of mammograms on page 277, copyright Richard D'Amico/Custom Medical Stock Photo

Chart, "What is your risk of acquiring an STD?" on page 336, adaptation of "Sex and Infection Risk," reprinted with permission of the Association of Reproductive Health Professionals

Photographs of malignant melanoma on page 685, courtesy of the American Academy of Dermatology

Library of Congress Cataloging-in-Publication Data
American Medical Association complete guide to women's health .
p. cm.
ISBN 0-679-43122-5
1.Women—Health and hygiene. I. American Medical Association.
RA778.A485 1996
613' .04244—dc20 96-33738

Produced by Alison Brown Cerier Book Development, Inc.
Random House website address:
http://www.randomhouse.com

Printed in the United States of America
on acid-free paper
9 8 7 6 5 4 3 2
First Edition

American Medical Association

Physicians dedicated to the health of America

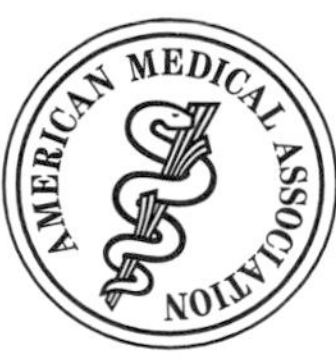

Foreword

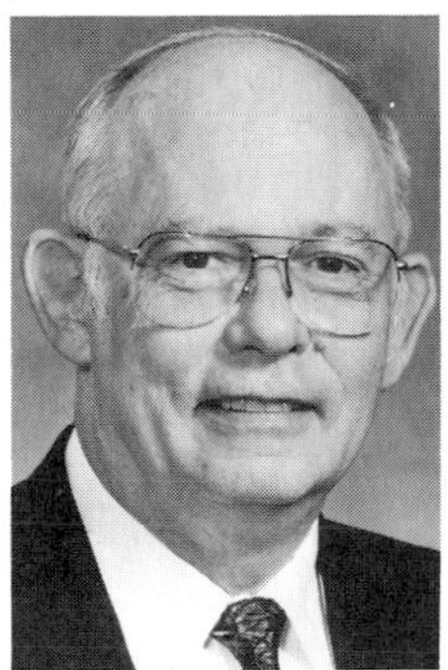

Women today have access to more information than ever before about health, including the basic knowledge they need to live a healthier, longer life. Medicine has made great strides in its understanding of how to prevent some of the most serious diseases that many women face—including heart disease (the number-one killer of American women), diabetes, osteoporosis, and some forms of cancer.

The ***American Medical Association Complete Guide to Women's Health*** can help you determine the steps you need to take—whether you are a teenager or a senior citizen—to feel better today and avoid serious illness in the future. In these pages, you will also find detailed information about a wide variety of disorders. The more knowledge you have about an illness that affects you or a loved one, the more effectively you will be able to work with your doctors to make informed decisions about treatments.

This book guides you through routine health care; complicated subjects, such as cancer and genetics; and difficult issues, such as domestic violence and rape. We at the American Medical Association hope that the ***American Medical Association Complete Guide to Women's Health*** becomes a useful reference for you, your family, and friends when you are seeking medical information or are faced with important medical decisions.

P. John Seward, MD
Executive Vice President

The American Medical Association

	P. John Seward, MD	*Executive Vice President*
	James F. Rappel	*Group Vice President, Business and Management Services*
	Larry Jellen	*Vice President, Marketing*
	M. Frances Dyra	*Director, Product Line Development*
Editorial Staff	Ramona I. Slupik, MD	*Medical Editor*
	Dorothea Guthrie	*Managing Editor*
	Donna Kotulak	*Senior Editor*
	Robin Fitzpatrick Husayko	*Editor*
	Debra Smith	*Editorial Assistant*
Acknowledgments	Alan Guttmacher Institute	
	Alzheimer's Association	
	American Cancer Society	
	American Diabetes Association	
	American Heart Association	
	American Lung Association	
	Centers for Disease Control and Prevention	
	March of Dimes	
	National Cancer Institute	
	National Institute of Mental Health	
	National Osteoporosis Foundation	
	USDA Human Nutrition Research Center on Aging	
Alison Brown Cerier Book Development, Inc.	Alison Brown Cerier	*Book Developer and Editor*
	Kathleen Cahill Allison	*Writer*
	Sharon Ellis	*Illustrator*
	Michaelis/Carpelis Design Associates, Inc./ Elizabeth Norton	*Designers/ Art Director*
	Chris Hendel	*Medical Researcher*

Medical Consultants

Bruce Berkson, MD	*Urology*
Steven N. Blair, PED	*Epidemiology*
Charles F. Burant, MD, PhD	*Endocrinology*
Paul J. Chaiken, DDS	*Dentistry*
Priscilla Clarkson, PhD	*Exercise physiology*
David Cugell, MD	*Pulmonary medicine*
Arthur W. Curtis, MD	*Otolaryngology*
Noel A. DeBacker, MD	*Internal medicine/Geriatric medicine*
Nehama Dresner, MD	*Psychiatry*
Jerome Garden, MD	*Dermatology*
Larry S. Goldman, MD	*Psychiatry*
Donald Goldstein, MD	*Obstetrics and gynecology*
Karyn Grimm Herndon, MD	*Obstetrics and gynecology*
Allen Horwitz, MD, PhD	*Genetics*
Alan M. Jaffe, PhD	*Psychology*
Perry L. Kamel, MD	*Gastroenterology*
Ralph Kazer, MD	*Reproductive endocrinology*
Jennifer Knopf, PhD	*Psychology*
Gary S. Lissner, MD	*Ophthalmology*
John R. Lurain, MD	*Gynecologic oncology*
Stephanie Marshall, MD	*Dermatology*
Lane J. Mercer, MD	*Obstetrics and gynecology*
Thomas A. Mustoe, MD	*Plastic surgery*
Gary Noskin, MD	*Infectious diseases*
David Orentlicher, MD, JD	*Medical ethics*
Janis M. Orlowski, MD	*Nephrology*
Barbara V. Parilla, MD	*Maternal/Fetal medicine*
Anthony Reder, MD	*Neurology*
Domeena C. Renshaw, MD	*Psychiatry/Sexual dysfunction*
Carol Saffold, MD	*Obstetrics and gynecology*
Anthony J. Schaeffer, MD	*Urology*
Lisa Schilling, MD	*General internal medicine*
Joanne G. Schwartzberg, MD	*Geriatric medicine*
Vesna Skul, MD	*Internal medicine*
Matthew Sorrentino, MD	*Cardiology*
Mark Stolar, MD	*Endocrinology*
Linda Van Horn, PhD, RD	*Nutrition*
Gerald I. Zatuchni, MD	*Obstetrics and gynecology*
Howard J. Zeitz, MD	*Allergy and immunology*

Contents

Quick reference lists

Practical guides

These illustrated, two-page features give you the facts you need to take action on important health concerns.

Symptom charts

These charts lead you through a question-and-answer format to help you find the possible causes and significance of many common symptoms.

How to use this book

The *American Medical Association Complete Guide to Women's Health* provides up-to-date information that will enable you to adopt healthy habits that you can follow throughout your life. The emphasis is on achieving an optimal level of health and vitality, and on preventing illness.

In clear, easy-to-understand language, this book describes how different body systems work, answers many questions you may have about common diseases and disorders, and explains how many of these conditions can be prevented. The book guides you in making important decisions about your health based on the latest medical information. You will learn how to work effectively with your doctor and become a more active, informed participant in your health care. The book's comprehensive medical information can benefit a woman of any age—yourself, all the other women in your family, and your friends.

WHERE TO START

At the beginning of the book is a section called What You Can Do for Your Body Now. It speaks directly to women in four different age groups—puberty to 18, 18 to 40, 40 to 60, and 60 and over. In four concise pages, you will learn about the top health priorities for a woman your age. Like many people, you may feel overwhelmed by the amount of health information that reaches you through newspapers, magazines, books, and television programs. This section will help you cut through information overload and focus on the health-enhancing lifestyle choices that are most important for you right now. You can learn more about any topic by following the page references you'll find throughout the book.

After you get an overview from What You Can Do for Your Body Now, read part 1, Staying Healthy for Life, which describes the many things you can do—including eating a nutritious diet and exercising regularly—to stay healthy and reduce your risk of developing chronic disorders. This part will answer your questions about nutrition, fitness, body weight, and stress management. It also covers preventive health care, including the examinations and tests most helpful to you at every stage of life. You will also learn how to change behaviors such as smoking that put your health at risk.

LOOKING UP YOUR HEALTH CONCERNS

The remaining chapters cover sexual and reproductive health, pregnancy, and major disorders of every system of the body. Included are the most common serious disorders that affect more women than men and disorders that affect women differently than men.

If you are experiencing symptoms, three features will help you determine whether to call your doctor. The information about specific disorders includes a description of typical symptoms. To look up a specific disorder, consult the index at the back of the book. For many serious disorders, separate boxes called Warning Signs highlight symptoms that require immediate medical attention. Symptom charts suggest the possible causes and significance of many common symptoms, such as chest pain or headache. Each chart is located near related disorders. You will find a quick-reference guide to symptom charts on page 14.

Throughout the book are two-page features, called Practical Guides, that present the essential facts about health concerns that are especially important for women—from early detection of breast cancer to recognizing the signs of a heart attack. You will find a quick-reference guide on page 14.

puberty to 18

Your body is undergoing dramatic changes as it begins to produce female hormones—chemicals that control your growth, development, and reproductive system. This period of change is called puberty. The first noticeable sign of puberty is a gradual increase in the size of your breasts. Female hormones stimulate an increase of fat on other parts of your body as well, mostly on your hips, thighs, and buttocks. Inside your body, your reproductive organs are beginning to mature. At some time during this process, you will start having periods. Once you begin menstruating, even if your periods are irregular, you can become pregnant.

Your top health priorities

As a teenager, you are making choices that will affect the rest of your life. It may be difficult to imagine that a bad habit you start now can make you seriously ill many years later, or that misjudging a single situation could cause you serious harm. Your power to make decisions, both good and bad ones, gives you a lot of control over your future health and the kind of life you will have. Here are some guidelines:

- ✔ Don't smoke (see page 152)
- ✔ Eat healthy foods (see page 44)
- ✔ Build strong bones (see page 553)
- ✔ Exercise (see page 78)
- ✔ Don't drink or take drugs (see page 160)
- ✔ Drive safely (see page 176)
- ✔ Wait until you're ready before you have sex (see page 173)
- ✔ If you have sex, have only safe sex (see page 337)
- ✔ Don't get pregnant until you're ready to be a parent (see page 174)
- ✔ Protect your skin from the sun (see page 671)

See page 134 for a schedule of the medical examinations and tests you should have.

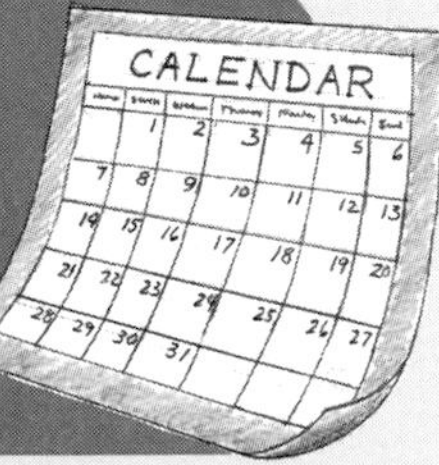

The best time for building strong bones

Your teenage years are the best time to build up your bone to its maximum strength and density. It will be harder to do after 20, and, after 35, your body will begin to lose more bone than it builds. You have probably seen many older women with a curved spine, which has resulted from the bone-thinning disease osteoporosis. The more bone you build now, the less likely you will be to develop osteoporosis later.

To make your bones as strong and healthy as possible, you need to take in 1,200 to 1,500 milligrams of calcium (see page 58) every day. Exercise can help build bones, just as it builds muscles. Menstruating regularly is also essential for maintaining the strength of your bones. If you are older than 16 and have never menstruated, or if you have begun to menstruate but have missed periods for 2 or 3 months, see a doctor immediately. Your body may not be producing enough of the important bone-strengthening hormone estrogen and you can begin to lose bone. Lack of estrogen dramatically increases your risk of osteoporosis. Your doctor can tell you about hormone therapies that can reestablish regular menstruation and keep your bones strong.

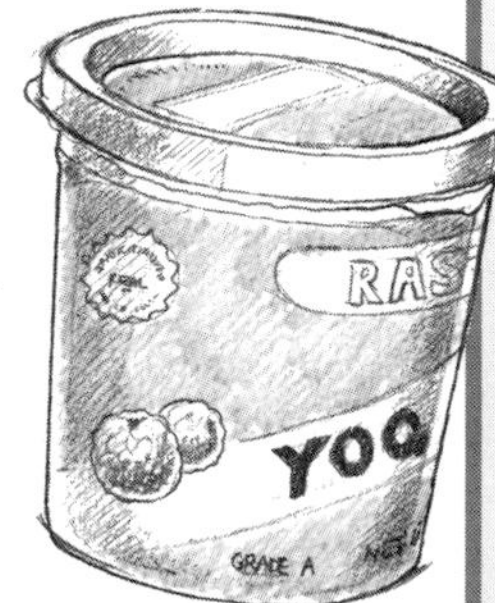

Your first gynecologic exam

If you have never had sex, you should have your first pelvic examination when you are 18. If you are under 18 and have had sexual intercourse, you should have your first pelvic examination as soon as possible and then have follow-up examinations every 6 to 12 months as your doctor recommends. Pelvic examinations are especially important if you continue to have sex because of the risk of sexually transmitted diseases (STDs; see chapter 12). STDs, many of which cause no noticeable symptoms, can increase your risk of cervical cancer (see page 250) and infertility. Having regular examinations can help prevent both of these.

You should have a pelvic examination if you experience any of the following symptoms at any age:

- Irregular periods after your first year of menstruation
- Any unwanted sexual contact or sexual abuse
- Unusual discharge from your vagina
- Sores, bumps, or lumps around your vagina
- Soreness, itching, or burning in your genital area
- Pain in your upper thigh, groin, or lower abdomen

No one looks forward to her first pelvic examination, but the reality is not nearly as bad as you imagine. Many women, especially younger women, feel scared or embarrassed about having a pelvic examination until they realize it is an important part of staying healthy. The examination is painless. Your doctor examines your reproductive organs to make sure their size, shape, and position are normal. He or she will take a sample of cells from your cervix (the opening into your uterus) to test for abnormal changes that could lead to cancer. This test is called a Pap smear (see page 127). Tell your doctor if you are sexually active (he or she will keep this information confidential) so that he or she can also test you for sexually transmitted diseases. For a complete description of a gynecologic examination, see page 124.

Here are some common reasons girls give for not having a pelvic examination, and reasons why they should:

- **"I don't want my parents to know I'm having sex."**

Call your local board of health or a local branch of the national organization Planned Parenthood. Planned Parenthood has offices in many communities that provide reproductive services to women and men for smaller-than-usual fees. Any doctor or other health care provider you see for birth control or STDs is legally obligated to keep your visit confidential; your parents need not know about it.

- **"I'm afraid it will hurt."**

A pelvic examination is painless and lasts for only a few minutes. Make sure you tell the doctor that it is your first gynecologic examination and ask questions throughout the exam so you know what is happening.

- **"I'm afraid I might find out I have an STD or that I'm pregnant."**

Ignoring a problem does not make it go away. If you don't know you have an STD, you cannot have it treated. If you are pregnant, finding out as early as possible enables you to make important decisions about whether you want to continue the pregnancy or have an abortion.

An obsession with thinness

Many young women dream of having the idealized body of a fashion model. In reality, few adult women have this figure naturally. It is important to develop healthy habits now that you can follow the rest of your life. It's OK to watch your weight, as long as you are realistic about how thin you need to be. Food is not your enemy; your body needs nutrients to grow to its appropriate adult height and weight. Some young women become so focused on being thin that they jeopardize their health. If you (or a friend) are dieting all the time, forcing yourself to throw up after you eat, using laxatives, or exercising excessively, you may have a serious illness called anorexia or bulimia. Both are eating disorders. Eating disorders can cause lifelong health problems. If you think you may have an eating disorder, get help immediately. Talk to a parent, school counselor, or doctor. For more about eating disorders, see page 610.

Feeling down

The teenage years are full of change and stress. You may feel that your parents do not understand you or are not there when you need them. You're expected to take on more and more adult responsibilities, compete for good grades to get into college, and succeed socially. At the same time, you do not yet have complete control over your own life. The result can be confusion, anxiety, and depression.

Everyone feels down from time to time, but, if your blues last more than a few weeks and are affecting your ability to function, you may have a disorder called depression (see page 594). Depression is common among teenage girls. The good news is that depression can be treated successfully in the vast majority of cases. Don't try to ignore it and hope it will go away on its own. It seldom does.

The signs of depression in teenagers include feelings of sadness, helplessness, hopelessness, loneliness, and emptiness; abuse of alcohol or other drugs; changes in sleeping and eating habits; withdrawal from friends and family; a drop in grades; or thoughts of suicide. If you recognize these signs in yourself, get help immediately. People are there for you. Here are some suggestions:

- ◆ Talk to your parents; explain your problems and tell them you need help.
- ◆ If you cannot talk to your parents, talk to another relative or a close friend you trust.
- ◆ Seek out a sympathetic adult, such as your family doctor or pediatrician, a school counselor, teacher, or social worker, who can help you. Ask about support groups in your school or community. In a support group, you can talk with and share your problems with other teenagers who are having similar difficulties. All discussions that take place among people in these groups are confidential.
- ◆ Get help immediately if a friend talks with you about making a suicide pact, or has taken steps to end his or her own life. Call a suicide hotline, a crisis hotline, or a local hospital emergency room and ask for help. Don't worry that your taking action may harm your friendship. You could be saving a life, which is much more important.

How to resist alcohol and other drugs

Alcohol and other drugs can harm your health and have serious consequences for the rest of your life. Drugs impair your judgment and lead you to take dangerous risks. They can reduce your chances of completing your education or having a productive, happy life. Don't let yourself be a victim of peer pressure. You have the power and the right to make decisions for yourself—and your friends should respect you for that. Here are some ways to turn down offers of alcohol or other drugs:

- ◆ Say, "No thanks, I'm not interested."
- ◆ Say, "It makes me feel sick."
- ◆ Leave the situation.
- ◆ Ignore the person who is offering the drugs and go talk to someone else.
- ◆ Laugh it off, tell a joke, or change the subject.
- ◆ Suggest doing something else.

A suntan: damage to your skin

You may think a suntan makes you look healthy, but the change in the color of your skin is actually the visible damage from ultraviolet radiation from the sun. Sun damage will make your skin wrinkle permanently—at a younger age than usual. Excessive exposure to the sun can also cause skin cancer, the most common cancer of all. The deadliest form of skin cancer—malignant melanoma (see page 684)—is increasing at a faster rate than any other cancer in the US because people are spending more time in the sun and are developing the cancer at increasingly younger ages.

To keep your skin healthy, always protect it by using a sunscreen that indicates on the label that it protects against both ultraviolet A (UVA) and ultraviolet B (UVB) rays. Make sure it has a sun protection factor (SPF) of at least 15. Wearing hats and dark, long-sleeved clothing can also help block your exposure to radiation from the sun.

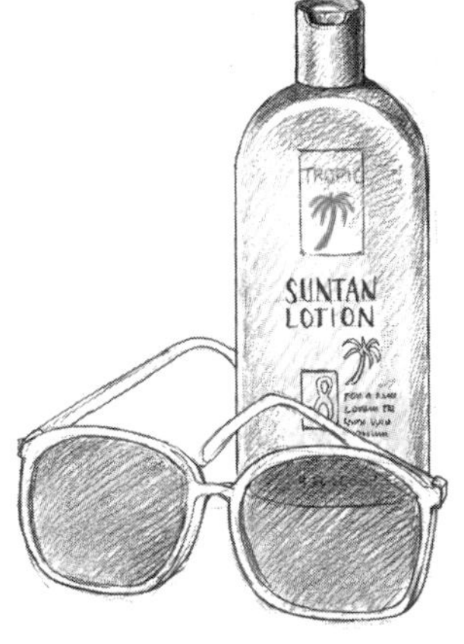

THE FACTS ABOUT SEX AND PREGNANCY

If you are sexually active and you do not use a reliable method of birth control, such as a latex condom with spermicide or birth-control pills, you are very likely to become pregnant. Here are some reasons girls have given for becoming pregnant unintentionally and information that could have helped them avoid it:

Mistaken thinking:	Important facts:
"I didn't think I could get pregnant the first time I had sex."	After your first period, you can get pregnant any time you have sexual intercourse, including the first time.
"I didn't know where to go to get birth control and I couldn't afford it."	A variety of safe, reliable, inexpensive contraceptives, such as condoms, are readily available at most drugstores. Go to your doctor or a local office of Planned Parenthood.
"I was too embarrassed to ask my boyfriend to use a condom."	You need to be able to speak openly with and trust a person you are going to have sex with. Otherwise, a better choice is to not have sex.
"My boyfriend promised he would withdraw his penis in time or not actually enter my vagina."	You can get pregnant even if your partner withdraws his penis before he ejaculates or even if his penis doesn't enter you but he ejaculates near your vaginal opening.

ARE YOU READY FOR SEX?

If you are considering becoming sexually active, think about whether you are prepared to:

- Help protect yourself from sexually transmitted diseases by using a latex or polyurethane male condom or a female condom with spermicide every time you have sex—even if you are using another method of birth control. For how to convince your boyfriend to use a condom, see page 21.
- Help protect yourself from pregnancy by using a reliable contraceptive every time you have sex.

Don't let persuasion or promises from a boyfriend, peer pressure, or your sexual urges lead you into a sexual relationship you are not ready for. You have the right to refuse to have sex if you don't feel you are ready, and your feelings should be respected. There is no reason to rush into sexual activity; you have the rest of your life to have sexual relationships. Keep in mind that you have much more than sex to offer as a person.

Smoking: it's not cool

Many teenagers start smoking because they see their friends doing it and they think it's cool and makes them look grown up. They also think they can quit any time they want. But your body becomes addicted to nicotine, the powerful chemical in cigarettes, and you continually crave more. Most adult smokers started when they were teenagers. Consider the following consequences of smoking:

- It causes lung cancer and other fatal lung diseases. Lung cancer kills more women than any other type of cancer, including breast cancer.
- It makes you five times more likely than a nonsmoker to have a heart attack in your 30s or 40s.
- It makes your breath, hands, hair, and clothes smell bad.
- It makes your teeth yellow.
- Most teenage boys say they would prefer to date a girl who doesn't smoke.
- Your skin will wrinkle at a younger age than your friends who don't smoke.
- It decreases your ability to perform athletically because your lungs can't get enough oxygen during exertion.
- It's very expensive.

18 to 40

The years from 18 to 40 are sometimes referred to as the reproductive years because most pregnancies occur in women these ages. If you are planning to become pregnant, you should get your body into the best condition possible to help ensure a healthy pregnancy and a healthy baby. If you are not planning a pregnancy, following a healthy lifestyle will still help you feel better and look better. Good habits—especially eating a nutritious, well-balanced diet and exercising regularly—can also help you avoid chronic, debilitating illnesses as you get older. It is just as important to avoid harmful habits—including smoking cigarettes, drinking excessive amounts of alcohol, or taking illegal drugs.

Your top health priorities

Now is the time to continue the healthy habits you have already established and develop new ones you can continue for the rest of your life. Here is a list of your top health priorities if you are between 18 and 40:

- ✔ Quit smoking (see page 156)
- ✔ Eat a healthy diet (see page 44)
- ✔ Exercise regularly (see page 78)
- ✔ Practice safer sex (see page 337)
- ✔ Don't abuse alcohol or other drugs (see page 160)
- ✔ Examine your breasts every month (see page 276)
- ✔ Plan your pregnancies (see page 370)
- ✔ Protect your skin from the sun (see page 671)

See page 135 for a schedule of the medical examinations and tests you should have.

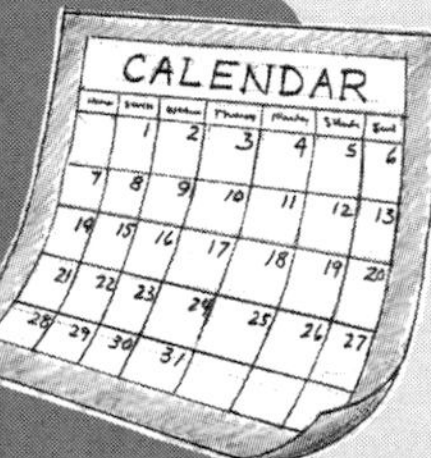

Breast self-exams

There is no known way to prevent breast cancer. Your best hope is to detect a cancer at an early stage, when a cure is more likely. Most breast lumps are discovered by women themselves during regular, monthly breast self-examinations or by chance during bathing or dressing. Most lumps in the breast are not cancerous, but you should tell your doctor immediately about any lump you find.

Ask your doctor when you should start having regular mammograms. Most doctors recommend that women begin in their 40s. If you have a family history of breast cancer—especially in a close relative, such as your mother or sister—your doctor may recommend that you start having mammograms at a younger age. Even if you have regular mammograms, it is important to do a monthly examination of your breasts by feeling with your hand and looking in the mirror for any changes in their shape or contour (see page 276).

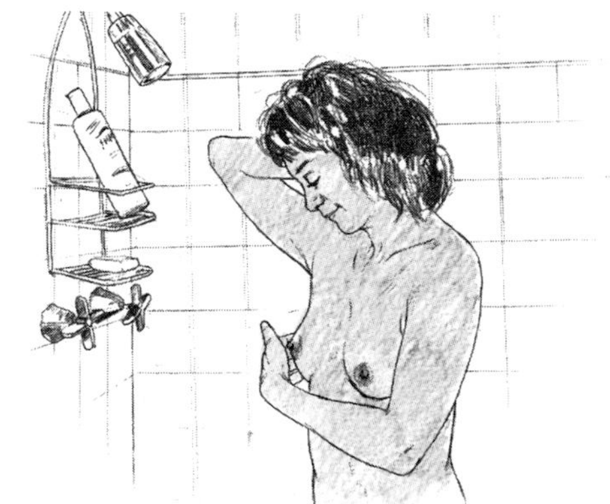

Guidelines for safer sex

It can happen to anyone. Women of every age and every socioeconomic, educational, ethnic, and racial group get sexually transmitted diseases (STDs)—whether they have many sexual partners or one. Here are some steps you can take to help protect yourself from STDs:

- Think twice before beginning sexual relations with a new partner. Limiting your sexual activity to only one partner who is having sex only with you reduces your exposure to disease-causing organisms.
- When you have intercourse, use a male condom made of latex or polyurethane (not natural materials) or a female condom (which is made of polyurethane). For instructions on how to use a male condom correctly, see page 172; for how to use a female condom, see page 319.
- In addition to a condom, always use a spermicide, which provides additional protection against STDs. Some condoms are already lubricated with spermicide. You can also insert spermicidal gel or foam into your vagina for extra protection.
- A female condom protects part of your external genitals as well as your vagina. Use a female condom if your partner will not use a male condom.
- During oral sex, help protect your mouth by having your partner use a condom; use a female condom to help prevent your partner from acquiring an STD from you.
- Ask your partner to wash his genitals before and after you have sex.
- Do not douche after intercourse. It does not protect you from STDs and, in fact, may spread an infection farther into your reproductive tract. Douching can also wash away spermicidal protection.
- Have annual Pap smears and tests for STDs.
- If you are involved in an intimate relationship but are concerned about STDs, you might try sexual activities other than intercourse or anal or oral sex. Consider mutual lovemaking techniques that do not involve the exchange of body fluids or contact between mucous membranes (such as those in the vagina, anus, and mouth).

When he won't use a condom

It's not easy to talk with a new sex partner about using a condom. It may help to practice responses like these ahead of time:

He: I don't need a condom because I don't have any diseases.

She: That's good to know. As far as I know, I don't either, but we still need to use a condom because either of us could have an infection and not know it. This way, it's safer for both of us.

He: It doesn't feel as good when I use a condom.

She: I know there is a little bit less sensation for some men, but it will feel better than no sex at all. I can help you put it on so we can make it part of our lovemaking. I've read that some men even like using a condom because it helps them last longer and prolongs their pleasure.

He: Let's not use a condom just this once.

She: Just once is all it takes. Most people don't even know when they're infected with an STD or that they're passing it on to someone else.

He: I just won't use one.

She: Then we'd better just kiss and cuddle for now. If we're not ready to use a condom then we're not ready for sex.

Quit smoking

Smoking is the most preventable cause of death. If you smoke, quitting is the most important thing you can do for your health. Quitting substantially reduces your risk of lung cancer and other cancers (including cancers of the esophagus, mouth, pancreas, bladder, and cervix), heart disease, and stroke.

Recognizing gynecologic symptoms

Vaginal bleeding and discharge are a normal part of your menstrual cycle. However, if you notice anything unusual, talk to your doctor. Some symptoms can result from mild infections that are easy to treat but that, if not treated, can lead to infertility or kidney damage. Vaginal symptoms can also be a sign of more serious problems—from sexually transmitted diseases (STDs) to cancers of the reproductive tract.

Recognizing the symptoms early and seeing a doctor right away increase the likelihood of successful treatment. Some women, when they notice a discharge or feel itchy or sore, treat themselves with over-the-counter medications. If you have had yeast infections before and you recognize the symptoms, this is safe to do. But if you have never had a yeast infection or if you have any doubt about your symptoms, see your doctor immediately. You could have something much more serious than a yeast infection. See your doctor if you have any of the following symptoms:

- Sores or lumps in your genital area
- Abnormal vaginal bleeding, particularly during or after intercourse
- Vaginal discharge with an unpleasant or unusual odor or of an unusual color
- Itching, burning, swelling, redness, or soreness in your vaginal area
- Pain or discomfort during intercourse
- Frequent and urgent need to urinate or a burning sensation during urination
- Pain or pressure in your pelvis that differs from menstrual cramps
- Bleeding between periods
- Increased vaginal discharge

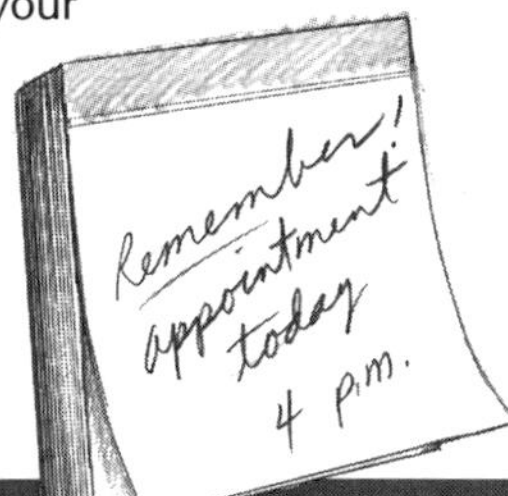

Managing the stress in your life

Many women face difficult challenges and responsibilities—as working women, mothers, or caregivers for aging parents. These roles may overlap or conflict, causing overwhelming stress that can affect their health. Emotional stress can lead to high blood pressure, increased susceptibility to substance abuse and illness, and depression. Here are some things you can do to help reduce or manage the stress in your life:

- **Eat a healthy diet and exercise regularly** A nutritious, well-balanced diet and exercise can keep your body fit and able to resist disease. Exercise is also an excellent way to elevate your mood.
- **Talk about it** Confide in someone you trust—a friend, relative, or member of the clergy. Sometimes just talking about your problems and concerns can help you put them into perspective and give you insights into ways to deal with them.
- **Stay organized** Good organization can help you manage your time more efficiently, which can reduce much of the time-related stress in your life. For example, make a list of things you need to do and complete each task one at a time. Break large projects into smaller, easy-to-manage parts. Carry a datebook with you for keeping track of important appointments, projects, deadlines, and phone and fax numbers.
- **Ask for help** No one can do it all alone. Let family members, friends, or coworkers know that you feel overloaded and ask them for help with specific tasks. People often don't realize you need help until you ask for it. And they will be less demanding of your time if they are aware that you have little to spare.
- **Learn how to relax** Relaxation techniques (see page 190) are quick, easy methods for calming your mind and body. Do them whenever you need a little stress reduction.
- **Get professional help if you need it** If you feel so overwhelmed by your responsibilities that you are having difficulty functioning normally, talk to your doctor. He or she will be able to recommend treatment or refer you to a qualified psychiatrist or other mental health specialist (see page 194).

Your diet: limited fat, lots of fruits, vegetables, and calcium

The healthiest changes you can make in your diet are to reduce the amount of fat you eat and increase your intake of fruits, vegetables, whole grains, and calcium-rich foods. Too much dietary fat can raise your cholesterol level and increase your risk of high blood pressure, heart disease, diabetes, stroke, and some forms of cancer. Eating lots of fruits, vegetables, and whole grains can help reduce your risk of heart disease, stroke, and cancer. Calcium is essential for maintaining the strength and density of your bones. You should take in 1,000 to 1,500 milligrams of calcium each day (see page 554). One 8-ounce glass of skim milk has 300 milligrams of calcium. For other good sources of calcium, see page 58.

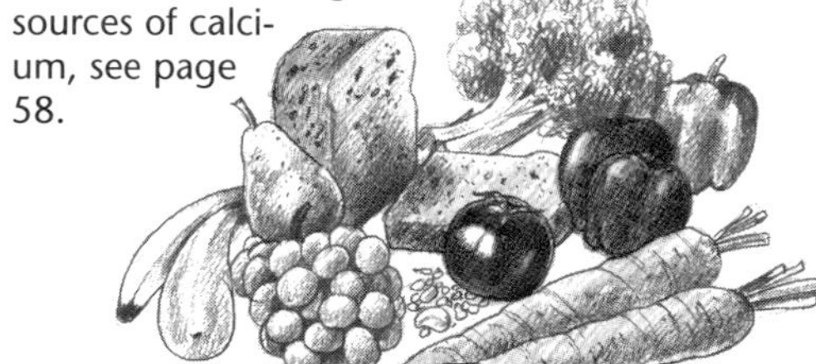

Violence against women

Violence against women is widespread and increasing. Most violence occurs in the home and is usually inflicted by a husband or boyfriend. Violence against women can take various forms, including physical abuse, emotional abuse, or sexual assault. No woman deserves to be abused; you have a right to be safe. Get help if you are involved in a violent relationship. For information about how to protect yourself from abuse, see page 721. For information about getting help if you are a victim of abuse, see page 723.

Before you become pregnant

The best time to prepare your body for a healthy pregnancy is long before you make a decision to become pregnant. Doing the following can help ensure a healthy pregnancy:

- See your doctor several months before you plan to become pregnant. Have a physical examination and blood tests for Rh factor and immunity to rubella, hepatitis B, and toxoplasmosis (see page 370). Talk to your doctor about any health conditions you have (such as high blood pressure or diabetes) that could affect your pregnancy.
- If you are over 35, have a family history of a genetic disorder, or are adopted and do not know your family health history, ask your doctor to refer you to a genetic counselor. A genetic counselor can evaluate your risk of having a child with a birth defect.
- Prepare your body for pregnancy by eating a nutritious diet and maintaining a healthy weight. At least 3 months before you become pregnant, you need to begin taking a daily multivitamin supplement containing 400 micrograms (0.4 milligrams) of the B vitamin folic acid. This nutrient helps prevent birth defects that can occur in the first 3 months of pregnancy—before many women know they are pregnant.
- Start exercising now so you can continue moderate exercise during your pregnancy. Exercise provides health benefits for both you and your fetus.
- Do not smoke cigarettes, drink alcohol, or use illegal drugs, all of which can harm a developing fetus (see page 413). Don't use over-the-counter drugs without talking to your doctor. If you are taking a prescription medication for a medical condition, tell your doctor that you are trying to become pregnant.
- Some sexually transmitted diseases (STDs), especially herpes and HIV (the AIDS virus), can be passed on to a fetus or can complicate labor. If there is a possibility you have an STD, have tests before you become pregnant. If you are infected with HIV, you can take a medication during your pregnancy that can significantly reduce your risk of transmitting the virus to your fetus (see page 345). Do not have sex without using a condom during pregnancy if there is any chance your partner has an STD.

40 to 60

Your ovaries will stop producing the hormone estrogen at some time during your 40s or 50s, and you will stop menstruating. This stage of life is called menopause. The average age of menopause is 51, but it can vary from 40 to 55. For several years before you actually stop menstruating, your ovaries release eggs less regularly and gradually produce less estrogen and other hormones. Your periods may begin to change and you are less fertile at this time. However, up until menopause you can still become pregnant, so you must continue to use birth control.

The lack of estrogen after menopause has effects on many parts of your body. You may experience symptoms such as hot flashes, vaginal dryness, or night sweats. In some women, symptoms are hardly noticeable; in others, they are severe and bothersome. Without estrogen, your bones will begin to lose density and become thinner, weaker, brittle, and more prone to fracture. The lack of estrogen also decreases your level of heart-protecting high-density lipoprotein (HDL) cholesterol and raises your level of harmful low-density lipoprotein (LDL) cholesterol. This change in cholesterol levels dramatically increases your risk of heart disease, making it equal to that of a man. Taking hormone replacement therapy (HRT) to provide the estrogen your body no longer produces can help prevent or reverse these and other symptoms of menopause.

Your top health priorities

Your doctor may be able to detect early signs of disorders that can become more serious as you grow older. Regular medical checkups and tests to diagnose diseases at an early, more treatable stage are especially important. Here are your top health priorities:

- ✔ Consider hormone replacement therapy at menopause (see page 359)
- ✔ Don't ignore chest pain—you could be having a heart attack (see page 465)
- ✔ Know your cholesterol level (see page 131) and blood pressure level (see page 126)
- ✔ Have regular mammograms (see page 127)
- ✔ Maintain your bone strength and density (see page 553)
- ✔ Have an annual test for colon cancer (see page 130)
- ✔ Maintain a healthy weight (see page 96)
- ✔ Exercise regularly (see chapter 2)

See page 136 for a schedule of the medical examinations and tests you should have.

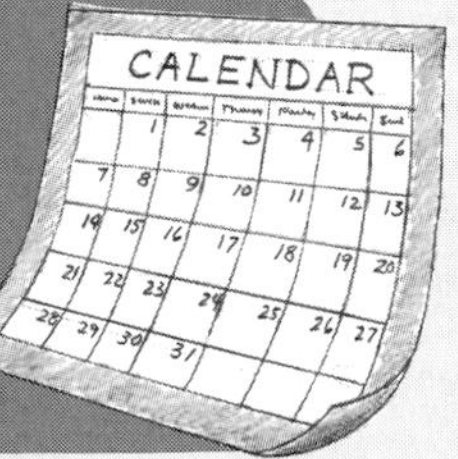

Watch your weight

During these years, controlling your weight becomes more important and even more difficult. Your body burns calories more slowly because it has less muscle. Eating in moderation and exercising regularly can help you maintain a healthy weight and significantly reduce your risk of illness.

Heart disease: the number-one killer of women

The estrogen your body produces helps protect you from heart disease. When your ovaries stop producing estrogen at menopause, you lose this protection and your risk of heart disease increases dramatically. After menopause, you are as likely as a man to have a heart attack. You may not have given much thought to preventing heart disease before now, but consider the following:

- **Your family history** If you have any close relatives who have had heart disease or a heart attack or stroke, especially before age 50, your risk of heart disease is increased. You need to be especially diligent about reducing your other risk factors, such as high blood pressure and a high total cholesterol level.
- **Your blood pressure** High blood pressure is a powerful risk factor for heart disease. The only way to know if you have high blood pressure is to have your blood pressure measured regularly (see page 126). If it is high, your doctor will recommend treatment—such as weight loss, exercise, or medication—to bring it under control.
- **Your cholesterol profile** Know your total cholesterol level and your levels of protective high-density lipoprotein (HDL) cholesterol and harmful low-density lipoprotein (LDL) cholesterol. If your total cholesterol level is high or your HDL level is low, your doctor will recommend measures to improve them. These measures may include a low-fat, high-fiber diet, regular exercise, or medication.
- **A heart-healthy lifestyle** The single most important thing you can do for your heart is not to smoke. Smoking is responsible for one out of four cases of heart disease. (For how to quit, see page 157.) Eat a well-balanced, low-fat diet that is rich in fruits and vegetables, exercise regularly, maintain a healthy weight, and try to reduce the stress in your life.
- **Hormone replacement therapy** Replacing the estrogen your body no longer produces after menopause can cut in half your risk of heart attack and stroke. Ask your doctor about taking estrogen.
- **The significance of chest pain** Women are more likely than men to experience angina (see page 465)—pain, tightness, or pressure in their chest that occurs with exertion. If you have angina, consider it a warning that you have heart disease. See your doctor immediately if you have chest pain.
- **The signs of a heart attack** A heart attack can feel different to different people. Learn about all the possible signs of a heart attack (see page 471) and get emergency medical attention if you experience any—even if you only think you may be having a heart attack. For more about heart attacks, see page 472.

Should you take hormone replacement therapy?

Most doctors believe that most women could benefit from taking estrogen in hormone replacement therapy (HRT) at menopause and for the rest of their life. Studies about the effects of estrogen on a woman's risk of breast cancer are conflicting. Most studies find no increased risk. When making a decision about whether or not HRT would be beneficial for you, you and your doctor will carefully weigh your personal risk factors for heart disease, osteoporosis, and breast cancer.

HRT significantly reduces your risk of heart disease and stroke and protects against the debilitating bone-thinning disorder osteoporosis. The average woman is 10 times more likely to die of heart disease or stroke than breast cancer and much more likely to develop osteoporosis than breast cancer.

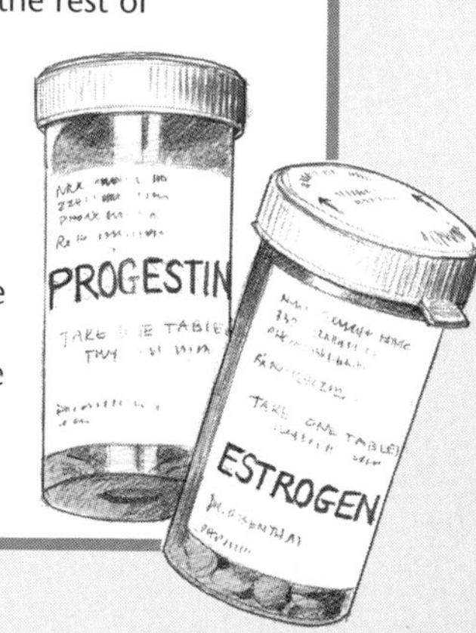

Testing for diabetes

Type II diabetes (see page 621) occurs most often after 40. Millions of people have type II diabetes and do not know it because the disease seldom causes symptoms in the early stages. Talk to your doctor about being tested for diabetes if any of the following risk factors apply to you:

- You have a family history of type II diabetes (parent or sibling with the disease).
- You are more than 20 percent over your ideal weight (see page 99).
- You are Native American, Hispanic, or black.
- You have one or more of the preceding risk factors and you are over 40.
- You have been diagnosed with a condition called impaired glucose tolerance (see page 623).
- You have high blood pressure or a high total cholesterol level.
- You have a history of diabetes during a pregnancy (called gestational diabetes, see page 418) or you have delivered a large baby (9 pounds or heavier).

If your glucose level is elevated, your doctor will recommend further testing to make an accurate diagnosis. You may be able to restore your glucose to a normal level by losing weight and exercising regularly, or your doctor may prescribe glucose-lowering medication or insulin injections.

Testing for colon cancer

Have an annual test for colon cancer (see page 130). Colon cancer is the third most common cause of cancer death in women—after cancers of the lung and breast. Eating a fiber-rich diet with lots of fresh fruits, vegetables, and whole grains, exercising regularly, and taking estrogen after menopause can help protect you from colon cancer. Have a fecal occult blood test (see page 130) every year after 40 to detect blood in your stool, which is an indication of possible colon cancer.

Controlling your weight

Even a 5- to 10-pound weight gain can increase your risk of high blood pressure, type II diabetes, heart disease, and some cancers. Maintaining a healthy weight is especially important if you or a close family member has had:

- Heart disease
- Type II diabetes
- Stroke
- High blood pressure
- Cancer of the uterus, gallbladder, kidney, stomach, breast, or colon
- A high total cholesterol level

If your weight is not in the healthy range for your height and build (see page 99), the best course for losing weight is to set a reasonable goal. Develop a healthy pattern of eating and exercising that you can follow for the rest of your life. Your weight loss should be slow and gradual. Here are some helpful tips for maintaining a healthy weight:

- **A calorie is a calorie** Although some foods have more calories than others (high-fat foods generally have more calories than foods that are high in carbohydrates or protein), the bottom line for losing weight is to eat fewer calories than you burn each day.
- **Exercise burns calories** Both aerobic exercise and strengthening exercise burn calories by increasing your heart rate.
- **Eat when you're hungry, stop when you're full** Many people eat for reasons other than hunger. Get into the habit of taking smaller portions, and never go back for seconds.
- **Focus on fruits and vegetables and other low-fat foods** Besides being low in fat and calories, fruits and vegetables help reduce your risk of heart disease, stroke, and cancer. You can usually eat a larger quantity of foods that are low in fat as long as they are also low in calories (check labels).

40 to 60

Mammograms: benefits increase as you age

It's time to start having regular mammograms. Your risk of breast cancer increases as you get older. You should have a mammogram every 1 to 2 years between ages 40 and 49 and every year after 50. Mammograms can be lifesaving. A mammogram does not replace the need for a monthly breast self-examination, but mammograms can detect cancerous tumors many times smaller and at a much earlier stage than those you can feel by hand. For more about mammograms, see page 276.

Warning signs of skin cancer

Your risk of skin cancer increases as you age because the damaging effects of exposure to the sun's radiation accumulate over the years. Preventing skin cancer is simple, but not necessarily easy. All you have to do is shield your skin from the sun's ultraviolet (UV) rays. Wear protective clothing and hats and always use a sunscreen that blocks both UVA and UVB rays (check the label) and has a sun protection factor (SPF) of at least 15.

Check your body regularly for signs of skin cancer—especially your face, chest, arms, legs, and back. Have your doctor or your partner examine the areas you cannot see easily. Like all cancers, the earlier skin cancer is detected, the more successful treatment is likely to be. For more about skin cancer, see page 683. For information about how to examine your body for skin cancer, see page 683.

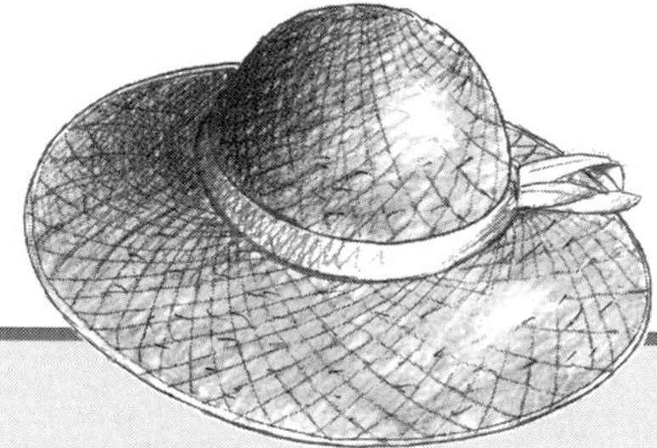

Should you have a bone density test?

Your doctor can help you determine your risk of developing osteoporosis by taking your medical history and asking about your family health history or by performing a bone density test. A bone density test can measure the strength and density of your bones as you approach menopause and, if the test is repeated a year later, can determine how quickly you are losing bone. Some women are at greater risk of osteoporosis than others. If the results of your bone density test show that you have osteoporosis or are at increased risk of developing it, you could benefit greatly from taking estrogen in hormone replacement therapy (HRT). Discuss HRT with your doctor.

If you have one or more of the following risk factors, a bone density test may be useful:

- You have already experienced a bone fracture that may be the result of thinning bones.
- Your mother, grandmother, or another close relative has had osteoporosis or bone fractures.
- Over a long period of time, you have taken medication that accelerates bone loss, such as corticosteroids for treating rheumatoid arthritis (see page 645) or other conditions, or some antiseizure medications (see page 583).
- You have low body weight, a slight build, or a light complexion.
- You have a history of cigarette smoking or heavy drinking.

For more about osteoporosis and risk factors, see page 552.

60 and over

Many older women remain vital well into their later years. If you have followed a healthy lifestyle, you are likely to continue to enjoy good health. Although your body will continue to undergo changes, healthy habits can prevent them from limiting your independence.

One of the biggest challenges facing many older women is bone thinning, which accelerates naturally at menopause and after, when your body no longer produces the bone-strengthening hormone estrogen. If you have been working to keep your bones strong throughout your life, you have reduced your risk of the common disorder osteoporosis and bone fractures. Talk to your doctor about taking estrogen or a nonhormonal medication to prevent further bone loss. Estrogen can also significantly reduce your risk of heart disease or stroke.

Your top health priorities

At this stage of your life, regular tests and medical examinations are very important. Your top priority is to stay as healthy and independent as possible.

- ✔ Continue to exercise or start now (see page 78)
- ✔ Take a daily vitamin/mineral supplement
- ✔ Have regular medical tests (see page 126)
- ✔ Have your vision, hearing, and teeth checked regularly (see page 140)
- ✔ Take chest pain seriously (see page 465)
- ✔ Monitor your blood pressure (see page 481)
- ✔ Get mammograms and perform breast self-examinations regularly (see page 276)
- ✔ Continue having Pap smears (see page 127)
- ✔ Get shots for flu and pneumonia (see page 138)
- ✔ Continue to protect your skin (see page 671)
- ✔ Take care with all medications (see page 139)

See page 137 for a schedule of the medical examinations and tests you should have.

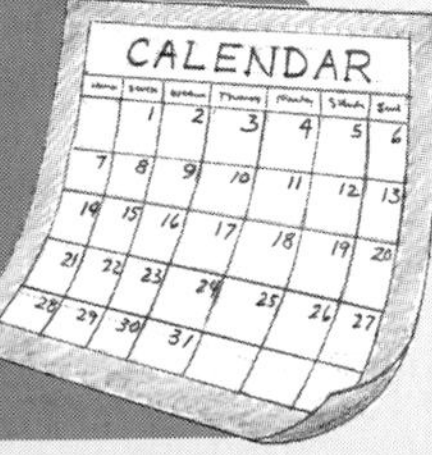

Good nutrition

Loss of appetite and poor nutrition are common problems for older women. They can lead to weight loss, headaches, lightheadedness, disorientation, and fatigue. Talk to your doctor about your eating habits. He or she can help you develop a plan that will make it easier for you to eat a well-balanced diet—one that is rich in fruits, vegetables, and whole grains. A healthy diet provides numerous benefits, including lowering your risk of illness and maintaining your energy level and the strength and density of your bones. Your doctor is also likely to recommend that you take a multivitamin/mineral supplement every day to help ensure that you are getting all the essential nutrients your body needs. For more about nutrition, see chapter 1.

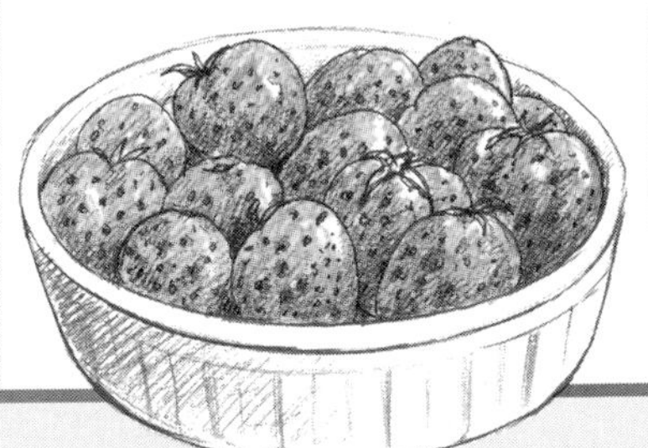

Exercise is still necessary for good health

The many benefits of exercise as you age cannot be overstated. Regular, moderate physical activity helps reduce your risk of illness—including high blood pressure, heart disease, stroke, and type II diabetes. Exercise helps lower your blood pressure and total cholesterol level. Without exercise, muscles and joints stiffen and weaken with age. Regular exercise keeps them limber and strong, which helps you avoid falls and injuries. Exercise also has powerful psychological benefits; it can boost your self-esteem and reduce anxiety and stress.

Even if you have been sedentary for most of your life, it is not too late to start exercising. The best exercise for you is a combination of weight-bearing aerobic exercise, such as walking, and strengthening exercises, such as weight lifting. Strengthening exercises can build muscle strength and bone density and increase your mobility and ability to function. Before you begin an exercise program, check with your doctor. He or she may recommend a program of aerobic and strengthening exercises you can do at home, or suggest signing up for weight-training classes at a local YMCA or health club.

If your mobility is limited by injury or illness, a physical therapist can design an exercise program for you. Even if you use a wheelchair or walker, exercise is essential for maintaining your body's strength and ability to function. Make it an integral part of your daily routine.

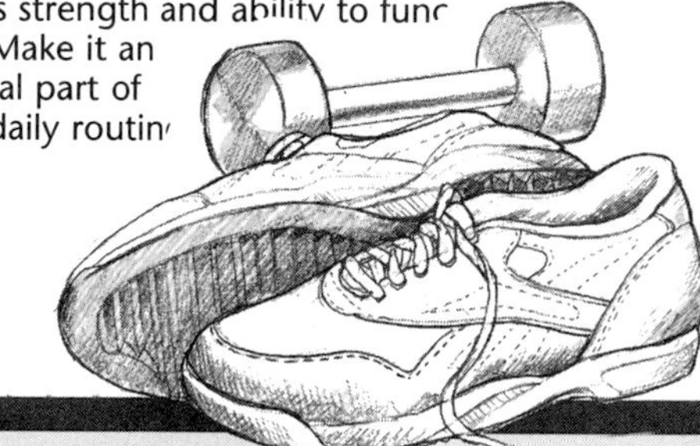

Avoiding disabling fractures

Bone fractures are much more serious when you are older. Although the immediate cause of a broken wrist or hip is usually a fall, the underlying cause is the gradual thinning and weakening of your bones over the years. Bone loss speeds up dramatically in the few years after menopause, when your body stops producing estrogen. Here are some things you can do to maintain your bone density and strength and avoid disabling fractures:

- **Consider hormone replacement therapy** Estrogen is essential for maintaining bone strength and density. Taking estrogen in the form of hormone replacement therapy (HRT) for the rest of your life is the single most effective way to slow or stop the natural loss of bone that occurs at your age. HRT substantially reduces bone fractures in older women. Ask your doctor about it.
- **Get enough calcium and vitamin D** Calcium and vitamin D are essential for helping maintain strong bones. Take in 1,500 milligrams of calcium every day (1,000 if you are on HRT and are under 65) and 600 international units (IU) of vitamin D. Nonfat or low-fat dairy products are good sources of calcium; fortified dairy products are good sources of vitamin D. If you do not get sufficient amounts of these minerals in your diet, take supplements.
- **Exercise** Stay active. Putting weight on your bones with activities such as walking can help you maintain your bone density and strength. Strengthening exercises such as lifting weights can help preserve strength in your upper body, spine, and arms.
- **Avoid falls** Because your bones may not be as strong as they used to be, a fall at your age can be disabling. Taking precautions—such as using a walker or cane when necessary and making your home safe from falls—can help you avoid falls. Have your vision tested regularly because poor eyesight can lead to a fall. For more about avoiding falls, see page 179.

Get your shots for flu and pneumonia

Influenza and pneumonia are common causes of death in people over 60. Ask your doctor about getting shots to guard against these serious illnesses. If you are healthy, one shot will protect you permanently against a common type of pneumonia caused by bacteria. You need to have a flu shot every year. Flu shots are usually given in the fall after health officials have determined which strain of the influenza virus is likely to cause the most widespread infection during that season.

Recognizing depression

Major depression is a common disorder that is often not diagnosed in older women. Many older women face serious challenges, including their own declining health or the death of a spouse or friends. Coping with these changes can be difficult. If your feelings of sadness become overwhelming, you may be experiencing depression. In most people, depression can be treated successfully, usually with a combination of antidepressant medication and psychotherapy. Many people who are depressed do not realize that they need treatment, or they feel unable to ask for help. If a relative or close friend is encouraging you to see your doctor for depression, do so.

If you have any of the following symptoms of depression and they do not go away within a few days or weeks, see your doctor:

- Loss of interest and pleasure in activities that you used to enjoy
- Persistent anxiety or irritability
- Persistent feelings of sadness or numbness
- Difficulty falling asleep or staying asleep
- Feelings of hopelessness and helplessness
- Poor appetite
- Loss of energy; fatigue

For more about depression, see page 594.

Going it alone

Most women will live some of their later years alone. You should plan ahead for this likelihood. If you are married now, make sure you have a will and an organized list of all of your and your husband's financial assets, insurance policies, deeds, and loan documents; know where to find them. If you do not manage your family's financial matters, learn as much as you can about them so you'll be able to manage on your own.

If you become a widow, it will take time to adjust to the loss of your partner (see page 711). Here are some guidelines that may help ease your transition:

- Don't move out of your home or make any major financial commitments in the first several months.
- Explore all possible sources of income that may be owed to you, including social security payments, tax benefits, debt relief, insurance policies, veteran's benefits, or civil service benefits.
- Revise your will.
- Maintain relationships with family and friends and try to develop new relationships and interests.
- Be wary of people who approach you with ideas for financial investments, loans, or business opportunities. Some unethical people take advantage of newly widowed women, knowing that they may be looking for financial advice.
- Choose financial advisors carefully, based on recommendations of people you trust.
- You will eventually want to plan for your future living arrangements. Educate yourself about all the options (see page 143) and don't make any quick decisions.
- Look into making a living will and other advance directives (see page 708).

Are you drinking too much?

Little by little, moderate drinking can become excessive drinking. Older women who live alone may find themselves using alcohol to help them forget their problems. They may not realize how much alcohol they are consuming until it begins to interfere with their ability to function. Alcohol-related health problems frequently put older people in the hospital, often because they are taking prescription medications that interact with alcohol.

Over time, excessive alcohol consumption damages your liver. It also is the leading cause of vitamin and mineral deficiencies that can result in numbness or tingling in the hands and feet, nerve damage, immobility, memory loss, and impaired vision. Alcohol increases your risk of falling and having a disabling injury. Talk to your doctor if you have any concerns or questions about your consumption of alcohol. For more information about alcohol and its effects, see page 160.

60 and over

Managing your medications

If you're taking several medications, managing them becomes a complicated daily task. Make sure you understand the exact dose and timing of each medication your doctor has prescribed. Tell all of your doctors about each medication you are taking; carry a list with you at all times. At home:

- Write out your daily schedule for taking your medications. Be sure to update the schedule every time your medication changes.
- Take the exact dosage your doctor recommends and carefully follow the time schedule.
- If you are taking several different medications daily, it may help to put your pills in a pill organizer at the beginning of each week. This will help ensure that you are getting the right dose at the right time.
- Store all your medications in their original container (except for those you put in an organizer). The labels contain important information such as dosage and expiration dates.
- Take the complete course of treatment your doctor prescribes. Never discontinue a medication on your own; some medications must be stopped gradually to avoid complications.
- If the medication is making you feel sick or causing side effects that you find difficult to tolerate, talk to your doctor. He or she may be able to adjust the dose or change the medication. Do not stop taking the medication on your own.
- Do not take medication in the dark; you might take the wrong medication or too much.
- Never take a drug that was prescribed for someone else.
- Be aware that alcohol can interact with many different kinds of drugs. Ask your doctor whether it is safe to drink alcohol with any new medication he or she prescribes.
- If children or grandchildren are around, keep containers out of reach, particularly if you choose lids that are not childproof.
- If you have medication left over after your doctor has told you to discontinue it, dispose of it immediately. It is safest to flush medicines down the toilet. You should also dispose of a medication if its expiration date has passed.

Getting help for urinary incontinence

Declining estrogen levels at menopause can cause the muscles of the lining of your urinary tract to lose their strength and tone. The result can be incontinence, the involuntary leaking of urine. Fear of having accidents causes many women to limit their social activities and stop exercising. If you have this problem, you need not suffer in silence and embarrassment. Incontinence can be successfully treated. Talk to your doctor; having your condition treated can significantly improve the quality of your life. For more about incontinence and treatment, see page 538.

When to be concerned about Alzheimer's disease

Many older people panic when they forget something—they think they have Alzheimer's disease. They forgot things when they were younger too, but it didn't cause them any concern then. Most memory loss is a normal part of aging. However, the symptoms listed below may be an indication of Alzheimer's disease. See a doctor if you or a loved one experiences any of the following:

- Severe memory loss
- Inappropriate behavior
- Change in personality
- Impairment in judgment, insight, and intellect
- Confusion or disorientation
- Inability to perform daily activities such as dressing, eating, or using the toilet

Atlas of the body

This anatomical atlas contains illustrations of the major systems and organs of the female body. Accompanying photographs show how imaging techniques can help doctors view the structures of internal organs. For more about the body systems and the diagnosis and treatment of specific medical problems, consult the index at the back of the book or follow the page references you'll find throughout the text.

THE TORSO

The upper part of the torso, the chest, contains the heart and lungs. The lower part of the torso, the abdomen, contains the digestive system and the urinary system. Between the chest and abdomen is the diaphragm, a dome-shaped sheet of muscle.

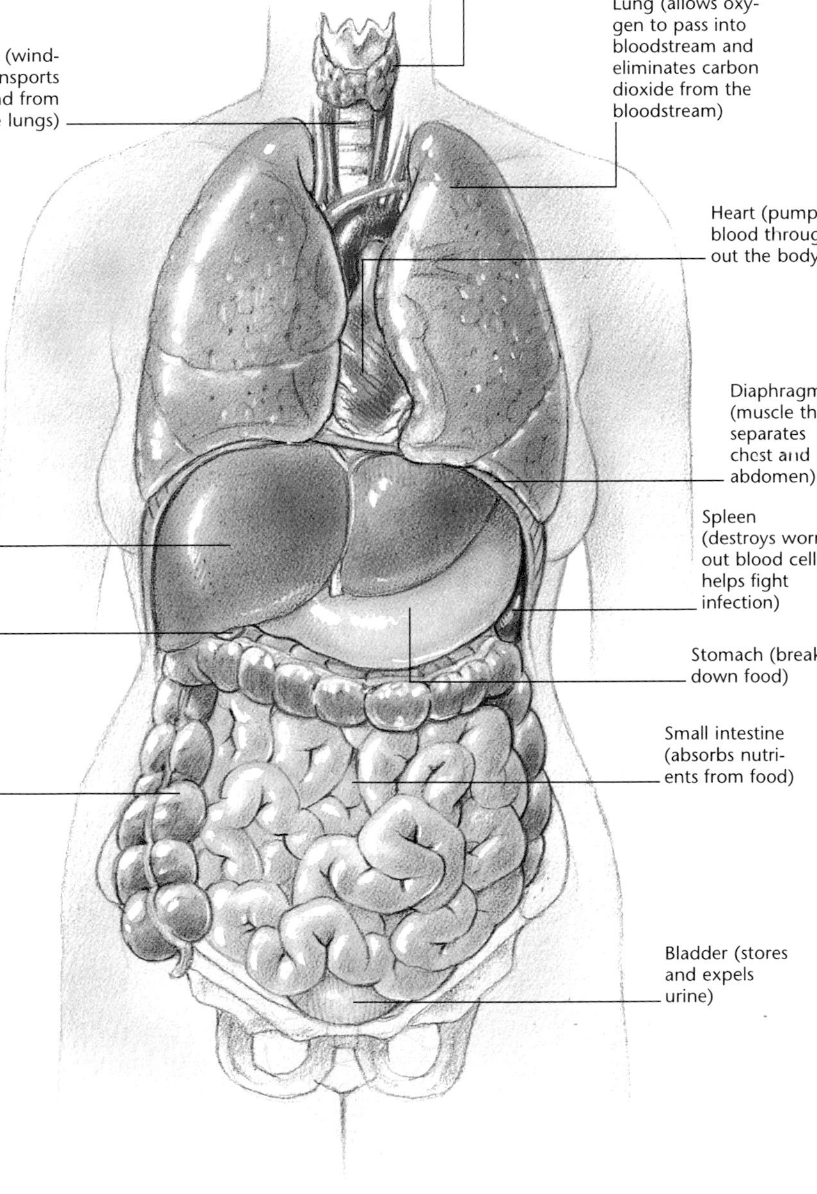

Bones and muscles

Your bones and muscles work together to support your body and enable you to move. To learn more about your bones, and especially how to keep them strong to avoid the bone-thinning disorder osteoporosis, see page 552. For information about building strength in your muscles, see page 84.

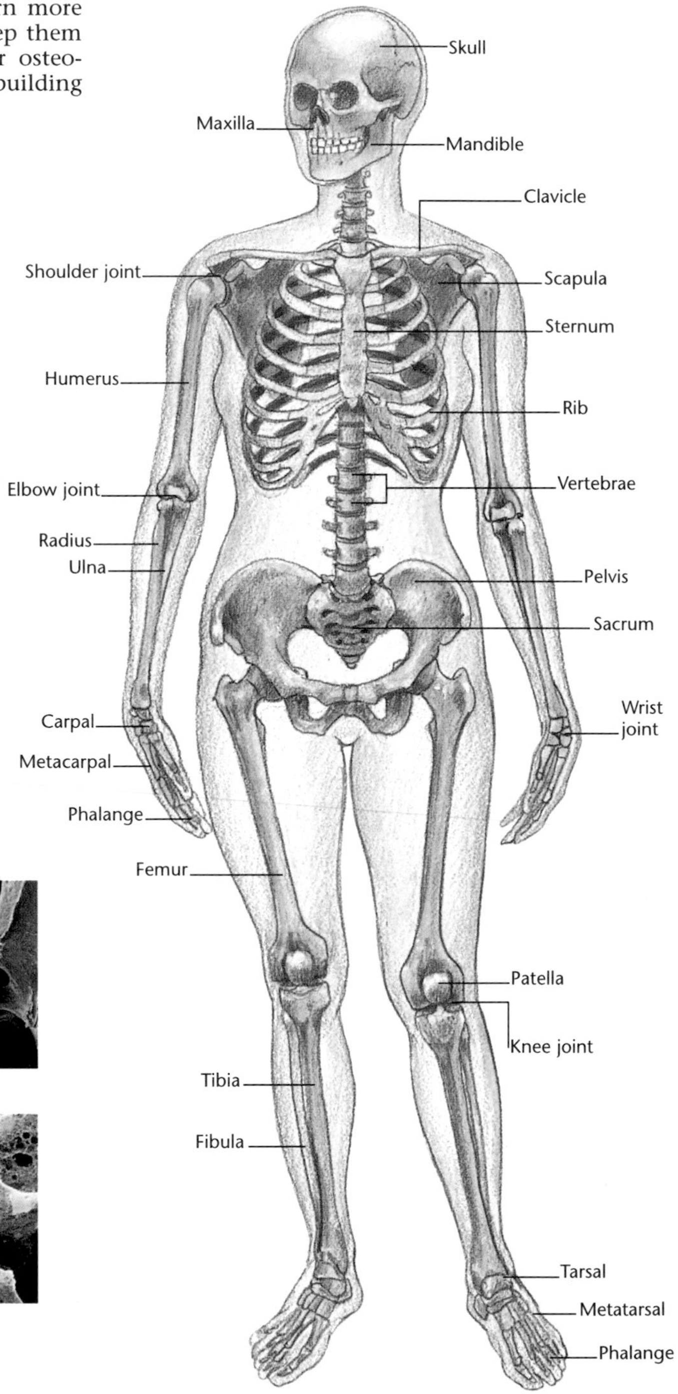

Skull
Maxilla
Mandible
Clavicle
Shoulder joint
Scapula
Sternum
Humerus
Rib
Elbow joint
Vertebrae
Radius
Ulna
Pelvis
Sacrum
Carpal
Wrist joint
Metacarpal
Phalange
Femur
Patella
Knee joint
Tibia
Fibula
Tarsal
Metatarsal
Phalange

BONES AND JOINTS

The 206 bones of your body protect and support your organs and allow movement. Bones are living, changing structures that require adequate calcium and weight-bearing exercise to build and maintain their density and strength. Bones are joined together by different types of joints: fixed joints (as in the skull), hinged joints (as in the fingers), and ball-and-socket joints (as in the shoulders and hips). The male and female skeletons are not quite identical. Females have lighter bones in their arms and legs, their elbow joint has a different angle, and the female pelvis is broader and has a larger space in the middle to allow a baby to pass through during childbirth.

OSTEOPOROSIS

Healthy bone consists of different kinds of cells, the structural protein collagen, and dense deposits of calcium, which give bone its strength. In osteoporosis, bone gradually becomes more porous, like a sponge with tiny holes that grow larger. This process makes the bone thin, weak, and prone to fracture.

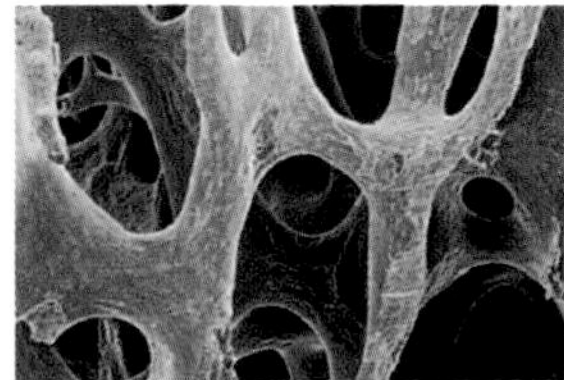

Healthy bone

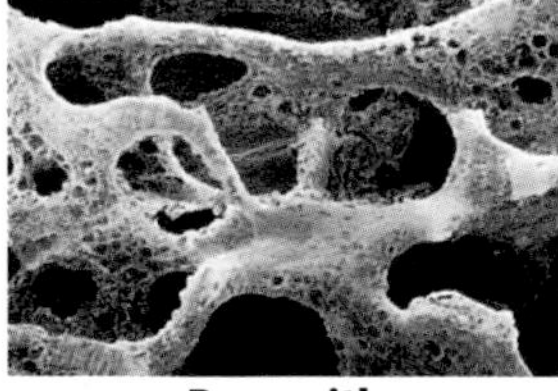

Bone with osteoporosis

MUSCLES

The more than 600 muscles in your body are composed of bundles of interlocking fibers that have the ability to contract and relax. The skeletal muscles are attached (directly or with a tendon) to two or more bones; when the muscle contracts, the bones move. A group of muscles often work together—one contracts, another relaxes, and nearby muscles provide stability.

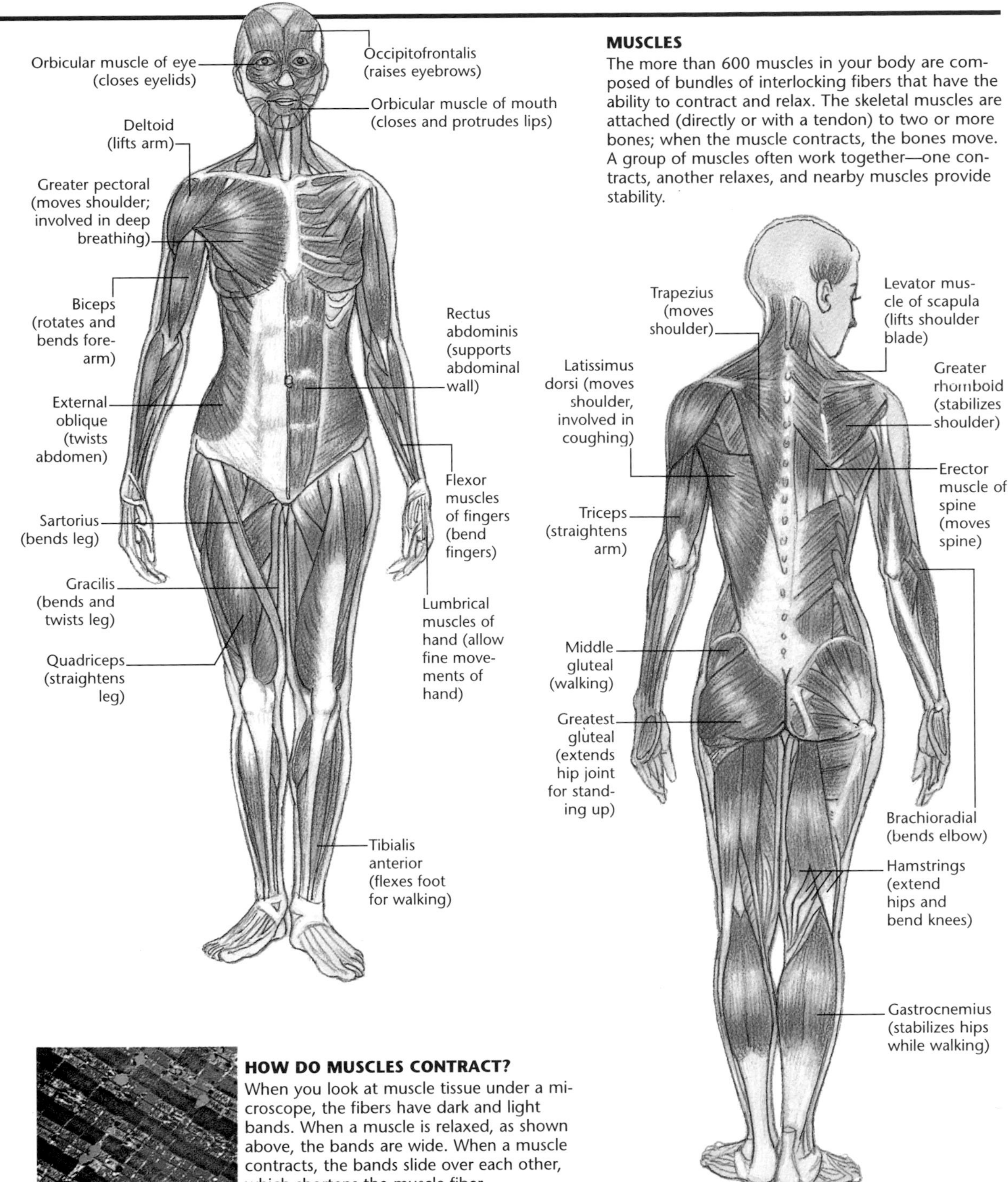

HOW DO MUSCLES CONTRACT?

When you look at muscle tissue under a microscope, the fibers have dark and light bands. When a muscle is relaxed, as shown above, the bands are wide. When a muscle contracts, the bands slide over each other, which shortens the muscle fiber.

The heart and circulatory system

Your heart pumps blood to every organ and tissue in your body. Although the heart functions the same way in both men and women, some conditions, such as mitral valve prolapse (see page 485), are more common among women. For more information, see chapter 17.

THE HEART

The heart is a muscular organ the approximate size and shape of a fist. It consists of two side-by-side pumps. The right side sends blood from the veins into the lungs, where the blood receives fresh oxygen. The oxygen-rich blood then enters the left side of the heart, which pumps it through the aorta and out to the entire body.

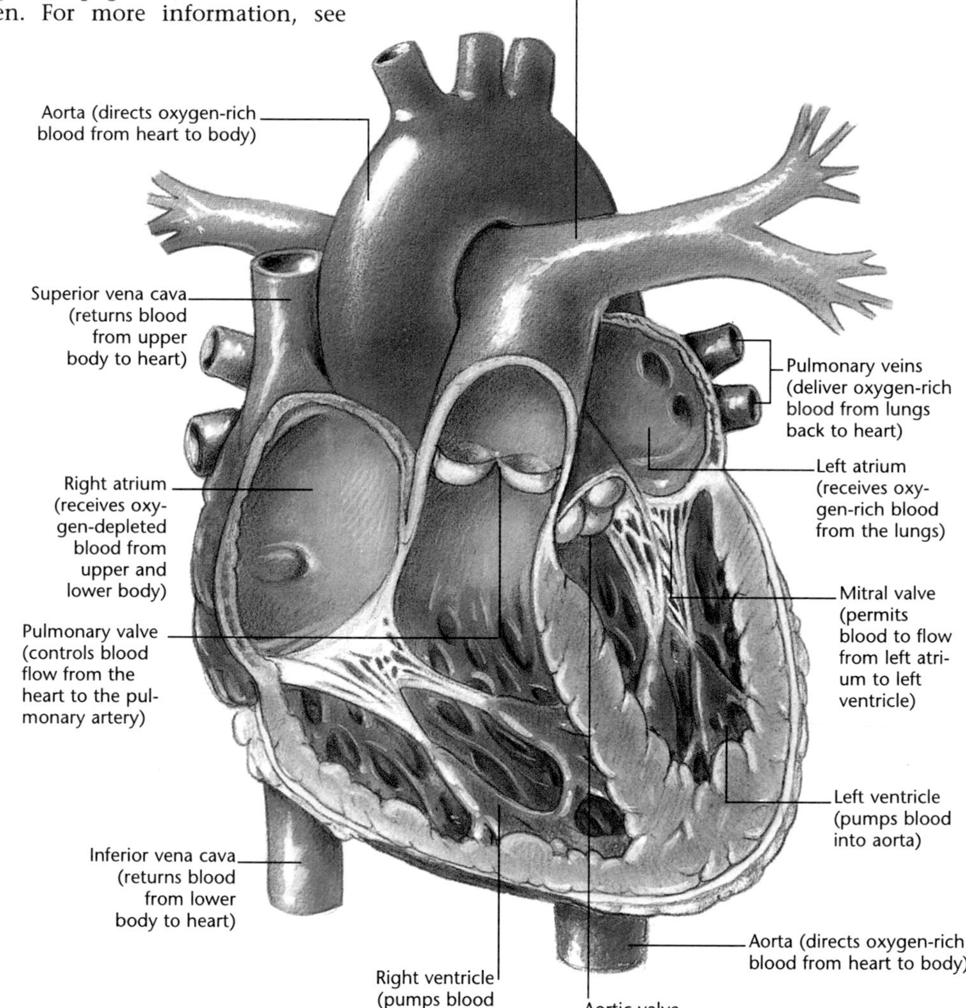

CORONARY ANGIOGRAM

In a coronary angiogram, dye is injected through a thin tube into the major arteries of the heart, making the arteries visible on an X-ray (see page 470). An angiogram is used to diagnose narrowing of the arteries and damage to heart tissues.

THE CIRCULATORY SYSTEM

Your circulatory system is made up of the heart and blood vessels, which continuously supply your body with oxygen and nutrients and remove carbon dioxide and other waste products. Arteries carry oxygen-rich blood away from the heart; veins return oxygen-depleted blood to the heart.

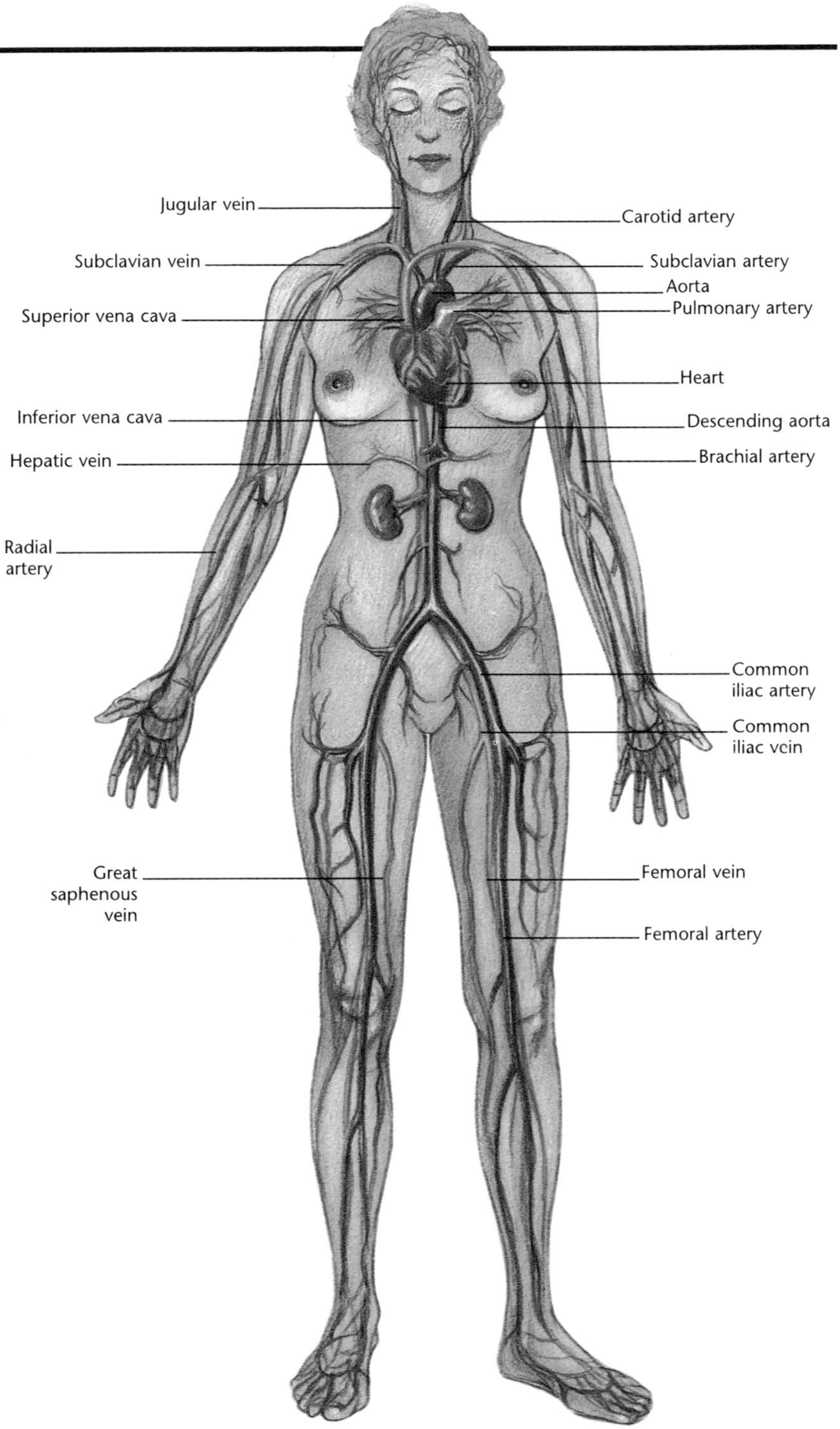

Jugular vein
Carotid artery
Subclavian vein
Subclavian artery
Aorta
Superior vena cava
Pulmonary artery
Heart
Inferior vena cava
Descending aorta
Hepatic vein
Brachial artery
Radial artery
Common iliac artery
Common iliac vein
Great saphenous vein
Femoral vein
Femoral artery

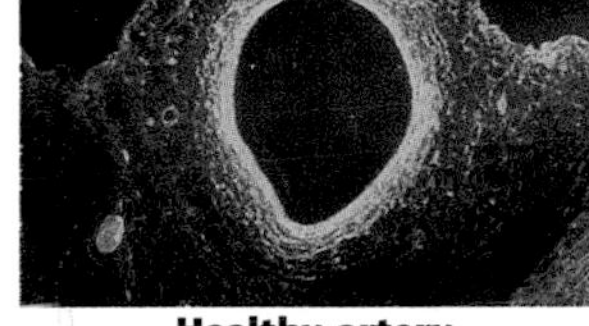

Healthy artery

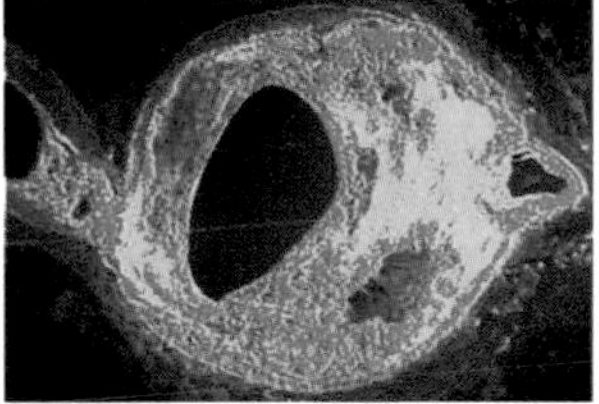

Narrowed artery

ATHEROSCLEROSIS

Atherosclerosis is the buildup of fatty deposits called plaque inside artery walls. This buildup can narrow the arteries and block the flow of blood to the heart or brain, causing a heart attack or stroke. For more about atherosclerosis, see page 468.

Female reproductive system, breasts, and urinary tract

Your reproductive organs and breasts are parts of a system designed to fulfill your sexual and reproductive needs. Your urinary tract filters and removes wastes from your body. For more about these important organs, see chapters 7, 8, 9, and 20.

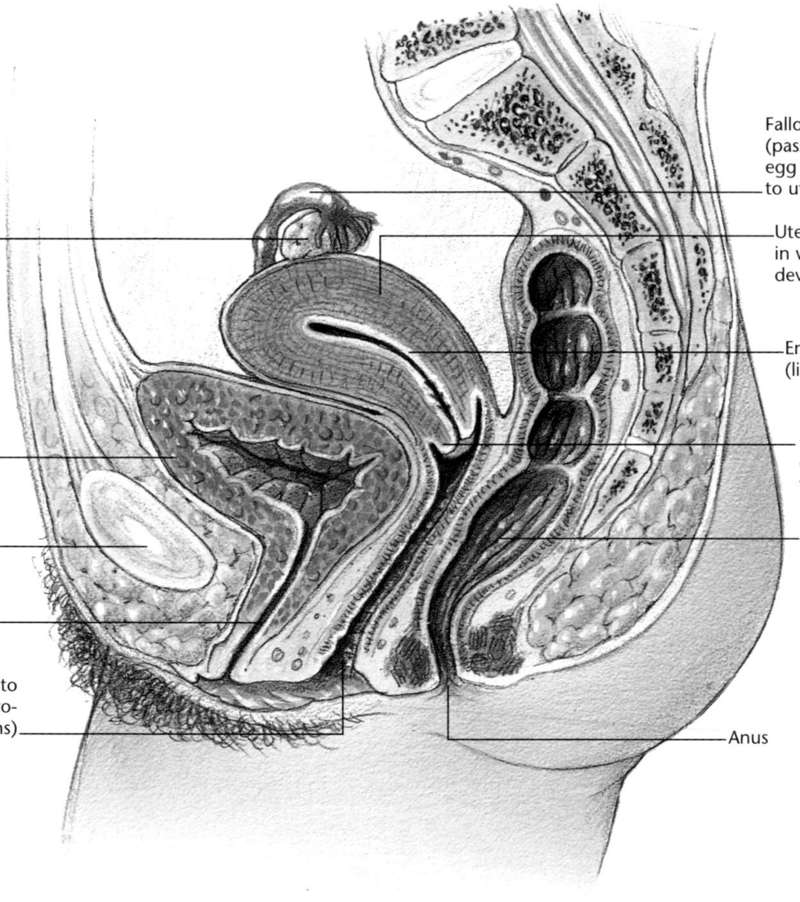

Fallopian tube (passageway for egg from ovary to uterus)

Ovary (stores and nurtures eggs)

Uterus (organ in which fetus develops)

Endometrium (lining of uterus)

Bladder

Cervix (opening of uterus into vagina)

Pubic bone

Rectum

Urethra

Vagina (passageway to and from internal reproductive organs)

Anus

INTERNAL REPRODUCTIVE ORGANS AND URINARY TRACT (SIDE VIEW)

Throughout your reproductive years, your reproductive system regulates your menstrual cycle, enabling you to become pregnant and bear a child. Many of the organs of your urinary system, including the bladder, are located in your lower abdomen, in close proximity to the reproductive organs.

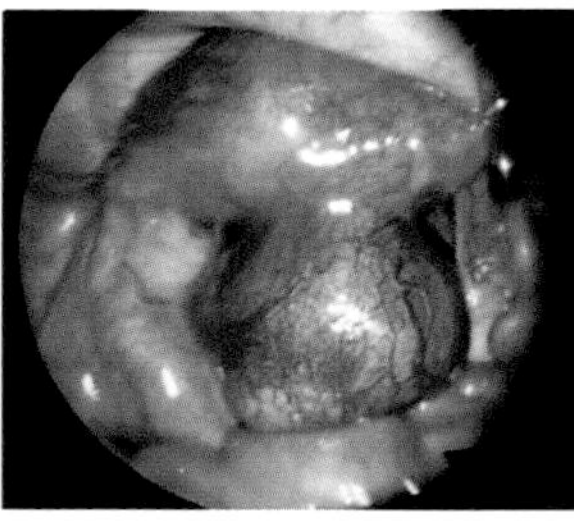

FIBROID

Fibroids are noncancerous growths that develop in or on the uterus. Fibroids are common; one in five women over age 35 has them. They can affect women differently; some women have no symptoms, while others experience pain or abnormal bleeding. For more about fibroids, see page 221.

THE URINARY TRACT AND REPRODUCTIVE ORGANS (FRONT VIEW)

Your kidneys filter excess water, calcium, salts, and waste products from your blood. These wastes are then propelled down two delicate tubes called ureters into your bladder, a muscular organ that stores urine until you feel the urge to urinate. You expel urine through a narrow, short tube called the urethra, which exits your body near your vaginal opening.

Inferior vena cava (delivers blood from lower body to heart)

Aorta (directs blood from heart to body)

Kidney (filters excess water and waste products from the blood)

Ureter (transports wastes from kidney to bladder)

Uterus

Fallopian tube

Ovary

Bladder (stores and expels urine)

Urethra (drains urine from bladder)

Fatty tissue

Pectoral muscle (chest muscle that moves arm across body)

Milk gland (secretes milk)

Milk duct (transports milk from gland to nipple)

Nipple (contains tiny openings through which milk can pass)

BREAST

The female breasts can provide milk to nourish a baby. The breasts are also sexually responsive. The size and shape of your breasts can vary with age, day of menstrual cycle, pregnancy, or breast-feeding.

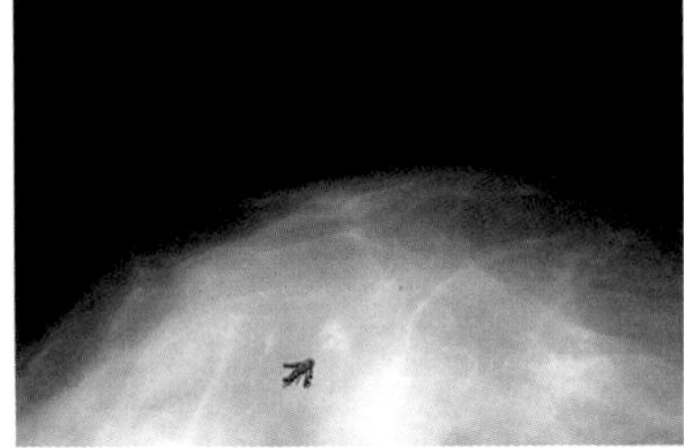

MAMMOGRAM

A mammogram, a low-intensity X-ray, can detect a cancerous tumor (arrow) in the breast that is too small to feel by hand. For a description of this procedure, see page 127.

Pregnancy

Pregnancy is a time of astonishing changes in both the pregnant woman and her fetus. These illustrations show the moment of conception, a developing fetus, and a pregnancy at full term. For more information, see chapters 14, 15, and 16.

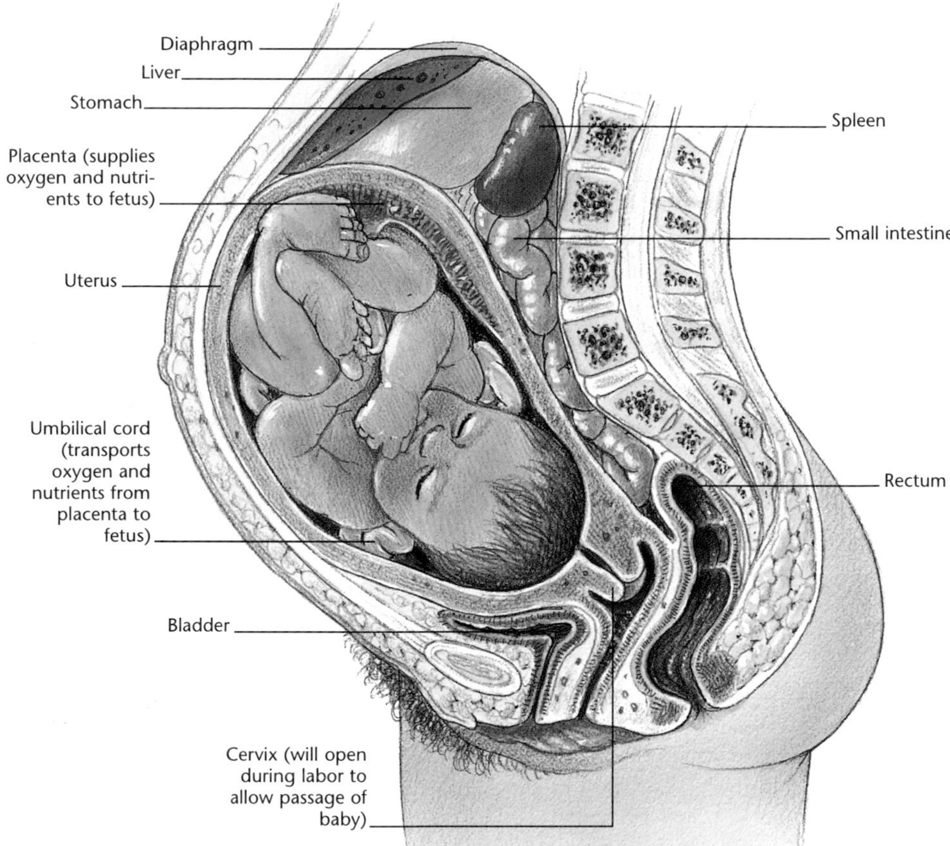

FETUS
This illustration shows a fetus during the ninth month of pregnancy in the most common position before labor begins, with head down and arms and legs curled in front.

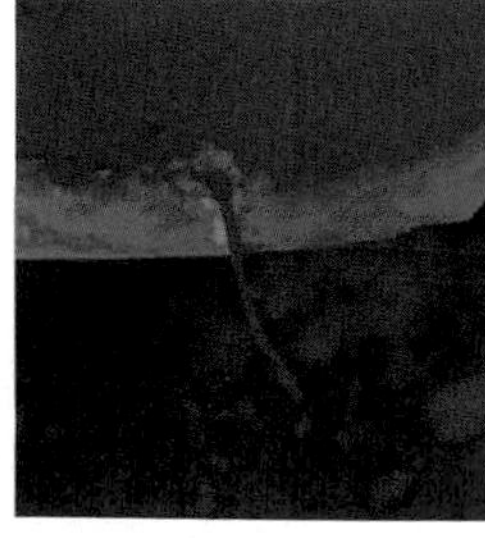

CONCEPTION
Pregnancy begins with conception—when a sperm penetrates a mature egg. This process, also called fertilization, quickly changes the egg's outer covering, preventing other sperm from entering. The fertilized egg begins to divide rapidly and will develop into a fetus.

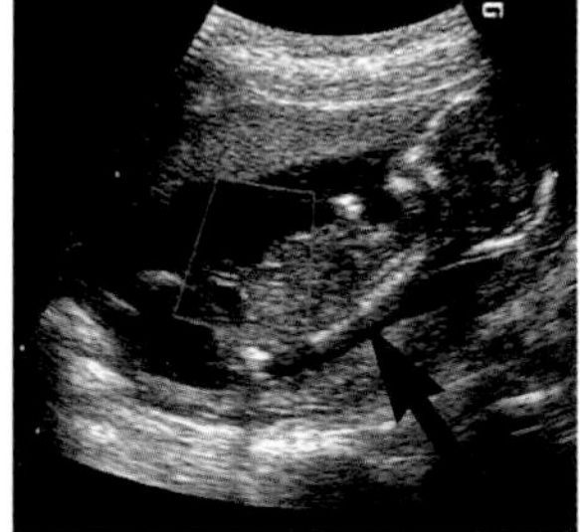

ULTRASOUND IMAGE OF FETUS
An ultrasound examination is a painless, safe, diagnostic procedure that uses sound waves to create an image on a computer screen. This image shows a healthy fetus in the fifth month of pregnancy (arrow points to the fetus's spinal cord). The colored areas reflect the flow of blood through the umbilical cord into the fetus.

·1·

Staying healthy for life

CHAPTER 1

Nutrition

Contents

Eating a well-balanced, nutritious diet is one of the most important things you can do for your health. A lifelong practice of healthy eating can reduce your risk of illness, increase your energy level, and improve your well-being.

Doctors have discovered that the link between diet and health is stronger than they previously thought. Of the 10 most common life-threatening diseases in the US, at least six—heart disease, cancer, stroke, diabetes, chronic liver disease and cirrhosis, and atherosclerosis (fat buildup in arteries)—are influenced by what people eat or drink. Many other conditions, which range from annoying to debilitating, are influenced by diet as well. Although other factors—most importantly, your genetic makeup—can influence your risk of disease, a healthy diet can help prevent a genetic susceptibility to a disease from becoming a reality.

Guidelines for healthy eating

Like most people, you are probably confused by the conflicting reports about foods that are either good for you or bad for you or sometimes both. The problem is not bad foods but rather the poor eating patterns that many people have. The key to a healthy diet is eating a balance of foods throughout the day and throughout the week.

Healthy foods are relatively easy to recognize. Vegetables, fruits, and whole grains are the best choices. Other foods, including protein-rich items such as meat, should be eaten in moderation. An occasional bowl of ice cream is OK, even though it is heavy in sugar and fat, as long as your overall diet contains mostly fruits, vegetables, and whole grains.

THE FOOD GUIDE PYRAMID

The Food Guide Pyramid developed by the US Department of Agriculture (USDA) shows you the relative amounts of the different foods you should include in your diet every day.

The pyramid places foods into six groups, showing how many servings from each group you should eat each day. Eat the greatest amounts of foods at the bottom of the pyramid (its broad base) and the smallest amounts of foods at the top (its peak).

The bottom layer of the pyramid contains grain products—breads, cereals, rice, and pasta. This group has the largest number (6 to 11) of recommended servings. That may seem like a lot, but it's easy to meet this goal. For example, a bowl of whole-grain cereal at breakfast, two slices of hearty whole-grain bread at lunch, a crusty hard roll with dinner, ½ cup of rice or pasta, and a bran muffin can fulfill the requirement. You probably eat more than this when you add in

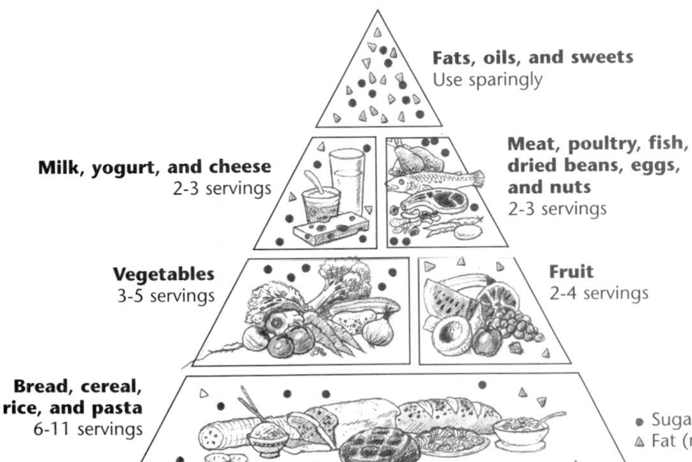

THE FOOD GUIDE PYRAMID
For good health, the US Department of Agriculture recommends a balanced diet that includes a number of servings from each of six food groups every day. Eat more servings of foods at the bottom of the pyramid and fewer of the foods at the top. Eating so many servings from each group may seem like a lot, but serving sizes are small—for example, a single carrot or a cup of pasta is one serving. Women usually require less food than men, so use the lower number of suggested servings.

Daily food choices

To help you make good choices, the chart below divides foods from each group into "more frequent," "less frequent," and "seldom" foods. "More frequent" foods can be eaten more often and regularly. "Less frequent" foods should be limited to less than once a day and only in moderate amounts. "Seldom" foods should be viewed as an occasional treat and eaten only in limited amounts.

FOOD GROUP	"MORE FREQUENT" FOODS	"LESS FREQUENT" FOODS	"SELDOM" FOODS
FATS, OILS, AND SWEETS (and substitutes)	Fat-free mayonnaise; fat-free salad dressings	Sugar; hard candies; vegetable oils; olives; pickles; soy sauce*; low-fat mayonnaise; salad dressings; squeeze or tub margarines	Butter; stick margarine; candy bars; chocolate; lard
MILK, YOGURT, AND CHEESE (two to three servings)	Skim or 1-percent milk; fat-free cheese; fat-free sour cream; fat-free cottage cheese; fat-free cream cheese; nonfat yogurt; frozen, fat-free desserts; sorbets	Buttermilk; 2-percent milk; low-fat cheese; light sour cream; low-fat cream cheese; part-skim or low-fat cottage cheese; low-fat yogurt; part-skim mozzarella; part-skim riccota; light ice cream; sherbert; puddings made with skim or low-fat milk	Whole milk; yogurt made with whole milk; cream cheese; hard cheeses such as cheddar, Swiss, or American; ice cream; cheesecake
FISH, MEAT, POULTRY, NUTS, AND EGGS (two to three servings; most meats trimmed and cooked with no added fat)	All fresh fish, seafood, and shellfish; tuna or salmon canned in water; chicken or turkey breast or drumstick without skin; lean ground chicken or turkey; low-fat poultry cold cuts; beef top or eye of round, sirloin, top loin, or tenderloin; 98-percent fat-free ground beef; pork tenderloin or loin; 98-percent fat-free hot dogs; egg whites or egg substitutes	Smoked fish; tuna or salmon canned in oil; chicken or turkey breast or drumstick with skin; breaded and fried chicken or turkey nuggets; ground chicken or turkey; chicken or turkey roll; beef tip, bottom round, chuck arm pot roast, flank, or T-bone steak; veal loin; pork loin (except blade); lamb sirloin; seeds and nuts (except macadamia nuts); peanut butter	Fried seafood; chicken thigh or wing with skin; hot dogs; untrimmed beef, pork, lamb, or veal; beefsteaks, roasts, or ribs; regular or lean ground beef; veal rib; ground veal; pork loin blade; bacon; ham; bologna; salami; liver and other organ meats; egg yolks; macadamia nuts
VEGETABLES (three to five servings)	Fresh, frozen, or canned* vegetables; no-sodium or reduced-sodium vegetable juices; all varieties of legumes (beans and peas)	Coleslaw; fried potato dishes; avocado (including guacamole); potato salad; vegetable juices*	Vegetables with high-fat sauces or butter; onion rings; au gratin potatoes; fried vegetables
FRUITS (two to four servings)	All fresh, frozen, or canned fruit (with juice); 100-percent fruit juices	Dried fruit; canned cranberry sauce; cranberry and other fruit cocktails; canned fruit in syrup; fruit drinks that are low in actual fruit juice	Coconut
BREAD, CEREAL, RICE, AND PASTA (6 to 11 servings)	Whole-grain breads; bagels; English muffins; breadsticks; air-popped popcorn; unsalted pretzels; rice cakes; corn tortillas*; low-fat tortilla chips*; low-fat crackers; rice; bulgur; couscous; kasha; pasta (not egg enriched); most whole-grain breakfast cereals (not heavily sweetened); low-fat or no-fat waffles; angel food cake	Biscuits; sweetened breakfast cereals; egg noodles; low-fat crackers; low-fat cookies such as fig bars; gingersnaps; graham crackers; pancakes; waffles	Fried pies; cakes (except fat free); oil-popped or buttered popcorn; bread stuffing; pastries; croissants; doughnuts; granola bars

*May be high in sodium—check label

grain-based snacks such as pretzels. But make sure that any grain-based snacks you eat (such as corn chips or oatmeal cookies) are not so packed with fat that you get more calories from the fat than from the grain.

The next largest level of the pyramid recommends two to four servings of fruits and three to five servings of vegetables each day. Eating five to nine servings of fruits and vegetables in a single day may seem impossible and, indeed, few of us eat even half that amount. But it's easier than you may think. A 4-ounce glass of orange juice counts as one serving and so does 1/4 cup of raisins, 1 cup of salad greens, or 1/2 cup of tomato sauce for pasta. These are some of the nutrient-rich foods to choose whenever you are preparing meals or having snacks.

The next step up the pyramid includes two food groups—dairy products (including milk, yogurt, and cheese) and a group that contains meat, fish, poultry, eggs, nuts, and dried beans. The USDA recommends two to three servings a day of foods in each of these two groups. A serving of meat is only 2 to 3 ounces—a quarter-pound hamburger counts as two servings (and is also often high in fat). If you add a handful of nuts as a snack, you've had your three servings from this group for the day. Choose the leanest meats and low-fat or nonfat dairy products to help cut down on excessive fat and calories. Dairy products provide lots of calcium, which you need to keep your bones strong. Having a 6-ounce glass of calcium-fortified orange juice; 1 cup of low-fat yogurt; two 8-ounce glasses of skim milk; and 1 ounce of low-fat cheese fulfills your daily calcium requirement of 1,000 to 1,500 milligrams.

At the top of the pyramid are fats, oils, and sweets. The USDA does not recommend a number of servings for this group because these foods are not essential to good health, and most of us eat too many of them. In addition to the obviously high-fat foods such as butter, ice cream, and candy bars, this group includes other foods that derive most of their calories from fat, including mayonnaise, salad dressings, pastries, and sauces.

Together, fruits, vegetables, and grains should comprise most of the calories (55 percent or more) you eat each day. These foods contain complex carbohydrates, which contribute the fiber, vitamins, and minerals that are essential to good health. The pyramid illustrates the relative importance of the food groups, but you still need good judgment when selecting foods from each group. For example, it is a good idea to drink three glasses of calcium-rich skim milk each day, but it would not be wise to eat three servings of cream cheese, which is high in fat.

Most women need to limit their calorie intake to avoid weight gain. One easy and healthy way to control calories is to limit your fat intake. By choosing low-fat or nonfat versions of foods, you will get all the nutrients you need—without the saturated fat, cholesterol, and extra calories you don't need.

NUTRITION GUIDELINES

The National Academy of Sciences—the group that sets the Recommended Dietary Allowances (RDAs) for nutrients—has developed specific goals for people who want to eat healthfully. These guidelines are a lifetime eating plan designed to reduce your risk of developing such chronic, debilitating diseases as heart disease.

■ **Reduce fat intake to no more than 30 percent of your total calories. Reduce saturated fats to less than 10 percent of total calories. Reduce cholesterol intake to less than 300 milligrams daily.** If you eat about 1,800 calories each day, your total daily fat intake should be less than 60 grams. American women eat more fat than this—an average of 36 percent of their total calories. The limit of 30 percent is the upper end, and less is better. However, you should not eliminate fat entirely because some unsaturated fat is essential for growth and development.

Overconsumption of saturated fat, found mostly in meat and dairy products, can increase your risk of heart disease, the number-one killer of American women. Saturated fat raises levels of cholesterol (see page 59) in the blood, causing fatty deposits to build up on artery walls, narrowing the artery. This narrowing increases blood pressure and the risk of heart attack and stroke. On an 1,800-calorie-a-day diet, you should limit saturated fat to less than 20 grams per day. You can accumulate that much saturated fat just by having one glass of whole milk, a 3-ounce steak (the size of a deck of cards), and a 1-ounce piece of cheddar cheese. But simply by replacing an 8-ounce glass of whole milk with a glass of skim milk, you can reduce your fat consumption from 8.5 grams to virtually no fat and cut your calories in half.

Like saturated fat, hydrogenated fat (which is found in margarine and canned shortening) may also raise cholesterol levels. Try to avoid hydrogenated fat or eat it only in moderation. Unsaturated fats (which are found in most vegetable oils) do not raise blood cholesterol. In fact, they help lower it. These cholesterol-lowering oils include olive, canola, safflower, soy, and corn oils. But, like all oils, they contain 120 calories per tablespoon and derive 100 percent of their calories from fat, so you need to limit your consumption.

The risk of obesity from eating a high-fat diet is another important reason to limit your fat intake. A high-fat diet is also linked to some types of cancer, particularly colon cancer, prostate cancer, and, possibly, breast cancer.

■ **Eat five or more servings of a combination of vegetables and fruits daily, especially green and yellow vegetables and citrus fruits. Increase your daily intake of starches and other complex carbohydrates by eating six or more servings of a combination of breads, cereals, and legumes.** These foods are rich in complex carbohydrates, fiber, and nutrients and should dominate your diet—accounting for at least 55 percent of your daily calories. An average serving of vegetables, fruits, and grains is equal to ½ cup.

■ **Eat a reasonable amount of protein, maintaining your protein consumption at moderate levels.** For women, the RDA for protein is 50 grams. Most women eat much more than that. Meat is a good source of protein, but you should eat smaller servings than typical in the American diet. Limit your intake to less than 6 ounces of lean meat per day. Nonfat dairy products, such as skim milk and nonfat yogurt, provide good quality protein. There are 28 grams of protein in a small chicken breast, 17 grams in a 3-ounce red snapper fillet, 8 grams in an 8-ounce glass of skim milk, and 12 grams in 1 cup of low-fat yogurt.

■ **Balance the amount of food you eat with the amount of exercise you get to maintain a healthy body weight.** When you take in more calories than you burn, you gain weight. Excess weight is associated with a variety of chronic diseases including heart disease, high blood pressure, diabetes, some cancers, and arthritis. Regular exercise is an important way to burn off calories. Women are especially prone to gaining weight as they age because they have a greater proportion of body fat to muscle compared with men. Without exercise, that proportion of body fat will increase with age.

■ **Drinking alcohol is not recommended. If you do drink, limit the amount in a single day to no more than one 12-ounce glass of beer, one 5-ounce glass of wine, or one cocktail (with 1½ ounces of hard liquor). Pregnant women should not drink alcohol at all.**

Although moderate alcohol intake is associated with a reduced risk of heart disease, doctors do not recommend drinking alcohol as a way to prevent heart disease. The risk of alcohol addiction is too great (see page 160).

Heavy drinking increases the risk of heart disease, high blood pressure, chronic liver disease, neurological diseases, nutritional deficiencies, birth defects, and many other disorders. Alcohol is also a major contributor to accidents, suicides, homicides, and other violent behavior.

■ **Limit the amount of sodium (salt) you eat to less than 6 grams (slightly more than 1 teaspoon) per day.** Limit your use of salt in cooking and avoid adding it to food at the table. Salty foods—including highly processed foods, salt-preserved foods, and salt-pickled foods—should be eaten sparingly, if at all. Foods in cans or boxes, frozen dinners, and convenience foods are usually high in sodium. So are condiments such as mustard and catsup. In some people, a high consumption of salt can increase blood pressure—a major risk factor for heart disease.

■ **Get an adequate amount of calcium.** Calcium is especially important for women, because women are susceptible to developing the bone-thinning disorder osteoporosis. Calcium should be an important part of a woman's diet throughout her life, beginning in early childhood. A woman's bones reach their peak strength and density by the time she is 20, so it is especially important for girls and young women between ages 11 and 24 to consume an adequate amount of calcium—1,200 to 1,500 milligrams a day. The recommendation for women over 24 is 1,000 milligrams a day (1,200 milligrams if you are pregnant or breast-feeding). You can get more than 1,200 milligrams of calcium in a day by having a 6-ounce glass of calcium-fortified orange juice (217 milligrams of calcium), an 8-ounce glass of skim milk (300 milligrams), a cup of plain low-fat yogurt (468 milligrams), a 1-ounce slice of part-skim mozzarella cheese (207 milligrams), and a cup of broccoli (42 milligrams). Adding nonfat milk powder to casseroles, soups, sauces, puddings, pie fillings, and dips and combining it with milk in recipes are easy ways to increase your consumption of calcium. After menopause, when bone loss accelerates, you need 1,500 milligrams of calcium per day. (If you are taking estrogen, you need 1,000 milligrams.) If you are not getting enough calcium from your diet, take a calcium supplement (see page 57) to reach the recommended amount.

Nutrients and your health

Most things we eat or drink fall into one of several categories—carbohydrates, fiber, fats, protein, vitamins, minerals, or water. Each serves useful functions and none is by nature unhealthy. However, the phrase "too much of a good thing" can apply to any one of them.

People crave foods that are sweet, fatty, or salty, but most are not getting enough exercise to burn off an excessive number of calories. Eating too many of the foods that we crave not only makes us gain weight but can keep us from eating the nutrient-rich foods that our body needs.

Following are descriptions of the essential nutrients, including their roles in maintaining your health.

CARBOHYDRATES

Carbohydrates—starches and sugars found in fruits, vegetables, and grains—are the body's best energy source. Carbohydrates contain less than half the calories of the same amount of fat. You should get at least 55 percent of your daily calories from carbohydrates.

There are two kinds of carbohydrates—complex carbohydrates and simple carbohydrates. Starchy foods (such as pasta, whole-grain bread, dried beans, rice, and potatoes) contain complex carbohydrates. Simple carbohydrates—also called simple sugars—are found in table sugar, corn syrup, honey, and fruit. Both kinds of carbohydrates contain the same number of calories, but complex carbohydrates are better for you. Unlike simple sugars, complex carbohydrates provide fiber and a variety of vitamins and minerals. Simple or refined sugars are considered to be empty calories—they provide no nutrients.

Sugar has been blamed for a variety of ailments but, other than cavities in teeth, sugar does not contribute to any health problems—not even hyperactivity in children. The problem with sugar is that our craving for it often leads us to overindulge in such high-fat, high-calorie foods as cake, candy, cookies, ice cream, and chocolate.

Artificial sweeteners Aspartame is the most commonly used sugar substitute. The FDA has set a safe limit for aspartame, which is much more than most

Starches and weight loss

It is a myth that, to lose weight, you need to eliminate pasta, rice, bread, potatoes, and other starches from your diet. These are excellent foods to include in your weight-loss diet (as long as you stay away from high-fat, high-calorie toppings). Although starch has the same number of calories as protein, starchy foods have almost no fat, unlike some high-protein foods such as meat and some dairy products.

Hidden sugars

Sugar is empty of calories, with no nutritional value. Food manufacturers often try to hide the high sugar content of a food by referring to the sugar by many different names on the label. The government requires that ingredients be listed in descending order by weight. When two or more forms of sugar are used in the same product, a manufacturer can list them separately—that way, each sugar will be further down the list than if all the forms of sugar were counted together. For example, a box of cereal might list wheat flour as the first ingredient, followed by corn syrup and fructose, which are two forms of sugar. If the two sugars were combined, they would be listed first as the most abundant ingredient.

Here is a list of names for sugar you will see on food labels. If you see two or more of these on a label, the food probably has more sugar than you need:

- corn syrup
- dextrose
- fructose
- glucose
- honey
- lactose
- malt syrup
- maltodextrin
- maltose
- mannitol
- maple syrup
- molasses
- sorbitol
- sucrose

people would consume—the equivalent of drinking about 17 cans of a diet soft drink in a day.

Because aspartame may cause brain damage in children with a genetic disorder called phenylketonuria (PKU), products containing the sugar substitute carry a warning on the label. Flavored seltzer water is a safe alternative to diet soft drinks for people who have PKU.

FIBER

The term "fiber" refers to many different substances in food that are not digestible. Fiber provides no vitamins, minerals, or calories, but it has a variety of important functions and is a vital part of a healthy diet. In addition to providing the bulk that helps your digestive system run smoothly, fiber may help protect against a variety of diseases including cancer, heart disease, and diabetes. Fiber helps prevent a variety of bowel disorders ranging from constipation to irritable bowel syndrome (see page 526) and diverticulosis (see page 528). The foods that provide fiber—fruits, vegetables, and grains—offer numerous nutritional benefits as well.

Fiber comes in two forms—insoluble and soluble. Insoluble fiber is found in most foods that contain complex carbohydrates, such as whole-wheat breads, wheat bran, and fruit and vegetable skins. Insoluble fiber provides the bulk that makes you feel full and protects against disorders of the bowel, including colon cancer.

Soluble fiber comes primarily from fruits; vegetables; and barley, dried beans, and oats (oat bran and oatmeal are good sources). The soluble fiber found in oats, barley, and dried beans, especially in conjunction with a low-fat diet, can help lower your cholesterol level, thereby protecting against heart disease.

Psyllium is a grass that is high in soluble fiber and is used in various over-the-counter stool softeners and laxatives. Psyllium is added to wheat-based cereals as well (oat- and barley-based cereals are naturally rich in soluble fiber). Always talk to your doctor before taking laxatives. Taken improperly, laxatives can cause bloating and may reduce your body's ability to absorb nutrients.

If you follow the dietary guidelines in this chapter, you are almost guaranteed a diet naturally high in fiber. The National Cancer Institute recommends that people eat 25 to 30 grams of fiber each day. The average American woman gets only half that amount. You can get 30 grams of fiber simply by eating a high-fiber bran cereal for breakfast, an apple as a snack, and an ear of corn and a carrot at dinner. Bran cereals provide the most concentrated source of fiber. Whole-grain, enriched breads are also good sources, although they are not as fiber-rich as bran cereals. White breads contain almost no fiber.

Increase your fiber intake gradually because an abrupt change may cause

Good sources of fiber

All fruits, vegetables, and grains provide some fiber. To get a good daily dose (25 to 30 grams) of fiber, eat oatmeal, bran cereal, or whole-grain bread, and plenty of fruits, vegetables, and dried beans. Read labels to find out which foods contain the most fiber in a serving—high-fiber foods are those with at least 2 grams per serving.

FOOD	SERVING SIZE	TOTAL FIBER (grams)
FISH, MEAT, POULTRY, DRIED BEANS, NUTS, AND EGGS		
Pinto beans (cooked)	1/2 cup	7.4
Navy beans (cooked)	1/2 cup	6.5
Kidney beans (cooked)	1/2 cup	5.7
Chickpeas (cooked)	1/2 cup	4.4
VEGETABLES (COOKED UNLESS OTHERWISE SPECIFIED)		
Artichoke	1 medium	6.5
Green peas	1/2 cup	4.4
Brussels sprouts	1/2 cup	3.8
Sweet potato	1 medium	3.4
FRUITS		
Raisins	12 tablespoons	4.7
Apple with skin	1 medium	3.7
Orange	1 medium	3.1
Prunes	4	2.4
BREAD, CEREAL, RICE, AND PASTA		
Ready-to-eat wheat-bran cereal	1/2 cup	3.9
Whole-wheat bread	2 slices	3.9
Oat-bran cereal (cooked)	1/2 cup	2.9

bloating, nausea, or flatulence. Drinking lots of water can help reduce these side effects, which will naturally taper off as your system adjusts to the increase in fiber. Fiber supplements are seldom recommended because they do not provide the other health benefits that fruits, vegetables, and grains do.

PROTEIN

Protein is an important part of the structure of every living cell and is essential for development and growth. Some proteins form structures in your body such as muscles, bone, and skin. Other proteins—including infection-fighting antibodies and some hormones—reside in your body's fluids, which carry them wherever they are needed.

The protein building blocks of your body are supplied and replenished by protein from the food you eat. The protein you get from your diet is also a source of energy. Meat, fish, dried beans, and dairy products are rich sources of protein. Vegetarians can get an adequate amount of protein by eating combinations of dried beans, peas, lentils, whole grains, eggs, and dairy products.

Protein deficiency is rare in developed countries where even vegetarians consume a wide variety of foods and get enough of each of the nine essential amino acids (the basic structural units of protein) from their diet. In fact, most people eat more protein than they need. It is recommended that about 10 to 15 percent of your total daily calories be in the form of protein. For women, this is about 50 grams per day—the amount in a small chicken breast, a glass of skim milk, and a cup of low-fat or nonfat yogurt.

Athletes sometimes assume that, because protein is used to build muscles, eating more protein will give them stronger muscles. But, an overabundance of protein is converted into body fat or excreted in the urine.

FATS

Fat is a source of stored energy. It has more calories per unit than any other food. Unsaturated fats, such as olive oil, provide essential nutrients called fatty acids, so no diet should be completely fat-free. But fats are also the major source of extra calories and some kinds of fat can contribute to heart disease by boosting the level of cholesterol in the blood.

Saturated fats—those found in meats, dairy products, and tropical vegetable oils (such as palm and coconut oils)—raise your cholesterol level. The foods that are highest in saturated fats include red meats, poultry skin, butter, whole milk, ice cream, and cheese.

Unsaturated fats come primarily from vegetable oils and do not increase your cholesterol level. They do, however, contain the same number of calories per unit as saturated fats. Unsaturated fats are divided into two groups—polyunsaturated fats (which are found in safflower oil, corn oil, and soybean oil) and monounsaturated oils (found in olive oil and canola oil).

Neither type of unsaturated fat raises a person's total cholesterol level. But both types affect the two kinds of cholesterol in the blood in different ways. Doctors worry most about the "bad" cholesterol called low-density lipoprotein (LDL). This is a type of fat that carries cholesterol through the bloodstream, unloading it onto artery walls where it can build up and block the flow of blood to the heart. This process is called atherosclerosis. High-density lipoprotein (HDL) is the "good" cholesterol that sweeps up the fatty debris left by LDL cholesterol and carries it to the liver, where it is broken down into harmless products. Polyunsaturated oils lower total cholesterol, but eating too much may lower the good HDL cholesterol as well. Monounsaturated oils lower only LDL.

When vegetable oils are turned into solid stick margarine or shortening used in baked goods, they become hydrogenated oils. These oils can raise the level of harmful LDL cholesterol. Soft, whipped, or liquid margarines are less hydrogenated. Check the ingredients list for hydrogenated oils when you buy baked goods. Some liquid vegetable oils are a better choice (especially canola and safflower oils).

Unlike saturated fat, which is found in animal products and in some oils,

Converting fat grams to calories

There are 9 calories in a gram of fat. A serving of ice cream with 24 grams of fat contains 216 calories of fat.

(24 fat grams x 9 calories per gram = 216 calories of fat)

Figuring fat

The best way to find out how many grams of fat you are eating each day is to record everything you eat. Look up the amount of fat per serving in a nutrient counter or read food labels. A good rule of thumb for packaged foods is to choose those that limit the fat to less than 3 grams for every 100 calories.

Your goal is to limit the total number of calories from fat to less than 30 percent of the total number of calories you eat each day.

To figure your average daily calorie intake, write down everything you eat for 1 week, adding up total calories at the end of each day. Or, for a quick estimate of your daily calorie intake, use the following formula. Your body needs about 12 calories per pound per day to maintain a certain weight. For example, if you weigh 150 pounds, your body requires 1,800 calories (150 X 12 = 1,800). If you are under 25 or very active, add up to 4 calories per pound before calculating your daily calorie intake.

Once you know your daily calorie total, you can find your daily fat allowance in the table below. But keep in mind that if you want to gain or lose weight, you must still compare the number of calories you eat with the number of calories you burn.

Daily calorie intake and fat allowance

CALORIES	FAT (grams)
1,200	40
1,400	46
1,600	53
1,800	60
2,000	66
2,200	73
2,400	80

Vitamins and minerals

The best way to get the vitamins and minerals you need is by eating a varied, balanced diet, rich in fruits, vegetables, and whole grains. This table describes the health benefits of the most important vitamins and minerals and the foods you can eat to get those nutrients. Vitamins are divided into two categories—fat soluble and water soluble. **Fat-soluble vitamins** are found in fats and oils in foods and they are stored in body fat. **Water-soluble vitamins** dissolve in water and mix easily in the blood. Your body stores only small amounts of them and they are excreted in urine. Some vitamins are **antioxidants**—chemicals that prevent damaging changes in cells and may help protect against cancer, heart disease, and aging.

VITAMIN OR MINERAL	BEST SOURCES	HEALTH BENEFITS
	FAT-SOLUBLE VITAMINS	
Vitamin A	Animal sources such as milk, eggs, cheese, butter, chicken, liver	Antioxidant; essential for growth and development; maintains healthy vision, skin, and mucous membranes
Vitamin D	Fortified milk	Essential for formation of bones and teeth; helps the body absorb and use calcium
Vitamin E	Vegetable oils, whole grains, wheat germ, nuts, leafy green vegetables	Antioxidant; helps form blood cells, muscles, and lung and nerve tissue; boosts the immune system
Vitamin K	Dark green leafy vegetables, liver, egg yolks	Essential for blood clotting
Beta carotene	Orange and deep yellow vegetables and fruit (carrots, sweet potatoes, winter squash, cantaloupe, pumpkins, mangoes); the body converts beta carotene in yellow and orange vegetables and fruits and some dark green leafy vegetables (spinach, broccoli) into vitamin A	Antioxidant; used by the body to make vitamin A
	WATER-SOLUBLE VITAMINS	
Vitamin C	Citrus fruits, vegetables (tomatoes, green peppers, cabbage), leafy green vegetables	Antioxidant; necessary for healthy bones, teeth, and skin; helps in wound healing
Thiamin (vitamin B_1)	Whole grains, enriched breads and cereals, pork, liver, peas	Helps convert food into energy
Riboflavin (vitamin B_2)	Meats, fish, whole grains, milk products, dark green vegetables, enriched breads and cereals, enriched pasta	Helps in energy production and other chemical processes in the body; helps maintain healthy eyes, skin, and nerve function
Niacin (vitamin B_3)	Whole grains, milk products, meat, poultry, fish, nuts, broccoli, green peas, green beans	Helps convert food into energy; helps maintain proper brain function
Vitamin B_6	Whole-wheat products, meat, fish, nuts, green beans, bananas, green leafy vegetables, potatoes	Helps produce essential proteins; helps convert protein into energy

VITAMIN OR MINERAL	BEST SOURCES	HEALTH BENEFITS
Vitamin B_{12}	Dairy products, eggs, liver	Helps produce the genetic material of cells; helps convert carbohydrates into energy; helps with formation of red blood cells and maintenance of central nervous system; helps make amino acids (the building blocks of proteins)
Folic acid (folate)	Dark green leafy vegetables, fruits, dried beans and peas, liver	Necessary to produce the genetic material of cells; essential in first 3 months of pregnancy for preventing birth defects; helps in red blood cell formation; protects against heart disease
MINERALS		
Calcium	Dairy products, sardines (with bones), salmon, dark green leafy vegetables	Essential for building bones and teeth and maintaining bone strength; important in muscle function
Chromium	Whole grains, brewer's yeast, nuts, dried beans	Works with insulin to convert carbohydrates and fat into energy
Copper	Whole grains, nuts, liver, oysters	Essential for making hemoglobin (oxygen-carrying protein in red blood cells) and collagen (a protein in connective tissue); essential for healthy functioning of the heart; helps in energy production; helps in absorption of iron from digestive tract
Iron	Meat, poultry, fish, dried beans, nuts, dried fruits, whole-grain and enriched grain products	Helps in energy production; helps to carry oxygen in the bloodstream and to transfer oxygen to muscles
Magnesium	Leafy green vegetables, nuts, whole grains, dried peas and beans, dairy products, fish, meat, poultry	Essential for healthy nerve and muscle function and bone formation; may help prevent premenstrual syndrome (PMS)
Phosphorus	Meat, dairy products, poultry, fish, grain products	Essential for building strong bones and teeth; helps in formation of genetic material; helps in energy production and storage
Potassium	Fruits, vegetables, nuts, grains, seeds	Essential for maintaining balance of body fluids, transmitting nerve signals, and producing energy
Selenium	Fish, meat, whole-grain breads and cereals, milk	Antioxidant; essential for healthy functioning of the heart muscle
Sodium	Table salt, vegetables, animal foods, some bottled waters	Essential for maintaining normal blood pressure and balance of body fluids and for transmitting nerve signals
Zinc	Meats, poultry, oysters, eggs, legumes, nuts, milk, yogurt, whole-grain cereals	Essential for cell reproduction, normal growth and development in children, wound healing (tissue repair and growth), and production of sperm and the male hormone testosterone

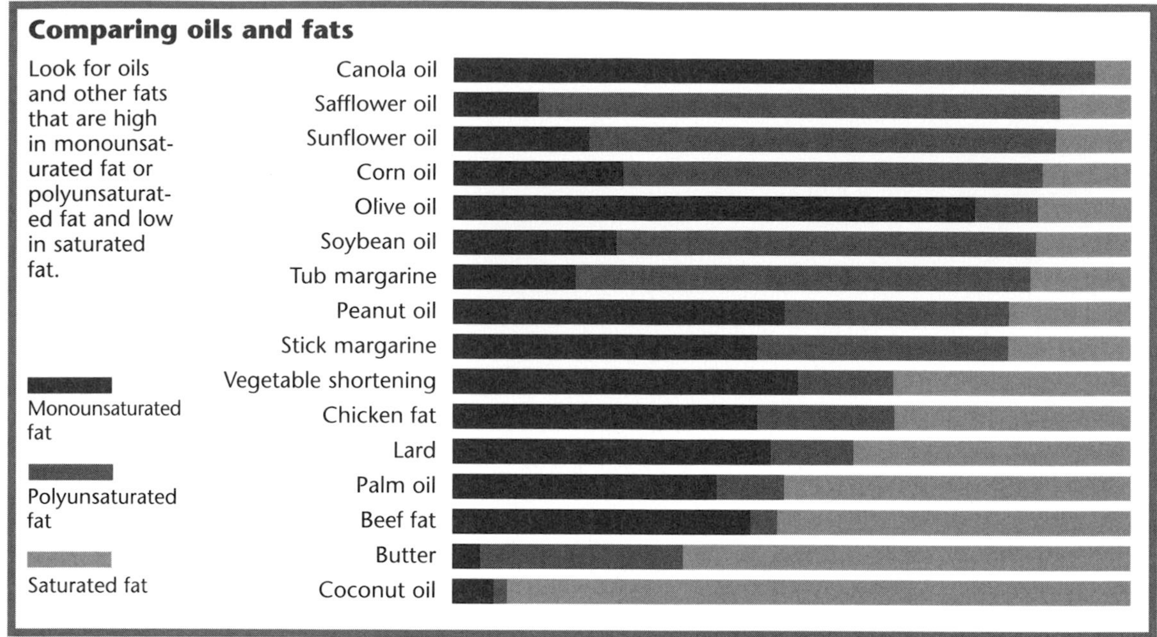

cholesterol in food is found only in animal products (meat, fish, dairy products, poultry, and eggs). Fish and poultry usually contain less cholesterol than red meats (beef, pork, and lamb). The saturated fat that people eat is the main culprit in raising the level of cholesterol in their blood.

VITAMINS AND MINERALS

Your body needs vitamins and minerals to function properly. Vitamins regulate the chemical processes inside your body and are essential for maintaining your immune system. Minerals help build structures such as bones and red blood cells. Vitamins and minerals also play a role in preventing heart disease, stroke, and some cancers.

There are two kinds of vitamins—water soluble and fat soluble. Eight B vitamins and vitamin C make up the nine water-soluble vitamins. Most of these are not stored well by your body and are washed away in urine. They need to be replenished daily.

The four fat-soluble vitamins—A, D, E, and K—are stored in your body's fat cells. They remain in your body until they are broken down. This means that, if you take too much of any of these vitamins, they can build up in your body and have harmful effects.

Many people take vitamin and mineral supplements. Nutritionists and other scientists are not sure if some of the vitamins in supplements are absorbed as effectively by the body as the vitamins and minerals in foods. That's why most doctors emphasize the importance of eating a well-balanced, high-fiber, low-fat diet rich in fruits, vegetables, and whole grains. Taking a vitamin pill cannot make up for the adverse effects of a poor diet. Nor can vitamin supplements

Don't chew vitamin C... eat oranges instead

Chewing vitamin C supplements may erode the surface enamel of your teeth. When chewed, vitamin C makes saliva more acidic. If you are taking vitamin C in chewable form, consider switching to tablets you can swallow. Better yet, eat fruits and vegetables—such as oranges, tomatoes, and cabbage—that are rich in vitamin C.

supply the fiber that your body needs. However, for many people who do not get all the nutrients they need from food (such as pregnant women, people on a calorie-restricted diet, and older people), a daily vitamin and mineral supplement that contains 100 percent of the RDAs for those nutrients can be helpful.

Many doctors recommend that, under some circumstances, women take supplements of specific vitamins or minerals. For example, women who are planning a pregnancy should take 400 micrograms (0.4 milligrams) of folic acid daily. Folic acid prevents birth defects that can occur during the first few months of pregnancy, before a woman knows she is pregnant. If you have difficulty getting a sufficient amount of calcium (see page 58) from your diet to keep your bones strong, you should take a calcium supplement.

Huge doses of vitamins will not make you healthier and, in fact, large doses of some vitamins may actually harm your health. The role of specific vitamins and minerals in preventing disease is discussed in detail later in this chapter. For more about disease prevention and nutrition, see page 56.

WATER

Unlike fat, carbohydrates, and protein, water supplies no energy or calories. However, like vitamins and minerals, water plays a vital role in your body's ability to perform its chemical interactions. You might even consider water your body's most important nutrient. We can survive for long periods without other nutrients but we can live for only a few days without water.

Water makes up one half to two thirds of your body. It carries nutrients and oxygen to all parts of your body through the bloodstream and lymphatic system. Water helps maintain body temperature through perspiration and removes wastes from your body in urine. It lubricates all of your joints and gives shape to each of your cells.

The average adult needs 2 to 3 quarts of water daily. Thirst is one indicator of when you need to drink but, because the sense of thirst is not completely reliable, nutritionists recommend drinking six to eight large glasses of water every day. Athletes and people who live in warm climates or high altitudes also need to be especially conscientious about getting enough water, because they lose more through perspiration.

Most of the fluids we drink consist primarily of water. But alcohol and, to a lesser extent, caffeine are diuretics—they stimulate your body to expel water (in urine) rather than absorb it. Therefore, alcohol and caffeine beverages are not adequate replacements for the same amount of water.

Special nutritional needs of adolescents and older women

Throughout your life, good nutrition is mostly a matter of eating a variety of foods and making sure that you eat generous portions of fruits, vegetables, and whole grains each day. But very young women and older women have some additional nutritional requirements for maintaining optimal health.

ADOLESCENTS

The main nutritional goal for teenage girls is to learn the basics about eating a balanced diet. The Food Guide Pyramid shown at the beginning of this chapter is designed to help you do this.

Although in moderation no food is bad for you, it is important to balance your diet and not eat too much of any one food. Even potato chips, as high in fat and salt as they are, can fit into a balanced diet as long as the chips do not take the place of lunch or exceed your limit of calories, fat, or salt.

Calcium and iron are two nutrients that are particularly important for teenage girls. Calcium is essential for building strong bones. Your bones reach their maximum level of strength and density by the time you are 20. After 35, your body will lose more bone than it builds. Like putting money in a bank, getting lots of calcium when you are young is a critical investment in the future strength of your bones.

You should take in 1,200 to 1,500 milligrams of calcium each day. You can do this with a combined total of four to five servings of skim milk, nonfat yogurt, and calcium-fortified orange juice. Consuming this amount of calcium throughout adolescence can increase your bone strength and may provide significant protection against a common, serious bone-thinning disorder called osteoporosis later in life.

Iron deficiency is common among teenage girls, especially after they begin to menstruate. When you menstruate, you lose iron-rich blood. In most cases, the iron can be replaced by eating foods that are high in iron, such as lean meats, iron-fortified cereals, whole grains, and dried beans. (For good sources of iron, see the chart on page 66.) If you are not getting enough iron from your diet, your doctor may recommend iron supplements.

OLDER WOMEN

Older people need fewer calories. The rate at which you burn calories (your metabolism) begins to slow down after 50. You will probably find that your appetite diminishes as you age. This pattern can set you up for health problems. When you eat less in general, you are likely to be getting fewer of the nutrients you need. Also, as you get older, your body becomes less efficient at absorbing nutrients.

Few adults between the ages of 55 and 74 eat even the minimum recommended five servings of fruits and vegetables each day. Many Americans over age 65 suffer from poor nutrition. Weight loss, lightheadedness, disorientation, and lethargy, which are warning signs of inadequate nutrition, are often mistaken for symptoms of illness.

Exercise can help boost your metabolism, and stimulate your appetite as well. Make it a point to go for a walk every day, and try lifting weights (see page 84) while you watch television. Many older women are not getting sufficient amounts of some important vitamins and minerals.

Vitamin B_{12} and another B vitamin called folic acid (also called folate) assist in maintaining the genetic material inside cells. The two nutrients are crucial for keeping nerve cells and brain cells from deteriorating. Symptoms of a low level of vitamin B_{12} may include numbness and tingling in the legs, decreased alertness, and memory impairment.

Calcium is important for maintaining strong bones. If your body is not getting enough calcium from your diet, it will take what it needs from the calcium that is stored in your bones. The resulting depletion of calcium can lead to the bone-thinning disorder osteoporosis and a high risk of bone fractures.

Vitamin D helps your body absorb calcium, which helps maintain strong bones. Exposure to sunlight contributes further to vitamin D absorption. Several minutes a day of exposure to sunlight stimulates your body to produce vitamin D.

Vitamin C aids in the body's absorption of calcium and iron; helps maintain connective tissues, bones, and teeth; and is important in wound healing. The vitamin may also help prevent cataracts or slow their progression and reduce the risk of cancers of the mouth and throat in people who smoke.

Drinking six to eight glasses of water daily is especially important when you are older because you are less likely to feel thirsty when your body needs water.

Disease prevention and nutrition

Doctors have linked diet to many of the most common chronic diseases—including heart disease, high blood pressure, some cancers, diabetes, osteoporosis, chronic liver disease and cirrhosis, and atherosclerosis (the buildup of fatty deposits on artery walls). In women, there is a relationship between a deficiency of iron and anemia, a deficiency of calcium and osteoporosis, and between diet and premenstrual syndrome (PMS).

Your diet can interact with other risk factors to affect your health. These influences include your genetic makeup; lifestyle factors such as smoking, lack of exercise, and excessive alcohol intake;

and environmental factors such as air pollution.

When designing your own eating plan, use your family health history (see page 120) to help you identify areas of nutrition that are especially important for you. For example, if you have a family history of osteoporosis, you need to be conscientious about getting adequate amounts of calcium and vitamin D (see below). These nutrients work together to keep bones strong.

DIET AND OSTEOPOROSIS

Osteoporosis is a disease in which bones become weak, porous, and prone to fracture. Osteoporosis affects millions of Americans, mostly older white or Asian women. Most women 75 and older and many women who are approaching menopause have symptoms of osteoporosis. One in three women who live to be 90 years old will fracture a hip, usually as a result of osteoporosis. At this age, a hip fracture is debilitating and can permanently limit a woman's ability to function independently.

Bone loss in women usually results from depletion of the female hormone estrogen at menopause, an insufficient amount of weight-bearing exercise, such as walking, and an inadequate intake of calcium throughout a lifetime. Inadequate consumption of vitamin D, which helps the body absorb calcium, also contributes to bone thinning.

Calcium and osteoporosis Although osteoporosis primarily affects older women, it has its roots in the eating habits they developed during their childhood, adolescence, and young adulthood. Throughout your life, calcium is constantly being added and withdrawn from your bones. During childhood and adolescence, more calcium is added than withdrawn. (Bones reach their maximum strength and density by about age 20.) But, after 35, more calcium is withdrawn than is added to your bones.

In the first few years after menopause, when a woman's ovaries stop producing the bone-strengthening hormone estrogen, bone loss accelerates. During this time, a woman can lose from 2 to 5 percent of her total bone density each year, possibly weakening her bones to half the strength they were when she was 20. Depending on how strong a woman's bones are when she enters menopause, this bone loss can put her at risk of developing osteoporosis. The stronger your bones are as you enter menopause, the less likely you will experience debilitating bone fractures as you get older.

To ensure maximum bone strength and density, it is essential for children, adolescents, and young adults to get adequate calcium—from 1,200 to 1,500 milligrams each day. In order to maintain your bone density, you need to continue taking in a sufficient amount of calcium for the rest of your life. After 24, you need 1,000 milligrams each day until you go through menopause, when you should increase your intake to 1,500 milligrams each day (1,000 milligrams if you are taking estrogen in hormone replacement therapy).

You can get adequate calcium from food (see page 58) by, for example, drinking four to five glasses of milk every day. But doing so is difficult for many women. In fact, most women get only 500 milligrams daily of calcium from their diet—far below the recommended amount for any age group. For this reason, many doctors recommend taking calcium supplements to bring your total daily consumption of calcium to the recommended level. Calcium supplements contain different forms of calcium in different amounts. Make sure you read the label to find the amount of elemental calcium in each tablet; this is the actual amount of calcium you are getting in each tablet.

Vitamin D and osteoporosis Vitamin D plays an important role in preventing bone loss and keeping your bones strong by helping your body absorb and use calcium. The recommended dietary requirement (RDA) for vitamin D is 400 international units a day. An 8-ounce glass of milk contains 100 international units of vitamin D. Skim milk, low-fat milk, and whole milk contain the same amounts of vitamin D and calcium; but skim milk has no fat and far fewer calories. Although your body manufactures vitamin D when your skin is exposed to the sun, you are unlikely to get a sufficient amount of the vitamin without drinking fortified milk or taking a multivitamin/mineral supplement.

Which supplement is best?

Calcium carbonate is the most concentrated form of calcium used in supplements. Most calcium carbonate supplements contain more elemental calcium in each tablet than other forms of calcium and are generally the most economical.

Good sources of calcium

Calcium is essential for developing and maintaining strong bones and teeth as well as for healthy functioning of your nerves and muscles. Getting calcium from whole-milk products such as cheese and whole milk gives you more fat and calories than you want. The low-fat and nonfat versions of these foods—such as skim milk and nonfat yogurt—provide as much or more calcium as well as less fat and fewer calories.

RECOMMENDED* FOR WOMEN

11 to 24 years:
1,200 to 1,500 milligrams (mg)

25 years and older:
1,000 mg

Pregnant or breast-feeding:
1,200 to 1,500 mg

Menopause and after:
1,500 mg; 1,000 mg if you are on hormone replacement therapy

*Consensus requirements from the National Institutes of Health

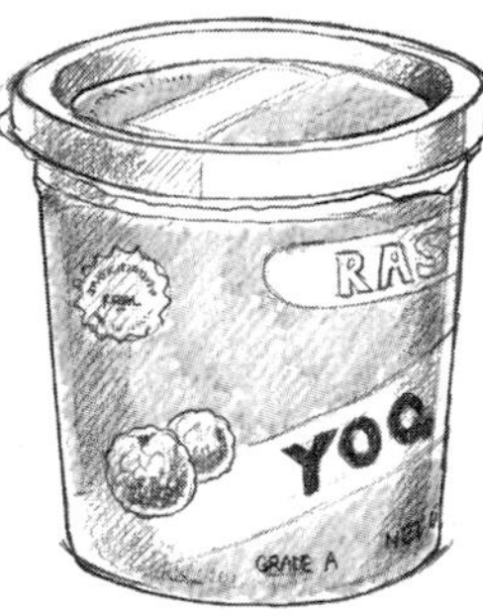

FOOD	SERVING SIZE	CALCIUM (milligrams)
MILK, YOGURT, AND CHEESE		
Nonfat or low-fat plain yogurt	1 cup	468
Ricotta cheese, part skim	1/2 cup	335
Skim or low-fat milk	1 cup	300
Swiss cheese	1 ounce	272
Provolone cheese	1 ounce	207
Mozzarella cheese, part skim	1 ounce	207
Cheddar cheese	1 ounce	148
Parmesan cheese	2 tablespoons	138
Cottage cheese	1/2 cup	63
FISH, MEAT, POULTRY, DRIED BEANS, NUTS, AND EGGS		
Sardines with bones, canned	3 ounces	324
Salmon with bones, canned	3 ounces	181
Tofu (firm)	3 ounces	177
Black beans (cooked)	1 cup	128
Ocean perch (broiled)	3 ounces	117
Blue crab	3 ounces	89
Chickpeas, canned	1 cup	80
VEGETABLES (COOKED UNLESS OTHERWISE SPECIFIED)		
Kale (fresh)	1 cup	102
Mustard greens	1/2 cup	99
Turnip greens (fresh)	1 cup	75
Bok choy (fresh)	1 cup	74
Broccoli (fresh)	1 cup	42
Rutabaga	1/2 cup	41
FRUITS		
Calcium-fortified orange juice	6 ounces	217
Figs, dried	5 medium	135
Orange	1 medium	58
Raisins	1/2 cup	38
Apricots, dried	1/2 cup	29
BREAD, CEREAL, RICE, AND PASTA		
Tortillas, flour	2	106
English muffin, plain	1	99
Corn muffin	1 large	95

DIET AND HEART DISEASE

Most people think heart disease is primarily a problem for men. In fact, heart disease is the major cause of death in American women, killing more women every year than all types of cancer combined. A woman who has a heart attack is twice as likely as a man to die of it, often because it is diagnosed at a later stage in the disease, when fewer treatment options are successful. Heart disease affects women about 10 years later than men, usually after menopause.

A stroke (damage to brain tissue caused by blockage or leaking of a blood vessel) results from many of the same problems that cause heart disease. Atherosclerosis (the buildup of fatty deposits in artery walls) and high blood pressure are related to both heart disease and stroke.

Fat and heart disease Too much saturated fat and cholesterol in the diet and obesity (being 20 percent or more over your ideal weight) are the major contributors to high total cholesterol level, which is a major risk factor for heart disease. Foods that are high in saturated fat (the kind found in red meat and whole-milk products) raise your cholesterol level much more than foods that are high in cholesterol.

These harmful dietary fats (and obesity) increase the level of low-density lipoprotein (LDL), the "bad" cholesterol that streaks the inside walls of arteries with fat. This buildup of fatty deposits causes a narrowing of the blood vessels, which sets the stage for a heart attack or stroke. For every 1-percent increase in your total cholesterol level, your risk of heart attack increases 2 to 3 percent.

Obesity is a major cause of high blood pressure, which is a powerful risk factor for heart disease and stroke. Losing weight and exercising regularly can reduce your blood pressure and increase your level of "good" HDL cholesterol. HDL cholesterol protects against heart disease by mopping up harmful LDL cholesterol in the bloodstream and carrying it back to the liver, which breaks it down and eliminates it.

Soluble fiber and heart disease Some forms of soluble fiber—such as that found in oatmeal, oat bran, barley, and dried beans—can help lower your cholesterol level and reduce your risk of heart disease and stroke.

Insoluble fiber, the type found in whole-wheat breads and many bran cereals, does not have the same cholesterol-lowering effect. But you should still eat both types of fiber—insoluble fiber for keeping your lower digestive tract running smoothly and soluble fiber for reducing your cholesterol level.

Antioxidants and heart disease Although reducing fat has long been thought to be the most important component of a heart-healthy diet, eating lots of fruits and vegetables also provides protection against heart disease. Especially important are those fruits and vegetables that contain antioxidant vitamins and other nutrients.

Antioxidants help protect your body from molecules called oxygen free radicals, which are by-products of the body's normal chemical processes. Oxygen free radicals lack an essential component called an electron. They become harmful when they steal an electron from another molecule in the body, causing damage to cells and the cells' genetic material. This process, called oxidation, is the same process that causes your car to rust. Damage from free radicals contributes to a variety of disorders—including heart disease, stroke, cancer, and cataracts—as well as the aging process.

Vitamin E is an antioxidant that may help prevent heart disease. The vitamin neutralizes free radicals and prevents them from damaging LDL cholesterol—the "bad" cholesterol. This free radical damage to LDL is what causes it to build up on artery walls.

The roles of other antioxidants—such as vitamins A and C, and beta carotene—in protecting against heart disease are being investigated. Women who eat lots of antioxidant-rich fruits and vegetables may cut their risk of stroke significantly compared with women who eat few fruits or vegetables. Scientists do not yet know if the protective effect comes from antioxidants or from other substances in the foods. Determining specific health benefits from specific foods is difficult because people who eat more fruits and vegetables often also eat less total fat, saturated fat, and cholesterol. This overall pattern is always the most beneficial.

Most doctors and nutritionists stop short of advising people to take antioxidants or any other specific nutrient supplements to prevent heart disease or other illnesses. No one knows the amounts of nutrients that are needed over and above a well-balanced, nutritious diet to provide optimum health benefits. A safe bet is to maintain a low-fat, high-fiber diet with lots of antioxidant-rich foods and take a multivitamin supplement once a day, sticking with the RDAs until more specific recommendations are available.

Alcohol and heart disease If you don't drink alcohol, don't start now. Although studies have shown that moderate alcohol consumption may be associated with a lower overall death rate from diseases of the heart and blood vessels, no one recommends using alcohol as a means of preventing heart disease. The risk of alcohol addiction is too high, and alcohol is involved in a large percentage of

Good sources of vitamin A

Vitamin A is essential for the development of healthy eyes, skin, hair, teeth, and gums. It increases your resistance to infection and it may protect against kidney stones and some forms of cancer.

RDA FOR WOMEN

11 years and older:
4,000 international units (IU)

Pregnant:
4,000 IU

Breast-feeding (first 6 months):
6,500 IU

Breast-feeding (second 6 months):
6,000 IU

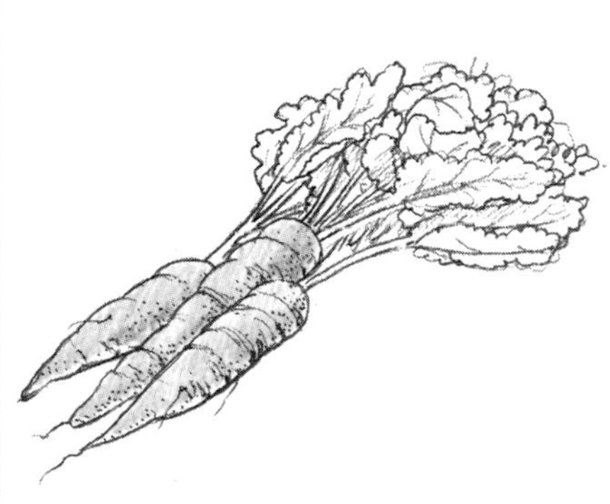

FOOD	SERVING SIZE	VITAMIN A (international units)
MILK, YOGURT, AND CHEESE		
Low-fat ricotta cheese	1/2 cup	536
Low-fat or skim milk	1 cup	500
Muenster cheese	1 ounce	318
Cheddar cheese	1 ounce	300
Low-fat yogurt	1 cup	150
Parmesan cheese, grated	2 tablespoons	70
Low-fat cottage cheese, 1%	1/2 cup	42
Nonfat yogurt	1 cup	16
VEGETABLES (COOKED UNLESS OTHERWISE SPECIFIED)		
Pumpkin, canned	1/2 cup	26,908
Sweet potato (baked)	1 medium	24,877
Carrot (raw)	1 medium	20,253
Spinach	1/2 cup	7,371
Winter squash	1/2 cup	3,628
Red pepper, sweet (raw)	1/2 cup	2,850
Romaine lettuce (raw)	1 cup	1,456
Broccoli	1/2 cup	1,099
FRUITS		
Mango	1/2 medium	4,030
Cantaloupe	1/2 cup	2,579
Apricots, canned	4 halves	1,629
Watermelon	1 cup	585
Peach	1 medium	465
BREAD, CEREAL, RICE, AND PASTA		
Ready-to-eat cereal, fortified	1 ounce	1,250-5,000
Oatmeal, instant (cooked)	3/4 cup	1,000

automobile accidents and violent incidents each year. Alcohol is also high in "empty calories"—it has very little nutritional value.

However, drinking a moderate amount of alcohol (one drink a day for women) can provide some health benefits. Moderation is the key. People who drink moderately live longer than people who do not drink at all or those who drink excessively.

A moderate amount of alcohol raises the level of high-density lipoprotein (HDL), the "good" cholesterol in the blood. Alcohol also reduces the blood's tendency to clot, lowering the risk that a blood clot in an artery will cause a heart attack. For the same reason, moderate drinking may also help prevent the most common kind of stroke—ischemic stroke (see page 573)—which is caused by blockage of an artery in the brain.

Sodium and heart disease Your risk of developing high blood pressure (hypertension) has a lot to do with your genes. Environmental factors, including your diet, play an important role as well.

Good sources of vitamin C

Vitamin C helps maintain healthy bones, teeth, and connective tissue. It assists in the body's absorption of folic acid and iron.

RDA FOR WOMEN*

18 years and older:
60 milligrams (mg)

Pregnant:
70 mg

Breast-feeding (first 6 months):
95 mg

Breast-feeding (second 6 months):
90 mg

*Smokers should consume more—at least 100 mg daily.

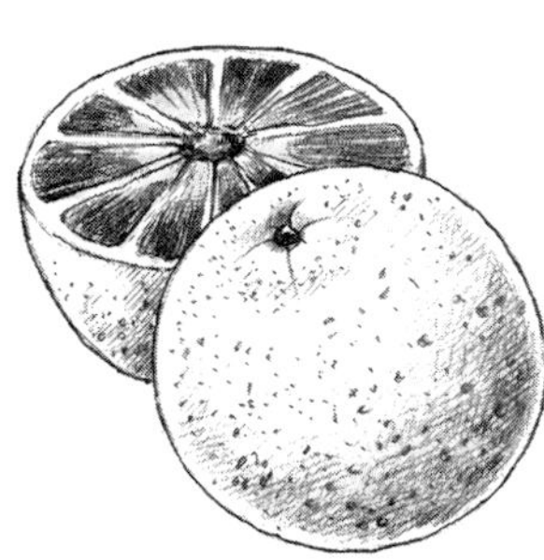

FOOD	SERVING SIZE	VITAMIN C (milligrams)
FISH, MEAT, POULTRY, DRIED BEANS, NUTS, AND EGGS		
Clams (steamed/boiled)	3 ounces	18.8
Mussels (steamed/boiled)	3 ounces	18.8
VEGETABLES (COOKED UNLESS OTHERWISE SPECIFIED)		
Red peppers, sweet (raw)	½ cup	95
Green peppers, sweet (raw)	½ cup	44.7
Snow peas (raw)	½ cup	38.3
Broccoli	½ cup	36.9
Brussels sprouts	½ cup	35.4
Tomato juice, canned	¾ cup	33.5
Tomato (raw)	1 medium	23.5
Potato with skin (baked)	1 medium	15.7
Red cabbage	½ cup	15
FRUITS		
Kiwi	1 medium	74.5
Orange juice	6 ounces	72.6
Orange	1 medium	69.7
Grapefruit juice	6 ounces	54
Grapefruit	½ medium	46.9
Watermelon	1 cup	46.4
Strawberries	½ cup	40.8
Cantaloupe	½ cup	33.8
Mandarin oranges	½ cup	30

Individuals vary widely in their response to sodium. Blood pressure in some people is strongly influenced by the amount of sodium they eat, while, in others, sodium seems to have no effect. Even among the people who already have high blood pressure, only about half appear to be sensitive to sodium.

Despite the variability in blood pressure response to sodium intake (often called salt sensitivity), many experts recommend that all people limit the sodium in their diet to less than 2,400 milligrams per day (the equivalent of 1½ teaspoons of table salt). Most people get more than 10 times the amount their body requires. Read labels when buying processed foods such as soups and sauces—many contain excessive amounts of sodium. You can get almost half your daily allowance of sodium from a single bowl of some commercially prepared soups. Other high-sodium foods include olives, pickles, catsup, mustard, lunch meats, baking powder, soy sauce, and monosodium glutamate (MSG).

It takes only a few weeks without salt to train your taste buds not to expect a salty flavor in everything you eat. See page 72 for flavoring ideas that can help replace salt in your diet and enhance the inherent flavors of foods.

Good sources of vitamin E

Vitamin E helps to form blood cells, muscles, and lung and nerve tissue. It boosts the immune system and protects tissue against the damaging effects of oxidation. It helps the body use vitamin K.

Many foods rich in vitamin E are also high in fat. For this reason, supplements may be a more healthful way of increasing your vitamin E intake.

RDA FOR WOMEN

18 years and older:
8 milligrams (mg)

Pregnant:
10 mg

Breast-feeding (first 6 months):
12 mg

Breast-feeding (second 6 months):
11 mg

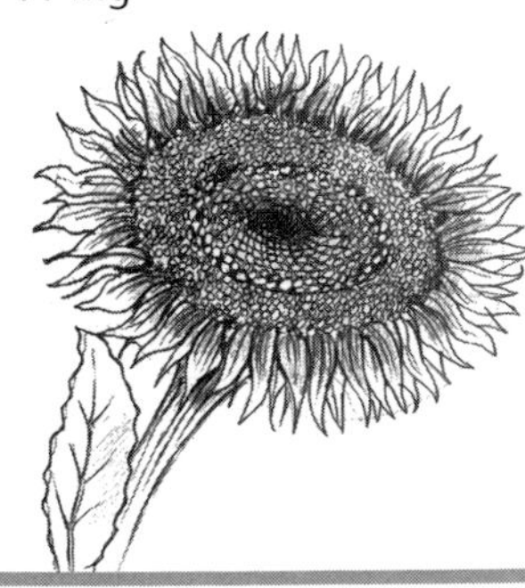

FOOD	SERVING SIZE	VITAMIN E (milligrams)
FATS, OILS, AND SWEETS		
Wheat germ oil	1 tablespoon	26.2
Safflower oil	1 tablespoon	4.7
Corn oil	1 tablespoon	2.9
Olive oil	1 tablespoon	1.6
FISH, MEAT, POULTRY, DRIED BEANS, NUTS, AND EGGS		
Sunflower seeds	¼ cup	18.1
Hazelnuts (filberts)	¼ cup	8.1
Peanuts	¼ cup	2.7
Peanut butter	2 tablespoons	2.6
Mackerel (broiled)	3 ounces	1.9
Clams (steamed/boiled)	3 ounces	1.7
Salmon (broiled)	3 ounces	1.6
VEGETABLES (COOKED UNLESS OTHERWISE SPECIFIED)		
Pumpkin, canned	½ cup	1.3
Green cabbage	½ cup	1.2
Sweet potato (baked)	1 medium	.5
FRUITS		
Avocado	1	2.7
Peaches, canned	½ cup	1.9
BREAD, CEREAL, RICE, AND PASTA		
Ready-to-eat cereal, fortified	1 ounce	20.1

DIET AND CANCER

More than half of all cancers in women are related to diet. Your genetic makeup can make you susceptible to some kinds of cancer, but how you eat can play a major role in increasing or reducing your risk of cancer.

Studies consistently show a relationship between a high-fat diet and cancer, particularly for colon cancer and breast cancer. A high-salt diet—one heavy in pickled vegetables or meats preserved by salting—has been linked to an increased risk of cancers of the stomach, esophagus, nose, and throat.

The strongest link between diet and cancer is between a low-fiber diet and cancers of the colon and rectum. Fiber protects against cancer by adding bulk to stool, helping it retain water and speeding its movement through the colon. These processes work together to dilute any cancer-causing substances that may be present in the colon and reduce their contact with the wall of the colon.

It now appears that eating lots of fruits and vegetables can help prevent many kinds of cancer, including cancers of the lung, colon, stomach, mouth, cervix, and, possibly, breast. A diet rich in fruits and vegetables is associated with a lower risk of lung cancer. It is not yet known whether the protective effect comes from fiber or other substances in the vegetables or from the replacement of higher-fat foods in the diet.

Antioxidants and cancer Among the substances in fruits and vegetables that have a protective effect against cancer are antioxidants, which include vitamins A, C, and E and beta carotene. People whose diets are rich in antioxidant-containing foods have a lower incidence of most types of cancer, including cancers of the lung, cervix, colon, and stomach. Antioxidants are thought to protect against cancer by slowing the formation of molecules called oxygen free radicals that can damage the genetic material inside cells. Over time, this damage can trigger the development of cancer.

The antioxidants vitamin A and beta carotene (which is converted into vitamin A in the body) are abundant in dark green and yellow vegetables such as sweet potatoes, carrots, winter squash, and spinach. These foods may also contain related cancer-fighting substances that you cannot get from vitamin supplements.

Vitamins E and C may play a protective role against cancer by boosting your immune system, rallying its defenses against cancer. The vitamins may also prevent nitrites (chemicals used to preserve food) from turning into cancer-causing substances inside the stomach.

Most experts recommend getting your daily supply of antioxidants by eating lots of fruits and vegetables. By doing so, you are also boosting your intake of fiber and probably reducing your consumption of fat. A high-fiber, low-fat diet is known to reduce your risk of cancer. For good sources of foods that contain these antioxidant vitamins, see charts on pages 60 to 62.

Fat and cancer The association between diet and colon cancer is clear. Eating a diet low in fat and high in fiber can reduce your risk of colon cancer, the third most common cancer killer of women after cancers of the lung and breast. By-products of fat digestion may stimulate the development of polyps, which are tiny growths in the intestine that can become cancerous. A substance inherent in fat itself may also contribute to cancer. Saturated fat—the kind found in red meat; butter, cheese, and other whole milk products; eggs; and tropical oils such as coconut and palm oils used in many commercially baked goods—is the most harmful kind.

The exact causes of breast cancer are not yet known. Breast cancer probably results from the interaction of a woman's genetic susceptibility and her diet and other environmental factors. A low-fat, high-fiber diet, which is linked to prevention of other cancers, appears to provide some protection against breast cancer as well. Eating lots of fruits and vegetables and other fiber-rich foods such as whole grains to replace fat in your diet can help reduce your risk of breast cancer.

Another way in which fat in your diet may increase your risk of cancer is by increasing your risk of obesity (being 20 percent or more over your ideal weight). Women who are obese die of cancer more often than women of normal weight. The most frequent cancers in obese women are cancers of the breast, cervix, endometrium, uterus, ovaries, and gallbladder. For ways to reduce your fat intake, see page 51.

Fiber and cancer A high-fiber diet may help protect against several forms of cancer, particularly colon cancer. A number of factors may contribute to this protective effect. By speeding food through the intestines, fiber reduces the time the intestinal lining is exposed to any cancer-causing substances (carcinogens) that may be present in the food. Fiber attracts water to the stool, which dilutes the carcinogens and reduces their cancer-causing potential. Fiber may also alter the normal bacteria and acidity in the digestive system, reducing the production of carcinogens.

It may be that fiber itself does not protect you against cancer, but high-fiber foods may replace less healthful high-fat foods in your diet. Other substances in high-fiber foods may be beneficial. Many doctors recommend that people who are at high risk for colon cancer increase their daily fiber intake to at least 35 grams a day.

Alcohol and cancer Alcohol intake increases the risk of some cancers. Alcohol may damage the genetic material inside cells and cause changes that can lead to cancer. Long-term heavy drinking increases the risk of liver cancer. There is a direct link between drinking and cancers of the mouth, throat, esophagus, and larynx, especially when combined with cigarette smoking. Alcohol and smoking work together to increase a person's risk of these cancers.

There also may be a link between alcohol and breast cancer. Although the evidence is not conclusive, the risk of breast cancer may increase with the amount of alcohol consumed. For some women, having only one to two drinks a day may increase this risk.

DIET AND DIABETES

Maintaining a healthy weight can significantly reduce your risk of type II diabetes (see page 621). (There is no known way to prevent the other form of the disease—type I diabetes, see page 617). For people who are diagnosed with type II diabetes, weight loss is often the first treatment that doctors recommend.

Because heart attacks are the leading cause of death in people who have diabetes, doctors recommend that people with the disease reduce their fat intake. If you are diagnosed with either form of diabetes, your doctor (often working with a dietitian) will design a meal plan to fit your needs. Carefully following your recommended eating program can help you control the level of sugar in your blood and reduce your risk of long-term complications (see page 619).

DIET AND LIVER DISEASE

Your liver plays an extremely important role in your body—it absorbs fats, makes proteins, stores and releases energy, and eliminates harmful substances. Alcohol can cause severe damage to your liver. Excessive consumption of alcohol can cause three different kinds of liver disease—fatty liver, alcoholic hepatitis, and cirrhosis of the liver.

Most heavy drinkers develop a fatty liver, in which the liver becomes enlarged and engorged with fat. Stopping drinking can reverse this process. In alcoholic hepatitis, the liver becomes inflamed and tender, causing fever, fatigue, and jaundice (yellowing of the skin and whites of the eyes). In many cases, alcoholic hepatitis can be cured by quitting drinking.

The most devastating, potentially fatal, alcohol-induced liver disease is cirrhosis, in which the liver becomes scarred. This damage to the liver is permanent. Although quitting drinking cannot reverse the liver damage from cirrhosis, it can prevent further damage.

DIET AND THE IMMUNE SYSTEM

Vitamins B_6 and C and the mineral zinc play a role in regulating the immune system. Some vitamins may help boost the immune system and fight off disease. Vitamins E, A, and C and beta carotene are antioxidants—they protect against the effects of cell-damaging molecules called oxygen free radicals. This damage to cells can lead to cancer. Because few Americans are eating even the minimum recommended servings of fruits and vegetables each day, many doctors recommend a daily multivitamin/mineral supplement. This is especially important for older people, who tend to eat less and, therefore, get fewer nutrients.

Caffeine and health

Despite years of controversy and hundreds of studies on caffeine's potential role in health and disease, no evidence has shown that caffeine in moderation contributes in any significant way to disease.

However, caffeine is not completely harmless, nor is it nutritious. In some people, caffeine causes irritability, nervousness, and sleeplessness. Most people build up a tolerance for caffeine and these symptoms taper off with regular moderate consumption. (Moderate consumption is the equivalent of two to three cups of brewed coffee per day.) Caffeine can cause stomach upset or heartburn in some people by stimulating the secretion of stomach acids. Caffeine can also contribute to dehydration, especially in older people, because it is a diuretic (a substance that increases urine output). Excessive consumption of caffeine during pregnancy may result in a baby with a lower weight at birth. To be safe, doctors recommend that all pregnant women limit their intake to the equivalent of two cups of coffee per day.

Many people experience caffeine withdrawal symptoms when they stop drinking their usual two cups of coffee or several cans of cola a day. These symptoms—which include headache, depression, dizziness, or anxiety—usually last only a few days. Besides coffee and cola drinks, caffeine is found in chocolate, tea, and some over-the-counter pain relievers, diet aids, and cold remedies.

BEVERAGE OR FOOD	SERVING SIZE (ounces)	CAFFEINE CONTENT (milligrams)
Brewed coffee	6	105
Instant coffee	6	57
Cola	12	37
Espresso coffee	2	35
Tea	6	35
Dark chocolate	1	20
Hot chocolate	6	3-12
Milk chocolate	1	6
Decaffeinated coffee	6	2

DIET AND PREMENSTRUAL SYNDROME

Premenstrual syndrome (PMS) is a group of emotional and physical symptoms that recur in the days preceding a woman's period, usually beginning in her 20s. Symptoms vary from woman to woman but may include fluid retention, enlarged and tender breasts, bloating, headache, joint or muscle pain, and heart palpitations. Other symptoms include depression, irritability, lethargy, panic attacks, poor concentration, food cravings, crying for no reason, and even violent or suicidal episodes.

Although it is not known if specific foods or beverages cause PMS, some substances can worsen symptoms a woman already has. For example, if you are feeling edgy or irritable, consuming caffeine or alcohol will make you feel more so. If you are bloated, eating foods that are high in fat or salt will cause your body to retain even more water. Eating simple sugars such as those found in candy bars may give you a short-term energy boost, but can leave you feeling tired and drained. Exercise can help relieve many of the symptoms of PMS, including fluid retention, and may also raise the level of the "feel-good" chemicals in your brain called endorphins.

IRON DEFICIENCY

Because women eat less food overall and they lose iron through menstruation, they are more susceptible than men to iron deficiency. Iron deficiency in young women often results from a combination of low iron consumption, heavy periods, constant dieting, and inadequate intake of vitamin C (which helps your body absorb iron). The RDA for iron is 15 milligrams a day. The average American diet supplies only about 6 milligrams per 1,000 calories—too little for the average woman who eats 1,800 to 2,000 calories per day. For good sources of iron, see page 66.

People who need to make sure they are getting enough iron include:

- **Women who have heavy periods** You lose iron each month when you menstruate. If you have unusually heavy periods, you may need extra iron. Menstruating teenagers who are still growing are at even greater risk of iron deficiency, particularly if they are dieting.

Good sources of iron

Iron is important for healthy red blood cells, which deliver oxygen throughout your body.

RDA FOR WOMEN

18 to 50 years:
15 milligrams (mg)

51 years and older:
10 mg

Pregnant:
30 mg

Breast-feeding:
15 mg

FOOD	SERVING SIZE	IRON (milligrams)
FISH, MEAT, POULTRY, DRIED BEANS, NUTS, AND EGGS		
Clams (steamed)	3 ounces	23.8
Oysters	3 ounces	10.2
Mussels (steamed/boiled)	3 ounces	5.7
Soybeans (cooked)	1/2 cup	4.4
Lentils (cooked)	1/2 cup	3.3
Sirloin steak (broiled)	3 ounces	2.9
Shrimp (boiled)	3 ounces	2.6
Red kidney beans (cooked)	1/2 cup	2.6
Chickpeas (cooked)	1/2 cup	2.4
Black beans (cooked)	1/2 cup	2.3
Turkey, dark meat only (roasted)	3 ounces	2
Sardines	3 ounces	1.2
VEGETABLES (COOKED UNLESS OTHERWISE SPECIFIED)		
Potato with skin (baked)	1 medium	1.6
Spinach	1/2 cup	1.4
Lima beans	1/2 cup	1.2
FRUITS		
Apricots, dried	1/4 cup	1.5
BREAD, CEREAL, RICE, AND PASTA		
Ready-to-eat cereal, fortified	1 ounce	1-18
Bagel, plain	1	2.4
Pasta	1 cup	2
Oatmeal (cooked)	3/4 cup	1.2
Whole-grain bread	1 slice	1

- **Pregnant women** As blood volume increases in pregnant women, so does the need for iron. If you are pregnant, your doctor will recommend that you take a prenatal multivitamin/mineral supplement daily. Some pregnant women may also need to take an iron supplement.
- **Women who are breast-feeding** You need adequate iron to produce breast milk.
- **Vegetarians and others who do not eat red meat** Your body does not absorb iron from vegetables, beans, and grains as easily as it does the iron from red meat.
- **Dieters** The less you eat, the less likely you are to be getting enough iron. Ask your doctor if you should take an iron supplement.
- **People who are preparing for or recovering from surgery** An ample supply of iron is needed to replace iron that may be lost in blood during surgery.
- **People with some illnesses** When you have some illnesses—including cancer, anemia (see page 493), or infections—your body needs more iron to help deliver oxygen to weakened tissues and help them heal faster.

The early stages of iron deficiency seldom cause symptoms. Mild iron deficiency is not as great a health problem as previously thought. But, as the iron level in the blood drops, less iron reaches the bone marrow, reducing its ability to produce new blood cells. A decrease in the number of oxygen-carrying red blood cells reduces the amount of oxygen that is delivered from your lungs to all of your cells, making you feel tired. This condition is called iron-deficiency anemia.

A severe iron deficiency can make you feel weak or short of breath (especially during exertion), look pale, lose your appetite, and become susceptible to infection. These symptoms disappear as soon as a healthy level of iron in your blood is restored. Because these symptoms can result from other conditions as well, including internal bleeding from the intestines (a sign of cancer), you should talk to your doctor if you experience any of them.

To increase your iron intake, you must eat more iron than the RDA calls for because your body absorbs only a small percentage of the iron from your diet. Iron is best absorbed from animal foods, such as lean beef. Some foods enhance your body's absorption of iron, while others block it. Foods containing vitamin C speed iron absorption. For this reason, it is a good idea to eat a food rich in vitamin C at the same meal with an iron-rich food. Coffee and tea contain substances that inhibit iron absorption.

Iron supplements and toddlers

A number of children have died after eating iron tablets that were left within their reach. Iron supplements often have brightly colored sugar coatings that attract children. Vitamins and mineral supplements should be treated like any medication and kept out of the reach of children.

Food selection and preparation

Knowledge about nutrition is essential for maintaining good health. The food labels on packaged foods, which give you important and useful information about the calorie, nutrient, and fat values of foods, can help you make wise food choices. The practical information in the following pages can help make your selection and preparation of food both easy and healthful.

READING LABELS

The FDA requires that labels on packaged foods list ingredients in descending order of relative amounts. The labels also provide useful information about the amounts per serving of fat, cholesterol, dietary fiber, and nutrients. Everything you need to know to compare foods and their overall nutritional quality is available on the label. To make this comparison easier, food labels have standardized serving sizes. Here are some words you might see on labels and what they mean:

- **Light** The term "light" can refer to calories, fat, or sodium content of a food. When used in reference to the number of calories or the fat content, a light food must contain one-third fewer calories or half the fat of the original food. When used to refer to the amount of sodium, a light food must have no more than half the sodium of the original food. The word can also be used to describe the texture, color, or flavor of a food as long as the label makes it clear—such as in "light brown sugar" or "light and fluffy."
- **Free** The term "free" means that the product contains none or insignificant amounts of one of the following—fat, saturated fat, cholesterol, sodium, sugar, or calories. Remember that a product that is "cholesterol free" may contain a great

What's a gram?

A gram is the metric unit of measure that you see on food labels to indicate nutrient quantities. There are 4 grams in a teaspoon, so a food with 12 grams of fat contains 3 teaspoons of fat. Cholesterol and sodium are listed in milligrams. There are 1,000 milligrams in a gram.

Fat packs the most calories, gram for gram. There are 9 calories in 1 gram of fat; 4 calories in 1 gram of carbohydrate or protein; and 7 calories in 1 gram of alcohol.

What you can learn from a food label

Frozen
MIXED VEGETABLES

Net. Wt. 16oz. (456g)
Ingredients: Carrots, Peas, Lima Beans, Corn

Nutrition Facts
Serving Size 1/2 cup (91g) — 1
Servings Per Container about 5

Amount Per Serving	
2 — Calories 58	Calories from Fat 0
	% Daily Value*
3 — **Total Fat** 0g	**0%**
Saturated Fat 0g	**0%**
Cholesterol 0mg	**0%**
Sodium 45mg	**2%**
Total Carbohydrate 12g	**4%**
Dietary Fiber 3g	**12%**
Sugars 3g	
Protein 3g	

(4: % Daily Value column)

5 — Vitamin A 92%	•	Vitamin C 16%	
Calcium 2%	•	Iron 5%	

* Percent Daily Values are based on a 2,000-calorie diet. Your daily values may be higher or lower depending on your calorie needs:

	Calories	2,000	2,500
6 — Total Fat	Less than	65g	80g
Saturated Fat	Less than	20g	25g
Cholesterol	Less than	300mg	300mg
Sodium	Less than	2,400mg	2,400mg
Total Carbohydrate		300g	375g
Dietary Fiber		25g	30g

Calories per gram:
7 — Fat 9 • Carbohydrate 4 • Protein 4

8 — *Many factors affect cancer risk. Eating a diet low in fat and high in fiber may lower risk of this disease.*

9 — ■ GOOD SOURCE OF FIBER
■ LOW FAT

1. To make it easy for you to compare different brands of a particular food, all serving sizes are required to be the same.
2. This line shows the total calories in one serving and also how many calories you are getting from fat in that serving.
3. This section indicates the amounts of different nutrients in one serving (expressed in grams or milligrams). With this information, you can compare the nutrient content of similar products, and add up your total daily consumption of each nutrient.
4. The Percent Daily Values (which are the same as the RDAs) are shown for each nutrient listed. Percent Daily Values are based on a daily diet of 2,000 calories. (There are no Percent Daily Values for sugars or protein because no dietary requirements have been set for them.)
5. This section gives the Percent Daily Values for vitamin A, vitamin C, calcium, and iron.
6. This section helps you determine your daily allowance of fats (total fat, saturated fat, and cholesterol), sodium, carbohydrates, and fiber. The allowances are given for diets totaling either 2,000 or 2,500 calories a day.

   Note: The fat allowances are based on limiting your intake of total fat to less than 30 percent of your total calories each day. The limit for saturated fat (the kind that can raise your cholesterol level) is less than 10 percent of your total calories.
7. This section provides general information about the number of calories in 1 gram of fat, carbohydrate, and protein.
8. The federal government has approved the use of some health claims on packaged foods. The following are examples of health claims that you might see on labels:
   - A diet low in fat and rich in fruits and vegetables may reduce your risk of some cancers.
   - A diet rich in fruits, vegetables, and grains may reduce the risk of coronary heart disease.
   - Eating a high-fat diet increases the risk of some cancers.
   - Low intake of calcium is one risk factor for osteoporosis.
9. Words such as "low," "high," and "free" on food labels must meet legal definitions. For example, a food described as "high" in a particular nutrient must contain at least 20 percent of the Daily Value for that nutrient.

deal of saturated fat, which can raise your cholesterol level more than eating a food that contains dietary cholesterol. Always check the label to find the true values of these components.

■ **Low** The term "low" is used with foods that can be eaten frequently without exceeding dietary guidelines for one or more of these components—fat, saturated fat, cholesterol, sodium, or calories.

"Low fat" means 3 grams or less total fat per serving. "Low saturated fat" means 1 gram or less per serving. "Low sodium" means less than 140 milligrams per serving. "Very low sodium" means less than 35 milligrams per serving. "Low calorie" on a label means the food has 40 calories or fewer per serving. Synonyms for "low" include "little," "few," and "low source of."

HEALTHFUL TIPS FOR EATING OUT

Many people find it difficult to keep up their good eating habits when they go out to a restaurant. Here are some tips for helping you make healthy menu choices when eating out.

Appetizers

■ Skip the cocktail, or limit yourself to one wine spritzer or light beer. Dry wines have about half the calories of sweet wines. A healthful drink is sparkling or plain water with a slice of lemon or lime or iced tea.

■ Have seafood (cooked any way but fried), raw vegetables, or fruit. Avoid rich sauces, dips, and batter-fried foods.

Fast-food facts

With the popularity of fast-food restaurants, many Americans are consuming more fat and calories in one meal than they might realize. Between 40 and 55 percent of the calories in a typical fast-food meal come from fat. Many fast-food chains now offer more nutritious selections including broiled meats, baked potatoes, and salads. Those are good as long as you avoid such high-fat, high-calorie extras as bacon, cheese, and sour cream. Plain hamburgers or cheeseburgers have fewer calories and less fat than the sandwiches with mayonnaise-based sauces; "junior" sandwiches have fewer calories still. Skipping the french fries and milkshake can eliminate up to 600 calories and 35 grams of fat.

Here are some numbers to think about the next time you're ordering a fast-food meal.

FOOD	CALORIES	FAT (grams)	SODIUM (milligrams)
Single hamburger	260-360	11-18	290-630
Double hamburger	394-560	21-28	543-718
Single cheeseburger	309-525	13-20	650-825
Double cheeseburger	478-650	27-37	827-980
Bacon cheeseburger	510-724	28-46	730-1,307
Chicken sandwich	320-690	10-27	500-1,423
Fish sandwich	400-490	20-27	520-1,013
Roast beef sandwich	312-500	12-28	590-826
Hot dog	280-520	16-27	830-1,365
Pizza (thin crust, 1 slice)	170-220	3-11	330-540
Regular french fries	200-280	8-17	30-180
Large french fries	320-406	16-22	120-306
Onion rings	274-382	16-23	140-655
Milkshake (10-12 ounces)	300-490	6-13	180-300

■ Eat bread (whole-grain types are the best) without the butter or margarine. Croissants and biscuits are higher in fat than other breads; many crackers are high in both fat and sodium.

Entrées
■ Ask about serving sizes. Are half portions available?
■ Choose an appetizer as a main dish, share a dish, or have an appetizer and a salad.
■ Stop when you are full; don't be embarrassed to take leftovers home.
■ When deciding on a main course, look for terms on the menu that indicate low-fat preparation—such as steamed, broiled, grilled, roasted, baked, poached, or simmered. Choose or request skinless cuts of poultry.
■ Watch for terms that indicate higher fat—such as buttered, fried, creamed, gravy, cheese sauce, au gratin, scalloped, rich, pastry, or cooked in oil.
■ The following terms may indicate higher salt content—smoked, pickled, broth, barbecued, cocktail sauce, tomato sauce, mustard sauce, soy sauce, teriyaki, or marinated.

Vegetables and salads
■ The salad bar is always a good choice—as long as you avoid the calorie- and fat-laden add-ons, including hard-boiled eggs, cheese, and bacon bits.
■ For salad dressing, use vinegar and oil, vinegar alone, lemon juice, or diet dressing. Ask to have your dressing served on the side. Avoid mayonnaise-based salad dressings, such as thousand island and ranch.
■ Look for vegetables seasoned with lemon, herbs, or spices rather than fat and salt. Instead of fries or chips, ask for a tossed salad or baked potato (try low-calorie dressing on the potato instead of butter or sour cream).

Desserts
■ Look for fruit on the dessert menu. If you don't see it on the menu, ask the waiter or waitress if it is available.
■ Order a light, low-fat dessert such as sherbet, sorbet, or fruit ice.
■ If you decide on a richer dessert, share it with your companions.
■ Have a cup of coffee, tea, or cappuccino made with skim milk while the others at your table are having dessert.

FOOD SAFETY

While much of the public's concern about food safety focuses on food additives and pesticides, contamination from bacteria and other microorganisms is a far more common and serious problem. Millions of Americans get some form of food poisoning each year, with symptoms ranging from nausea to diarrhea, fever, and dehydration. Young children and older people are the most vulnerable.

To avoid food poisoning, take extra caution when handling any of the following foods:

Chicken and other poultry Poultry is much more prone than other meats to contamination with salmonella bacteria. Store chicken in the back of the refrigerator where it is coldest. Cook poultry within 2 days of purchase and rinse it before cooking. The safest way to thaw frozen chicken is in the refrigerator overnight or, if you plan to cook it the same day, in the microwave. Do not refreeze poultry once it has been thawed. When cooking poultry, make sure it is cooked completely by checking that the meat near the bone is not pink. Thoroughly wash (with hot, soapy water) your hands and knives, cutting boards, and other surfaces that have been touched by raw poultry during preparation.

Eggs Salmonella bacteria can also be found in raw eggs. Throw away any eggs that are cracked. Be careful about eating dishes that are made with raw eggs, such as homemade eggnog, key lime pie, and Caesar salad dressing. Buy these foods already prepared or make them using egg substitutes.

Ground beef Ground beef is more likely than other forms of beef to be contaminated with bacteria because surface bacteria can be spread throughout the meat during the grinding process. The USDA recommends cooking ground beef to a temperature of 160°, leaving none of the meat pink. Ground poultry or any uncooked meat has the same potential for contamination.

Pork Trichinosis (an illness produced when the larvae of a tiny worm found in pork hatch in a person's intestine) is

Handling food safely

Here are some guidelines for avoiding food poisoning:

- Never leave foods (cooked or uncooked) at room temperature for more than 2 hours. Keep foods refrigerated at a temperature below 40°.
- Rinse all meat, fish, and poultry before cooking.
- Wash hands, utensils, and cutting surfaces with hot, soapy water before and after food preparation.
- Thaw frozen foods in the refrigerator or in the microwave, not on the counter.
- Keep cooked foods hot on the stove or cold in the refrigerator until you are ready to serve them.
- When cooking large batches of food, divide leftovers into small batches to refrigerate; the temperature will drop more quickly to a safe level.
- Refrigerate leftovers immediately after finishing a meal.

much less common than it once was. However, it is still recommended that you cook pork to at least 160°, leaving no traces of pink. Freezing meat for 20 days also kills the worm. When microwaving, cover the meat and turn it regularly to make sure that it is cooked thoroughly, paying particular attention to meat near the bones.

Fish and shellfish In the market, whole fish can be safely stored directly on ice, but fish fillets and steaks should be placed on a metal tray to prevent them from coming into direct contact with the ice. Choose fish that smell sweet, not fishy. Choose fillets that are moist and firm. Refrigerate fish immediately and cook it as soon as possible—fish can spoil within a day or two.

Fish carry a variety of parasites. Oysters on the half shell and cherrystone clams, both served raw, carry the risk of causing illness. They are harvested from coastal waters that may be contaminated with raw sewage. Eating contaminated raw shellfish can result in gastrointestinal infections, causing diarrhea, nausea, abdominal cramps, and vomiting. Eating steamed clams can also be dangerous—they are usually cooked only to the point at which their shells open, not long enough to kill any bacteria. Cook clams and other shellfish for at least 6 minutes. If you are pregnant, you should not eat raw fish or meat of any kind.

IMPROVING YOUR DIET

It is easy to say that a healthy diet consists of lots of vegetables, fruits, and grains and very little fat. However, if you are not used to it, you may think that eating that way is impossible. Here are some tips to help you get started:

Stocking up Replace some of the foods in your refrigerator and cabinets with healthier choices. First, get rid of the worst offenders—foods with saturated fat. Replace high-fat meats and lunch meats with lean poultry, fish, beans, and other proteins. Buy reduced-fat or nonfat dairy products instead of whole milk, butter, or cheese.

Make sure your refrigerator is always full of high-quality fruits and vegetables that are ready to eat whenever you have an urge to snack. Keeping peeled carrots, broccoli, cherry tomatoes, and other cleaned vegetables in bite-size amounts in the refrigerator and keeping a well-stocked fruit bowl within easy reach are good ways to increase your intake of these nutritious foods.

Aim for a diet that includes only small portions of meat (about the size of the palm of your hand, or 3 or 4 ounces). Eat lots of pasta with low-fat sauces, pizza with low-fat toppings, and meals based on grains, rice, and dried beans with vegetables and flavorful herbs.

Here are some other healthy foods to have on hand:

- **Egg substitutes** They contain no cholesterol and are lower in fat than eggs. In fact, egg substitutes are only egg whites with food coloring added. Use them instead of eggs for baking and for scrambled eggs and omelettes, sauces, and salad dressings. You can also substitute two egg whites for each whole egg a recipe calls for.
- **Dried beans or legumes (such as peas and lentils)** Use beans liberally with a small amount of meat to create a hearty main-course stew. Puréed beans make a smooth, thick base for soups and sauces and they make a nutritious vegetable dip. For quick and easy preparation, buy canned beans.
- **Grains** Try the many varieties of rice (brown, wild), couscous (a cracked-wheat grain), bulgur (a type of cracked wheat), and pasta in all shapes and sizes.

Cooking methods Low-fat cooking means steaming, microwaving, grilling, sautéing, or stir-frying your food with little or no oil. Deep-fat frying adds a large amount of fat to whatever you are cooking.

Using nonstick pans and cooking sprays, you can eliminate oil or butter when sautéing or stir-frying meats and vegetables and, when baking, you don't have to grease the pan. A vegetable steamer allows you to cook with no oil or fat and, at the same time, preserve many of the nutrients that leach into the water during boiling.

In moderation, grilling is a good way to cook meat and poultry because it allows the fat to drip away from the meat. Because of concern about cancer-causing substances called nitrosamines that form during grilling or any other high-temperature cooking of meat, it is recommended that you partially cook meat in the microwave before grilling it. Avoid charring or overcooking meat.

Enhancing flavor Instead of using butter or salt to improve the flavor of foods, try these alternatives:

- Prepared spice combinations that do not contain sodium
- Dried and fresh herbs
- Cooking wine
- Dried tomatoes
- Low-sodium broths
- Prepared mustards
- Vinegars
- Oil sprays
- Fruit preserves

Similar foods, big differences in fat and calories

Replacing high-fat foods in your diet with low-fat ones is usually a good way to reduce calories as well.

INSTEAD OF . . .	FAT (grams)	CALORIES	CHOOSE . . .	FAT (grams)	CALORIES
Croissant	19	324	English muffin	1	140
Doughnut	13	235	Bagel (1 medium)	1	157
Granola (1 ounce)	6	133	Bran flakes (1 ounce)	1	90
French fries (10)	7	129	Baked potato with skin	0	133
Ham (2 ounces)	6	105	Turkey breast without skin (2 ounces)	2	90
Ice cream (1/2 cup)	7	135	Frozen yogurt (1/2 cup)	1	98
Corn chips (1 ounce)	9	155	Pretzels (10 small sticks)	0	10
Mayonnaise (1 tablespoon)	11	100	Nonfat mayonnaise (1 tablespoon)	0	10
Whole milk (1 cup)	8	150	Skim milk (1 cup)	0	85
Chocolate cake (1 slice)	12	264	Angel food cake (1 slice)	0	125
Sour cream (1 tablespoon)	3	25	Nonfat yogurt (1/4 cup)	0	34
Egg (1 large)	6	74	Egg substitute (1)	0	25
Salad oil (1 tablespoon)	14	125	Flavored vinegar (1 tablespoon)	0	2

CHAPTER 2

Fitness

Contents

The National Institute on Aging says that if exercise could be packed into a pill, it would be the single most widely prescribed and beneficial medicine in the nation. Four out of five Americans are not getting enough exercise. It is now known that even moderate exercise can provide substantial health benefits. You should try to accumulate at least 30 minutes of moderate exercise throughout the day, most days of the week.

Simply fitting more activity into your daily routine can help keep you healthy. Time spent (even for 5 to 15 minutes) taking the stairs instead of the elevator, walking all or part of the way to and from work, walking the dog, or gardening can add up to your daily workout. Vigorous exercise is even more beneficial.

Why exercise is good for your health

Higher levels of fitness are associated with lower rates of death from all causes. In addition to the major benefit of exercise—protection against heart disease—physical activity may provide protection against many other chronic diseases, including type II diabetes, high blood pressure, osteoporosis, and some types of cancer. Physical activity can also raise your self-esteem and improve the quality of your life by helping you keep your weight down and your muscles and bones strong, and helping to reduce emotional stress, depression, and anxiety.

The best time to develop a lifelong habit of regular physical activity is during childhood and adolescence. At any age, increases in your level of activity can improve your health and well-being. Exercise may also help you live longer.

EXERCISE AND HEART DISEASE

Exercise plays a major role in preventing heart disease—the number-one killer of American women. Physical inactivity is a major risk factor for heart disease—along with cigarette smoking, high blood pressure, type II diabetes, and a high cholesterol level.

Women who are physically inactive are three times more likely to die prematurely of a heart attack than women who are active. People who have already had a heart attack live longer afterward if they exercise even moderately.

Regular exercise lowers the level of harmful low-density lipoprotein (LDL) cholesterol in the blood—the kind that causes fatty deposits to build up along artery walls. Exercise raises the level of helpful high-density lipoprotein (HDL) cholesterol, which prevents fat buildup inside arteries. The buildup of fatty deposits called plaque in artery walls (a process called atherosclerosis) is a major cause of heart attacks. Exercise can also reduce blood pressure and control sugar levels in the blood. Regulation of sugar in the blood helps prevent type II diabetes, which is another major cause of heart disease.

The best heart-strengthening activities are aerobic exercises, which increase the amount of oxygen your muscles use by increasing your heart rate. Walking, jogging, biking, and swimming are aerobic activities. Aerobic exercise boosts the power of your heart and blood vessels, gradually training your heart to pump more blood with less effort. When you first start exercising, you huff and puff because your heart and lungs have to work hard to supply oxygen to your muscles. Regular exercise improves the transport and use of oxygen throughout your body because your heart is able to pump more blood with each beat, reducing the hard breathing. This is called the "training effect."

EXERCISE AND HIGH BLOOD PRESSURE

High blood pressure, called hypertension, improves with exercise. High blood pressure increases your risk of heart disease and stroke. Lack of regular exercise is a major risk factor for high blood pressure. If you have mildly elevated blood pressure (see page 482), regular exercise (at least 20 minutes a day, 3 days a week) can be enough to bring your blood pressure to a healthy level. People who have high blood pressure that requires treatment with medication can dramatically reduce their need for medication by exercising regularly.

EXERCISE AND STROKE

Physically active people who do not smoke are much less likely than other people to have a stroke (see page 569). Stroke results from either a blockage of a blood vessel in the brain or leaking of a blood vessel in the brain. A stroke can damage brain tissue, which often leads to partial paralysis and loss of speech.

Even moderate activities such as brisk walking can have a preventive effect. Exercise may provide protection against stroke by preventing narrowing of the carotid artery in the neck, which provides oxygen-rich blood to the brain. This narrowing is caused by atherosclerosis, the buildup of fatty deposits in artery walls. Narrowing of the carotid artery contributes to the occurrence of a stroke by reducing blood flow to the brain.

Exercise can also reduce the risk of stroke by lowering blood pressure. High blood pressure (see page 480) is a major risk factor for stroke. Exercise can help you burn calories and lose weight, which, in turn, can significantly reduce your blood pressure.

Doctors now recommend exercise as an important part of the rehabilitation process after a person has had a stroke. Regular exercise has been shown to reduce a person's risk of having another stroke.

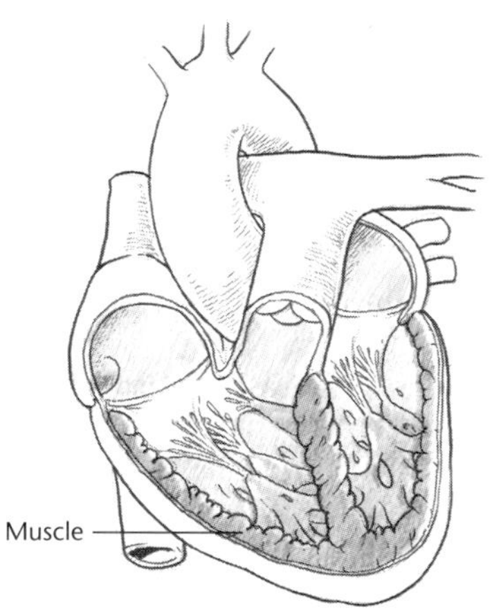

Heart of an inactive person

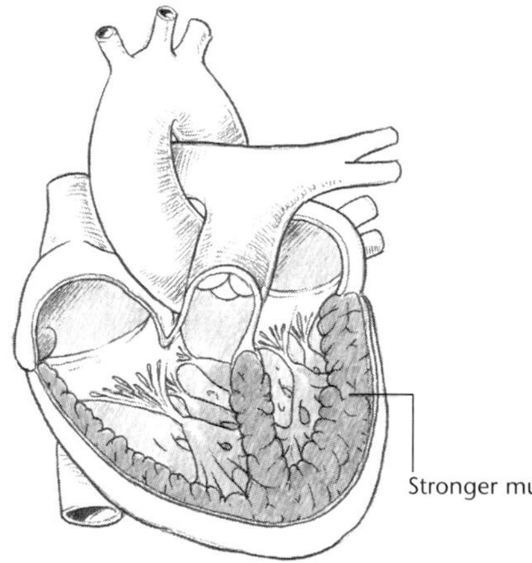

Heart of an active person

HOW EXERCISE AFFECTS THE HEART
Your heart is a muscle. Like any muscle, it becomes stronger when you exercise it. The heart of a physically inactive person (far left) has thinner walls than the heart of a physically active person (left). The thicker, stronger walls of an exercised heart enable it to pump more blood more efficiently throughout the body.

HOW EXERCISE AFFECTS THE CORONARY ARTERIES
The coronary arteries deliver blood and oxygen to the heart muscle itself. An inactive lifestyle encourages the buildup of fatty deposits called plaque on the inside of artery walls. Physical activity helps keep your arteries open. A total blockage of a coronary artery cuts off the oxygen supply to the heart muscle, causing a heart attack.

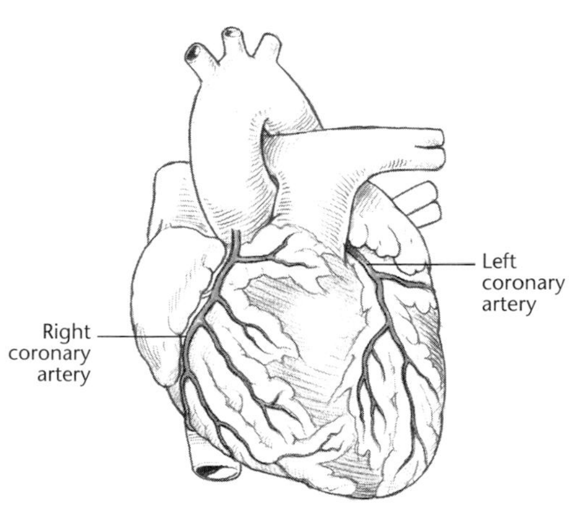

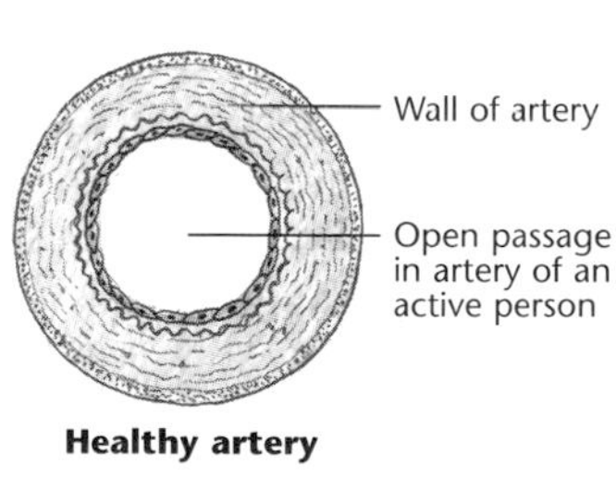

Healthy artery

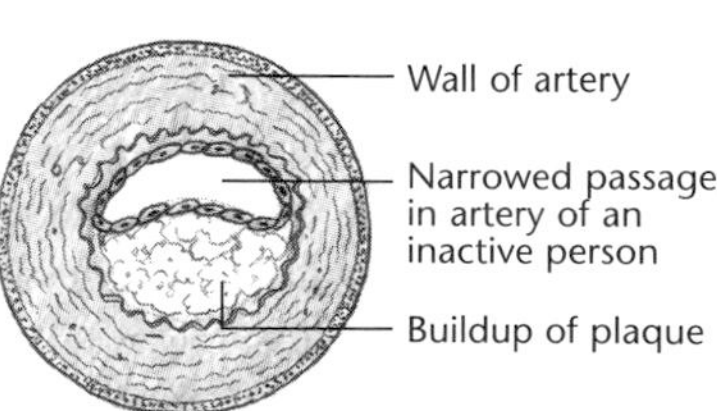

Unhealthy artery

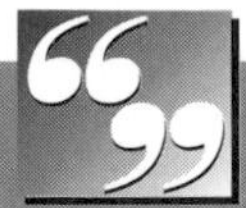

One woman's story
Exercise: her life depends on it

My first heart attack took everyone by surprise, especially my doctor. I was only 42, I had two kids, and I was running around like crazy from my job as a social worker, then home to make dinner for my kids or chauffeur them to all their many activities. My cholesterol level was normal and my blood pressure was only mildly high. I didn't smoke and I was only a few pounds overweight. I had none of the usual risk factors for heart disease—except one. My mother died of a heart attack when she was 54, but I didn't think it would happen to me.

I had never exercised. I thought I led an active life, with my demanding job and all the responsibilities of juggling motherhood and a career. But I was actually doing a lot of sitting all day, first at my job and then in the car. It took two more heart attacks in the next 4 years plus bypass surgery to convince me I had to change my life. My children might be left without a mother and I would miss seeing them grow up. I had a lot to live for.

"My mother died of a heart attack when she was 54, but I didn't think it would happen to me."

Eight weeks after surgery, I joined a cardiac rehabilitation program. In addition to eating a low-fat, low-salt diet as my doctor advised, I began an exercise program. For an hour, four times a week, I walked on a treadmill, rode a stationary bike, and worked on weight machines to improve my strength. I hated it at first. I wasn't used to pushing myself physically. Just staying on that treadmill took a huge amount of self-discipline. I resented having to do it and it was hard to carve out the time for it. But, as I built up my endurance and strength, I got to like the routine and I enjoy the feeling of being strong and healthy. Also, I no longer get tired as easily.

I've drastically reduced the amount of fat in my diet and in the food I make for my kids. Because they are also at an increased risk of heart disease, I want to do everything I can to help them develop healthy habits—especially regular exercise—that they will follow the rest of their life. I'm glad they're involved in sports both in and out of school.

I began working out at home after my health insurance coverage for the cardiac rehabilitation center ran out. I walk outdoors now on nice days and, when the weather is bad, I do an aerobics workout with a videotape. I don't know what the future holds in terms of my heart condition. But so far all the signs look good. My blood pressure is down, my weight is down, and my HDL cholesterol, the good kind, is up. Exercise has changed my life and I'm not about to quit. My life depends on it.

EXERCISE AND DIABETES

The most common type of diabetes—type II diabetes—affects twice as many women over age 45 as men the same age. You can reduce your risk of type II diabetes, especially if you are overweight and have a family history of the disease, by exercising regularly. (There is no known way to prevent type I diabetes.) In a person with type II diabetes, cells are resistant to the action of insulin, the hormone that helps the body use the sugar glucose for energy. When cells do not take in glucose, it builds up in the blood. Regular exercise has a similar effect on the body as insulin—it helps muscle cells take up glucose from the bloodstream and use it for energy.

Being overweight is a major risk factor for type II diabetes—three out of four people with the disease are substantially overweight. Body fat, especially fat stored in the abdominal area, increases cells' resistance to insulin and may make it more difficult to control the level of glucose in the blood. Exercise can help you reduce that risk by helping you reduce body fat and increase muscle. Muscle uses glucose more efficiently than fat does.

Regular exercise can also benefit people who already have diabetes (of either type). Active people with diabetes tend to require less medication, have more control over the level of sugar in their blood, and may have fewer long-term complications from the disease (see page 619). If you have diabetes, you should talk to your doctor before beginning an exercise program.

EXERCISE AND OBESITY

People who exercise are more likely to have a healthy body weight. You gain weight when you eat more calories than your body burns. Physical activity is half of the equation for losing weight; the other half is restricting the number of calories you eat each day.

While evidence has shown that many obese people exercise little, it has not been proven that a low level of activity causes obesity. It appears that obesity results from a complex interaction of a person's genetic makeup and lifestyle factors. However, physical exercise, particularly aerobic exercise, which burns fat efficiently, can reduce your risk of becoming overweight and is an important part of any weight-loss program.

Physical activity is especially helpful for maintaining a healthy weight. Excessive weight has been linked to heart disease, high blood pressure, a high cholesterol level, and diabetes. (For more about how to lose weight, see page 106.)

EXERCISE AND OSTEOPOROSIS

Exercise helps young women build strong, healthy bones and helps older women maintain their bone strength and density. Active people of all ages have higher bone density than people who are sedentary.

To build strong bones, you need to do weight-bearing exercises such as walking, jogging, climbing stairs, skiing, or aerobic dancing. Activities that put stress on your bones, including lifting weights, stimulate new bone growth. Activities such as swimming (in which the water is supporting your weight) or biking (in which the bicycle is supporting you) are less likely to help maintain or increase your bone density, although they are excellent forms of exercise. Plan to be physically active for the rest of your life because the positive effects of exercise are lost after you stop exercising.

Weight-bearing exercise can help girls and young women increase their bone density during the critical years (up to age 20) when 95 percent of their bone is being built. Bone density reaches its natural peak at about age 20 and gradually decreases from age 35 until menopause, when it drops sharply. At menopause, your ovaries stop producing the bone-strengthening hormone estrogen. The more reserve you have built up during childhood and adolescence, the more protection you will have against osteoporosis and debilitating fractures later in life.

But it's never too late to start exercising. Even after menopause, walking 45 minutes a day several days a week may help slow bone loss in your spine. Doing moderate weight-lifting exercises can help you maintain the strength and density in your muscles and bones, improving your ability to do everyday tasks.

If you are at increased risk of osteoporosis (see page 555), your doctor can evaluate your bone density. If you are diagnosed with osteoporosis, your risk of bone fractures is extremely high. Your doctor may recommend that you stick with low-impact exercises such as walking and moderate weight lifting, and avoid activities—such as golf, bowling, tennis, or racquetball—that involve a high degree of twisting or unbalanced movement.

EXERCISE AND CANCER

Overall cancer rates decrease as physical activity increases. Exercise may help prevent some types of cancer, including colon cancer, endometrial cancer, and breast cancer. Exercise can reduce your risk of obesity, which is a major risk factor for all three of these cancers.

Endometrial cancer and breast cancer are associated with increased estrogen levels in the body. Exercise may help reduce the risk of these cancers by reducing the amount of fat on the body (fat cells produce estrogen).

Exercise may also reduce the risk of colon cancer by helping speed waste through the colon, reducing the time that any cancer-causing substances present are exposed to the lining of the colon. This contact may encourage the growth of tiny precancerous tumors called polyps.

EXERCISE AND EMOTIONAL WELL-BEING

People who exercise regularly say they feel better—not just physically, but emotionally and mentally as well. Exercise can help relieve stress and reduce your risk of depression or anxiety. This is especially important for women because they are much more likely than men to experience depression.

Aerobic exercise stimulates your body to produce chemicals called endorphins, which act on your brain to reduce pain and brighten mood. Most people feel calm, relaxed, and happy after they exercise. People who exercise also tend to sleep better. Lack of sleep can make you irritable, less able to cope with everyday problems, and unable to enjoy relationships with family and friends.

How the body responds to regular aerobic exercise

Aerobic exercise is physical activity, such as walking or swimming, during which your heart rate increases and your body meets your muscles' increased demand for oxygen. Regular exercise directly benefits many important functions of your body.

- Your heart will gradually become stronger as it works to pump more blood. Your heart rate when you are not exercising, called your resting heart rate, will be lower because each heart beat is stronger and pumps more blood.
- Your blood vessels will be less likely to narrow and your blood pressure will lower as your circulation improves.
- Your muscular endurance will improve. Your ligaments and tendons (which support your muscles and bones) will become stronger and tighter.
- Your bones will maintain their strength and density, reducing your risk of the bone-thinning disorder osteoporosis.
- Your body fat will likely decrease because your metabolism increases during exercise, burning more fat calories. Your level of "good" cholesterol will increase and your level of harmful cholesterol will decrease.
- Your intestinal tract will work more efficiently, absorbing nutrients and eliminating waste more quickly and easily, helping to reduce your risk of colon cancer.
- Your brain may be stimulated to produce more chemicals called endorphins, which will make you feel better. You may also experience reduction in stress, anxiety, and depression.

Starting an exercise program

If you do not exercise regularly, you have probably thought about it at some time or even tried it, but were discouraged by the time or physical demands you think it involves. Try increasing your level of physical activity in very small amounts at first. Your goal is to start a habit that fits comfortably into your lifestyle.

HOW MUCH EXERCISE IS ENOUGH?

For sedentary people, just the act of getting up and moving around can provide health benefits. Increasing your level of activity gradually will help you get used to it and help avoid frustration and discouragement. You will be more likely to stick with it. Even if you have a disability or condition that makes physical activity difficult, you can make changes in your daily routine that can contribute to your overall health and the quality of your life. It is simple—moving around is good for you. Do it as much as you can.

Everyday activities such as housework, caring for children, and walking may be sufficient exercise to provide protection against illness. An increase in daily activity can have substantial long-term benefits, especially if you are sedentary, sit at a desk all day, and drive home, eat dinner, and watch TV at night. Climb a few flights of stairs at the office each day instead of taking the elevator. Walk part of the way home from work or running errands. (See Everyday fitness, page 80.)

While any increase in activity provides health benefits, to achieve cardiovascular fitness—that is, to train your heart and lungs to deliver oxygen more efficiently throughout your body and to improve your endurance—you need to develop a regular program of aerobic exercise. That means walking, jogging, bicycling, dancing, swimming, playing tennis, or any repetitive activity that makes your heart work harder and become stronger. For the best cardiovascular effect, you need to accumulate at least 30 minutes of vigorous aerobic activity most days of the week.

How fit are you?

To get a general idea of your level of fitness, take the following simple 1-mile walking test. All you need is a pair of comfortable shoes, and a stopwatch or a watch with a second hand to time your walk and measure your pulse rate after the test. Here is how to take the test:

1. After warming up (walking slowly) for 5 minutes, walk briskly for 1 mile at a steady pace. If you are using a quarter-mile track, walk the 4 laps using the inside lane.
2. Determine your time in minutes and seconds using your watch or stopwatch, jot it down, and immediately take your pulse for exactly 15 seconds and write down this number. You can take your pulse on the inside of your wrist or along the carotid artery at the side of your neck, as shown below. Practice taking your pulse before the test so that you will be able to find it easily and quickly.
3. After recording your 15-second pulse, continue walking slowly for 5 minutes to allow your heart rate and blood pressure to return to normal.
4. Multiply your 15-second pulse count by 4 to get your heart rate in beats per minute. For example, if your 15-second pulse count was 32 beats, your heart rate was 32 X 4, or 128 beats per minute.
5. For every 10 pounds over 125 that you weigh, add 15 seconds to your time before looking at the chart. For every 10 pounds under 125 that you weigh, subtract 15 seconds from your walking time before checking the chart. These calculations are required because the information provided at right is based on fitness levels for a woman who weighs 125 pounds.
6. Read down the far left-hand column in the chart to the right until you come to your age group. Find your heart rate from the walking test in the column titled "heart rate." (If you do not find your exact heart rate, round it off to the nearest 10. For example, round off a rate of 128 to 130 and a rate of 144 to 140.) Then, read across the row to determine which fitness category your 1-mile walk time falls into.

TAKING YOUR PULSE
Don't use your thumb because the pressure can slow your heart rate.

Fitness test results

If your walk time is more than the higher number, your fitness level is low; if it is less than the lower number, your fitness level is high; if it is in the range shown here, you have an average fitness level.

AGE	HEART RATE	WALK TIME (min:sec}
20-29	110	19:08-20:57
	120	18:38-20:27
	130	18:12-20:00
	140	17:42-19:30
	150	17:12-19:00
	160	16:42-18:30
	170	16:12-18:00
30-39	110	17:52-19:46
	120	17:24-19:18
	130	16:54-18:48
	140	16:24-18:18
	150	15:54-17:48
	160	15:24-17:18
	170	14:55-16:54
40-49	110	17:20-19:15
	120	16:50-18:45
	130	16:24-18:18
	140	15:54-17:48
	150	15:24-17:18
	160	14:54-16:48
	170	14:25-16:18
50-59	110	17:04-18:40
	120	16:36-18:12
	130	16:06-17:42
	140	15:36-17:18
	150	15:06-16:48
	160	14:36-16:18
	170	14:06-15:48
≥ 60	110	16:36-18:00
	120	16:06-17:30
	130	15:37-17:01
	140	15:09-16:31
	150	14:39-16:02
	160	14:12-15:32
	170	13:42-15:04

EVERYDAY FITNESS

REGULAR PHYSICAL ACTIVITY is one of the most important things you can do for your health. Besides strengthening your bones, muscles, and heart, exercise can reduce your risk of illness and increase the quality and length of your life. You can achieve many of these benefits in less time and at lower levels of activity than you might think. The key is to incorporate physical activity into your daily life, even if it's only a few minutes at a time.

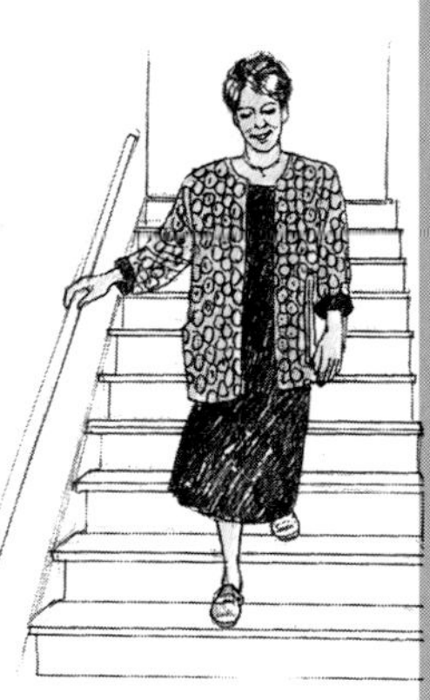

MAKE EXERCISE PART OF YOUR LIFE
Look for ways to incorporate exercise into your daily routine. Take the stairs instead of the elevator or escalator, walk all or part of the way to work, take a walk at lunchtime, ride your bike, or walk the dog.

What regular exercise can do for you

You've heard many times that exercise is good for you, but you may be surprised to learn how it can benefit you. Regular exercise can:

- Build strong muscles and bones
- Strengthen your heart
- Reduce your risk of chronic diseases, including heart disease, osteoporosis, type II diabetes, and high blood pressure
- Help control your weight
- Reduce your risk of some cancers, including colon cancer
- Slow the aging process
- Raise your level of helpful HDL cholesterol and lower your level of harmful LDL cholesterol
- Reduce stress
- Reduce symptoms of premenstrual syndrome (PMS)
- Relieve menstrual pain
- Improve your self-image
- Relieve depression
- Improve the quality of your sleep
- Improve your posture
- Improve the quality of your life, particularly as you age

Physical intensity of activities

MODERATE

Sweeping floors
Grocery shopping
Mopping floors
Pushing power mower
Walking (brisk)
Swimming (slow)
Weeding garden
Painting house

HARD

Cycling
Planting garden
Scrubbing floor
Pushing hand mower
Shoveling snow
Tennis (singles)
Skating
Hiking (without a backpack)

VERY HARD

Aerobic dance (high impact)
Skiing (cross country or downhill)
Soccer
Basketball
Running (slow)
Dancing (fast)
Climbing stairs

When not to exercise

Exercising when you are ill can worsen your condition. Do not exercise if you are experiencing any of the following symptoms:

- Fever
- Sore throat
- Cough that produces phlegm
- Abnormal genital discharge
- Heavy menstrual bleeding
- Painful urination
- Pain in your muscles and joints

Fitness benefits of exercise

Different physical activities provide different kinds of health benefits—aerobic fitness, bone strength, muscle strength, flexibility, and weight loss or maintenance. Fitness experts agree that you should try to achieve all five of these goals by engaging in a variety of alternating activities. The benefits you gain from a particular exercise or activity are indicated by an "X."

Activity	Aerobic fitness	Bone strength	Muscle strength	Flexibility	Weight loss or maintenance
Walking	X	X	X		X
Running	X	X	X		X
Swimming	X		X	X	X
Bicycling	X		X		X
Aerobic dancing	X	X	X	X	X
Stair climbing	X	X	X		X
Free weights		X	X		
Weight machines		X	X		
Yoga				X	
Stretching				X	
Tennis	X	X	X		X
Racquetball	X	X	X		X
Volleyball	X	X	X		X
Shoveling snow	X	X	X		X
Vacuuming	X	X	X		X
Raking leaves	X	X			X
Carrying groceries		X	X		
Square dancing	X	X	X		X

Fitting physical activity into your daily life

Think about ways to build exercise into your regular activities. Here are some ideas:

- Walk to the store.
- Park your car far from your destination and walk the rest of the way.
- Walk your dog.
- Do your own yard work—rake the yard, mow the lawn, shovel snow.
- Play active games with your children or grandchildren.
- When you get together with a friend, suggest taking a walk instead of just sitting together to talk.
- Ride your bike to the store, to classes, or to work.
- Take a walk with your child or grandchild in a stroller.
- On weekends, make time for active outdoor activities. Go swimming, hiking, canoeing, biking, or cross-country skiing.
- Walk up a few flights of stairs before getting on the elevator.

Starting out

If you have been physically inactive until now, see your doctor before you begin an exercise program. Here are some tips for getting started:

- Choose a low-impact exercise such as walking, swimming, or cycling.
- Begin slowly, just enough to get your muscles and joints accustomed to the increased activity.
- Build up gradually, starting with a few minutes, three times a week.
- To increase the health benefits, exercise longer and more vigorously.

Should you see a doctor before exercising?

If you answer "yes" to any of the following questions, it is a good idea to talk to your doctor before beginning an exercise program.

- Have you been physically inactive for a long time?
- Has a doctor ever said you have heart trouble?
- Do you have chest pains frequently?
- Do you often feel faint or have spells of severe dizziness?
- Have you ever had a reading of high blood pressure?
- Are you taking prescription medication for heart problems, high blood pressure, or diabetes?
- Have you ever had bone or joint problems such as arthritis?

Although you can get plenty of health benefits by simply increasing your daily activities, there are good reasons to begin a more formal program of regular exercise. Regular exercise boosts your immune system, reducing your risk of cancer and other illnesses; improves your emotional well-being; and may even lengthen your life. Arranging a time and place to exercise regularly makes it more likely that you will follow through and stick with it.

If you are also interested in weight control, making exercise a regular part of your life can be beneficial. Many people who exercise say they don't need to watch their calories so closely—an especially nice benefit for anyone who loves to eat.

STICKING WITH IT

Half of the people who begin an exercise program drop out during the first 3 to 6 months. Your goal is to develop a fitness program you can follow for the rest of your life. Choosing activities that you enjoy will make it easier for you to stay with it. Brisk walking is popular because it is easy to do and convenient and you can do it with a friend.

You shouldn't limit yourself to only one form of exercise. In fact, alternating activities is a good idea. Doing too much of one exercise can cause injuries, as many longtime runners know. Walk one day and swim the next. If you exercise at a fitness club, use the stair-climbing machine one day and work out with weights the next day.

Three kinds of fitness

The three kinds of fitness—aerobic fitness, strength, and flexibility—are achieved with different kinds of exercise. You attain aerobic fitness from exercises—such as walking, running, and cycling—that make your heart work harder and more efficiently. The best exercises for maintaining and building strength in your muscles and bones are resistance exercises, such as lifting weights and doing push-ups. Exercises for flexibility, such as stretching, improve the range of motion in your muscles and joints and help prevent injuries.

AEROBIC FITNESS

Aerobic exercise is defined as exercise that makes your heart rate increase to deliver more oxygen to your working muscles. Aerobic exercise involves any repetitive motion of large muscles, such as those in your legs, that can be sustained for a long period of time. Walking, jogging, cycling, swimming, aerobic dancing, rowing, and stair climbing are aerobic exercises. Aerobic exercise provides many health benefits, including protection against heart disease, high blood pressure, type II diabetes, and cancer. To also be protected against the bone-thinning disorder osteoporosis, do aerobic exercises in which your bones are supporting your weight, such as walking and jogging (swimming and biking are not weight-bearing exercises).

Aerobic exercise is also called endurance training because it improves your muscles' endurance as well as their strength. It is an efficient way to burn fat. Regular aerobic exercise changes your body composition by reducing the proportion of fat and increasing the proportion of muscle.

Any amount of aerobic activity will help you condition your heart and lungs. Exercising at any level over your normal, resting heart rate is good for your heart—and three 10-minute sessions can provide the same fitness effects as one 30-minute session.

A good heart rate level when exercising is between 60 and 75 percent of your maximum heart rate (the fastest your heart can beat). This is called your target heart rate. When you first start exercising, aim for the lower end (60 percent); you will gradually build up to the higher end (75 percent) after several months of exercising. Experienced exercisers often go as high as 90 percent of their maximum heart rate, but you do not have to exercise that hard to stay in good condition. For how to find your target heart rate, see below right.

The benefits of aerobic exercise do not stay with you if you do not keep it up. The longer you have been exercising, the more slowly you will lose your conditioning if you stop exercising for a period of time.

Starting a walking program The only equipment you need to start a walking program is a pair of well-cushioned walking shoes with adequate room in the toe. Wear loose, comfortable clothing that is appropriate for the weather. Many regular walkers who hate to miss their daily walk do not let a light rain stop them. Other walkers prefer the controlled climate and safety of a shopping mall. Many malls sponsor walking clubs and open their doors early to allow walkers a clear path.

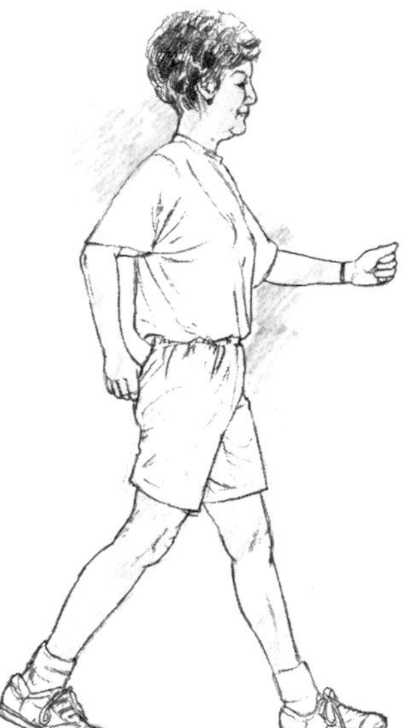

TAKE A WALK
Walking is one of the best exercises you can do. It builds cardiovascular fitness as well as bone and muscle strength, burns fat, feels good, and requires only a pair of well-cushioned shoes. Walk as often as you can.

Walk briskly, landing on your heels and rolling forward to push off with your toes on each step. Keep your shoulders relaxed. Bend your arms and swing them next to your body, keeping your elbows close to your waist. Relax your hands.

If you are a beginner, try walking 10 to 15 minutes a day three times a week. If that feels comfortable, increase it to 5 days a week. After a month, begin adding 5 minutes to your total daily walking time each week until you reach a goal of at least 45 minutes a day, 5 days a week. Remember that it is not necessary to do all your walking in one session—you can spread it out in short walks throughout the day. If you want to increase your heart rate even more and improve your upper body conditioning, use hand weights while you walk.

Guidelines for aerobic exercise To get the most out of any aerobic exercise you choose—walking, swimming, biking, aerobic dancing, stair climbing, or a

Finding your target heart rate

You can easily determine your target heart rate to help you judge whether your workout is appropriate and effective. Let's say you are 40 years old.

1. Subtract your age from 220 to get your maximum heart rate (220 - 40 = 180).
2. Find 60 percent of your maximum heart rate in beats per minute (180 X .60 = 108).
3. Find 75 percent of your maximum heart rate (180 X .75 = 135). Your target heart rate zone while exercising is 108 to 135 beats per minute.
4. Immediately after exercising take your pulse for 15 seconds (see page 79). Multiply the number of beats by 4 to find your heart rate in beats per minute.
5. If you are below your target zone, work a little harder the next time; if you are above your target zone, slow down a little next time.

combination of two or more exercises—use the following guidelines. These guidelines apply even if you do your exercising at home with a video.

- Exercise 3 to 5 days a week.
- Warm up for 5 minutes before you begin your exercise session. Gently stretch (see page 87)—don't bounce—before doing anything. After stretching, any slow repetitive motion (walking or using a stationary bicycle, for example) that raises your heart rate slightly is a good warm-up.
- Exercise hard enough to reach your target heart rate (see page 83) for 20 to 60 minutes each time or accumulate that amount of time over the day.
- Gradually decrease your level of activity to cool down; then stretch for a few minutes.
- To lose weight, do aerobic activity for at least 30 minutes, 5 days a week.

STRENGTH

Weight training is just as beneficial for your health as aerobic exercise. Strengthening exercises help condition your heart and build strength in your muscles and bones. Women do not accumulate as much muscle naturally as men because of their smaller size and their hormones, so they have to keep their muscles strong through some form of resistance exercises.

Strength-building exercises are often referred to as resistance exercises because they require your muscles to push against or resist an object. Weight lifting, using either free weights or machines, is a common and efficient form of strength-building exercise. Many people, not just those who are trying to lose weight, use weight machines for toning their muscles or as an alternative form of exercise. Calisthenic exercises such as sit-ups, push-ups, or leg lifts also build strength. In calisthenics, your body is pushing against gravity or against its own weight.

Exercise that strengthens muscles and bones is especially important for older women, because they lose muscle and bone as they age. By age 75, picking up a bag of groceries or getting up unassisted from a low chair becomes difficult for many women.

But it's never too late to increase your strength. Even if you are in your 80s or 90s, lifting weights of as little as 1 to 5 pounds three times a week can more than double your muscle strength and improve your ability to do daily tasks. You will also be less likely to experience a disabling fall.

By building up your strength, weight-bearing exercise, such as walking, reduces your risk of osteoporosis and bone fractures. Putting weight on your bones can increase your bone density and help reduce the amount of bone you lose naturally as you age (see page 554).

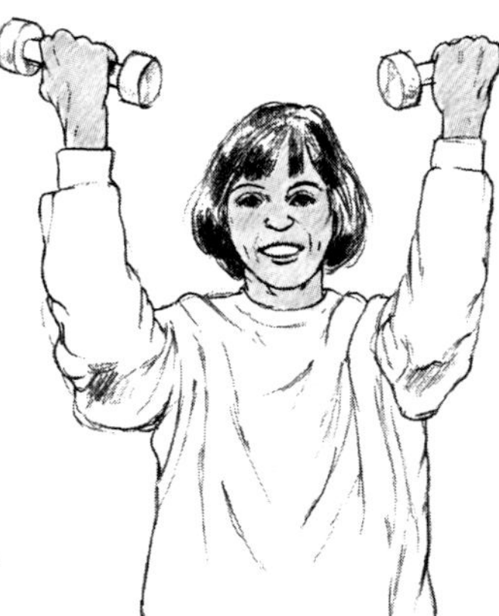

WEIGHT LIFTING
Lifting weights can help you build strength at any age.

Building more strength If you are just starting out, try the exercises on page 85. If you want more intensive strength building or if you are already fit, one of the safest and most effective ways to increase your strength is to use weight machines at a fitness center. But first make sure you are trained by an instructor in the proper use of the machines.

For optimum strength building, choose a weight heavy enough that you can lift it only six to eight times without difficulty. Lighter weights will build muscular endurance but not strength. Many weight lifters repeat the set of six lifts two or three times, resting in between, but this is not necessary in the beginning. Doing one set strengthens your muscles nearly as much as doing multiple sets.

You probably do not need to do as much weight lifting with your legs if you are doing weight-bearing aerobic exercises such as walking or jogging. Lifting leg weights can, however, help inactive people walk longer distances and prevent leg and hip injuries.

Strength building at home

If you are an exercise novice, or you want to build muscle strength at home without using a weight machine, the following program can help you get started. It is good to alternate strengthening exercises with aerobic exercise. Walk one day, for example, and do strength-building exercises the next.

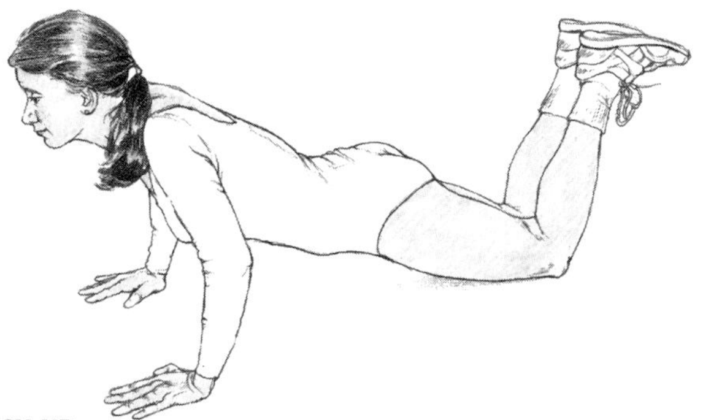

PUSH-UP

For women (who on average have about half the upper body strength of men), the modified push-up is the best overall upper body strengthener. Lie on the floor facedown with your palms next to your shoulders. Push off with your hands, raising your upper body from your knees, keeping your back straight. Push up until your arms are almost straight but not locked at the elbows. Lower your body until it almost touches the ground and repeat as many times as you can without straining.

If these push-ups are too hard at first, start with standing push-ups. Face a wall with your toes about 12 inches from the wall, arms bent, and your palms flat against the wall at shoulder height. Push away from the wall. Keep your back straight, not arched. If you can do 12 repetitions, increase the resistance by standing 18 inches from the wall.

PARTIAL SIT-UP

Lie on your back with your knees bent and your arms straight at your sides. Press the small of your back into the floor. Lift your head and upper body until most of your upper back is off the ground. Hold for a count of two. Lower your body to the floor. Keep the small of your back pressed into the floor to avoid straining your back. Once you can do 12 repetitions, increase the resistance by lifting farther off the ground, exercising on an incline in which your buttocks are higher than your head, or by holding a small weight on your chest while sitting up. A more difficult way to do sit-ups is with your hands placed lightly on the back of your neck.

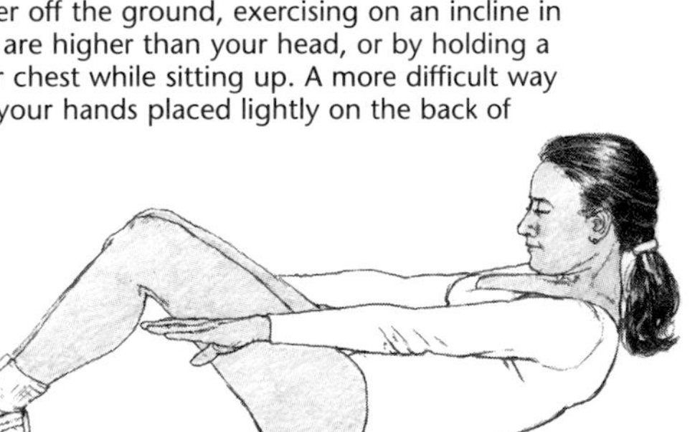

PUMP UP

Stand with your back straight, knees slightly bent, and feet slightly apart. Hold the weights in front of your thighs, palms facing inward. Raise the weights slowly to chest level without turning your palms. Your elbows should go straight out to the sides. Lower the weights slowly to thigh level. When you can repeat the exercise 12 times, increase the weights by 1 pound.

BICEPS CURL

Use two small hand weights (begin with 1-pound weights). Stand with your back straight, knees slightly bent, and feet slightly apart. Hold the weights in your hands in front of your thighs, palms turned out. Slowly bring the weights up and in toward your chest. Lower them slowly to thigh level again. When you can repeat the exercise 12 times, increase the weights by 1 pound.

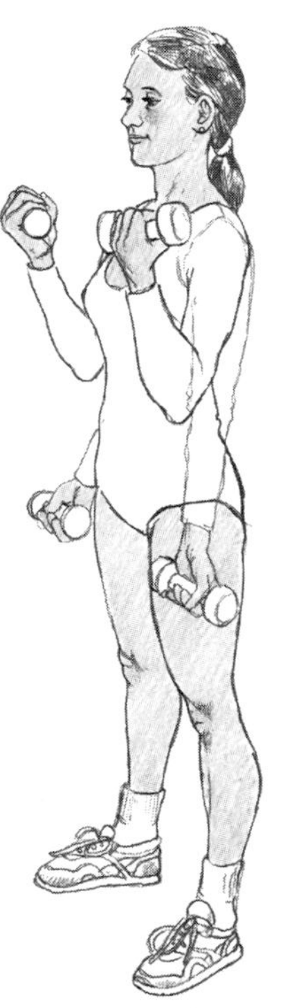

How flexible are you?

Some of your joints may be more flexible than others. For example, you may have tight hamstrings but flexible shoulder joints. These three tests will give you an idea of how flexible you are in different joints. Walk around a while first to warm up.

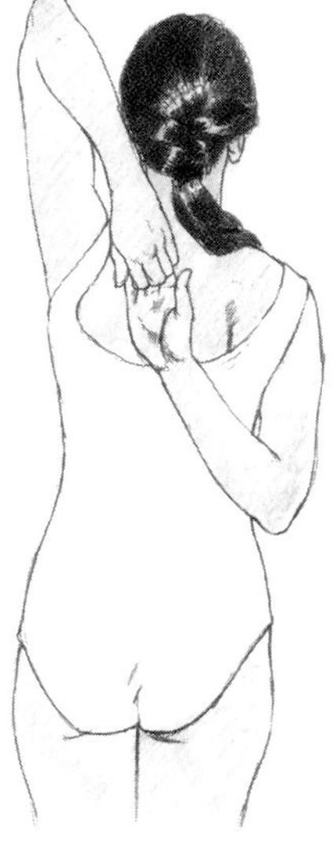

SHOULDER FLEXIBILITY

Lift your left hand over your head and reach down your back. Put your right arm behind your back and reach up to meet your left hand. Perform the same movements with the opposite arms. If your hands overlap, you are reasonably flexible in your shoulder joints. If your hands do not touch, you lack some flexibility in your shoulders.

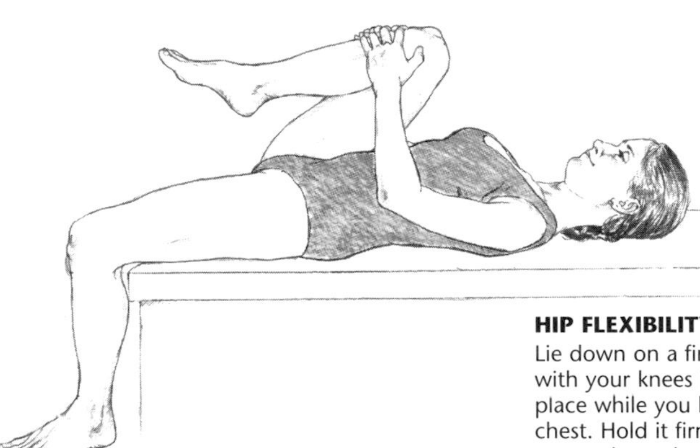

HIP FLEXIBILITY

Lie down on a firm, raised surface, such as a firm bed, with your knees bent over the edge. Leave one leg in place while you bend the other and pull it toward your chest. Hold it firmly with both hands. Switch legs. If you cannot keep the lowered leg in place or if you feel tingling or twitching in your pelvic area, you have little flexibility in your hip joint.

HAMSTRING FLEXIBILITY

To test the flexibility in your hamstrings (the muscles in the back of your thighs), use a step or a sturdy box 8 to 12 inches high. Tape a ruler to the top of the step with the end extending 6 inches out from the step toward you. Sit with your feet flat against the step, about 4 inches apart. Reach forward slowly toward the step as far as you can without bending your knees. Note the point at which your fingertips touch the ruler. You may not be able to reach the step. If you reached more than 12 inches, the flexibility in your hamstrings and lower back is excellent; reaching 9 to 12 inches is good, 4 to 8 inches is fair, under 4 inches is poor.

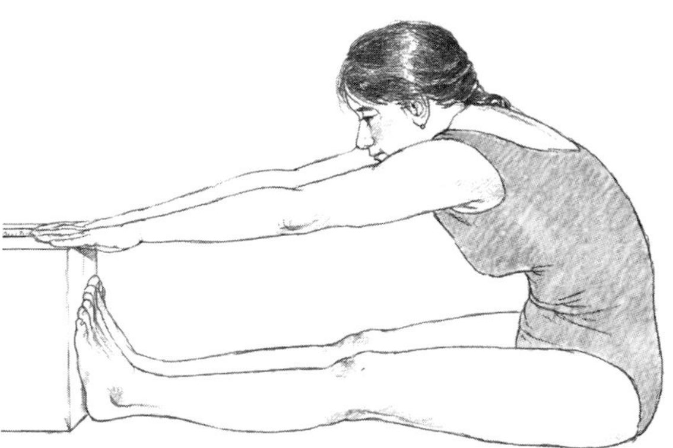

Flexibility program

If you tried the flexibility tests on page 86 and had some difficulty, the stretches shown here will help you gain some flexibility in your joints. The best time to do these stretches is during your warm-up and cool-down sessions before and after exercising. Walk around a while first to warm up. It is important to do these stretches slowly and gently. Do not bounce. Hold each stretch for 30 seconds. The following stretches are particularly good to do before and after aerobic exercises—including walking, jogging, biking, stair climbing, and aerobic dancing—in which you use your leg muscles.

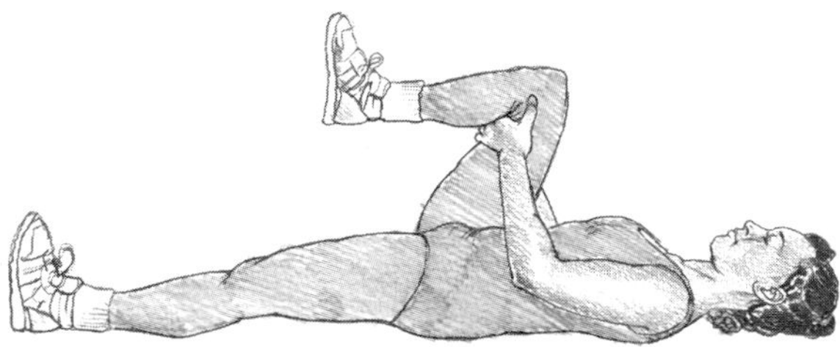

LOWER BACK AND BUTTOCKS STRETCH
Lie on your back on the floor with your left leg stretched out straight and your right leg bent. Press your lower back gently into the floor. Point your toes toward the ceiling. Hold your right leg behind your knee and pull it slowly toward your chest. Hold it for a count of 5 and release. Repeat with the other leg.

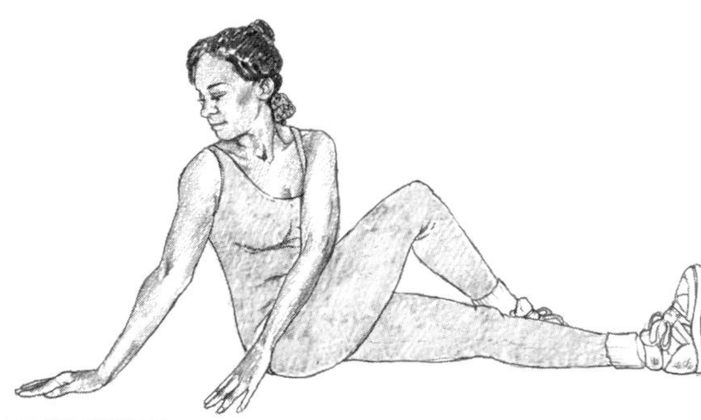

BACK TWIST
Sit up and cross one leg over the other, placing your foot on the floor. Gently turn your body in the opposite direction, rotating your hips to the side and looking over your shoulder. Keep your back straight and buttocks on the ground. Hold the position for a count of 5. Repeat on the other side.

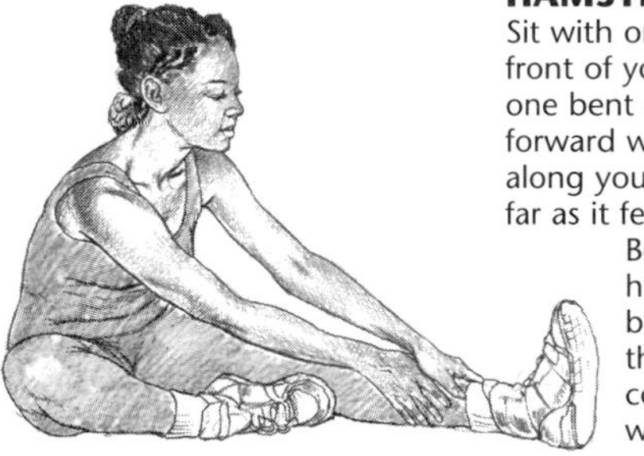

HAMSTRING STRETCH
Sit with one leg extended in front of you and the other one bent as shown. Reach forward with both hands along your extended leg as far as it feels comfortable. Bend from your hips, keeping your back straight. Hold the position for a count of 5. Repeat with the other leg.

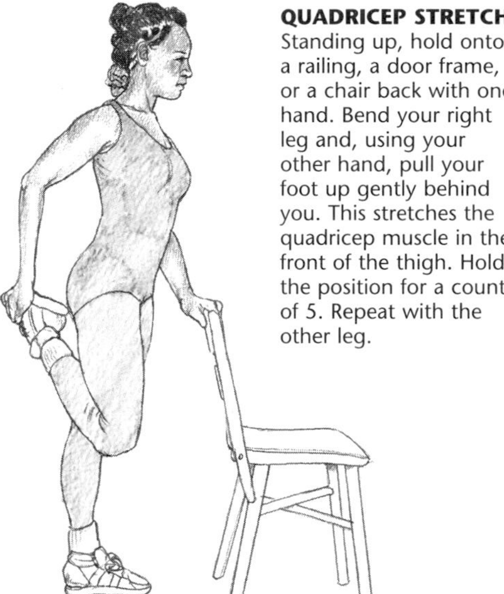

QUADRICEP STRETCH
Standing up, hold onto a railing, a door frame, or a chair back with one hand. Bend your right leg and, using your other hand, pull your foot up gently behind you. This stretches the quadricep muscle in the front of the thigh. Hold the position for a count of 5. Repeat with the other leg.

CALF STRETCH
Stand about 2 to 3 feet from a wall and place your palms on the wall. Step forward with one foot. Bend your rear leg while keeping both feet flat on the ground and toes pointed straight ahead. Lean forward, keeping your back straight. Feel your calf muscle stretch. Hold the position for a count of 5. Repeat with the other leg.

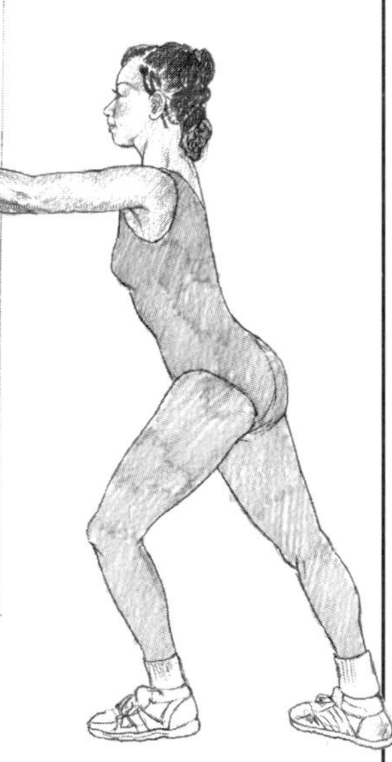

FLEXIBILITY

Flexibility is the ability to move your muscles and joints through their full range of motion. Some people are naturally more flexible than others. If you have never been able to bend over and put your palms flat on the floor, it does not mean you are not fit. Your hip joint may not have a particularly wide range of motion when it flexes forward. You may, however, find that you are able to bend other joints farther than other people can.

If you improve your flexibility, you will find that everyday activities are easier and you will help protect your muscles against pulls and tears. For example, if you slip and fall on your side, and your leg shoots out as you fall, you are less likely to pull a leg muscle if your hip, knee, and ankle joints are flexible. Because exercise tends to shorten and tighten muscles, it is a good idea to pause for a few minutes before and after you exercise to do a series of slow, gentle stretches. Warm up with 5 or 10 minutes of walking.

Stretching can also help relieve some kinds of pain. For example, stretching the hamstring and lower back muscles can help relieve lower back pain. Calf stretches can help prevent painful cramping in your calf muscles.

We all begin life with flexible joints. Just watch an infant put a foot to his or her mouth with ease. Children remain relatively flexible until puberty when their bones begin to grow rapidly and their muscles tighten and strengthen. As they reach middle age, many women become less active, which causes their muscles to weaken and their joints to become tighter and more rigid. Staying as active as you can throughout your life will help you maintain your strength and flexibility.

Good posture

Good posture is not just a matter of appearance. Sitting and standing put considerable pressure on your lower back. When you are standing, you are putting five times more pressure on your back than when you are lying down. Good posture helps relieve that pressure by strengthening the muscles that support your back.

To evaluate your posture, stand normally with your back and buttocks against a wall. Slide your hand into the space between the wall and the small of your back. It should slide in easily but touch both the wall and your back. If there is extra space, it means you are standing in a swayback position, which puts added stress on your lower back. To correct it, pull in your stomach and tilt your hips to reduce the area between the wall and your lower back. Hold your head and shoulders high. When you walk away, try to maintain that posture.

When sitting, keep your shoulders back with your head centered above them. Your feet should be flat on the floor. Do not hunch over because doing so puts strain on your upper back and neck. Hold in your stomach. When you are sitting for extended periods of time, use a chair with lower back support. Arm rests are good because they help keep some of your weight off your spine.

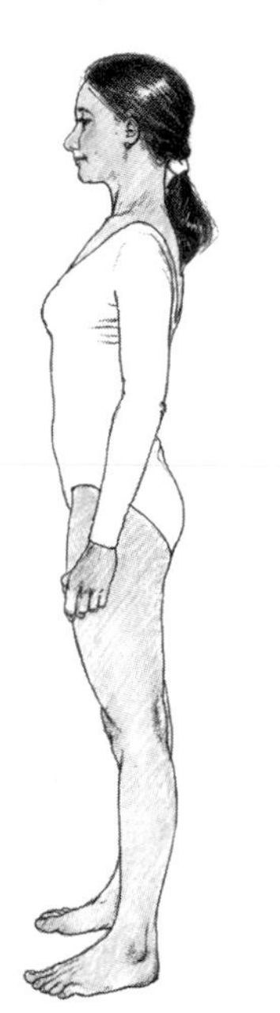

While you exercise

Taking some simple measures when you exercise can significantly reduce your risk of injury. One of the best things you can do is to wear athletic shoes that are designed for the particular activity you engage in. It is also important to drink plenty of water to replace the fluids your body loses during exercise.

DRINK PLENTY OF FLUIDS

When you exercise, be sure you drink plenty of water and other liquids. Fluids help prevent dehydration and heat stress that can result from exercising intensively or in the heat. Your blood needs a sufficient amount of water because blood transports oxygen to working muscles. Before you exercise, have a glass of water, juice, or a sports drink. If you are trying to lose weight, water is the best choice because fruit juices and sports drinks contain enough sugar (and calories) to offset the calories you burn exercising. You should not drink caffeinated drinks such as coffee or colas before or during exercise because caffeine is a mild diuretic, which actually makes your body lose water by increasing the output of urine.

If you exercise vigorously, such as running 5 or more miles a day or participate in intensive aerobics classes or other activities that result in significant sweating, you need to increase your fluid intake. You cannot rely on thirst alone to tell you when to drink. If you exercise intensely or are a competitive athlete, drink one or two glasses of water about 15 minutes before you exercise or compete. Drink one glass of water every 20 minutes while you are exercising. Make an effort to drink water throughout the day, even when you are not exercising.

WEAR A GOOD ATHLETIC SHOE

Good shoes are your best protection against injury during exercise. A shoe that fits poorly or is not designed for a particular activity can result in a variety of problems ranging from blisters and calluses to knee or hip problems.

The qualities of a good athletic shoe include:

- **Cushioned insoles** Cushioning in the soles of your shoes absorbs shock and reduces jarring to your joints. A good cushion should spring back to its original shape after each step. Shoes should be replaced when the cushioning begins to wear out, which often happens before the outside of the shoe shows much wear.
- **Heel counter** The heel counter of a shoe is the hard cup that encircles and stabilizes your heel and cushions the back of your ankle. The heel counter is often notched in the middle to allow for more ankle movement.
- **Sole** The outer sole of the shoe should be flexible and rugged enough to withstand wear and tear from whatever surface on which you walk, run, or play a sport. It should also be waterproof and insulated and provide adequate traction. Different types of soles are designed for different activities and surfaces.
- **Upper** The upper is the outer covering of the upper part of the shoe and is usually made of leather or a synthetic material. An upper should be flexible but also help stabilize the foot. Uppers often have air vents to allow your feet to breathe. Uppers are designed for specific activities.

Choose your shoes to fit your activity. A variety of athletic shoes are available that have specific qualities that provide protection against the types of injuries that are most likely to occur from a particular activity. You can buy shoes for walking, running, aerobic dancing, or playing tennis. You can even buy shoes, called cross trainers, that are designed for people who engage in more than one activity or sport.

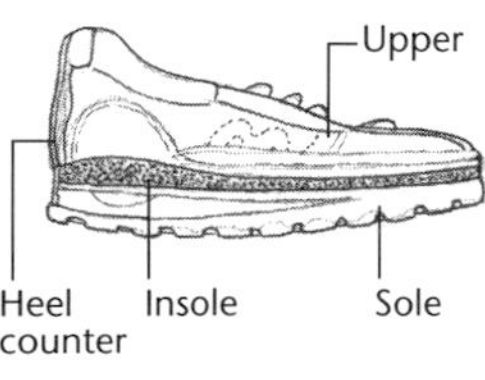

PARTS OF AN ATHLETIC SHOE

Shoe-shopping tips

In addition to having the appropriate athletic shoe for a particular activity, it's important to have shoes that are the right size. When you shop for athletic shoes:

- Have both feet measured. Choose the size that fits your larger foot.
- Wear the same type of socks you wear when you exercise.
- Test the fit by standing on one foot at a time, wiggling your toes, and then standing on tiptoe. If you are buying walking or running shoes, walk or run around the store.
- Check to make sure you have a thumbnail's width of room between your big toe and the front of the shoe.
- Make sure the widest part of your foot fits comfortably into the widest part of the shoe.
- Shop for shoes in the middle or later part of the day because your feet tend to swell gradually throughout the day.

BREAST SUPPORT

It is a good idea to wear a bra when you are doing any kind of exercise, including weight lifting. Jogging or doing high-impact aerobics without a sports bra can stretch the ligaments supporting your breasts, which may eventually cause your breasts to sag.

Highly elastic sports bras compress the breasts and immobilize them during high-impact activities such as running. To find if a bra is right for you, try it on and move around in it; imitate the action you will be performing when you exercise. Choose a bra that doesn't ride up or twist when you move. Make sure that the wide shoulder straps and the band at the bottom of the bra do not cut into your skin. For the same reason, do not wear a bra that has "bones" or underwires when you exercise.

Special fitness concerns

If you are training strenuously, are in your teens, are pregnant, or are over 50 years old, you should take some precautions that can help you exercise more safely. You may also want to talk to your doctor to make sure your exercise program is suitable for you and is not compromising your health in any way.

ATHLETES

For female athletes, prolonged exercise sometimes causes irregular periods or a complete stop of menstruation (amenorrhea). The explanations for this effect of exercise include a drop in weight and body fat that often accompanies strenuous exercise, and the reduced calorie intake that some athletes impose on themselves. It may also result from the associated stress of the exercise itself or the competition. The more intensely a woman trains, the more likely she is to stop menstruating.

Excessive dieting and exercising can affect the pituitary gland and hypothalamus, areas of your brain that regulate hormone production by your ovaries. Changes in the levels of hormones that these glands produce can disrupt ovulation (release of an egg from an ovary) and menstruation. If your periods have stopped, it may indicate that your ovaries are not producing either of the two hormones—estrogen or progesterone—that controls your menstrual cycle.

If your body is not producing estrogen, you need to be extremely concerned about losing bone density, which increases your risk of fractures and other injuries. Not getting enough calcium (1,000 to 1,500 milligrams daily) increases that risk further. Even the weight-bearing exercise you are doing in your sport cannot protect you against bone loss. Each year that you are not menstruating, you can lose about 4 percent of your total bone density.

If you have stopped menstruating, see your doctor immediately. The only way to determine if exercise is the cause is by excluding other possibilities. Lack of periods can result from pregnancy, menopause, a high level of male hormones in your blood, or a more serious problem such as a pituitary gland tumor (see page 628) or an underactive thyroid gland (hypothyroidism, see page 624).

After ruling out these other causes, your doctor may recommend that you reduce your level of activity and increase your weight. These measures are often enough to stimulate the ovaries to begin producing estrogen again, which will stop further bone loss. If these measures do not restore a normal menstrual cycle within 6 months to a year, your doctor may recommend that you take estrogen and other hormones to restore a normal cycle and prevent further bone loss. (For more about amenorrhea, see page 210.)

TEEN ATHLETES

A young girl who participates in sports may find that the changes in her body as she reaches puberty affect her ability to perform athletically. At puberty, estrogen production increases and growth in height stops. At this stage, girls begin to add fat to their hips, buttocks, and breasts. Carrying the additional fat requires greater exertion and may affect a girl's ability to perform athletically. Some previously athletic girls tend to drop out of sports at this point.

But the development that occurs during puberty also brings benefits to an athlete. Although estrogen slows growth in height, it helps to increase bone and muscle strength. This is the stage at which girls develop their adult physique, including strong bones. A slight rise in the male hormone testosterone also promotes the development of bones and larger muscles. The increase in hormones actually makes girls better equipped for athletics than they were before they began menstruating. Coordination usually improves at this stage.

Menstruation often begins later in athletes than in other girls. The onset of menstruation occurs at an average age of 12.8 years in the US. Among athletes, it occurs 1 to 3 years later. The energy drain from strenuous exercise affects the area of the brain that switches on puberty (the hypothalamus), causing a delay in onset of puberty.

Late onset of menstruation most often occurs in girls who participate in activities—such as marathon running, gymnastics, and ballet—in which low body weight and low percentage of body fat are considered ideal for peak performance. Menstruation usually begins once these girls reduce their level of activity and gain some weight.

Delayed onset of menstruation is not harmful as long as it occurs by age 16. After that age, it can indicate a below-normal level of estrogen. A low level of estrogen can contribute to thinning and weakening of the bones, which increases the risk of injury. A young woman who has not menstruated by the age of 16 should see a gynecologist for a pelvic examination. So should a young woman who has not begun to develop breasts, underarm hair, or pubic hair by age 14. A lack of estrogen may compromise a young woman's ability to achieve peak bone strength and density during her teens, which can put her at increased risk of the bone-thinning disorder osteoporosis (see page 552) later in life.

PREGNANT WOMEN

Moderate exercise during pregnancy is beneficial for both the pregnant woman and the developing fetus. Along with maintaining or improving your fitness during pregnancy, exercise can help make labor easier and speed recovery after delivery. Exercise during pregnancy can also improve your self-image and emotional well-being.

The key to exercising safely is to be in shape before you decide to become pregnant. If your body is used to exercise, it is probably safe to continue during pregnancy, slowing down in the last trimester; ask your doctor to be sure. Avoid exercising too strenuously. If you have not exercised before, pregnancy is not the time to learn a new sport or begin a vigorous exercise program. However, a moderate walking program is beneficial for anyone. (For more about exercise and pregnancy, see page 410.)

OLDER WOMEN

Many women who are over 50 believe that exercise is dangerous to their heart or joints. In fact, most people tend to reduce their physical activity as they age. But slowing down can actually be dangerous to your health—it can lead to weakness and debilitation.

The drop in estrogen levels after menopause increases your risk for several debilitating conditions, including osteoporosis and heart disease. Exercise can significantly reduce your risk of both of these disorders.

Osteoporosis Estrogen helps your bones retain calcium, which helps keep them dense and strong. Once estrogen production tapers off at menopause, bone loss accelerates. You can lose up to 30 percent of your bone mass in the first 5 to 7 years after menopause. But even simple exercise—such as walking 45 minutes 4 days a week—can slow this bone loss after menopause. Weight-bearing exercise may even increase bone density in older women. Walking, jogging, aerobic dancing, stair climbing, weight lifting, and resistance exercises (such as push-ups) are good bone-strengthening exercises. However, exercise is most effective if you are also getting sufficient calcium (1,500 milligrams daily; 1,000 milligrams if you are on hormone replacement therapy) from your diet or supplements. Stay with your exercise program because, as soon as you stop exercising regularly, your bones will begin to lose their strength and density.

Heart disease You lose your natural protection against heart disease after menopause, when your ovaries stop producing the heart-protecting hormone estrogen. This lack of estrogen is likely to increase your blood pressure and alter your cholesterol profile (see page 131). Your level of harmful low-density lipoprotein (LDL) cholesterol increases. At the same time, your level of protective high-density lipoprotein (HDL) cholesterol decreases. These factors significantly increase your risk of heart disease, especially after 65. The heart-conditioning effects of exercise, along with a nutritious, low-fat diet, are more important than ever. Regular exercise can also raise the level of beneficial HDL cholesterol in your blood, which helps prevent the buildup of fatty deposits inside your arteries, a major cause of heart attack. It is never too late to start exercising—whether you are in your 70s or your 90s.

However, to avoid injury, make sure you build up the level of intensity gradually and always warm up and cool down before and after exercising.

Exercise guidelines for older women

If you are over 50:

- Check with your doctor before you start an exercise program.
- Choose weight-bearing exercises—such as walking and low-impact aerobics—that reduce your risk of injury.
- Increase the activity gradually to avoid injury.
- If you experience light-headedness, chest pain, or shortness of breath during exercise, stop; see your doctor immediately.
- Stop exercising if you experience any pain.

Preventing and treating exercise-related injuries

Exercise involves a risk of injury, but the many health benefits of exercise far outweigh the risks. Instead of avoiding exercise for fear of injury, take precautions, such as doing stretching exercises (see page 87) regularly, to prevent muscle strain and other injuries. If you do get injured, allow time for recovery before you resume your activity.

The main cause of exercise-related injury is a sudden change in the type of activity or its intensity or duration. For example, if you normally walk a couple of miles a day, it is not a good idea for you to suddenly decide to run a 5-mile race. Work up to that 5-mile run by increasing the distance you walk. Then combine walking and running until you can run most of the distance. If you decide you like running, give yourself time to condition your body by running several miles before you enter a marathon or other competitive run.

If you do get injured, you do not have to stop exercising altogether and lose the conditioning you have developed. After the pain subsides, temporarily switch to a different exercise or activity that does not put stress on the injured part of your body.

WEAR-AND-TEAR INJURIES

Most exercise-related injuries in women are wear-and-tear injuries, also known as overuse injuries. The following are the most common injuries of this kind. If you have an injury that does not get better, see your doctor.

Shin splints Pain in your shin (the front of your lower leg) is usually referred to as a shin splint. Shin splints are often caused by strained muscles or, sometimes, the tearing away of a muscle's attachment to a bone. To treat shin splints, use RICE (see page 93). Stop doing the exercise that caused the injury until the pain stops. Doing exercises to strengthen the muscles in the front of your leg and stretching for longer periods before and after exercising can help you avoid shin splints.

First aid for athletic injuries

The standard prescription for most athletic injuries is known by its acronym "RICE", which stands for rest, ice, compression, and elevation. If you are in any doubt about the severity of your injury, see your doctor.

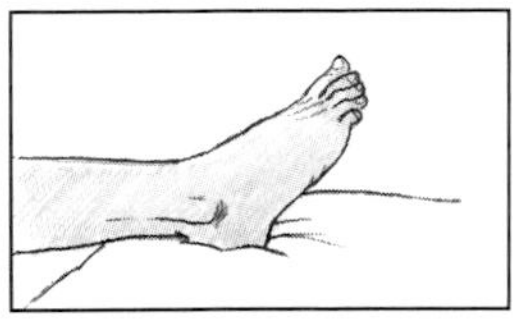

REST

If you feel pain, immediately stop the activity that is causing the pain. If you continue running on an injured foot or ankle, for example, you can make it worse.

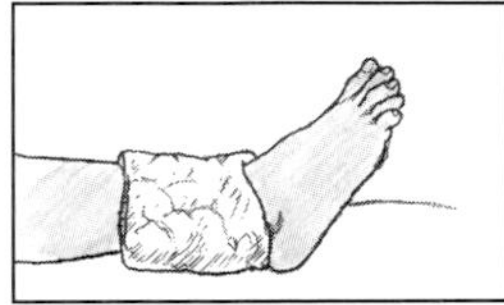

ICE

Apply an ice pack or a chemical cold pack to the injury to help narrow the blood vessels and limit swelling. The less the swelling, the quicker the injury will heal.

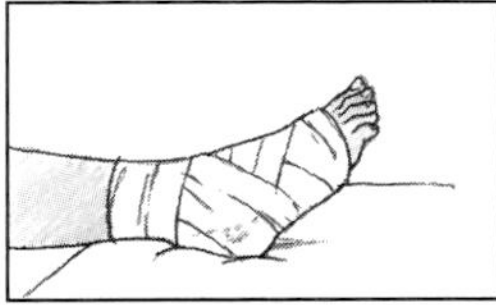

COMPRESSION

Wrap an elastic bandage around the injured area to help limit the swelling. Be careful not to wrap it too tightly; you should be able to slip your finger under the bandage.

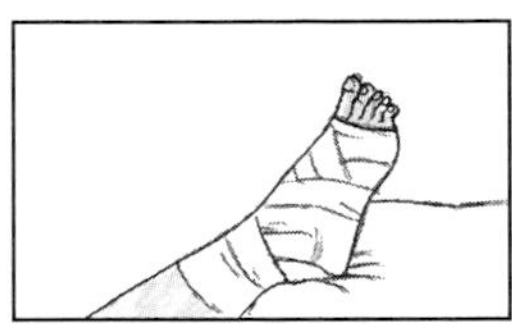

ELEVATION

Keep the injured area elevated above the level of your heart to prevent blood and other fluids from collecting at the injury, thereby reducing swelling.

Plantar fasciitis Plantar fasciitis is a long name for a common problem—pain and inflammation in the bottom of your heel that hurts more when you stand up on your toes. The injury results when the band of protective tissue (called the plantar fascia) that runs from your heel along the bottom of your foot to the base of your toes detaches slightly from your heel. Place an ice pack on your heel to relieve swelling and pain. If the pain is so severe that you cannot put weight on your foot, see your doctor immediately. To relieve the symptoms, stop or reduce the activity that caused the problem. Try activities such as swimming or rowing that do not put stress on your feet. Arch supports or flexible shoes may also help. If the pain persists, see your doctor.

Stress fractures of the small bones of the foot Stress fractures are small cracks on the surface of bones that result from injury. The most common site of stress fractures is the bone just behind your fourth toe. Stress fractures can result from repetitive pounding of your feet on the ground. People who have inflexible ankles and high arches are more susceptible than others to stress fractures. Place an ice pack on the injury as soon as possible. If the pain is so severe that it is difficult to walk, see your doctor. A stress fracture usually heals on its own if you temporarily switch to a different activity. Always wear shoes that have good cushioning.

Achilles tendinitis When you injure your Achilles tendon (the tendon that runs along the back of your leg from your calf muscle into your heel), you might feel pain anywhere along the tendon. It usually hurts most when you first get up in the morning or when you start to exercise. If your Achilles tendon is injured, stop the activity that caused it. Use RICE (see above) to treat the injury. If the pain is severe or you cannot walk, see your doctor immediately. When the injury starts to heal, strengthen the tendon with exercises such as rising up on your toes from a standing position several times every day. Stretching before you exercise can help prevent an injury to your Achilles tendon.

Hamstring pull You can pull or tear your hamstring (the large muscle in the back of your thigh) with a sudden motion such as sprinting or leaping, or with a gradual pull during a long distance run or walk. RICE (see above) is the best treatment for a hamstring pull. Rest the muscle and, when it begins to heal, do strengthening exercises. Lie facedown on the floor and flex your leg at the knee. Repeat with the other leg (it may help

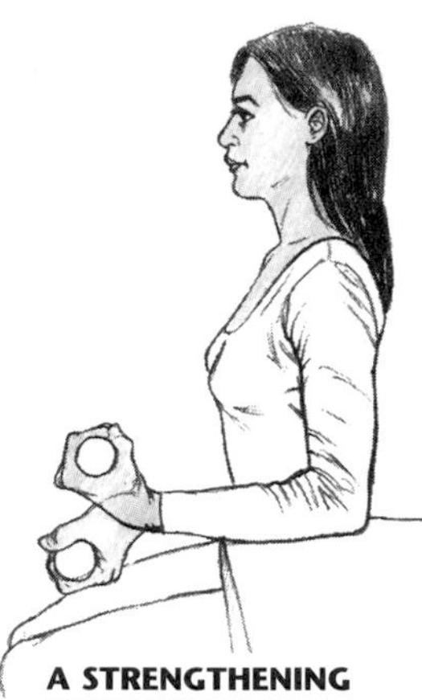

A STRENGTHENING EXERCISE TO PREVENT TENNIS ELBOW
1. While sitting or standing, lay your arm on a table next to you, palm facing down, wrist and hand hanging over the side. Hold a 1-pound weight in your hand and slowly raise it and lower it by bending and straightening your wrist. Stop if you feel any pain. Raise and lower the weight 10 times. Rest and then repeat the set two more times.
2. Turn your hand over so your palm is facing up. Repeat the exercise, lifting the weight up and down 10 times. Rest, repeat the set two more times.
3. As the exercises get easier, increase the weight to 2 pounds.

How to avoid injury during exercise

By taking these few precautions, and listening to your body, you can help protect yourself from injury during exercise:

- Wear well-cushioned athletic shoes and socks.
- Warm up. Begin your exercise program at an easy, undemanding pace. Do stretching exercises (see page 87).
- Build up gradually. Increase your distance or pace by no more than 10 percent a week.
- Alternate. Go easy and then hard. Work out intensely one day and more easily the next to give your body a chance to recover. Or exercise one day and skip the next.
- Listen to your body. If it hurts, stop doing it.
- Vary your program. Don't stop exercising altogether if something hurts—switch to a different activity that doesn't cause pain.
- If you are engaged in an activity, such as tennis, that requires twisting and turning, try to avoid jerky or sudden twisting motions.
- Protect your bones. Avoid exercising on hard surfaces. If you are an older woman with the bone-thinning disorder osteoporosis, you are at risk of fractures. Choose activities such as walking or water aerobics that are less likely to result in falls. Walk at a mall during the winter when the sidewalks are icy.

prevent a hamstring pull in that leg). Do a few repetitions every day.

Lower back pain Lower back pain is a common and chronic problem. It can be caused and worsened by many different factors, including exercise, lifting heavy objects, and pregnancy. If the pain is intense, see your doctor. He or she can rule out a serious condition such as a herniated disc or a broken bone in your back. Rest can help relieve the pain.

Once the pain has subsided, ask your doctor what you can do to avoid lower back pain in the future. The following measures can be helpful:

- Do abdominal muscle-strengthening exercises, such as sit-ups, regularly; strong abdominal muscles help support your lower back.
- Do not stand in a swayback position—it puts pressure on your lower back. For an illustration of proper posture, see page 88.
- Squat to pick up objects off the floor; do not bend at your waist.
- Avoid wearing high heels.
- When you drive a car, make sure that the back of the seat is not inclined too far back.
- Sit in chairs with a back support and arm rests.
- Ask your doctor or exercise instructor how to avoid straining your back during exercise.

Tennis elbow Tennis elbow is tearing of the tendons of your forearm at the place where they attach at your elbow. You can get tennis elbow from bowling, pitching a softball, opening a jar, or pulling on a stuck door, as well as from playing tennis. The injury makes it painful to move your wrist. If you have pain in your elbow, see your doctor to rule out joint damage, a pinched nerve, or a torn ligament. If you have tennis elbow, stop the activity that caused it. Doing exercises (see illustration upper left) regularly to strengthen the tendons of your forearm can help you avoid tennis elbow.

CHAPTER 3

Body weight

Contents

Millions of American women who are a normal, healthy weight think they should be thinner. On the other hand, many women are carrying excess weight that is jeopardizing their health, and they need help losing it. The information in the following pages will help you evaluate your weight and determine whether it is healthy for you (based on your body frame and height) or threatening to your health.

If your weight is within the healthy range for your height and body frame (see page 99), and you still want to lose weight to improve your appearance, it is best to set modest goals. Aim for a long-term, slow weight loss based on a balanced, nutritious diet and regular exercise. This approach will make it easier for you to keep the weight off.

Are you overweight?

Determining if you are overweight is more complicated than merely standing on a scale. The amount you weigh is not as important as the proportion of your body that is made up of fat—something a scale can't tell you. The way in which fat is distributed on your body may be an important factor in determining your health risks. For example, people who gain excess fat in their upper body, particularly in the abdominal area, are at a greater risk of heart disease, stroke, and type II diabetes than are people who gain weight mainly in their hips and thighs.

BODY COMPOSITION

The best measure of the healthiness of your weight is not only how much you weigh, but also the percentage of your body that is made up of fat. The health risks associated with obesity come not only from being overweight but from being overly fat.

Women have more body fat naturally than men. The female hormone estrogen causes you to add fat, particularly in your hips and thighs, beginning at puberty.

Your body composition is the proportion of lean tissue to fatty tissue. Lean tissue is made up mostly of muscle and bone. Your body composition is partially determined by your genetic makeup. We are each predisposed to have a fat range that is normal for us, but it is difficult to determine exactly what that level is for any one person. It is also difficult to precisely measure body fat percentage. The various ways of measuring it require skill and technical training to perform accurately. For this reason, you may best judge how much fat you have on your body by considering your level of activity. The more active you are, the less your percentage of body fat is likely to be.

BODY MASS INDEX

Because of the difficulty in evaluating percentage of body fat, it is more practical for people to refer to established tables to determine the relative healthiness of their weight. Because these tables are based on information most of us already know—our height and weight—they are easy to read. One such table is the body mass index (BMI), which gives a score that indicates the healthiness of a person's weight.

Although the BMI does not indicate body fat percentage itself, for most people it has a correlation with the amount of fat they carry. The exceptions are people, such as football players and body builders, whose BMI is high but whose bodies are obviously mostly muscle. For most people, the BMI is an indication of their risk of health problems that are related to being overweight. Even being moderately overweight—by 5 or 10 pounds—can increase your risk of developing heart disease, high blood pressure, and type II diabetes.

Determine your BMI from the chart on the facing page. You are at lowest risk of heart disease if your BMI is between 18 and 21. Most people exceed this. If your BMI is between 22 and 25, you are moderately overweight and should try to shed those extra pounds. A BMI over 27 indicates obesity. If your BMI is 25 or over, see your doctor. Together, you and your doctor can design a weight-loss and exercise program that will help you reach a healthier weight and maintain it.

Body mass index

To determine your body mass index (BMI) on the chart below, find your height in the left-hand column and read across the row to your weight; the number at the top of that column is your BMI.

	BODY MASS INDEX (kilograms per square meter)													
	19	20	21	22	23	24	25	26	27	28	29	30	35	40
HEIGHT	BODY WEIGHT (pounds)													
4′10″	91	96	100	105	110	115	119	124	129	134	139	143	167	191
4′11″	94	99	104	109	114	119	124	129	133	138	143	148	173	198
5′	97	102	107	112	118	123	128	133	138	143	148	153	179	204
5′1″	100	106	111	116	122	127	132	137	143	148	153	158	185	211
5′2″	104	109	115	120	126	131	136	142	147	153	158	164	191	218
5′3″	107	113	118	124	130	135	141	147	152	158	163	169	197	225
5′4″	111	116	122	128	134	140	145	151	157	163	169	174	204	233
5′5″	114	120	126	132	138	144	150	156	162	168	174	180	210	240
5′6″	118	124	130	136	142	148	155	161	167	173	179	186	216	247
5′7″	121	127	134	140	147	153	159	166	172	178	185	191	223	255
5′8″	125	131	138	144	151	158	164	171	177	184	190	197	230	263
5′9″	128	135	142	149	155	162	169	176	183	189	196	203	237	270
5′10″	132	139	146	153	160	167	174	181	188	195	202	209	243	278

WAIST-TO-HIP RATIO

Are you shaped like an apple or a pear? Do you gain weight around your waist or add pounds to your hips and thighs? If you tend to store fat around your waist and abdomen (an apple shape), you may be at higher risk of heart disease, diabetes, or cancer than a woman who weighs the same amount but carries most of her weight in her hips and thighs (giving her a pear shape). Fat distribution—determined by a person's waist-to-hip ratio—is an important indicator of health risk. Waist-to-hip ratio may predict health risks even better than your body mass index, especially if you are past menopause.

Younger women have a waist-to-hip advantage over men and older women. Before menopause, most women gain weight in their hips and thighs. After menopause, however, women begin to add fat around their waists, as most men do at all ages.

Apple-shaped people tend to have higher levels of low-density lipoprotein

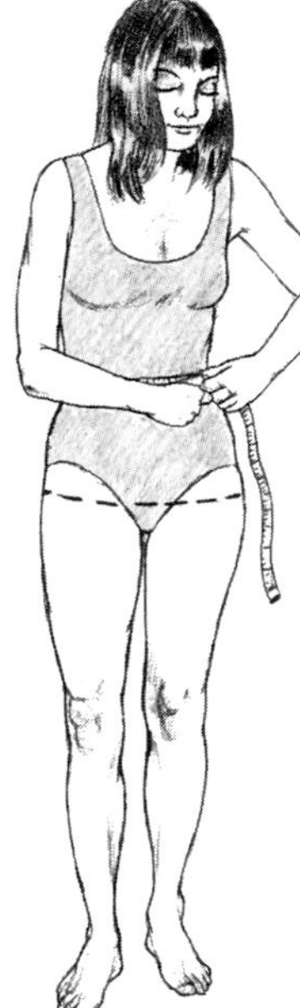

MEASURING YOUR WAIST-TO-HIP RATIO

To determine your waist-to-hip ratio, first measure around your waist at the narrowest part, keeping your stomach muscles relaxed. Next, measure around your hips or buttocks at the widest part. Divide your waist measurement by your hip measurement. If the number you get is higher than 0.80, you may be at increased risk of heart disease, type II diabetes, high blood pressure, or some cancers. You can significantly reduce those risks by losing weight and exercising regularly.

(LDL) cholesterol, the harmful cholesterol that raises the risk of heart disease. LDL cholesterol causes fatty deposits called plaque to build up in artery walls

By contrast, people who store fat in the lower part of their bodies—pear-shaped people—have higher levels of heart-protecting high-density lipoprotein (HDL) cholesterol. HDL cholesterol cleanses the arteries of fat. Women who have apple-shaped bodies are at increased risk of developing type II diabetes (see page 621). However, exercise and weight loss can help reverse the process and prevent a person from developing diabetes.

Genetics plays an important role in determining where fat collects on your body. But, with weight loss and regular exercise, you can limit or reduce the amount of fat that accumulates on your body. If you have an apple shape, you may be able to reduce your health risks by shedding as few as 12 pounds. Drinking alcohol only in moderation and avoiding cigarette smoking—both of which increase fat accumulation in the abdominal area—can also reduce those risks. The one advantage apple-shaped women have over their pear-shaped counterparts is that it is easier to lose fat from the abdomen than from the hips or thighs.

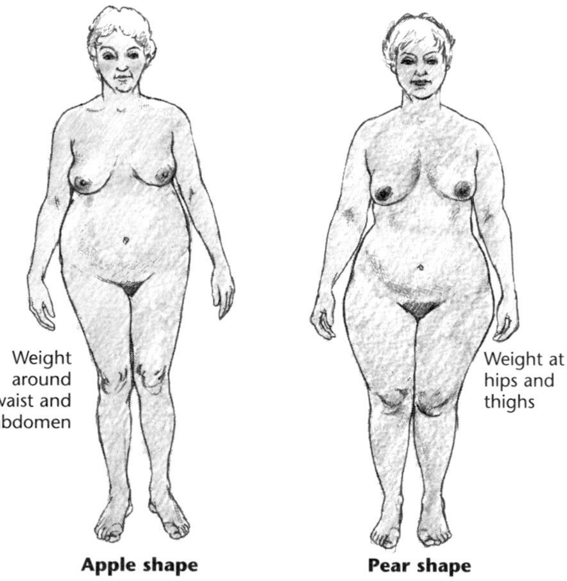

ARE YOU SHAPED LIKE AN APPLE OR A PEAR?
If fat tends to accumulate around your waist and abdomen, you have an apple shape. If you accumulate fat in your hips and thighs, you have a pear shape. People with an apple-shaped body are at increased risk of heart disease, type II diabetes, high blood pressure, and some forms of cancer.

CHECKING YOUR WEIGHT

Gaining even 10 pounds during early and middle adulthood may significantly increase your risk of heart disease. If you have a family or personal history of diseases that are related to excess weight—such as type II diabetes, heart disease, or colon cancer—you should try especially hard to keep your weight in the healthy range for your body frame and height, as shown in the chart on page 99.

However, it is not a good idea to get obsessive about your weight or try to reach a weight that is unrealistically low for your height and frame. Here are some tips for keeping track of your weight:

- Weigh yourself at about the same time of day each time.
- Do not wear shoes or clothes when you weigh yourself.
- Keep your scale on a level surface.
- Periodically check the accuracy of your scale; home scales can be imprecise or lose their accuracy over time.

Eating salty foods, such as processed foods, can make you retain water, which may show up on the scale as an additional pound or two. Some women's weight may fluctuate normally by 2 to 3 pounds during their menstrual cycle, in the week or so before their period. This is normal.

Healthy weights for women

Find your ideal weight in the chart below. A variety of charts give broader weight ranges. However, many doctors believe that the lower weight ranges shown in this table are the healthiest for most people.

Note: All height figures are without shoes; all weight figures are without clothing. Most people have a medium frame.

HEIGHT	BODY WEIGHT (pounds)		
	SMALL FRAME	MEDIUM FRAME	LARGE FRAME
5′	98-106	103-115	111-127
5′1″	101-109	106-118	114-130
5′2″	104-112	109-122	117-134
5′3″	107-115	112-126	121-138
5′4″	110-119	116-131	125-142
5′5″	114-123	120-135	129-146
5′6″	118-127	124-139	133-150
5′7″	122-131	128-143	137-154
5′8″	126-136	132-147	141-159
5′9″	130-140	136-151	145-164
5′10″	134-144	140-155	149-169

DO YOU NEED TO LOSE WEIGHT?

Considering the various measures of weight together can help you determine if your current weight is healthy.

Determining your frame size To determine your frame size have a ruler or measuring tape handy. Hold one of your arms out in front of you and bend it up at the elbow at a 90-degree angle with the palm of your hand facing you. Place the thumb and forefinger of your other hand on the two prominent bones on either side of the bent elbow. Keeping your fingers the same width apart, place them over the ruler and measure the space between them. Look at the chart below right, which shows elbow widths of women of different heights who have a *medium frame*. If the measurement of your elbow is greater than that listed for your height, you have a large frame; if it is less than that listed here, you have a small frame.

- Know your risk factors. If you have a personal history or a family history of heart disease, type II diabetes, high blood pressure, high cholesterol level, or cancer, all of which are linked to excess weight, maintaining a healthy weight is especially important for you.
- Know your body mass index (BMI). You can find it on the chart on page 97. If your BMI exceeds 27, you are at increased risk of the health problems mentioned above.
- Find your waist-to-hip ratio (see page 97). If it is higher than 0.80, your health risks are increased.
- Check your weight on the table above. Consider losing weight if your weight exceeds the limit for your height and frame size.

If you find you are in a healthy range on all of the above points, you do not need to lose weight.

Medium frame size

HEIGHT	ELBOW WIDTH
4′10″-4′11″	2¼″-2½″
5′-5′3″	2¼″-2½″
5′4″-5′7″	2⅜″-2⅝″
5′8″-5′11″	2⅜″-2⅝″

How your body changes with age

Wide variations from these examples are still considered normal.

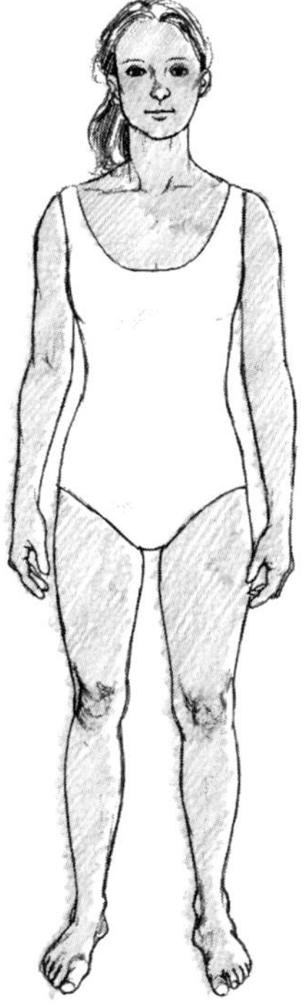

AGE: 12-24
Height: 5′5″
Weight: 126 pounds
BMI*: 21

The hormonal changes and growth spurt (increase in height) during puberty cause girls to gain from 20 to 30 pounds during their teenage years. This weight gain is normal for a girl who is within the healthy weight range for her height and frame size (see page 99). For all girls, but especially for those whose weight exceeds the healthy range, adolescence is a good time to develop a pattern of nutritious eating and regular exercise. A young woman at this age is adding both fat and muscle.

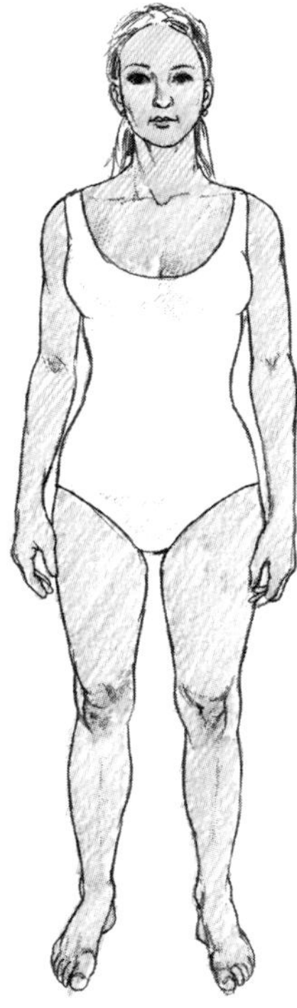

AGE: 25-34
Height: 5′5″
Weight: 136 pounds
BMI: 22

Many women gain weight during these years, mostly in their hips and thighs, usually because they become less active, often sitting at desk jobs all day. Some women retain extra weight after pregnancy. These years are a good time to improve your diet by eating less fat and more fruits, vegetables, and whole grains. Maintain the exercise program you started when you were younger. If you have not been active before, start exercising regularly now and plan to make it a habit for the rest of your life.

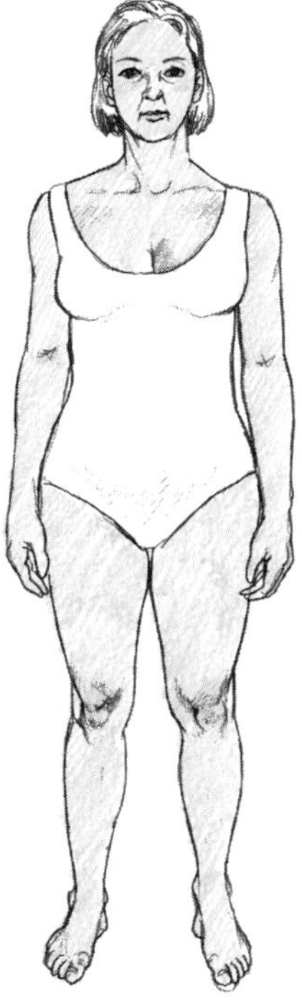

AGE: 35-44
Height: 5′5″
Weight: 138 pounds
BMI: 23

At this age, the proportion of lean body tissue (muscle and bone) on your body will decrease and the proportion of fat will increase. The rate at which you burn calories begins to slow, so eating and exercising the same amount as before can cause you to gain weight. Even a modest weight gain of 5 to 10 pounds can increase your risk of health problems. Make a conscious effort to maintain a healthy weight by raising your level of activity and eating fewer calories and less fat each day.

*BMI = body mass index, a figure based on height and weight used to determine the healthiness of a person's body composition. For women, a BMI below 25 is considered healthy (see page 97).

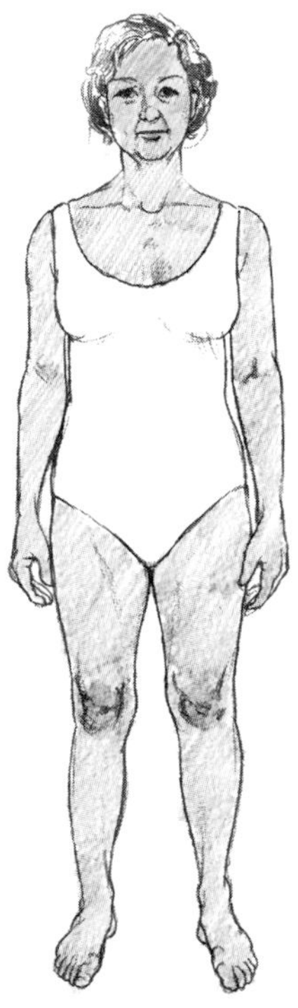

AGE: 45-54
Height: 5'5"
Weight: 144 pounds
BMI: 24

At menopause, your body stops producing the hormone estrogen, which causes fat to be redistributed to your abdominal area. Many women need about 50 fewer calories a day at age 50 than they did at 40. The drop in estrogen production at menopause sharply increases your risk of heart disease. Talk to your doctor about taking estrogen. A gain in weight can also increase the risk of heart disease. Try to maintain a healthy weight. Continue exercising, making sure to include strengthening exercises (such as weight-lifting) to maintain strength in your muscles and bones and help prevent osteoporosis. Strength-building exercises can also help reduce your risk of type II diabetes.

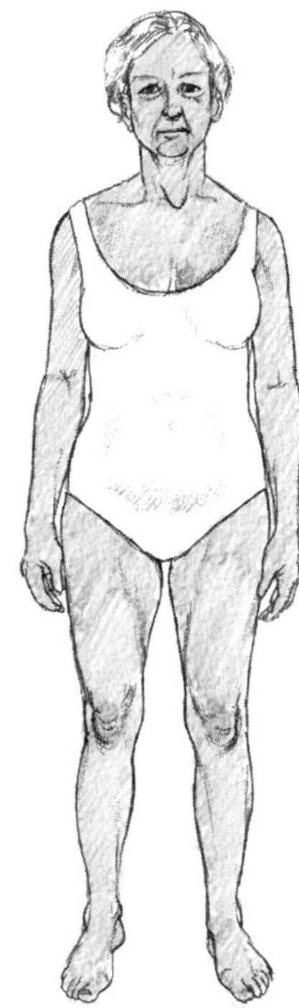

AGE: 55-64
Height: 5'5"
Weight: 146 pounds
BMI: 24

Weight gain usually slows during this decade of life. Risk of heart attack increases. You may carry excess weight, particularly in your abdominal area, which increases your risk of heart disease, type II diabetes, and high blood pressure (a major risk factor for heart disease and stroke). Concentrate on eating a high-fiber, low-fat diet. Exercise is critical at this age to prevent many age-related disorders, including osteoporosis. Take a walk every day, do strength-building exercises, and continue the activities (such as swimming, biking, and tennis) that you have always enjoyed. Talk to your doctor about taking estrogen to reduce your risk of heart disease and osteoporosis.

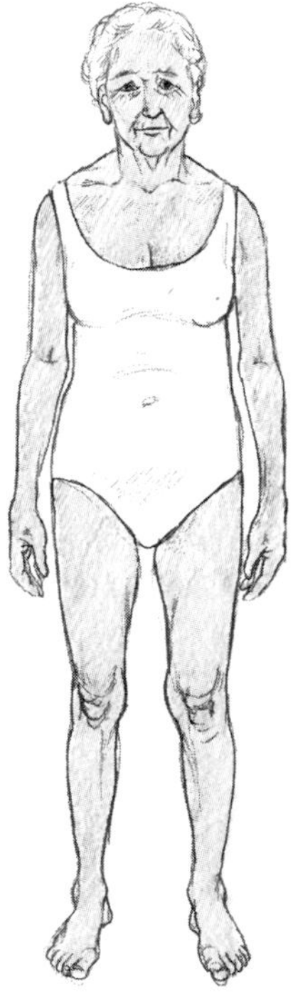

AGE: 65 AND OLDER
Height: 5'4"
Weight: 140 pounds
BMI: 24

You will probably lose a few pounds as you get older. Your appetite may diminish and you may not be eating enough to get all the nutrients your body needs. You will continue to lose strength in your muscles and, unless you are taking estrogen, your bone density will continue to decrease. It is a good idea to take a multivitamin/mineral supplement in addition to a calcium supplement (which helps keep your bones strong) to help ensure that you get all the essential nutrients. Exercise is critical for helping you maintain strength in your muscles and bones. Weight-bearing exercise, such as walking, and strengthening exercises, such as weight lifting, are especially beneficial.

Influences on your weight

CALORIE IMBALANCE

Eating more calories than you burn each day is the primary cause of weight gain. When the number of calories you eat equals the number of calories you burn (see illustration at right), your weight stays the same. Even a small increase in calorie consumption without a corresponding increase in activity, or calories burned, will result in a gradual weight gain (see illustration at far right).

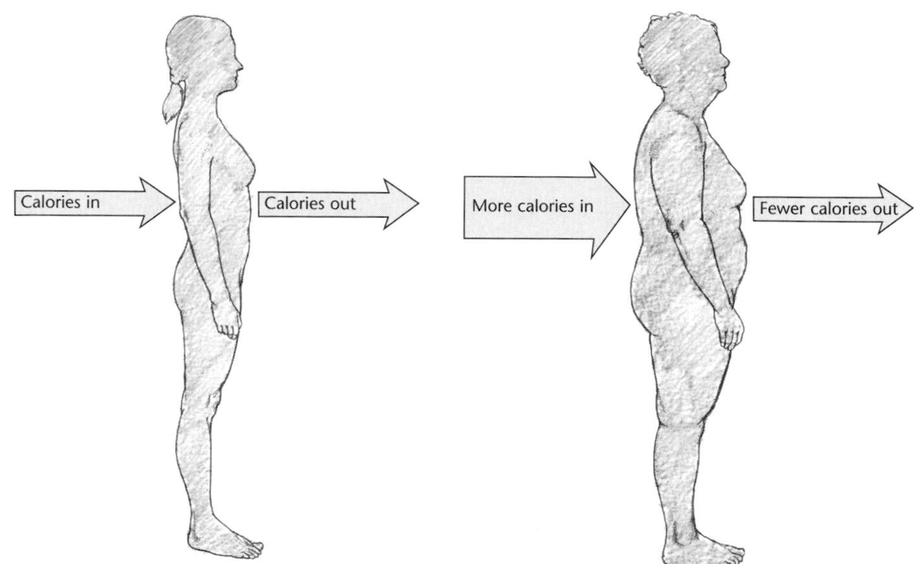

In simple terms, you gain weight when you eat more calories than your body uses. These extra calories are stored as fat. Even a small daily excess of calories can lead to substantial weight gain over months or years.

In spite of our society's obsession with thinness, most Americans are overeating and underexercising and, as a result, becoming overweight. Americans burn up far fewer calories in physical exercise today than they did in 1900. Most jobs do not require physical labor. In addition, we are getting more of our calories from fat. High-fat foods contain more than twice the calories of foods that are high in carbohydrates and proteins. Many people eat processed foods and fast foods, which are convenient but most are loaded with fat and calories.

Given these circumstances, why are some people able to maintain a normal weight while others keep gaining? Your weight is influenced by the complex interaction of a number of factors, including your genetic makeup, eating habits, level of physical activity, metabolism, and hormones.

YOUR GENES

Studies of adopted children have shown that their weight more closely resembles the weight of their biological parents than that of their adoptive parents. This observation suggests that genes have a stronger influence than family environment on a person's weight. Other evidence showing that genes exert a significant influence on body weight comes from observations of identical twins. Twins tend to gain weight at approximately the same rate and the weight is distributed on their bodies in the same way, whether or not they are raised in the same home.

Some people who have a tendency to gain weight may have inherited traits, such as a slow metabolism, that cause them to accumulate fat more easily than other people.

APPETITE REGULATION

Your brain has a short-term and a long-term way of knowing when to eat and when your body has had enough. The short-term response is the craving you have when you see or smell something tasty to eat. Whether you choose to eat or not and how much you eat depend on the response of the hypothalamus, an area in your brain that is stimulated when the stomach is full or empty. Fat cells release a chemical called a satiety factor, which tells your brain that you are full and should stop eating. Some people inherit a deficiency of the satiety factor and, therefore, lack the control mechanism that tells them when to stop eating.

The hypothalamus also regulates your body's long-term eating controls. It stimulates you to eat until you accumulate a certain amount of body fat. However, your thinking brain can override those controls. You can decide not to eat even when you are hungry or to eat when your body tells you not to. Compulsive overeaters tend to override their body's signals because of an emotional rather than physical need to eat.

METABOLISM

You burn most of your calories every day doing nothing. Your body's normal processes—such as breathing, pumping blood, and digesting food—burn most of those calories to provide you with energy. The rate at which you burn calories while at rest is called your resting metabolic rate. A person with a slow metabolism burns fewer calories at rest than a person with a fast metabolic rate. Some overweight people have a slower metabolic rate than people of normal weight, giving them a tendency to gain weight. Metabolic rate appears to be inherited, which may help explain why obesity tends to run in families.

You can increase your metabolic rate with exercise. Exercise helps speed up metabolism by building muscle. Muscle burns more calories than fat; therefore, the more muscle you have, the higher your metabolic rate.

LEVEL OF PHYSICAL ACTIVITY

The increase in obesity in the US may at least partly result from a decrease in physical activity. Changes in the work force from farms and factories to offices have made people much less active. Appliances and new technologies in the home have further curtailed the amount of energy we expend every day.

You will gain weight if you stop exercising without reducing your calorie consumption at the same time. You need to carefully balance your food intake with your current reduced level of physical activity to maintain the same weight.

As you age, staying active can help prevent your metabolism from slowing down. Alternating between aerobic exercises, such as walking or jogging, and strengthening exercises, such as lifting weights and doing push-ups, is an excellent way to control your weight. Exercise can also help you maintain strength in your muscles and bones and reduce your risk of illness as you get older.

CALORIE INTAKE

All people gain weight when they eat too many calories for their level of activity. Many of us underestimate the amount of food we eat. Keeping a journal is one way to keep track of that handful of tortilla chips and the last bite of your child's grilled-cheese sandwich. Try writing down everything you eat every day for 1 week. Add up the calories at the end of each day. You may be surprised to find how much you are eating. A rule of thumb: women need 12 to 15 calories a day for every pound they weigh to maintain their weight. The older you are and the less active you are, the fewer calories you need—closer to 12 per pound.

HORMONE IMBALANCE

In some cases, obesity results when a person's body makes too little or too much of a particular hormone. For example, a deficiency of thyroid hormone (a condition called hypothyroidism, see page 624) can cause obesity. Thyroid hormone is manufactured in the thyroid gland and released into the bloodstream. Thyroid hormone regulates your metabolic rate. A deficiency of the hormone lowers your metabolic rate, which can cause fatigue. A reduced metabolic rate, combined with a reduction in physical activity caused by the fatigue, leads to a buildup of fat. Other signs of hypothyroidism include weight gain, irregular periods (either skipped or lengthened), constipation, and fluid retention. A blood test at your doctor's office can determine if you have a deficiency of thyroid hormone, which can be treated by taking the hormone in pill form.

SYMPTOM CHART

Overweight

If you weigh more than the ideal weight for your height (see page 99), you are overweight and may be endangering your health.

START

Have you been overweight most of your life?

YES → Are both of your parents overweight?

YES → A tendency toward being overweight can run in families. See Influences on your weight, page 102. See also Obesity and its effects on health, page 110.

NO → You are probably overweight because you eat more calories than your body burns. See Changing your diet, page 107, and Getting more exercise, page 108.

NO → Did you recently quit smoking?

YES → Many people gain weight when they quit smoking, usually because they overeat. See How to quit, page 157.

NO → Did you gain an excessive amount of weight during a pregnancy or are you planning a pregnancy and are concerned about gaining too much weight?

YES → Many women gain too much weight during pregnancy and have difficulty losing it after the baby is born. See Losing weight, page 106, and Starting an exercise program, page 78. See also Nutrition and weight gain during pregnancy, page 408.

NO → Did you put on weight at a time when you were depressed?

YES → Many people overeat when they are depressed or gain weight when they take some antidepressant medications. Talk to your doctor. See Depression, page 594.

NO → continued on next page

Maintain a healthy weight

Being even moderately overweight can affect your health. Excess weight can alter your metabolism—your body's ability to burn calories and use them for energy. This alteration can cause your body to work harder and less efficiently, increasing your risk of high blood pressure, type II diabetes, and heart disease.

continued from previous page

Did you gain weight after a change in your lifestyle, such as switching from an active job to a sedentary one?

YES → Make a conscious effort to exercise more and eat more healthful foods. See Losing weight, page 106, and Starting an exercise program, page 78.

NO ↓

Have you noticed any of the following symptoms since you began to put on weight?

- Feeling cold more than you used to
- Thinning or brittle hair
- Dry skin

YES → *Call your doctor.* You may have an underactive thyroid gland, which slows the rate at which your body burns calories. See Hypothyroidism, page 624.

NO ↓

Have you been taking corticosteroid drugs for a problem such as asthma or rheumatoid arthritis?

YES → Corticosteroids can cause weight gain. Talk to your doctor; he or she may be able to change your prescription.

NO ↓

Are you over 40?

YES → People often gain weight as they age because they are exercising less and eating more food than their body needs.

NO ↓

Have you gained weight suddenly, for no apparent reason?

YES → *Call your doctor.* A sudden, unexplained weight gain can be a sign of a serious disorder.

NO ↓

If you are unable to make a diagnosis from this chart, talk to your doctor.

Tips for losing weight:

- Eat fewer calories.
- Exercise more.
- Reduce the fat in your diet.
- Eat more fruits, vegetables, and whole grains.

Losing weight

Although many women are dieting unnecessarily, many others are carrying excess weight that is a serious threat to their health. For them, losing weight is essential. If you are overweight and want to lose weight, your efforts are more likely to be successful if you follow the weight reduction and maintenance methods that are most appropriate for you and your lifestyle.

All successful weight-loss programs have the same premise, whether they say so or not: You must burn more calories than you eat if you want to lose weight. You can do this by eating fewer calories or by increasing your level of activity or, most effectively, by doing both.

Reducing the proportion of fat in your diet, and increasing the proportion of low-fat, high-fiber foods such as fruits, vegetables, and whole grains, can be an important part of losing weight. The calories you get from fat are more likely to be stored as fat on your body. Because carbohydrate calories require more energy to burn, they are less likely to be stored as fat.

The problem with almost all weight-loss programs is that, for a large percentage of people, the weight returns after they finish the program. Most of the good programs now focus on ways to help people keep the weight off in the long term. The slower you lose weight, the more likely you are to keep it off.

People who are the most successful in keeping lost weight off are usually those who design their own program of diet and exercise. Instead of thinking of your diet as a short-term program to lose weight, consider it a lifetime habit of nutritious eating. The four most commonly used methods for losing weight—change in diet, exercise, behavior modification, and drug treatment—are often done in combination.

AVOIDING YO-YO DIETING

Nine out of 10 dieters gain back most or all of their lost weight within 5 years. Many regain it faster than they lost it. In the process of losing and regaining weight, dieters are programming their body to do exactly what they don't want it to do—store fat. Fluctuating up and down in weight, or yo-yo dieting, may also increase your risk of heart disease.

Severely restricting the number of calories you eat each day may help you lose weight faster than a more moderate approach, but it can also make it harder for you to keep the weight off. Fasting (defined as eating fewer calories than your body needs at rest) causes your metabolism to slow down.

The drop in metabolic rate produces a frustrating plateau in weight loss midway through a diet. Once you return to your normal diet, your reduced metabolic rate will make you put on weight even faster than you would have before you started the diet. Each time you go on a diet, your metabolic rate may drop even more quickly and lower than it did the last time, making it even more difficult for you to lose weight.

Severe or prolonged fasting can cause your resting metabolic rate (your body's need for calories when at rest) to drop to as low as 500 calories a day. At that rate, you are not burning enough calories to keep warm, even in summer. Other side effects of a severely reduced metabolic rate can include fatigue, dry skin and hair, constipation, and depression.

A healthy weight-loss program

The average woman consumes between 1,900 and 2,200 calories a day. Very active women can eat more than inactive women to maintain their weight and can usually lose weight faster. It is easiest to lose weight with a combination of exercise and diet. If you have been very inactive, build up gradually (see page 78).

To eliminate calories, reduce the amount of fat in your diet. Switch to nonfat salad dressings and avoid commercially prepared baked goods such as muffins, cookies, and croissants. Eat smaller portions of meat. Eat more vegetables, fruits, and whole grains, which will make you feel full. For healthy weight loss, it is better to exercise more than to eliminate so many calories that you are not getting enough of the nutrients your body needs.

Slow weight reduction is best because you are more likely to stick with it and keep the weight off permanently. Make eating a low-fat diet and exercising habits you will follow for the rest of your life. If you return to your former eating habits and lack of activity, you will quickly regain the weight.

Besides decreasing your ability to lose weight, yo-yo dieting may be bad for your heart. People who repeatedly gain and lose weight have a higher risk of heart disease than those who maintain a more stable weight, even if that stable weight is higher than normal. The larger the amount of weight you lose and regain, the greater your risk of heart disease and death from all causes.

The health risks associated with losing and regaining large amounts of weight underscore the importance of maintaining a healthy weight once you reach it. The most reasonable course is a slow, long-term weight loss based on a nutritious, balanced, low-fat diet and regular exercise, followed by a lifetime weight maintenance program. If your thighs are a little thicker than you would like them to be, exercising to improve muscle tone may do more for your appearance than trying to lose too much weight. Exercise provides many health benefits as well.

CHANGING YOUR DIET

Changing their diet is the most common and most successful weight-loss strategy people use. The methods range from a simple reduction of calories and fat to a new eating pattern. Eating small amounts of food throughout the day is a better way to control your weight than eating one large meal at the end of the day. The most effective strategy for losing weight is to reduce the calories and fat in your diet and increase your activity.

Proponents of some diets claim that eating certain foods or food combinations will burn fat more efficiently. When people lose weight on these diets, it is because they are reducing calories, not because of a particular combination of foods.

Dieting without exercising is a slow process with a high potential for failure. Most people who diet without exercising gain two thirds of the lost weight back within 1 year and almost all of the weight within 5 years.

Diets that rely on calorie restriction are referred to as low-calorie diets and very low–calorie diets. Low-calorie diets are about 1,000 to 1,500 calories a day and

Losing weight by counting fat grams

When you are trying to lose weight, counting fat grams is sometimes easier than counting calories. When you eliminate fat from your diet, you are often reducing calories at the same time. Here are some steps to take to help you reach your desired weight:

- Estimate your daily calorie limit by multiplying the weight you want to reach by from 12 to 15 calories, depending on your level of activity. For example, if you are inactive and you want to weigh 140, multiply 140 by 12 to get your total daily calories (140 X 12 = 1,680). If you are very active, you can consume more calories and still reach your weight-loss goal (140 X 15 = 2,100).
- Decide whether you want to limit your fat intake to 20 percent, 25 percent, or 30 percent of your total daily calories.
- Check the chart at right to find your daily limit of fat grams based on your calorie intake. If you weigh 140 and are inactive, you should limit fat grams to less than 53 per day. If you are active, eat fewer than 69 fat grams per day.
- Read food labels and your nutrient counter to determine both fat grams and calories in the foods you eat.

Daily fat gram limit

	FAT ALLOWANCE (as percent of calories)		
TOTAL CALORIES	20%	25%	30%
1,200	26	33	40
1,400	31	38	46
1,600	35	44	53
1,800	40	50	60
2,000	44	55	66
2,200	48	61	73
2,400	53	66	80

often include some form of structured commercial program and prepackaged food products. At 800 calories a day, very low–calorie diets are usually conducted under a doctor's supervision and are recommended only for people who are dangerously overweight. This type of diet often relies on a liquid formula drink. Because very low–calorie diets can cause serious health problems, you should never follow such a calorie-restricted diet except under a doctor's supervision.

You can improve your eating habits in some basic ways to help control your calorie consumption and your body's tendency to store fat.

- Eat only when you're hungry.
- Stop eating when you're full.
- Eat three meals every day and healthy snacks in between. You are less likely to gain weight eating several small meals than one or two large ones.
- Don't skip meals. Going for long periods without food can lower your body's metabolic rate and slow the rate at which you burn calories. Eating a sensible breakfast sparks your metabolism and helps you burn calories more efficiently throughout the day.
- Avoid alcohol. Ounce for ounce, alcohol contains almost as many calories as fat does and alcohol provides no essential nutrients.
- Get most of your calories from starchy foods—complex carbohydrates—such as grains, breads, pasta, and potatoes. Carbohydrate-rich foods are broken down by your body more slowly than other foods and are less likely to be stored as fat.
- Watch your appetite when dining with friends and family. People tend to eat more when they are eating with others than they do when eating alone.

GETTING MORE EXERCISE

Exercise is an essential part of any weight-loss program and is critical for helping you maintain a healthy weight. Exercise without dieting is not as effective in helping you lose weight as dieting without exercise. It takes a lot of exercise to burn enough calories to shed pounds. But combining regular exercise with a calorie-restricted diet can increase the number of pounds you drop and shorten

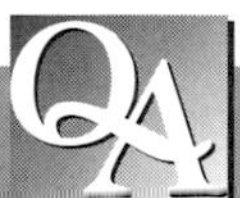

QUESTIONS WOMEN ASK
EXERCISE AND WEIGHT LOSS

Q I've been doing sit-ups to reduce my waistline and leg lifts to make my thighs smaller, but I haven't seen much improvement. Why not?

A These exercises are good for toning your muscles, but they will not reduce fat in those areas. Spot reduction of fat on specific parts of the body is not possible. To see improvement in any one area of your body, you need to reduce your weight and overall body fat by doing aerobic exercises such as brisk walking, biking, or swimming.

Q If I lift weights, will my muscles get large like a man's?

A No. Male hormones make a man's muscles large. Because women have only small amounts of male hormones, it would be extremely difficult for you to build up your muscles that much. Lifting weights in a supervised program is an excellent way to maintain strength in both your muscles and bones.

Q I exercise more and eat less than my friend. Why is she thinner?

A In addition to diet and exercise, another factor that influences your weight is your metabolic rate (the rate at which your body burns calories), which is largely determined by your genes. If your friend really does eat more than you do and exercises less, she probably has a higher metabolic rate than you do—her body naturally burns more calories. Continue with your exercising.

the amount of time it takes to do so. An ideal goal is to lose 2 pounds per week.

Although exercise increases the body's metabolic rate only during the exercise period and shortly after, it may help prevent the drop in metabolic rate that often accompanies dieting. When metabolic rate slows, as it often does in dieters who skip meals, it takes the body longer to burn calories, which slows weight loss.

Exercise increases muscle strength. People who follow weight-loss regimens that emphasize calorie limitation and ignore exercise usually lose muscle. Your muscles are your body's furnace—they burn the calories you eat. The more muscle you have, the higher your metabolism and the faster and more efficiently your body burns calories.

Both aerobic exercise—such as brisk walking, jogging, and cycling—and strengthening exercises—such as weight lifting—are effective for helping you lose weight and keeping it off. Strengthening exercises are also good for building muscle. You can purchase a small set of hand weights to use at home (see page 84).

Besides helping you lose weight, exercise provides many important long-term health benefits. It reduces your cholesterol level, increases your cardiovascular fitness, and helps prevent some of the health problems associated with obesity—including heart disease, type II diabetes, high blood pressure, and some cancers. By keeping your bones strong, exercise also helps prevent the debilitating bone-thinning disorder osteoporosis.

CHANGING YOUR BEHAVIOR

Most supervised weight-loss programs include so-called behavior modification techniques that help you change the habits that led to your weight problem. In such a program, a counselor will review your pattern of eating and exercising, and help you set specific goals. The aim is usually to change poor eating patterns and, at the same time, increase your knowledge about good nutrition. The best eating pattern for weight control is to eat breakfast and distribute your calorie intake throughout the day. Most Americans skip breakfast, eat a small lunch, and consume a huge dinner—an eating pattern that is likely to promote weight gain.

The most successful behavior change programs are those based on realistic goals that combine calorie reduction and exercise for a slow and steady weight loss. Successful programs also help you learn to deal with situations in which you are likely to overeat, such as at times of emotional stress. You are taught to recognize triggers that make you snack—such as watching TV, clearing off the children's dinner plates, or talking on the phone.

When behavior modification is used alone (without calorie reduction or exercise), the program usually lasts about 18 weeks and a person loses an average of 1 to 1½ pounds per week. Most people gain back most of the weight within 5 years. Only a small percentage of people are able to maintain the weight loss for longer periods.

DIETING WITH DRUGS

For many people, the idea of a pill that can help them lose weight has immense appeal. But no magic pill exists. Even those drugs, both over-the-counter and prescription, that have been found to be effective in helping take weight off often produce side effects and do not help keep the weight off over the long term. Although prescription medication is usually provided only to people who have been diagnosed as clinically obese (20 percent or more overweight), over-the-counter pills are readily available and are often misused by people who take excessive amounts. Young women, particularly teenagers, are the most frequent abusers of over-the-counter diet aids.

Phenylpropanolamine Most over-the-counter appetite suppressants contain a chemical called phenylpropanolamine (PPA) that acts as a mild stimulant. PPA may help you lose weight for a short time, but it loses its effectiveness after about 8 to 12 weeks. In that time, you can develop a tolerance for the chemical so that it no longer stimulates your metabolism.

In high doses, PPA can cause anxiety, sleeplessness, headache, irregular heartbeat, convulsions, and circulation problems. If you have high blood pressure, heart disease, diabetes, or a thyroid condition, you should not use the drug without talking to your doctor.

Questions to ask about a weight-loss program

If you are considering joining an organized weight-loss program, make sure its goals are for long-term rather than quick weight loss. Evaluate the cost of the program and find out if a lower-cost program is available in your area. Call a local hospital, fitness center, or university for recommendations. Look for the following characteristics of a good program:

- A diet based on foods from all levels of the food pyramid (see page 44)
- A diet based on limiting fat consumption to less than 30 percent of total calories
- Emphasis on an eating pattern of regular, small meals and nutritious snacks throughout the day (rather than one large meal)
- Emphasis on developing eating and exercise habits that will last a lifetime
- A weight-loss goal of no more than 1 to 2 pounds a week
- Individualized attention to a person's eating and exercise patterns and health problems
- Education about the benefits of good nutrition, exercise, and behavior changes
- A good track record—the percentage of people in the program that lose weight, how much they lose, and how long they keep it off
- A weight-maintenance program a person can follow after the weight loss
- No advertisements with inflated claims or personal testimonials as evidence of overall success
- Weight-loss goals that do not depend on the purchase of a particular brand of expensive, packaged foods (by reading the nutrition labels on any packaged food before you make your choice, you can fit most foods into your program)
- Medical supervision or a health screening to detect possible health risks

Benzocaine An over-the-counter weight-loss aid called benzocaine temporarily deadens receptors on your tongue, which reduces your ability to taste, especially sugar. This effect can reduce a person's desire to eat. Benzocaine is often included in chewing gums and candies that are sold as appetite suppressants. However, doctors warn that the chemical is similar to cocaine and can be addictive.

Guar gum In 1990 the Food and Drug Administration (FDA) ruled that guar gum was neither safe nor effective as a nonprescription weight-loss aid. But it is sometimes marketed as a health food. If you see a food with a guar gum content of more than the 2 to 3 percent allowed as an additive, do not buy it. Guar gum can obstruct your esophagus (the tube leading from your mouth to your stomach).

Fenfluramine and phentermine Two prescription medications—fenfluramine and phentermine—when taken together over a period of several years have helped many obese people take excess weight off and keep it off. Fenfluramine increases the level of a chemical messenger in the brain called serotonin, which makes a person eat less and more slowly. Phentermine increases the levels of two other chemicals in the brain—dopamine and norepinephrine—that also make a person eat less. The side effects of all of these drugs can include dry mouth, diarrhea, and irritability. The effects of long-term use of these drugs for weight control are not yet known.

Obesity and its effects on health

Being seriously overweight can compromise your health and shorten your life. Overweight people—particularly those who were overweight during their young adult years—die earlier than people of average weight. Obesity (being 20 percent or more over your ideal weight) is a risk factor for 5 of the 10 leading causes of death in the US—heart disease, stroke, some types of cancer, type II diabetes, and atherosclerosis (buildup of fatty deposits inside arteries). Obesity also increases your risk of many other health problems, including gallstones, arthritis, and back pain.

Obesity works its adverse effects on the body over time. The sooner you take off the extra pounds with a slow, sensible weight-loss program (see page 106), the better for your health. It's much easier to lose 20 pounds than 50 and it's easier to keep the weight off over the long term if the weight loss is reasonable. To determine whether you are overweight to the extent that your health is in danger, see page 99.

DIABETES

More than three out of four people with type II diabetes (see page 621) are at least 15 percent over their ideal weight. Excess weight contributes to the development of diabetes by making cells more resistant to the effects of insulin. Insulin is a hormone that acts like a messenger in the body, telling muscle cells and fat cells that calories are on the way, and preparing them to absorb the calories. In an obese person, the fat cells are already packed with sugar (in the form of glucose) and fat and, therefore, do not respond to insulin's signal. As a result, sugar and fat remain in the bloodstream. The pancreas—the organ that secretes insulin into the bloodstream—reacts by increasing the amount of insulin it produces to overcome the cells' resistance. In people with diabetes, the pancreas cannot produce enough insulin to overcome this resistance and the level of sugar continues to rise in their blood.

Type II diabetes is more common among blacks, Native Americans, and Hispanics than whites. In all groups, the risk increases with age, being overweight, or having a family history of the disease. If you have any of these risk factors, ask your doctor if you should be tested (see page 623). For many people who are at risk of type II diabetes, exercising and regularly losing weight can prevent the onset of symptoms.

HIGH BLOOD PRESSURE

High blood pressure, or hypertension, is a major risk factor for heart disease and stroke. Blood pressure tends to increase with weight gain and with age. More than half of all women over age 55 and two thirds of women over 65 have high blood pressure.

It is not clear why obesity is a major cause of high blood pressure. It may be because blood needs to be under greater pressure to circulate through a larger body. Or it may be that a high level of insulin in the blood—which is common in people who are obese—causes a rise in blood pressure. If you have high blood pressure, losing weight may help you lower it. A weight loss of as little as 7 pounds can reduce blood pressure to a safe level in overweight people who have moderately high blood pressure.

UNHEALTHY CHOLESTEROL LEVELS

Obesity can raise your total cholesterol level and alter your cholesterol profile. Many women face a double risk as they age because both weight and cholesterol level tend to rise with advancing age. More than half of women 55 and older have elevated levels of cholesterol.

People who are overweight have lower levels of high-density lipoprotein (HDL) cholesterol, the protective cholesterol that reduces your risk of heart disease, and normal-to-high levels of the harmful cholesterol, low-density lipoprotein (LDL). These relative proportions of cholesterol types—low HDL and normal-to-high LDL—increase your risk of heart disease. Losing weight and exercising regularly can raise your level of heart-protecting HDL and reduce your level of damaging LDL, which can significantly reduce your risk of heart attack or stroke.

Obesity can also cause fat to build up in your liver, enlarging it. If you also drink an excessive amount of alcohol and eat a poorly balanced diet, fat buildup in your liver can lead to severe liver damage. (For more about cholesterol's role in disease, see page 131.)

HEART DISEASE

More than one third of cases of heart disease in women are linked to being overweight. The more overweight a woman is, the higher her risk of developing heart disease. Women who are more than 30 percent over a healthy weight are three times more likely than other women to develop heart disease. But even a weight gain of 10 pounds can increase your risk.

Excess weight is linked to heart disease mainly because it raises blood pressure and cholesterol level and can lead to type II diabetes. High blood pressure, high cholesterol level, and diabetes are major risk factors for heart disease. The way in which fat is distributed on your body also affects your risk. Women who accumulate fat around their waist are at greater risk of heart disease than are women who accumulate fat on their hips and thighs (see page 97).

If you are overweight, losing as few as 12 pounds may reduce your risk of developing heart disease. You can lower your risk even more if you also exercise regularly. Regular exercise can raise your level of helpful HDL cholesterol. This type of cholesterol protects against heart disease by cleansing the arteries of fat and lowers your level of harmful LDL cholesterol (which causes fat to build up in the blood).

STROKE

Most strokes are caused by the same narrowing of the arteries that causes a heart attack. A stroke is damage to the brain that results from a blockage in an artery that supplies blood to the brain. A less common form of stroke is caused by rupture of a blood vessel in the brain that usually occurs after the blood vessel has been weakened by high blood pressure. Both high blood pressure and fat buildup in artery walls (atherosclerosis) are made worse by obesity. The distribution of fat around the waist and in the abdominal area (see page 97) may also increase the risk of stroke. (For more about stroke, see page 569.)

CANCER

Women who are significantly overweight are at increased risk of cancer of the endometrium (the lining of the uterus). If you are obese and your periods are irregular, it is important for you to have regular gynecologic checkups to rule out endometrial cancer. In some women who are obese, hormones released by the pituitary gland in the brain (to help regulate the menstrual cycle) and the female hormone estrogen do not fluctuate normally during the menstrual cycle. This hormone imbalance can prevent ovulation (release of an egg from an ovary). If you do not ovulate, your body does not produce the balancing hormone progesterone, which limits the growth of the endometrium and causes it to break down and leave your body in the form of menstrual blood.

If you are not ovulating and your periods are irregular, the endometrium may continue to grow abnormally. This abnormal growth can cause abnormal cell changes that could lead to cancer if they are not detected at an early stage and treated. If your periods become more frequent or less frequent or abnormal in any other way, see your doctor. (For more about anovulation, see page 210.)

GALLSTONES

Obesity causes the liver to secrete excessive amounts of a fluid called bile, which is stored in the gallbladder. Bile is necessary for the body to digest fats. But an overproduction of bile sets the stage for the formation of gallstones (solid lumps of various sizes inside the gallbladder). Gallstones occur three to four times more frequently in people who are overweight than in people of normal weight. The incidence rises with advancing age and increasing weight.

Gallstones are sometimes painless and cause no symptoms. But when the stones block the exit of bile through the bile ducts into the intestinal tract, they can cause symptoms of indigestion or severe abdominal pain. If you have chronic pain in the right upper part of your abdominal area, especially after eating a high-fat meal, talk to your doctor. He or she may recommend an ultrasound scan to help determine if you have gallstones (see page 532).

INFERTILITY

Obesity sometimes leads to changes in hormone levels that can result in a failure of the ovaries to release eggs regularly. This abnormality, called anovulation, is associated with irregular or absent periods and infertility.

Anovulation can also result in excessive production of male hormones by the ovaries, which may cause symptoms such as acne and excessive hair growth. (For more about infertility and treatment, see page 382.)

JOINT PROBLEMS AND BACK PAIN

Excess weight puts extreme pressure on your joints, sometimes causing inflammation in the joints (known as arthritis). Obesity is also a factor in osteoarthritis—a form of arthritis that is caused by wear and tear on the joints. Osteoarthritis primarily affects the weight-bearing joints of the knees, hips, spine, and ankles.

Excess weight, especially in the abdominal area, can put strain on one of your body's most vulnerable parts—the spine. Lower back pain is especially common in people who are obese. The best treatment for lower back pain is weight loss and exercises that strengthen the muscles that support the lower back.

TREATING OBESITY

In severe, life-threatening cases of obesity, doctors sometimes recommend surgery—such as closing off a portion of a person's stomach or narrowing the digestive tract, as a way to help people lose weight. However, these techniques have a low rate of success and a high rate of complications. Most doctors recommend a conservative, gradual approach to weight loss—a combination of eating a nutritious, well-balanced, low-fat diet, exercising regularly, and making changes in behavior that a person will continue for a lifetime.

A regular exercise program is an essential part of any weight-loss program. However, excess weight can put strain on your joints and muscles, increasing your risk of sprains and strains. If you have arthritis, exercise may worsen it. Talk to your doctor before you start an exercise program. The following guidelines can help you get started:

- Choose a low-impact exercise such as walking, swimming, or cycling; avoid running or high-impact aerobics.
- Begin at a low intensity, just enough to get your muscles and joints accustomed to moving.
- Build up gradually, starting with 5 to 10 minutes per session.
- Begin by exercising three times a week and gradually build up to exercising every day.
- To increase the number of calories you burn, exercise for longer periods rather than at a faster pace.
- Don't count on the scale to tell you the whole story. Because muscle weighs more than fat, you may very well be getting fitter and thinner without a corresponding loss of pounds.

Extreme underweight and its effects on health

For some women, particularly young women, losing weight and staying model-thin is an obsession—an obsession that can be life threatening. These women have an intense fear of being fat and a distorted perception of their body weight and image. They see themselves as fat even when they are thin or of normal weight.

This abnormal body image can lead to an eating disorder, such as bulimia or anorexia nervosa. Early treatment of eating disorders is vital. If untreated, they can result in severe health problems. Most people with eating disorders cannot stop their self-destructive behavior without professional help. If you or a loved one needs help for an eating disorder, talk to your doctor. Treatment usually consists of individual counseling and psychotherapy that includes the family, as well as counseling about nutrition, behavior modification, and participation in support groups.

BULIMIA

The eating disorder bulimia is characterized by episodes of binge eating followed by purging. Immediately after consuming enormous amounts of food, people with bulimia force themselves to vomit or they use excessive amounts of laxatives or diuretics to rid (or purge) their body of unwanted calories.

The symptoms of bulimia often begin during the teenage years but can continue unrecognized for years. People who have bulimia often maintain a normal weight but may engage in frequent eating binges—eating huge quantities of food in one sitting. Between binges, many fast excessively. Because many women who have bulimia are of normal weight, the disorder often is unnoticed by family and friends and, therefore, goes undiagnosed.

The constant purging that goes along with bulimia can upset your body's balance of important chemicals. This chemical imbalance can cause fatigue, seizures, irregular heartbeat, and thinning bones. Repeated vomiting can damage the linings of your stomach and esophagus and erode the enamel on your teeth. (For more about bulimia and treatments, see page 610.)

ANOREXIA

People who have anorexia nervosa drastically limit their food intake, often to the point of severe malnourishment that requires hospitalization. Anorexia usually starts during the teenage years but can begin at any age. The incidence among 8- to 11-year-old girls is increasing dramatically. These young girls may avoid eating with the family or, when they do, spend most of mealtime pushing the food around on their plate.

Besides severely limiting their food intake, people who have anorexia often exercise excessively. Severe weight loss and excessive exercise can cause menstruation to stop. In young adolescents, anorexia can prevent the onset of menstruation. Absence of menstruation (amenorrhea, see page 210) is serious because it indicates that a woman is not producing the important female hormone estrogen. A lack of estrogen can cause bones to thin and weaken, increasing a young woman's risk of developing the bone-thinning disorder osteoporosis (see page 552).

Anorexia can also cause a drop in blood pressure, breathing rate, and body temperature. In severe cases, anorexia is fatal. (For more about anorexia and treatments, see page 610.)

CHAPTER 4

Preventive health care

Contents

Traditionally, American medicine has focused on treating and curing disease. But today, doctors consider helping people stay healthy to be equally important. During an office visit, your doctor may spend time talking to you about lifestyle factors—including diet and exercise, smoking, and drinking—that can either improve or harm your health. Because of the growing knowledge about the important role that genes play in a person's susceptibility to many of the most common chronic, debilitating diseases—including heart disease, cancer, diabetes, and osteoporosis—your doctor will probably ask you to complete a family health history. (For how to compile your history, see page 120.) Knowing which diseases you are at risk of may encourage you to make important lifestyle decisions—such as quitting smoking—to reduce your risk of actually developing the diseases.

Getting regular checkups, tests, and immunizations is essential for protecting your health. For example, tests such as the Pap smear for cervical cancer and the mammogram for breast cancer can help detect cancers at an early, more curable stage.

Choosing your health care provider

Your primary care physician is the doctor you go to regularly for physical examinations, tests, advice about staying healthy, and treatment of minor illnesses and injuries. In many health plans, the primary care physician serves as a gatekeeper, deciding which conditions and diseases you need to be tested for and determining if you should see a specialist. It is important to find a primary care physician you feel comfortable with—a doctor who communicates openly with you in language you can understand. You need to have confidence in your doctor and feel that he or she is responsive to your questions and concerns.

CHOOSING YOUR PRIMARY CARE PHYSICIAN

Although most people go to a family physician or an internist, many women choose a gynecologist as their primary care physician. If you have a specific medical condition, such as heart disease, you may want your primary care physician to be an internist who specializes in a particular area, such as cardiology.

Choose a doctor who is certified by the American Board of Medical Specialties. Directly ask a doctor in what specialties he or she is board certified. Find a doctor you trust and have confidence in.

Some women feel more comfortable with a female doctor, especially for gynecologic problems. If a female doctor is your preference, you have a broader choice than ever before, because of a rapid increase in the number of female doctors in the US.

There are many ways to find a good doctor. If you are in a health plan that limits your choice of doctors, you will be given a list of doctors to choose from. To narrow down the list, it's a good idea to talk with the administrators of the health plan to find the doctors' credentials and areas of expertise. Find out how long a doctor has been at an institution. Talk to other people who are in the same health plan to find out about their experiences.

If you have an insurance plan that gives a large number of doctors from which to choose, develop your own list by talking with friends and relatives. Call hospitals in your area, university medical centers, or the local medical society for recommendations. Make sure the doctor you choose is covered by your insurance plan.

Once you have a short list, check all the doctors' credentials. If your health plan supplied you with a list of doctors, it can also give you their credentials. Some plans routinely provide this information; with others, you have to ask. If you are choosing from a longer list of doctors, call the hospitals with which they are affiliated or their office to find out their credentials. Ask where they attended medical school and did their internship and residency. Ask whether they are board certified in a specialty.

The final step is an interview with the prospective doctor. (You may be charged for this visit.) Although many insurance plans do not cover such a visit, the

Qualities to look for in a doctor

Your doctor should:

- Take the time to talk with you and ask you questions
- Take the time to listen to you and answer your questions thoroughly
- Welcome your input and involvement
- Know your health history
- Keep informed of the latest medical advances
- Be available by phone without excessive delay
- Have a system to handle emergencies 24 hours a day
- Be aware of any medication you are taking and prescribe new medication carefully
- Tell you when you need to have screening tests

When to get a second opinion

Getting a second opinion is not an insult to your doctor. In many situations it is standard practice and is often required by insurance companies before such procedures as major surgery. Tell your doctor you would like to get a second opinion under the following circumstances:

- Your doctor is unable to diagnose your problem within a reasonable length of time—for example, two or three office visits
- Your doctor says you have a serious, chronic, or fatal condition
- Your doctor recommends surgery as part of the treatment of a disorder or as part of a complicated diagnostic procedure
- Your doctor diagnoses a very rare illness
- Your doctor tells you your illness is emotional, not physical

information you gain may be worth it to you. If you belong to a health maintenance organization (HMO), preferred provider organization (PPO), or other closed health plan, you will probably be charged only a minimal fee or a co-payment for your initial visit, the same fee you pay for any office visit under the plan.

The goal of the interview is to meet the doctor and determine whether he or she is easy to talk to, is willing to communicate freely with you about your health, and will welcome your participation concerning your own health and any recommended treatment plan. Find out the average waiting time for appointments. Is the support staff friendly and helpful? How often are you likely to see a nurse practitioner or other health care professional instead of the doctor? Ask how many doctors are in the group and if there is a backup doctor you can see if yours is away. How many patients does the doctor see per hour? If an office books ten patients per hour, a doctor can spend only 6 minutes with each. If you prefer a doctor who takes time with patients, look for one who sees fewer patients. If you have special concerns (such as the role of nutrition in staying healthy), ask the doctor's opinion about them.

Talk to the doctor or one of the support staff about fees and other practical matters. How much will you be charged? How much will you be expected to pay, when, and how? What kind of access to medical care is available on nights and weekends? What do you do in the case of an emergency or if your doctor is out of town?

SELECTING A HEALTH PLAN

The emergence of managed care health plans that offer a package of health care services provided by a limited number of doctors who are members of the plan has limited the choice of doctors for most people. In some cases the doctors and other health care professionals are staff employees of the plan; in other cases they are contracted by the plan to provide services for a previously agreed-upon fee. If you belong to a managed care plan such as a health maintenance organization (HMO) or a preferred provider organization (PPO), you have access only to the doctors and other health professionals that belong to the plan. Health care plans now offer a wide variety of choices with varying deductibles, co-payments, and coverage. Here are some guidelines for choosing a health care plan that is right for you. There are three basic types of health plans—the traditional fee-for-service plans, HMOs, and PPOs.

Fee-for-service Fee-for-service is the traditional form of health insurance that has become more expensive and less common. The insurance company pays fees to doctors and other health care providers for services they provide to members of the plan. Fee-for-service insurance plans give you an unlimited choice of doctors and other health care professionals and hospitals. You are usually required to pay a deductible (a specified amount you must pay before the insurance coverage takes over) and you pay a percentage of the cost of each visit or service. The plan is also likely to have standard or maximum fees that it will pay for specific services. If your doctor charges more than the standard fee, you are required to pay the difference. Preventive care (such as physical examinations, immunizations, and tests) is usually not covered by fee-for-service plans. This type of plan offers you the widest choice but requires the most paperwork; you have to fill out and submit claim forms to the insurer. If the doctor requires payment at the time of service, you will probably have to wait to be reimbursed by your insurance company.

Questions to ask about a fee-for-service plan:

- What does the policy cover? Does it cover prescription drugs? Home care?
- Will a health problem that has already been diagnosed (a so-called preexisting condition) be covered by the plan? If it recurs, is there a waiting period before it will be covered?
- What is the yearly deductible? Can I lower my monthly premium by choosing a larger deductible?
- What percentage of the bill will I have to pay (the coinsurance rate)?
- What is the maximum I will have to pay each year?
- Is there a maximum amount of coverage (a "lifetime cap") after which I won't have to pay any more?

Health maintenance organization A health maintenance organization (HMO) is a prepaid health plan that provides comprehensive coverage, usually for a lower monthly premium than a fee-for-service plan. In an HMO, you use only the doctors, services, and hospitals that are under contract with the HMO. Your choice of doctor is limited. However, in some cases, you may be allowed to see a doctor outside of the plan—such as in emergencies or when an unusual medical problem requires a specialist with expertise in a particular area. In an HMO, you are usually required to pay a small co-payment for each visit or service. HMOs usually cover at least some preventive care and tests. It is in the financial interest of the plan to keep people healthy and diagnose illnesses early—before they become more serious and difficult to treat. HMOs do not require patients to fill out claim forms for office visits or hospital stays. Instead, the doctor's office staff submits claims to the HMO. Some people who belong to HMOs find that they may have to wait longer to get appointments with their doctor than people who are in a traditional fee-for-service plan.

Questions to ask about an HMO:

- How many doctors can I choose from?
- Are most of the doctors now accepting new patients?
- Will I see the same doctor each time or different ones?
- Will I always be able to see a doctor or will I sometimes see a nurse practitioner or other health professional?
- How far in advance must I schedule an appointment?
- What preventive services—such as mammograms, Pap smears, and cholesterol tests—does the HMO provide?
- Where is the facility located?
- What happens if I have an emergency while I am out of town?
- What is the monthly premium?
- What is my co-payment per office visit, prescription, and emergency room visit?
- Are prescriptions covered?

Preferred provider organization A preferred provider organization (PPO) combines the qualities of a fee-for-service plan and an HMO. Most PPOs give you a broader list of doctors and hospitals to choose from than HMOs. In some PPOs, when you see a doctor, the visit is covered by the plan and you usually pay a small co-payment. You do not have to fill out forms; the staff in the doctor's office do the paperwork. Other PPOs are more like fee-for-service plans; you fill out forms for your doctor visits and send them to the PPO for reimbursement. Some PPO plans may have a deductible. As with an HMO, your primary physician may serve as a gatekeeper who refers you to specialists. The primary physician may be an internist, a family practice doctor, or, in some cases, an obstetrician/gynecologist. In some PPOs, administrators manage your use of services in a system called managed care. Most PPOs cover preventive care, including Pap smears and mammograms. Unlike HMOs, PPOs usually allow you to use doctors outside the plan, but in this case, you are required to pay a larger proportion of the bill yourself.

Questions to ask about a PPO:

- How many doctors can I choose from?
- How many doctors on the list are currently accepting patients?
- How does the plan handle referrals to specialists?
- What hospitals are covered by the plan?
- In case of an emergency, can I go to the nearest hospital and be covered?
- What preventive services—such as Pap smears, mammograms, and cholesterol tests—are covered?
- What is the monthly premium?
- What is my co-payment per office visit, prescription, and emergency-room visit?
- How much will I have to pay per visit if I choose a doctor who is not in the plan?
- Are prescriptions covered?

Medicare and Medicaid Women over age 65 who are eligible for Social Security are also eligible for Medicare, the federal health plan for older people. Medicare provides coverage for inpatient hospital treatment. Many older people also have private health insurance to cover regular doctor's visits, screening tests, and co-payments and deductibles not covered by Medicare. Older people who have a lower income and do not have private health insurance often have to pay a much higher percentage of their own health care costs. Medicaid is available to help cover medical expenses for those older people who meet the income requirements.

Medicare is designed to cover acute (sudden, severe) illnesses or major surgical procedures. Chronic, long-term diseases that are common in women, such as osteoporosis and the long-term aftereffects of heart attack or stroke, are not covered by Medicare unless they require hospitalization. Many of these diseases are treated on an outpatient basis.

If you are soon to be eligible for Medicare, make sure you apply to your local Social Security Administration office well in advance to avoid delays in your coverage. Medicare covers only services and doctors that it approves. The hospitals and doctors must agree to care for patients for the fees that have been set by Medicare. Ask in advance if the doctor or office you plan to visit accepts Medicare coverage. Ask if the office will bill Medicare directly or expects you to pay at the time of the visit. If you pay at the time of your visit, you will have to fill out the forms and submit them to Medicare for reimbursement.

Knowing your family health history

The health history of your family—your parents, grandparents, aunts and uncles, brothers and sisters—is important for your doctor to know because of the role of genetic factors in most diseases. Some relatively rare but life-threatening diseases, such as cystic fibrosis (which affects the lungs) and sickle cell anemia (which affects blood cells), are passed on from parents to children in a single gene. For now, there is no known way to avoid a disorder of this type if you inherit the disease-causing gene. But the vast majority of the most common diseases and disorders result from the interaction of a person's genetic makeup and environmental factors. These environmental influences include smoking, lack of exercise, a poor diet, drinking, and exposure to pollutants.

Because you can inherit susceptibilities to particular diseases, knowing the disorders that have occurred in your family can help you evaluate your own risks. Once you understand these risks, you can make healthful lifestyle choices and get appropriate screening tests that can help you avoid those diseases.

Your Family Health History

USE THIS QUESTIONNAIRE to get a useful health history from your blood relatives. The health histories of your parents, grandparents, and brothers and sisters are the most important ones for you to know. For relatives who have died, ask someone who was close to them to answer as many questions as possible. Once you have completed the questionnaire, use the information to make a family health history tree like the one on the next page.

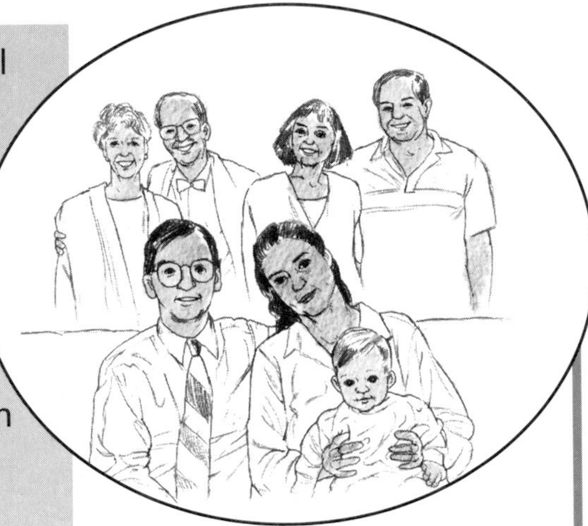

Health questionnaire

Name of relative ______________________ Relation to you ____________

❑ Male ❑ Female Year of birth_______ Year of death _______ Cause of death ____________

If the person was ever diagnosed with any of the following health problems, note his or her age at the time of the diagnosis.

❑ Heart attack
❑ High blood pressure
❑ High cholesterol level
❑ Angina (chest pain that may precede a heart attack)
❑ Coronary bypass surgery
❑ Heart disease
❑ Stroke
❑ Breast cancer
❑ Lung cancer
❑ Colon cancer
❑ Other cancer (type?)
❑ Diabetes
❑ Allergies, including reactions to medications
❑ Miscarriages, abortions for medical reasons, stillbirths, infant deaths, and birth defects
❑ Depression or other mood disorders
❑ Schizophrenia
❑ Alcoholism or other drug addiction
❑ Psychiatric treatment for other disorders

Lifestyle factors—such as smoking, lack of exercise, a poor diet, or excessive drinking—can also influence a person's risk of dying prematurely. Try to find out the following about the lifestyle of each of your relatives who have died:

Weight Overweight ________ Healthy weight ________ Underweight ________

Smoking Smoked (How many years?) ________________ Never smoked ________

Drinking Heavy ________ Moderate ________ Never drank ________

Other strategies

To find or verify the cause of death of a relative, contact the health department of the town in which your relative lived. For a small fee, you can get a copy of the death certificate. If you have no living relatives or if you are adopted, refer to the chart on page 122 for your risk of disease based on statistics from the general population.

Does it run in the family?

The following are indications that a particular disease may run in your family:

- The disease has occurred largely or completely on one side of your family.
- The disease occurs in a relatively young family member. Because it often takes decades for environmental factors to cause illness (for example, it usually takes many years of cigarette smoking to cause lung cancer), early onset of disease suggests a strong genetic influence.
- The same disease occurs at about the same age in more than one member of the family. A mother and a daughter who each develop breast cancer in their 40s are likely to have the inherited form of the disease.
- Cancer occurs in more than one location in the body, such as tumors in both breasts; this pattern may indicate an inherited form of cancer.
- The disease occurs despite a family member's healthy lifestyle. A marathon runner who develops heart disease probably has inherited a strong genetic susceptibility to it.

Sample family health history tree

Susan and her sister (below) are at high risk of breast cancer because their mother died of breast cancer at an early age—41. Breast cancer that is diagnosed before a woman has gone through menopause may indicate a genetically inherited form of the disease. Their maternal grandmother also died of breast cancer. It is important for the two sisters and any daughters they have to do monthly breast self-examinations beginning in their 20s. Both sisters should begin having mammograms when they are about 10 years younger than their mother was when her cancer was first detected.

Heart disease and stroke have occurred on both sides of Susan's family, putting some family members at increased risk of these conditions. Lifestyle factors—such as not smoking, getting plenty of exercise, drinking only moderately (if at all), eating a low-fat diet, and taking estrogen during and after menopause—can help reduce this risk.

Alcoholism is also seen on both sides of the family, which may increase the sisters' susceptibility. For them, the safest course is to avoid drinking, or drink only moderately.

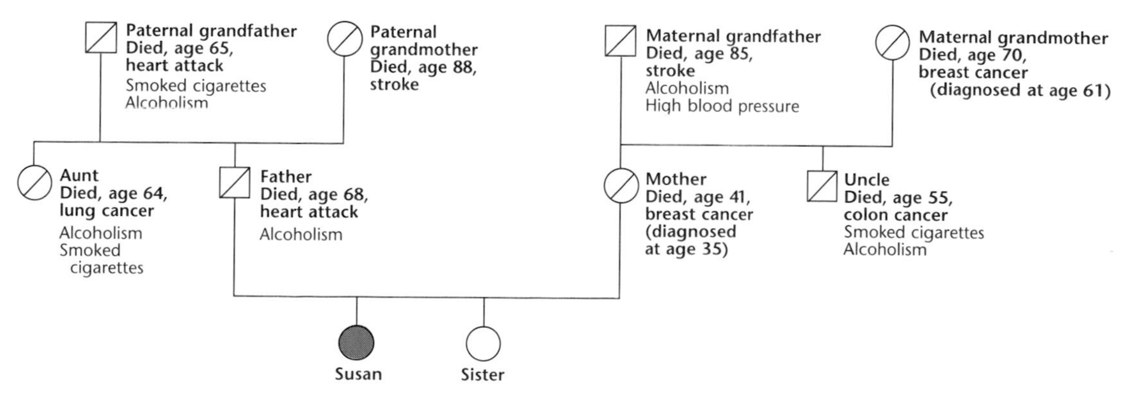

For example, if you have a family history of heart disease, you can lower your risk by not smoking and by exercising regularly and eating a low-fat diet. Other potentially heart-protecting measures include keeping your cholesterol and your blood pressure at healthy levels.

Protective measures for cancer are less obvious. However, it is known that you are much less likely to get lung cancer if you never smoke. You are less likely to get colon cancer if you eat a high-fiber diet that is rich in fruits and vegetables and low in fat (see page 44).

Your doctor may ask if there is a history in your family of heart disease, diabetes, cancer, or high blood pressure; the forms you fill out at your first office visit will ask similar questions. (If you were adopted and do not know your birth parents' health histories, tell your doctor.) It is a good idea to research and prepare your family health history before your office visit and bring it with you. Find out all you can about the health of your parents, grandparents, aunts, uncles, sisters, and brothers. Ask if they have been treated for any major illnesses—such as cancer, heart disease, or diabetes—that have a genetic component. Find out the cause of death of relatives and the disorders they may have had. For help gathering this information, see Your family health history, page 120.

Genetic risk of major disorders

The second column in the table shows the average risk a woman has of contracting one of the major disorders shown in the first column during her lifetime. The third column shows the increased risk of a woman who has one parent with the disorder.

DISORDER	AVERAGE RISK	INCREASED RISK
Alcoholism	2%	10% to 20%
Alzheimer's disease	2% to 5%	19%
Asthma	4%	26%
Breast cancer	13%	26%*
Colon cancer	4%	10%
Ovarian cancer	2%	5%
Uterine cancer	4%	9%
Diabetes	2%	5% to 19%
Duodenal ulcer	10%	30%
Glaucoma	2%	4% to 16%
Manic depression	1%	25%
Migraine	5% to 10%	45%
Schizophrenia	1%	8% to 18%

*Risk may be as high as 39% if mother's breast cancer was diagnosed before she reached menopause.

Your doctor's appointment

Most doctors no longer recommend a regular annual checkup that includes a complete physical examination and a battery of laboratory tests. Besides seeking treatment for an illness, visits to the doctor should be based on getting the counseling, medical tests, and immunizations you need to stay healthy, depending on your personal risk factors. Once you and your doctor have determined your risk factors, your doctor can recommend steps you can take to reduce those risks, including following a healthy lifestyle.

The following procedures and tests have proved to be the most valuable for preventing and detecting disease:

- Blood pressure reading
- Breast examinations and mammograms
- Pap smear (to test for cervical cancer)
- Skin examination for melanoma (a life-threatening form of skin cancer)
- Listening for a heart murmur (an abnormal heart sound that may indicate a heart problem)
- Regular dental checkups

PREPARING FOR YOUR VISIT TO THE DOCTOR

Prepare for a visit to your doctor by writing down any unusual symptoms you may have and a list of questions you want to ask. Bring a list of all the medications you are currently taking, including vitamins. Writing down the subjects you want to discuss with your doctor can help you stay focused during the visit and prevent you from forgetting anything important.

If this is your first visit to a new doctor, call his or her office ahead of time to make sure that copies of your medical records have been sent from your previous doctor. When you move to another city or state, it is a good idea to bring the medical records yourself to your new doctor.

If you will be having a pelvic examination (which is likely if you have not had a Pap smear within a year or if you are having vaginal discharge or discomfort), do not douche or insert any vaginal creams or suppositories for at least 24 hours before the visit. (Douching is generally not recommended because it can increase your risk of vaginal and pelvic infections.)

TALKING WITH YOUR DOCTOR

Good communication between you and your doctor is probably the most important factor in your health care. You need to feel comfortable enough with your doctor to discuss anything, no matter how embarrassing, that you think might affect your health. Do you smoke? Are you concerned about your drinking? Are you depressed? Have you or your sexual partner had other sexual partners recently? Are you experiencing pain during intercourse? Don't hesitate to tell your doctor such important information.

At the same time, you should expect your doctor to be able to communicate openly with you. Tests and examinations may be routine to your doctor, but you should feel free to ask as many questions as you want about what is going on. Your doctor needs to explain clearly why he or she is recommending a particular test or procedure or prescribing a medication. Ask your doctor to repeat any instructions you don't understand and take notes so you will have the information on paper when you get home. Some doctors may be abrupt when they are pressed for time but you should be persistent about getting the information you need.

If your primary care physician is a gynecologist, make sure he or she knows that you are not seeing any other doctor. That way, he or she will know to include in your visits all the recommended tests of general health, such as blood pressure and cholesterol.

If you go to your doctor with a specific health problem or set of symptoms, make sure you provide the following information:

- When the symptoms first began to bother you.
- The order in which the symptoms first occurred.
- A clear description of how you feel. Do you have stabbing pain, a dull ache, burning, tingling, or a sensation of pressure or squeezing?
- The intensity of your symptoms when they began. Did they recently become more intense?
- How often the symptoms occur. Are they constant or sporadic?
- The things that seem to trigger or worsen the symptoms. Certain activities? Certain foods? When you are in certain positions?
- Whatever you do that seems to make the symptoms better.
- A brief description of any lifestyle changes (such as diet or a new exercise program) that you made around the time the symptoms developed. Did you recently begin taking a new medication? Do you have a new sexual partner? Do you have a new job? Are you under unusual stress?

General symptoms to report to a doctor

Watch for these symptoms, and report them to your doctor. Many diseases (such as heart disease, high blood pressure, osteoporosis, and the early stages of most forms of cancer) have no symptoms. For this reason, screening tests and regular physical examinations are extremely important.

- Weight loss of 10 pounds or more for no apparent reason
- Abnormal or unusual-smelling vaginal discharge
- Two or three missed menstrual periods
- Irregular vaginal bleeding between periods
- Vaginal bleeding after menopause
- Nipple discharge that is persistent, occurs without squeezing the nipple, or occurs in only one nipple
- A sore on the skin or in the mouth that doesn't heal
- A change in the shape, color, or size of a mole or raised patch of skin, including bleeding
- A lump that appears under the skin
- A recurrent headache accompanied by vomiting
- A headache that persists for several hours despite taking over-the-counter pain relievers
- Loss of consciousness, fainting, or dizziness for no apparent reason; fainting followed by numbness and tingling anywhere on the body
- Sudden changes in vision, sensitivity to light, blurred vision, appearance of flashing lights or black dots, or loss of part of your field of vision
- Difficulty swallowing, possibly accompanied by rapid weight loss
- Persistent cough, hoarseness, or loss of voice
- Coughing up blood
- A change in regular bowel movements (to either diarrhea or constipation)
- A change in the appearance of stools (black stools can indicate the presence of blood; pale stools can indicate other problems, such as liver disease)
- Urine that is pink or stained with blood
- Painful urination
- Hair loss
- Unusual mood swings or other psychological problems including anxiety, depression, or inability to concentrate
- Change in sleep patterns

GYNECOLOGIC EXAMINATION

When you enter the examining room before having a gynecologic examination, you may be asked to provide a sample of urine. In any case, it's a good idea to empty your bladder before the examination. You will be asked to undress completely, put on a gown or sheet, and sit on the examining table. The doctor or nurse will ask if you have been experiencing any unusual problems or symptoms. If this is your first gynecologic examination, say so; ask the doctor to explain each step to you.

Your doctor will look at your breasts for signs of lumps and may ask you to raise your arms. He or she will feel for any abnormal growths, compressing the breast tissue between his or her fingers and your chest wall underneath. The doctor will feel the tissue up under your arms and try to detect enlarged lymph nodes that can be a sign of infection or breast cancer. The doctor may ask you to lie down while he or she repeats the manual examination of your breast tissue. He or she may squeeze your nipple to check for a discharge. If your nipples are inverted, the doctor may gently try to bring the nipples out to examine them.

You will be asked to place your heels in metal stirrups at the end of the examining table to enable the doctor to check your genital area. He or she will look for any abnormalities, including changes in

MANUAL PELVIC EXAMINATION

A manual pelvic examination is a regular part of a gynecological checkup. The doctor inserts one or two fingers into the vagina and presses on the abdomen with the other hand to feel for normal placement and size of the uterus, ovaries, and fallopian tubes.

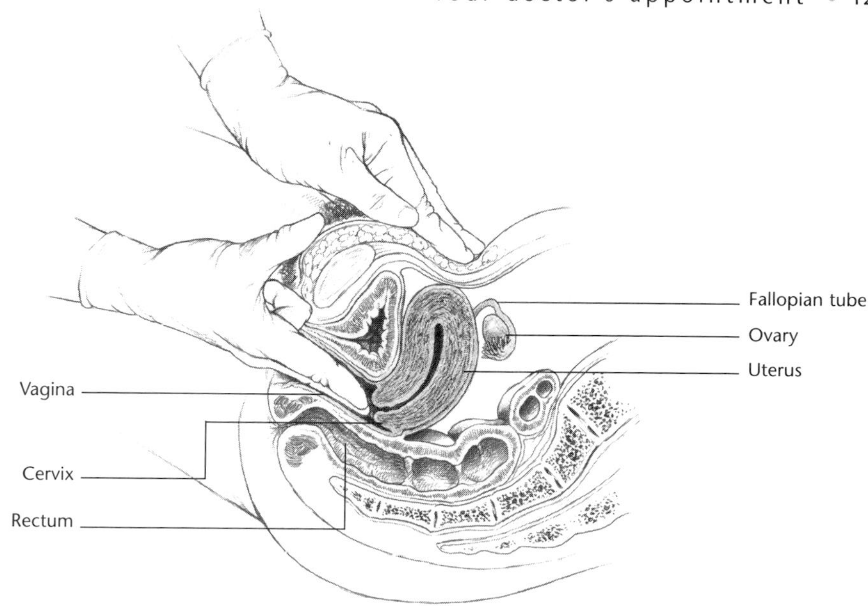

the skin, signs of irritation, swelling, or "bumps" on your vulva (the outer genital area), and any unusual vaginal discharge. The doctor may ask if you ever leak urine when you cough or sneeze.

The doctor will then insert an instrument called a speculum into your vagina to open it and examine the vaginal walls. Some women feel pressure in their bladder or rectum when the speculum is inserted. Emptying your bladder before the examination and trying to relax your muscles may help. If you are uncomfortable, ask your doctor to adjust the speculum or try a different size. In addition to examining the walls of the vagina, the doctor usually checks the cervix (the opening into the uterus). He or she is likely to perform a Pap smear, a procedure in which a small sample of cells is taken from your cervix. You may feel a slight pinch or a mild cramp when this is done. The sample will be sent to the laboratory to be examined for cancer cells.

The final step in the gynecologic checkup is a manual (by hand) internal

What to expect during a gynecologic examination

- Your doctor or an assistant will ask about your personal and family health histories.
- Your doctor will ask about your menstrual history; make sure to tell him or her about irregular periods, bleeding between periods, or heavy periods.
- Your blood pressure will be taken.
- Your weight will be compared to previous weights.
- Your urine will be tested for signs of infection.
- A visual and manual examination of your breasts (for lumps) will be done. The doctor may recommend that you have a mammogram, depending on your age and your personal and family health histories.
- Your doctor will visually examine your external genitals. Then he or she will insert a device called a speculum into your vagina to visually examine the internal walls of the vagina and the cervix.
- A Pap smear, a procedure in which a sample of cells is taken from your cervix, will be done to test for cervical cancer.
- In the internal examination, the doctor inserts two fingers into your vagina and simultaneously presses on your lower abdomen to check the size and shape of your uterus and ovaries and to feel for abnormal growths.
- If you are over 40, you will have a rectal examination along with the pelvic examination.

pelvic examination. While you are still lying on your back, the doctor stands between your legs and inserts the index and middle fingers of one hand into your vagina and places the other hand on your abdomen. You should try to relax as much as possible, even though you may feel uncomfortable. Lifting up your cervix with the fingers and pressing your abdomen with the outside hand, the doctor can feel the size, shape, and position of your uterus and ovaries. At the same time, he or she notes any tenderness you may feel. (For more about the reproductive organs, see page 198.)

If, after examining your uterus or ovaries, your doctor suspects any abnormalities, he or she may recommend an ultrasound (see page 405). An ultrasound is a computerized image of internal body structures made from reflected high-frequency sound waves. In most cases, ultrasounds are not required for a regular physical examination.

Your doctor may continue to examine your uterus, ovaries, and lower pelvic area by placing a finger in your rectum and compressing your abdomen. The doctor will also feel for growths in your rectum and take a stool sample to check for blood. Blood in the stool can be an indication of either rectal or colon cancer. A manual rectal examination is standard for women over 40 because the risk of cancers of the colon and rectum increases with age.

Your doctor will discuss the results of the examination with you. He or she will tell you of any unusual or abnormal findings. Make sure you ask any questions you may have. It is easier to do then than later by telephone.

Tests you might have

Don't hesitate to ask your doctor about the purpose of any test or diagnostic procedures you might have. Following are descriptions of the medical tests and procedures your doctor is most likely to recommend. A number of tests, such as blood pressure and cholesterol tests, are recommended for everyone at some time. The information from these tests helps your doctor monitor the state of your health and your risk of disease and detect disorders at an early stage.

BLOOD PRESSURE

Blood pressure is the force created in your bloodstream when your heart pumps blood into your arteries and throughout your body. A blood pressure reading measures how hard your circulating blood is pushing against the walls of your arteries. To take your blood pressure, an inflatable cuff is wrapped around your upper arm and inflated. When inflated, the cuff compresses a large artery in your arm, briefly stopping the flow of blood. The person measuring your blood pressure releases the air in the cuff while listening through a stethoscope placed over an artery on the inside of your arm. When the blood starts to pulse through the artery, it makes a sound that can be heard until the pressure in the artery exceeds the pressure in the cuff, when the sound stops.

While listening to the sound, the person watches a gauge and records two measurements. The first, higher number is called the systolic pressure; it indicates the pressure in your blood vessels when your heart beats and pumps blood into the circulation. The second number, the diastolic pressure, indicates the pressure when your heart rests between beats and fills with blood. Your blood pressure is recorded as the systolic pressure over the diastolic pressure—for example, 120/80.

The harder it is for your blood to flow, the higher both numbers will be. High blood pressure is defined as a reading higher than 140/90. Because high blood pressure can, over time, damage major organs and lead to heart attack and stroke, it is extremely important that you work with your doctor to keep it under control. If you are diagnosed with high blood pressure, your doctor may recommend medication to lower it. Depending on how high your blood pressure is, you may be able to lower it by exercising regularly, losing weight, or cutting back on your consumption of salt. (For more about the health effects of high blood pressure, see page 481.)

PAP SMEAR

A Pap smear is a test for cancer of the cervix (the opening into the uterus). Pap smears can also detect some sexually transmitted diseases. For a Pap smear, which is usually a painless procedure, a sample of cells is taken from your cervix during a pelvic examination and sent to a laboratory for examination under a microscope. The doctor collects the cells by wiping a tiny brush or a cotton swab and a narrow plastic or wooden spatula over the entire surface of your cervix and inside the cervical canal. Regular Pap smears are recommended for all women 18 and older or for any girl or woman who has ever had sexual intercourse.

A negative (normal) result on a Pap smear means that your cervix is probably healthy. However, a positive (abnormal) result on a Pap smear does not prove that you have cancer. Your doctor may tell you that some of your cells show "precancerous" changes (also called cervical dysplasia, see page 218). This means that, if not treated, these abnormal cells could become cancerous. Your doctor will recommend further testing to confirm the presence of abnormal cells and determine if treatment is necessary.

You are at increased risk of cervical cancer if you first had sexual intercourse before age 18, you have had many sexual partners and have not used condoms, or you have had the sexually transmitted diseases genital herpes (see page 342) or genital warts (see page 341). You are also at increased risk of cervical cancer if you are 24 or older and your mother took a synthetic hormone called diethylstilbestrol (DES) while she was pregnant with you. Tell your doctor if you have any of these risk factors. Make sure you have Pap smears as frequently as your doctor recommends.

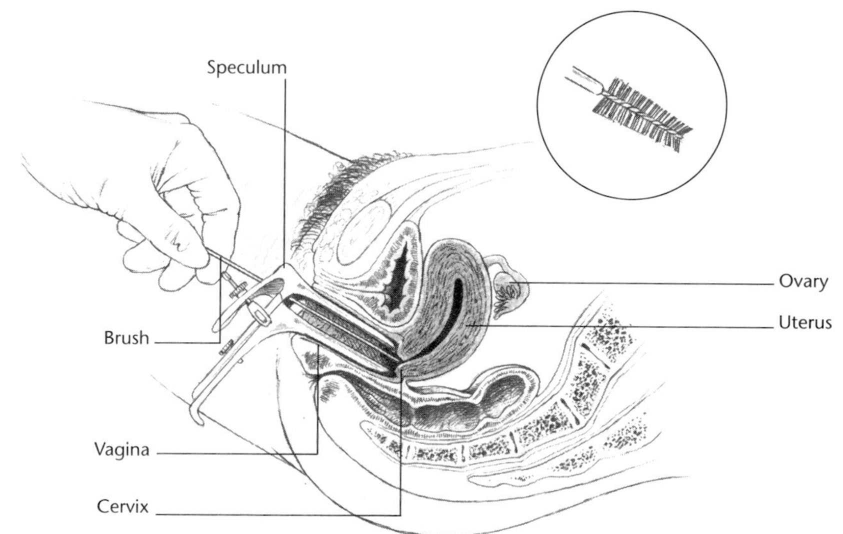

PAP SMEAR

A Pap smear is a sample of cells taken from the cervix, the opening into the uterus from the vagina. For a Pap smear, the doctor inserts a device called a speculum into your vagina to examine it. Using a tiny brush (inset) or swab and a spatula, the doctor takes a sample of cells for examination under a microscope. The test is used to detect cervical cancer, precancerous changes in cells, and some sexually transmitted diseases. The test is recommended for all women 18 and older or anyone who is sexually active.

MAMMOGRAM

A mammogram is a low-intensity X-ray taken to detect cancer or precancerous changes in the breast. Mammograms can detect breast cancer at an early stage, when it is easier to treat and more likely to be cured. But mammograms do not detect all cancers. They are most effective when performed in conjunction with a woman's monthly breast self-examinations and annual breast examinations by a doctor.

Because breast cancer is rare in younger women, most women do not need to have their first mammogram until 40. However, if you are at increased risk because of a strong family history of breast cancer or other factors (see page 272), talk to your doctor. Together you can decide when you should start having mammograms. If you have no family history of breast cancer or other risk factors, have a mammogram every 1 to 2

MAMMOGRAM

For a mammogram, the breast is compressed between two plates and a low-intensity X-ray is taken. The image helps doctors detect cancerous tumors in the breast at an early stage. Because your risk of breast cancer increases with age, it is especially important to have a mammogram every year after age 50.

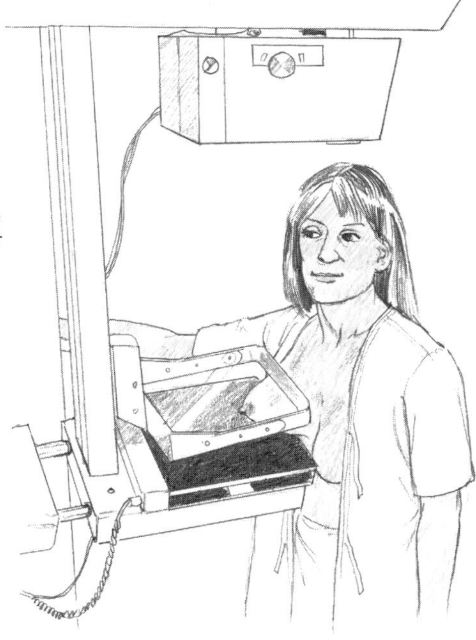

years between the ages of 40 and 49. After 50, you should have one every year because your risk of breast cancer increases as you age.

Before your mammogram, you will be asked not to use any talcum powder, lotion, or deodorant because they contain substances that can interfere with the X-ray image. When having your mammogram, you will be asked to disrobe to the waist and given a gown to put on. A health care professional will ask you to stand at the mammography machine and place your breast on an X-ray plate. She may assist you in making sure your breast is in the proper position. An upper plate will push down on your breast, flattening it out to get a clearer picture of the cells. Two views of each breast usually are taken. Some women experience mild discomfort. Many women schedule their mammograms during the week after their period, the time of the menstrual cycle when their breasts are less likely to be swollen or tender. (For more about early detection of breast cancer, see page 274.)

TESTS FOR SEXUALLY TRANSMITTED DISEASES

Many sexually transmitted diseases (STDs) are harder to detect in women than in men because they cause no noticeable symptoms. Some STDs that go undetected can spread to your fallopian tubes, causing a condition called pelvic inflammatory disease (PID; see page 232), which can scar and block the tubes. PID is the most common preventable cause of infertility in American women. It is estimated that PID develops in more than 1 million women each year, usually as the result of undetected and untreated STDs.

To determine if you need to be tested for STDs, tell your doctor about any unusual symptoms such as abnormal vaginal discharge, itching or discomfort, or the presence of a sore or growth on your genitals. If you have a new sex partner or you or your partner have had other partners recently, your doctor may recommend that both you and your partner be tested for STDS.

Although more than 50 different diseases are known to be transmitted sexually, here is a list of the most common ones and the tests that are used to diagnose them. (For more about STDs, see chapter 12.)

Chlamydia Chlamydia is a bacterial infection that can be diagnosed from a sample of discharge from the cervix. The sample is examined in the laboratory for the presence of chlamydia bacteria.

Trichomoniasis Trichomoniasis is an infection caused by an organism that can be identified by examining a sample of vaginal discharge under a microscope. It is sometimes detected on a Pap smear.

Gonorrhea Gonorrhea is a bacterial infection that can affect the cervix, urethra, or rectum. The bacterium can be detected in a sample of cells from vaginal discharge. The cells are examined in the laboratory under a microscope.

Syphilis Syphilis is a bacterial infection that can spread throughout the body. The disease can be diagnosed by a doctor's evaluation of the symptoms, visual examination of a sore, and a blood test.

Genital warts Genital warts are painless, fleshy growths in the genital area caused by a virus. If the virus is present on the cervix, it can be detected on a Pap smear.

Genital herpes Genital herpes is a viral infection that produces painful, blister-like sores on the genitals. Laboratory examination of a swab from an open sore is necessary to diagnose herpes. Blood tests can detect antibodies that your body produces to fight the virus; these antibodies indicate exposure to the virus even if you do not have a visible infection.

Hepatitis B Hepatitis B is a viral infection that attacks the liver. The virus can be diagnosed by a blood test. The blood test may detect the virus itself or antibodies that the body produces to fight the virus.

AIDS AIDS is a collection of symptoms caused by a type of virus that progressively destroys the immune system's ability to fight infections and cancer. The virus—human immunodeficiency virus (HIV)—is diagnosed from a blood test for antibodies that the body produces to fight it.

TESTING FOR OVARIAN CANCER

Ovarian cancer (see page 249) is less common than some other kinds of cancer that affect women. But ovarian cancer is deadlier than most—fewer than 10 percent of cases are cured. Early detection is crucial for successful treatment of this cancer.

There is no completely reliable way, short of surgery, to detect ovarian cancer. Because the tests that are available are costly and not completely reliable, screening of all women for ovarian cancer is not recommended. During a regular pelvic examination, your doctor feels for cysts or tumors on the ovaries. However, this method can detect only the largest tumors.

A blood test called CA-125 and a vaginal ultrasound examination may be recommended for women with symptoms such as bloating, pelvic discomfort, abdominal swelling, or the presence of a growth in the pelvic area.

CA-125 CA-125 is a test in which a sample of your blood is examined in the laboratory for the presence of an antigen called CA-125. Antigens are chemical markers on the surface of cells that can distinguish cancer cells from healthy ones. An elevated level of CA-125 (a positive result) can indicate ovarian cancer, but the antigen has also been found at elevated levels in women with noncancerous conditions such as fibroid tumors (see page 221) and pelvic infections. Elevated levels of CA-125 may also indicate some conditions, including hepatitis and colon cancer, that are not gynecologic. Another problem with the test is that some types of ovarian cancer do not produce an elevated level of CA-125. For these reasons, doctors must use other tests and procedures along with the CA-125 to diagnose ovarian cancer.

Vaginal ultrasound A vaginal ultrasound is an imaging method used to detect abnormalities of the reproductive system. Vaginal ultrasound produces an image of a woman's reproductive organs using energy in the form of sound waves. During the procedure, which is painless, a long thin wand called a transducer is inserted into the vagina. The transducer sends out sound waves that bounce off the ovaries, producing an image on a video screen. Doctors can determine if the size or shape of an ovary is abnormal and if a growth on an ovary is solid, liquid, or both. In some cases, transvaginal sonography can help doctors distinguish between noncancerous (benign) growths and cancerous ones.

The technique is also used to determine the location of a pregnancy at a very early stage. A pregnancy that occurs outside the uterus, called an ectopic pregnancy (see page 233), is life threatening if not treated immediately.

ENDOMETRIAL BIOPSY

Endometrial cancer—cancer of the lining of the uterus—is the fourth most common type of cancer in women after cancers of the breast, lung, and colon and rectum. You are at increased risk of endometrial cancer if you are obese (20 percent or more over your ideal weight), have diabetes, have a family history of the cancer, experience recurrent abnormal bleeding from your uterus, or do not ovulate (see page 210). Other factors that may increase your risk of endometrial cancer include taking hormone replacement therapy (see page 360) after menopause with estrogen alone (without the balancing hormone progestin) or undergoing treatment for breast cancer using the drug tamoxifen.

If you have any of these risk factors and symptoms such as abnormal vaginal bleeding, your doctor may recommend taking a sample of tissue from your endometrium. The procedure, called an endometrial biopsy or endometrial tissue sample, usually does not require anesthesia. Using a speculum to open the vagina, the doctor stabilizes the cervix with a clamp. You may feel a slight pinching sensation. Then the doctor inserts a thin, flexible hollow tube into your uterus to remove a small piece of tissue. You may feel a brief cramping sensation. The tissue is examined under a microscope for abnormal changes or signs of cancer.

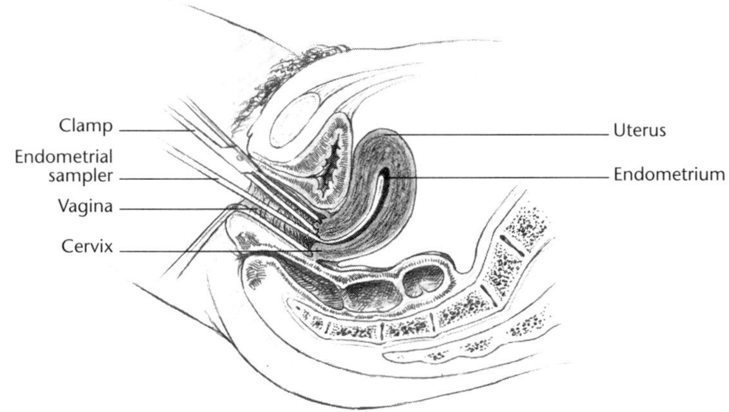

ENDOMETRIAL BIOPSY

An endometrial biopsy is a procedure in which a doctor takes a sample of tissue from the endometrium (the lining of the uterus). The tissue is examined for signs of cancer. To perform the procedure, the doctor stabilizes the cervix with an instrument and inserts a long, thin, flexible tube called an endometrial sampler into the uterus to take the sample of tissue.

FECAL OCCULT-BLOOD TEST

Blood in the stool can indicate colon or rectal cancer as well as less serious problems such as hemorrhoids (see page 522). The test for detecting blood in the stool is called a fecal occult-blood test. Your doctor may take a stool sample during a pelvic examination. Alternatively, your doctor may ask you to take a stool sample at home, put it on a special card, and return it to his or her office. The sample is sent to a laboratory to be examined under a microscope for traces of blood.

A fecal occult-blood test is recommended every year starting at age 40.

SIGMOIDOSCOPY

Sigmoidoscopy is a visual examination of the lower part of the colon and of the rectum, using a tubular instrument called a sigmoidoscope to look for signs of cancer. Colon cancer (see page 529) is the third most common cancer in women, after breast cancer and lung cancer. You should have your first sigmoidoscopy at age 50, or at age 40 if you have a family history of the cancer. Have sigmoidoscopy 1 year later and, if both tests are negative, you should have the test every 3 years, depending on your doctor's recommendation. Sigmoidoscopy can detect colon cancer at an early, curable stage.

Before you have sigmoidoscopy, you may be given one or two prepackaged enemas to empty your bowel in the doctor's office or at home before you go to

SIGMOIDOSCOPY

In sigmoidoscopy, a small, flexible, lighted tube is inserted into the lower part of the colon. Looking through the viewing piece at the other end, the doctor checks for small growths (polyps) that may or may not be cancerous.

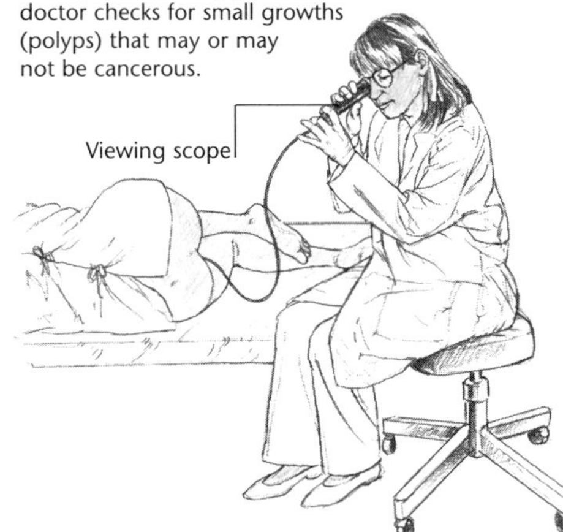

the doctor's office. The test lasts about 10 minutes and may be mildly uncomfortable but not painful. While you are lying on your side with your knees drawn up toward your chest, the doctor inserts the small lubricated tip of the scope into your rectum and guides it through the lower portion of your colon. The doctor then gradually withdraws the scope while viewing the inside of your colon, looking for bleeding, polyps (tiny growths that may or may not be cancerous), and other abnormalities. An attachment on the end of the instrument allows the doctor to take a sample of tissue for examination if necessary. If any polyps are found, your doctor will recommend a colonoscopy (see page 530), a procedure in which the whole colon is examined.

BLOOD TESTS

Because blood travels throughout your body and interacts with nearly every organ, a disease or malfunction anywhere in your body is often reflected in changes in your blood. Following are descriptions of the 11 most common blood chemistry tests and what they may indicate about the state of your health.

Complete blood cell count A complete blood cell count measures the main components of blood, including red cells, white cells, and platelets. Red blood cells transport oxygen from the lungs to body tissues; white blood cells fight infection; platelets help blood to clot. This test can provide much helpful information. For example, a low level of red blood cells indicates anemia and an elevated level of white blood cells indicates the presence of infection.

Cholesterol level A cholesterol test is a measurement of the level of fats in your blood. A person's total cholesterol level is used as an indicator of his or her risk of heart disease. If your total cholesterol level is below 200, you are considered to be at low risk for heart disease. A total cholesterol level between 200 and 239 is considered borderline; you are at moderate risk for heart disease, depending on the presence or absence of other risk factors such as smoking, obesity, diabetes, or a family history of heart disease. A total cholesterol level above 239 is abnormal and indicates increased risk of heart disease.

If your total cholesterol level is above 239, ask your doctor how you can lower it. Lifestyle changes such as limiting fat in your diet and getting regular exercise can help reduce your cholesterol level. Your doctor will want to analyze the various components of your total cholesterol reading to better evaluate your risk of heart disease.

Cholesterol is made up of different types of fat. One type, called low-density lipoprotein (LDL), is the "bad" kind of cholesterol that causes fat to build up in artery walls, narrowing them and raising the risk of heart attack and stroke. Another type, called high-density lipoprotein (HDL), is the "good" cholesterol that sweeps up the debris left by LDL and carries it back to the liver, where it is broken down.

Total cholesterol levels in women tend to rise after age 45. Doctors now think that your level of protective HDL cholesterol and the ratio of your total cholesterol level to your HDL level are more important indicators of your risk of heart disease than your total cholesterol level. For example, if your total cholesterol level is 230 and your HDL level is 65, your total cholesterol to HDL ratio is 3.5 (230/65=3.5). A ratio under 4.5 is desirable. Your risk of heart disease is reduced because you have a high level of HDL. You can raise your level of protective HDL with weight loss and regular exercise.

Glucose A normal range is 70 to 110 milligrams per deciliter (mg/dL). A blood glucose test measures the level of the sugar glucose in your blood. Your body uses glucose for energy. Elevated levels of glucose in the blood can indicate diabetes (see page 617). If your glucose level is found to be elevated, further testing is necessary to determine the cause.

Bilirubin A normal range is 0.1 to 1.2 milligrams per deciliter (mg/dL). Bilirubin is an orange-yellow pigment in bile, a liquid secreted by the liver to remove waste products and break down fats during digestion. An abnormal level of bilirubin can indicate liver disease or obstruction of the bile duct (the tube that carries bile from the liver) that can result from a gallstone (see page 532) or a

What do your cholesterol levels mean?

Here are the numbers to look for on your cholesterol profile and what they may indicate about your risk of heart disease. Your total cholesterol/high-density lipoprotein ratio should be under 4.5.

LEVEL (in milligrams per deciliter)	RISK OF HEART DISEASE
TOTAL CHOLESTEROL	
Less than 200	Low
200 to 239	Borderline
More than 239	High
HIGH-DENSITY LIPOPROTEIN (HDL)	
More than 50	Low
LOW-DENSITY LIPOPROTEIN (LDL)	
Less than 130	Low
130 to 159	Moderate
More than 159	High

pancreatic tumor. The accumulation of bilirubin in the skin gives it a yellow color, a condition called jaundice.

Lactic dehydrogenase A normal range is 60 to 120 international units per liter (IU/L). Lactic dehydrogenase is an enzyme (a protein that promotes chemical reactions) that is found in many body tissues. Its level rises when a tissue is injured. Along with the results of other tests, elevated levels may indicate a heart attack, liver disease, or lung problems.

Creatinine A normal range is 0.7 to 1.5 milligrams per deciliter (mg/dL). Creatinine is a waste product that is normally filtered out by the kidneys and excreted in urine. Elevated levels of creatinine or another waste product in the blood called blood urea nitrogen indicate impaired kidney function.

Potassium A normal range is 3.5 to 5.5 milliequivalents per liter (mEq/L). Potassium is a mineral called an electrolyte that is necessary for normal heart rhythm, the body's water balance, the conduction of nerve impulses, and muscle contraction. Low levels of potassium may result from excessive loss of water from sweating, vomiting, or diarrhea. High levels of potassium may indicate kidney failure or insufficient production of hormones that regulate the body's water balance.

Sodium A normal range is 136 to 142 milliequivalents per liter (mEq/L). Sodium is a chemical with functions similar to those of potassium. High levels of sodium may indicate dehydration (excessive loss of water) or congestive heart failure (see page 492).

Chloride A normal range is 95 to 105 milliequivalents per liter (mEq/L). Chloride maintains the body's water balance and the acid/base balance of body fluids. Low levels of chloride can indicate infection, an obstruction in the intestine, or severe diabetes.

Carbon dioxide A normal range is 20 to 30 milliequivalents per liter (mEq/L). Carbon dioxide is a waste product of normal metabolism. The lungs capture carbon dioxide and eliminate it through breathing. An elevated level can indicate the presence of diseases that impair the lungs, such as pneumonia (see page 509) or emphysema (see page 502). An elevated level can also indicate a problem with the hormone-producing adrenal glands, which control metabolism. Low levels may indicate severe, uncontrolled diabetes, kidney failure, or severe diarrhea.

Calcium A normal range is 9 to 10.5 milligrams per deciliter (mg/dL). Calcium is essential for strong bones and teeth and for nerve and muscle function. A high level may indicate a late stage of some types of cancer or overactivity of the parathyroid gland, which regulates the calcium level in the blood. A low level may indicate poor absorption of calcium by the intestines.

ELECTROCARDIOGRAM

An electrocardiogram, often called an ECG, is a painless test that measures the electrical activity of the heart muscle. An ECG can reveal early signs of heart disease (such as narrowing of the arteries). If you have two or more risk factors for heart disease, including a family history, high blood pressure, high cholesterol, diabetes, or cigarette smoking, you should have an ECG at age 40.

An ECG cannot always detect injury to the heart. The reading is normal in about 50 percent of people who have chest pain, including those whose arteries are, in fact, blocked.

When you have an ECG, a jellylike substance is rubbed onto areas of your chest. Electrodes are placed over these areas. The electrodes feed into a machine that records the electrical activity of your heart muscle. The electrical waves from the heart's four chambers are recorded on paper. Looking at the printout, a doctor can determine if your heart rhythm is regular and originates from the normal place, or if there are signs of injury to or enlargement of the heart muscle.

In some cases, an ECG may be combined with an exercise stress test (see page 469) to determine if the heart is getting a sufficient amount of oxygen during increased activity or stress. To do the test you walk on a treadmill until you reach a predetermined heart rate based on your age and physical condition. An ECG combined with an exercise stress test can detect early signs of heart disease that may not be apparent during a resting ECG. If an ECG is abnormal, a doctor will usually recommend further testing before making a diagnosis. (For more about how an ECG is used to help doctors diagnose heart disease, see page 465.)

SKIN CANCER CHECK

A visual examination of your skin by your doctor once every 3 years is a good way to check for possible signs of skin cancer (see page 683). The doctor simply looks at the skin all over your body for any changes or abnormalities. If there is any doubt in a doctor's mind about whether or not a skin abnormality is cancerous, he or she will perform a biopsy. For a biopsy, the doctor removes a tiny piece of the affected skin and sends it to a laboratory for examination under a microscope for cancer cells.

Having a thorough skin examination is particularly important for people who are at increased risk of skin cancer such as those who have fair skin that burns easily. You are also at increased risk of skin cancer if you have a family history of the cancer, you have spent an excessive amount of time in the sun and have had severe sunburns, or your skin shows evidence of abnormal changes that could lead to cancer.

Most skin cancers are detected by people themselves. Check your skin regularly for changes (see page 685) and report anything unusual to your doctor immediately. The earlier skin cancer is detected, the better the chance for a cure.

TUBERCULIN SKIN TEST

In the second half of the 20th century, a dramatic drop in the incidence of tuberculosis (TB; see page 510) made doctors hopeful that the disease was nearing extinction in the US. But a resurgence in the incidence of this highly contagious respiratory infection began in the late 1980s. New strains of the disease-causing bacterium have developed that are resistant to the standard antibiotics used to treat the infection. These new resistant bacterial strains have produced more complicated and difficult-to-treat forms of the disease.

As a result, doctors recommend testing for people who are at increased risk of TB. High-risk groups include health care professionals and others who are likely to come into contact with infected people; the very young and very old; people who live in group settings such as nursing homes, college dormitories, or homeless shelters; and people whose immune system is weakened by alcohol or drug abuse, cancer, AIDS, or chronic illnesses such as diabetes.

Many doctors recommend that you have a tuberculin skin test as part of a general physical examination and then have the test at periodic intervals, depending on your risk of exposure to the disease. You should definitely be tested for TB if you have a close friend or relative with the infection.

The most common test for TB involves a pinprick injection of a tiny amount of TB bacterium on the skin of your arm. A reaction in the form of swelling and redness at the site indicates you have been exposed to or infected with the bacterium. In this case, further testing (such as a chest X-ray) is done to make an accurate diagnosis and determine treatment. The infection can remain in an inactive state for many years and then suddenly be reactivated.

Women's health care calendar

Following are general guidelines for the tests, procedures, and immunizations your doctor is likely to recommend. Depending on your risk factors, your doctor may suggest that you have some tests more frequently.

PUBERTY TO AGE 17

TEST OR PROCEDURE	WHO NEEDS IT?	HOW OFTEN?
PHYSICAL EXAMINATIONS		
General physical exam (including blood pressure and lifestyle counseling)	Everyone	Every 3 years
Pelvic exam	Girls under 18 who are sexually active, have menstrual problems, abnormal vaginal discharge, or pelvic pain	Every 6 to 12 months
Dental exam	Everyone	Every 6 months
Eye exam	Everyone	Every 2 years
LABORATORY PROCEDURES		
Pap smear	Anyone who has ever been sexually active	Every year
Blood cholesterol	Everyone	Every 5 years (if first test was normal); as recommended by doctor if level is elevated
Tests for sexually transmitted diseases	Anyone who is sexually active	Every 6 to 12 months or as recommended by doctor
Tuberculin skin test	Anyone who is at increased risk (see page 133)	Every year or as recommended by doctor
IMMUNIZATIONS		
Tetanus booster	Everyone	Every 10 years
Diphtheria booster	Everyone	Every 10 years

Women's health care calendar, continued

AGES 18 TO 39

TEST OR PROCEDURE	WHO NEEDS IT?	HOW OFTEN?
PHYSICAL EXAMINATIONS		
General physical exam (including blood pressure and lifestyle counseling)	Everyone	Every 3 years
Pelvic exam	Everyone	Every year
Dental exam	Everyone	Every 6 months
Eye exam	Everyone	Every 1 to 2 years
Breast exam*	Everyone	Every year
Breast self-exam	Everyone	Every month
Skin cancer check	Everyone (particularly those with a family history of skin cancer, heavy exposure to sunlight, or evidence of abnormal skin changes)	Every 3 years
LABORATORY PROCEDURES		
Pap smear	Everyone	Every year
Blood cholesterol	Everyone	Every 5 years (if first test was normal); as recommended by doctor if level is elevated
Tests for sexually transmitted diseases	Anyone who is sexually active	Every 6 to 12 months or as recommended by doctor
Tuberculin skin test	Anyone who is at increased risk (see page 133)	Every year or as recommended by doctor
IMMUNIZATIONS		
Tetanus booster	Everyone	Every 10 years
Diphtheria booster	Everyone	Every 10 years

* Women with a family history of breast cancer (a mother, grandmother, sister, daughter, or aunt with the disease) that was diagnosed before the relative went through menopause should begin having mammograms earlier than 40; talk to your doctor.

Women's health care calendar, continued

AGES 40 TO 60

TEST OR PROCEDURE	WHO NEEDS IT?	HOW OFTEN?
PHYSICAL EXAMINATIONS		
General physical exam (including blood pressure and lifestyle counseling)	Everyone	Every year
Pelvic exam	Everyone	Every year
Dental exam	Everyone	Every 6 months
Eye exam	Everyone	Every year
Breast exam	Everyone	Every year
Breast self-exam	Everyone	Every month
Skin cancer check	Everyone	Every 3 years
Rectal exam	Everyone	Every year
LABORATORY PROCEDURES		
Pap smear	Everyone	Every year
Blood cholesterol	Everyone	Every 3 years (if first test was normal); as recommended by doctor if level is elevated
Mammogram	Everyone	Every 1 to 2 years between 40 and 49; once a year after age 50
Tests for sexually transmitted diseases	Anyone who is sexually active	Every 6 to 12 months or as recommended by doctor
Electrocardiogram (ECG)	Anyone with two or more of the following risk factors for heart disease: family history, smoking, high cholesterol, diabetes, high blood pressure	Every 3 to 5 years
Sigmoidoscopy	Anyone over 50	Every 3 years
Fecal occult-blood test	Everyone	Every year
Tuberculin skin test	Anyone who is at increased risk (see page 133)	Every year or as recommended by doctor
IMMUNIZATIONS		
Tetanus booster	Everyone	Every 10 years
Diphtheria booster	Everyone	Every 10 years

Women's health care calendar, continued

AGES 61 AND OLDER

TEST OR PROCEDURE	WHO NEEDS IT?	HOW OFTEN?
PHYSICAL EXAMINATIONS		
General physical exam (including blood pressure and lifestyle counseling)	Everyone	Every year
Pelvic exam	Everyone	Every year
Dental exam	Everyone	Every 6 months
Eye exam	Everyone	Every year
Hearing exam	Everyone	Every year
Breast exam	Everyone	Every year
Breast self-exam	Everyone	Every month
Skin cancer check	Everyone	Every year
Rectal exam	Everyone	Every year
LABORATORY PROCEDURES		
Pap smear	Everyone	Every year
Blood cholesterol	Everyone	Every year
Mammogram	Everyone	Every year
Electrocardiogram (ECG)	Anyone with two or more of the following risk factors for heart disease: family history, smoking, high cholesterol, diabetes, high blood pressure	Every 3 to 5 years
Sigmoidoscopy	Everyone	Every 3 years
Fecal occult-blood test	Everyone	Every year
Tuberculin skin test	Anyone who is at increased risk (see page 133)	Every year or as recommended by doctor
IMMUNIZATIONS		
Tetanus booster	Everyone	Every 10 years
Diphtheria booster	Everyone	Every 10 years
Pneumococcal pneumonia vaccine	Everyone	Once
Influenza vaccine	Anyone over 65	Every year

Immunizations

Most people associate immunizations against disease with childhood, but adults need to have some vaccinations too, depending on their risk of specific diseases. Don't rely totally on your doctor to remember when you need your next vaccination; keep a record and bring it with you when you see your doctor.

RUBELLA (GERMAN MEASLES)

All women should be tested for immunity to the rubella virus before they get pregnant. A rubella infection during pregnancy can cause serious birth defects in a fetus. A blood test can determine whether or not you need the vaccination (which offers lifetime protection). If you do get vaccinated, you need to use a reliable method of birth control for the next 3 months. Because the vaccine contains altered but live virus particles, there is a slight possibility that the fetus could be affected if the virus crosses the placenta.

TETANUS/ DIPHTHERIA

It is recommended that everyone have the combined vaccination for tetanus and diphtheria every 10 years throughout life. People often associate tetanus with puncture wounds from sharp objects such as rusty nails, but tetanus can also result from a prick by a rose thorn or a scratch in the garden. Any wound that allows entry of the disease-causing organisms, which are often present in soil, can cause a tetanus infection.

Diphtheria is a serious bacterial infection that usually strikes children. As a result of large-scale immunization programs that began in 1922, diphtheria is now extremely rare in the US.

MEASLES

Anyone born after 1956 who has not had measles or been immunized should have the vaccination. Most people born before 1957 have been exposed to the virus and have developed lifelong immunity to it. If you were vaccinated between 1957 and 1967, you may need another vaccination because some of the vaccine used during that time was found to be ineffective. Do not get vaccinated if you are pregnant or planning to become pregnant in the next 3 months. If you do get vaccinated, use birth control for 3 months afterward. There is a slight possibility that the fetus could be affected if the virus crosses the placenta.

HEPATITIS B

Hepatitis B (see page 534) is a virus carried in body fluids, including blood, that can cause severe liver damage. People at risk of infection with the virus include those who are sexually active and those whose sexual partners are intravenous drug abusers. People such as health care workers, whose job brings them into contact with blood, and people who receive frequent blood transfusions are also at risk. It is recommended that all children be vaccinated against hepatitis B.

INFLUENZA

Every year, thousands of people die needlessly because they were not immunized against influenza. An annual flu shot is strongly recommended for people 65 and older, as well as people with heart, liver, or kidney disease, diabetes, AIDS, or any type of lung disorder. The shot is also recommended for health care workers and people who are undergoing treatment for cancer. Even if you are in perfectly good health, you should consider having an annual flu shot. You need to get a flu shot every year because new strains of the influenza virus develop each year.

PNEUMOCOCCAL PNEUMONIA

If you have any of the risk factors for complications from influenza (see above), you should also be vaccinated against a common bacterial form of pneumonia call pneumococcal pneumonia. One vaccination provides lifelong protection. Ask your doctor about being immunized against pneumonia.

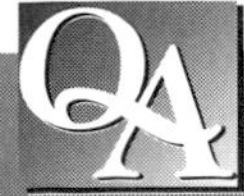

QUESTIONS WOMEN ASK
FLU VACCINES

Q My friend said she got a flu shot and was sick for the next 2 weeks. Can a flu shot make you sick?

A Many people think it is possible to get sick from a flu shot, but this is not true. Years ago some flu vaccines were less pure and caused side effects such as fever and headache. Today, side effects from flu shots are rare. You may experience some soreness at the vaccination site. You should not have a flu shot if you are allergic to eggs because the vaccine is made with eggs.

Q Why are flu shots always given in the fall?

A In the United States, flu season is between December and March but it can start as early as October. It is a good idea to get your flu shot in September because it can take up to 2 weeks for your body to build up immunity to the influenza virus.

Q I'm 35 and healthy. Should I get a flu shot this season?

A There is no reason you should not get a flu shot. Even if you are not in the high-risk groups of people (see page 138) for whom flu shots are strongly recommended, you can benefit by getting the shot and significantly reducing your risk of being sick with the flu. Ask your doctor about having the shot.

Medications

Before your doctor can safely prescribe a new medication, he or she needs to know what other medications you are taking, including over-the-counter vitamins and birth-control pills. Because some prescription drugs can cause problems when they are combined with alcohol or other drugs, make sure you tell your doctor if you drink alcohol or use any illegal drugs.

Make a list of all the medications you are taking (along with their dosages) and bring the list with you when you visit your doctor. This precaution is especially important if you are seeing more than one doctor and more than one doctor is prescribing medication for you. Your doctor may ask you to bring in the medicine bottles themselves to avoid any confusion, especially if you are taking several different medications. For more about misuse of prescription drugs, including sleeping pills, tranquilizers, and pain killers, see page 166.

QUESTIONS TO ASK ABOUT MEDICATION

Learn as much as you can about each medication you are taking. Your doctor or pharmacist can answer any questions you may have. Take notes so you have a written record of the information when you get home. Here are some questions to ask:

- What are the brand name and generic name of the medication?
- Is the drug's generic form as effective as the brand-name form?
- Are there any foods, substances such as alcohol or caffeine, or other medications that I should avoid when taking this medication?
- How will the medication improve my condition?
- How long does it take for the medication to have an effect?
- How often should I take it?
- What time of day should I take it?
- Should I take it with food or on an empty stomach?
- How should the medication be stored?
- Should I save the unused portion for future use?

Safety tips for taking and storing medicines

- Store all medications in the containers in which they come or ask your pharmacist for a convenient travel package. Some people find child-resistant containers difficult to open. If this is the case for you, ask your pharmacist for easy-to-open containers.
- Store medicines away from heat and direct sunlight.
- Do not store medicines in the bathroom medicine cabinet; heat and moisture may cause them to break down.
- Prevent liquid medicines from freezing.
- Keep all medicines out of the reach of children.
- Read labels carefully.
- Keep a chart, marking off when you take your medicine each day. This procedure is especially important if you are taking more than one medication. Or try using a day-of-the-week and time pill organizer.
- Never take medicine in the dark; you want to be sure you know what you're taking.
- Shake all liquid medicines before pouring.
- Drink enough water with pills to swallow them completely and to prevent throat irritation. Your doctor or pharmacist will tell you if you need to drink a larger quantity of liquid with a particular medication.
- If you realize you have taken the wrong medicine or the wrong dosage of a medicine, call your doctor right away.
- Check the expiration dates on medications. When the drugs are too old to use, flush them down the toilet.

- Will I need to have the prescription refilled? If so, how many times?
- Are there any potential side effects of the medication I should be aware of?
- What precautions should I take, such as not driving, when I use the medication?
- I am taking several different medications. Are all of them necessary?

Vision, hearing, and dental examinations

Taking care of your vision and hearing, as well as your dental health, can significantly improve your sense of well-being and the quality of your life. Taking care of minor problems as they come up can help you prevent more serious, potentially permanent problems from developing later.

VISION TESTING

Young adults who do not need corrective lenses and have neither a family history of an inherited form of eye disease such as glaucoma, nor any symptoms of eye disease, should have an eye examination once every 2 to 3 years. If you wear corrective lenses, an examination every 1 to 2 years is usually sufficient. You should have more frequent eye examinations after age 40 because your risk of an eye disorder called glaucoma (see page 649) is greater. If not treated, glaucoma can lead to loss of vision.

An optometrist can test you for corrective lenses, but only an ophthalmologist (a medical doctor trained in all medical and surgical aspects of eye care) can provide complete health care for your eyes. Like your primary care physician, your ophthalmologist will want to know your health history as well as your family health history. Many eye disorders, including glaucoma, can be inherited. If you have diabetes, make sure your ophthalmologist knows about it. It is especially important for you to have regular yearly eye examinations because diabetes can lead to blindness.

A typical eye examination includes the following:

Vision test To test your ability to see at a distance, you will be asked to read a chart several feet away from you with rows of letters of different sizes. You will read first with one eye covered and then the other. To test your near vision, you will be asked to read a text held close to you. Your doctor will ask to see your glasses, if you wear any. He or she will compare the prescription of your glasses with the result of the vision test you just took.

Physical exam The ophthalmologist will look at the overall anatomy of each eye and the surrounding area. He or she will pull your eyelids down and, using a light and magnifying lens, examine the inner surface of your lids. Your eyes will be observed for any signs of abnormalities and to determine if your pupils react normally to light.

Eye muscle tests Your doctor will perform a series of tests to make sure your eyes work together normally. Do both eyes move in coordination in all directions? Do you see the same thing with each eye? A special pair of glasses with a red lens over the right eye and a green lens over the left is often used to determine if the person is using both eyes correctly.

Checking the surface of the eye Using a lighted magnifying instrument called a biomicroscope, the doctor examines the surface of your eyeball. He or she is looking for signs of a cataract (a clouding of the lens that can impair vision) or scratches on the surface of your eyes.

Vision correction The ophthalmologist may dilate your pupils with eye drops. When your pupils are enlarged, it may be easier for the doctor to see light reflected from the inside of your eye; this enables him or her to estimate your vision correction. Using an instrument with a variety of lenses, the doctor can determine the correct prescription for lenses.

Eye pressure test for glaucoma To test for glaucoma, the doctor will do a procedure called tonometry to measure the pressure inside your eye. A buildup of pressure in the eye is an indication of glaucoma. In glaucoma, fluid in the eye does not drain normally, causing pressure to build up. This extra pressure can damage the optic nerve and result in permanent loss of vision. When detected early, glaucoma can be treated with medications, laser surgery, or surgery to preserve vision.

To do the pressure test, the ophthalmologist will anesthetize your eye and apply a bright orange dye to make observations and check the eye pressure. You should have the pressure test regularly, especially if you are over 40, have a family history of glaucoma, or have signs of glaucoma.

HEARING TESTS

Hearing tests are usually not necessary before age 50 unless you notice a decrease in your ability to hear. However, people, such as musicians, who are regularly exposed to loud noises should have regular hearing examinations.

Hearing tests are usually performed by an audiologist, a person trained in the measurement of hearing. During the test, an audiologist evaluates the degree of any hearing loss by testing your ability to hear sounds of different frequencies and volumes. A machine called an audiometer is used to generate sounds of varying frequency and intensity.

An audiologist also determines the cause of a hearing deficiency. One type of hearing loss, called conductive hearing loss, results from insufficient transmission of sound waves through the outer or middle ear. Sensorineural hearing loss is caused by damage to the inner ear, to the acoustic nerve (the nerve that transmits sound signals to the brain), or to hearing centers in the brain. (For more about hearing loss and hearing aids, see page 656.)

Some types of hearing loss are treatable, especially if they are diagnosed at an early stage.

DENTAL EXAMINATIONS

Women have special dental needs. The fluctuation in hormone levels that accompanies puberty, menstruation, pregnancy, breast-feeding, and menopause can cause problems with tissues in the mouth, setting the stage for dental problems. For example, high levels of the hormone progesterone can make your gums more susceptible to the harmful effects of bacteria in your mouth, which can lead to an infection of your gums and the bone supporting your teeth. Gum disease—called gingivitis (see page 662) or, in an advanced stage, periodontitis (see page 663)—is a major cause of tooth loss.

If you already have problems with gum disease, you may find that it gets worse during pregnancy. Many women develop red, tender, or bleeding gums during pregnancy.

Some medications can make you more susceptible to gum disease. For example, birth-control pills cause hormonal changes that make your gums more sensitive to the effects of plaque (soft accumulations on the teeth that can lead to gum disease if not removed). Some drugs that are used to treat diabetes, epilepsy, depression, and heart problems can make you more susceptible to gum disease. Make sure to tell your dentist about any medications you are taking. Depending on the medication, he or she may recommend that you have more frequent checkups.

The hormonal changes that occur during menopause (see page 352) sometimes reduce the production of saliva, causing dryness in the mouth and a decreased sensation of taste. A lack of protective saliva may also lead to gum disease. Decreased estrogen production at menopause can cause bone loss, which may affect the jawbone and, possibly, lead to tooth loss.

To prevent potential problems with your teeth and gums, see your dentist for a checkup and cleaning once every 6 months. To diagnose gum disease, your dentist takes X-rays of your jawbone and probes your gum line for evidence of bacterial infection and other early signs of gum disease. If you have gum disease, your dentist will recommend checkups and cleanings at intervals more frequent than every 6 months.

Along with the diagnosis and treatment of gum disease and tooth decay, the dental checkup will include an examination of your mouth for signs of oral cancer or disorders of the jaw joint (the temporomandibular joint). For reasons that are not understood, temporomandibular disorders (see page 664) are much more common in women than in men.

Make sure you ask your dentist for detailed explanations of all possible treatments. The explanation should include a discussion of expected results, potential complications, the expected longevity of a filling or other restoration, and estimated costs.

Choosing a dentist Here are some helpful tips for choosing a good dentist:

- Call the local or state dental society for a list of dentists practicing in your area.
- Ask friends their opinion of their own dentist.
- If you know a dental specialist such as an orthodontist, a periodontist, or a dental surgeon, ask for the name of a good dentist.
- If you're moving and have been satisfied with your current dentist, ask for a referral to a dentist in your new area.

Keeping your mouth healthy

To avoid dental injuries and tooth decay:

- Brush your teeth twice a day and floss at least once a day.
- Replace your toothbrush every 3 months.
- Have regular dental checkups. All problems can be treated more easily and less expensively in the early stages.
- Have X-ray examinations when your dentist recommends them; X-rays enable your dentist to detect hidden problems at an early stage.
- Eat a balanced diet to avoid tooth decay.
- Do not use your teeth as tools.
- Do not bite on pens or other hard objects or chew ice—such habits can fracture teeth or damage fillings and other restorations.
- Wear a mouth guard when playing sports to protect your teeth from injury.
- Do not smoke or chew tobacco. Tobacco contributes to gum disease and can cause oral cancer.
- Do not drink excessive amounts of alcohol. Heavy alcohol consumption is a risk factor for oral cancer.
- Do not chew vitamin C tablets or suck on acidic citrus fruits such as lemons and limes; the acid can erode tooth enamel.
- Have missing teeth replaced with bridges, dentures, or implants to avoid additional loss and drifting of teeth.

■ Do not rely on television or radio advertisements. The dentists who have paid for the ads are not necessarily the best qualified.

Here are some qualities to look for when evaluating a dentist:

■ A good dentist should listen. A dentist who listens to your concerns or problems is likely to be better at diagnosing and treating mouth disorders and helping you prevent them.

■ At the initial visit, your dentist should ask about your medical history and perform a complete examination of your head and neck, including your teeth, gums, jaw, facial muscles, and the inside of your mouth.

■ A good dentist talks to you about keeping your teeth and gums healthy; he or she does not just take care of problems as they occur.

■ The dentist should tell you beforehand what the cost of a procedure will be. Don't be afraid to ask. You should receive an itemized bill after treatment.

■ A good dentist respects your tolerance for pain and will give you a stronger anesthetic or a sedative pain-relieving medication if you need it.

■ A good dentist allows you to relax your jaw occasionally during a prolonged period of drilling or other treatment.

■ When a restoration such as a filling or crown is finished, your bite should feel natural, your tongue should not catch on the edge of any fillings, and you should be able to floss between your teeth without difficulty.

Living arrangements as you age

As you get older, the kind of home that is right for you may change. As your general health and physical abilities change, you may be faced with important decisions about where to live in your later years.

If you have a serious chronic or terminal illness, you will probably need continuing help and care. Even if you are in relatively good health now, your ability to take care of yourself may change as you get older. You may need to make adjustments in your living situation, such as moving or arranging for nurses or other caregivers to come to your home. Depending on your personal situation and preference, you can choose from numerous options for care and assistance. The best time to make these decisions is long before you actually need to.

Call your local or state department on aging for listings and information about the many different housing options for people who need some kind of assistance in their daily life. The yellow pages of your phone book may also have a listing of social service organizations in your community. It is a good idea to gather as much information as you can about the different housing options available and consider them all, including those described here.

STAYING IN YOUR OWN HOME

Increasing numbers of older people are choosing to stay in their own home. Family, friends, aides from home health care agencies, or volunteers from community organizations provide them with any necessary help. This arrangement allows greater freedom and independence than other types of housing.

Home health care Home health care provides services such as part-time nursing care; physical therapy; occupational therapy; and assistance with daily activities such as dressing, bathing, meal preparation, grocery shopping, light cleaning and laundry, and other household chores. Some nursing and medical services are covered by Medicare, Medicaid, or private health insurance. But other services are usually not covered by any kind of health insurance.

Many communities offer a wide variety of services to older people who live at home but need some assistance with daily tasks. For example, there are agencies that deliver nutritious meals to a person's home. Some organizations serve noon meals at a local site, such as a senior citizen center, which provides people an opportunity to socialize as well as eat a nutritious meal.

In many areas, volunteer programs provide transportation for shopping and other tasks. Some services provide escorts who accompany older people on errands and help them accomplish their tasks. Telephone reassurance programs provide a daily contact for people who live alone and are worried about their safety or have health problems that may require monitoring. With this program, the person checks in with a central switchboard at an agreed-upon time during the day. The community you live in may offer more programs than these or fewer. Check with your local or state department on aging to find out which services are available in your area.

Hospice Hospice programs provide comfort and care to dying people in their own home or sometimes in a special unit in a hospital. The goal of a hospice is to make a person's final days, weeks, or months as comfortable as possible. Different hospice programs provide different levels of care—ranging from sophisticated medical services and successful control of pain and other symptoms to social support, psychological counseling, spiritual counseling, and help with everyday activities. Some hospices offer bereavement counseling to family members after the death of their loved one.

Your doctor will recommend a hospice program that is appropriate to your needs. Most hospice programs will not accept a person until a doctor has certified that his or her illness is terminal and the person's life expectancy is less than 6 months. At this point, the burden of further therapy outweighs the benefits, and medical treatment to try to cure the illness is stopped.

Hospice care is directed to the person and his or her physical and emotional suffering—not to the illness itself. The emphasis is on controlling symptoms, such as intolerable, chronic pain, and helping the person achieve as much

Caring for a loved one at home

If you choose to be the primary caregiver of a member of your family or a close friend, you will probably feel overwhelmed at first or even afraid. The challenge is daunting, particularly if you have a job, family, or other responsibilities. At the same time, you may feel comforted to know that you are doing everything you can for your loved one on a daily basis.

The best way to cope with your new role and to avoid becoming overwhelmed is to get help early. You do not have to do it all yourself. Home health services or hospice programs are good sources of guidance and information. For example, a nurse from a home health service can teach you practical skills, such as how to bathe or dress a person who cannot do so. A nurse can also teach you how to move the person properly to avoid hurting your back. Home health personnel can also share in the day-to-day care. You can hire a private health aide through a home health service or by advertising in your local newspapers. Always ask for references and make sure you call the referring person to get his or her evaluation of the candidate.

If you just need someone who can step in for you every now and then to give you some time to yourself, call local volunteer agencies or your church or synagogue. Many hospice programs also have volunteers who can help you care for your loved one. In many communities, day-care facilities are available for people with degenerative mental conditions, such as Alzheimer's disease (see page 584). Although day-care facilities can vary, most provide transportation to and from the facility, where the person spends the day. Trained staff at the facility engage the person in activities geared to his or her needs.

If your loved one requires considerable care for a prolonged period, you may become exhausted or experience frequent illnesses or depression. You will need to get help for your own needs to avoid harming your health. At some point, it may become necessary to make the decision to move your loved one into an assisted living community or nursing home. For more about being a caregiver, see page 585.

Coping with a disabling illness

Many chronic illnesses, including arthritis or a stroke, can impair your ability to perform activities of daily living, such as bathing, dressing, eating, or walking. Many helpful devices are available to enable you to continue to do things for yourself and remain in your own home. For example, if you have arthritis in your hands, you can obtain special devices to help you open jars and packages and turn handles. If a stroke has left you paralyzed on one side of your body, you can use implements that enable you to do tasks, such as cutting your food, with one hand. A computerized system can help a person in a wheelchair open doors, turn on lights, or control the heat and other aspects of his or her home environment.

If your ability to function independently is impaired, an occupational therapist from a home health agency can evaluate your condition and your home environment and recommend equipment that would be helpful for you. Most states have an assistive technology program that can provide information about the various devices that are available to help people remain independent for as long as possible.

quality of life as possible in his or her final days. In many cases, hospice programs give a person greater control over the dying process and the opportunity to come to accept death as a natural part of life. Hospice care is usually covered by Medicare, Medicaid, and some private health insurance plans.

OTHER HOUSING OPTIONS

When you are looking for housing specifically designed for older people, it is important to carefully evaluate both the services provided and the cost, which can vary greatly. It is also important to plan ahead. Many facilities, especially good ones, have long waiting lists and you may have to wait months or years for available housing.

Apartment complexes or retirement communities that offer continuing care or assisted living can provide some help with cooking, housework, personal care (such as dressing or bathing), or transportation. These types of living arrangements make it possible for an older person who does not have a serious illness to live independently. They also provide access to a higher level of medical care should it become necessary.

Continuing care retirement communities Continuing care retirement communities offer a complete range of housing and care in one setting—from independent living to 24-hour nursing care. To join a continuing care community, you must be healthy. You pay a substantial entrance fee and then monthly rent and medical fees. You have your own apartment or townhouse within the community and may receive a specified number of meals, a limited amount of personal and nursing care, and cleaning services, according to your needs and desires. Many communities have areas set aside for recreational and social activities and a library, beauty shop, and other conveniences.

As your health needs fluctuate, you may move between your apartment or townhouse, an assisted living facility (see below), or a nursing home within the complex or nearby. In some places, the monthly fee for living in the nursing home is the same as that for your apartment.

Assisted living facilities An assisted living facility (sometimes called sheltered care) is recommended for a person who needs help with personal care, such as dressing and bathing, but does not require 24-hour nursing care. This arrangement enhances the person's independence, often delaying his or her need for institutional care. Assisted living facilities are also called personal care homes, residential care facilities, or adult care homes.

An assisted living facility that is not part of a continuing care community does not require an entrance fee, but the monthly fee, which can vary greatly from one complex to another, may be higher than that of a continuing care community. Many assisted living facilities provide meals and laundry and recreational and transportation services. Assisted living facilities may not have an

A PRACTICAL GUIDE TO SUCCESSFUL AGING

AGING IS A NATURAL part of life that you can anticipate with enthusiasm and optimism. Growing older may present some challenges to your health, but there are things you can do that will enable you to live your later years with vigor and in good health.

Although many of the symptoms associated with aging are partly determined by your genes, they are also influenced by lifestyle choices that you make. Healthy habits that you adopt early in your life can help postpone or reduce many of the symptoms of aging, and can profoundly influence the length and quality of your life.

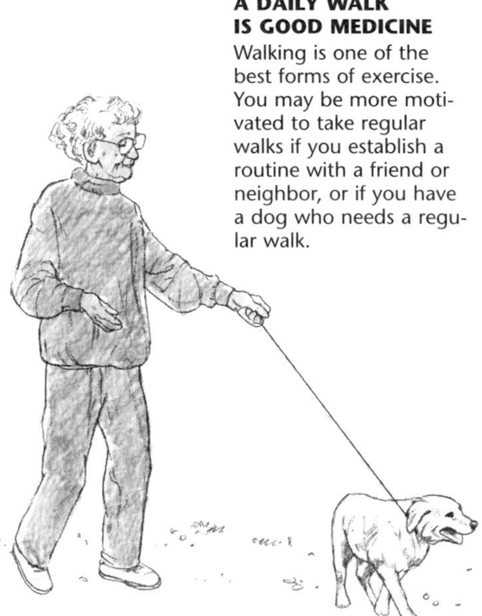

A DAILY WALK IS GOOD MEDICINE
Walking is one of the best forms of exercise. You may be more motivated to take regular walks if you establish a routine with a friend or neighbor, or if you have a dog who needs a regular walk.

Staying vigorous at any age

No matter what your age, you can live longer and better if you exercise regularly, do not smoke, eat a diet low in fat and high in fruits, vegetables, and whole grains, and see your doctor for regular examinations and tests (see page 126).

- **Preserve your muscles** From age 20 to 70, people lose about 30 percent of their total muscle, resulting in loss of strength. No matter what your age or physical condition, you can maintain or regain strength through exercise.

- **Burn more calories** Smaller muscles and an inactive lifestyle can slow the rate at which an older person burns calories. Regular exercise can build muscle and increase the burning of calories.

- **Keep your body fat low** Most older people have a greater percentage of fat on their body, even if their weight has not increased. Fat around the abdomen is especially dangerous (see page 97). A low-fat diet and regular exercise can reduce body fat.

- **Exercise aerobically** Your body delivers oxygen to your muscles less efficiently as you age. Regular aerobic exercise, such as walking, boosts your aerobic capacity.

- **Prevent diabetes** Your risk of developing type II diabetes (see page 621) increases with age. You can reduce this risk by maintaining a healthy weight and exercising regularly.

- **Watch your cholesterol level** Cholesterol levels tend to worsen with age. Know your cholesterol profile (see page 131). Following a low-fat diet, maintaining a healthy weight, exercising regularly, and not smoking will improve your cholesterol profile and reduce your risk of heart disease.

- **Control your blood pressure** Most people experience a steady increase in blood pressure as they age. To lower your blood pressure (see page 481), exercise regularly, maintain a healthy weight, eat a low-salt diet, and take medication if your doctor prescribes it.

- **Keep your bones strong** To help prevent your bones from thinning after menopause, get 1,000 to 1,500 milligrams of calcium daily (see page 58) and do weight-bearing exercises (see page 84). Consider hormone replacement therapy at menopause.

Keeping your memory sharp

Memory loss is not necessarily a part of aging. While the ability to retrieve specific information from memory slows to some degree, older people often benefit from the many strategies they've developed over the years for keeping track of details and jogging their memory.

Many older people panic when they forget things; they assume they have Alzheimer's disease (see page 584). It is normal to forget where you put your car keys; it may be a sign of Alzheimer's disease if you forget what the car keys are for. Most people in their 80s do not have Alzheimer's disease. Some other, less serious problems—including an underactive thyroid gland, reduced levels of the hormone estrogen, anxiety, fatigue, stress, mild depression, as well as some medications and excessive use of alcohol—may cause varying degrees of memory loss. Talk to your doctor if you notice a significant change in your ability to remember.

Here are some tips for keeping your memory sharp:

- Make mental pictures of the object, person, place, or number you want to remember.
- When you want to concentrate, eliminate distracting background noise, voices, television, or radio.
- Restate in conversation the information you want to retain.
- Keep lists and write things on your calendar; refer to them often.
- Remember that it's OK to forget and that you probably forgot a lot of things when you were younger too.
- Have your hearing checked regularly and get a hearing aid if you need one. You can't remember what you don't hear.

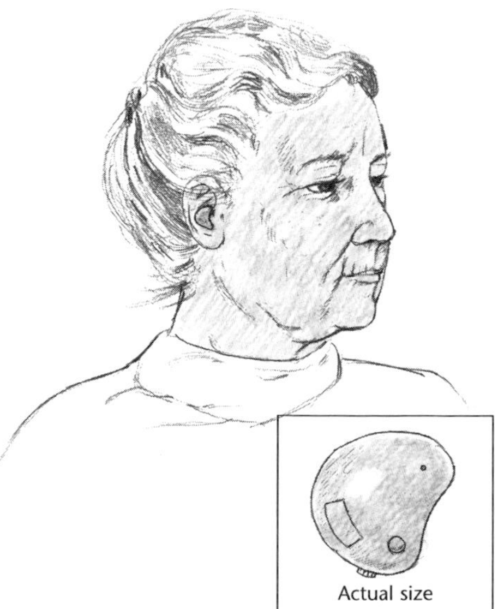

Actual size

HEARING AIDS: SMALLER THAN YOU THINK

Don't put off a hearing test or the chance to improve your ability to hear because you think a hearing aid will be unattractive. Hearing aids today are smaller and less conspicuous than they used to be. The most common type of hearing aid fits into the outer ear. Another type fits inside the ear canal, almost completely out of sight. Hearing aids are custom-made to precisely fit in your ear. For more about hearing tests and hearing aids, see page 656.

Taking care of your emotional health

Here are some practical steps you can take to help make your life happier and more rewarding, now and in the years to come.

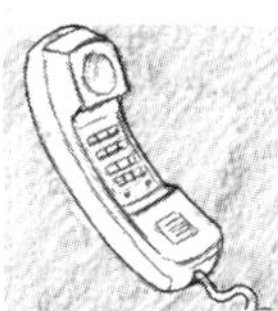

Maintain relationships At all ages, mental health is enhanced by forging ties with others. Work at maintaining relationships with your family and friends, and take the initiative to meet new people. Volunteer, join groups and clubs, and take classes.

Plan your lifestyle Do you plan to move away when you retire or stay near your family? Will you work part time? Do you plan to travel extensively? Think about your priorities now and make decisions with clear goals in mind.

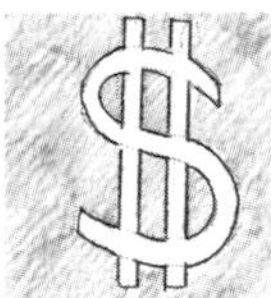

Plan your finances When you live on a fixed income, finances can affect every aspect of your life. If you have complicated financial matters, seek qualified professional help. (Ask a trusted friend for a recommendation.) Even if you are in perfect health, write a will to ensure that your assets will go where you want them to after your death.

Expand your interests Don't give up the interests and activities you already have, and try to develop new ones. Divide your time between solitary activities—such as reading or playing the piano—and group activities—such as a water aerobics class. Engaging in intellectually stimulating activities may delay the onset of Alzheimer's disease.

Be prepared for change No matter how much you plan ahead, unexpected developments can change your life. Consider that while change is often stressful, it can also bring new experiences and make your life more interesting.

on-site nursing home, but they are usually affiliated with a nearby nursing home that charges more than you are paying for your apartment. Be sure you are guaranteed access to the nursing home should it become necessary.

In both continuing care and assisted living communities, monthly fees may rise each year. Some communities specify a maximum annual increase, or cap, in the contract; most do not. In addition, some people may require more care than is provided in the monthly fee. The hourly fee for additional services may be high. Residents may have to hire private health aides when they begin to need more in-home care.

Evaluating community living arrangements When choosing a continuing care or assisted living community, look carefully at the contracts before making a decision. It is a good idea to have a lawyer review the contracts. Consider the following questions when you are making your decision:

- What are the entrance fees or purchase prices for the community? Are they fully or partially refundable if you have to leave the community?
- After your death, does some or all of the entrance fee or purchase price revert to your estate?
- Does the community require that you carry supplemental private health insurance (in addition to Medicare)? If so, how much do you need?
- What services does the monthly fee include? How many hours of service are provided in the fee before you are charged an hourly rate?
- How often and by how much can the monthly fee be increased? Look for increases that are no more frequent than yearly and that have an upper limit.
- What happens if you run out of money? Some communities guarantee that you will not be asked to move out.
- If access to a nursing home is provided, will you and your doctor have the authority to decide when you should transfer to it, or does some group within the community decide? What kinds of medical conditions or behaviors can be handled before transfer to a nursing home is deemed necessary?
- If you or your spouse is transferred to an on-site nursing home while one of you remains in the apartment, will your monthly fee cover both expenses?
- Will the community's transportation service take you to places you need to go (such as your doctor's office), or will it go to only a limited number of places or a limited number of miles?

Nursing homes A nursing home, also called a skilled nursing facility, provides around-the-clock nursing care and supervision to people who require it. Some people stay for a short time in a nursing home while they recover from a serious illness; others live there permanently. If you are looking for a nursing home for a loved one who is mentally sound, make sure to include him or her in every step of the process. Pay close attention to his or her needs and preferences.

Nursing homes can range in quality from excellent to poor. Good nursing homes often have a long waiting list, so begin the process of looking for a nursing home early—long before you or your loved one actually needs to move in. Ask for recommendations from family members and friends, as well as from local social service agencies, doctors, senior citizen administrators, and community or church groups. A good nursing home should have well-trained aides and should give residents some privacy and the freedom to express their individuality in their room and belongings.

When evaluating a nursing home, make an appointment with the home's administrator or director of nursing and social services. Ask about the home's history, philosophy, and licensing. Stay for a couple of hours and see as much of the facility as you can. Stay through a meal so you can evaluate the food. Make an unannounced visit on another day to make sure the home is just as nice when you are not expected. Every nursing home is required to have a document called the residents' bill of rights; ask to see it because it is likely to raise some issues you may not have considered.

Evaluating a nursing home Here are some questions to consider when you are looking for a good nursing home:

- What services are included in the contract, and what will be extra? Most homes have basic rates that do not cover doctors' fees, medication, physical therapy, diagnostic tests, or personal services.
- Does the home accept people with

Medicare or Medicaid? Medicare pays only a fraction of the cost of a nursing home, usually for up to 100 days. Medicaid pays the long-term expenses of people who have little or no money, but you become eligible for Medicaid only after your own funds are depleted.

- Will you need to switch from your own doctor to a doctor associated with the nursing home? How often can you see the doctor, and what steps will be taken if an urgent medical problem arises? Ask about guidelines for cardiopulmonary resuscitation (CPR; see page 471) and other lifesaving techniques that may be necessary in an emergency, which you may or may not want.
- Does the home require you to sign over your assets or your social security or Medicare checks or put your money into an escrow account? Be extremely skeptical of any nursing home that requires this.
- What is the typical resident in the home like? You may prefer to live among people of the same religious, ethnic, or educational background so you have something in common.
- What kinds of medical conditions or disorders do residents have? You may feel more comfortable in a place where residents have disorders similar to yours. The nursing home may have specific areas or floors set aside for people who require various levels of care.
- Does the building look and smell clean? Is it neat and uncrowded? Are there nice touches that help make it feel like a home?
- Does the home have safety features, such as handrails, grab bars, and emergency call buttons in the bedrooms and bathrooms?
- Do the residents like the staff, the food, and the facilities? Would they recommend it to a friend? Make contact with as many residents as possible and ask questions.
- What kinds of activities and classes are available to the residents? Are there any trips away from the home? How often?

Alternative living arrangements A number of other living arrangements are available for people who need some help with daily tasks but do not require full-time nursing care. In one alternative living arrangement, you can choose to remain in your own home and share it with another person. An agency can help

Insurance for long-term care

As increasing numbers of older people live in nursing homes at some time in their life, the cost of such care becomes a serious consideration for many families. Currently, government programs pay only a fraction of the costs of long-term care—whether it is provided in a nursing home, in your own home, or in a community living arrangement. You must pay for the rest.

Many private insurance companies now offer long-term care insurance for nursing home care. Some plans also provide coverage for in-home care. The premiums are high and, like any insurance policy, you must study the plan carefully to be sure you understand what is covered and what the limitations are. You will find big differences in the dollar benefits, in definitions of covered facilities, in the length of time benefits are paid, and in eligibility for benefits.

The age at which you buy long-term care insurance is an important factor in whether or not the policy pays off for you. The premiums increase sharply at about age 60, but most people do not think about purchasing long-term care insurance until they are 65 or older. If you are considering purchasing a long-term care insurance policy, read consumer magazines that compare specific policies, work with a salesperson you trust, or ask friends with similar policies for advice.

Each state has its own laws and regulations governing all types of insurance. State departments of insurance are responsible for enforcing these laws and providing information about insurance and companies that sell insurance. Your local agency on aging can also give you information about insurance. Ask for the toll-free number of your state's insurance counseling service, which can answer your questions and direct you to other sources of help.

you find someone to live with you who can either pay full rent or partial rent in addition to providing you assistance with housekeeping or other services. Or you may chose to move into a group home in which several older people live together, with or without a housekeeper. Each person has a private room and, possibly, a private bathroom but they share common areas, such as the kitchen, dining room, and living room. These arrangements offer opportunities for socializing that many older people who live alone do not have. If you are interested in learning about these options and finding out how you can participate, contact your local agency on aging or a private agency for the elderly.

CHAPTER 5

Avoiding risky behavior

Contents

Every day you make choices that can lead to a lifetime of good health, or that can ultimately put your health or your life at risk. These lifestyle choices may involve risky behaviors—such as smoking cigarettes and drinking excessively—that adversely affect your health. Making choices that safeguard your health can do more for your quality of life than the most advanced medical technology.

Most disability and chronic diseases that women experience are the direct consequence of their behavior and lifestyle—choices they make throughout their life. Along with a poor diet and lack of exercise, risky behaviors (such as cigarette smoking, abuse of alcohol and other drugs, unsafe sexual practices, and failure to wear seat belts) contribute substantially to all 10 of the leading causes of death among American women—including heart disease, cancer, diabetes, and death and disability resulting from injury, violence, and suicide. Half of these deaths and most chronic disorders could be prevented if people changed their harmful behaviors.

Smoking

Tobacco is the most widely abused drug in the US. It is extremely addictive. Each year more than 300,000 Americans die of smoking-related illnesses, including lung cancer, emphysema, and heart disease—and all of those deaths are entirely preventable. If you smoke, read this section carefully and give some real thought to quitting. If you have children, make sure they understand that smoking cigarettes is a deadly habit.

Although the total number of people who smoke is declining, the decline is slower among women than men. Women are starting to smoke at increasingly younger ages. Most start before age 18; nearly all start before 21. Teenage girls are the only group showing a significant increase in smoking.

Underestimating the risks from smoking can be fatal. Learning how to quit can save your life.

HEALTH EFFECTS OF SMOKING

With an increase in the number of women who smoke has come a dramatic increase in lung cancer deaths. In 1986, lung cancer surpassed breast cancer as the leading cancer killer of American women. It now appears that women who smoke heavily are more than twice as likely to develop lung cancer as men who smoke heavily. Doctors believe that women may be more susceptible to lung cancer because their lungs are generally smaller than men's and, therefore, they may be getting a more concentrated dose of tobacco smoke at the same level of smoking. Smoking also plays a role in the development of other forms of cancer, including cancers of the cervix, larynx, oral cavity, esophagus, pancreas, and bladder.

Smoking is a major risk factor for the most common cause of death in American women over 50—heart disease. Women between 30 and 55 who smoke a pack of cigarettes or more a day are five times more likely to die of a heart attack than nonsmokers. Women over 35 who smoke and use birth-control pills (see page 156) increase their risk of heart attack still more.

Smoking contributes to heart disease by lowering the level of high-density lipoprotein (HDL), the "good" cholesterol in the blood that helps protect against heart disease. The female hormone estrogen also provides protection against heart disease. Because smoking lowers the level of estrogen, women smokers tend to go through menopause 1 to 2 years earlier than nonsmokers. Lack of estrogen and early menopause increase the risk of heart disease in smokers. Because estrogen also keeps bones strong, smokers face a greater risk of developing the bone-thinning disorder osteoporosis (see page 552).

Smoking causes a number of respiratory disorders that range from such infections as influenza, pneumonia, and bronchitis to emphysema and declining lung function.

If you are a smoker, consider these facts:

- If you have a persistent cough, tire easily, are short of breath, or have problems sleeping, you are experiencing the health effects of smoking.

- You are at greater risk of the bone-thinning disorder osteoporosis because smoking interferes with the formation of new bone tissue. Osteoporosis increases your risk of debilitating bone fractures.
- You are likely to go through menopause an average of 1 to 2 years earlier than a nonsmoker.
- Your skin will wrinkle prematurely, making you look older than you are.
- Smoking contributes to heart disease, lung cancer and other cancers, narrowing of the blood vessels in the legs, and numerous respiratory disorders, including emphysema and bronchitis, pneumonia, and other infections.
- If you get cancer, you are more likely than a nonsmoker to have a recurrence of the cancer after treatment.
- It's never too late to quit. Even long-term smokers affected by smoking-related diseases benefit from quitting.

WHAT MAKES TOBACCO SMOKE DANGEROUS?

Tobacco smoke contains at least 47 substances that are linked to cancer. These substances are quickly absorbed by the lungs and transported to all parts of the body through the bloodstream. Here is a short list of some of the most dangerous components of tobacco smoke.

Nicotine Nicotine is a chemical that occurs naturally in the tobacco leaf. Nicotine is a powerful addictive substance because it can cause both physical and psychological dependence. The most unusual characteristic of nicotine is its ability to act as both a stimulant and a relaxant.

The brain is especially sensitive to nicotine. The chemical provides a "hit" as soon as it reaches your brain, triggering a wide range of responses throughout your body.

Nicotine affects your brain less than 6 seconds after you inhale. It triggers the release of stress hormones (such as adrenaline) which raise your heart rate and blood pressure and constrict your small blood vessels. Nicotine can have a stimulating effect on mood, ability to concentrate, learning, and performance. When the nicotine level drops and the stimulation subsides, a smoker reaches for another cigarette to regain that

Some good reasons to give up smoking

The health-related reasons for quitting smoking are compelling:

- Your body immediately begins to repair itself. Your circulation improves. The small blood vessels expand, bringing more blood to your brain and other tissues. The tiny, hairlike cilia in your lungs grow back, improving your lungs' ability to filter out impurities and reducing your risk of infection.
- If you quit before 50, your risk of dying in the next 15 years is half that of people who continue to smoke.
- After 1 year of not smoking, your risk of heart disease is cut in half. After 15 years, your risk is similar to that of people who have never smoked.
- Your risk of developing lung cancer is cut in half 10 years after quitting and continues to decline with each additional year.
- Former smokers have fewer days of illness, fewer health problems, and reduced rates of bronchitis and pneumonia.
- Your risk of stroke is reduced to normal levels within 2 to 4 years of quitting.
- If you quit before getting pregnant or during the first 3 months of pregnancy, your risk of giving birth to a baby with low birth weight is reduced to that of a nonsmoking woman.

In addition to reducing your risk of heart disease, stroke, and various cancers, quitting smoking can improve your life in a number of ways, including the following:

- Your physical stamina will improve.
- Your sense of taste and smell will improve.
- You will save money usually spent on cigarettes.
- Your persistent cough will go away.
- You won't have dangerous secondhand smoke, a stale smell, or messy ashtrays in your home or work environment.
- You will avoid the social conflict that arises when you smoke in public places.
- You will be less likely to wrinkle prematurely and look older than your age.
- You will no longer have "nicotine breath"; smelly hands, hair, and clothes; or yellow teeth.

heightened state. Nicotine can also enhance the brain activity pattern associated with relaxation and stimulate the release of endorphins, the body's natural tranquilizers.

Carbon monoxide Carbon monoxide is a deadly, odorless gas present in cigarette smoke. Carbon monoxide displaces the oxygen molecules in red blood cells, making oxygen less available to the heart, brain, muscles, and all the other organs. It also damages the lining of arteries. As a result, the heart must pump harder to deliver a sufficient amount of oxygen to cells—one reason smokers become out of breath faster than nonsmokers. Carbon monoxide's harmful effects are partly responsible for smokers' dramatically increased risk of having a heart attack and dying of it.

Hydrogen cyanide Hydrogen cyanide is a poisonous gas found in cigarette smoke. It slows down the motion of microscopic hairlike projections in the lungs called cilia that sweep out foreign particles. When the cilia are not working properly, a smoker is more susceptible to respiratory infections.

Tars The small particles of tar that escape even from filtered cigarettes also destroy the cleansing action of cilia in the lungs and make the lungs more susceptible to respiratory infections. Smokers have a significantly higher incidence of bronchitis, influenza, emphysema, and sinus conditions than nonsmokers.

Nitrosamines Precisely which of the many harmful substances found in tobacco smoke cause cancer has not been

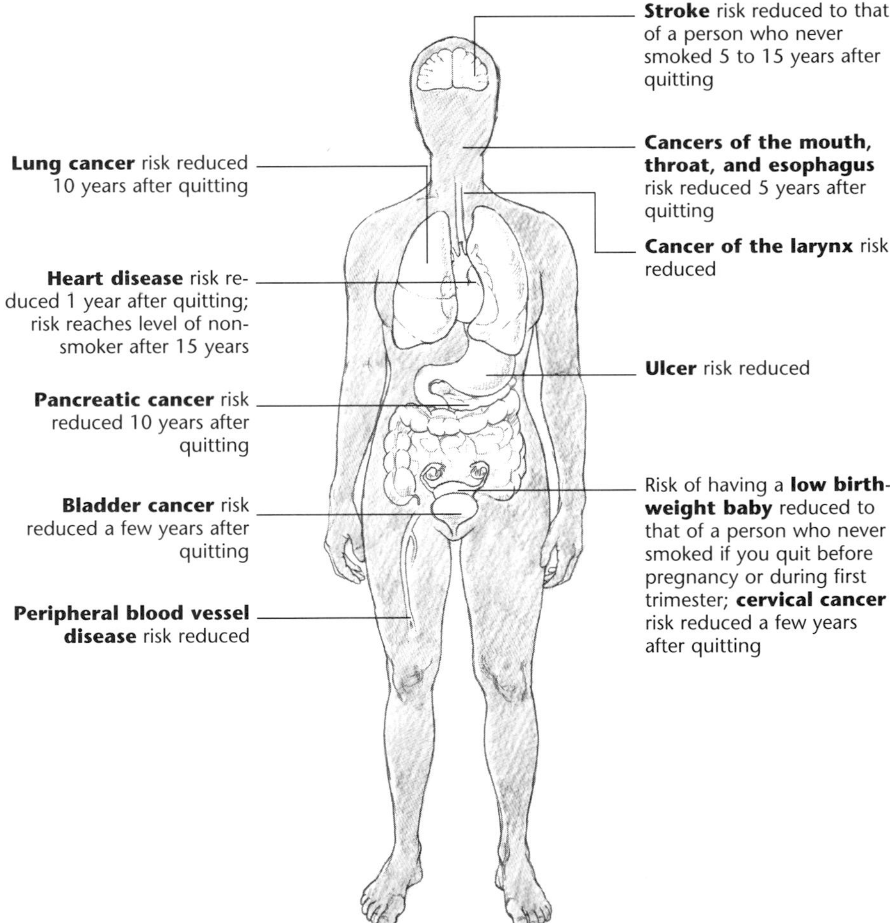

THE BENEFITS OF QUITTING SMOKING
It doesn't take long before the damaging effects of smoking begin to reverse themselves. Even people who have been smoking for years can benefit greatly from quitting.

established. But eight different nitrosamines, chemicals that are known to cause cancer in animals, are the most likely culprits. The high percentage (85 percent) of people with lung cancer who are longtime smokers offers overwhelming proof of a direct connection between smoking and lung cancer.

SECONDHAND SMOKE

Even if you have never smoked a cigarette, several years of breathing in smoke from someone else's cigarette can threaten your health. Exposure to this so-called secondhand, or passive, smoke is a significant preventable cause of heart disease, stroke, lung cancer, and respiratory infections.

Two different types of smoke enter the air when a person smokes—that which he or she exhales and the more dangerous type of smoke that comes directly from the cigarette. This second type, which comprises most of the smoke in a smoke-filled room, has a higher concentration of some of the most harmful compounds of tobacco smoke. If exposed to secondhand smoke over a period of several years, a nonsmoker may experience many of the same health problems that smokers do.

Secondhand smoke is especially harmful to infants and young children. Smoking by parents can worsen the chronic lung disorder asthma (see page 635) in children and even trigger asthma attacks. Children without asthma whose parents smoke have far more respiratory illnesses—including coughs, colds, middle ear infections, pneumonia, and bronchitis—than children of parents who do not smoke. The more a parent smokes, the more respiratory infections his or her child has.

TEENS AND SMOKING

Nearly one out of three American women between the ages of 18 and 44 is a smoker. Tobacco industry advertising targets teenagers to encourage them to take up smoking. The advertisements promise teens that smoking will make them thin, successful, glamorous, independent, and attractive. Many young women are already worried about their weight and obsessed with being thin; many teen smokers say they smoke to help control their weight.

For teenagers, the harmful effects of smoking may seem to lie in the distant future. But smoking at any age begins the damaging path toward heart disease, lung cancer, emphysema, and other smoking-related illnesses. If you start smoking as a teenager, you are five times more likely than a nonsmoker to have a heart attack in your 30s or 40s.

Most teenagers think that they can quit easily any time they want. But they are underestimating the powerful addictive hold of nicotine. Nearly all long-term smokers became addicted to cigarettes when they were teens or young adults. Four out of five teenagers who smoke say they have tried to quit at least once and failed. Keep trying; most long-term quitters make several attempts before they succeed.

SMOKING AND PREGNANCY

Smoking during pregnancy narrows the blood vessels in the placenta, reducing the amount of nutrients such as oxygen and sugar that the fetus gets. This lack of nutrients interferes with the fetus's normal development, increasing the risk of miscarriage, bleeding during pregnancy, premature birth, premature separation of the placenta, stillbirth, and low birth weight. Babies with a low birth weight are more likely to die in infancy than are babies of normal weight. The more a woman smokes, the lower the average birth weight of her baby. Smoking during pregnancy accounts for up to 14 percent of premature births.

The long-term health effects on children of smokers include delayed physical growth and intellectual and emotional development. Their lungs may not develop fully, which may increase their risk of frequent respiratory infections during childhood. Children of women who smoked two packs a day during pregnancy are twice as likely as the children of nonsmoking women to have significant behavior problems.

The best time to quit smoking is before you get pregnant. But quitting at any time during your pregnancy can provide benefits to your baby. Babies of women who quit smoking before they get pregnant have the same average birth weight as do babies of women who never smoked. Even infants of women who quit later in pregnancy, up to the eighth month, have a higher birth weight than infants of women who smoke throughout their pregnancy. (For more about smoking during pregnancy, see page 413.)

GIVING UP CIGARETTES

Quitting smoking is the single most important step you can take to improve your health and the quality of your life and to live longer. Even if you have been smoking for many years, it is never too late to improve your health by quitting. The health benefits are immediate and substantial for people of all ages, even those who have smoking-related illnesses.

Most smokers say they want to quit. But for many people, quitting smoking is extremely difficult—primarily because of a powerful physical and psychological addiction to nicotine.

Nicotine is the chemical in tobacco that induces and reinforces a person's desire to smoke. Smokers develop a tolerance to nicotine; that is, they need increasing doses to achieve the desired effect. Eventually, they reach a set number of cigarettes they need each day to feel satisfied. Many smokers who switch to low-nicotine cigarettes end up smoking more cigarettes per day to maintain their usual level of nicotine.

Being addicted to nicotine means that your body gets used to having the substance in it. When you quit smoking, the nicotine is no longer available and your body has to readjust. This chemical readjustment causes withdrawal symptoms. Not every person who stops smoking has the same symptoms. However, most people experience a few of the following symptoms:.

- Craving for cigarettes
- Restlessness
- Anxiety
- Irritability
- Mood changes (including depression)
- Difficulty concentrating
- Change in appetite
- Craving for sweets
- Difficulty sleeping
- Tremors
- Light-headedness
- Drowsiness during the day
- Headaches
- Gastrointestinal discomfort
- Decreased heart rate

Nicotine is usually cleared from your body within a few days after you stop smoking. For most people the symptoms are most intense in the first 1 to 2 days after quitting and usually subside rapidly during the following weeks. Some former smokers continue to have occasional cravings for a cigarette several years after quitting, but the cravings are mild compared to those they have the first week.

Because people become physically addicted to nicotine to varying degrees, knowing how addicted you are can help you decide which approach to quitting smoking is likely to work best for you. If you answer "yes" to any of the following four questions, you may be addicted to nicotine.

- Do you have a cigarette within 30 minutes of waking up in the morning?
- Do you smoke one pack of cigarettes or more each day?
- Do you smoke even when you are so ill that you are in bed most of the day?
- Do you smoke a cigarette with a high tar content (more than 1 milligram)? Check the tar content on your cigarette pack.

If you are physically addicted to nicotine, you might be a good candidate for nicotine substitution therapy to help you quit. Aids such as nicotine patches applied to the skin or nicotine gum (see page 159) can help reduce withdrawal symptoms in people who have a strong physical addiction. Talk to your doctor;

Smoking and the birth-control pill

Women over 35 who smoke more than half a pack of cigarettes a day should not use birth-control pills (also called oral contraceptives). Taking birth-control pills alone does not increase your risk of heart disease, but combining them with smoking can increase the risk tenfold if you are over 35. The combination of cigarette smoking and the hormones contained in birth-control pills increases the risk of the formation of dangerous blood clots. These clots are life threatening when they travel to vital areas such as the arteries supplying blood to your heart or brain, where they can cause a heart attack or stroke.

If you want to use the birth-control pill for contraception or are already using the pill, you must stop smoking. If you cannot stop smoking, you need to stop taking birth-control pills.

he or she can give you a prescription for the patch or gum. These aids are most effective when they are combined with a structured program that emphasizes the behaviors you need to change to quit smoking successfully. A structured program helps you understand the triggers that make you reach for a cigarette and teaches you ways to avoid them.

As strong as the physical addiction to nicotine can be, the psychological addiction can be even stronger. It is responsible for the majority of failed attempts to quit. After making it through the physical withdrawal symptoms of quitting, many people cannot resist a long-term, intense craving for cigarettes. The psychological addiction may make it more difficult for many women to quit than for men. Women tend to smoke to help them relax or cope with stress and to relieve feelings of emotional discomfort. They often smoke when they are angry, under stress, lonely, tired, bored, or sad.

Women who smoke usually develop daily routines involving smoking, such as having a morning cup of coffee, talking on the telephone, or meeting with friends during a break at work. Those are often the cues that make you want to smoke after you have quit. For this reason, it is a good idea to change your routine when you quit—for example, give up your morning cup of coffee in the early stages of quitting, limit your time on the telephone with friends (or play with a pencil or sketch while on the phone), or take a walk during your break or lunch hour.

Despite the difficulties, millions of American smokers have quit. Most smokers try to quit three or four times over a period of 5 to 8 years before finally succeeding, so don't be discouraged if your first attempt fails. Try again as soon as possible. If quitting on your own has not worked for you, consider one of the many self-help and group programs offered by organizations such as the American Lung Association, the American Cancer Society, and the American Heart Association. Many hospitals and community centers also offer low-cost programs to help you quit smoking. Ask your doctor for a recommendation.

HOW TO QUIT

If you are a smoker, quitting smoking is the single most important thing you can do for your health. Millions of people have quit smoking on their own—9 out of 10 have done so by stopping "cold turkey." Other people have successfully quit with help and support from a variety of structured methods and programs. Nicotine substitutes (such as the patch and gum), hypnosis, behavior modification, medication, and support groups are all helpful methods.

Plan in advance when you will quit. This is a better approach than impulsively throwing away your cigarettes. If you live with a smoker, quitting together will be easier for both of you. Here are some tips to help get you started:

- Talk with people who have successfully quit smoking. Find out how they overcame difficulties during the process of quitting. Ask them how they felt.
- Pick a day to quit and stick to it. Try to make sure it will not coincide with other stressful events such as a deadline at work. Some people choose to quit during a vacation when they are away from the everyday activities that trigger a craving to smoke.
- Make a list of your reasons for quitting. Make sure to include the health risks you are most afraid of. Place the list on your desk at work or on your refrigerator where you are most likely to see it and think about it.
- Before quitting, keep a record of your smoking habits and routines. Determine which three cigarettes you enjoy the most each day and note where and when you smoke them. Think of something else to do instead of smoking those three cigarettes and try to avoid the triggering situations.
- Begin a moderate exercise program such as walking for at least 20 minutes every day.
- Go on the record. Tell friends and family members that you're quitting and rely on their support. "Going public" can give you extra incentive to keep up your willpower.
- Talk with your doctor. Even a brief conversation about the health effects of smoking can increase your chances of successfully quitting. If you decide that the nicotine patch or gum would be helpful, your doctor can give you a prescription and discuss the proper use of

Tips for controlling your weight when you quit smoking

A major barrier for women who want to give up cigarettes is the fear of gaining weight. Women are more likely than men to use cigarettes as appetite suppressants. You may gain from 6 to 8 pounds when you quit smoking, but focus on the most important goal—giving up cigarettes. Concentrate on quitting smoking and then deal with controlling your weight. Once you have successfully quit, use the self-control you developed for quitting to help you shed those extra pounds.

Here are some tips for helping you avoid weight gain:

- Drink six to eight large glasses of water or low-calorie drinks each day.
- Keep tempting, high-calorie, high-fat foods out of the house.
- Have sugarless gum, hard candy, or low-calorie snacks such as fresh fruit or raw vegetables available for whenever you crave a cigarette.
- Reduce the fat in your diet. Eat low-fat or nonfat versions of salad dressing, yogurt, cheese, and other products.
- When you are finished with a meal, get up and do something; it will keep you from missing that after-a-meal cigarette and from overeating.
- Exercise regularly; walking for 20 minutes or more most days of the week can help you control your weight and relieve stress.

these aids. Never smoke while using a nicotine patch or nicotine gum.

When you quit:

- Get rid of all the cigarettes in your home, in your car, and at work. Eliminate all ashtrays, lighters, and matches.
- Think about your reasons for quitting and do alternative activities at the times you most like to smoke. Walking for a couple of blocks can kill the desire to smoke.
- Remember that any physical symptoms of withdrawal you experience, such as headaches, will last only a week or two. After that, the hardest part is coping with the psychological addiction. Overcoming the uncomfortable feelings and cravings can give you confidence that you have gained control over your life.
- Treat yourself. Eat a good meal, go to a movie, take a long bath. Buy some favorite magazines or some new makeup or cologne. Remind yourself that this is the money you otherwise would have spent on cigarettes.
- Avoid situations in which you know people will be smoking. Sit in the nonsmoking area of restaurants. If you have to go to a function at which people will be smoking, consider ahead of time how you will deal with your craving for a cigarette. As difficult as it is, avoid seeing friends who smoke. The old desire to smoke together may be almost impossible to overcome at this early stage.
- Avoid alcohol. Smoking and drinking often go hand in hand. Alcohol can weaken your willpower too.
- Avoid coffee, at least in the early stages of quitting, if drinking coffee makes you want to have a cigarette.
- Watch your weight by having low-calorie snacks handy at your office and at home. Try not to eat more than usual at meals. If you do gain some weight, it is still healthier than smoking. In fact, you would have to gain as much as 75 pounds to harm your health as much as smoking does.
- Exercise regularly. Regular exercise burns calories and can also help reduce the stress caused by quitting.
- Stick with it. It gets easier each day.

For many people, the craving for a cigarette never goes away completely. Beware of having even one cigarette. Although some people seem to be able to smoke occasionally without it becoming a habit, most people cannot. Having one cigarette usually makes it easier to have another, and then another. Don't get discouraged if you return to smoking after your first attempt to quit. You can always quit one more time. The majority of former smokers tried at least once unsuccessfully before finally quitting for good.

AIDS FOR QUITTING

Some people have difficulty quitting smoking on their own. A variety of methods—including the use of nicotine gum or the nicotine patch, hypnosis, and medication—are available to give you the extra help you may need. Talk to your doctor; he or she can give you advice about finding the technique that will work best for you.

Support groups Participating in a group program to quit smoking can increase your chances of success by providing you with support from other people

A quick fix

When you have an urge for a cigarette, take three deep breaths. Hold the last breath for a few seconds and exhale slowly. This will relax you and help keep you from reaching for that cigarette.

who are also trying to quit. Organizations such as the American Lung Association, the American Cancer Society, and the American Heart Association offer programs for low fees, with trained instructors and an emphasis on health education. Commercial programs are generally more expensive. Although the programs can differ greatly in structure, content, and cost, most consist of a series of classes or regular meetings. The success of the programs also varies greatly, often depending on the skills of the group leader.

Ask your doctor to recommend a program that has been successful for his or her patients, or call a local hospital or branch of the organizations listed above. In looking for a reputable program, consider the following questions:

- Who runs the program? Make sure the group is reputable.
- What is the program's structure? Is it mostly educational? Is it unstructured or does it present a strict plan for quitting? Find a program that fits your needs.
- Does the program provide follow-up sessions in case you start smoking again?
- What are the program's success rates? Find out how many people quit smoking through the program and how many are still not smoking 1 year later.
- How much does the program cost? Although there are many good, inexpensive programs, some people are more motivated if they have made a major financial commitment.
- Does the program use practical and effective techniques? Ask other people who have used a particular program and instructor.

Nicotine patch Nicotine patches, available only by prescription, help reduce the physical symptoms of withdrawal from nicotine. You apply a nicotine-containing patch to a different location on your skin each day. It releases a continuous stream of nicotine through the skin into your bloodstream. Because the patch helps only with the physical dependence on nicotine, it is most effective when combined with a structured behavioral program to help you quit smoking. The doctor who prescribes the patch will instruct you on how to use it and help you develop a plan for quitting.

The patches come in a variety of strengths. Usually, a stronger patch is used for the first 6 weeks and then patches with successively smaller doses of nicotine are used for 2 to 4 weeks each. Some people have mild itching, burning, or redness for a few minutes after they first apply the patch. Some people have insomnia or nightmares. For these people, patches designed to be removed at night may work better. The only dangerous side effect from nicotine patches occurs in people who smoke while they are using the patch. Smoking while using the patch increases your risk of a heart attack by giving you an extra dose of nicotine. Never smoke while using the patch.

Nicotine gum Like the nicotine patch, nicotine gum is available only by prescription and is designed for smokers who are highly physically dependent on nicotine. When you chew the nicotine-containing gum, nicotine is absorbed into your bloodstream through the lining of your mouth. The gum is most effective when combined with a structured program for quitting smoking. Never smoke while using the gum because you could be taking in a harmful level of nicotine.

It can take up to 20 minutes for the nicotine from the gum to be absorbed by your body, so you need to try to anticipate your craving for a cigarette. (Nicotine from a cigarette gets into your body in less than 10 seconds.) The method can help you delay and then control your urge for a cigarette. Chewing the gum longer than 30 minutes can cause nausea and burning in your mouth and throat. Avoid drinking coffee, juices, or carbonated beverages just before and while you are chewing the gum; they can interfere with your body's absorption of the nicotine.

You should not use the gum for longer than 6 months because you can become physically dependent on it. Taper off gradually when you are ready to stop using the gum.

Hypnosis The most common form of hypnosis therapy for quitting smoking uses a technique called self-suggestion. The purpose of self-suggestion is to help a smoker develop a positive, receptive attitude toward giving up cigarettes. A hypnotist teaches you, usually in one or two sessions, to use the technique on your own several times a day. In self-hypnosis, you use motivating suggestions to interrupt and reduce your craving for a cigarette, to envision a healthy life without cigarettes, and to create positive images of yourself. You develop a way to impose confident thinking that will overpower your urge to have a cigarette. Then you practice seeing yourself as a proud, confident, sociable nonsmoker with a healthy body. The positive suggestions are meant to replace the negative attitudes that kept you smoking.

If you are interested in trying hypnosis to help you quit smoking, talk to your doctor about finding a good program. It is important to find a reputable program administered by properly licensed health professionals who are trained in hypnosis techniques.

Alcohol

Because alcohol is so widely available and socially acceptable, it's easy to forget that it is a drug with many harmful physical and psychological effects.

If you have any doubt about your level of alcohol consumption or your ability to control it, consider these questions:

- Has a friend or your spouse or another family member ever expressed concern about your drinking?
- Has such concern annoyed you?
- Do you frequently drink alone?
- Do you drink to relax, relieve stress, overcome shyness, or go to sleep?
- Have you ever felt the need to cut down on your drinking?
- Have you ever felt guilty for drinking?
- Do you ever have a drink first thing in the morning?
- Have you ever missed or been late for work because of a hangover?
- Have you gotten into arguments when you have been drinking?
- Have you ever had an automobile accident or even a close call when you have been drinking?
- Have you sprained an ankle or had other injuries while drinking?
- After drinking, have you had sex with someone you would not have had sex with if you were sober?
- Have you hit your children or spouse while drinking?
- Have you gotten sick when drinking?

If you answered yes to any of these questions, you may be addicted to alcohol. Addiction is a serious risk you take when you begin to drink, even in moderation. If you have any concern at all about your drinking, talk to your doctor.

Heavy drinking by women often goes unnoticed, even by family members and friends. Their doctors are also unlikely to know. Many women who drink do so secretly but regularly at home.

Alcoholism is thought to have a genetic component. If you have a family history of alcoholism, you may be at higher risk of becoming addicted to alcohol than women who do not have a family history of the disease. If you have one or more close blood relatives—parents, aunts, uncles, grandparents, brothers, or sisters—who are or have been addicted to alcohol, you may want to avoid alcohol altogether. (For information about alcohol addiction and treatment, see page 164.)

HEALTH EFFECTS OF DRINKING

Alcohol has a more potent effect on women than it does on men. Drinking the same amount of alcohol, a woman is affected more easily and more quickly than a man. Women experience the health effects of long-term, heavy drinking sooner than men do and they die sooner than men from those effects. In part, this is because women are usually smaller and weigh less than men. But it is also because women's bodies metabolize, or process, alcohol more slowly than men's bodies. Women have lower levels than men of the stomach enzymes that neutralize alcohol before it is absorbed into the bloodstream. As a result, more alcohol goes directly into a woman's bloodstream, raising her blood-alcohol level more quickly than in a man.

Women are more susceptible than men to liver damage from heavy drinking. They show signs of cirrhosis of the liver after only 13 years of heavy drinking compared with 22 years for men. Other alcohol-related health problems—including high blood pressure, obesity, anemia, and malnutrition—also affect women years earlier than men. Heavy drinking may increase a woman's risk of stroke.

Excessive consumption of alcohol increases a woman's risk of the bone-thinning disorder osteoporosis (see page 552). Excessive use of alcohol may damage the cells that make bone and reduce the intestine's ability to absorb calcium, which is essential for strong bones. Heavy alcohol intake may also contribute to poor eating habits, which can prevent a woman from getting sufficient calcium from her diet.

Drinking may also have a harmful effect on a woman's reproductive system. Heavy drinking is linked to infertility, irregular menstrual cycles, and severe premenstrual syndrome (PMS), and may contribute to premature menopause. Alcohol may also be associated with an increased risk of breast cancer. For reasons that are not clear, even moderate drinking (one to two drinks per day) may increase the risk of breast cancer in some women.

Moderate alcohol consumption has been found to reduce a person's risk of heart disease. For women, having one drink a day decreases the buildup of fatty deposits in the arteries that supply blood to the heart and brain. The buildup of fat in arteries is a major risk factor for heart attack and stroke. One drink is usually defined as half an ounce of alcohol—the equivalent of a 12-ounce can of beer, a 5-ounce glass of wine, or 1½ ounces of 80-proof liquor.

Despite the potential protection of moderate drinking against heart disease, no doctor recommends that a nondrinker start drinking to prevent heart disease. Most of the effects of long-term, heavy consumption of alcohol are harmful and the risk of addiction is too great.

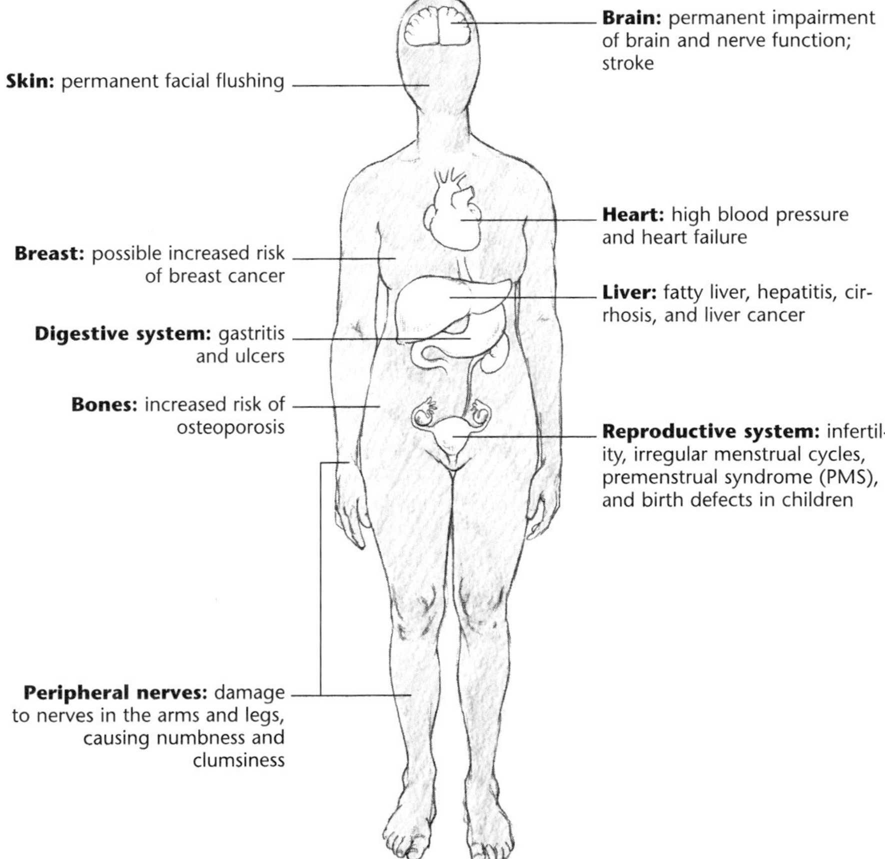

LONG-TERM EFFECTS OF DRINKING
Heavy drinking (more than two drinks a day for women) can cause a number of physical changes and serious health problems.

If you drink, drink wisely

While it's true that a little alcohol is good for you, too much can be devastating. The most sensible course is to limit yourself to one drink a day. Here are some tips for keeping your drinking under control:

- All drinks are not equal. The alcohol content of drinks can differ greatly. The alcohol in beer and wine is more diluted than that in hard liquor—but the average serving of beer or wine produces the same effects as a mixed drink.
- Don't drink on an empty stomach. Eating before drinking helps slow the entry of alcohol into your bloodstream.
- Drink slowly—never have more than one drink per hour.
- Know your capacity and don't exceed it. Don't let friends talk you into drinking more than you know you can handle. The smaller you are, the more affected you will be by alcohol.
- Dilute your drink. Adding lots of ice, water, mixer, or juice to your drink will make it last longer. Add sparkling water and ice to a glass of white wine. Better yet, switch to a mixer by itself after your first drink.
- Alcohol is a drug. Never mix it with over-the-counter or prescription medications. Mixing alcohol with other drugs can cause serious problems.
- Do not drink alone. Try other ways to unwind at the end of a hard day—call a friend, get some exercise, or absorb yourself in a good book.
- Learn to say no. If you don't want to drink, but you want to appear social, order a glass of sparkling water with a twist of lemon or lime. Or order water, juice, or your favorite soft drink. Try nonalcoholic beer, wine, or champagne—they have the same flavor without the alcohol.
- If you think you may have a drinking problem, see page 165 for information about how to seek help.

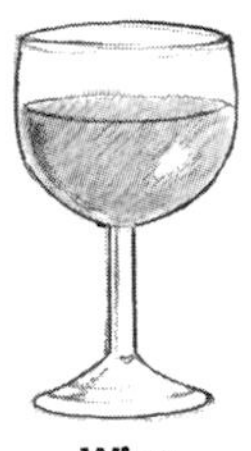
Wine
5 ounces

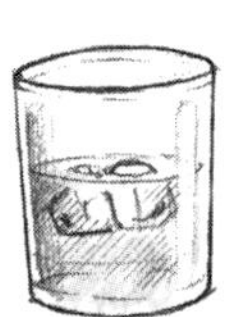
Hard liquor
1½ ounces

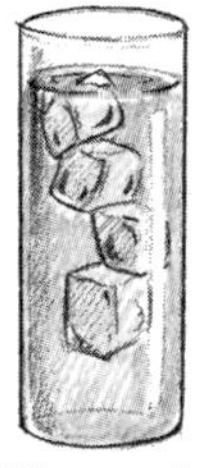
Wine cooler
12 ounces

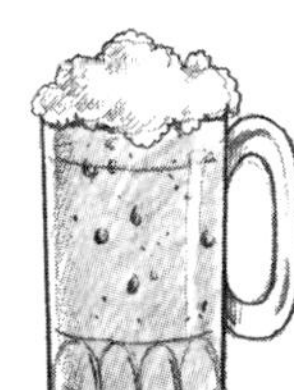
Beer
12 ounces

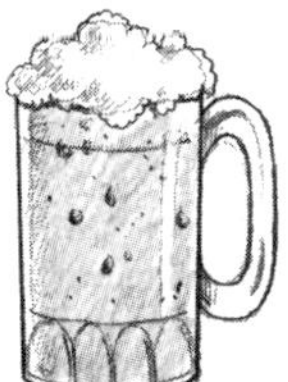
Light beer
12 ounces

DIFFERENT DRINKS: SAME AMOUNT OF ALCOHOL
Ounce for ounce the alcohol content varies widely from one alcoholic beverage to another. A 5-ounce glass of wine contains about the same amount of alcohol as a 12-ounce glass of beer or a mixed drink with 1½ ounces of 80-proof liquor.

DRINKING AND DRIVING

Never drink and drive. And never ride with a driver who has been drinking. More than 40,000 Americans are killed in automobile accidents every year; nearly half of these fatal accidents involve alcohol use. In most states the legal limit for alcohol level in the blood for driving is 0.1 percent. Driving skills begin to deteriorate at a level half that—0.05 percent—or even lower. Most women reach a blood alcohol level of 0.05 percent after having two drinks.

The safest course is not to drink if you are going to drive. Even one drink can

How alcohol affects behavior

The same number of drinks has a stronger effect on a 100-pound woman than on a 175-pound man. Only a few drinks can impair your judgment, making an activity such as driving dangerous.

	WEIGHT (pounds)				BLOOD ALCOHOL (%)	EFFECTS
	100	125	150	175		
DRINKS PER HOUR*	1-2	1-2	2-3	2-3	0.05-0.1†	Euphoria, impaired judgment
	2-4	2-4	3-6	4-7	0.1-0.2	Lack of coordination and judgment
	4-6	5-7	6-9	7-10	0.2-0.3	Staggering, slurring, confusion
	6-8	7-9	>9	>10	0.3-0.4	Unconsciousness, memory lapses

*One drink equals 1½ ounces of 80-proof liquor, 12 ounces of beer, or 5 ounces of wine.
†The legal limit for driving in most states is 0.1 percent.

affect your judgment. If you are out with a group of people, choose a designated driver who agrees not to drink and make sure he or she sticks to the plan. Take a cab or public transportation if you are in a situation in which there is no non-drinking driver. Make sure your children do the same.

ALCOHOL AND OTHER DRUGS

Alcohol can interact with more than 100 different prescription and over-the-counter medications. Alcohol is particularly harmful when combined with drugs that depress the central nervous system, such as sedatives, sleeping pills, anticonvulsants, antidepressants, antianxiety drugs, and some painkillers.

Excessive drinking often goes hand in hand with the abuse of drugs—including cocaine, heroin, sedatives, opiates, hallucinogens (such as LSD), and marijuana. Whether using illegal drugs is the consequence of heavy drinking or whether people who are addicted to alcohol are predisposed to use other drugs as well is not completely understood. The relationship appears to vary from person to person and may result from the interaction of a person's genetic makeup and environmental factors.

If you are having a problem with alcohol and other drugs, talk to your doctor. He or she can recommend a medically supervised substance abuse program to help you overcome your addiction. (For information about treatment for alcohol addiction, see page 164.)

ALCOHOL AND PREGNANCY

Because doctors do not know if there is a minimum safe level of alcohol consumption during pregnancy, they recommend that women avoid alcohol altogether even before they get pregnant.

Drinking alcohol during pregnancy is the most common preventable cause of mental retardation in children. Heavy drinking or even a single episode of heavy drinking during the critical first 3 months of pregnancy may be enough to cause permanent harm to a fetus. All of a fetus's major organs—including the brain and heart—are formed during the first 3 months. A common result of heavy drinking during pregnancy is a collection of serious abnormalities called fetal alcohol syndrome. These abnormalities include mental retardation, growth retardation, and defects of the heart, genitals, bones, and joints. (For more about alcohol and pregnancy, see page 413.)

If you are used to drinking socially, substitute an alcohol-free beer or wine for an alcohol-containing drink on social occasions.

ALCOHOL AND RISKY SEX

Alcohol lowers inhibitions and often causes people to be less restrained in their sexual behavior. Women under the influence of alcohol are more likely to engage in unprotected sex, exposing themselves to the dual risk of an unwanted pregnancy and sexually transmitted diseases, including AIDS.

Limit your alcohol consumption while socializing. Alcohol can impair your judgment to the degree that you might have sex with someone you wouldn't have chosen if you were sober. After drinking, women are less likely to use any protection against pregnancy or sexually transmitted diseases. Always carry your own protection with you in the form of latex or polyurethane male condoms or female condoms, and always use them. Don't be embarrassed about insisting that your partner use a condom—it only takes one exposure to contract a sexually transmitted disease, including AIDS. (For how to use a male condom, see page 173; for how to use a female condom, see page 319.)

OLDER WOMEN AND ALCOHOL

Alcoholism can be hard to detect in older women, in part because they often live alone, but it can be more physically devastating. Excessive drinking late in life usually follows decades of moderate drinking. Alcohol-related medical problems put older people in the hospital more often than heart attacks. Excessive alcohol consumption can impair vision, sexual function, and circulation.

Heavy drinking in older people can also lead to malnutrition because they are less likely to eat a balanced diet. Drinking may be the primary cause of nutritional deficiencies, particularly of vitamin B_{12}, in older people. The effects of a vitamin B_{12} deficiency can range from mild numbness and tingling in the hands and feet to severe degeneration of nerve and brain cells that can result in immobility, dementia, and impaired vision. If you have any of these symptoms, see your doctor.

Liver damage from long-term heavy drinking, including cirrhosis (scarring of the liver), is not reversible. However, stopping drinking can slow or stop the cell-damaging process in the liver.

Another serious alcohol-related problem for older women is the risk of injury from falls. Because older women tend to have thinner, weaker bones, they are at increased risk of disabling fractures. This risk is increased further because older women generally take more prescription medication than younger people. Combining drugs with alcohol can be dangerous.

If you are taking prescription medication and you drink, discuss it with your doctor. He or she can tell you if the medication you are taking causes a reaction when combined with alcohol. Confide in your doctor if you have any doubts about your alcohol intake. He or she may be able to detect alcohol-related health problems, such as liver damage, through a blood test. If necessary, he or she can refer you to an addiction specialist for treatment.

TREATMENT FOR ALCOHOL ADDICTION

The first, and sometimes most difficult, step in getting treatment for alcohol addiction is admitting that you have a problem and that you need help. Alcohol dependence is not a sign of weak character or personal failure; it is a common but serious medical condition that can be managed and controlled.

Once you have accepted that you have a problem with alcohol and need help, talk to your doctor. He or she may be able to recommend treatment options, such as counseling, support groups, or a supervised addiction program, depending on the severity of your addiction. Talk with trusted friends and family members about your concerns and ask for their support in helping you overcome your problem.

Your doctor may refer you to an experienced counselor, who can help you resolve issues that may be contributing to your drinking. Self-help groups such as Alcoholics Anonymous (AA) or support groups run by hospitals are helpful for many people. You may want to participate in a group with women only because women's drinking patterns often differ from those of men. Learning about other women's experiences with drinking and the coping strategies they developed to help them quit can help you sort out your own feelings and develop your own strategies for quitting.

Treatment programs Some people choose to enter a formal substance abuse treatment program—either on an outpatient or an inpatient basis at a hospital or clinic. If you are severely addicted to alcohol, your treatment will start with a detoxification program to end your physical addiction to alcohol. Detoxification is the elimination of alcohol from your system under medically supervised conditions in a hospital. The detoxification process usually takes from 4 to 7 days. Some people experience withdrawal symptoms when they stop drinking, such as nausea, fever, and chills. If you have withdrawal symptoms, you will be given medication to help relieve them. You will also be treated for any medical problems associated with your alcohol consumption, such as high blood pressure, increased blood sugar levels, liver disease, or heart disease. A nutritionist will help you correct any dietary deficiencies that have resulted from your drinking.

Most people do not need to go through the detoxification process when they stop drinking and do not experience withdrawal symptoms. Even though they have been drinking excessively for a long time, they have not become physically addicted to alcohol. For most people who are trying to stop drinking, treatment includes education about addiction and its effects on their life and their health. You are taught ways to avoid the situations (triggers) that cause you to drink.

Support groups and individual counseling are part of most alcohol treatment programs. The goal is to help you realize how much you have to lose by continuing to drink. A good alcohol treatment program will help you evaluate your life, identify the good things that you have, and understand how continuing to drink can interfere with them. The ultimate goal of treatment is to help you abstain from alcohol for the rest of your life.

Some alcohol treatment programs include training in life skills, which helps you develop ways to meet the challenges of your life without alcohol or other

Learning new ways to relieve stress

People who are dependent on alcohol usually need the support of other people to help them recover. But you also can help yourself by developing new ways to deal with the stresses of everyday life. Instead of relying on alcohol to relieve stress, try the following:

- Think about the situations or difficulties that make you want to drink. Develop positive ways to deal with specific problems or sources of stress in your life.
- Often just talking openly with a caring, trusted friend or relative can help ease your stress and make life seem more manageable.
- Regular exercise, a healthy diet, and sufficient sleep will reduce stress, improve your overall health, and boost your self-esteem.

How to get help for a drinking problem

If you suspect that you or someone you love has a drinking problem, seek help immediately. No matter how long you have been drinking, stopping will significantly improve your health and your life. Here is how you can get help:

- Ask your doctor for the name of an internist, psychiatrist, or psychologist who specializes in the treatment of alcohol dependency.
- Call a major hospital and ask if it has an alcohol addiction program. Ask if the hospital provides an evaluation and diagnosis and a recommendation of a program that would be effective for you.
- Call a local mental health center and ask if it provides a program for alcohol addiction.
- Ask friends who successfully quit drinking how they did it.
- Call the local chapter of Alcoholics Anonymous (AA), a support group of alcoholics who meet regularly to help each other stop drinking and stay sober.
- If you are concerned about the drinking of a family member or friend, call the local chapter of Al-Anon, a support group for relatives and friends of alcoholics. Al-Anon provides tips for coping with a relative's drinking problem and for helping him or her stop drinking.

drugs. Once your treatment program is complete, it is a good idea to attend regular meetings of sobriety support groups such as Alcoholics Anonymous (AA) or Rational Recovery. For many people who have a problem with alcohol, these support groups are essential for helping them remain abstinent.

Drug abuse

Tobacco and alcohol are the most commonly abused drugs, but abuse of prescription and illegal drugs by women is a significant problem. While women abuse illegal drugs less than men, they abuse prescription drugs more, and often do so in combination with alcohol.

Many drugs can have a stronger effect on women than on men. Drugs are usually eliminated from a woman's body more slowly than from a man's. Some medications, including sleeping pills and tranquilizers, are stored in fat cells, of which women have more. Therefore, the effects of the drugs may last longer, making them potentially more harmful and their adverse effects worse—especially when combined with alcohol.

ADDICTIVE PRESCRIPTION DRUGS

Prescription drugs that alter a person's mood—including sleeping pills, tranquilizers, and painkillers—are particularly likely to be abused. When people use these drugs for reasons other than those for which they were prescribed, they often take more than was prescribed. Taking the drugs in large doses can lead to physical and psychological addiction.

This does not mean that you should avoid all mood-altering prescription drugs. Together, you and your doctor can weigh the benefits of a particular drug—short-term relief from pain, anxiety, or sleeplessness—against the drug's potential side effects and the risk of addiction. If you are already addicted to alcohol, you are at increased risk of becoming addicted to another substance. The many potentially harmful effects of combining other drugs with alcohol can be life threatening.

If you think you have a problem, talk to your doctor. Describe your symptoms clearly to help him or her differentiate between an emotional problem, such as anxiety, and a physical one. Make sure you understand the reason a particular medication has been prescribed, especially in the case of tranquilizers and other mood-altering drugs. Methods other than taking medication are often more effective in helping people deal with emotional problems over the long term. Your doctor may recommend talking with a psychiatrist or psychologist, or joining a support group of people who are experiencing problems similar to yours.

If you have problems with any of the following medications, talk to your doctor.

Sleeping pills Sleeping pills act by chemically shutting down some areas of the brain. Although they work well at first, after a few days the same amount of the drug may no longer have the same effect. Continually increasing the dose can lead to physical addiction. Sleeping pills can also lead to subtle disorders of thinking and judgment during waking hours, which can be particularly dangerous while driving. People can become psychologically addicted to sleeping pills, continuing to take them long after the drugs have stopped having any sleep-inducing effect. For more about sleeping pills, see page 609.

Tranquilizers Tranquilizers are prescribed to relieve the symptoms of anxiety and stress experienced during emotional crises such as divorce or the death of a loved one. They are meant to be used as a short-term bridge to other forms of therapy such as counseling and support groups. Tranquilizers have an effect on the brain similar to that of alcohol. A small amount brings pleasant feelings and relaxation; larger amounts can cause intoxication. As the effect of the drug wears off, a person often feels nervous and irritable. Over the long term, increasing doses are often needed to attain the same effects, potentially leading to addiction.

If you are or have been addicted to alcohol or other drugs, you should not use tranquilizers because you are at increased risk of becoming addicted to tranquilizers too. Withdrawal from tranquilizers after long-term use can cause symptoms that include dizziness, headaches, restlessness, and upset stomach. For this reason, you may need a doctor's supervision to gradually reduce your usage of the drug before stopping completely. If you think you may be addicted to a prescribed medication, talk to your doctor. He or she will probably refer you to a trained substance abuse counselor.

Painkillers If you are suffering from pain that is so severe it is not helped by over-the-counter pain relievers (analgesics), such as aspirin, your doctor may prescribe stronger painkillers. Many prescription painkillers contain narcotics such as codeine and morphine. Doctors usually prescribe painkillers for a limited amount of time and for short-term conditions, such as pain following surgery. Under normal circumstances, you should not need more refills than your doctor prescribes.

In addition to their pain-relieving effects, these drugs also cause a feeling of relaxation and well-being. It is this mood-enhancing effect to which people can become addicted; they continue taking the drug even after the original symptom of pain is no longer a problem. If you still feel pain after your prescription has run out, your doctor may recommend that you have further testing and reevaluation to find the cause. However, if your condition is improving, your doctor may substitute a milder, less habit-forming painkiller.

You should never borrow prescription medications from your friends. If you or your doctor feels that your dependency on prescription pain relievers has become a problem, your doctor may recommend that you enroll in a specialized treatment program, which can help you withdraw from the drug under medical supervision.

Doctors are sometimes reluctant to prescribe painkillers even to people in severe pain because of the risk of addiction. Many people are reluctant to take painkillers for the same reason, and many mistakenly equate pain with healing. In reality, people who take narcotics to relieve chronic pain rarely become addicted to the medication. Chronic pain can be debilitating; do not hesitate to ask your doctor for medication when you need it.

ILLEGAL DRUGS

Illegal drugs are widespread. For the individual, the price is steep—addiction, emotional and social problems, financial ruin, health risks, involvement with illegal activity, and death. Society also pays a price—each year, thousands of babies are born to women who used drugs during pregnancy. Most people who begin using drugs are unaware of the danger of addiction and the harmful effects of the drugs themselves. The safest course with all illegal drugs is to never try them in the first place.

The most commonly used illegal drugs and their effects are described in the following pages. If you are using any of these drugs—or are addicted—you need to get help. Talk to your doctor; he or she can recommend a drug rehabilitation program that might be helpful for you. (For more about drug addiction and treatment, see page 169.)

Cocaine Cocaine is sold on the street as a fine white powder that is usually sniffed into the nose. More recently, cocaine is being used in a stronger, more addictive form called crack, which is smoked. Cocaine acts as both a stimulant and a local anesthetic (an agent that causes loss of sensation). Cocaine produces a rush of euphoria and energy and can also suppress the appetite. Because its effects wear off quickly, users often feel a strong urge to take another dose shortly after the last one. Regular use often causes nervousness, insomnia, inability to concentrate, fatigue, depression, or anxiety. In some people, cocaine use has been linked to aggression and violence. Cocaine can cause seizures, hallucinations, abnormal heart rhythm, stroke, coma, heart attack, and death.

When a pregnant woman uses cocaine, it can deprive the fetus of oxygen and cause the placenta to bleed, which can be fatal to the fetus. Cocaine use by a pregnant woman can damage the delicate blood vessels of the fetus's brain, causing bleeding into the brain tissue itself. This bleeding can cause severe brain damage in the fetus or, in some cases, death.

Even in women who stop using the drug during the last trimester of pregnancy, cocaine use is associated with premature separation of the placenta from the lining of the uterus and premature birth.

Babies born to women who are addicted to cocaine are at risk of birth defects affecting the spine, such as spina bifida, and birth defects affecting the intestinal tract and bladder. Because cocaine stimulates a fetus's central nervous system, an affected newborn is often unusually irritable and may have seizures.

Heroin Heroin is a white, odorless compound that is derived from opium, a powerful natural narcotic. A narcotic is a drug that dulls the senses, relieves pain, and induces deep sleep. Excessive doses of heroin can lead to convulsions, coma, and death. Injecting small doses of heroin just under the skin or into a vein, or snorting the drug through the nose produces immediate effects that last from 3 to 4 hours.

The complications of heroin addiction are caused by the side effects of the drug itself and the manner in which it is introduced into the body. An overdose of heroin can induce coma, respiratory failure, shock, and convulsions. The injection of heroin into a vein with a used hypodermic needle carries with it the risk of exposure to HIV, the virus that causes AIDS (see page 344), and hepatitis (see page 534), which can also be fatal. Intravenous injections of heroin can also introduce bacteria directly into the bloodstream, potentially causing serious infections of the heart and heart valves (called endocarditis), tetanus, and lung abscesses.

Heroin use during pregnancy increases the risk of premature birth. Pregnant women who are addicted to heroin have babies who are also addicted to the drug. The babies experience withdrawal symptoms such as irritability, trembling, and seizures in the first few days of life. These babies also tend to gain weight slowly, which further compromises their health.

While withdrawal symptoms from heroin addiction are severe and difficult to endure, many people have overcome their powerful addiction. Some drug rehabilitation programs rely on the use of a drug called methadone to treat heroin addiction and withdrawal symptoms. Methadone blocks the effects of heroin. Although methadone is also addictive, it does not produce the feeling of euphoria that heroin does.

Marijuana Marijuana, a drug that comes from the leaves of the hemp plant, is usually smoked. It produces a variety of effects—from mild relaxation to a sense of detachment and an altered sense of time. In some people the drug can cause paranoia (excessive generalized fear), mild hallucinations, and anxiety that can turn into panic. Because smoking marijuana can impair your memory, your ability to think logically, and your coordination, driving while under the influence is dangerous. Never drive while under the influence of marijuana and never ride with a driver who has been smoking it.

Marijuana affects the lungs in a manner similar to that of cigarettes. As with cigarette smoking, smoking marijuana impairs the lung's defenses against infection and inhaled foreign substances. Regular long-term marijuana smoking can also cause bronchitis and emphysema. Occasional use of marijuana has not been shown to permanently affect the nervous system or affect a normal heart. However, occasional use of the drug can pose a threat to people with high blood pressure and heart disease because it places additional stress on the heart and cardiovascular system.

Heavy, chronic use of marijuana can cause a psychological addiction that can lead to loss of energy, ambition, and drive. People who are psychologically addicted to marijuana tend to be underachievers and have difficulty dealing with normal, everyday stress.

LSD LSD (lysergic acid diethylamide) is a powerful hallucinogen made from an acid found in a fungus that grows on rye and other grains. Although LSD, or "acid," is not considered to be addictive like cocaine or heroin, its potent mood-altering effects can easily lead to abuse. The colorless, odorless, and tasteless drug is sold on the street in tablet, capsule, or, occasionally, liquid form and is usually taken by mouth.

The effects of LSD are unpredictable and depend on the amount and strength of the drug taken. However, it is impossible to know the exact dose of the drug you are getting. The effects of LSD are also influenced by the user's personality, mood, and expectations and the surroundings in which the drug is used. The physical effects of using LSD include dilated pupils, increased heart rate and blood pressure, sweating, loss of appetite, sleeplessness, dry mouth, and tremors. The emotional effects are more dramatic—the user may feel several different emotions at once, or swing rapidly from one emotion to another. In a large dose, the drug produces delusions, hallucinations, and changes in senses. For example, a user may have the feeling of "hearing" colors or "seeing" sounds. These changes can be frightening and often cause panic. Some users experience terrifying thoughts and feelings of despair, fear of losing control, and fear of insanity and death.

A single dose of LSD can last for 12 to 18 hours, and many users experience flashbacks (recurring memories of some aspects of their experiences) more than a year after they stop taking the drug. As with all illegal drugs, the only safe course with LSD is to never try it in the first place.

DRUGS AND PREGNANCY

Almost all drugs that a pregnant woman takes, including alcohol, cross the placenta and enter the fetus's bloodstream. The most serious effects for the fetus include premature birth, stillbirth, and low birth weight. Babies born too small are at increased risk of dying in the first month of life. A pregnant woman who uses drugs puts herself at increased risk of bleeding, miscarriage, and nutritional deficiencies. Because women who use alcohol often use other drugs, it is difficult for doctors to determine precisely which drugs are responsible for which of the many resulting problems these women have during pregnancy.

Many women do not stop taking drugs or drinking until after they find out they are pregnant. By that time, the fetus has been exposed to any drugs they have taken during the most critical early weeks of pregnancy when the fetus's major organs—including the brain, heart, and lungs—are developing.

If you are planning to get pregnant, you should stop using drugs, including tobacco and alcohol. Even if you are not actively planning a pregnancy but are not using a reliable method of birth control (and are therefore likely to get pregnant), it is wise to avoid alcohol and drugs.

TREATMENT FOR DRUG ADDICTION

If you abuse illegal drugs or prescription medications, you may be afraid to admit to your family, or even to yourself, that you have a problem. You may feel isolated and not know where to turn for help. You may feel powerless to change. But asking for help from other people is the first step in helping you overcome your addiction. Talk to friends and family members first and ask for their support. You should also talk to your doctor or see a counselor who is trained in helping people who are addicted to drugs. Call local hospitals and ask if they have a substance abuse program.

The kind of treatment you need will depend on the severity of your addiction. Treatment programs for drug addiction are similar to programs for alcohol addiction (see page 165). In many cases, the two programs are combined. You may be able to overcome the addiction with counseling and participation in a support group of other people who have similar problems. You may need to spend several days in a hospital detoxification program, which helps you discontinue your drug use with a minimum of side effects or withdrawal symptoms. Drug addiction can cause a variety of mental and physical problems, for which you may also need to be treated.

If you have children, you may be worried about who will care for them while you attend a drug treatment program. You may even be afraid that authorities will take your children away from you; they won't. By getting treatment, you are being a responsible, loving parent. Your children will benefit as much as you will. Some centers allow mothers to bring their children with them, and others provide child care.

Most drug treatment programs involve counseling, education, and support groups. You may attend sessions during the day at a local hospital or at night after work. Depending on your addiction, your doctor may recommend a drug rehabilitation program in which you live at the center or hospital for a period of time. No matter which program you go through, you may have a relapse at some point during your recovery, as many people do. If you have a relapse, don't consider yourself a failure. Accept the fact and go on with your recovery. You will succeed eventually.

Risky sexual practices

Sex, one of life's greatest pleasures, also presents risks and responsibilities. With the development of the birth-control pill in the 1950s, women were given sexual freedom and an effective, safe, and easy way to protect themselves against pregnancy. The pill gave them the power to control conception, allowing them to choose to have or not to have children and to plan their lives and their families. Reliable contraception has given women opportunities to pursue careers and to decide at what point in their lives they are ready to have children.

But along with these liberating choices has come a dual threat—skyrocketing rates of sexually transmitted diseases (STDs) and unplanned and unwanted pregnancies. Both STDs and pregnancy discriminate biologically against women. Not only do women carry the burden of pregnancy but their anatomy makes it easier for them than men to contract some STDs. STDs are harder to diagnose in women because the symptoms are often vague or nonexistent or confused with less serious conditions, such as yeast infections. Many STDs produce no symptoms at all in women. In addition, the long-term complications from STDs, which include infertility, occur more frequently and are more serious in women.

SEXUALLY TRANSMITTED DISEASES

More than 20 well-known diseases can be transmitted through sexual contact. The incidence of many of them is increasing rapidly in the US. More than 12 million new cases of sexually transmitted diseases (STDs) are diagnosed each year, most of them in people under 25. Many more cases go undetected because several STDs cause no noticeable symptoms, especially in women. If you are sexually active, you are at risk of acquiring an STD, regardless of the number of sexual partners you have. It only takes one exposure to become infected.

STDs range from diseases caused by bacteria (such as gonorrhea, syphilis, and chlamydia), which can be cured—to those caused by viruses (such as genital herpes), which are incurable but not fatal—to HIV, the virus that causes AIDS, which is both incurable and fatal.

Many of the fastest-growing STDs are caused by viruses and cannot be cured. More than one in five Americans—an estimated 56 million people—are infected with incurable STDs that are caused by viruses, such as genital herpes, genital warts, or hepatitis B. With the dramatic increase in the number of people who are infected with STDs, women who have unprotected sex with a new partner or women whose partner has sex with other people are putting themselves at serious risk.

Few people consider themselves to be personally at risk of STDs—even those who are sexually active with more than one partner. The more people you have sex with, the greater your risk of acquiring an STD.

Many STDs have more severe health consequences for women than men. Women are the fastest-growing group infected by HIV. In some US cities, AIDS is the leading cause of death in women aged 25 to 44. Other STDs can also be deadly. More than 4,500 women die each year of cervical cancer, which is associated with several strains of a sexually transmitted virus called the human papillomavirus (HPV). The virus causes genital warts, one of the most common and fastest-spreading STDs.

Many STDs cause no symptoms in women and are, therefore, difficult to detect. Undetected and untreated, STDs can lead to serious health problems for women and their children. Undetected STDs (especially chlamydia and gonorrhea) are responsible for an estimated 1 million cases of pelvic inflammatory disease (see page 232) in American women each year; up to 150,000 of those infections lead to infertility. The infection causes the fallopian tubes to fill with pus, which gradually blocks them completely and causes abscesses to form in the ovaries. The rupture of these abscesses can be life threatening.

STD-related pelvic infections are also a major cause of ectopic pregnancies (see page 233)—pregnancies that develop outside the uterus, usually in a fallopian tube—which are fatal to the fetus and life threatening to the pregnant woman.

A woman infected with an STD can transmit the infection to her fetus during pregnancy or childbirth. An infection during pregnancy can also cause miscarriage, stillbirth, premature delivery, and birth defects such as blindness and mental retardation.

Avoiding STDs The most effective way to avoid STDs is to abstain from sex. After abstinence, the next safest course is to use a latex or polyurethane male condom or a female condom with spermicide correctly each time you have sex (see page 172). Some people find satisfying alternatives to intercourse, such as kissing, touching, mutual masturbation, and use of vibrators and other sexual props.

Lesbians also need to take precautions in sexual relationships. They should not assume they are 100-percent safe from STDs, particularly if their partner has been bisexual at one time. In addition, some STDs can be transmitted through oral sex.

Because many STDs, including AIDS, cause either no symptoms or symptoms that do not show up for months or years, your partner may not even know he is infected. For this reason, if either you or your partner has recently had sex with another person, you are both at risk of AIDS and other STDs. Talk to your doctors about having a blood test to detect HIV (the virus that causes AIDS) and other STDs. A single negative HIV test does not guarantee, however, that you are not infected with the virus; you may have had the test before your immune system produced antibodies to fight the virus. It usually takes the immune system 3 to 6 months after exposure to the virus to produce HIV antibodies. Nor does a negative HIV test guarantee that you and your partner are free of other STDs. Unless you are in a long-term, stable, mutually monogamous relationship (both you and your partner are having sex only with each other) and you know you are both free of STDs, make sure you always use a condom. (For a discussion of the major STDs and their symptoms, treatments, and health effects, see chapter 12.)

In a perfect world, women would have one device that would protect them against both STDs and pregnancy. For now, there is no one method that is

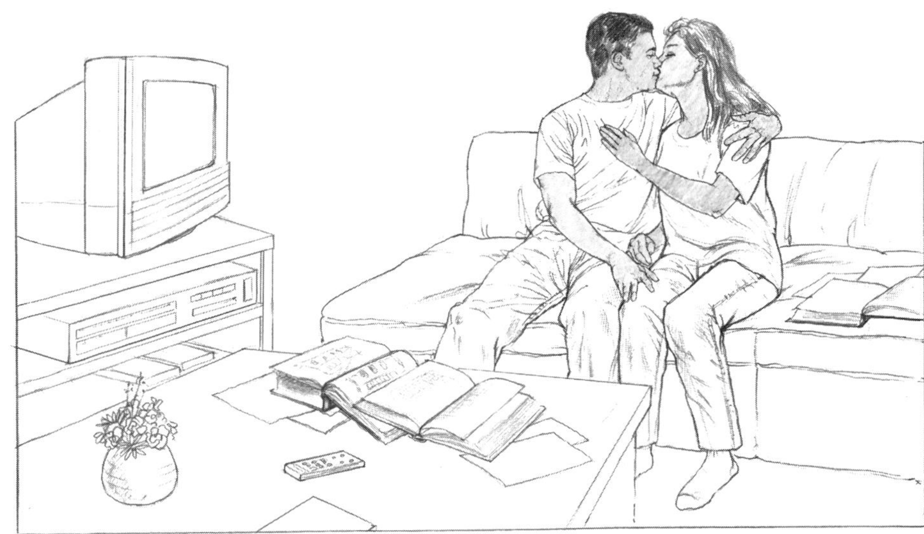

DON'T LET SEX TAKE YOU BY SURPRISE

Having sex is an intensely emotional, pleasurable experience but it requires responsibility or it can have long-lasting and serious consequences. The best time to consider how you will protect yourself against pregnancy and sexually transmitted diseases (STDs) is before you have sex. It takes only one act of sexual intercourse to get pregnant. It also takes only one sexual encounter to acquire an STD.

highly effective against both. The male condom with spermicide provides the best protection against STDs (the female condom may be as effective), but its protection against pregnancy is not as good as the birth-control pill. A condom's protection against pregnancy is improved when it is used with a barrier method of birth control such as the diaphragm. To be reliable, a condom must be used correctly and consistently.

If you are sexually active, here are some guidelines for reducing your risk of acquiring or transmitting an STD:

- Have only one sexual partner who has sex only with you.
- Use a latex or polyurethane male condom or a female condom for vaginal intercourse. Use a male condom for anal intercourse.
- In addition to a condom, use spermicidal jelly, cream, or foam containing the spermicide nonoxynol 9, which may provide additional protection against some STDs. Using a barrier method of birth control such as a diaphragm or vaginal spermicide (in a gel, foam, or suppository), in addition to a male or female condom, can also provide extra protection against some STDs and pregnancy.
- Use water-based lubricants only; oil-based lubricants, such as petroleum jelly, can damage latex condoms.
- Make sure the condom is in place before you have any direct sexual contact.
- Avoid situations in which you are under the influence of alcohol or other drugs—they can impair your judgment.
- If you notice any sores on your partner's genitals or discharge from his penis, refrain from having sex.
- Abstain from sex if either you or your partner has symptoms of an STD or is being treated for one.
- After having sex, urinate to eliminate any bacteria that may have entered your urinary tract. Wash your genital area with mild soap and water. Do not douche—douching can force semen up into the cervical canal, increasing your risk of pregnancy and STDs.

Using condoms correctly Condoms are inexpensive and available in most drugstores, supermarkets, and convenience stores. Buy male condoms made of latex or polyurethane. All female condoms are made of polyurethane. Condoms made of natural materials such as lambskin tend to be more porous and may allow microscopic organisms, including HIV, the AIDS virus, to pass through. Carry a latex or polyurethane male condom or a female condom with you at all times, even if you are not expecting to have sex.

Using a condom correctly and consistently can significantly reduce your risk of acquiring an STD. For information about how to use a female condom, see page 319. Follow these guidelines for using a male condom:

- Talk to your partner about using a condom before you even begin any sexual activity (see page 21). If your partner objects to using a condom, do not have sex with him.
- Before any contact between your partner's penis and your genital area, you or your partner should put the condom on his penis. The penis must be erect.
- Before putting on the condom, make sure you know in which direction it will unroll. Place the condom over the tip of

STDs: When to see a doctor

Because the symptoms of some STDs are not always obvious, especially in women, it is important that you have annual pelvic examinations and Pap smears. Tell your doctor you are sexually active and would like to be tested for STDs—particularly if you have had sex with more than one partner or if you think your partner may have had sex with other people. Don't be embarrassed to talk to your doctor; he or she is there to help you. And don't let feeling guilty get in the way of your health.

Not all of the following symptoms always accompany an STD and some may be symptoms of other, nonsexually transmitted infections. See your doctor if you notice any of these symptoms:

- Sores, bumps, lumps, warts, or blisters around the outside or just inside your vagina or anus
- Itching, burning, soreness, or redness in or around your vagina or anus
- Unusual or unpleasant-smelling discharge from your vagina
- Burning during urination
- Sore throat
- Swollen lymph glands in your groin
- Pain, pressure, or other discomfort in your upper thigh, pelvic area, or lower abdomen
- A rash, including one on your palms or the soles of your feet

FAILURE OF CONDOMS IS USUALLY CAUSED BY INCORRECT USE

When putting on a condom, make sure to leave a space at the tip to accommodate semen. Squeeze the tip to make sure there is no air inside. Roll the condom all the way down the base of the penis.

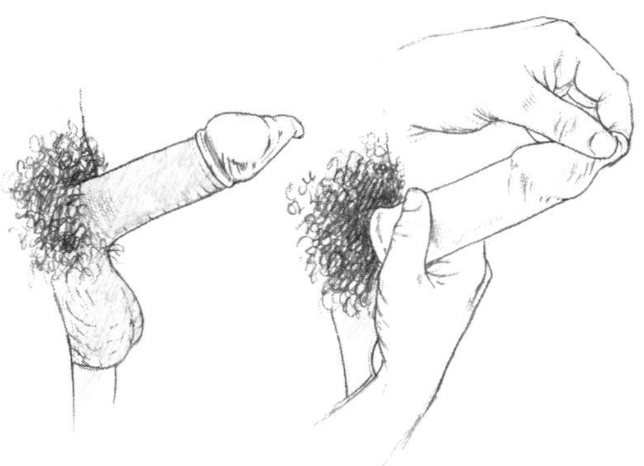

the penis, lubricated side out, and, squeezing the tip of the condom with one hand, with the other hand roll the condom downward as far as possible toward the base of the penis. Make sure some space is left at the tip of the condom for semen. If you don't leave space in the tip, the condom is more likely to tear, putting you at risk of both infection and pregnancy.

- If insertion is difficult because you are not lubricated sufficiently, stop your sexual activity. Friction is another major cause of tearing of a condom. A longer period of foreplay and direct manual or oral stimulation of your genitals can help promote lubrication. Lubricating jellies can be helpful too; they can usually be found in the same section of the pharmacy as contraceptives. But make sure the water-based type you buy is safe to use with latex condoms. Never use oil-based lubricants, which can damage latex.
- Your partner should withdraw his penis immediately after intercourse to prevent the condom from slipping off as the penis loses its erection. He should hold the rim firmly to the base of the penis to prevent semen from leaking into your vagina. Remove and dispose of the condom; never reuse a condom.

TEENAGE PREGNANCY

Along with skyrocketing rates of sexually transmitted diseases, unsafe and irresponsible sexual practices have produced a dramatic increase in the number of unplanned and unwanted pregnancies, mostly among teenagers. An unplanned pregnancy can confront a woman with difficult decisions that can have a permanent impact on her life. Taking responsibility for practicing birth control is the single best way to ensure that you have a child only when you want to and when you are fully prepared for the challenges of parenthood.

The US has the highest rate of teenage pregnancy of any developed country. More than one third of American teens become pregnant at least once during their adolescence. Half of these pregnancies occur within the first 2 months of first having intercourse. The vast majority of teen pregnancies are neither planned nor wanted. The heavy responsibilities of early parenthood can make it difficult for a young woman to complete her education and pursue a career. Pregnancy does not discriminate—it happens to girls in the inner city and girls in the suburbs and to girls of all racial and ethnic groups.

If you are a teenager, think about whether you are ready for the adult responsibilities of a sexual relationship—from both a physical standpoint (protecting yourself from pregnancy and STDs) and an emotional one (adding sex to a friendship can produce complicated and intense emotional changes).

Remember that not having sex is an option—you don't have to do it and there are plenty of good reasons not to. Many girls choose not to have sex until later in their life, when they feel better prepared for the responsibility.

The high rate of teenage pregnancy in the US appears to result from denial of

A myth about withdrawal

Some women mistakenly believe that they cannot get pregnant if their partner withdraws his penis before ejaculating. But small amounts of semen usually seep out of the penis before a man reaches sexual climax and ejaculates. Many women have become pregnant by wrongly assuming that, if their partner withdraws before ejaculating, no sperm will be left inside their vagina.

the risk of becoming pregnant ("it won't happen to me"), a lack of basic knowledge about reproduction and birth control, early sexual activity, and peer pressure. Most sexually active teenagers report that they do not use any form of contraception regularly.

If you are sexually active, there are several forms of contraception to choose from, including the birth-control pill, hormone injections or implants, the male condom, the female condom, the diaphragm, the cervical cap, and spermicidal jellies and foams. At different times in your life, different methods of contraception might work better for you than other methods. To determine which one is best for you, see the description of

One woman's story
Teen pregnancy: it changed my life

I never thought it could happen to me. I guess that's why it happened. I was a senior in high school, I had been accepted at my number-one college choice, and I could hardly wait to go.

Tom and I had been dating since sophomore year in high school. We never talked about having sex because he knew it was something I didn't feel ready for. But one night things went a little too far and we did it. I figured, since it was the first time, we didn't have to worry about my getting pregnant. Things like that don't happen to people like me.

Well, a month later it dawned on me that I had missed my last period. My breasts were really sore too. But it never occurred to me that I might be pregnant until I missed another period.

I panicked. I didn't know what to do. I couldn't talk to my parents and I was too ashamed to tell my friends. I stopped eating because I thought that I could keep it a secret longer if I didn't gain any weight. I didn't want to go to our family doctor because I thought she would tell my mother.

I was scared to death. I knew I could never have an abortion because of the way I was brought up. I kept thinking about how my parents would respond and how angry and disappointed they would be. What would I do about college? I didn't want to stay home and get some job just to support myself and my baby. There was no way Tom and I were going to get married.

I knew it was just a matter of time before I would be forced to tell my parents. When I finally did, it wasn't nearly as bad as I thought it would be. They tried hard to be supportive and helpful even though I knew they were crushed. They made sure I went to the doctor right away to start getting the right kind of care. Before I left, the doctor told me to start thinking about what kind of birth control I would use after the baby was born. That made me feel so old all of a sudden.

My baby was born healthy and I love him more than anything. But we're still living with my parents, which is hard on everyone. I'm working at a department store downtown and trying to save as much money as I can. I'm going to a community college, but because I work I can only take one course at a time. It seems like it will be forever before I finish. My mother takes care of the baby while I'm at work and I feel bad when I think about all the things she could be doing if she weren't helping me out all the time. I had never thought much before about what it would be like to have a baby. I didn't know that you have to think about a baby every minute of your life.

When I look back at that last year in high school, I can't believe how careless Tom and I were. We didn't connect sex with having a baby. We should have stopped things before they went too far. It was just stupid to have sex without using at least a condom.

I think about how much better my son's life would be if he had a father at home and a mother who was through school and wasn't always worrying about money. If I ever have another child, I'm going to do things differently. I want to make sure both the father and I are ready to be parents and are excited about it. Children deserve all the time and care you can give them.

"If I ever have another child, I'm going to do things differently. I want to make sure both the father and I are ready to be parents and are excited about it."

each of these methods beginning on page 308. Birth-control pills are often used by women who have sex on a regular basis. The pill is popular because it is both highly effective and very convenient. However, the pill provides protection only against pregnancy—it does not protect against sexually transmitted diseases (STDs).

Because you have to take a birth-control pill every day whether you are sexually active or not, many women who have sex less frequently choose barrier methods of contraception. Barrier contraceptives work by preventing sperm from reaching an egg. Barrier contraceptives, such as the diaphragm, are inserted shortly before you have sex. Latex or polyurethane male condoms and female condoms provide the most effective protection against AIDS and other STDs. You must use a condom every time you have sex in order to be protected from STDs. Most spermicidal jellies and foams do not provide nearly as much protection against STDs as the male and female condoms. Spermicides are most effective when they are used together with condoms.

If you have had sex without using any means of contraception, or if you have been the victim of sexual assault, you have the option of obtaining the morning-after pill (see page 317) from a doctor or a family planning clinic within 72 hours. Even though it is called the morning-after pill, it is actually a series of four birth-control pills that prevent a fertilized egg from implanting in the wall of the uterus. The first dose must be taken within 72 hours of the unprotected intercourse. The side effects of the morning-after pill are minor and may include mild nausea, breast tenderness, and light vaginal bleeding. The method is highly effective in preventing pregnancy but should not be used as a regular means of birth control.

If you have missed a period and you think you might be pregnant, see a doctor immediately or tell an adult you trust or call the local office of Planned

Questions Women Ask
Preventing Early Pregnancy

Q I have an older boyfriend who says that since I recently started having my period, I'm ready to have sex. Am I too young to get pregnant?

A Any woman who menstruates can become pregnant but having your period has nothing to do with being ready to have sex. If you don't feel ready, tell your boyfriend. He needs to consider your feelings. If you have only recently started having your period, you are probably too young to handle the heavy responsibilities that go along with a sexual relationship, such as protecting yourself from pregnancy and sexually transmitted diseases. If you do choose to have sex, use a latex or polyurethane male condom or a female condom with spermicide every time. Ask your doctor about other birth-control methods.

Q I'm too embarrassed to carry condoms. My boyfriend might think I'm sleeping around. How can I protect myself?

A To keep from getting pregnant, a hormonal birth-control method such as the pill or hormone implants might be a good choice for you. But to protect yourself from sexually transmitted diseases, you and your boyfriend must use a condom every time you have sex.

Q How often do you have to have sex to become pregnant?

A You can get pregnant even if you have sex only once. The more often you have sex without contraceptive protection, the more likely you are to become pregnant. Prepare yourself for the next time. Go to your doctor and choose a reliable method of birth control.

Parenthood. If you make a decision to terminate the pregnancy (have an abortion), the earlier you take action, the safer and easier the procedure will be. More women die each year from complications related to pregnancy and delivery than from having an abortion during the first 3 months of pregnancy.

Driving

Even though the rate of injury and death from automobile accidents has gradually declined over the past few decades, more than 40,000 Americans die in traffic accidents in the US each year and many more are injured. The reasons for the decline include improved driver education, stricter laws against drunk driving, an increase in seat belt use, use of child safety seats and air bags, improved steering assemblies and anti-lock brakes in cars, and improved highway safety design.

The following guidelines can help keep you safe from injury while driving:

- Wear lap and shoulder seat belts every time you drive or ride in a car. Most accidents occur within 5 miles of home.
- Never drive after drinking alcohol or taking other drugs that might impair your judgment. Nearly 50 percent of drivers who are killed every year consumed alcohol before the accident.
- Drive within the speed limit. Drive slower than the speed limit in bad weather or when road conditions are unsafe. Slower is nearly always safer. If you are in an accident, the probability that you will be seriously injured is three times greater if you are driving 55 miles per hour than if you are driving 25 miles per hour.
- Keep your child in a safety seat appropriate for his or her age at all times. The most dangerous thing you can do is hold a child on your lap. In an accident, the weight of your body can crush and kill a child.
- Drive defensively; even if you are driving safely, other people may not be. Maintain adequate distance between your car and the car in front of you (see page 177)—the faster you are traveling, the greater the distance should be. Never assume another driver will yield the right-of-way. If another driver cuts in front of you and makes you angry, do not respond in any way. Stay well behind any car that is driving erratically.
- Make sure everyone in the car you are driving wears a seat belt. A passenger thrown from the back seat can injure front-seat passengers.
- Whenever possible, do not drive when weather conditions are unsafe (in heavy rain or snow) or very late at night.
- Don't drive if you are emotionally upset; you may be too distracted to drive safely.

SEAT BELTS AND AIR BAGS

Wearing a seat belt significantly improves your chances of surviving a car crash—the majority of people killed in crashes were not wearing seat belts. There are two collisions in a car accident. The first occurs when the car is hit and comes to a stop. The second—the "human collision"—occurs a fraction of a second later when unbelted passengers are thrown through a windshield, door, or window or collide with someone else or something in the car. At 30 miles an hour, the impact is the same as falling from a three-story window. A seat belt works by spreading the force of the impact over your hips and shoulders, slowing you down with the car, lessening the force of the second collision, and preventing you from being hurled forward.

To make sure your seat belt works the way it is supposed to, wear it correctly each time you get into a car. Make sure your children and other passengers wear theirs too. Here's how:

- Wear the lap belt under your abdomen and across your upper thighs (see page 412), never over your abdomen. If the belt is too high, a sudden stop can damage internal organs.
- Sit up straight. Slumping down in your seat can cause the belt to ride too high.
- Wear the shoulder strap between your breasts and across your shoulder. Never wear it under your arm or across your neck. Your chest and shoulder muscles are strong enough to withstand a heavy impact, but your neck and abdomen are not.

- Keep the belt as tight as possible yet still comfortable. A loose belt can cause broken ribs or injure your abdomen.
- Wear a seat belt throughout your pregnancy (see page 412).

Air bags, which provide additional protection in an accident, are becoming more common in new cars. An air bag is a cloth bag that is usually concealed in the steering wheel or dashboard. When activated by a crash sensor, the bag inflates with harmless nitrogen gas to cushion the driver and front-seat passenger on impact. The bag deflates within a second. Because air bags are only activated in a front-on crash, you must still always wear your seat belt. A seat belt holds you in position, making the air bag more effective and protecting you in any kind of crash.

The 2-second rule for safe following distance

Many accidents occur because drivers fail to give themselves enough room behind the car in front of them to stop quickly. To make sure you're at a safe distance, follow these simple steps:

1. Look for a stationary object, such as a signpost, along the side of the highway.
2. When the back bumper of the car in front of you is even with the signpost, start counting in seconds (one-one-thousand, two-one-thousand, etc).
3. Your front bumper should be even with that signpost only after you have counted at least 2 full seconds.
4. Add 1 second for *each* condition that might make it more difficult for you to stop in enough time to avoid an accident—rain or snow, an icy or wet road, driving at night, the vehicle in front of you is a small car or motorcycle (they stop faster than bigger cars or trucks), or you are driving a big car or truck.

WHEN TO CONSIDER GIVING UP DRIVING

Giving up driving in a society that is dependent upon the automobile is no small decision. Many older people fear becoming isolated in their home, especially if they live in an area without access to public transportation. But if you have any doubt at all about your ability to drive, you may be putting yourself and others in danger every time you get behind the wheel of a car.

Consider the following when evaluating your own ability to drive. If you have any doubts at all, talk to your doctor.

Vision See an ophthalmologist once a year for a regular eye examination (see page 140); see him or her immediately if your vision has worsened.

Musculoskeletal problems If a disorder that affects your muscles or bones, such as osteoporosis, impairs your ability to sit properly in a car and see clearly, adjust the seat, sit on pillows, or use wide-angled mirrors to get a better view of the road. See your doctor.

Seizures, dizziness, and other attacks In general, any driver who has a condition that may cause lack of consciousness, such as a seizure disorder (see page 578), should refrain from driving. If treatment of the condition successfully eliminates the attacks, ask your doctor about your ability to drive.

Impaired perception or judgment Mental impairment caused by disorders that affect the brain, such as dementia, stroke, and Parkinson's disease, must be evaluated by a doctor. He or she can determine to what degree the impairment would affect your ability to drive and put you and others at risk.

Medications Do not drive when you are taking any medication that can affect your driving skills. Some over-the-counter medications can affect your ability to drive as much as prescription drugs. Ask your doctor about driving while you are taking a particular medication and make sure you check all labels carefully for instructions or warnings about driving. It's a good idea to refrain from driving until you have taken the first few doses of a new medication to see what, if any, effect it has on you.

Alcohol and other drugs Never drive after consuming any amount of alcohol. Alcohol can be especially lethal if you have combined it with another drug or medication. (For more about drinking and driving, see page 162.) You should never drive after you have used any illegal drugs.

Other risks

You may not think of a sunburn as a health risk, but excessive exposure to the sun is the main cause of skin cancer, which is increasing dramatically in the US. You may not think of the loud noises around you as dangerous, but they can gradually impair your hearing. If you are older, you may not realize the importance of reducing your risk of a disabling fall. By recognizing and reducing these risks, you can protect yourself from serious, disabling health problems in the future.

FALLS

For many women, especially older women, falls are the most common cause of serious injury and disability. Older women are at increased risk of fractures because their bones have thinned, mostly in the first few years after menopause. At menopause, the ovaries stop producing the bone-strengthening hormone estrogen. The lack of estrogen makes your bones weak and porous and, therefore, prone to fractures. Taking estrogen at menopause and after can prevent this rapid bone loss. Your bones will weaken further if you reduce your level of physical activity.

Many women become so fearful of falling that they cut down drastically on their activities and become sedentary. But being sedentary can cause even more problems; without use, muscles and bones become weak. The more inactive you are, the more likely you are to become physically frail and to be at greater risk of a fall and serious injury. Many older women become physically frail.

But physical frailty in older people is both preventable and treatable—not an inevitable consequence of aging. Increasing your level of activity and doing regular weight-bearing exercises such as walking and weight lifting, even if you are in your 80s or 90s, can maintain strength in your muscles and bones and substantially reduce your risk of falls and injuries.

SUN EXPOSURE

In spite of the amount of negative publicity sunbathing has received in recent years, many people still spend much time and money trying to get a tan. Although you may think a tan makes you look healthy, it is the evidence of damage to your skin from ultraviolet radiation from the sun. Sun exposure is the single most common cause of skin cancer—including the deadliest kind, malignant melanoma (see page 684). Malignant melanoma is increasing in the US and is occurring at younger ages.

Wrinkles are also caused primarily by the sun. Most people think that wrinkles are an inevitable part of aging, but sun exposure is a much more significant factor. All you have to do is compare the skin on different parts of your body. The skin on your breasts and buttocks, which has probably not been exposed to the sun over the years, looks smoother, softer, and younger than the sun-damaged skin on your face and hands.

The best protection against the sun is clothing. Hats are an effective means of preventing exposure to the sun. Sunscreens are a good alternative when it is too warm for much clothing. Use a sunscreen with a sun protection factor (SPF) of at least 15. Get into the habit of putting on sunscreen before you go out. Whenever possible, apply sunscreen half an hour before you go out in the sun to allow time for it to be absorbed into your skin. Make sure you apply sunscreen liberally; a thin layer does not provide sufficient protection.

Fair-skinned people are more vulnerable to skin cancer and wrinkles caused by the sun. If you've always had difficulty tanning or if you tend to burn easily, you should never go out in the sun without protection. Many women use a daily moisturizer or makeup base that contains sunscreen.

Preventing falls

In addition to increasing your activity and doing strengthening exercises (see page 84) to reduce your risk of a serious fall, here are some things you can do to make your home safer:

- Make sure that light switches are in reach of doorways so you don't have to cross a dark room to turn on a light. Lighting that is too dim or too bright can impair your vision, causing falls.
- Carpets and rugs should have slip-resistant backing or be tacked down to prevent trips and slips. Get rid of unnecessary loose rugs.
- Arrange your furniture so that you have clear, unobstructed pathways from one place to another. Eliminate furniture that you do not use. Keep telephone cords and electrical cords out of pathways. Keep hallways uncluttered.
- Make sure chairs and tables are sturdy, stable, and balanced in case someone leans on them for support.
- Have a lamp within reach of your bed. Have a night-light along the path between your bedroom and bathroom.
- Setting the heat at a warm temperature (at least 72°) can help keep your joints from stiffening.
- A wet or waxed kitchen floor is a hazard. Place a rubber mat on the floor in the sink area and wear rubber-soled shoes in the kitchen. Clean up spills on the floor immediately.
- In the bathroom, put a rubber mat or nonskid adhesive strips on the tub or shower floor to prevent slips. Install handrails on the wall next to the toilet and along the bathtub. Do not use towel racks to steady yourself because they are not strong enough for this purpose.
- Don't lock the bathroom door, or make sure the lock can be opened by someone on the outside, in case you fall and are unable to get up. Use a night-light in the bathroom.
- Handrails should be installed on both sides of a stairway, 30 inches above the stairs, and they should extend the full length of the stairs. Place nonskid treads on all bare steps. Provide enough light to see each stair. Do not put loose area rugs at the top or bottom of stairways.
- Outdoors, wear sturdy shoes with soles that grip the pavement. Use a cane when necessary. Stay indoors, if possible, when streets and sidewalks are icy. Spread sand or salt on icy surfaces.

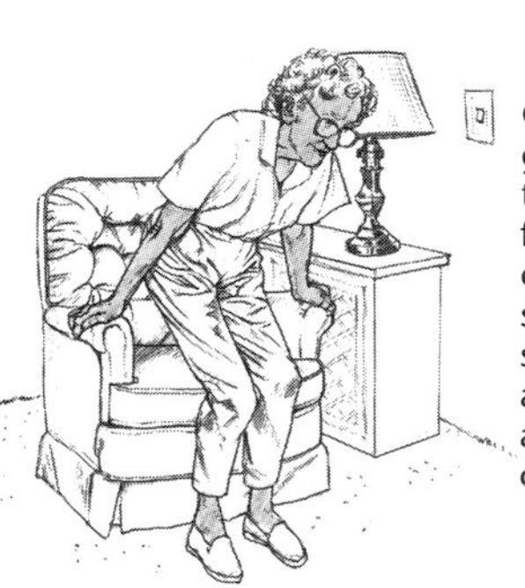

Chairs are easier to get in and out of if the armrests come forward to the edge of the seat. Make sure rugs are flat and secured to the floor, and furniture is arranged to allow a clear walking path.

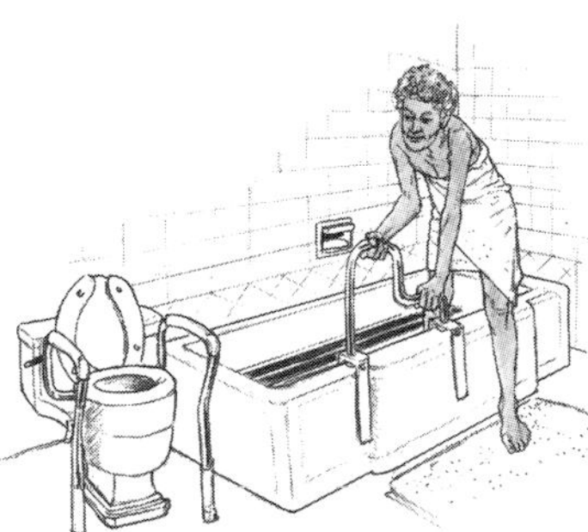

In the bathroom, install handrails to help you get in and out of the tub. For some people, an elevated toilet seat is easier to use.

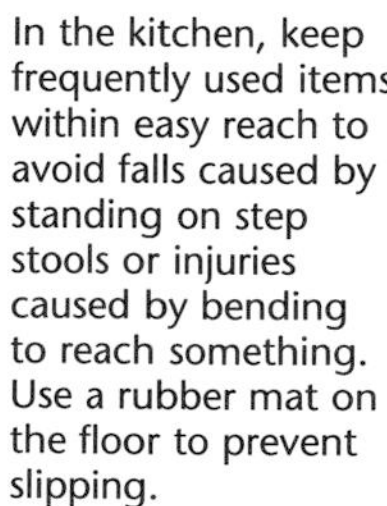

In the kitchen, keep frequently used items within easy reach to avoid falls caused by standing on step stools or injuries caused by bending to reach something. Use a rubber mat on the floor to prevent slipping.

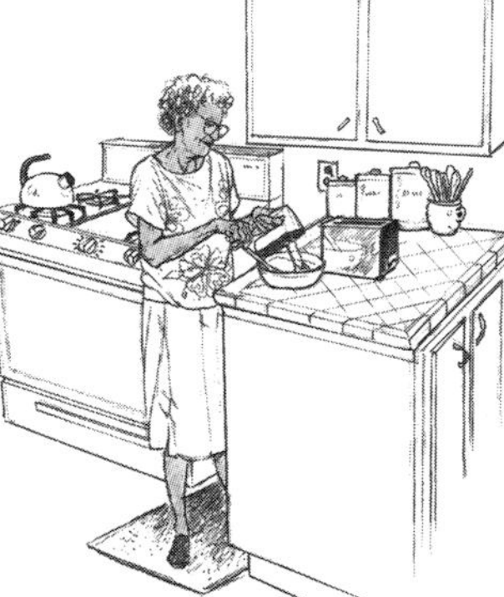

Outdoors, wear sturdy walking shoes with good traction, use a cane if you need to, and do not hesitate to get help from someone else whenever necessary.

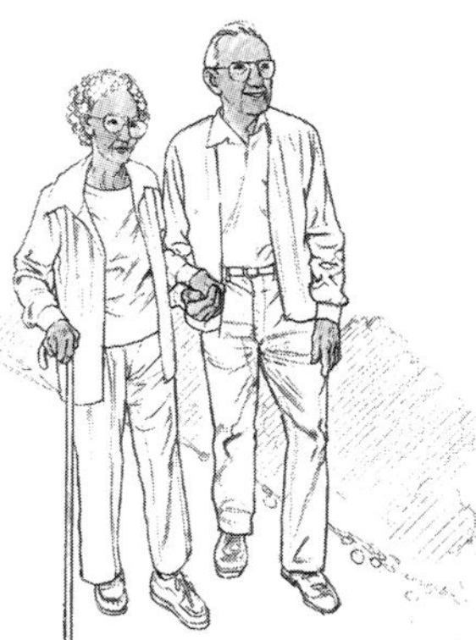

EXPOSURE TO LOUD NOISE

Most of us do not think about noise as a danger. But exposure to loud noise throughout your life can gradually impair your hearing. Loud noise kills the tiny hair cells in your inner ear (see illustration below) that signal the auditory nerve to send sound messages to your brain. Once these cells die, they never grow back.

It doesn't take much to lose your hearing. Even listening to loud music, either live or from speakers or headphones, can reduce your ability to hear. Without realizing it, you may have already lost some of your hearing. A majority of college students show some signs of hearing loss, usually from listening to excessively loud rock music.

Your hearing may be in danger if you have any ringing in your ears, if sounds seem muffled or distorted, or if you find yourself shouting to communicate. Another indication that you may have a hearing problem is if someone mentions that you have the TV on very loud or if friends ask you if you can hear them. When you come out of a noisy environment, such as a loud rock concert, you may notice that things sound strange and subdued. This effect is a sign of hearing damage. When listening to music, the rule of thumb for protecting your hearing is to keep it low enough that you can hear other sounds above it. When you can't avoid loud noise, wear earplugs.

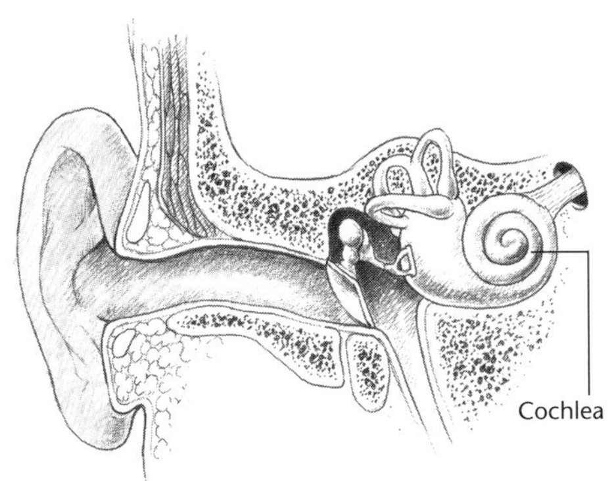

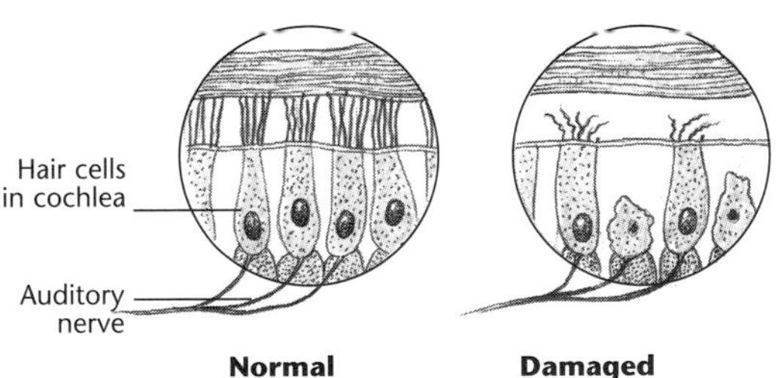

HOW LOUD NOISES DAMAGE THE EAR

Repeated exposure to loud noises gradually destroys the hair cells that line the cochlea, an organ in your inner ear that transmits sound vibrations via the auditory nerve to your brain.

Protect your hearing

Noise is measured in units called decibels. Try to avoid extended exposure to sound above 80 decibels or, if you can't avoid it, wear earplugs. You can damage your hearing after only half an hour of listening to your stereo headphones at full blast.

SOUND	DECIBELS
Alarm clock	80
Lawn mower	90
Snowmobile, chain saw, video arcade	100
Rock music concert, stereo headphones at full blast	110
Jet plane takeoff	120
Jackhammer	130
Firearms, air raid siren	140

CHAPTER 6

Well-being and stress management

Contents

Your physical and emotional health are closely linked. Exactly how the mind can influence the health of the body is only beginning to be understood. Some specific personality types and psychological or emotional conditions have been linked to specific illnesses. For example, people who have a hostile or aggressive "type A" personality are more susceptible to heart disease.

People who have a positive outlook on life are generally healthier and live longer than people who have a negative outlook on life. Major life events, both good and bad—including marriage, divorce, childbearing, changing or losing jobs, and the death of a spouse—can increase your risk of becoming ill. Even everyday stress, if not managed effectively, can cause health problems such as headaches, difficulty sleeping, and digestive disorders.

Your mental state also influences how you see yourself, what path you choose in life, and how other people perceive you. Your sense of who you are, your level of self-esteem, and your ability to manage stress all influence your experiences and your relationships with other people. This chapter offers suggestions for improving your emotional health and sense of well-being.

A woman's emotional health

Many women understand that physical well-being is only part of the equation for leading a healthy life. Recognizing emotional problems and finding ways to deal with them appear to come more naturally to women than to men. Women are twice as likely as men to seek help for a variety of psychological problems, including depression. The ability to ask for help, to reach out and connect with others, makes it more likely that women will get help when they need it.

To develop a healthy personality, or sense of identity, a young woman must become gradually more self-sufficient, independent, and autonomous as she matures. But just as crucial to personality development is the need and desire to connect with others. Women tend to focus on creating and sustaining relationships in their lives, beginning with their parents and moving on to close friendships in adolescence and intimate friendships and sexual relationships in adult life.

The ability to nurture relationships and seek social support from others can benefit both your physical and mental health. People who have strong supportive relationships with others are less likely to become ill than people who do not have supportive relationships. If they do become ill, they usually recover more quickly. People with strong social supports also fare better after a stressful life event than people who are more isolated.

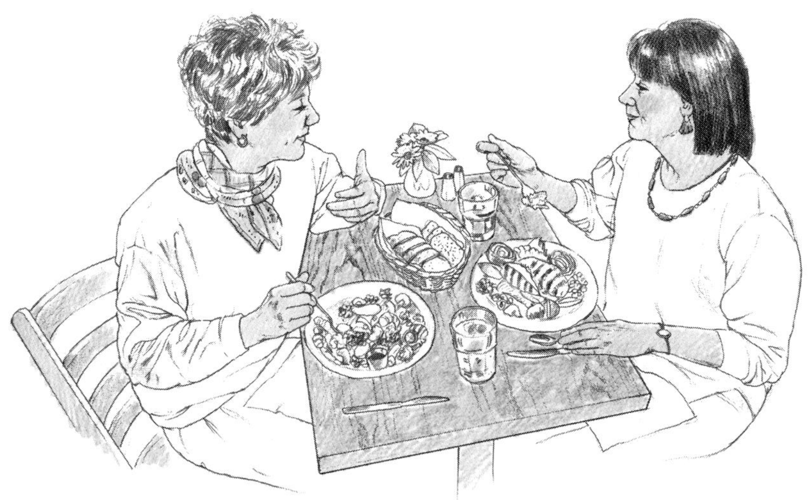

MAKING CONNECTIONS

A woman can benefit from her ability to form and maintain relationships. The tendency of women to nurture connections with others and to ask for help when they need it is important to their sense of fulfillment. Healthy relationships are an effective means of managing the stress in life.

Self-esteem

Self-esteem is essentially the value we attach to ourselves—a self-appraisal based on our beliefs and convictions about ourselves. It defines our character and guides our behavior. For example, your choice of a mate and a career are heavily influenced by how highly you think of yourself and, therefore, how high you have set your goals.

A person with high self-esteem can tolerate small failures by downplaying them, seeing them as a small part of a brighter, bigger picture. People with low self-esteem may be devastated by failure and blame themselves. They may become detached or distant in order to avoid the painful possibility of disappointment.

Whether or not you have high self-esteem was largely determined early in your life. Most psychologists believe that self-esteem is acquired from childhood experiences, the judgment of others, and positive identification with family members and friends. Once a person develops low self-esteem, it often reinforces itself. For example, children who form a low opinion of their abilities often lack self-confidence and eventually come to expect little of themselves.

In school, children who believe they are not intelligent are less likely to put effort into learning than are children who believe they can do well. Teachers then interpret this lack of effort as evidence of disinterest or lack of ability and treat these children accordingly—by placing them in a lower learning group, for example, where less is expected of them. Their low expectations of themselves are confirmed, and their already poor self-image is reinforced.

Parents can encourage a positive sense of self in their children by giving their children unconditional love, by respecting their individuality and talents and encouraging them to develop those talents, by praising their successes, and by allowing them to make some of their own choices. It is also important for parents to set clearly defined rules of behavior for their children—and enforce them consistently and fairly.

While both girls' and boys' self-esteem drops in early adolescence, the drop is much greater for girls. In elementary school, nearly two out of three girls say they are happy the way they are. By the time girls reach high school, only one out of three feels good about herself. One reason for the decline in self-esteem may be that, as girls mature, they are bombarded by changes—hormonal changes that affect them physically and emotionally and developmental changes that cause them to focus on relationships and be more affected by social acceptance or rejection. Especially during their early teens, many girls are more sensitive and concerned than boys about how other people perceive them; they may misread a normal social exchange as a slight or rejection or take constructive criticism as a personal insult.

IMPROVING YOUR SELF-ESTEEM

The effects of low self-esteem are complex. Low self-esteem is thought to be a major cause of depression. It can also affect other areas of your life, including the way you present yourself in a job interview, your tendency to put other people's needs before your own, and your ability to form and maintain relationships.

Your manner of speaking says a lot about how you feel about yourself. If you tend to put yourself down or take the blame for situations, you are sending a message that you do not think highly of yourself. As a result, other people may come to accept your view of yourself as less than competent. Try to avoid self-defeating language by eliminating such phrases in your speech as "I'm probably wrong but..." or "It's only my opinion but...." Instead, state your opinions firmly through positive statements such "I think" and "I feel." Don't back down easily; instead say "You may disagree, but I still believe...."

Your body language can also project a negative image. Slumped shoulders, fidgeting hands and feet, chewed-off fingernails, arms crossed protectively in front of your chest, and downcast or averted eyes may indicate to others that you are insecure. Instead, make a conscious effort to appear confident. For example, when you are talking to others, make eye contact and speak clearly and directly.

Make time for yourself Like many women, you may take care of everyone else's needs before your own. Nurturing and caring for others is a major part of a woman's identity. But it is important to learn to balance your own needs with the needs of others.

If you are a mother, you may be accustomed to thinking of your children first and never getting around to doing what you need to do or want to do for yourself. It is hard to be good at mothering if you are unhappy or if your own needs are not being met. You will help your children more by also fulfilling your own needs. You will be setting a good example for your children if you develop your own talents and pursue your own goals and interests.

Encourage yourself To boost your self-esteem, it's important to recognize your strengths and good qualities. Look for things you do well. Ask family members, colleagues, and friends what they think you do well. Their answers may surprise and please you. Write them down and look at the list frequently.

For some people, low self-esteem is deeply ingrained. Simply making a list of

Think positively about yourself

Do you expect yourself to be perfect? Do you assume it is your fault if something goes wrong? Such negative thinking can lower your self-esteem. Look at the chart below and consider how you might replace the negative approaches listed on the left with the positive ones on the right. Doing so will improve your image of yourself and the quality of your life.

NEGATIVE APPROACHES	POSITIVE APPROACHES
■ **Perfectionism:** You see yourself as a failure if your performance falls short of perfection. You put off decisions and tasks to avoid the possibility of a less-than-perfect outcome.	■ **Tolerance:** You accept that some of your abilities are stronger than others and your performance might not be perfect every day or on every task. You have realistic expectations of yourself and others.
■ **Negative thinking:** You ignore your accomplishments and dwell on your faults or failures.	■ **Positive thinking:** You concentrate on your achievements and successes and look for supportive and nurturing personal contacts.
■ **Negative assumptions:** Without real evidence, you assume that people are critical of you.	■ **Positive assumptions:** You assume that you are competent and accepted. If you do receive criticism, you use it constructively to improve yourself.
■ **Generalizing:** A single failure becomes a symbol of general failure and incompetence. You attribute failures to your personal flaws.	■ **Focusing:** You apply criticism to the specific task or experience being addressed, not to yourself as a person.
■ **Pessimism:** You assume that the worst will happen and don't consider possible positive outcomes.	■ **Optimism:** You are hopeful about your ability to meet challenges. You think about the gratification you will get from a positive outcome, such as doing a job well.

their talents may not be enough to overcome the difficulties caused by a poor self-image. If you are concerned about your poor self-image, you may want to see a psychiatrist, psychologist, or other mental health specialist. A therapist can help you learn more about the reasons you may have low self-esteem and teach you techniques for coping and for improving your self-image.

Recognizing and managing stress

Stress is the tension and heightened awareness you feel when you are challenged physically or emotionally. Stress has been given a bad name but, in reality, most stress is normal and healthy. Stress drives you to act, challenges you to think, and makes your life interesting, productive, and meaningful. For example, a job promotion can be stimulating and exhilarating but is also stressful because it requires you to change your life to some degree to make the adjustment. Many other happy events in your life, including getting married and having a child, are stressful for the same reason—they are major changes.

The way in which you deal with stress determines whether it affects you positively or negatively. We all react to stress in different ways. What is challenging and exhilarating to one person may be overwhelming and debilitating to another. What is stressful to you at one time in your life may be exciting at another. For example, a pregnancy that is unplanned can be stressful, while one that occurs when you are ready to have a family is a joyous event.

Stress that takes hold of your life can affect your health. The body's "fight-or-flight" response to an immediate danger is a vivid illustration of how high levels of stress can affect the body. In response to danger, the body releases adrenaline and other stress hormones into the bloodstream, causing a cascade of physiological changes, including increased heart rate, blood pressure, and muscle tension. These responses give you the short-term energy to face or escape the source of stress. But, over the long term, unrelieved stress—and the persistently elevated levels of stress hormones that result—are linked to high blood pressure, diabetes, heart disease, cancer, and susceptibility to infections.

Stress can affect your health in other ways as well. It can interfere with your sleep, making you tired and irritable during the day and even more likely to react

Warning signs
Stress

Stress can affect you physically and emotionally. Stress can also influence your behavior. If you have any of the symptoms below, see your doctor. He or she can rule out a medical cause and, if necessary, refer you to a qualified mental health professional such as a psychiatrist or a psychologist.

- **Physical:** Bowel and stomach disorders, including irritable bowel syndrome (a condition characterized by alternating bouts of constipation and diarrhea), nausea, abdominal pain, heartburn, and ulcers; loss of appetite; heart palpitations; headache; back pain; elevated blood pressure; weakened resistance to disease, resulting in frequent infections
- **Behavioral:** Eating disorders, such as compulsive overeating, anorexia, or bulimia; substance abuse; tendency to have frequent minor accidents; impaired performance on the job or at school; family conflict; interpersonal problems; social withdrawal
- **Emotional:** Feelings of anxiety, irritability, anger, or depression; insomnia; difficulty concentrating; fatigue; negative thinking

negatively to everyday events. Many people resort to harmful ways of coping with stress—"quick fixes" such as cigarettes, alcohol, and other drugs. Such negative coping mechanisms have serious, potentially fatal, consequences.

Unabated stress may make you feel helpless and cause you to withdraw from friends and family when you need them the most. Isolating yourself can make you feel even more anxious and helpless. A more positive way of coping with stress is to reach out for help from relatives, trusted friends, a member of the clergy, your doctor, and, if needed, a mental health professional.

SELF-HELP FOR STRESS

Stress affects people in different ways. Most people can learn to manage stress, at least to some extent, on their own. There are many things you can do to keep stress from escalating and affecting your life in a negative way. For example, stopping what you are doing and just sitting back, relaxing, shifting your thoughts, and taking a few deep breaths may help you relieve tension. But if stress begins to interfere with your ability to function on a daily basis, you should talk to your doctor. He or she may recommend a therapist or suggest that you join a support group of other people who are experiencing similar problems.

Everyday stress Daily stress can build up. Here are some positive steps you can take to control the stress in your life:

- Talk about your problems. Get support wherever you can—from friends, relatives, coworkers, your doctor, teachers, counselors, or support groups.
- Eat a healthy diet. A nutritious, well-balanced diet (see page 44) is especially important when you are under stress because stress increases your metabolism, which raises your energy needs. Avoid caffeinated drinks and foods—they can make you more nervous.
- Exercise regularly. Regular exercise is one of the best ways to reduce stress. Fit it into your daily routine (see page 80).
- Get plenty of sleep. Fatigue can reduce your ability to deal with stress.
- Learn to relax. Take at least a few minutes every day to sit back, close your eyes, relax your body, and clear your mind (see page 190).
- Make lists. Writing things down and setting priorities each day helps you gain control of your workload and prevents needless stress.
- Set realistic goals. Being practical about what you can accomplish will avoid frustration, disappointment, and guilt.
- Set priorities. Concentrate your time and energy on doing essential tasks. Delegate whatever responsibilities you can.
- Avoid too many changes at once. Whenever you can, plan major life events, such as changing your job or moving, so they do not occur at the same time.
- See your doctor if the stress in your life becomes overwhelming. Ask him or her to recommend a therapist.

Stress in relationships In many cases, long-term, persistent stress develops in a relationship because a woman (usually unknowingly) has selected a partner who does not meet her needs in a positive way. Women sometimes enter unhealthy relationships, repeating harmful patterns from their past or having their needs met in less than beneficial ways. In this type of relationship, long-standing, unresolved tensions or arguments can lead to depression, anxiety, low self-esteem, or an overall feeling of inadequacy. A stressful relationship can also interfere with a woman's ability to function day-to-day, especially on the job or in other relationships.

Most relationships, casual or serious, short-term or long-term, involve some tension or stress. Choosing a partner who can contribute to your overall emotional well-being will help reduce much of that stress. Learning how to communicate and then making the effort to keep the lines of communication open can be one of the best ways to improve your relationship. Here are some tips:

- Make your relationship a priority. Enjoy at least part of your leisure time together and create time to be alone with each other.
- When making a request of your partner, be specific about what you are asking. Express your message in a way that your partner can understand. Do not expect your partner to be a mind reader.
- Listen actively. Summarize or paraphrase the message you heard to make

sure you understand what your partner said.

■ Do not assume that you know what your partner is thinking or feeling. Ask.

■ Timing is everything. If you are discussing something important, make sure both you and your partner have the energy and time necessary to consider the matter thoroughly.

■ Show appreciation regularly—even for everyday common kindnesses. Let your partner know whenever he or she has done something that has helped you or made you happy. Many relationships fail because people feel taken for granted.

■ Prevent the escalation of a disagreement into a damaging confrontation—it will reduce the possibility of badly hurting your partner's feelings.

■ In disagreements, don't engage in character assassinations, blaming, or name-calling. Focus on the specific behavior, not the person.

■ Concentrate on one problem at a time. Don't confuse the issue at hand with additional problems. Avoid bringing up old conflicts.

■ Think about what you can do constructively to improve a situation. It is far easier to change your own behavior than to change your partner's.

■ Do not use accusatory terms such as "you always" or "you never." They put the other person on the defensive.

■ Acknowledge and respect your partner's right to his or her feelings, whether or not you agree with those feelings. How feelings are expressed is what is most important.

■ If an argument is heating up and escalating to an unproductive point, either partner can step away and take a time-out to allow the situation to cool down. Make sure your partner knows you are putting the argument on pause and not abandoning him or her. You can always approach the topic again at a later time when cooler heads prevail.

■ If your partner compromises or gives in a little, make a compromise yourself.

■ Don't try to win an argument or have the last word. Remember that your goal is to come to some mutual understanding. If either partner loses, the relationship loses.

If you are experiencing problems in your relationship that seem persistent and resistant to change, you and your partner may want to seek professional counseling (see page 194).

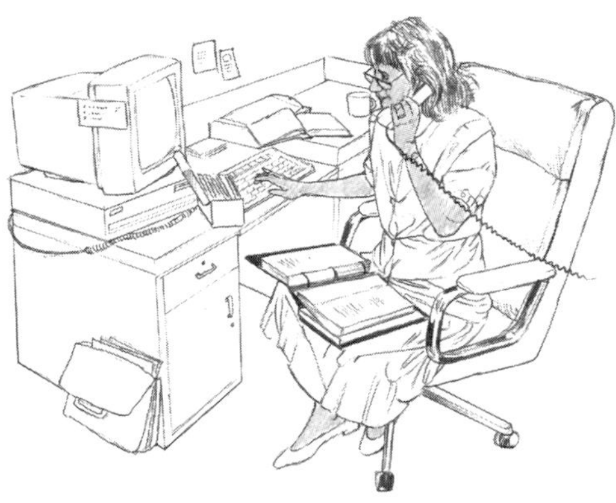

JOB STRESS
A persistently heavy workload is a common source of stress at work. Balancing a demanding or stressful job and personal responsibilities requires good time management skills and a positive attitude.

Stress at work Like any other stress, job stress can build up and affect the quality of your life. If on-the-job difficulties spill over into your personal life, they can affect your relationships and your ability to enjoy life. If you feel that your job is affecting your life in a negative way, the following suggestions may help you regain control of your life.

■ Identify your problems. Make a list of the things that interfere with your ability to work or prevent you from completing assignments.

■ If you think your boss is overloading you with assignments you cannot possibly complete on time, tell him or her. Perhaps you can work out a schedule that is acceptable to you both.

■ Budget your time and set priorities. Spend time each day organizing your work and assigning priorities to tasks.

■ Don't procrastinate. Get assignments done as quickly as you can.

■ Turn unwelcome tasks into challenges and reward yourself for doing a good job.

■ Tackle the most difficult task first.

■ Divide overwhelming projects into manageable chunks. That way, you can feel a sense of accomplishment each time you complete a part.

■ Take regular breaks. Taking a short break from a difficult task can refresh your mind and relieve frustration.

■ Build a network of friends. During lunch hours and breaks you can discuss your difficulties with them. Talking through problems can be one of the best ways to reduce stress.

■ Don't isolate yourself. When you keep everything to yourself, you tend to blow

Coping in times of crisis

If you have experienced a major crisis, such as a death or the loss of a job, the following guidelines can help you cope:

- Friends are good medicine. Choose a person close to you who has a sympathetic ear and talk to him or her about your feelings, no matter how bad. If you have no one you feel you can confide in, talk to your doctor or a qualified mental health professional.
- Break up your time into manageable chunks. If looking ahead to the next few weeks seems overwhelming, plan the coming day. If a full day seems like too long, think about what you will do in the next hour.
- Take action. If someone or something needs your attention, give it. Activity may help you feel more competent.

things out of proportion, which makes them seem worse than they are.

- Don't let your job interfere with your social and family lives.
- Improve your working environment. If you have a desk job, make sure your chair is the right height and your work materials and equipment are where you won't strain your back or your eyes. Personalize your work space by displaying objects that give it a warm feeling.
- If all else fails, explore the possibility of changing jobs while you are still working in the one you have. Networking is the best way to search; call people you know and ask them about positions that may be open at their place of work. Consider retraining for a new career. Many colleges have a wide range of evening classes for adults.

Stress as a parent Nothing can fully prepare you for the role of being a parent. Parenting can provide challenges as well as joys. While the dynamics of family life produce stress for everyone involved, much of that stress is normal and healthy. The way in which you handle difficulties can make the difference—it can strengthen family bonds or break them apart.

Having a child changes your life forever. Whether you are a full-time mother or you work outside the home, are married or single, your energies are focused on meeting the needs of a person who is totally dependent on you. You find little time for yourself. The needs of children demand immediate attention whenever they arise, and every child needs almost 24-hour care to keep him or her happy, healthy, and safe. When your children are very young, you may find it difficult to get enough sleep, which can make you feel tired and irritable most of the time.

Juggling parenting with work outside the home can be especially challenging. Many women who are doing both have a persistent feeling of guilt—they feel they are not doing a good enough job in either role. If you are a single mother, it is especially important to form a network of caring relatives and friends who are there when you need help caring for your children. This benefits everyone; you are sharing the joys of parenting and giving your children opportunities to develop relationships with other adults they can trust. Talking over difficulties with experienced parents can help you learn different ways of dealing with everyday problems and conflicts.

To take on the responsibilities of family life, it is necessary to recognize that there will be stressful situations. Knowing that difficulties are likely to occur can help you deal with them. Sometimes all it takes is better organization and management of your time. Working to solve problems as they come up can strengthen your skills as a parent and bring your family closer together. For example, if money is a source of stress in your family life, get everyone involved in planning a budget and agreeing on how the money should be spent. Show your children that saving—even one dollar a week—is a rewarding habit. Turning stressful events into learning situations can help you focus on the rewards of parenting rather than the problems.

The overall rule for dealing with problems in a family is to concentrate on the stresses you can control and learn to live with the others. Here are some things you can do to help make your experience as a parent a rewarding one:

- Plan for your future needs long before the baby's arrival. If you have a job, think about whether you will continue working or will stay at home to raise your child. Allow yourself some flexibility; give yourself permission to change your mind.
- If you plan to continue working, invest some time in finding a day-care arrangement that makes you feel confident.
- Get all the help you can. Consider trusted friends and relatives valuable

resources—you will benefit and so will your children.

- Share household responsibilities with your partner and your children.
- Learn to say no.
- Set priorities. It is more important to read a bedtime story to your child than to finish the laundry.
- Don't feel guilty about occasionally sitting down with a good book or pursuing another activity you enjoy.
- Leave part of your day unscheduled so that you can accommodate unexpected events or tasks.
- Establish rules for your children and make sure you enforce them. A lack of discipline can cause stress for everyone in the family.
- Teach your children about safety. Make sure they understand they should never talk to strangers.
- Get your children involved in activities—such as playing sports or learning a musical instrument—that they enjoy and can do well. They will take pride in their achievement. Children can become bored, unchallenged, or mischievous when they have too much free time.
- Have realistic expectations of your children. If you expect too much of a child, you will constantly be disappointed and your child will feel he or she can never measure up.
- Stock up. Having things on hand that you know you need can limit time-consuming trips to the grocery store.

Stress as a caregiver Women who care for sick relatives or close friends may find that their own emotional and physical health begins to suffer. Most people who care for aging relatives show signs of emotional distress and depression that cause physical ailments as well. You need occasional relief from the responsibilities of caregiving to take care of your own needs and replenish your energy. The only way to get help when you need it is to ask for it. Here are some steps you can take to relieve some of the pressures of caregiving:

- Take care of your own needs first; you'll then be better prepared to take care of someone else's needs.
- Actively seek out a small number of people who will be reliable, consistent helpers when you need them.
- Look for groups in your community that offer support and help for caregivers—including home nursing or day care for people with Alzheimer's disease. Many such groups have volunteers that can relieve you of some daily tasks, such as meal preparation.
- Accept offers of meals and other favors from friends and neighbors.
- Ask a relative or friend to stay with your loved one while you take care of your own affairs.
- Ask for help finding alternative sources of care when you can no longer provide adequate care at home. (For more about being a caregiver, see page 585.)

When to seek help

Everyone feels down from time to time, especially after a loss or disappointment. In some people, overwhelming stress can cause symptoms similar to those of depression (see page 594). There is no clearly defined line between mild depression or feeling bad about a normal everyday problem and major depression that becomes incapacitating. But here are some clues to help you distinguish between a temporary setback or blue mood and more serious depression for which you may need professional help. Talk to your doctor if you experience any of the following:

- A low mood that feels severe and painful and lasts for more than a month or recurs frequently
- A mild depression that won't lift after several months
- Suicidal thoughts
- A low mood that is accompanied by symptoms such as loss of appetite, sleeping problems, loss of sexual desire, or inability to concentrate or make decisions
- Inability to live your life normally or enjoy activities that you used to find pleasurable
- Feelings of worthlessness, helplessness, hopelessness, or guilt

RELAXATION TRAINING

For some people, learning techniques to induce relaxation can help reverse many of the physical effects of stress—including increased heart rate, blood pressure, and muscle tension. Relaxation training can also help prevent normal, everyday stress from becoming overwhelming.

Relaxation training can be helpful in reducing pain for people who have migraine and tension headaches and in reestablishing normal sleeping patterns for people who have sleep disorders. Couples with infertility problems often find that stress can interfere with their treatment; for many of these couples, relaxation therapy may improve the odds of conception. For people who are undergoing chemotherapy or radiation therapy for cancer, relaxation therapy may help relieve the anxiety and depression that often accompanies these treatments.

Learn to relax

A state of relaxation can counteract the potentially harmful effects of being under stress. When you are relaxed, your breathing and heart rate slow, your need for oxygen is reduced, and the electrical activity of your brain changes to a characteristic resting pattern.

Learning to make yourself relax is easy to do. Try to find at least 10 to 20 minutes in your day to relax—twice a day is even more effective. Here's how:

- Sit in a comfortable position in a quiet place. Close your eyes and relax your muscles.
- Choose a single word or short phrase to focus on. Choose a word or phrase with some personal meaning to you. You can even choose a neutral word such as "one" or "love."
- Breathe slowly in a comfortable rhythm, repeating your word silently as you exhale. Try to keep your mind blank except for the word. When other thoughts enter your mind, don't worry about them—just go back to concentrating on the focus word.
- Choose a length of time—10 to 20 minutes—and stick to it. You may open your eyes every now and then to check the time, but don't use an alarm, because the noise can be too startling.
- When you are finished, sit quietly for a few minutes with your eyes closed and then with your eyes open to ease out of your relaxed state.

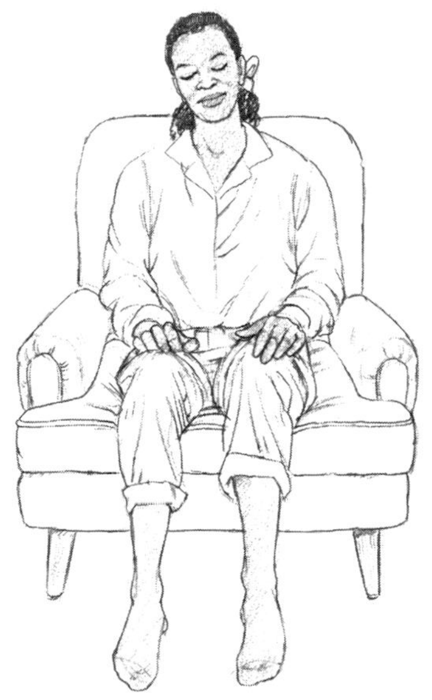

Exercise is good for your mind

Exercise is good for both your body and your mind. Most people who exercise say that, in addition to improving their physical fitness, it makes them feel healthier and happier and helps them sleep better. Exercise is one of the most effective stress relievers. It can lift mild depression and boost self-esteem. Exercise affects the brain by boosting levels of endorphins, brain chemicals that make you feel good and that act as natural painkillers. Regular exercise can also instill a feeling of accomplishment and achievement.

The physical improvement that comes from exercise, including a reduction in fat and increase in muscle strength and fitness, can give you a more positive self-image and greater self-confidence. Exercise can also raise mental and intellectual capacities such as alertness. When you exercise, your brain receives more blood, which delivers oxygen and other nutrients to brain cells. Regular exercise may help prevent the gradual mental decline that sometimes occurs with age.

You do not have to exercise as vigorously as experts once thought to obtain physical and psychological benefits. People who are the most sedentary have the most to gain in terms of improving their health from introducing even moderate exercise into their daily life. (For more about fitness, see chapter 2.)

Getting a good night's sleep

Getting enough hours of sound sleep is important for your health and well-being. A lack of sleep can affect you both physically and mentally. Sleep deprivation can reduce the effectiveness of your immune system, making you more susceptible to colds and other illnesses, and can interfere with your memory and concentration. People who do not get enough sleep may have trouble coping with minor irritations, completing necessary tasks, or enjoying family and social relationships. Lack of sleep may make you fall asleep suddenly during the day under inappropriate or even dangerous circumstances. People who fall asleep while driving are responsible for a large percentage of accidents.

Sleep deprivation has a number of causes. Many people have some degree of insomnia, a sleep disorder characterized by difficulty falling or staying asleep. If you have insomnia, see your doctor. Do not try to treat the problem yourself with alcohol or drugs. (For more about insomnia and its treatment, see page 609.)

Sleep deprivation can also result from taking some medications, working nights or changing shifts, or from simply not setting aside enough hours for sleep. Some illnesses—such as depression, incontinence, or painful arthritis—can also interfere with sleep. For self-help tips for getting a good night's sleep, see the box below.

Self-help tips for improving your sleep

If you have difficulty getting a good night's sleep, changing your habits can sometimes help. Try the following:

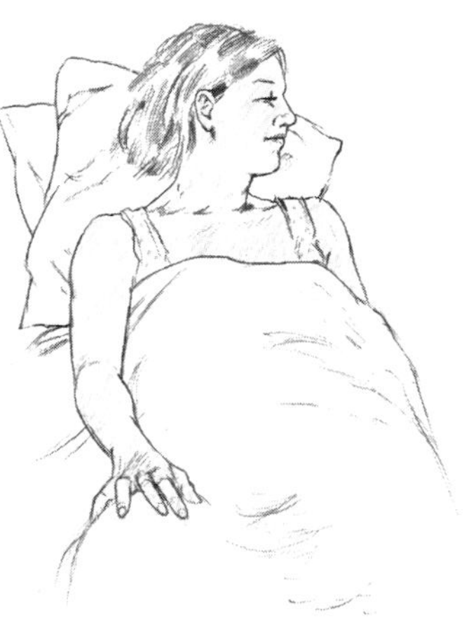

- Try to go to bed and get up at the same time every day; doing so can help program your body's biological clock.
- Set aside enough hours for sleep each day.
- Limit naps. A short nap at the same time each day can be refreshing, but you should allow that much less time for sleep at night.
- Make your bedroom comfortable for sleeping. Do not use it for other activities such as watching TV, eating, reading, or finishing work.
- Wind down before you go to bed. Do some relaxation exercises (see page 190), listen to soft music, or read a good book—whatever you find relaxing.
- Although regular exercise will help you sleep, exercising right before bedtime can make it more difficult to fall asleep. Exercise increases metabolism and alertness.
- Do not drink alcohol late in the evening. Even one drink can make you sleep less soundly.
- Do not drink caffeinated beverages or smoke cigarettes before going to bed. Caffeine and nicotine are stimulants that can keep you awake.
- Don't go to bed either hungry or on a full stomach. A light carbohydrate snack before bedtime can help you sleep.

SYMPTOM CHART

Difficulty sleeping

Frequent problems either falling asleep or staying asleep during the night (also called insomnia).

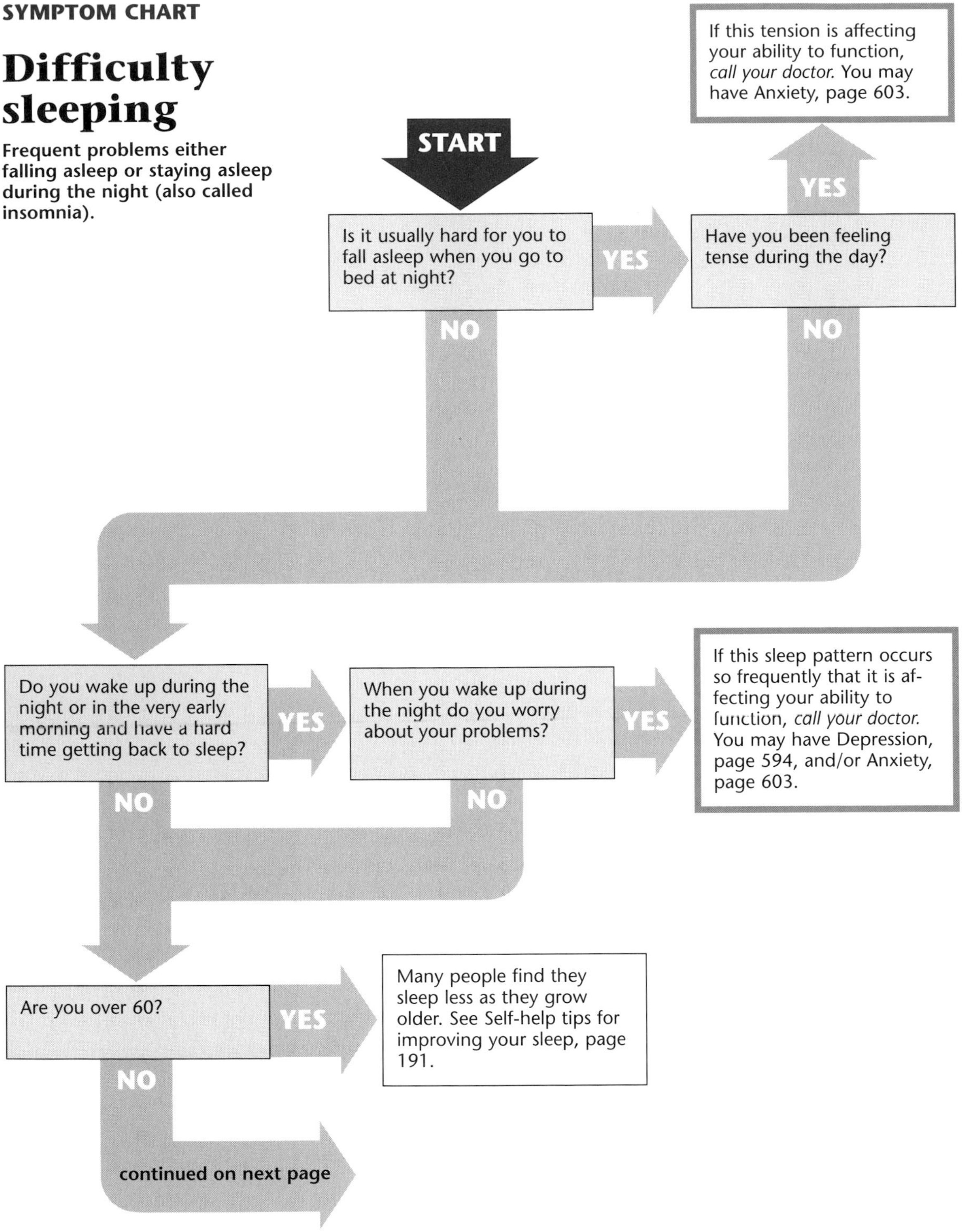

START

Is it usually hard for you to fall asleep when you go to bed at night?

YES → Have you been feeling tense during the day?

YES → If this tension is affecting your ability to function, *call your doctor.* You may have Anxiety, page 603.

NO (to either question) → Do you wake up during the night or in the very early morning and have a hard time getting back to sleep?

YES → When you wake up during the night do you worry about your problems?

YES → If this sleep pattern occurs so frequently that it is affecting your ability to function, *call your doctor.* You may have Depression, page 594, and/or Anxiety, page 603.

NO (to either question) → Are you over 60?

YES → Many people find they sleep less as they grow older. See Self-help tips for improving your sleep, page 191.

NO → **continued on next page**

continued from previous page

On nights when you have difficulty sleeping, have you had more caffeine-containing coffee, cola, or tea than usual?

YES → Try to avoid caffeine or drink only small amounts in the late afternoon and evening. Try switching to decaffeinated beverages. See Caffeine, page 65.

NO ↓

On nights when you have difficulty sleeping, have you eaten a late, heavy meal or consumed a lot of alcohol?

YES → For many people, eating late at night or consuming a large amount of alcohol can disrupt sleep. Try eating your evening meal earlier and/or reducing your intake of alcohol.

NO ↓

Have you recently stopped taking, or reduced your dosage of, tranquilizers or sleeping pills?

YES → *Call your doctor.* Suddenly stopping or reducing your intake of sleeping pills can cause dizziness, headaches, and other symptoms. See Sleeping pills, page 609.

NO ↓

Do you have a sedentary job and get little exercise when you are not working?

YES → Getting more exercise may help you sleep better. See Starting an exercise program, page 78.

NO ↓

If you are unable to make a diagnosis from this chart, and the self-help suggestions do not work, call your doctor.

Don't self-medicate

If you are having difficulty getting enough sleep, do not try to solve your problem with over-the-counter sleeping pills or alcohol. They do not help you over the long term and may even contribute to other problems. Try the self-help tips on page 191 or talk to your doctor.

Getting professional help

When psychological or emotional problems become so severe that they interfere with your ability to function on a daily basis, you need to get help. Discuss your concerns with your doctor, who may be able to help you or can refer you to a qualified mental health professional. It is important to choose a therapist wisely—you need to feel comfortable talking with this person about your innermost thoughts and feelings and trust in his or her ability to help you.

There are a variety of mental health professionals—including psychiatrists, psychologists, and social workers—who differ primarily by their training. Psychiatrists are medical doctors (MDs) who have completed 4 years of medical school in addition to 3 or more years of training in the medical specialty of psychiatry. Psychiatrists are the only therapists who can prescribe medication. They tend to deal with more severe mental disorders—including major depression—that can be treated with medication. They are also more medically oriented than other therapists—they can evaluate the effect that a medical illness may have on a person's emotions and behavior. Psychiatrists can distinguish between stress-related physical symptoms and an accompanying medical illness.

Psychologists have a doctorate (PhD) in psychology and up to 2 years of supervised full-time clinical training. They must be licensed by the state in which they practice. Social workers usually have a master's degree; some have a PhD as well. Social workers must also pass a state licensing examination to practice. Psychologists and social workers often work in collaboration with a psychiatrist if a patient's symptoms are related to a medical illness that requires evaluation or medication. Some mental health professionals specialize in specific areas such as children, families, marriage counseling, or substance abuse.

PSYCHOTHERAPY

Most therapists—psychiatrists, psychologists, or other counselors—practice some form of psychotherapy. Psychotherapy is a general term for a variety of treatments that are used for helping people change their behavior and experience through talking. Besides discussion, psychotherapy includes techniques such as reinforcement, reassurance, and support. Most mental health professionals use one or more of these techniques, depending on the situation and the person's needs. The goals of psychotherapy, either with individuals or with groups, include changing behavior, improving relationships, resolving inner conflicts that may be causing problems, and improving a person's self-image.

Psychotherapy can also be effective in helping people recover more quickly from an illness and in reducing their risk of a relapse. Psychotherapy can help relieve some of the devastating emotional impact of being seriously ill. In some people, emotional issues or conflicts that are difficult to express verbally are expressed in the form of a physical symptom or condition.

Group therapy—a form of psychotherapy in which people with similar experiences share their thoughts and feelings—can be useful in situations in which emotions and physical illness interact. For example, following treatment for breast cancer, women who attend group therapy sessions with other women who have breast cancer can improve their chance of survival. In group therapy, people support and encourage each other by sharing their feelings and physical problems and experiences, such as coping with the loss of a breast. The effectiveness of support groups for people with serious health problems lies in their ability to help them relieve depression and sustain their interest in life.

·2·

Sexual and reproductive health

CHAPTER 7

The reproductive system and menstrual cycle

Contents

Your reproductive organs are part of an elegantly synchronized system that is designed to fulfill both your sexual and reproductive needs. Knowing how your reproductive system works, from before puberty to menopause and after, helps you plan your reproductive life, understand your sexual life, and recognize symptoms of possible problems.

The female reproductive system

Your reproductive system includes your vulva (external genitals) and internal reproductive organs—the vagina, cervix, uterus, fallopian tubes, and ovaries. All the reproductive and sexual processes that take place in these organs are carefully orchestrated by chemical signals from your brain.

EXTERNAL GENITALS

To see your external genital area, sit cross-legged with a small mirror between your legs. The vulva is the entire outer, visible genital area, including the mons pubis (the hair-covered mound over the pubic bone). Pubic hair runs the length of the vulva and, in some women, down the upper thighs or up the abdomen toward the navel. The amount of hair, which first appears during puberty, tends to increase as a young woman matures. The amount of pubic hair she ends up with as an adult can be heavy or sparse, both of which are normal.

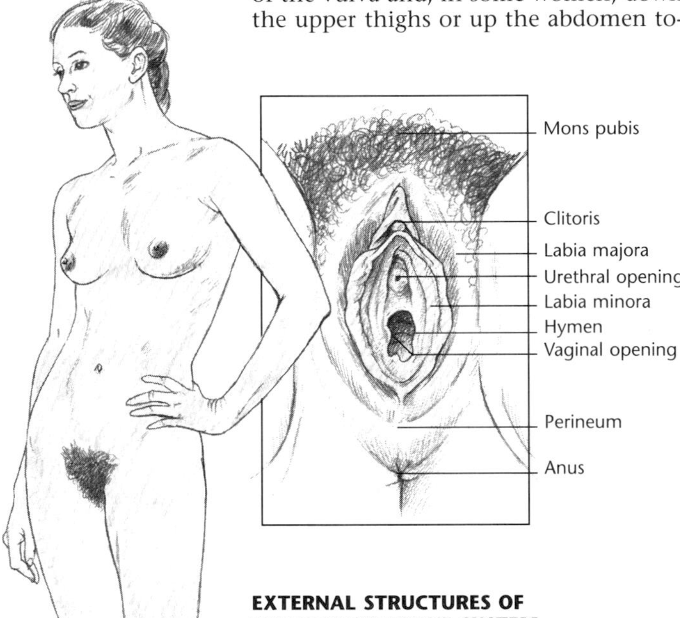

EXTERNAL STRUCTURES OF THE REPRODUCTIVE SYSTEM

Although much of a woman's reproductive system is internal, the genitals are visible. It's a good idea to familiarize yourself with the way your genitals look so you can identify any change that might warrant a visit to your doctor. See your doctor if you notice any swelling, irritation, change in color, or new lumps or bumps.

The vulva includes the labia majora, the outer, larger set of hair-covered "lips" that cover and protect the opening to your vagina. The labia majora lie close together in women who have not had children. After childbirth, they tend to separate slightly, making the labia minora (the smaller, inner lips) and the opening to the vagina easier to see. The labia minora, which lie just inside the labia majora, are hairless and very sensitive to touch. They also protect the opening to the vagina.

The clitoris lies at the junction where the labia minora meet at the top. The clitoris is a tiny (about the size of a pea) but extremely sensitive mound of tissue that plays a powerful role in a woman's sexual arousal (see page 291). During sexual arousal, the clitoris, the labia minora, the vagina, and the network of connecting blood vessels and muscles all swell with blood.

The urethral, or urinary, opening is located just below the clitoris. Urine from your bladder empties into a short tube called the urethra and out of your body through the urethral opening. The vaginal opening lies just below the urethral opening. The hymen is a delicate, elastic mucous membrane that surrounds the vaginal opening. The perineum is the area of skin and underlying muscle between the vagina and anus. The perineum stretches during childbirth to allow passage of the baby.

INTERNAL ORGANS

The vagina is the entrance to the internal reproductive system. Sperm travel through the vagina and cervix, into the uterus and on into one of the fallopian tubes, where one sperm may fertilize an egg. The ovaries produce eggs and release them one at a time in a monthly cycle into a fallopian tube. When an egg is fertilized in the fallopian tube, it then travels to the uterus and embeds itself in the lining (the endometrium), where it develops and grows into a fetus. An egg that is not fertilized disintegrates and is eliminated in menstrual blood.

INTERNAL ORGANS OF THE REPRODUCTIVE SYSTEM

The female reproductive organs are located in the lower abdomen. Each month, an ovary releases a mature egg, which moves through a fallopian tube into the uterus. If the egg is fertilized by a sperm, it will implant itself in the wall of the uterus (endometrium) and develop into a fetus. If the egg is not fertilized, it will be eliminated through the cervix and vagina in menstrual blood.

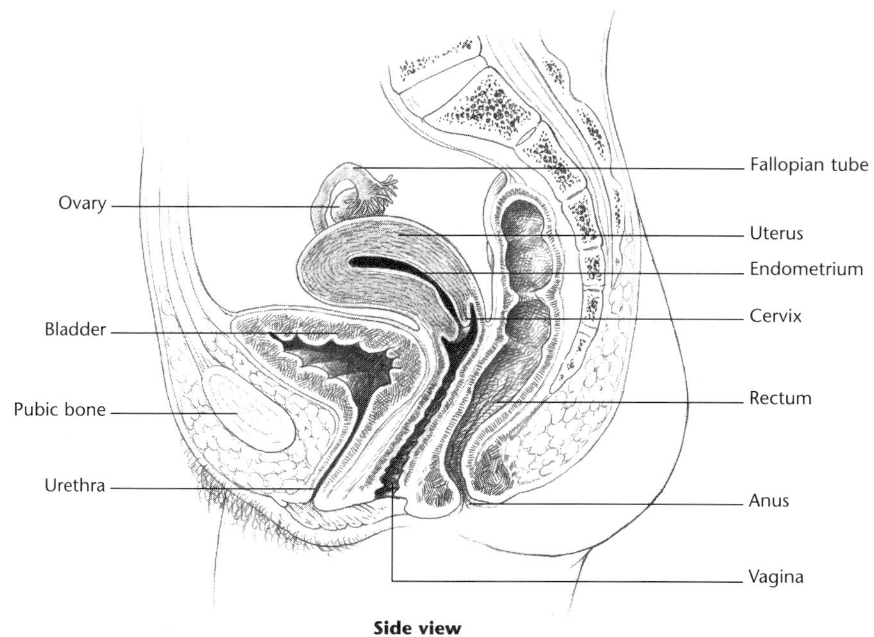

Side view

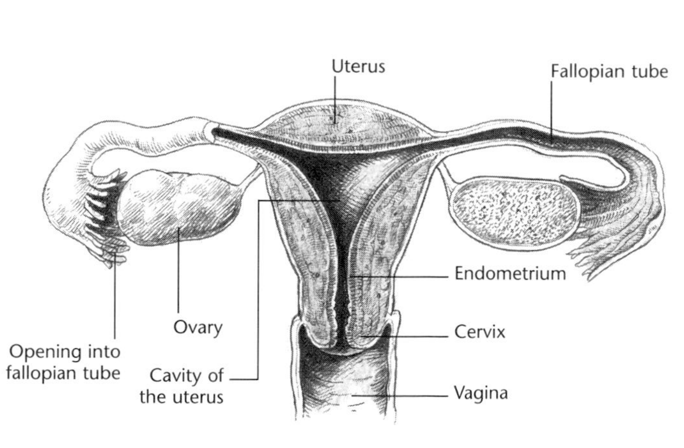

Front view

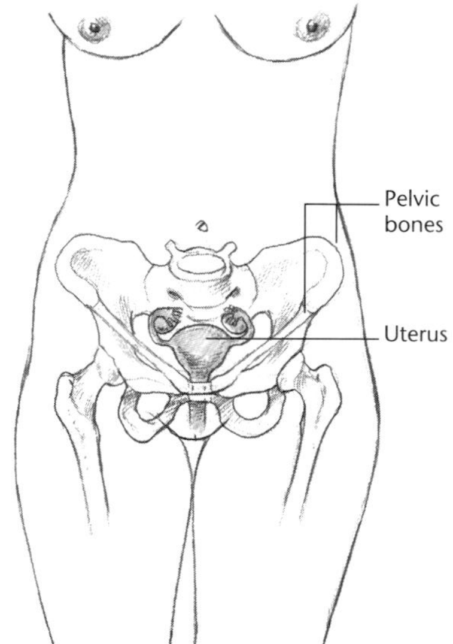

Location of reproductive organs in pelvis

Vagina The vagina is a muscular tube about 3 to 5 inches long. It is the entrance to your internal reproductive organs and accommodates a man's penis during sexual intercourse. If you insert your finger into your vaginal opening, you can feel ridges, which are rings of muscle inside your vagina. During intercourse, the vaginal muscles tighten around the penis, giving both partners increased sexual sensation. During labor and delivery, these muscles expand and stretch to allow passage of the baby.

The inside of the vaginal opening may be partially covered by a membrane called the hymen. During a woman's first experience of sexual intercourse, the penis stretches the hymen and sometimes tears it. Traditionally, the hymen has been considered an indicator of virginity. In fact, a woman "loses her virginity" only by having intercourse for the first time.

The vagina constantly produces secretions to maintain a naturally moist environment and a balance of helpful bacteria. During sexual arousal, the vagina secretes more fluids to provide lubrication during intercourse. Some vaginal discharge is normal for everyone. However, if these vaginal secretions cause irritation, have a strong or unpleasant odor, or increase significantly in volume, you should see your doctor. You may have a vaginal infection. (For more about vaginal infections, see page 216.)

Cervix The cervix is a small, cylindrical organ that makes up the lower portion of your uterus. The cervix is the opening into the uterus from the vagina. Glands inside the cervix produce cervical mucus, which increases in amount in the middle of your menstrual cycle.

Most of the time the cervix is covered by a mucous plug that prevents bacteria and other microbes from entering the uterus. The mucous plug dissolves every month to allow blood to flow out during menstruation.

Uterus The uterus is a small, hollow organ about the size and shape of a small pear in the center of the pelvis. Its thick, muscular walls are lined with endometrium, tissue that builds up and then sheds during each menstrual cycle.

In pregnancy, a fertilized egg implants itself in the lining of the uterus and grows into a fetus inside the uterus. The uterus is remarkably elastic, expanding to many times its original size to accommodate the growth of a fetus. Following pregnancy, it gradually returns to its original shape and size.

In most women, the uterus tips forward toward the bladder, but, in about one fourth of women, it tips backward. This backward tilt is a normal variation and not a cause of infertility or any other gynecologic disorder, nor does it affect a woman's ability to carry a pregnancy to term.

Fallopian tubes The fallopian tubes are two thin tubes, about 4 or 5 inches long, that extend from the uterus to the ovaries. The ends of the tubes nearest the ovaries flare out and are open to receive an egg. Each month, one egg is expelled by one of the ovaries and transported through the adjoining tube toward the uterus. If the egg is fertilized in a fallopian tube, this fertilized egg continues its journey to the uterus, where it will develop into a fetus. An egg that is not fertilized eventually disintegrates and is eliminated in menstrual blood.

When you hear of a woman having her tubes tied to prevent pregnancy, it is her fallopian tubes that are closed off (see page 327).

Ovaries You have two ovaries, one on each side of your pelvis, next to the opening of a fallopian tube. The ovaries are about the size of walnuts. You are born with hundreds of thousands of eggs inside each ovary; only about 500 of them ever develop into mature eggs. The eggs reside in tiny cavities called follicles inside each ovary. The cells that surround the egg nurture it. The follicle and supporting tissue manufacture the female hormones estrogen and progesterone as well as a small amount of male hormones called androgens, all of which play an important role in the reproductive cycle.

Between puberty and menopause, your ovaries release an egg each month. Each monthly cycle begins when the pituitary gland at the base of your brain releases a hormone called follicle-stimulating hormone (FSH), which signals one of your ovaries to begin forming a follicle. Midpoint in the cycle, the pituitary gland releases luteinizing hormone (LH),

Sex hormones

The sex hormones play key roles in the reproductive cycle. Their delicately balanced and timed release keeps the intricate reproductive system functioning smoothly.

- **Estrogen** Estrogen is the key female sex hormone, produced mostly in the ovaries. Estrogen has been present in most living organisms for millions of years. The hormone is incredibly versatile—it can carry different messages to many types of cells. In females, estrogen carries instructions for building and maintaining the reproductive system. In both males and females, estrogen plays a critical role in keeping brain cells healthy.
- **Follicle-stimulating hormone (FSH) and luteinizing hormone (LH)** FSH and LH are hormones that are produced by the pituitary gland in the brain in both men and women. In women, the hormones regulate the menstrual cycle by stimulating the ovaries to produce and release a mature egg in a cyclic process called ovulation. In men, FSH and LH regulate the production of sperm in the testicles.
- **Progesterone** Progesterone is produced in the ovaries during the second half of the menstrual cycle after ovulation has occurred. Progesterone causes the lining of the uterus (the endometrium) to become thick and spongy in preparation for a fertilized egg. During pregnancy, progesterone is essential for the healthy development of the fetus and for normal functioning of the placenta, the organ that develops around the fetus and links the blood supplies of the fetus and the mother. Progesterone is also produced in small quantities in the adrenal glands in both men and women and in the testicles in men.
- **Testosterone** Testosterone is a male hormone that is produced in small amounts in a woman's ovaries and adrenal glands. Testosterone plays a role in bone and muscle growth and in sexual development. The hormone is also involved in both male and female sex drive (libido).

which triggers the fully formed follicle to release an egg. The release of an egg is called ovulation. The egg normally travels through the fallopian tube to the uterus. Because the pituitary gland regulates the menstrual cycle, any damage to the pituitary gland can affect a woman's fertility.

Puberty

Puberty is a process, not an event. It is the body's natural transition from physical and sexual immaturity to maturity. The process of puberty can take from 1½ to 6 years and can begin anytime between ages 8 and 13. By the end of puberty, your ovaries are producing the female hormone estrogen, your reproductive organs are fully functioning, and you are capable of having children.

STAGES OF PUBERTY

The timing of puberty is different for everyone. Genes play a large role. Daughters tend to go through puberty at about the same age as their mother or the women on their father's side of the family. If your mother or female relatives began developing breasts at an early age, you may too.

Girls who begin to develop earlier than their friends may be worried about their body's rapid changes and may feel self-conscious. Girls who are "late bloomers" may feel just as self-conscious. But both patterns are normal. The age at which the breasts begin to develop or a girl has her first menstrual period can vary by several years (from ages 9 to 15) from one person to the next. Most girls, however, begin to develop breasts by age 13 and to menstruate by age 15 or 16.

In general, puberty progresses in the following stages:

Stage 1 (roughly ages 8 to 11) The first stage of puberty begins when the pituitary gland and hypothalamus in the brain and the ovaries begin producing hormones. The first thing you may notice is breast buds; your nipples become slightly elevated as a result of the growth of breast tissue underneath them.

At this time, you will begin to grow rapidly in height and weight. At about age 10, the average girl has reached about 80 percent of her adult height. She will make up the remaining height very quickly in the next few years. The growth spurt follows a distinctive pattern. First the head, feet, and hands begin to grow. Then the arm and leg bones grow longer and stronger, adding several inches of height. The trunk is the last area to reach adult proportions.

Weight also increases. After age 10, you will begin to gain weight rapidly. In females, fat increases in greater proportion to muscle and bone; a woman's body has a higher proportion of fat than a man's. The female hormone estrogen adds fat to a woman's body, while the male hormone testosterone builds muscle in a man's body.

Stage 2 (roughly ages 9 to 14) Breast growth is the first visible sign of sexual development. Pubic hair appears several months later. The growth of underarm hair begins about a year later, coinciding with an increase in sweat glands under the arms that cause a girl to perspire more. The inner and outer folds of the labia majora (the lips of the external genitals) enlarge somewhat; by the time menstruation begins, they will cover the vaginal opening. The vagina begins to grow longer and the uterus begins to grow into a strong, muscular organ about the size and shape of a small pear. The increased production of hormones triggers increased oil production in pores in the skin, especially those on the face, which can cause acne (see page 677).

Stage 3 (roughly ages 10 to 17) The breasts continue developing; the areola may protrude, forming a separate mound from the rest of the breast. Although still sparse, the pubic hair becomes thicker and darker, starting to fill in a characteristic triangle pattern. Height and weight increase gradually. The vagina and internal organs continue to grow, and the composition of vaginal fluids begins to change. A white, creamy discharge from the vagina often appears 6 to 12 months before menstruation begins. The discharge may be heavy or barely noticeable—both are normal. Wearing cotton underwear helps absorb the fluid. Any pain, soreness, or itching in the genital area may be a sign of infection. In this case, you should see your doctor.

Most girls begin menstruating during this stage. In the US, the average age for a girl to begin menstruating is about 12 years. Very thin girls may begin menstruating later than other girls because their body may not be producing as much estrogen. Although most estrogen is supplied by the ovaries, fat cells also produce the hormone. Therefore, the more fat cells a woman has, the more estrogen her body produces.

The ovaries continue to enlarge and begin releasing eggs each month. This process, called ovulation, may begin 3 to 12 months after menstruation begins. Once you start ovulating, you are able to become pregnant. It is safest to assume that you can become pregnant once you have started having periods. Ovulation becomes more regular and consistent in the next stage.

Stage 4 (roughly ages 14 to 18) In the final stage of development, a girl reaches physical and sexual maturity. She grows to her full height. Her menstrual periods and ovulation become regular. Her breasts reach full size, and the protruding areola becomes part of the contour of the breast. A rapid growth spurt or sudden weight gain may cause darkened lines called stretch marks to form on the skin of a girl's upper thighs, buttocks, or breasts; these marks will fade with time but never disappear completely.

EARLY DEVELOPMENT

Most girls who develop earlier than their peers fall within the normal range and there is no reason for concern. But when puberty begins before age 8, it is considered to be premature. For some reason, either the ovaries, or the hypothalamus and pituitary gland in the brain—which regulate the onset of puberty and sexual development—get an early signal to "switch on." If your daughter begins developing before age 8, you should take her to see a doctor to find the cause. He or she can rule out a tumor on an ovary or on the pituitary gland, a cyst on an ovary, or other medical condition. A tumor or cyst may be removed surgically.

How your body matures

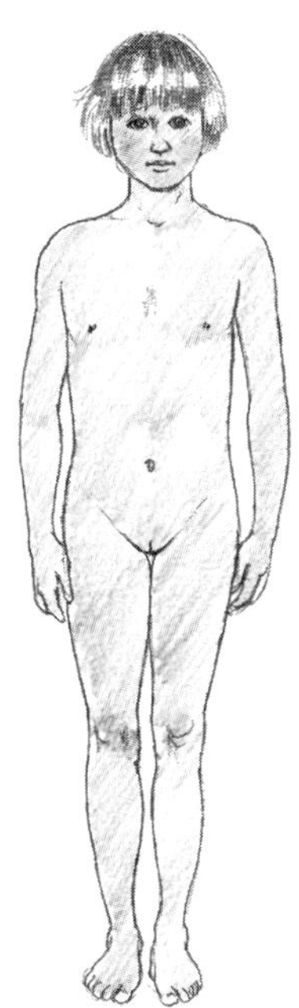

BEFORE PUBERTY
The breasts are flat and the hips are narrow. There is no underarm or pubic hair. The reproductive organs are small and not yet developed.

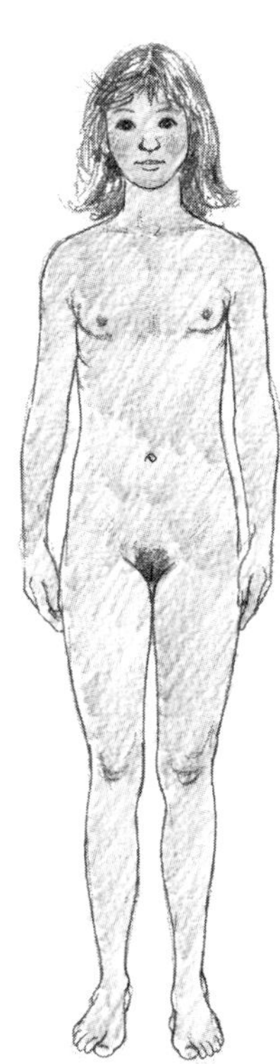

EARLY PUBERTY
Breast buds begin to emerge and the pelvis begins to widen. Fat accumulates on the hips. Pubic and underarm hair begins to grow. Growth spurts occur in the long bones, such as those in the legs, and in the head, hands, and feet. Internal and external sexual organs begin to grow. Menstruation may begin.

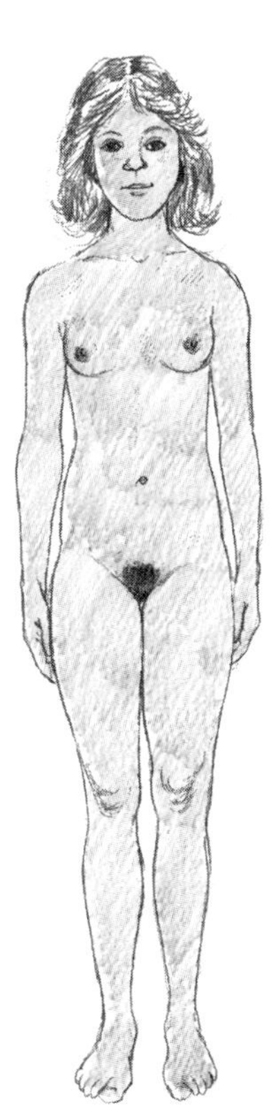

LATE PUBERTY
The breasts continue to grow. Pubic hair and underarm hair begin to thicken. The hips widen. Fat accumulates on the hips, buttocks, and breasts. Menstruation begins. The reproductive organs continue to develop. The ovaries begin to produce eggs (a process called ovulation). The long bones, such as those in the legs, continue to grow.

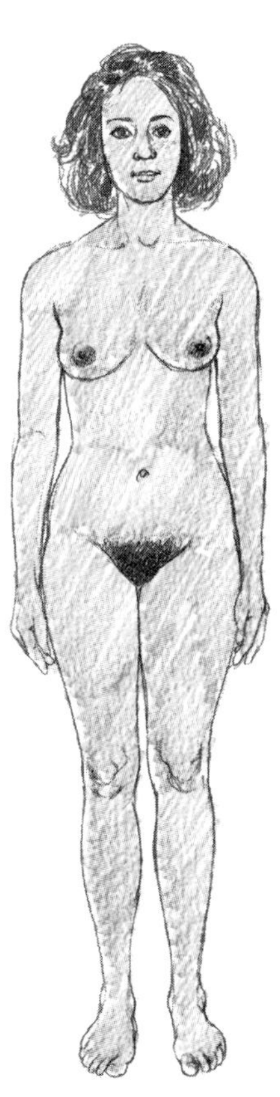

MATURATION
The body reaches full, rounded proportions. The bones have completed their growth. Menstruation and ovulation become regular.

In other cases, treatment with a hormone that decreases estrogen production may help slow sexual development.

A girl who begins to develop within the normal range but earlier than her peers may feel self-conscious around friends and classmates. She needs to be reassured that her development is normal and healthy. She is going through a stage that all girls go through; she is just going through it at an earlier age. It takes most girls a period of adjustment to feel comfortable with their own natural development. But it is equally important for girls who are reaching physical and sexual maturity to receive adequate information about what is happening to their body and to understand that sexual activity can result in pregnancy.

Why are girls beginning puberty at younger ages?

The average age at which puberty begins has gradually decreased in the US over the past century. Although the reasons for the increasing incidence of early puberty are not fully understood, onset of menstruation appears to be related to a girl's weight and percentage of body fat. As a result of improved nutrition in the 20th century, girls are physically maturing at a faster rate and, therefore, are beginning to menstruate at younger ages.

LATE DEVELOPMENT

Like early puberty, late puberty is influenced by genes. If a girl's mother or the women on her father's side of the family matured late, she may also. She and her parents need not be worried unless she shows no signs of sexual development, such as breast enlargement or the growth of pubic hair, by age 14 or if she has not begun to menstruate by age 16. In either case, she should see a doctor. He or she can determine the cause of her late development and recommend treatment, if necessary.

Girls who mature late may worry that they never will. They may feel different from the girls whose breasts have already developed and who have begun menstruating. In most cases, girls who mature late catch up to their peers by the time they are 18.

Menstruation

Whether or not you ever plan to have children, your body prepares for that possibility every month for 35 to 40 years between puberty and menopause. Each month, your reproductive system goes through a cycle of fertility that results in either conception (pregnancy) or menstruation. Menstruation is the cyclical shedding of the lining of the uterus, accompanied by bleeding. The menstrual cycle is intricately orchestrated by your brain and its hormone-signaling system. A woman's menstrual cycle is an essential process. Understanding your menstrual cycle can help you figure out when you are most likely to get pregnant—important information whether you want to get pregnant or avoid it.

THE CYCLE

The average menstrual cycle is 28 days long, but the length can vary by several days from woman to woman. The normal range is from 24 to 35 days, counting from the first day of one period to the first day of the next. Generally, the cycle progresses as follows:

- **Day 1** On the first day of menstrual blood flow, the lining of the uterus (endometrium) begins to leave your body through the vagina.
- **About day 5** Blood flow stops.
- **About day 9** The endometrium begins to thicken again.
- **About day 14** Ovulation occurs (an egg is released from an ovary). Your chance of becoming pregnant is greatest around this time.
- **About day 28** If the egg is not fertilized, the egg and the endometrium are shed. Menstrual blood flow begins a new cycle.

Every woman is born with hundreds of thousands of immature eggs inside her ovaries. Each egg is encased in a nest of cells called a follicle. At puberty, the pituitary gland in the brain begins producing follicle-stimulating hormone (FSH) in slowly increasing amounts each month. At the beginning of each menstrual cycle, this hormone stimulates the ovaries and causes a few eggs and follicles to develop. Usually only one follicle fully matures and grows—from being barely visible to the naked eye to measuring about three quarters of an inch across.

About 14 days before the start of the next menstrual period, the pituitary gland and hypothalamus release a surge of luteinizing hormone (LH). In response, ovulation occurs—the ovary releases the mature egg and its surrounding mass of cells. Usually only one egg is released from one of the ovaries, but occasionally two or more are released. The egg (or eggs) travels through the fallopian tube, where it may or may not be fertilized by a sperm, and into the uterus. The fertilization of two eggs results in nonidentical twins.

You are most likely to get pregnant while the egg is traveling through the fallopian tube. An egg lives for 12 to 24 hours after it is released from an ovary but sperm can survive for 2 to 3 days in the fallopian tube; for this reason, you can get pregnant having intercourse 2 or 3 days before ovulation or a day or two after ovulation. (For more about timing intercourse for pregnancy, see page 379; for more about timing intercourse to avoid pregnancy, see page 329.)

Before and after ovulation, the follicle produces hormones that help synchronize the entire menstrual cycle. Before ovulation, the follicle secretes hormones that signal the uterus to prepare to receive a fertilized egg. During this period, called the preovulatory or follicular part of the cycle, the follicle produces mainly the hormone estrogen.

After ovulation, the follicle continues to produce hormones that nourish the lining of the uterus. When an egg is released from an ovary, the follicle secretes the hormone progesterone, which makes the lining of the uterus (endometrium) receptive to a fertilized egg. The endometrium has already responded to the increased level of estrogen by thickening with additional supporting tissue and blood vessels. After ovulation, the presence of both progesterone and estrogen causes the endometrium to fully mature and swell.

If an egg has not been fertilized, the levels of estrogen and progesterone drop. The membranes holding the blood vessels in the endometrium disintegrate and the supporting tissue fills with blood. The uterus begins breaking down its rich lining and sheds it in the monthly flow of blood called menstruation. The first day of menstrual flow is considered the first day of a new cycle. After the bleeding stops, the lining of the uterus begins preparing for the next cycle and, with the next period, the process starts again.

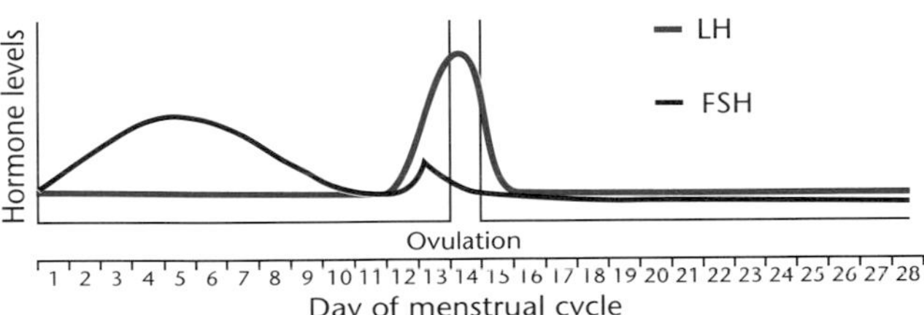

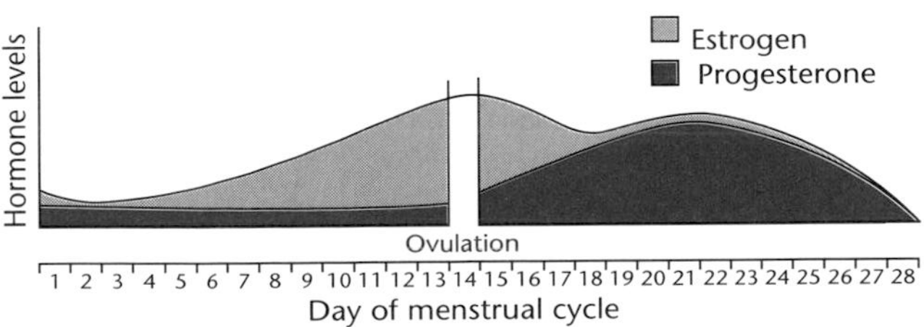

HORMONES AND THE MENSTRUAL CYCLE

Early in the menstrual cycle (top), increased levels of follicle-stimulating hormone (FSH) stimulate eggs to develop. On about day 14, a surge in luteinizing hormone (LH) causes an ovary to release an egg. Early in the menstrual cycle (bottom), estrogen production steadily increases, signaling the uterus to prepare for a fertilized egg. After ovulation, production of progesterone increases, further preparing the uterus for pregnancy. If the egg is not fertilized, hormone levels drop and menstruation occurs.

HOW OFTEN? HOW LONG?

Menstruation usually begins between ages 11 and 14. (The first period is referred to as menarche.) Your periods may be irregular for the first few years because ovulation (release of an egg from one of your ovaries) does not always occur. However, you should not think that you cannot become pregnant during these early years. As soon as you begin to menstruate, you are able to become pregnant. Most women have regular periods by age 18, or several years after they begin

The menstrual cycle

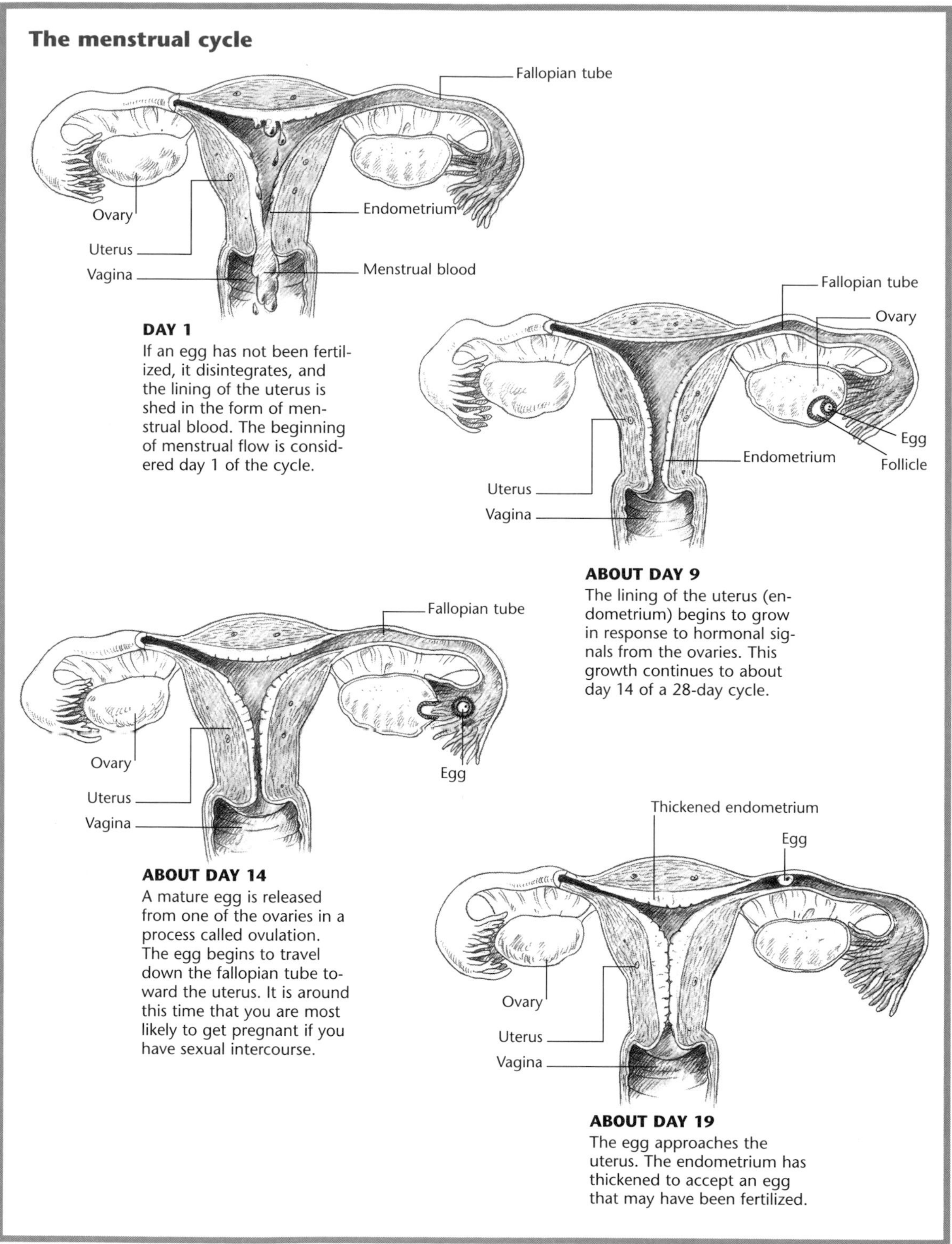

DAY 1
If an egg has not been fertilized, it disintegrates, and the lining of the uterus is shed in the form of menstrual blood. The beginning of menstrual flow is considered day 1 of the cycle.

ABOUT DAY 9
The lining of the uterus (endometrium) begins to grow in response to hormonal signals from the ovaries. This growth continues to about day 14 of a 28-day cycle.

ABOUT DAY 14
A mature egg is released from one of the ovaries in a process called ovulation. The egg begins to travel down the fallopian tube toward the uterus. It is around this time that you are most likely to get pregnant if you have sexual intercourse.

ABOUT DAY 19
The egg approaches the uterus. The endometrium has thickened to accept an egg that may have been fertilized.

Calculating the length of your cycle

The first day of your period is day 1 of your menstrual cycle. To keep track of your cycle, start counting on the day you see the first sign of blood. Your period will probably last from about 3 to 7 days.

At midpoint in your cycle—around day 14 or 15—hormones signal ovulation, the process in which one of your ovaries releases an egg into a fallopian tube. Some women feel mild discomfort in their pelvis when they are ovulating, but most women are unaware of it. If you have sexual intercourse at this time, you are most likely to get pregnant because the egg is most likely to be fertilized as it travels through the fallopian tube to the uterus.

About 5 days after ovulation, around day 20, if the egg has not been fertilized, your hormone levels drop and the egg begins to disintegrate in the fallopian tube or uterus. The lining of your uterus (endometrium) breaks down around day 28.

When the endometrium begins to shed, which you experience as menstrual bleeding, start counting your new cycle. If you keep track of your periods on a calendar, you will begin to see a pattern that tells you about how long your menstrual cycle is.

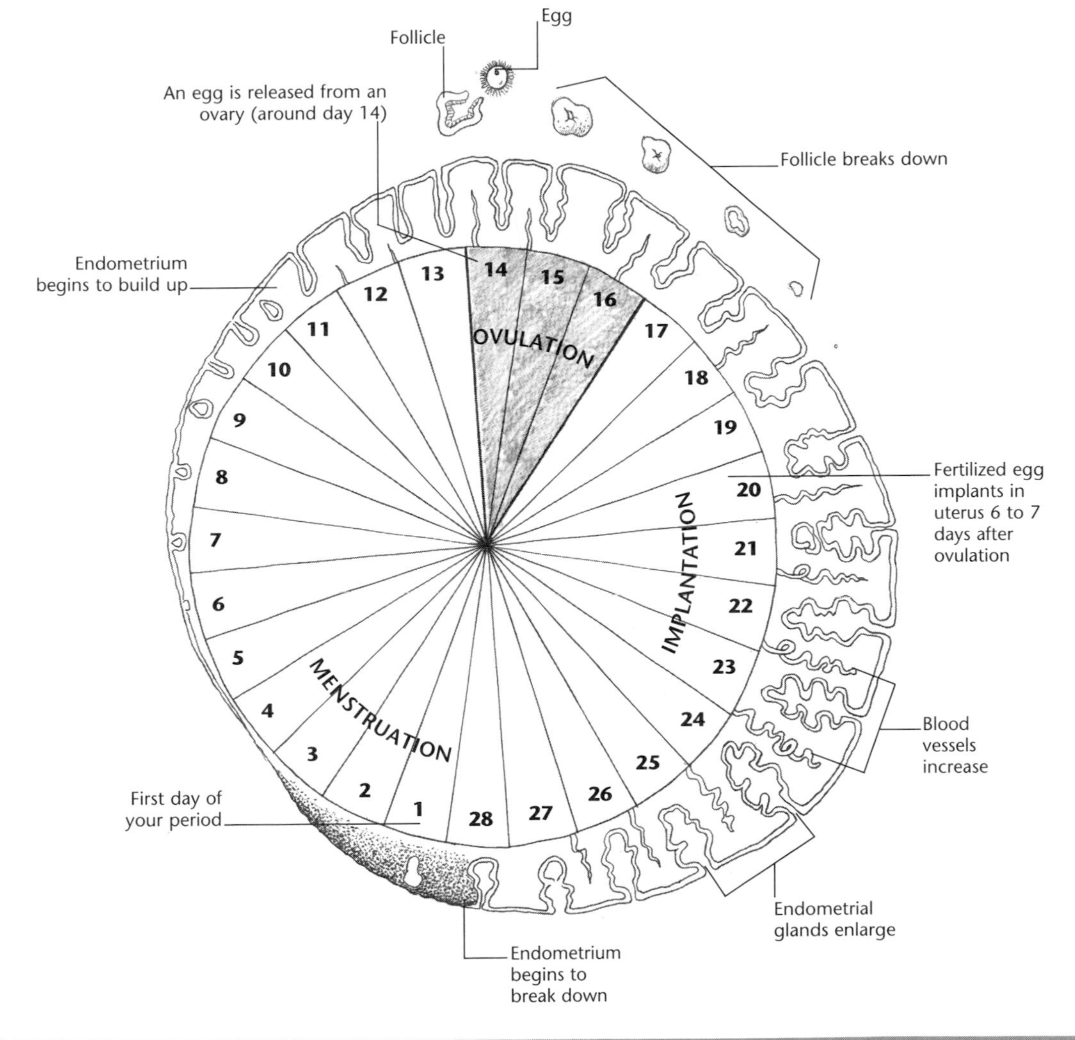

menstruating. Later in life, at about age 45, periods again become irregular until about age 51, when they stop altogether. The end of menstruation is called menopause (see page 352). Menopause is a process that occurs over a period of years and is experienced at different ages by different women.

The length of periods varies from woman to woman. A normal period may last from 1 to 7 days. In teenagers, the amount of blood may be small. Some girls may have some unusually heavy periods at first. The average monthly cycle is 28 days, but it can vary from 24 to 35 days in different women. A woman's own menstrual cycle may vary by 3 to 7 days each month. Talk to your doctor about any unusual change in your cycle or if your cycle is longer or shorter than the average.

It is a good idea to mark your calendar and calculate the length of your cycle so you know when to expect your period. You can also calculate approximately when you are ovulating and, therefore, when you are most likely to get pregnant. However, this is not a reliable means of planning a pregnancy or avoiding one. (For more about determining the exact day of ovulation, see page 379.)

A woman can miss a period for several reasons, most of which do not threaten her health. Pregnancy is the first and most important cause of a missed period. At-home pregnancy tests (see page 381) are generally reliable, as long as you follow the instructions on the package carefully. If you have any doubt about the results, call your doctor.

Other causes of missed periods include extreme stress, such as that caused by a death in the family or moving to a new home. Traveling through different time zones can disrupt the body's biological clock and cause a missed period. Many girls have irregular periods when they first start menstruating. Some medications, including corticosteroids taken for inflammatory conditions such as asthma, can cause a temporary disruption of a woman's menstrual cycle.

There are some more serious reasons for missing a period. If you miss a period after your periods have become regular, first determine whether you are pregnant by giving yourself an at-home pregnancy test. If you have missed one or more periods and you are not pregnant, see your doctor to rule out a health problem such as hypothyroidism (see page 624) or premature menopause. Girls and women with eating disorders such as anorexia nervosa (see page 610) sometimes stop menstruating, as do girls and women who exercise

Myths about menstruation

Misconceptions about menstruation are common. However, this natural process is not nearly as difficult to understand or burdensome as some of the myths suggest.

- **Myth: You should avoid exercising during menstruation.** There is no reason to avoid exercise when you are menstruating. Active women often have less menstrual discomfort than inactive women and many women find exercise helps relieve menstrual cramps.
- **Myth: You will lose your virginity if you use tampons.** The only way you can "lose your virginity" is to have sexual intercourse for the first time. Using a tampon does not damage the hymen, the thin membrane inside the vagina that has traditionally been associated with virginity. If you prefer to use tampons instead of pads during your period, find the size tampon that is comfortable for you. At first, try thinner tampons that are easier to insert.
- **Myth: It is impossible to get pregnant during your period.** You are not likely to get pregnant during your period, but it is still possible. If you want to avoid getting pregnant, always use a reliable method of birth control whenever you have intercourse.
- **Myth: It is unhealthy to have sex when you are menstruating.** There is no medical reason for avoiding sexual intercourse when you are menstruating. It is a decision entirely between you and your partner based on your personal preferences. Some women use their diaphragms (see page 321) to contain the menstrual flow while they have intercourse.
- **Myth: Menstrual discomforts are all in your head.** In the past, premenstrual problems and menstrual pain were sometimes dismissed as emotional reactions. But premenstrual syndrome (PMS; see page 214) and menstrual pain are well recognized and treatable conditions.

excessively. Excessive dieting or exercising can put so much stress on a woman's system that her body stops producing estrogen. A lack of estrogen can cause bone loss and increase the risk of the bone-thinning disorder osteoporosis (see page 552). See your doctor right away if you have stopped menstruating.

PAINFUL PERIODS

Many women experience some discomfort during their period. If you have intense menstrual pain, see your doctor to rule out possible underlying disorders and to discuss possible solutions.

Primary menstrual pain Doctors use the term primary dysmenorrhea for pelvic pain that is the normal result of having a period. Many women experience mild-to-intense pain during their period, although some women experience little or no discomfort. Menstrual pain can take the form of cramps or pain in the lower abdomen or lower back or a pulling sensation in the inner thighs. It can be accompanied by fainting, nausea, vomiting, constipation, diarrhea, dizziness, or headache. Much of this discomfort is caused by prostaglandins, substances that are produced abundantly by the body during menstruation. Prostaglandins stimulate contractions of the uterus and gastrointestinal tract, which can cause pain.

The most effective over-the-counter pain relievers for menstrual pain contain anti-inflammatory agents such as ibuprofen or naproxen that block the formation of prostaglandins, and thereby reduce contractions of the uterus and gastrointestinal tract. These medications work best when they are taken at the first sign of discomfort. Stronger prescription medications are also available, but they may cause stomach irritation or ulcers if they are taken in high doses for long periods.

Taking birth-control pills also reduces menstrual pain. Because the birth-control pill prevents ovulation, the lining of the uterus does not fully thicken in women who take it and, consequently, much less blood and tissue than normal are shed during menstruation. Fewer prostaglandins are produced to cause painful contractions. If you have severe menstrual cramps and also need reliable contraception, your doctor may recommend taking birth-control pills. They may be used safely with over-the-counter or prescription pain-relieving medications.

Secondary menstrual pain The term secondary dysmenorrhea refers to pain during menstruation that is caused by an abnormal process or condition—not by menstruation alone. Some of the most common causes of this secondary pain include endometriosis (see page 230), fibroids (see page 221), or pelvic inflammatory disease (see page 232). These conditions may occur at any age. If you start having pain during your periods that you have not had before, see your doctor.

Mid-cycle pain Pain can sometime occur during the middle of the menstrual cycle, at around the time of ovulation (day 14 or 15). When you ovulate and

Relieving menstrual pain

Although you may not be able to eliminate menstrual pain, some or all of the following techniques may help:

- Aerobic exercise (see page 82)—such as brisk walking, jogging, biking, or swimming—reduces menstrual pain in some women. Brain chemicals called endorphins, which are released during vigorous exercise, can boost mood and reduce pain.
- A warm bath or a heating pad may help relieve mild pain.
- Talk to your doctor. He or she may recommend a prescription or over-the-counter anti-inflammatory medication to help relieve the pain.
- For some women, limiting caffeine consumption helps reduce pain during periods.
- Limiting salt consumption can help reduce the amount of water your body holds, relieving discomfort caused by bloating.
- It is important to get adequate sleep before and during your period to avoid fatigue and increase your body's ability to tolerate discomfort.

the egg follicle, which has been nurturing a mature egg, ruptures and releases the egg, you may have a small amount of bleeding into the pelvic cavity. Occasionally, this bleeding may cause mild pain. Many women feel no discomfort during ovulation. An over-the-counter anti-inflammatory drug such as ibuprofen or naproxen can help relieve this discomfort.

INFREQUENT PERIODS

Some women menstruate less frequently than the usual 28-day cycle; their cycles may be as long as 35 days. Although every woman's periods become less frequent as she approaches menopause, some women have infrequent periods all their life. No one knows exactly why this occurs, but doctors believe it may have to do with an irregularity in the hypothalamus or pituitary gland in the brain, or in the ovaries—all of which produce hormones.

Infrequent periods do not endanger a woman's health and do not usually require treatment unless a woman is having trouble becoming pregnant. (For more about difficulty becoming pregnant, see page 382.)

If your periods become irregular, see your doctor for a pelvic examination and, possibly, tests to measure your hormone levels. Depending on how infrequent your periods are, your doctor may want to perform tests to evaluate the functioning of your thyroid gland (which can affect menstruation) or rule out approaching menopause. If you have additional symptoms such as acne or excessive hair growth, your doctor will measure your levels of male hormones. High levels of male hormones can cause irregular periods by interfering with the normal production of the hormones that regulate the menstrual cycle. If your ovaries are found to be producing too little estrogen, your doctor may prescribe estrogen to restore normal menstruation. A lack of estrogen increases your risk of the bone-thinning disorder osteoporosis (see page 552).

LACK OF PERIODS

Pregnancy is the most obvious cause of an absence of menstruation (called amenorrhea). If you fail to menstruate one month and there is any chance you may be pregnant, take a home pregnancy test (see page 381). Make sure that you follow the instructions on the package exactly. Or see your doctor, who can give you a pelvic examination and pregnancy test. Other causes of the absence of periods include excessive exercise, excessive dieting, eating disorders (see page 610), severe stress, or hormonal disorders such as hypothyroidism (see page 624) that are not directly related to the reproductive system.

See your doctor right away if you have missed three periods and you are not pregnant or if you have not begun to menstruate by age 16. Absence of menstruation can be caused by unusually low levels of estrogen, which can lead to bone depletion and osteoporosis (see page 552).

HEAVY PERIODS

Heavy periods are common, especially in young girls who are not yet ovulating regularly and in women in their 40s who are approaching menopause. However, heavy periods can occur at any time during a woman's reproductive years.

Sometimes, heavy periods reflect a disturbance of the hormone cycle such as lack of ovulation (anovulation). Anovulation causes a deficiency of the hormone progesterone. Without progesterone, the lining of the uterus becomes less stable and sheds in an unsynchronized, prolonged fashion.

Painful, heavy periods can also result from fibroids (see page 221), pelvic infection (see page 232), or, in rare cases, endometriosis (see page 230). Use of an intrauterine device (IUD; see page 324) can also cause heavy periods.

A single heavy period that occurs later in the menstrual cycle than expected may be an early miscarriage. If this occurs, see your doctor immediately. If the miscarriage is incomplete (that is, if some tissue remains in your uterus), your doctor may perform a dilation and curettage (D and C; see page 262), a procedure in which he or she gently removes the remaining tissue from your uterus by scraping or using suction.

SYMPTOM CHART

Painful periods

Pain, usually a dull ache or cramps in your lower abdomen, during your periods.

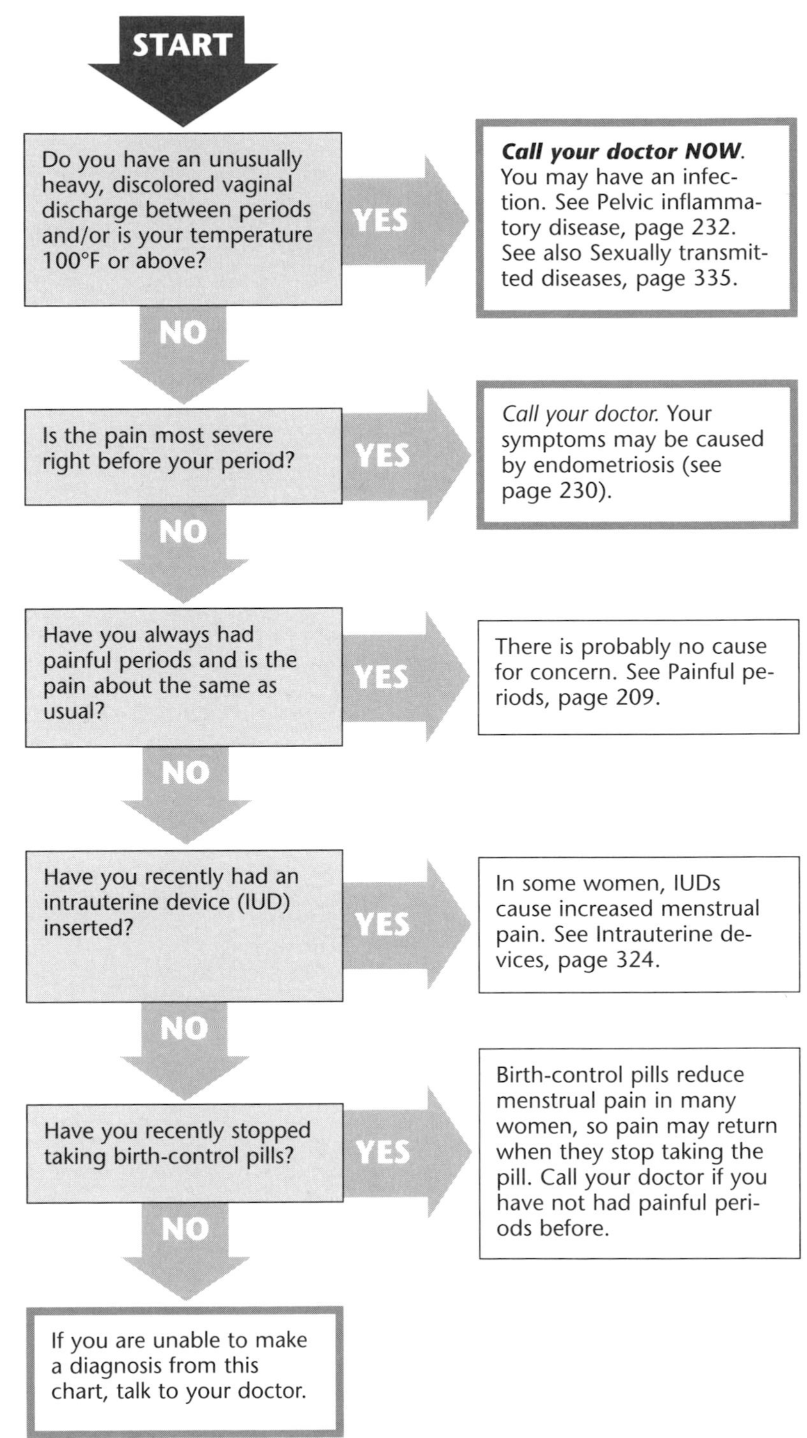

Relief from menstrual pain

Don't hesitate to seek help for painful periods. Your doctor can recommend over-the-counter or prescription medication. He or she may also give you tips for helping you control your pain in other ways, such as using a heating pad or drinking hot tea.

SYMPTOM CHART

Lack of periods

The absence of a menstrual period for at least 2 weeks after your period was due.

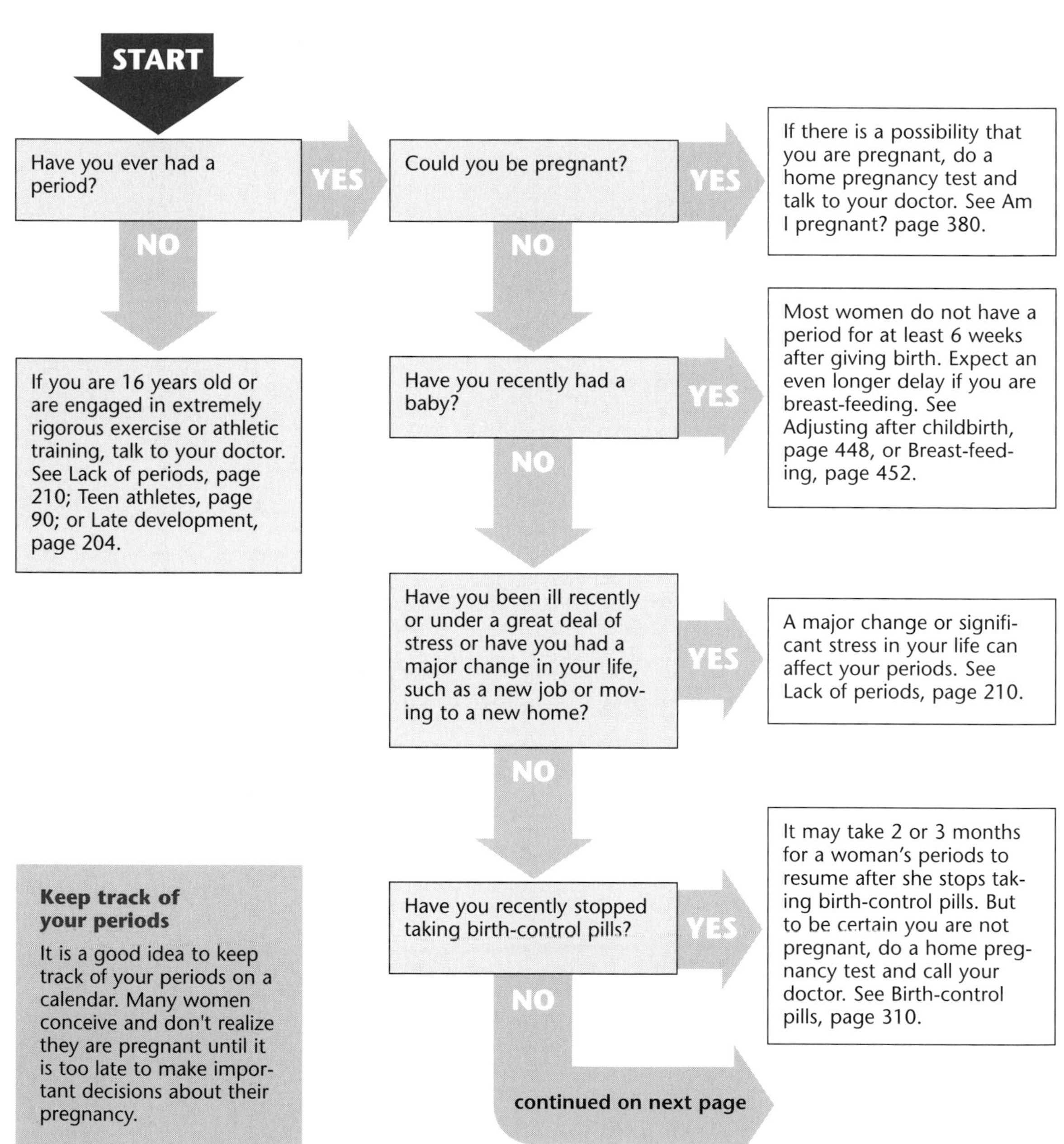

Keep track of your periods

It is a good idea to keep track of your periods on a calendar. Many women conceive and don't realize they are pregnant until it is too late to make important decisions about their pregnancy.

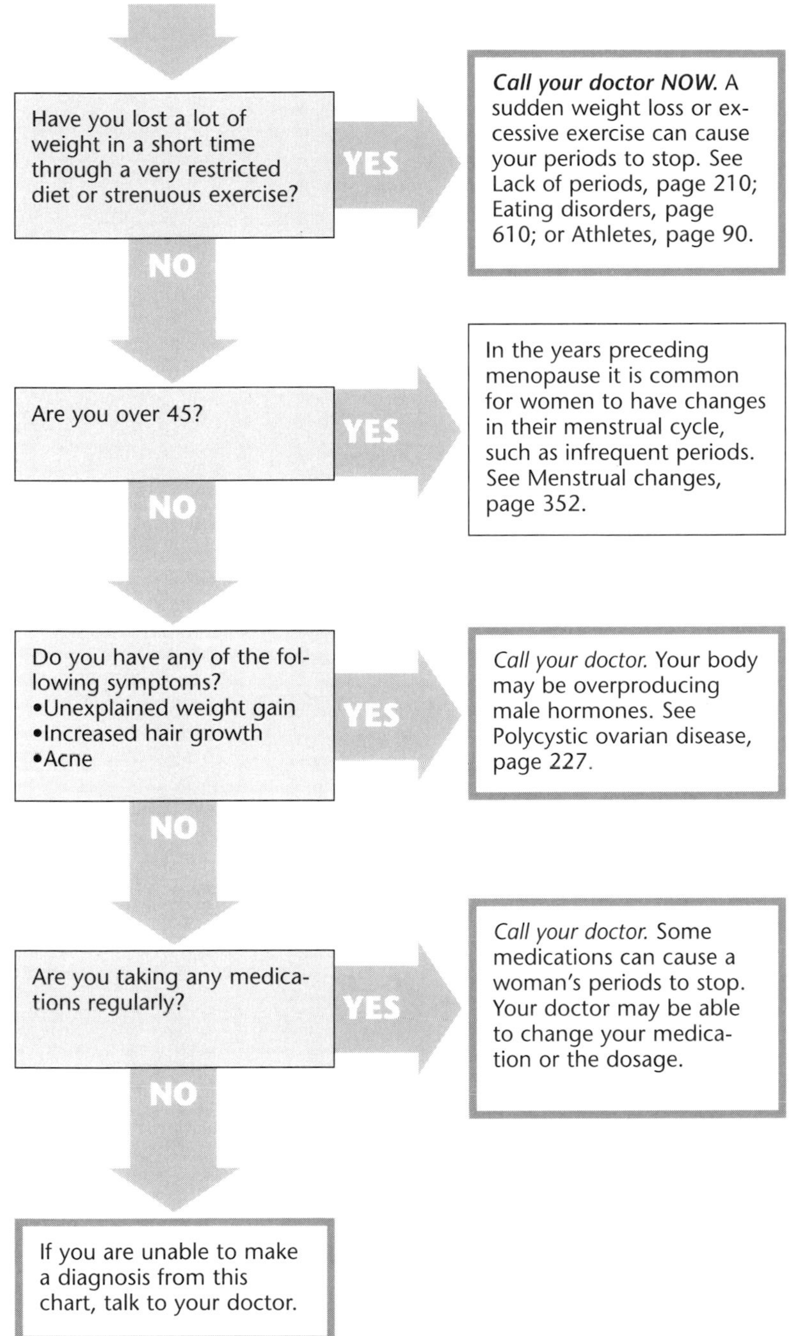

Lack of periods

A lack of periods can have serious health consequences. If your body is not producing important hormones, such as estrogen and progesterone, you may be at risk of serious disorders, such as osteoporosis (see page 552) or endometrial hyperplasia (see page 221).

If you have a single heavy period that is not late, and you have no reason to think you are pregnant, you probably do not need to see your doctor. In this case, simply reduce your activity until the bleeding subsides. If it does not lessen within 24 hours, call your doctor. A sudden, heavy flow can be unsettling if you are not prepared for it. If you are accustomed to using only tampons, try using a full-sized sanitary pad instead of (or in addition to) the tampon. If you have several heavy periods, see your doctor to be tested for iron-deficiency anemia (see page 493), a condition that can result from heavy blood loss.

PREMENSTRUAL SYNDROME

An estimated 20 to 40 percent of all women experience a range of physical and emotional symptoms in the 7 to 10 days preceding their period. This recurring cycle of symptoms is called premenstrual syndrome or PMS.

The nature and cause of PMS remain a mystery, but there is a growing recognition that it is a serious problem for many women. New treatments to lessen the symptoms of PMS are being developed. If you seek medical help for PMS, it is important to note the timing of your symptoms because this information can help your doctor track their cyclical nature and make a diagnosis.

PMS represents a wide variety of symptoms that can include any of the following: breast tenderness and swelling, weight gain, and bloating; emotional changes such as depression, crying, anxiety, nervous tension, mood swings, and irritability; and insomnia, headaches, food cravings (especially for sweets), increased appetite, and fatigue. These symptoms can range from mild to severe and vary among women.

The current method of treating PMS is to treat the most troublesome symptoms. For example, bloating and breast tenderness caused by water retention can be treated by limiting salt in your diet. If the bloating is severe, your doctor may prescribe diuretics, which cause the body to expel more water through urine. Mild diuretics are a component of many over-the-counter PMS medications. Three diuretic ingredients that you might see on over-the-counter package labels include caffeine, ammonium chloride, and pamabrom. But remember that, although caffeine acts as a diuretic and can also help relieve the fatigue that some women feel, too much caffeine can increase anxiety and nervousness, another symptom of PMS, and interfere with your sleep. Caffeine may also aggravate some premenstrual breast tenderness. Because over-the-counter medications can relieve only a few of the symptoms of PMS, see your doctor to determine the best treatment for you.

For women who have severe, disabling PMS, a doctor may prescribe an antidepressant medication (see page 595), such as fluoxetine. Your doctor may recommend taking the medication 7 to 10 days before your period or every day.

Toxic shock syndrome

Use of some types of highly absorbent tampons manufactured in the past has been linked to a bacterial infection called toxic shock syndrome. In some women, these tampons caused tiny breaks in the vaginal lining when left in for a long time, allowing staphylococcal bacteria to enter the blood circulation. The number of cases dropped sharply after the most absorbent type of tampon was taken off the market. Toxic shock syndrome is now rare.

The symptoms of toxic shock syndrome include fever, rash, aching in muscles and joints, and diarrhea. In extreme cases, the infection can cause dangerously low blood pressure and kidney, heart, liver, and blood-clotting problems. A small number of women have died of the resulting complications.

Because tampon-related cases of toxic shock syndrome result from leaving a superabsorbent tampon in the vagina for a long time, doctors recommend leaving a tampon in for no more than 4 to 8 hours. Some women switch to a pad at night. It is a good idea to make sure you don't have a tampon remaining in your vagina after your period. Because you cannot always feel a tampon, it is possible to forget to remove the last one.

CHAPTER 8

Disorders of the reproductive system

Contents

Nearly every woman, at some time in her life, will experience a problem with her reproductive system that requires medical attention. Each year millions of women visit doctors for problems ranging from vaginal infections that can be treated easily with medications to more serious conditions that require surgery. By recognizing the symptoms and knowing when to discuss them with your doctor, and by learning about your particular problem and treatment options, you can become a more active participant in your own health care. The more knowledge you have, the more effectively you will be able to work with your doctor to maintain or improve your reproductive health.

Disorders of the vagina

The vagina is a muscular tube that serves as the entrance to your internal reproductive organs. The vagina is the channel for the flow of menstrual blood during your periods. It can accommodate a man's penis during intercourse and is able to expand to allow the passage of a baby during birth. One of the most common gynecologic problems of all—vaginitis—affects the vagina.

VAGINITIS

Vaginitis—irritation, redness, or swelling of the vaginal tissues—is extremely common. It is responsible for more than half of all visits by women to the doctor's office. Vaginitis can cause a discharge, odor, burning, or itching. Infection—the multiplication of bacteria or other organisms in the vagina—is the most common cause of vaginitis. Other causes include irritation from chemical products such as soaps, and the lack of estrogen that accompanies menopause (see page 352).

Some women have recurring vaginitis. Because similar symptoms can arise from various causes, medication that works in one case may not work in others. When one medication does not clear up the problem, your doctor will recommend another treatment. Sometimes vaginitis recurs during pregnancy or when a woman takes antibiotics. These conditions can make the environment in the vagina conducive to the multiplication of disease-causing organisms. Some vaginal infections can be transmitted through sexual contact. Your sexual partner may be reinfecting you during intercourse. Ask your doctor if your partner should see his doctor too.

A healthy vagina always has some bacteria and other organisms living in it. The naturally acidic environment of the vagina usually keeps the number of organisms in check. However, if something decreases this acidity, these normally harmless organisms can multiply, causing irritation, swelling, and, possibly, a discharge. The natural acid balance in your vagina can be altered by such factors as having diabetes, taking antibiotics or birth-control pills, being overweight, being pregnant, or recently giving birth. Douching, wearing too many layers of clothing or clothing that is too tight (which restricts ventilation), or wearing underwear or panty hose without a cotton crotch can also alter the normal environment of the vagina.

One of the most common symptoms of vaginitis is abnormal discharge. Most women have some normal vaginal discharge that varies during their menstrual cycle, but increased discharge that has an unusual odor (particularly if it is accompanied by burning or itching) warrants a trip to the doctor. Because the causes of vaginitis vary, a doctor must examine the vaginal discharge to make a diagnosis. Do not douche or use vaginal creams or suppositories for a day before your visit.

It is important to get a diagnosis from a doctor before using over-the-counter medications. What appears to be an easy-to-treat yeast infection (see page 217) may be a sexually transmitted disease (see chapter 12) that can cause serious health problems and infertility.

Bacterial vaginosis Bacterial vaginosis is the most common vaginal infection. Symptoms include an unpleasant or fishy odor; increased vaginal discharge; or itching, burning, or redness in the vaginal area.

Bacterial vaginosis is caused by an overgrowth of one or more types of bacteria including *Gardnerella* (also called *Haemophilus*) *vaginalis, Mycoplasma* species, and *Mobiluncus* species. Although women who are sexually active are more likely to develop bacterial vaginosis, the infection is not necessarily a sexually transmitted disease.

Treatment options include applying a vaginal antibiotic gel or cream to your vagina or taking antibiotics. In severe or recurrent cases, oral antibiotics may be prescribed for both the woman and her sexual partner.

Yeast infection Yeast infections are the second most common cause of vaginal irritation. Yeast infections can be persistent, recurring repeatedly, even after treatment. The main symptoms of a yeast infection are intense itching, burning, and redness in the vaginal area. These symptoms are usually accompanied by a white, cottage cheese–like discharge. The infection can also cause pain during intercourse.

The most common yeast infection, candidiasis, is caused by an overgrowth of a fungus of the *Candida* species that is commonly present in the vagina. Contributing factors include pregnancy, diabetes, obesity, or taking antibiotics or birth-control pills. All of these factors can change the acid-base balance in the vagina, allowing the fungus to grow. Some of these factors may increase the amount of estrogen in the vagina, which sets up a nutrient-rich environment for the fungus. As a result, the fungus thrives and multiplies. Women with AIDS (see page 344), whose immune system is suppressed, are particularly susceptible to recurring yeast infections.

A doctor diagnoses a yeast infection by a physical examination and microscopic evaluation of the vaginal discharge or by taking a sample of the discharge for laboratory testing. If a laboratory test shows the presence of *Candida* organisms, the doctor will prescribe medication in the form of suppositories or a cream or gel to be used in the vagina. Over-the-counter medications are safe to use if you have had a yeast infection in the past and are now certain it is the same. See your doctor if you have any doubt whatsoever.

Trichomoniasis Trichomoniasis is the third most common vaginal infection after bacterial vaginosis and yeast infections. Symptoms of trichomoniasis may include an irritating, frothy, yellow-green discharge with an unpleasant odor, and burning, itching, and redness in the vaginal area. You may also experience irritation during urination.

Trichomoniasis is caused by a one-celled organism called *Trichomonas vaginalis*. The infection is usually transmitted during sexual intercourse. Both you and your partner need to be treated with an antibiotic taken by mouth to avoid reinfecting each other. For more about trichomoniasis, see page 349.

Atrophic vaginitis When a woman's ovaries stop functioning—because of menopause, for example, or because she has had her ovaries removed in a hysterectomy (surgical removal of the uterus)—the resulting decrease in estrogen can cause her vagina to become dry. The dryness can cause irritation, burning, or itching and a feeling of pressure that is uncomfortable and may affect a woman's enjoyment of sex. The same symptoms may occur after childbirth or during breast-feeding because of changing hormone levels.

The treatment for atrophic vaginitis involves taking estrogen in hormone

How to avoid vaginitis

Here are some steps to take to help you avoid vaginitis:

- Wash your genital area daily. Always wash from front to back to avoid spreading bacteria from the anal area to your genitals.
- Keep your genital area as dry as possible. Avoid tight clothing that traps moisture and does not allow air to circulate. Wear underwear or panty hose with a cotton crotch. Do not wear underpants to bed at night. Avoid excess layering of clothes, which can prevent ventilation.
- Do not douche or use harsh soaps, feminine hygiene sprays, perfumed toilet paper, or deodorant tampons or sanitary pads.
- See your doctor immediately when you first notice symptoms.

replacement therapy (HRT; see page 359) either in pills or in estrogen-containing vaginal creams. Vaginal lubricants and moisturizers can help make intercourse more comfortable. Avoid contact with irritating deodorants, deodorant panty liners, tight clothing, and underwear without a cotton crotch.

Disorders of the cervix

The cervix is a cylindrical organ that forms the opening between the vagina and the uterus. Cervical cancer was once the leading cancer killer of women. But today, widespread use of the Pap smear, a test that can detect cervical cancer at an early, curable stage, has made this type of cancer rare.

CERVICAL DYSPLASIA

Cervical dysplasia occurs when cells in the cervix change in abnormal ways and begin to resemble cancer cells. Dysplasia is not cancer. The cells look similar to early cancer cells under a microscope, but they do not invade underlying healthy tissues, as cancer cells do. However, these cells have the potential to become cancerous if they are not detected early and treated.

Because of the Pap smear (see page 127), which provides samples of cervical cells for laboratory study, more and more of these abnormal cell changes are being detected at an early stage and treated before they become cancerous. Although, for reasons that are not clear, more women are developing cervical dysplasia, the incidence of cervical cancer and the number of women who die of it are steadily decreasing.

The human papillomavirus (HPV; see page 341) is an extremely common sexually transmitted disease. Infection with some strains of HPV may be responsible for most cases of cervical dysplasia and cervical cancer. HPV causes some types of genital warts—small, raised bumps that appear on the genitals, inside the vagina, and on the cervix. If you have or have had genital warts, you should be especially diligent about having regular Pap smears. Some doctors recommend that you have a Pap smear and pelvic examination every 6 months if you have had genital warts.

Early, or mild, cervical dysplasia develops most often in women between ages 25 and 35; severe dysplasia, or a nearly identical condition called carcinoma in situ, is most common between ages 30 and 40. All forms of dysplasia can be treated successfully by the various methods described here.

Symptoms Symptoms of cervical dysplasia include abnormal vaginal bleeding, particularly during or after intercourse, and bleeding between periods.

Diagnosis When a Pap smear shows an abnormality in cells taken from the cervix, the doctor must confirm the presence of dysplasia, determine the degree of change in the cells, and identify their location in the cervix. To do so, he or she performs a biopsy (removal of a small piece of tissue for laboratory testing). To determine the best area from which to take a tissue sample, the doctor uses a lighted magnifying instrument called a colposcope to directly examine the vagina and cervix. This procedure is called a colposcopy. He or she may take a scraping of tissue from the cervical canal and a biopsy from the surface of the cervix. You may feel mild cramping when the tissue sample is taken.

Treatment If the abnormal cell changes are diagnosed as dysplasia, your doctor will discuss treatment options with you based on the degree to which your cells are abnormal. Some doctors recommend delaying treatment for mild dysplasia to see if it goes away on its own, which it sometimes does. However, your doctor will want to monitor it carefully in frequent follow-up visits (every 3 to 6 months) to make sure it does not progress to moderate or severe dysplasia or carcinoma in situ. Treatment is delayed only in cases of very mild dysplasia, in which the cell changes have not extended into the cervical canal and in women with no additional risk factors, such as previous dysplasia. Moderate and severe dysplasia and carcinoma in situ must be treated or they can develop into cancer.

All the following treatments for cervical dysplasia involve removing or destroying the abnormal tissue.

Cryosurgery Cervical dysplasia can be treated with cryosurgery—a procedure that destroys the abnormal tissue by freezing it. Cryosurgery is used when the area of abnormal cell changes is small and does not extend into the cervical canal. The procedure can be performed in the doctor's office. The doctor applies a cold metal probe to the cervix and holds it there for 3 to 5 minutes. You will feel mild menstrual cramps during and shortly after the treatment.

Most women experience a heavy, watery discharge for 2 to 4 weeks after having cryosurgery. You should avoid using tampons, douching, or having sexual intercourse for a week after the procedure. Although rare, complications include bleeding and infection. Your doctor will probably recommend a follow-up visit in 3 to 4 months.

If you have had cryosurgery for cervical dysplasia followed by normal ("negative") Pap smears for 2 to 3 years, your risk of cervical cancer is the same as that of any other woman. Having cryosurgery for cervical dysplasia does not affect your sex life or your ability to become pregnant.

What is a "precancerous" condition?

Subtle changes can occur in cells over a period of months or years. Sometimes cells can change in size and shape and begin to resemble cancer cells. They are not cancer cells but, if their growth is allowed to go unchecked, they have the potential to turn into cancer.

In a so-called precancerous condition, the abnormal cells do not spread to other tissues—they are limited to an isolated area. Doctors use tests such as the Pap smear (see page 127) to help them make a diagnosis at this early stage, because treatments are easier and more likely to be successful.

How doctors classify cell changes in the cervix

Doctors classify cervical dysplasia (abnormal changes in cells in the cervix) by the extent of the cell changes apparent from a Pap smear or a cervical biopsy (see page 220). They use either of two classification systems:

Cervical intraepithelial neoplasia (CIN) In CIN, intraepithelial cells are found in the cell layers of the surface of the cervix. Doctors classify mild dysplasia as CIN I, moderate dysplasia as CIN II, and severe dysplasia or carcinoma in situ (abnormal cells that are confined within the outer layer of the cervix) as CIN III. Doctors cannot clearly distinguish carcinoma in situ from severe dysplasia.

Squamous intraepithelial lesion (SIL) SIL is an alternative system for classifying cervical dysplasia. Squamous cells are found in the layers of the outer cervix. Mild dysplasia and cell changes linked to infection with a sexually transmitted disease called the human papillomavirus (HPV) are classified as low-grade SIL; moderate or severe dysplasia and carcinoma in situ are called high-grade SIL.

Laser surgery and LEEP/LLETZ Laser surgery or a procedure called by one of two names—loop electrosurgical excision procedure (LEEP) or large loop excision of the transformation zone (LLETZ)—is used when the abnormal cells occupy a large part of the cervix or extend into the cervical canal. (The transformation zone is the area containing the abnormal cells.) Both laser surgery and LEEP/LLETZ are performed in the doctor's office using a local anesthetic that is injected into the cervix to numb it. Because a doctor can remove a larger area of tissue with these techniques than with cryosurgery (freezing), abnormalities are less likely to recur.

A laser is a device that transforms light waves into a powerful beam that is used to destroy abnormal tissue. In laser surgery, the doctor destroys the area of abnormal cells on the outer part of the cervix and around the cervical canal.

In LEEP/LLETZ, which is performed more frequently than laser surgery, the area of abnormal cells is shaved off with a thin wire loop that is part of an electrocautery device. Electrocautery uses heat from a low-energy electric current to remove abnormal tissue. Because a local anesthetic has been injected into your cervix, you will not feel the heat or any pain. The heat also seals the blood vessels and prevents bleeding.

The advantage of LEEP/LLETZ is that the abnormal tissue is not destroyed as it is in cryosurgery or laser surgery, so it can be sent to the laboratory for examination. Laboratory examination can confirm that all the abnormal cells were confined within the area that was removed and rule out any unexpected findings, such as a hidden source of cancer.

Bleeding from the cervix is a potential complication of both laser surgery and LEEP/LLETZ. Any bleeding almost always occurs at the time of the procedure and is taken care of immediately by burning the tissue to seal the blood vessels. Rarely, a woman may experience bleeding several days after either of these procedures. Before you go home, your doctor will give you specific instructions about how to prevent bleeding, such as avoiding sexual intercourse, douching, or putting anything in your vagina (including tampons) for up to 4 weeks. You should not try to get pregnant for 3 months.

Cone biopsy In the past, a cone biopsy was often the recommended treatment for women with severe dysplasia or carcinoma in situ. In this type of biopsy, the doctor uses a scalpel to remove a cone-shaped piece of tissue, including the area of abnormal cells, from the outer cervix and cervical canal. A cone biopsy must be done in an operating room because it is more likely to cause bleeding severe enough to require stitches in the cervix and it requires spinal anesthesia (see page 260) or general anesthesia (see page 216).

If you have had a cone biopsy, your doctor will recommend that you not have sexual intercourse for about 4 weeks. After this time, having a cone biopsy does not affect your sex life in any way. However, in some cases, the cervix may be weakened, which can make it difficult to carry a pregnancy to term. If you have had a cone biopsy and you plan to become pregnant, make sure your doctor knows so that he or she can monitor you more closely throughout your pregnancy.

Today, fewer women are treated with cone biopsy because it has more potential complications than laser surgery or LEEP/LLETZ and it must be done in an operating room. However, a cone biopsy is still recommended in some circumstances, such as when laser surgery or LEEP/LLETZ fails to remove all the abnormal cells from the cervix.

Follow-up Follow-up visits with your doctor after any treatment for cervical dysplasia are extremely important because no treatment is completely successful for all women and the condition may recur. Follow-up involves pelvic examinations and Pap smears every 4 to 6 months, depending on the degree of dysplasia and the treatment you received. If you have an abnormal Pap smear during a follow-up visit, your doctor will perform another colposcopy (see page 218) and a biopsy to confirm whether the dysplasia has recurred and, if so, where it has recurred and to what degree. A biopsy helps the doctor determine the best course of treatment for you.

CERVICITIS

Cervicitis—inflammation of the cervix—can cause vaginal discharge, pelvic pain, and, sometimes, bleeding between periods or after intercourse. If you experience any of these symptoms, see your doctor.

The causes of cervicitis are varied and not always obvious. Infections resulting from chlamydia (see page 339) and gonorrhea (see page 340), which are transmitted sexually, are a major cause. In these cases, your doctor will identify the disease-causing organism through laboratory testing and treat the infection with medication.

Cervicitis can also result from a reaction to a foreign object such as an intrauterine device (IUD), a forgotten tampon, or a pessary (a device inserted into the vagina to temporarily support a uterus that has dropped down out of position; see page 235). Removing the object may be all the treatment that is necessary to clear up the symptoms.

POLYPS

Cervical polyps are small, red, teardrop-shaped growths on the cervix. The primary symptom is vaginal bleeding, particularly during and after intercourse. The usual treatment is to remove the polyp in the doctor's office. Although these polyps are almost always noncancerous, the removed tissue is usually sent to the laboratory to make sure it is benign.

Disorders of the uterus

The uterus is a hollow organ in which a fetus is nourished and grows during a pregnancy. The lining of the uterus, called the endometrium, builds up each month and is shed in menstrual blood if pregnancy does not occur. Disorders of the uterus often cause abnormal menstrual bleeding.

ABNORMAL BLEEDING

Any change in your period, such as unusually heavy bleeding or bleeding at unpredictable times in your menstrual cycle, should be reported to your doctor. Frequent, heavy bleeding can lead to anemia (see page 493) if it is not treated.

Medication is usually the first treatment for heavy bleeding. Because abnormal bleeding is often caused by an irregularity in hormone production by the ovaries, your treatment may involve the use of hormones—such as birth-control pills—that regulate your menstrual cycle. Birth-control pills contain small amounts of the female hormones estrogen and progesterone, which together synchronize the menstrual cycle. The pills are taken on a precise schedule—usually one pill a day for 21 days and then no pills for 7 days. Severely heavy bleeding may be treated with higher doses of the pills at first.

While you are on the pill, your ovaries do not produce any hormones. By providing continuous low-dose cycles of estrogen and progesterone, birth-control pills can correct a hormone imbalance and bring your menstrual cycle under control.

The most common type of hormone imbalance is failure to ovulate (release an egg from an ovary each month). The most common causes of failure to ovulate are severe physical or emotional stress, such as a serious illness, hospitalization, a job change, or a move. Other causes, which are more frequent in young women, include the eating disorders anorexia nervosa (see page 114) or bulimia (see page 610), strenuous exercise or athletic training, or polycystic ovarian disease (see page 227).

Endometrial hyperplasia If you do not ovulate in a given month, your ovaries are still producing estrogen. However, if you do not ovulate, your body is not producing the counterbalancing, stabilizing hormone progesterone. Without progesterone, the growth of the lining of the uterus (endometrium), which has been stimulated by estrogen, does not stop. In normal menstrual bleeding, which occurs at regular intervals, the endometrium is shed—it detaches from the uterus and is expelled in menstrual blood. If this regular menstrual bleeding does not occur, endometrial tissue may accumulate inside the uterus. As the tissue accumulates, its growth may become uncontrolled, resulting in a condition called endometrial hyperplasia. The symptoms include irregular, unpredictable, heavy bleeding, or less frequent periods.

To treat endometrial hyperplasia, your doctor may prescribe the hormone progesterone alone, to be taken a certain number of days each month. Progesterone limits the growth of the endometrium, thereby reducing the amount and number of days of bleeding and regulating the menstrual cycle.

FIBROIDS

One in five women over age 35 has fibroids, also called myomas. Fibroids are noncancerous growths in or on the uterus. Although some women with fibroids have no symptoms and require no treatment, others experience pain or abnormal bleeding.

Doctors do not know why fibroids develop. They grow from cells that make up the muscle in the wall of the uterus. They may be attached directly to the inside or outside wall, or they may hang from a stem (pedicle) inside or outside the uterus. Fibroids can also grow inside the wall of the uterus. Fibroids range from the size of a pea to the size of a grapefruit. In rare cases, fibroids have grown so large that they have been mistaken for a pregnancy.

The hormone estrogen promotes the development and growth of fibroids. For this reason, fibroids often grow larger during pregnancy (when estrogen production increases) and shrink afterward. The declining production of estrogen at menopause usually halts their growth and may even cause them to shrink or disappear.

Symptoms Fibroids can cause an increase in the amount, frequency, or duration of menstrual bleeding, pain ranging from mild to severe in the abdomen or lower back, or more frequent urination resulting from fibroids that press on the bladder.

Fibroids can also cause infertility, especially if they grow inside the uterus. If the normal surface of the cavity of the uterus is distorted by fibroids, a fertilized egg may not be able to implant itself in the wall of the uterus. A fibroid that blocks the entrance of a fallopian tube can cause infertility by obstructing the passage of sperm or a fertilized egg. Large fibroids that take up a lot of space in the uterus can block the growth of a developing fetus and cause premature labor. Very rarely, fibroids become cancerous. Cancerous fibroids occur most often after menopause.

Diagnosis When fibroids are discovered, either through symptoms or during a pelvic examination, the doctor may want to examine the tumors more closely using one of the techniques described here:

- **Ultrasound** (see page 405) creates an image of the pelvic organs.
- **Laparoscopy** (see page 263) enables the doctor to view the interior of the pelvis through a small, lighted viewing instrument that is inserted through a small incision in the abdomen.
- **Hysteroscopy** (see page 264) enables the doctor to insert a viewing instrument through the vagina and cervix to examine the interior of the uterus.
- **Hysterosalpingography** is a method of producing an X-ray image of the interior of the uterus and the fallopian tubes to determine if there are any changes in their size and shape.

Treatment Treatment is not always necessary for fibroids unless they cause excessive bleeding or pain or if the doctor is not sure if the growth is a fibroid or a cancerous tumor. When treatment is required for fibroids, the most common procedure is hysterectomy, removal of the uterus (and the fibroids with it).

Myomectomy Another treatment option is myomectomy, in which the doctor removes only the fibroids (myomas), leaving the uterus intact. Myomectomy is most often performed when a woman wishes to retain her ability to have a child.

Because myomectomy is a more complicated procedure than hysterectomy, it carries an increased risk of bleeding. The

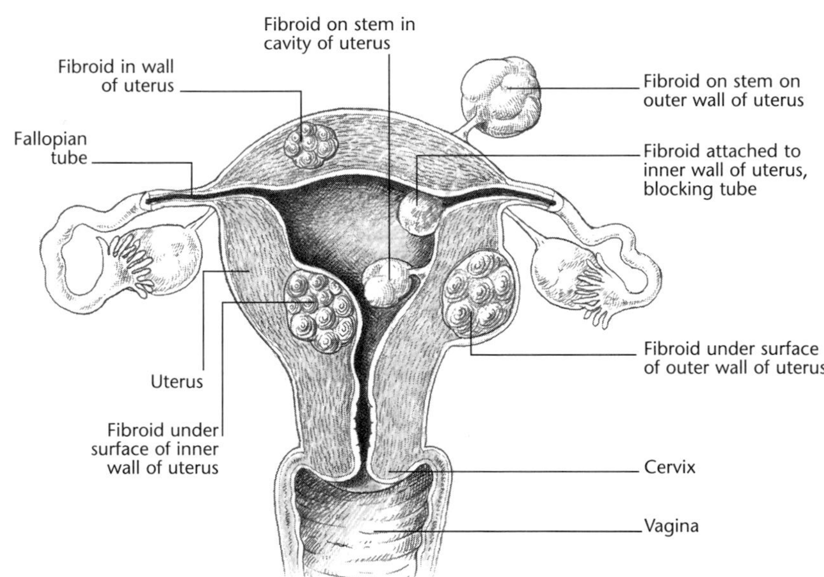

FIBROIDS
Fibroids cause pain and discomfort in some women and no symptoms at all in others. They grow from muscle cells in the wall of the uterus. They may grow on stems or remain part of the wall itself. Fibroids can range from pea size to the size of a grapefruit and can sometimes interfere with a woman's ability to become pregnant.

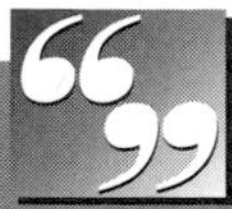

ONE WOMAN'S STORY
MAKING A DECISION ABOUT FIBROIDS

When I was 32 my doctor discovered I had fibroids in my uterus. I was having very painful periods, and the heavy bleeding was getting worse. I wasn't surprised to find that I had fibroids because they are very common. My friend had them too. I was scared because she had to have a hysterectomy. She had already had her children but I didn't have any yet, and I wanted to have a family.

My doctor said she might be able to do a myomectomy, a procedure to remove only the fibroids and save my uterus. I went to another doctor for a second opinion and he told me that a myomectomy was a more complicated and difficult operation than a hysterectomy and that fibroids often grow back after a myomectomy. The doctors also told me that sometimes a myomectomy causes scarring in or around the uterus that can make you infertile. But, since I wanted to have children, I decided that a myomectomy was the best choice for me.

"For me, being informed meant the difference between having an early hysterectomy and having a child."

It took until 3 years after the operation for me to get pregnant. It was a very stressful time because I kept wondering if the operation had made me infertile. But it finally happened. I was 36 when my daughter was born; I had to have a cesarean delivery because of the repair work that was done on my uterus during the myomectomy, but I was happy to have my daughter.

I never got pregnant again and then, gradually, the fibroids came back. One day I started bleeding so heavily that I got really scared. A blood test revealed I had anemia. My doctor told me the heavy bleeding caused the anemia and that the fibroids were so big that they were becoming dangerous to my health. She suggested that I have a hysterectomy because at my age, 44, I was not likely to have more children. She also recommended that both my ovaries be taken out at the same time because I had a family history of ovarian cancer. I decided to go ahead with it. We discussed the benefits and risks of going on hormone replacement therapy after the operation to give me the estrogen I would be lacking without my ovaries to produce it. I decided to take hormone replacement therapy.

Although it took several weeks to recover from the operation, that was less time than I had expected. My doctor said I recovered quickly because I started taking estrogen shortly after the surgery. She told me estrogen can prevent hot flashes and other symptoms of menopause and can help prevent heart attacks and osteoporosis.

One thing I have learned from all of this is that you need to educate yourself about your health. You need to read everything you can so you know what your doctor is talking about. That's the only way to make an informed decision. For me, being informed meant the difference between having an early hysterectomy and having a child.

procedure may also lead to the development of scars, called adhesions, that can interfere with a woman's future fertility or cause pain. If a woman becomes pregnant after having a myomectomy, she is more likely to need a cesarean delivery (see page 442). In 20 percent of women who have myomectomies, the fibroids recur, requiring another operation.

Sometimes doctors recommend hormone treatment before a woman undergoes a myomectomy or a hysterectomy. Hormone treatments with drugs called gonadotropin-releasing hormone (GnRH) agonists, which mimic menopause by blocking the production of estrogen, can help shrink the fibroids. This treatment is temporary and is given for 3 to 6 months before the hysterectomy or myomectomy. A woman takes the hormones in a monthly injection or uses a nasal spray daily.

Hormone treatment is usually given to women with large fibroids to reduce the risk of bleeding during surgery, or to shrink the fibroids enough to be able to do a hysterectomy through the vagina (see page 259) instead of through an incision in the abdomen (see page 259). This treatment is not an alternative to surgery because, as soon as the woman stops taking the drugs, her fibroids rapidly grow back to their original size.

The use of this hormone treatment for fibroids is limited because some women cannot tolerate the side effects. The side effects of treatment with GnRH agonists are similar to those of menopause—including hot flashes and vaginal dryness. Tell your doctor about any side effects that are bothering you.

ADENOMYOSIS

Some women develop abnormal menstrual pain when they are in their 40s. In some cases, the pain is caused by a condition called adenomyosis, in which glands in the lining of the uterus grow deeper and deeper into the muscle wall of the uterus as a woman ages. The glands may then bleed. In most cases, the bleeding can be controlled with hormonal medication, such as birth-control pills. But if the bleeding and pain cannot be controlled with medication, a doctor may recommend that the woman have a hysterectomy (see page 256).

Disorders of the ovaries

A woman is born with hundreds of thousands of eggs in her ovaries, which nurture the eggs as they mature. The ovaries are complex organs with many types of cells. These cells are continuously dividing as part of the normal menstrual cycle. Such constant activity can make ovarian cells vulnerable to genetic changes that can produce unusual growths such as cysts and tumors.

OVARIAN CYSTS

Ovarian cysts are small, fluid-filled areas that form on the ovaries. There are many different kinds of ovarian cysts.

Functional cysts Functional cysts are formed from tissue that changes in the normal cyclical process of ovulation, when the ovary releases a mature egg.

Follicular cysts Follicular cysts, the most common type of functional cyst, occur when a follicle that normally grows and releases an egg during ovulation does not rupture to release the egg. Instead, the follicle continues to grow. Follicular cysts usually cause no pain and disappear within a few months. A doctor may notice one during a pelvic examination.

Corpus luteum cysts The corpus luteum is a normal structure formed from a follicle that has ruptured and released an egg (ovulation). A corpus luteum cyst is a cyst that can persist abnormally after ovulation, and sometimes bleed within itself. Although it usually does not cause pain, this type of cyst may cause discomfort from about day 20 to day 26 of the menstrual cycle.

Your doctor may perform an ultrasound to look for a cyst, blood clot, or fluid. If the pain subsides, your doctor may recommend waiting another one or two menstrual cycles to see if the cyst goes away on its own. However, if the pain increases, or the cyst enlarges, your doctor may recommend removing it surgically through laparoscopy (see page 263).

Dermoid cysts Dermoid cysts are composed of different tissues such as skin, hair, and teeth. These cysts occur most often in women in their 20s. Although dermoid cysts are usually benign (not cancerous), they must be removed to confirm this.

Endometriomas An endometrioma develops when tissue similar to that which lines the uterus (endometrium) becomes attached to and grows inside an ovary, forming a cyst. An endometrioma is sometimes called a chocolate cyst because it is filled with thick, reddish-brown blood. Because this type of cyst is a form of endometriosis, it is treated in the same way. For treatment of endometriosis, see page 230.

Symptoms Ovarian cysts can cause symptoms such as severe pain in your lower abdomen, irregular or delayed periods, or a dull ache or feeling of pressure in your lower abdomen. You may also experience pain during intercourse.

Diagnosis An ovarian cyst is often discovered during a pelvic examination.

When a doctor detects an abnormal growth on an ovary, he or she usually performs tests to determine the size and nature of the cyst.

Your doctor may recommend an ultrasound to determine if the ovary is enlarged or whether a growth on the ovary is solid or filled with liquid. A solid growth or tumor needs to be examined further to rule out cancer. The doctor may also use laparoscopy (see page 263) to view the ovaries. Laparoscopy can be used to drain fluid from a cyst, stop bleeding, or take a tissue sample (biopsy) for laboratory testing.

Treatment In recommending treatment for an ovarian cyst, your doctor takes into consideration the size and type of cyst as well as your age and your plans for having children. If the cyst is small and not causing symptoms, the doctor is likely to wait 2 or 3 months to see if it goes away by itself. Most functional cysts less than 2 inches (5 centimeters) in diameter go away on their own in 1 to 3 months.

Birth-control pills are sometimes prescribed to help shrink a functional cyst. Because the pills contain hormones that prevent ovulation, they also help block the formation of new functional cysts.

If a cyst does not go away or does not respond to treatment with birth-control pills, it may have to be removed surgically. Surgery is usually recommended when a cyst is very large, appears after menopause, or is causing severe pain.

Growths on the ovary that occur after menopause are not, by definition, "functional" cysts, because the ovaries are no longer functioning and ovulation (release of an egg from an ovary) has stopped. These growths that occur after menopause are more likely to be cancerous or have the potential to become cancerous than cysts in younger women. For this reason, they require more immediate investigation and treatment.

Because the earlier a cyst is found the less extensive the surgery required to remove it, it is important to have regular pelvic examinations (at least once a year). A small cyst can sometimes be removed or drained without having to remove the entire ovary. For larger cysts, the entire ovary may have to be removed. Removal of both ovaries makes a woman of childbearing age infertile. For a woman with severe endometriosis (see page 230) or when cancer is suspected, more extensive surgery, such as a complete hysterectomy—which includes removal of the ovaries, fallopian tubes, and uterus—may be recommended. (For more about hysterectomy, see page 256.)

In some cases, the extent of surgery that is required is not apparent until the doctor can directly view the problem during the operation. Discuss the possibilities thoroughly with your doctor before the operation.

Twisting of an ovarian cyst Occasionally, a cyst or the ovary on which it originates

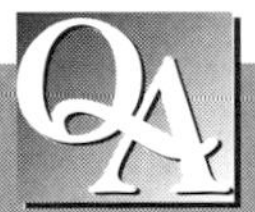

QUESTIONS WOMEN ASK
OVARIAN CYSTS

Q Does having an ovarian cyst make it more likely that I will get cancer?

A Most kinds of ovarian cysts are not linked to an increased risk of cancer. If you are past menopause, be sure to have an annual pelvic examination to detect any enlargement of the ovaries. Ovarian cancer is more common after 50.

Q I had an ovary removed several years ago because I had an ovarian cyst. What are my chances of conceiving with just one ovary?

A Your chances of conceiving are the same as those of a woman who has two ovaries. When one ovary is removed, the other ovary takes over all of its functions. As long as your remaining ovary is healthy, it will secrete normal amounts of the female hormones estrogen and progesterone (which are necessary for pregnancy) and release an egg every month.

Some common ovarian cysts

FUNCTIONAL CYST
A functional cyst results when an egg follicle grows but fails to rupture and release the egg or continues to grow after releasing the egg. This type of cyst often goes away on its own after one or two menstrual cycles.

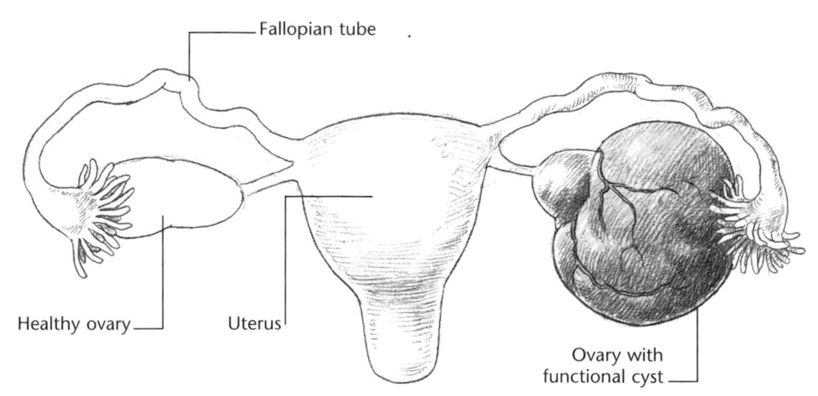

DERMOID CYST
A dermoid cyst is an unusual-looking cyst composed of various types of tissues such as hair, skin, or even teeth. It is usually not cancerous but must be removed surgically to make sure.

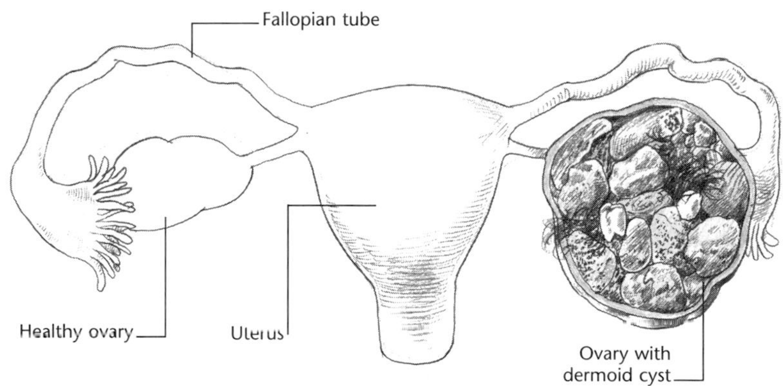

ENDOMETRIOMA
An endometrioma is a blood-filled cyst formed from tissue resembling the endometrium (the lining of the uterus). Endometriomas grow on the surface of an ovary and can be removed surgically.

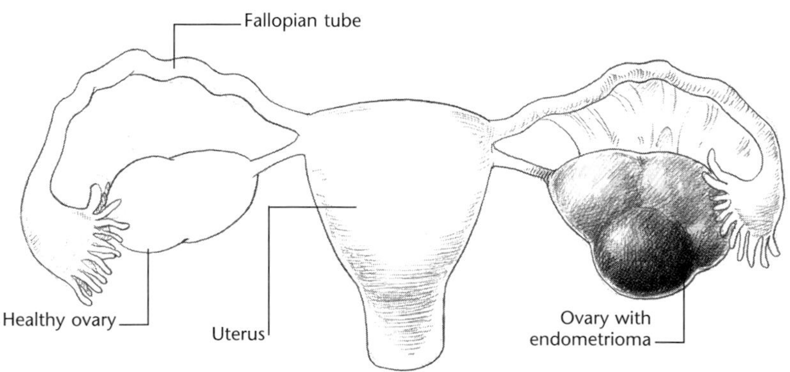

twists. In many cases, the adjacent fallopian tube also twists. Because this twisting, called torsion, is often accompanied by severe pain, nausea, and vomiting, it is sometimes mistaken for appendicitis or a bowel obstruction.

To diagnose and treat torsion, the doctor uses a procedure called laparoscopy (see page 263) to untwist the ovary and remove or drain the cyst, if one is present. If a cyst is unusually large, is bleeding, or has attached itself to adjacent organs, more extensive surgery called laparotomy (see page 264) may be required to remove it.

Polycystic ovarian disease Polycystic ovarian disease occurs as a result of an increase in the production of male hormones by the ovaries and the adrenal glands. The disease occurs most frequently in obese women. The ovaries become enlarged and contain many cysts. The increase in male hormones can also cause excess hair to grow on the face and body.

The increase in male hormones and an imbalance of the hormones that regulate menstruation cause a failure to ovulate (release of an egg from an ovary) and irregular menstrual cycles. Some women with polycystic ovarian disease may have little or no menstrual bleeding; other women have irregular heavy bleeding. In some cases, the condition is diagnosed during an investigation into the cause of a woman's infertility.

If you have polycystic ovarian disease, you should see your doctor regularly—every 6 to 12 months, or more frequently if you have symptoms such as severe bleeding. Because you are not ovulating, you are not producing the hormone progesterone, which balances and limits estrogen's effect on the endometrium (the lining of the uterus). Estrogen stimulates the endometrium to build up each month; progesterone causes it to shed in menstrual blood. The increase in estrogen without the counterbalancing effects of progesterone puts you at increased risk of endometrial cancer (see page 239) and breast cancer (see page 272).

Irregular menstrual cycles can be treated with either the hormone progesterone or with birth-control pills (see page 310) to create regular periods and limit the growth of the endometrium. Taking birth-control pills may also slow the growth of excess hair by lowering the levels of male hormones. If excess hair growth is the main problem, your doctor may also prescribe a medication that works with the birth-control pill to lower levels of male hormones; this treatment usually takes several weeks to slow excess hair growth. If you are obese, losing weight can also help correct your irregular menstrual cycles and slow down the growth of excess hair.

BENIGN OVARIAN TUMORS

The word "tumor" refers to an abnormal growth. A tumor may be benign (noncancerous) or malignant (cancerous). Eighty percent of ovarian tumors are benign. The symptoms can vary, depending on how long the tumor has existed, but can range from mild bloating to severe abdominal swelling and pain. Some tumors cause no symptoms at all and are only discovered during surgery for another problem.

Your doctor may suspect a tumor to be either benign or malignant based on characteristics found during a physical examination or on an ultrasound. An accurate diagnosis can be made only by removing part or all of the tumor and examining it under a microscope.

An ovarian tumor is more likely to be benign if it is less than 2 inches (5 centimeters) in diameter, is not attached to other organs, or looks (on an ultrasound) like it is filled with fluid. If you do not have any symptoms, such as pain, your doctor may decide not to remove the tumor right away and monitor it in follow-up visits.

On the other hand, if an ovarian tumor is larger than 2 inches (5 centimeters), attached to nearby organs, or looks solid on an ultrasound, your doctor may recommend surgically removing it right away, regardless of whether you are experiencing pain or other symptoms.

During surgery, a doctor cannot always determine by a tumor's appearance whether it is benign or malignant. To obtain a diagnosis quickly, while you are still under general anesthesia (see page 261), your doctor may perform a type of biopsy called a frozen section. In this procedure, a section of tissue is removed from the tumor and quickly frozen and analyzed under a microscope to rule out or confirm the presence of cancer. Making an immediate diagnosis prevents you from having to undergo a second operation.

If the tumor is malignant, the doctor checks to see if the cancer has spread by taking tissue samples from your lymph nodes (glands that can carry cancer cells to other parts of the body) for laboratory examination. The doctor then removes the tumor, the ovary, and any other organs to which the cancer has spread, including the uterus, other ovary, and both fallopian tubes. (For more about the treatment of ovarian cancer, see page 250.)

If the tumor is benign, the doctor removes only the tumor, leaving the ovary intact. Before you have any surgery for an ovarian tumor, ask your doctor about having a frozen section biopsy and ask about what your options will be if cancer is found.

BORDERLINE OVARIAN TUMORS

Borderline ovarian tumors are in a category of their own, occupying a position somewhere between clearly benign tumors and clearly malignant ones. If a doctor suspects that you have ovarian cancer, he or she will remove the tumor to examine it under a microscope.

In some cases, the tumor is found to be a borderline tumor. Borderline tumors have a small potential to become malignant even though they are not considered to be cancerous at the time of the initial surgery and diagnosis. If a woman has borderline ovarian tumors, is under 40, and still wants to have children, the doctor will remove only her affected ovary.

A small percentage of these tumors recur 10 to 20 years later. Most doctors encourage a woman with a borderline ovarian tumor to complete her childbearing as quickly as possible and then have surgery to remove the tissues in areas the tumor is most likely to recur, such as the uterus and the remaining ovary.

Disorders of the vulva

Vulva is the collective term for the external structures of your reproductive system. The vulva can be affected by disorders that range from relatively minor skin conditions, which are relatively easy to treat, to allergic reactions, which are often recurring and more difficult to treat.

BARTHOLIN'S GLAND CYSTS

The Bartholin's glands, located just inside the vaginal opening (one on each side), secrete a lubricating fluid during sexual arousal. When they become clogged because of infection, injury, or another cause, a cyst (fluid-filled sac) can form. If the cyst becomes infected, the watery fluid inside it turns into pus, creating an abscess. At the same time, the surrounding external tissue of the lips at the vaginal opening becomes firmer, redder, and painful.

To treat the cyst or abscess, a doctor may cut the area open to allow the fluid to drain. In some cases, a small, hollow, flexible tube (catheter) may be inserted into the incision to keep it open. The catheter allows more secretions to drain and helps prevent another blockage. The catheter is removed after a few days.

If the cyst recurs, the doctor may make a larger incision, turn the cyst wall inside out, and stitch it to the edge of the incision. This allows the cyst to drain well and heal in a permanently open position. When the incision heals, it looks like a small dimple. The gland still functions normally.

DYSTROPHIES OF THE VULVA

Dystrophy is a disorder that results when tissues do not function or develop properly because they are not being adequately nourished. Dystrophies of the vulva are conditions in which the skin of the vulva becomes either abnormally thickened or thinned out. The skin undergoes changes that can cause a variety of symptoms, depending on the type of dystrophy. Vulvar dystrophies can occur at any age but are most common after menopause. They are usually recurring and require long-term treatment. Because some cancerous conditions closely resemble vulvar dystrophies, your doctor may perform a biopsy (take a small tissue sample for examination in the laboratory) to rule out cancer and determine the type of dystrophy.

Atrophic dystrophy Atrophic dystrophy occurs as a result of reduced estrogen levels after menopause. The skin of the vulva atrophies—it thins out, shrinks, turns white, and becomes fragile. The shrinking causes the inner and outer lips around the opening to the vagina to flatten, and the vaginal opening to become smaller. The most common symptom of atrophic dystrophy is itching or irritation of the vulva.

Atrophic dystrophy can be treated by rubbing ointment containing the male hormone testosterone into the affected area. In some women, the testosterone ointment may cause mild irritation. If this occurs, your doctor will recommend using the medication less frequently than originally prescribed or alternating it with a milder medication such as hydrocortisone cream. In rare cases, atrophic dystrophy occurs in girls before puberty; it then is treated with a milder cream containing the female hormone progesterone.

Hyperplastic dystrophy Hyperplastic means that the number of cells in a tissue has increased, causing the tissue to thicken. Hyperplastic dystrophy usually appears as thickened white or red areas on the surface of the vulva. Itching is a common symptom. Treatment usually involves applying a corticosteroid-containing cream such as hydrocortisone to the area. Corticosteroids are natural or synthetic hormones that stabilize the functioning of cells. Once treated, hyperplastic dystrophy rarely recurs.

Abnormal cell changes, which could lead to cancer if not treated, may occur in areas of the vulva that are affected by hyperplastic dystrophy. If your condition does not improve after using the medication, your doctor will perform a biopsy of the tissue to rule out a precancerous condition.

Mixed vulvar dystrophy More than one type of dystrophy may occur at the same time. Because the symptoms and appearance may vary, a biopsy is required to make a diagnosis. Initial treatment usually involves applying a corticosteroid-containing cream. Continued treatment, which is always long-term, involves applying testosterone ointment alone or alternating it with corticosteroid cream.

Psoriasis and other conditions affecting the whole body In some cases vulvar conditions are caused by disorders that affect the whole body. For example, the skin disease psoriasis (see page 680), which causes red, thick, scaly, itchy patches to form on the scalp and other areas of the body, can also affect the vulva. Crohn's disease (see page 527), in which ulcers form along the gastrointestinal tract, may cause ulcers to form on the vulva also. In these cases, the disease—such as psoriasis or Crohn's disease—must be treated to clear up the symptoms on the vulva. To help relieve these symptoms, your doctor may recommend applying corticosteroid creams to the affected area, avoiding irritation caused by chemicals in soaps and deodorants, and wearing loose clothing.

Vitiligo Vitiligo (see page 682) is an inherited disorder in which the pigment of the skin of the vulva turns pale, even white. Vitiligo rarely causes other symptoms and seldom needs to be treated. However, vitiligo can occur in the presence of more serious disorders, such as some types of thyroid dysfunction or diabetes. These disorders do require treatment, so it is important to report this symptom to your doctor.

VESTIBULITIS

Vestibulitis is recurring inflammation of the vestibule, the area of the vulva just outside the vagina. Although it can occur at any age, vestibulitis occurs most often in sexually active women of childbearing age.

The most common symptoms of vestibulitis are a burning sensation around the opening of the vagina and pain during intercourse. Some women with vestibulitis are unable to insert tampons. The disorder may suddenly disappear and then reappear a few months later.

The most common causes of vestibulitis are chemical irritants such as strong soaps, shampoos, deodorants, fabric softeners, or bubble bath. Women with very sensitive skin may even have a reaction when they wear panty hose or noncotton underwear.

Vestibulitis is sometimes associated with the human papillomavirus (HPV; see page 341), a sexually transmitted virus that causes genital warts. Your doctor is likely to test you for the virus. If HPV is not detected, your doctor may test you for other infections. Depending on the specific disease-causing organism found from the tests, your doctor will prescribe an antibiotic or other medication.

In severe cases that do not respond to treatment, your doctor may recommend removing the affected tissue with traditional surgery or with laser surgery (which uses high-energy beams of light). Discuss the options thoroughly with your doctor. In some cases, surgery must be repeated if the condition recurs. For some women, treatment of this persistent condition can significantly improve their sex life because they no longer experience pain during intercourse.

Other disorders of the reproductive system

Some disorders affect more than one reproductive organ. Most of these disorders are relatively easy to treat if they are detected at an early stage. However, if left untreated, they can affect your fertility and may require major surgery. It is essential to see your doctor regularly even if you don't have any symptoms.

ENDOMETRIOSIS

The endometrium is the tissue that lines the uterus and swells with blood each month to prepare for a fertilized egg in the event of conception. If an egg is not fertilized, excess endometrial tissue is eliminated as menstrual blood each month. For reasons that are not fully understood, this type of tissue sometimes grows outside the uterus, on or near the ovaries or fallopian tubes, or in other areas of the abdominal cavity. This condition is called endometriosis. The term endometriosis also refers to the abnormal tissue that grows outside the uterus.

Many doctors believe that endometriosis is caused by a backup of some menstrual blood through the fallopian tubes and into the pelvic cavity. Like the endometrial tissue inside the uterus, this displaced tissue responds to the monthly hormonal signals by filling with blood. At the end of the menstrual cycle, this tissue sheds like the endometrium lining the uterus, but the blood and tissue have no place to go. Instead, they irritate surrounding tissues, causing scarring and adhesions (scar tissue that binds two tissues that are normally unconnected). This formation of scar tissue can lead to pelvic pain and infertility.

Endometriosis is one of the most common gynecologic disorders, affecting 1 of every 10 to 12 women of childbearing age. Although the disorder is most common in women in their 30s and 40s, it can also occur in teenagers.

Symptoms The symptom that brings most women with endometriosis to a doctor is pain that follows a certain pattern during the menstrual cycle—increasing pain and discomfort in the days preceding a period and during the first few days of a period. You might also experience a sharp pain deep in your pelvis during intercourse.

Endometriosis can make it more difficult for you to get pregnant. You may have spotting before your period or painful bowel movements. Many women have no symptoms so it goes undetected and untreated. If not treated, endometriosis can lead to infertility.

Diagnosis Although your symptoms may alert your doctor to the possibility of endometriosis, he or she must perform a procedure called laparoscopy (see page 263) in order to make a diagnosis. Laparoscopy is performed using local anesthesia (see page 260) but does not require a hospital stay. During the procedure the doctor will remove any endometriosis that he or she finds, either burning the tissue with a laser or with heat, or cutting it out. If tissue on the pelvic organs looks abnormal, but does not have the characteristic appearance of

POSSIBLE SITES OF ENDOMETRIOSIS

Endometrial tissue, which normally thickens inside the uterus each month to prepare for a fertilized egg, sometimes grows in other parts of the pelvic cavity. This displaced tissue thickens with blood during the menstrual cycle, as does the endometrium itself, which can cause pain and irritation. Common sites of endometriosis include the surface of the ovaries, uterus, bladder, fallopian tubes, colon, connective tissues inside the pelvis, and vagina.

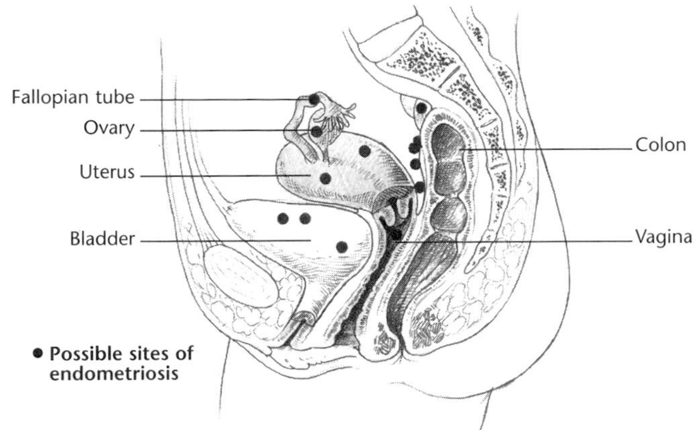

endometriosis, the doctor will take a sample for laboratory testing. Endometriosis is almost never cancerous. If the doctor cannot reach all of the endometriosis using laparoscopy, he or she will determine how much abnormal tissue was left behind, which will influence any decisions about further treatment.

Treatment Endometriosis is treated with hormones. Your doctor may prescribe birth-control pills that you take every day without the usual 7-day break during menstruation. This treatment suppresses the ovaries' normal production of the hormones that make the tissue of endometriosis grow and bleed, causing pain.

Your doctor might prescribe a different hormone treatment—injections of the hormone progesterone. The doctor injects the hormone into a large muscle (such as that in the buttocks) every 3 months.

In another treatment, you may be given a medication called danazol, which is a synthetic hormone derived from progesterone that you take in pills every day. Danazol suppresses menstruation and, therefore, the growth of endometrial tissue. The side effects of taking this hormone include acne, weight gain, and excessive hair growth.

A side effect of all three hormone treatments is irregular bleeding. These treatments are usually used only for mild cases of endometriosis or for women who cannot tolerate the side effects of more aggressive treatment, such as the use of stronger synthetic hormones called gonadotropin-releasing hormone (GnRH) agonists.

GnRH agonists stop the ovaries from producing estrogen. The lack of estrogen, which stops your periods altogether, helps prevent the endometriosis from growing anywhere in your pelvis. The side effects of this therapy include the same symptoms that often accompany menopause (see page 352)—such as hot flashes and vaginal dryness. However, the usual, short-term treatment (6 months or less) with GnRH agonists does not result in the bone loss that a lack of estrogen usually causes. Your periods will resume when the treatment is stopped.

If you have pain during or after treatment, your doctor may recommend additional laparoscopic surgery to remove abnormal tissue. In some women, the initial laparoscopy performed to make the diagnosis and remove the endometriosis may cause scar tissue to form. This scar tissue, called adhesions, can prevent an ovary from releasing a mature egg (ovulation) or a fallopian tube from picking up an egg, causing infertility. In this case, the doctor will do further surgery to remove the scar tissue.

Endometriosis can also be removed using a more extensive surgical procedure called laparotomy (see page 264), in which the doctor makes a larger incision than that needed for laparoscopy. He or she has access to a larger area in the pelvis and can use a wider range of surgical instruments to remove tissue.

Hysterectomy, the surgical removal of the uterus, is the most serious treatment for endometriosis. A hysterectomy may or may not include removal of one or both ovaries. However, if the ovaries are left intact, endometriosis may recur.

When both ovaries are removed, the monthly growth of endometrial tissue stops.

Removal of the ovaries causes immediate menopause because your body is no longer producing estrogen. Your doctor is likely to recommend that you take estrogen in the form of hormone replacement therapy (HRT; see page 359). (For more about hysterectomy, see page 256.)

PELVIC INFLAMMATORY DISEASE

Pelvic inflammatory disease (PID) is a term used to describe an infection in the upper reproductive tract—usually in the uterus, fallopian tubes, or ovaries. About 1 million American women are diagnosed with PID every year. The sexually transmitted diseases chlamydia (see page 339) and gonorrhea (see page 340) are common causes of PID. Chlamydia is extremely common in the US—there are 4 million new cases every year. Because chlamydia often causes no symptoms in women, it is often not detected or treated. If not treated, the infection can spread to the upper reproductive tract, causing PID.

One of the most devastating effects of PID is infertility caused by scarring and blockage of the fallopian tubes. Infertility occurs in about 12 percent of women after one episode of PID and in more than 50 percent of women who have had three or more episodes.

Salpingitis is the most common form of PID. Salpingitis is an infection of the fallopian tubes caused by bacteria or other disease-causing organisms that have entered the reproductive tract through the cervix, usually from sexual intercourse. Salpingitis can cause scar tissue to form in the fallopian tubes, blocking them. If the tubes are narrowed by a partial blockage, a life-threatening ectopic pregnancy (see page 233) may result. If you have had PID in the past and you become pregnant, it is important to let your doctor know you had PID. He or she will want to make sure that an ectopic pregnancy has not developed inside one of your fallopian tubes. Complete blockage of the tubes prevents sperm from reaching an egg, causing infertility.

Symptoms The symptoms of PID can vary and tend to be milder and less obvious when chlamydia is the cause of the infection. You may feel mild pelvic pain and pain in your lower back or pain that is noticeable only during intercourse. Your vaginal discharge may change in consistency (become thicker or thinner) or may increase slightly. Even though

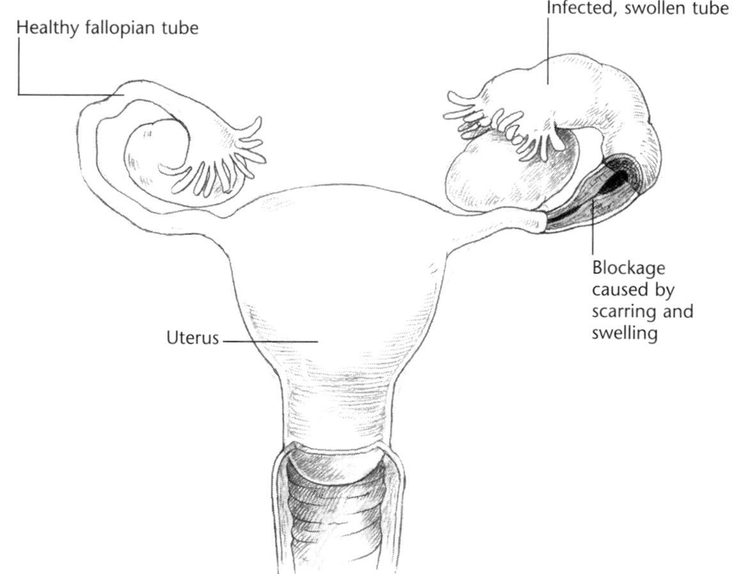

LONG-TERM EFFECTS OF PID

Pelvic inflammatory disease can have serious consequences, including infertility or even death. When a fallopian tube is infected, it can become inflamed, swollen, and scarred. This scarring can block the tube, keeping a sperm or egg from passing through, causing infertility by preventing fertilization. An egg that is fertilized in the fallopian tube may get trapped there, implant itself in the tube, and begin to grow, resulting in an ectopic pregnancy (see page 233). If the fertilized egg continues to grow inside the tube, the tube can rupture, which is life threatening.

these symptoms may be mild, the ultimate damage caused by PID can be severe. When gonorrhea is the cause of PID, the symptoms are more obvious. Severe pelvic pain, fever, and chills are common, as is increased vaginal discharge that may resemble pus. Vaginal bleeding may also occur in PID that results from a gonorrhea infection.

Diagnosis To diagnose PID, your doctor will ask about your symptoms and then perform a pelvic examination, looking for abnormal discharge and tenderness in the pelvic and vaginal areas. Taking a sample of cells from the cervix for laboratory testing helps identify the disease-causing organism. A blood test can also help determine if an infection is present. Because some signs and symptoms of PID may resemble those of appendicitis (see page 523) or an ectopic pregnancy, the doctor must rule these out before prescribing antibiotics to treat the PID.

Treatment Antibiotics are the first means of treating PID. If the symptoms are not severe, your doctor may give you an injection of antibiotics into a muscle and prescribe antibiotics in pills. If the infection is widespread, or if the prescribed antibiotics are not effective, you may need to have antibiotics administered intravenously in the hospital. Introducing the medication directly into the bloodstream delivers it to the site of infection more efficiently. More severe infections require a combination of antibiotics and may not respond to treatment for several days.

If the infection does not respond to intravenous antibiotics, or an abscess (a pus-filled sac) forms that does not show signs of shrinking, the doctor may decide to perform laparoscopy (see page 263). During laparoscopy, the doctor can drain the pus from the abscess, cut scar tissue, or take samples of any infected fluid in the pelvis for laboratory examination.

ECTOPIC PREGNANCY

An ectopic pregnancy is a pregnancy that occurs somewhere other than the normal location inside the uterus. Most ectopic pregnancies develop in a fallopian tube and are called tubal pregnancies. The ovaries, abdominal cavity, and cervix are less common sites.

Ectopic pregnancies can occur in a fallopian tube that has been damaged and narrowed, usually by a previous pelvic infection or surgery that was performed on the tube or surrounding area. Women at high risk of an ectopic pregnancy include those who have had a sexually transmitted disease (STD) of any kind (but especially chlamydia or gonorrhea) or pelvic inflammatory disease (PID), which can result from an STD.

Use of an intrauterine device (IUD) can increase the risk of an ectopic pregnancy if the IUD caused an infection in your fallopian tubes or pelvis. Women who have had surgery on a fallopian tube, such as a tubal ligation (in which the tubes are cut and tied to prevent pregnancy) or reversal of a tubal ligation, are also at increased risk of an ectopic pregnancy.

Any of these factors can result in scarring and narrowing of a fallopian tube. Although the tube may be open enough to allow a sperm to reach an egg and fertilize it, the fertilized egg is too large to travel down the narrowed tube to the uterus. Instead, the fertilized egg gets stuck in the narrowed segment of the tube and grows there. The embryo cannot develop normally because its growth is restricted by the size of the tube. The egg continues to divide and grow, causing the tube to swell until it can no longer accommodate the expanding embryo. The tube ruptures. A ruptured tube causes pain and bleeding and can be life threatening. For this reason, it is essential that an ectopic pregnancy be diagnosed as early as possible, before it ruptures.

Symptoms The symptoms of an ectopic pregnancy are a missed period, pelvic pain, or abnormal vaginal bleeding. Some women do not have any symptoms.

Diagnosis If the result of a pregnancy test is positive and your doctor suspects the pregnancy may be ectopic, he or she will ask about the timing of your last period. By the time your period is 2 weeks late, an ultrasound (see page 405) usually can show a pregnancy in the uterus. If the ultrasound does not show a pregnancy in the uterus, there are several possible explanations. Your pregnancy may not be as far along as you originally thought, the pregnancy may be in the fallopian tube, or you may have had a miscarriage (see page 422).

The next step in diagnosis depends on your symptoms. If you have no bleeding or pain, your doctor may simply schedule another ultrasound 7 to 10 days later to see if the pregnancy is then visible, and a blood test to measure the level of the hormone human chorionic gonadotropin (HCG). HCG is produced by the cells of the placenta in a developing pregnancy. In a normal pregnancy, the placenta has enough room to grow at the usual rate—doubling the amount of HCG every 1½ to 2 days. But in a tubal pregnancy, the placenta does not have enough space to expand normally and, therefore, the level of HCG does not increase as quickly. Performing a series of HCG blood tests enables your doctor to determine if your HCG levels are rising normally. These hormone measurements may alert your doctor to the possibility of an ectopic pregnancy before it is large enough to show up on an ultrasound.

Treatment If your doctor cannot detect a pregnancy in your uterus on an ultrasound, further investigation depends on whether or not you are experiencing bleeding or pain or are at risk of an ectopic pregnancy because of a narrowed tube. In either case, your doctor may recommend laparoscopy (see page 263). If, in laparoscopy, the doctor finds that an ectopic pregnancy has occurred, he or she will remove the developing egg by making an incision in the fallopian tube and scooping out the egg. If the tube is ruptured or bleeding, part or all of it may also be removed. Surgical removal of a fallopian tube is called a salpingectomy (see page 262). The removal of one fallopian tube does not affect the functioning of the other tube. If your remaining fallopian tube is healthy, you will still be able to get pregnant.

Before having any surgery for a suspected ectopic pregnancy, ask your doctor to explain the procedure and tell you which tissues may need to be removed. An ectopic pregnancy that has already ruptured and is bleeding may require more extensive abdominal surgery called laparotomy (see page 264).

In some cases, an ectopic pregnancy may be treated with medication. If the diagnosis is certain, the ectopic pregnancy is at an early stage and has not ruptured the tube, and the woman is not in pain or experiencing bleeding, a doctor may recommend treatment with a drug called methotrexate. Methotrexate breaks down the tissue of the abnormal pregnancy and the body absorbs it. Your doctor will monitor your condition carefully after this treatment to ensure the drug is working effectively and the fallopian tube does not rupture. In some cases, more than one dose of medication is necessary.

LOSS OF PELVIC SUPPORT

The pelvic organs—the uterus, bladder, urethra, rectum, and vagina—are held in place by ligaments, strong connective tissues called fascia, and muscles. These supporting tissues are attached to the sides of the pelvis, the pelvic organs, and the openings of the urethra, vagina, and anus. If the supporting tissues become stretched, they slacken, causing the organs they normally support to sag or bulge into the vagina. Occasionally an organ, such as the uterus or bladder, drops down so much that it protrudes out of the vagina. These pelvic support problems can cause urinary incontinence (see page 538) or difficulty urinating or having complete bowel movements.

Childbirth and aging are the primary causes of pelvic support problems. Vaginal childbirth stretches the supporting tissues—the ligaments, fascia, and muscles—and may weaken them. But pelvic support problems can also occur in women who have not had children. Some women are born with weak supporting tissues in their pelvis, and the problem only becomes apparent as they age. Diminishing levels of the hormone estrogen at menopause may cause these tissues to become thinner and weaker. Obesity can also contribute to pelvic support problems, as can a chronic cough or repeated heavy lifting.

Types of pelvic support problems

There are several types of pelvic support problems, and they often occur together. All pelvic support problems can be corrected with surgery. Other treatments may be effective for correcting mild or moderate problems.

Prolapse of the uterus When the uterus drops from its normal position, it may fall part way into the vagina or it may protrude into the vaginal opening and,

Prolapse of the uterus

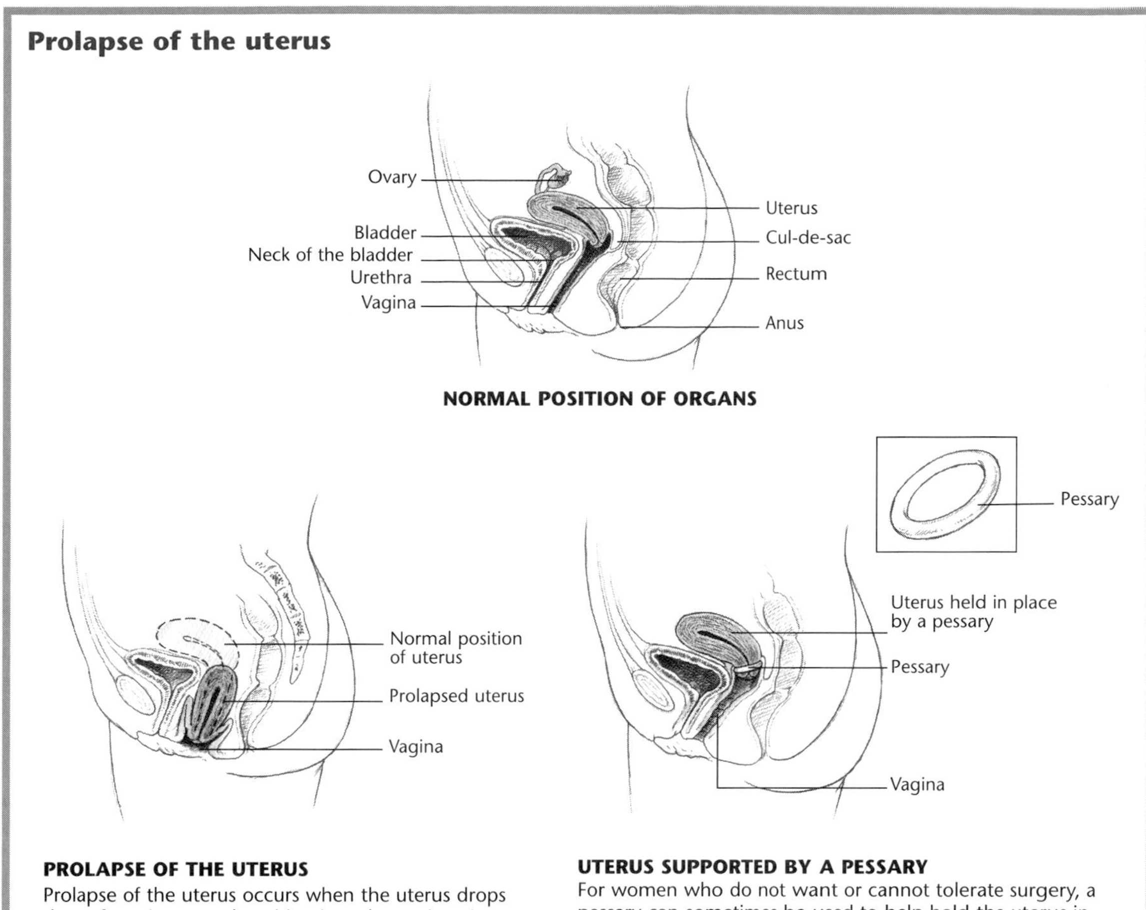

PROLAPSE OF THE UTERUS
Prolapse of the uterus occurs when the uterus drops down from its normal position into the vagina. A prolapsed uterus may occur as a result of pregnancy, vaginal childbirth, or aging. The uterus may protrude partly into the vagina or all the way into the vaginal opening. Surgery can correct this problem.

UTERUS SUPPORTED BY A PESSARY
For women who do not want or cannot tolerate surgery, a pessary can sometimes be used to help hold the uterus in place. A pessary is a rubber device shaped like a doughnut or cube that comes in a number of sizes and is worn inside the vagina to support the uterus. If the prolapse is very severe, a pessary may not provide enough support to hold the uterus in place.

in some women, partly out of the body. This displacement of the uterus often brings other pelvic organs down with it. Women with uterine prolapse commonly feel pressure in the pelvic area and sometimes a pulling in the groin or lower back. Because prolapse of the uterus moves the cervix lower in the vagina than it usually is, this condition can make intercourse painful.

Cystocele A cystocele results when the base of the bladder drops from its usual position into the vagina. In severe cases, a cystocele may create a sharp angle at the junction of the urethra and bladder that can temporarily close off the urethra during urination. In order to urinate, some women have to strain or lean forward. A cystocele may occur with a cystourethrocele (see below).

Cystourethrocele A cystourethrocele results when the tissues that hold up the upper half of the urethra and its connection to the bladder become weak. This weakening causes stress incontinence—leaking urine when you put pressure on your abdomen such as when you sneeze, cough, jump, or lift heavy objects. Your doctor will want to determine if you have stress incontinence (see page 540),

Pelvic support problems

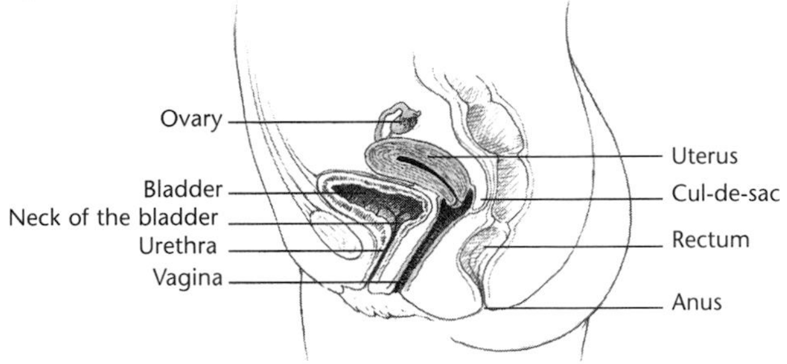

NORMAL POSITION OF ORGANS

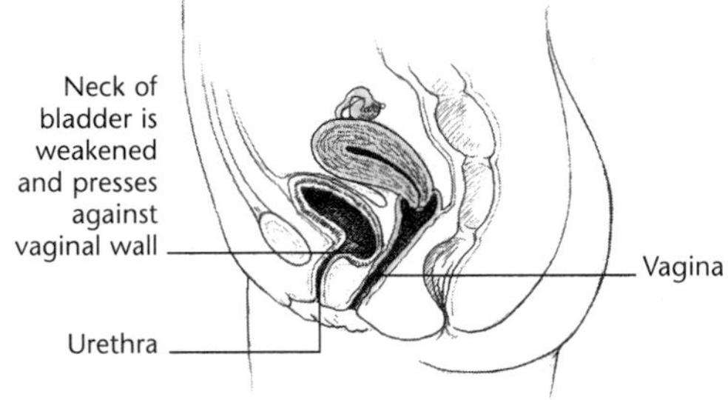

CYSTOURETHROCELE
The tissues supporting the urethra and bladder are weakened, sometimes causing urine to leak when you cough, sneeze, or jump.

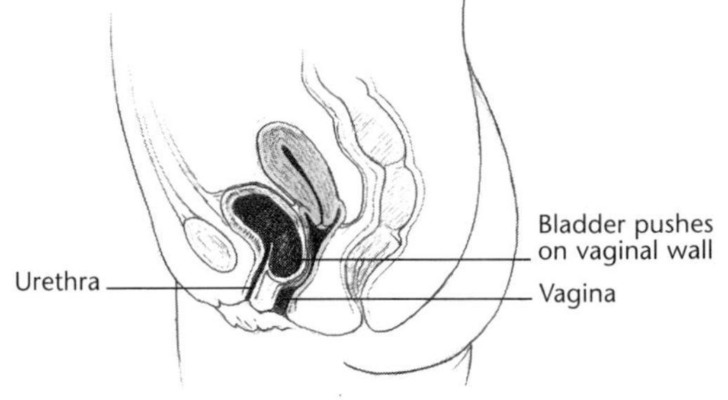

CYSTOCELE
The bladder descends from its normal position, pushing on the front wall of the vagina. The pressure may make urination difficult.

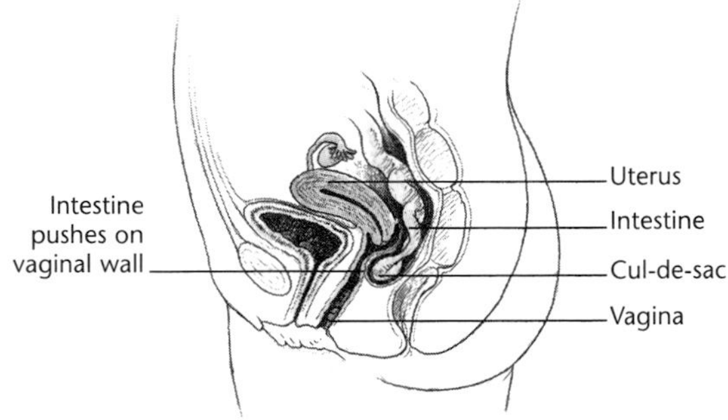

ENTEROCELE
A portion of the intestines bulges into the top of the vagina, sometimes causing recurring pain in the lower back.

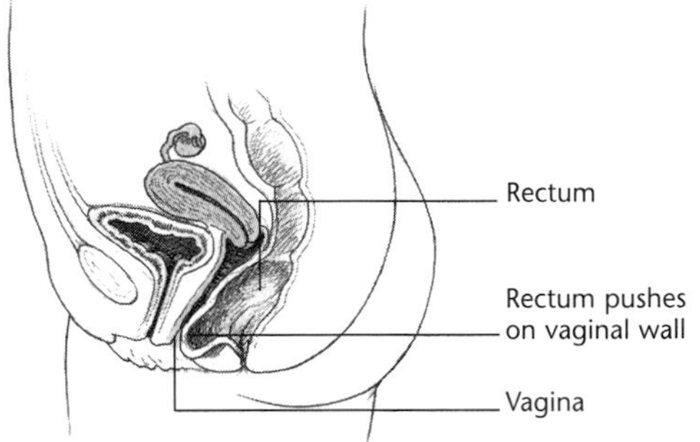

RECTOCELE
The rectum bulges into the vagina because the vaginal wall is weak, making bowel movements difficult.

because it can be treated surgically. Other types of incontinence are treated in different ways.

Enterocele An enterocele is formed when a portion of the intestine bulges into the top of the vagina through the tissues at the bottom of the cul-de-sac (the space between the uterus and the rectum). During a pelvic examination, a doctor can see an enterocele as a bulge in the top and upper back of the vaginal wall or feel it by examining you while you are in a standing position. An enterocele causes lower back pain and pressure in the pelvic area.

Rectocele A rectocele occurs when the rectum bulges into the vagina as the result of a weakened vaginal wall. The doctor can see and feel a rectocele close to the vaginal opening. A large rectocele may make it difficult to empty your bowels completely; constipation can make it worse. Some women have to put their fingers in their vagina to push the bulging tissue back in order to have a bowel movement.

Vaginal vault prolapse After a hysterectomy (surgical removal of the uterus), the top (vault) of the vagina can sometimes lose its support and collapse; this is called vaginal vault prolapse. The vaginal vault may drop part way into the vagina and remain there, or drop all the way or part way through the vaginal opening. Many women who have vaginal vault prolapse also have an enterocele (see above). Bladder problems may also accompany this condition. If the delicate tissue of the vagina remains outside of the body, it can become irritated, which may cause open sores (ulcers) and bleeding.

Symptoms Leaking urine when you cough, sneeze, or jump—called stress incontinence (see page 540)—is often the first sign that the supporting tissues of your pelvis have relaxed. Another common symptom is the feeling of pressure, as though something from your pelvis were falling out through your vagina. You may also have lower back pain or persistent, aching pain or discomfort in your lower pelvis or vaginal area. These symptoms often worsen with each childbirth and with age as tissues normally become thinner and weaker.

Diagnosis To diagnose pelvic support problems, which often occur together, your doctor will take your full medical history and perform a pelvic examination. He or she may have to perform examinations both while you are lying down and while you are standing.

If you are having trouble with leaking urine, the doctor may also perform other tests. Using a technique called urethroscopy, the doctor can view the inside of your urethra (the tubular passage through which urine drains from the bladder) using a small instrument similar to a telescope. A technique called cystoscopy (see page 540) uses a viewing instrument to examine the inside of the bladder. Cystometry (see page 540) is used to measure how much your bladder can hold and your ability to control the flow of urine. Uroflometry is used to measure urine flow. These tests are usually performed together to create a "urologic profile," which helps your doctor evaluate the extent of the problem and determine treatment.

Treatment Depending on the nature and severity of a pelvic support problem, a doctor may recommend exercises, hormone therapy, surgery, electrical stimulation to strengthen the pelvic muscles, collagen injections, or a combination of these.

Pelvic-floor exercises, also known as Kegel exercises, strengthen the muscles that surround the openings of the urethra, vagina, and anus. These exercises can help prevent the leaking of urine in mild forms of urinary incontinence and rebuild some pelvic support.

If you are past menopause, your doctor may prescribe estrogen in hormone

Preventing pelvic support problems

- Do pelvic-floor (Kegel) exercises (see page 238) every day to strengthen your pelvic muscles.
- Control your weight; extra weight puts increased pressure on your pelvic organs.
- Don't smoke; smoking can cause a chronic cough that can put pressure on your pelvic organs.

Pelvic-floor exercises (Kegel exercises)

Pelvic-floor exercises, called Kegel exercises after Arnold Kegel, the gynecologist who first described them, are used to both treat and prevent mild pelvic support problems. Doing these exercises every day—whether or not you have pelvic support problems—can help improve bladder control and maintain strength in your vaginal muscles. Pelvic-floor exercises are simple to do:

1. Identify the muscles you need to exercise. While urinating, practice stopping the flow in midstream. These are the muscles you will tighten. Stop and start the flow several times to get the feel of contracting the muscles.
2. You can do these exercises any time, while sitting, standing, or lying down. Start by holding the contraction for 2 to 3 seconds and gradually work up to 8 to 10 seconds. Repeat 10 times.
3. Repeat the set of 10 contractions several times throughout the day. To be effective, you need to do at least 50 contractions (5 sets of 10) every day.
4. Most importantly, make sure to hold the muscle tightly for several seconds. Don't just tighten and release quickly. The longer you can hold the contraction, the more effective the exercise will be.

You can do these exercises while you are in the shower, in your car waiting for a red light to change, at your desk, or at the playground with your child. No one but you will know when you are doing your Kegel exercises.

replacement therapy (see page 359) together with pelvic-floor exercises to help pelvic muscles regain some strength. Reduced production of estrogen after menopause causes vaginal and other pelvic tissues to thin and weaken.

Some doctors may recommend injections of collagen (a protein found in connective tissues such as ligaments) to help strengthen the tissues around the urethra. Collagen is injected through the vagina into the tissue around the urethral opening. This treatment is often effective for women with mild stress incontinence.

When exercises or other treatments are not effective in correcting pelvic support problems that cause urinary incontinence, surgery may be recommended. A procedure called an anterior repair is performed through the vagina to lift and strengthen the support of the bladder; this procedure can help correct a cystourethrocele. To correct stress incontinence (see page 540), a surgical procedure called retropubic suspension can be performed through an incision in the abdomen. In this operation, the supporting tissue around the upper urethra is lifted to its normal position behind the pubic bone and stitched in place.

Surgery can also be used to treat a rectocele. A rectocele can make it difficult to move your bowels when stool collects in the area where the rectum is pressing into the vaginal wall. Surgery can help tighten and flatten the wall of the vagina, eliminating the bulge of the rectum and allowing the stool to be passed more easily.

Surgery for prolapse of the uterus is likely to include hysterectomy (removal of the uterus; see page 256). If you choose not to have a hysterectomy and you want to have children, your doctor may recommend cesarean delivery (see page 442); a vaginal delivery puts extra strain on the pelvic muscles and can trigger a recurrence of a pelvic support problem such as a cystourethrocele or a rectocele.

For older women who have medical problems that reduce their ability to tolerate surgery, a device called a pessary, which is inserted through the vagina, may be used to hold the uterus in place (see page 235). A pessary must be fitted properly by your doctor. You must remove and clean your pessary regularly (every 1 to 2 weeks) with warm water and mild soap to avoid infection.

Another treatment option for pelvic support problems in women who cannot or prefer not to have surgery is electrical stimulation of the pelvic floor muscles. This stimulation is delivered by a small electrode (about the size and shape of a tampon) that is inserted into the vagina. The stimulation causes the pelvic muscles to contract, in much the same way they do during pelvic-floor exercises, which makes them stronger.

Your doctor will give you instructions about how to use the device at home. You begin by inserting the electrode into your vagina and leaving it in for 15 minutes twice a day, increasing the time to 30 minutes twice a day over a period of several weeks. This treatment can help make your pelvic muscles stronger and better able to withstand the stress of normal activity. However, electrical stimulation does not work for everyone; if the treatment does not have any effect after several weeks, talk to your doctor. He or she may recommend an alternative treatment.

Cancers of the reproductive system

After cancers of the breast, colon and rectum, and lung, reproductive tract cancers as a group are the most common cancers in women. These cancers most often involve the endometrium (the lining of the uterus), the ovaries, and the cervix (the neck of the uterus).

Cancer is a disease in which abnormal cells divide rapidly, grow without any order, and spread to other sites in the body (metastasize), invading and destroying tissues and organs. For more about cancer, see Understanding cancer, page 506.

Tumors are abnormal growths. Tumors that are composed of cancerous cells are described as malignant. Some tumors are benign (not cancerous)—they do not spread to other parts of the body and are seldom a threat to health. The earlier the stage at which a cancer is found—before it begins to spread—the more likely it is to be curable.

For some cancers of the reproductive system, the likelihood of cure is greater today than ever before. With the increasing use of the Pap smear (see page 127) to screen for cervical cancer, and endometrial biopsies (see page 129) to test for endometrial cancer, more of these cancers are being detected at an early, curable stage.

Cancer survival rates

If you or someone in your family is diagnosed with cancer, you will naturally be concerned about the outlook. Your doctor or another source of information may refer to the survival rate for the cancer—how long the average person who has this cancer lives. A 5-year survival rate does not mean that you can expect to live for only 5 years after treatment, nor that there is no chance of cure. You may be considered cured if you are free of symptoms 1 year, 3 years, 5 years, or more after treatment, depending on the type of cancer.

Keep in mind that these statistics are averages based on the long-term outcomes of large numbers of people who have undergone various types of cancer therapy. Your own prospects for recovery are influenced by many factors such as your age, general health, and your individual response to treatment. While no one can precisely predict outcome, your doctor will discuss your care with you in terms of your individual medical situation. Remember, millions of Americans are alive today who can be considered cured of cancer.

ENDOMETRIAL CANCER

Although cancer of the endometrium (lining of the uterus) is the most common reproductive cancer in women, it has a high rate of cure—more than 90 percent when it is detected and treated at an early stage. Although there is no test for endometrial cancer comparable to the Pap smear for cervical cancer, the increasing use of endometrial biopsy (see page 129) is enabling doctors to detect more endometrial cancers at an early, curable stage. Endometrial cancer is most common between ages 50 and 70.

Increased exposure to the female hormone estrogen may increase a woman's risk of endometrial cancer. Other risk factors for the cancer include:

- Obesity; fat cells produce more estrogen.
- Irregular ovulation or menstruation; estrogen is not counterbalanced by the other female hormone progesterone, which is produced at ovulation (release of an egg by an ovary).
- A history of infertility.
- Early menstruation or late menopause, resulting in a longer lifetime exposure to circulating estrogen in the body.
- A history of polycystic ovarian disease (see page 227).
- A history of abnormal thickening of the endometrium, called endometrial hyperplasia (see page 221), a condition marked by abnormal cell changes that can progress to cancer if not treated.
- A history of cancer of the ovary, breast, or colon.

SYMPTOM CHART

Abnormal vaginal bleeding

Any bleeding that occurs between regular periods, during pregnancy, or after menopause.

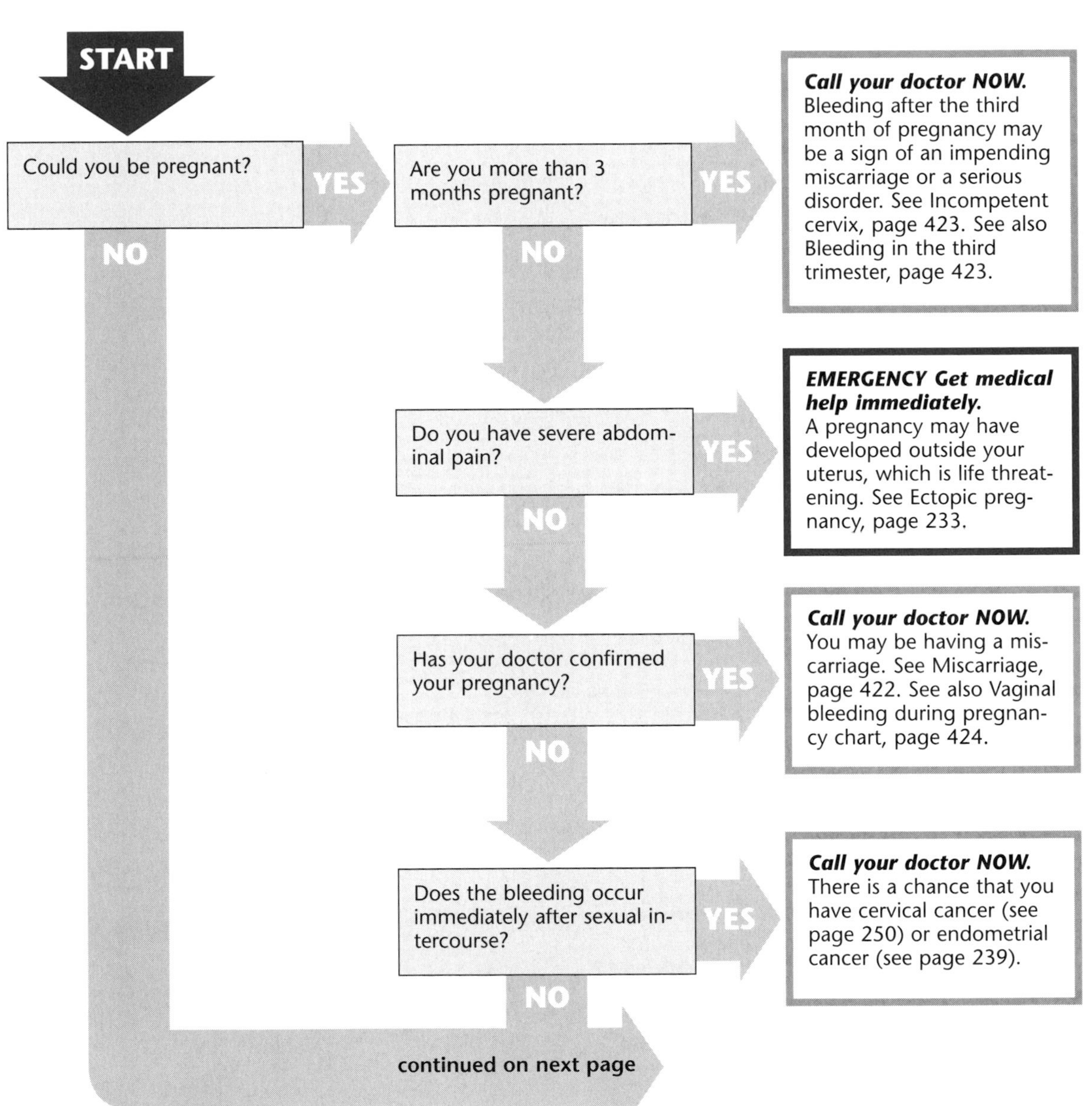

continued from previous page

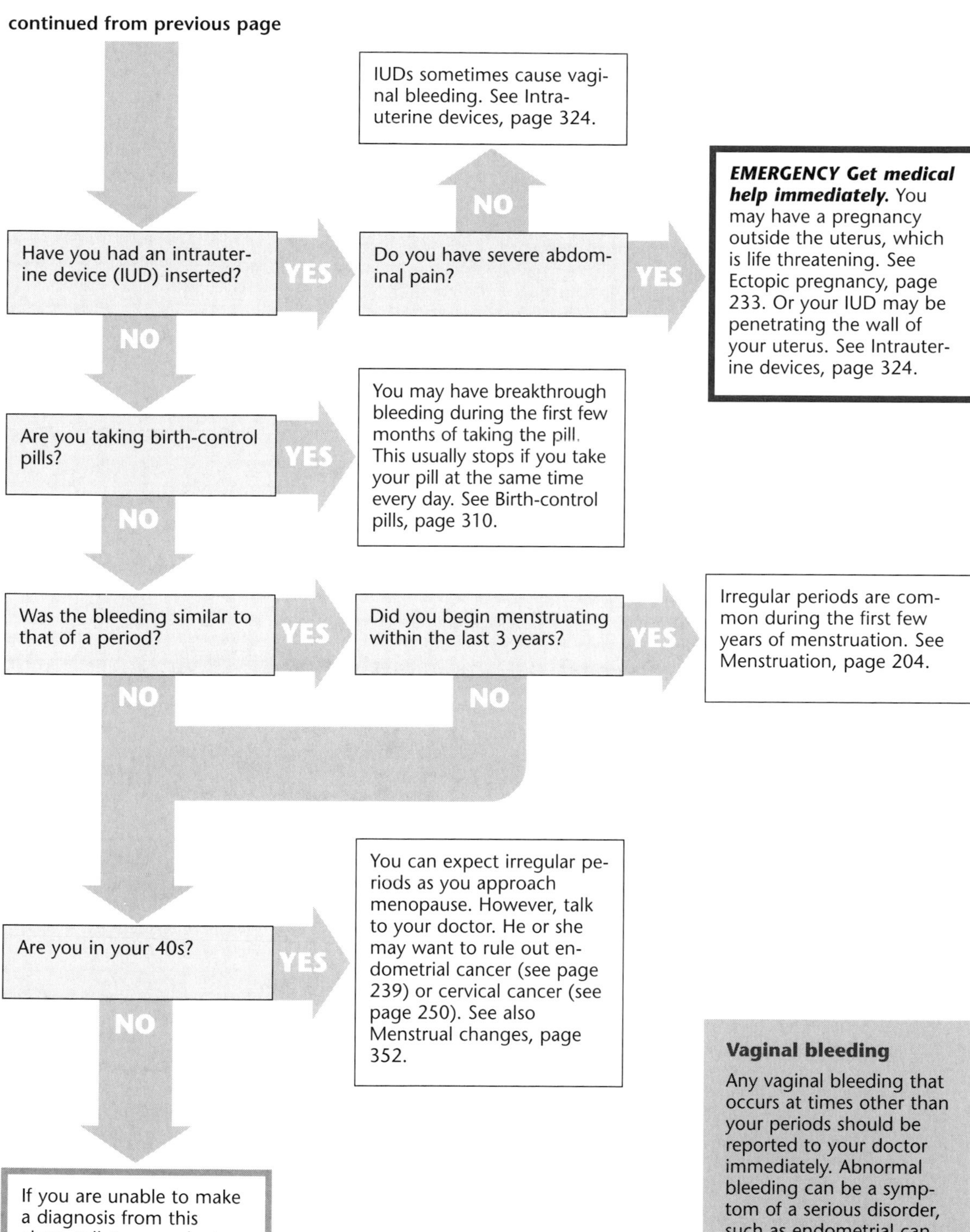

Vaginal bleeding

Any vaginal bleeding that occurs at times other than your periods should be reported to your doctor immediately. Abnormal bleeding can be a symptom of a serious disorder, such as endometrial cancer or cervical cancer.

SYMPTOM CHART

Pelvic pain

Any pain in your lower abdomen or pelvic area.

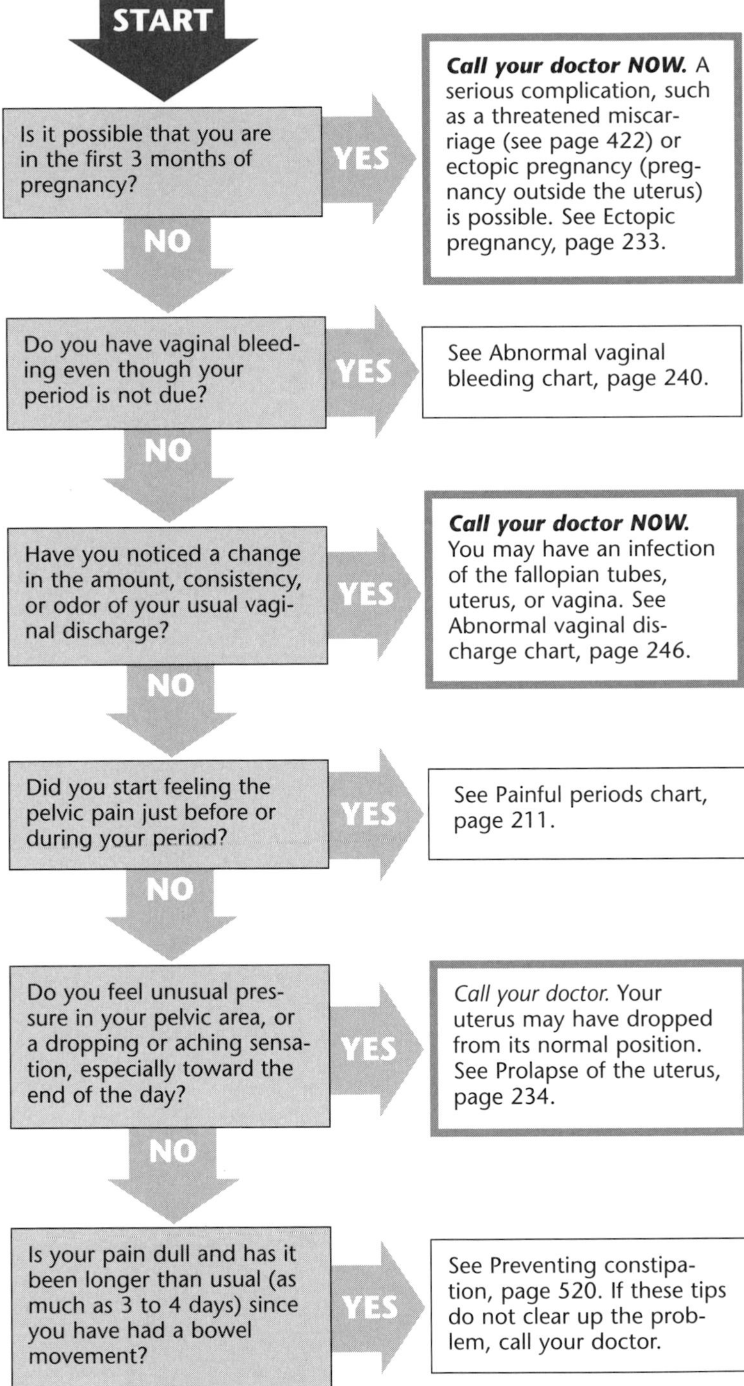

Waiting for medical attention

While waiting for medical help for pelvic pain, do not eat or drink anything, in case you need to have tests or surgery immediately. Do not take aspirin to relieve the pain or drink alcohol; aspirin and alcohol cause the blood to thin, which increases your risk of bleeding.

continued from previous page

Do you have an unusual bloating sensation not related to your period or do your clothes fit more tightly than usual?

YES → ***Call your doctor NOW*** to see if you should have a pelvic examination. See Disorders of the ovaries, page 224.

NO ↓

Is your pain cramping and do you have diarrhea?

YES → Gastroenteritis (inflammation of your stomach or intestines) can be caused by infection or food poisoning (see page 521). ***Call your doctor NOW*** if you notice blood or mucus when you have a bowel movement.

NO ↓

Is your pain severe and located mainly in your lower right side and/or have you had nausea or vomited?

YES → ***EMERGENCY Get medical help immediately.*** You may have appendicitis. Do not eat or drink anything before you get medical help. See Appendicitis, page 523.

NO ↓

Is your pain intermittent and cramping, especially in your lower left abdomen?

YES → ***Call your doctor NOW.*** You may have diverticulitis. See Diverticulosis, page 528.

NO ↓

Do you have a burning sensation when you urinate or are you urinating more frequently than usual?

YES → Do you also have fever and pain in the middle of your back?

- YES → ***Call your doctor NOW.*** You may have a kidney infection. See Pyelonephritis, page 544.
- NO → ***Call your doctor NOW.*** You may have a bladder infection. See Cystitis, page 543.

NO ↓

If you are unable to make a diagnosis from this chart, talk to your doctor.

Abdominal pain

Severe and continuous abdominal pain requires urgent medical attention in the following cases:

- It persists for more than 4 hours.
- It is accompanied but unrelieved by vomiting.
- Your abdomen is swollen and tender.
- It is accompanied by faintness, drowsiness, or confusion.
- You also have a fever.

SYMPTOM CHART

Painful intercourse

Pain or discomfort during or after sexual intercourse.

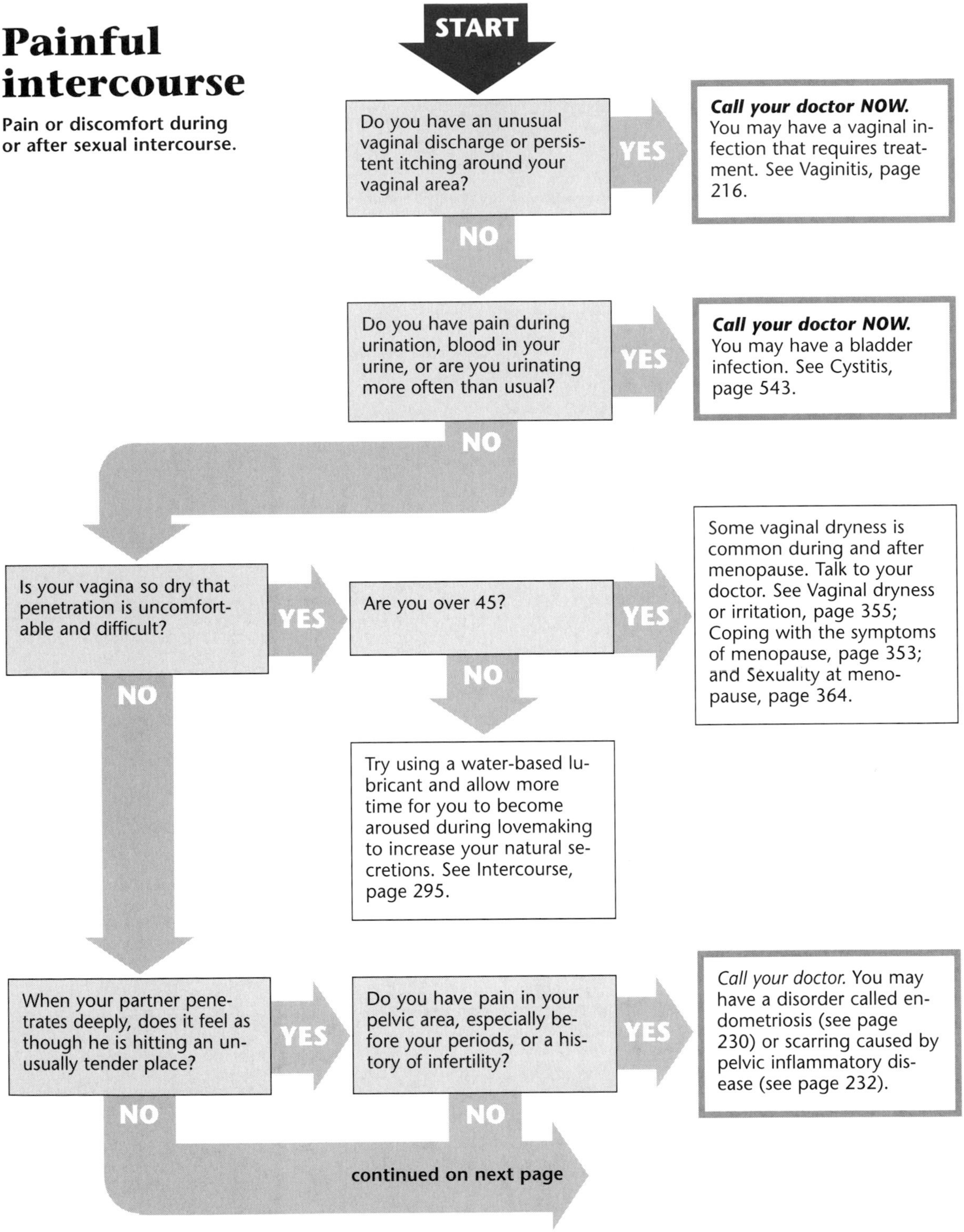

START

Do you have an unusual vaginal discharge or persistent itching around your vaginal area?

YES → ***Call your doctor NOW.*** You may have a vaginal infection that requires treatment. See Vaginitis, page 216.

NO ↓

Do you have pain during urination, blood in your urine, or are you urinating more often than usual?

YES → ***Call your doctor NOW.*** You may have a bladder infection. See Cystitis, page 543.

NO ↓

Is your vagina so dry that penetration is uncomfortable and difficult?

YES → Are you over 45?

YES → Some vaginal dryness is common during and after menopause. Talk to your doctor. See Vaginal dryness or irritation, page 355; Coping with the symptoms of menopause, page 353; and Sexuality at menopause, page 364.

NO ↓

Try using a water-based lubricant and allow more time for you to become aroused during lovemaking to increase your natural secretions. See Intercourse, page 295.

NO ↓

When your partner penetrates deeply, does it feel as though he is hitting an unusually tender place?

YES → Do you have pain in your pelvic area, especially before your periods, or a history of infertility?

YES → *Call your doctor.* You may have a disorder called endometriosis (see page 230) or scarring caused by pelvic inflammatory disease (see page 232).

NO ↓

NO ↓

continued on next page

continued from previous page

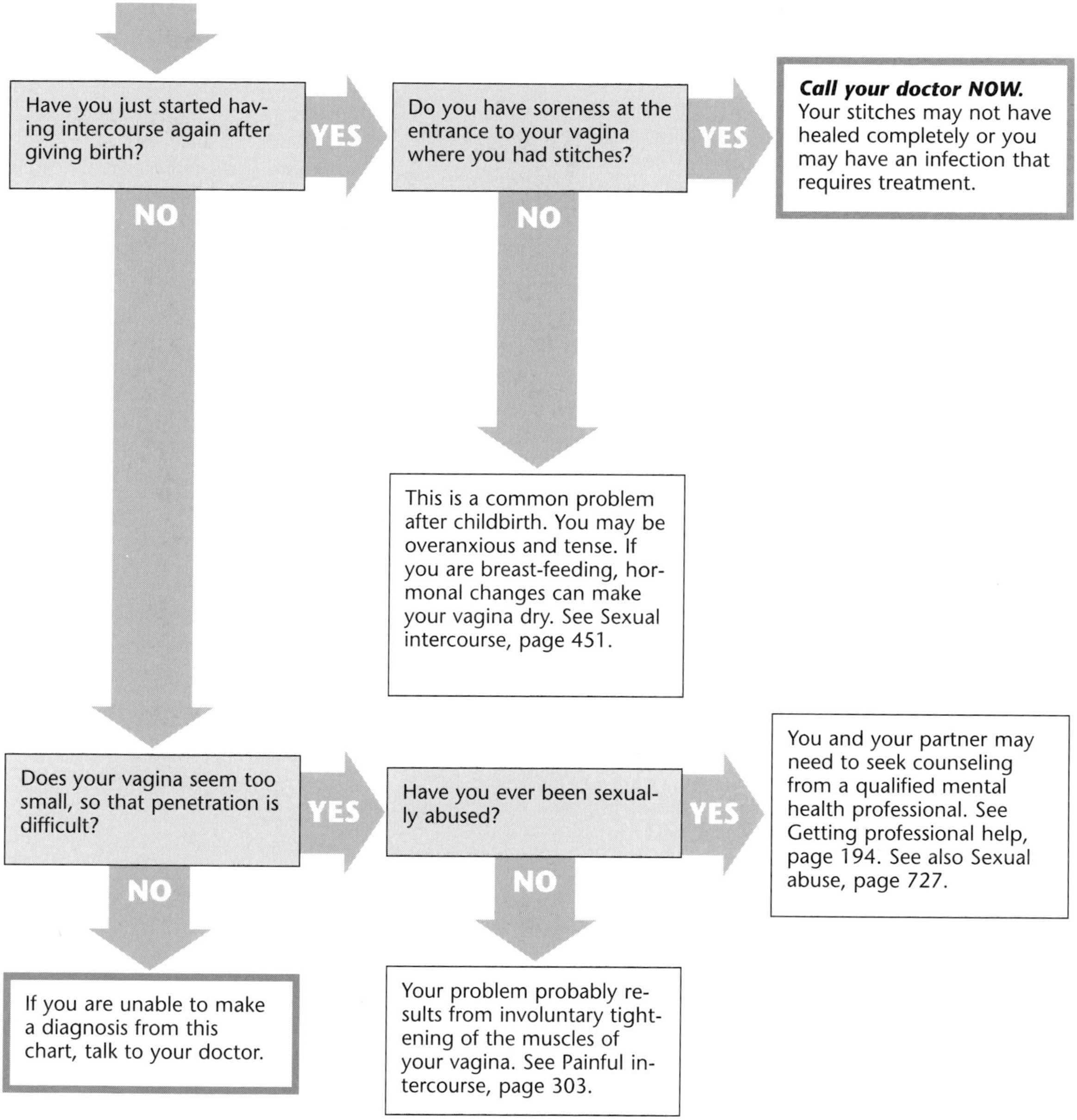

Have you just started having intercourse again after giving birth?

YES → Do you have soreness at the entrance to your vagina where you had stitches?

YES → **Call your doctor NOW.** Your stitches may not have healed completely or you may have an infection that requires treatment.

NO → This is a common problem after childbirth. You may be overanxious and tense. If you are breast-feeding, hormonal changes can make your vagina dry. See Sexual intercourse, page 451.

NO → Does your vagina seem too small, so that penetration is difficult?

YES → Have you ever been sexually abused?

YES → You and your partner may need to seek counseling from a qualified mental health professional. See Getting professional help, page 194. See also Sexual abuse, page 727.

NO → Your problem probably results from involuntary tightening of the muscles of your vagina. See Painful intercourse, page 303.

NO → If you are unable to make a diagnosis from this chart, talk to your doctor.

SYMPTOM CHART

Abnormal vaginal discharge

Fluid from your vagina that differs in color, consistency, and/or quantity from your normal discharge between periods.

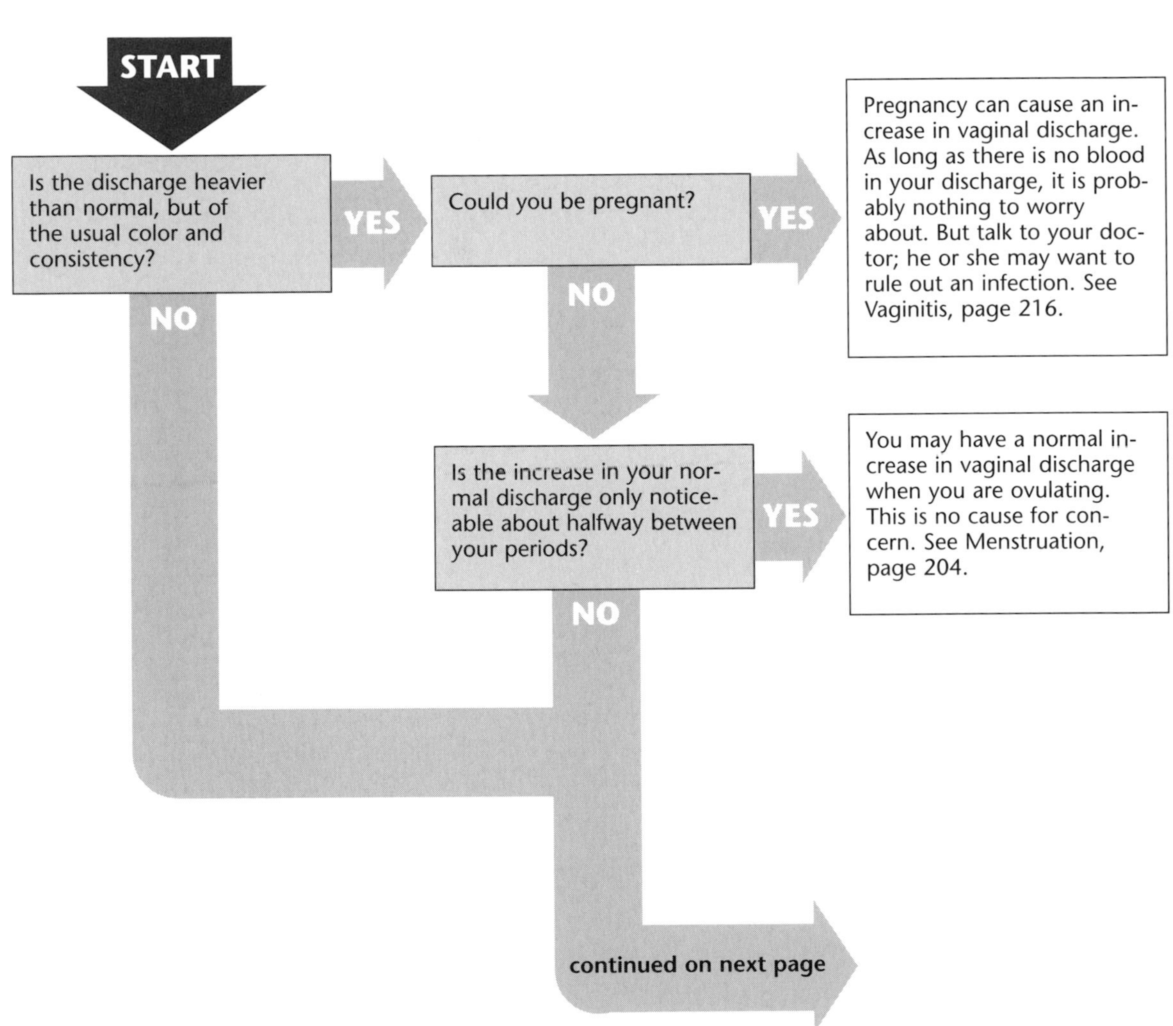

continued from previous page

Is the discharge thick, white, clumpy, and accompanied by itching in your vaginal area?

YES → You may have a yeast infection. See Yeast infection, page 217.

NO ↓

Is the discharge green or yellow and does it have an unpleasant odor?

YES → Do you have a fever or pain in your lower abdomen?

- **YES** → ***Call your doctor NOW.*** You may have an infection in your fallopian tubes or uterus. See Gonorrhea, page 340. See also Pelvic inflammatory disease, page 232.
- **NO** → *Call your doctor.* You may have a vaginal infection that requires treatment. See Bacterial vaginosis, page 216. See also Trichomoniasis, page 349.

NO ↓

Is the discharge tinged with blood and/or have you noticed occasional spotting of blood between periods?

YES → ***Call your doctor NOW.*** You may have a sexually transmitted disease that is infecting your cervix. See Chlamydia, page 339. See also Genital herpes, page 342.

NO ↓

If you are unable to make a diagnosis from this chart, talk to your doctor.

Vaginal discharge

Every woman has a certain amount of vaginal discharge throughout her menstrual cycle that is normal for her. But any change in your discharge can be a symptom of a problem that requires treatment. Tell your doctor about anything unusual you observe about your discharge.

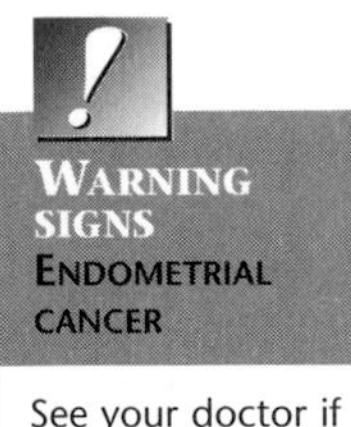

WARNING SIGNS
ENDOMETRIAL CANCER

See your doctor if you have any of the following symptoms:

- Abnormal vaginal bleeding or spotting
- Any vaginal bleeding or spotting after menopause

- Family history (mother, daughter, or sister with endometrial cancer).
- Use of the drug tamoxifen to treat breast cancer (see page 284); tamoxifen blocks estrogen's effects in the breast, but, in other organs, such as the uterus, the drug acts as a weak form of estrogen.
- Taking estrogen without the hormone progestin (which prevents the endometrium from building up).

Symptoms The most common symptoms of endometrial cancer are abnormal bleeding, spotting, and discharge from the vagina. After menopause, any bleeding or spotting is abnormal, no matter how small the amount—except for regular cyclical bleeding when you are taking hormone replacement therapy. Make sure to tell your doctor about any bleeding or vaginal discharge.

Diagnosis The first step in diagnosing either endometrial hyperplasia (abnormal thickening of the endometrium) or endometrial cancer is usually an endometrial biopsy (see page 129). In this procedure, which is performed in the doctor's office without anesthesia, the doctor takes a small sample of tissue from the endometrium for microscopic examination in the laboratory. You might feel a mild to moderate cramping during the procedure.

Sometimes, a woman who has a vaginal ultrasound (see page 129) for another reason is told that the test shows an abnormal thickening of the endometrium. When this occurs, her doctor performs an endometrial biopsy to investigate further. A doctor may do hysteroscopy (see page 264) to directly examine the inside of the uterus using an instrument called a hysteroscope, which resembles a thin telescope. The doctor can take a tissue sample from any area in the endometrium that looks abnormal.

Doctors sometimes perform a dilation and curettage (D and C; see page 262) to diagnose endometrial cancer. Tissue from the endometrium is scraped away for examination in the laboratory. A D and C is usually performed in a special procedure room or outpatient operating room using local anesthesia and, sometimes, a sedative to relax you.

A Pap smear is not a reliable test for endometrial cancer because the cells are taken only from the cervix, not from inside the uterus.

Treatment If you are diagnosed with endometrial cancer, surgery is required to remove the cancer and to determine whether or not it has spread to your lymph nodes or other organs. Further treatment depends on the degree of abnormal cell change and how far the cancer has spread. Most women with endometrial cancer have a total hysterectomy (surgical removal of the uterus and cervix) and removal of the fallopian tubes and ovaries. (For more about hysterectomy, see page 256.) During surgery, the doctor takes tissue samples from the lymph nodes in the pelvis and alongside the major blood vessels in the pelvic and abdominal areas to see if the cancer has spread.

Some cases of endometrial cancer require radiation therapy in addition to a hysterectomy. Internal radiation is administered by placing radioactive materials at the top of the vagina through a device inserted into the vagina. The material is left in place for 2 to 3 days, during which you remain in bed. A screen around you protects other people from the radiation; your contact with other people is restricted during this time. When treatment is completed, the radioactive materials are removed from your body. This treatment helps prevent the cancer from recurring in the pelvis. Radiation therapy is sometimes administered externally, using high-power X-ray beams directed at the pelvis from outside the body.

The side effects of radiation therapy depend on your age, health status, the number of radiation treatments you have, and the dose of radiation. You may feel unusually tired during the time of treatment. Other side effects may include diarrhea; frequent, painful urination; cystitis (inflammation of the inner lining of the bladder); or scarring of the vagina. Most of these side effects are temporary. However, some scarring that narrows the vagina may be permanent; it can usually be treated with medications and devices called dilators that stretch open the vaginal canal.

Hormone therapy (see page 284), chemotherapy (see page 284), or both are used when the cancer has spread or recurred after surgery and radiation. Side effects of hormone therapy are usually temporary and can vary, depending on the particular hormone used.

OVARIAN CANCER

Ovarian cancer is the second most common reproductive cancer in women after endometrial cancer. It is much more likely to be fatal than cancer of the cervix or endometrium because it is more difficult to detect at an early stage.

Ovarian cancer is most common in women 50 to 75, although it can occur at any age. The tendency to develop ovarian cancer may run in some families, but heredity is not a factor in the majority of cases.

Regular ovulation that is not interrupted by pregnancy or breast-feeding appears to play a major role in the development of ovarian cancer. In the process of ovulation, cells in the ovaries are continuously dividing. This constant cellular activity increases the possibility of genetic mistakes occurring in ovarian cells, which can lead to cancer.

The following factors increase a woman's risk of ovarian cancer:

- Never having children
- Having children at an older age
- Going through menopause late (after age 55)
- Never having taken oral contraceptives (which block ovulation)
- Having a family history of ovarian cancer
- Having a family history of cancer of the colon, breast, prostate, or lung
- Having a history of cancer of the breast, endometrium, or colon and rectum
- Being white

Symptoms Ovarian cancer has no symptoms in the early stages. The cancer is most often detected when a doctor feels an enlarged ovary during a routine pelvic examination (see page 124) or while he or she is investigating other problems in the reproductive tract. At more advanced stages, a woman with ovarian cancer may have vague intestinal problems, a sensation of fullness, and abdominal or pelvic pain or discomfort. (As the cancer progresses, it causes fluid to build up inside the abdomen.) Often a woman's first indication of a problem is noticing that her waistline is expanding for no apparent reason and her clothes don't fit.

Diagnosis Because there is no easy, completely reliable test for ovarian cancer (such as the Pap smear for cervical cancer), most women are not tested for it. Annual pelvic and rectal examinations in which the doctor feels for any abnormalities in the ovaries are the best ways to detect early signs of ovarian cancer in women with no symptoms or known risk factors.

After menopause, women who are at increased risk of ovarian cancer or who are experiencing symptoms may choose to have a yearly CA-125 blood test (see page 129) and, possibly, a vaginal ultrasound (see page 129). However, neither test is completely reliable for detecting the cancer.

CA-125 is a protein found on the surface of cells, including cells in the ovaries. Ovarian cancer can elevate the level of CA-125 in the blood. But the CA-125 test does not always detect ovarian cancer that is present (doctors call this a "false negative" test result), or the CA-125 level may be raised by a condition other than ovarian cancer (a "false positive" test result). CA-125 levels can be elevated because of noncancerous conditions including endometriosis (see page 230), fibroids (see page 221), pelvic infections, pregnancy, and menstruation. Other conditions that may raise CA-125 levels are hepatitis (see page 534) and colon cancer (see page 529). These factors cause positive readings in women who do not have ovarian cancer.

However, the test is useful for following the progress of a woman who has an elevated level of CA-125 and is found to have ovarian cancer. Under these circumstances, the test can determine the cancer's response to a particular treatment or detect a recurrence or progression of the cancer.

Vaginal ultrasound is also limited in its ability to detect ovarian cancer because it provides only a picture of the ovary. If the ultrasound scan does show a tumor, surgery is required to remove the tumor and rule out cancer. Most of the time, tumors in the ovary are found to be noncancerous.

A doctor may use laparoscopy (surgery performed through a small incision in the abdomen; see page 263) to diagnose ovarian cancer and determine the degree to which it has spread. However, it is usually necessary to perform more extensive surgery (called exploratory laparotomy) through a larger abdominal incision to establish the diagnosis and full extent of the cancer.

Some women at very high risk of ovarian cancer, such as those with more than one close relative (mother, daughter, aunt, or sister) with the disease, may choose to have their ovaries removed as a preventive measure. Women who make this choice usually have completed their childbearing and are nearing menopause. After surgery, they can replenish and maintain their supply of estrogen by taking hormone replacement therapy (see page 359).

Treatment About 80 to 85 percent of ovarian cancers start in the epithelial cells, which are cells that cover the surface of the ovaries. Epithelial ovarian cancer is most common in women over 40. Other types of ovarian cancer, including those that originate in the egg or the tissue in which the egg grows inside the ovary, tend to occur in women under 40.

Treatment depends on the type of cancer and how far it has spread. A woman's age, her general state of health, and whether or not she has completed her family are all considerations in the choice of treatment. For example, if a young woman has a tumor in a very early stage that is confined to one ovary, her doctor may remove only that ovary to preserve her ability to have children. However, the doctor may recommend removal of her other ovary and her uterus once she has completed her childbearing.

Surgical treatment for ovarian cancer usually consists of removing the ovaries, uterus, cervix, fallopian tubes, and the omentum (the fatty lining of the abdominal cavity). When your source of estrogen (the ovaries) is removed, you experience immediate menopause (see page 352) and its accompanying symptoms, such as hot flashes. The doctor may perform additional surgery to determine the extent of the cancer's spread beyond the ovaries or, if it has spread, to take out as much of the cancer as possible. In some cases, a portion of the intestine must also be removed.

Chemotherapy (see page 254) is usually given after surgery for ovarian cancers. Radiation therapy (see page 253) is occasionally used in addition to surgery to kill any cancer cells that remain in the pelvic and abdominal areas.

CERVICAL CANCER

Cervical cancer occurs when abnormal cells in the cervix (cervical dysplasia, page 218) become cancerous. The Pap smear (see page 127) is an easy, reliable test that can detect abnormal cells in the cervix at an early stage, before they progress to cancer.

The exact cause of cervical cancer is unknown, but it appears to be related to sexual activity. Women at increased risk of the cancer include those who had first sexual intercourse before 20, have been infected with the human papillomavirus (which causes genital warts; see page 341), or have had more than one sexual partner. Women who have never had sexual intercourse are the least likely to develop cervical cancer. Smoking cigarettes also increases the risk of cervical cancer.

WARNING SIGNS
CERVICAL CANCER

See your doctor if you have any of the following symptoms:

- Vaginal bleeding after intercourse
- Genital warts
- Vaginal bleeding between periods
- Abnormal vaginal discharge
- Pain during intercourse

Symptoms In its early stages, cervical cancer seldom causes symptoms, which is why it is so important to have your annual Pap smear and pelvic examination. In later stages, the cancer can cause vaginal bleeding after intercourse or a bloody vaginal discharge between periods. In very late stages, when the disease has spread, symptoms include painful intercourse, back pain, and weight loss.

Diagnosis Cervical cancer is diagnosed from a Pap smear or a biopsy of a visible abnormality found in a procedure called colposcopy (see page 218). If cancer is found, the doctor then must determine if it has spread. To do so, he or she performs a complete examination of the cervix and surrounding tissues. Blood and urine tests, a chest X-ray, and imaging of the pelvic organs help determine the extent of the cancer. Tests of the bladder, colon, and rectum show whether the cancer has spread to those organs.

In many cases of cervical cancer, the cells spread deep into the cervix and to nearby tissues; in more advanced stages, cells spread to distant organs. The more advanced forms of cervical cancer are most common in women between the ages of 40 and 60. The cancer can spread to the uterus and vagina and to the lymph nodes along the major blood vessels in the pelvis.

Treatment The treatment for cervical cancer depends primarily on the extent of its spread to other tissues. If the cancer has affected only the cervix, a hysterectomy is the usual treatment. Such surgery may include a total hysterectomy (removal of the uterus and cervix) or a radical hysterectomy (removal of the uterus, cervix, upper part of the vagina, and lymph nodes in the area). Surgery is more likely to be successful in removing cancers that are isolated and concentrated in a well-defined area.

If the cancer has spread to the tissues next to the cervix, uterus, or upper part of the vagina, treatment involves radiation therapy—both external and internal—without surgery. Surgery cannot successfully remove all the cancerous tissue once it has spread to tissues next to the cervix or to lymph nodes (tiny organs that lie along lymphatic vessels and blood vessels). From the lymph nodes, cancer cells can enter the lymphatic system and blood circulation and travel to sites throughout the body.

In external radiation therapy, high-powered X-ray beams are directed at the pelvis from the outside. When using internal radiation to treat cervical cancer, the doctor places radioactive materials inside the uterus and at the top of the vagina through a tube inserted through the vagina into the cervix. The material is left in place for about 1½ days, during which time you remain in bed. A screen around you protects other people from the radiation; your contact with other people is restricted during this time. When treatment is completed, the radioactive materials are removed from your body. The treatment may be repeated 2 weeks later.

The side effects of radiation therapy depend on your age, health status, number of radiation treatments, and dose of radiation. You may feel unusually tired during the time of treatment. Other side effects of radiation therapy are caused by irritation to local tissues and may include diarrhea; frequent, painful urination; cystitis (inflammation of the inner lining of the bladder); or scarring of the vagina. These side effects may occur during treatment or months later. Tell your doctor about any symptoms you are experiencing. Although most of the side effects are temporary, some scarring that can narrow the vagina may be permanent; it can sometimes be treated with lubricants or other medications or with devices called dilators, which stretch open the vaginal canal.

Radiation therapy slows hormone production by the ovaries, stops menstruation, and produces other symptoms of menopause (see page 353), such as hot flashes. Taking estrogen (see page 359) during treatment and after reduces these symptoms.

If cervical cancer has spread to the bladder, rectum, or distant parts of the body, or has recurred after surgery or radiation, treatment may include chemotherapy (see page 254) in addition to surgery or radiation.

CANCER OF THE VULVA

Cancer of the vulva (the external genital organs) occurs most often in women over 50, but can occur in younger women as well. The outlook for a woman with cancer of the vulva is usually good when the cancer is detected early and treated. However, some women delay seeking treatment because they are embarrassed about it. They may mistake their symptoms for those of an infection and try over-the-counter medications before talking to their doctor.

Symptoms The most common symptom of cancer of the vulva is itching or irritation in the vaginal area, although you may also find a lump. In more advanced stages of the cancer, these symptoms may be accompanied by open sores or bleeding.

Diagnosis Your doctor will take a sample of tissue from the vulva to be examined under a microscope for the presence of cancer cells. Further investigation will determine if the cancer has spread and, if so, how far. The doctor must determine how deep the cancer goes beneath the skin and whether it has spread to nearby tissues or organs such as the vagina, urethra, or rectum, or to the lymph nodes in the groin. This information is important in planning treatment.

Treatment Sometimes a biopsy does not reveal cancer, but shows changes in the cells that are abnormal and may eventually lead to cancer if not treated. The abnormal tissue can be removed surgically by cutting it out or destroying it with laser surgery.

For cancer of the vulva, the most common and effective treatment is surgical removal of the vulva (vulvectomy) and the lymph nodes in the groin. A simple vulvectomy involves removal of the skin and some underlying fatty tissue. A radical vulvectomy involves removal of all the tissue down to the muscle layer. The urethral opening, the rectum, and most of the vagina are usually preserved.

You can continue to have intercourse after a vulvectomy. Some women continue to experience orgasm while many others find they are no longer able to. The ability to achieve orgasm after a vulvectomy depends on many factors, including the amount of tissue removed from the clitoris (sexually sensitive tissue at the top of the vulva) and the extent of scar formation. Psychological factors, such as how you feel about yourself and your ability to handle the stress of surgery, can also play a role in how the procedure affects your sexuality.

CANCER OF THE VAGINA

Cancer of the vagina is rare, representing only 1 to 2 percent of all reproductive cancers. The risk of the cancer increases with age—it is most common in women over 50. Women who have been diagnosed with cancer of the cervix or vulva are at increased risk of developing cancer of the vagina. The daughters of women who used a medication called diethylstilbestrol (DES) during pregnancy in the 1950s and 1960s are at increased risk of having a rare form of cancer of the vagina called clear cell carcinoma. But even in these women the risk is small. The granddaughters of women who used DES are not at any increased risk of the cancer.

Symptoms The most common symptom of cancer of the vagina is abnormal bleeding or discharge. Any bleeding after menopause is abnormal and should be reported to your doctor immediately. Pain or frequent urination can be symptoms of vaginal cancer but usually occur only in advanced cases.

Diagnosis Cancer of the vagina is often discovered by a doctor during a routine pelvic examination or from a Pap smear. To confirm the diagnosis, the doctor performs a biopsy to analyze a sample of cells in the laboratory.

Treatment The treatment for cancer of the vagina is determined by how far the cancer has spread. Surgery is rarely performed to treat this type of cancer because it is extremely difficult to remove the vagina without harming surrounding organs such as the urethra, bladder, and rectum. Radiation therapy is the most common treatment—doctors usually use a combination of internal and external radiation. (For more about radiation therapy, see page 253.)

External radiation—high-power X-rays directed at the cancerous tissue from the outside—is used first to shrink the tumor. In internal radiation, capsules or needles containing radioactive materials are placed in the vagina next to the tumor.

You may feel unusually tired during the time of treatment. Other side effects of radiation therapy, which result from irritation to the tissue, include drying, itching, burning, and scarring of the vagina. The scarring is permanent and may make sexual intercourse difficult.

CANCER OF THE FALLOPIAN TUBES

Cancer of the fallopian tubes is one of the rarest cancers of the female reproductive tract, accounting for fewer than 1 percent of these cancers. Because the cancer is so rare, little is known about the risk factors except that it occurs more often in older women.

Symptoms The most common symptoms of cancer of the fallopian tube are a watery discharge from the vagina, irregular vaginal bleeding, and pelvic pain. However, many women with the cancer have no symptoms at all and it is discovered only incidentally during surgery for another medical problem in the pelvic area.

Treatment The treatment for fallopian tube cancer usually involves surgical removal of the uterus, ovaries, and fallopian tubes (see page 256). The surgery may also include removal of any neighboring tissues to which the cancer has spread and the omentum (the fatty lining of the abdomen). During the surgery, the doctor will also take tissue samples from the lymph nodes in the area and adjacent organs for microscopic examination to determine if the cancer has spread.

Further treatment will depend on how far the cancer has spread. Chemotherapy (see page 254) and radiation therapy (see below) are sometimes used to treat fallopian tube cancers that have spread to other parts of the body.

GESTATIONAL TROPHOBLASTIC DISEASE

Gestational trophoblastic disease is a pregnancy-related spectrum of conditions ranging from a hydatidiform mole to a type of cancer called choriocarcinoma. Trophoblasts are cells that make up one of the layers of the placenta, the organ that develops in the uterus during pregnancy and links the blood supplies of the mother and fetus.

A hydatidiform mole is an uncommon tumor that forms inside the uterus early in pregnancy, when an embryo has failed to develop normally. The tumor, which is sometimes called a molar pregnancy, resembles a cluster of grapes. The tumor arises from the swelling and abnormal growth of the chorionic villi, tiny fingerlike projections inside the placenta.

In rare cases, the mole (the abnormal mass) develops into a cancerous tumor called a choriocarcinoma. Less frequently, a choriocarcinoma develops from placental cells left behind after an abortion or after a normal or ectopic pregnancy. This cancer can rapidly invade the walls of the uterus and spread through the bloodstream to other organs such as the lungs and brain.

Symptoms Vaginal bleeding and excessive morning sickness early in pregnancy are the most common symptoms of a hydatidiform mole. During a physical examination, a doctor may find the uterus is larger than expected for the stage of pregnancy and may be unable to detect a fetal heartbeat. Urine and blood tests usually show higher-than-normal levels of a hormone called human chorionic gonadotropin (HCG), which is secreted by cells in the placenta.

Treatment The tumor is removed by suctioning out the contents of the uterus during a dilation and curettage (D and C; see page 262). In some cases, a hysterectomy may be recommended if the woman has completed her childbearing. After either procedure, the woman has blood tests for HCG every 1 to 2 weeks until the levels are normal and then at 3-month intervals for 6 to 12 months. This testing ensures that the tumor has been completely eliminated from the uterus.

In the case of choriocarcinoma, chemotherapy (see page 254) is used. Choriocarcinoma responds to chemotherapy better than any other tumor. Chemotherapy almost always cures choriocarcinoma, even when the cancer has spread widely.

There is a 1 in 100 risk that a trophoblastic disease will recur in a future pregnancy. You should wait at least a year after treatment before becoming pregnant again. If you become pregnant, see your doctor right away and make sure he or she is aware that you have had a trophoblastic disease in the past.

CANCER TREATMENTS AND THEIR SIDE EFFECTS

Before undergoing any treatment for cancer, the most important thing you can do is to educate yourself. Ask your doctor questions, learn about all the available treatment options for your cancer, understand how a recommended treatment works, and find out what side effects you can expect. Knowing what to expect and taking an active role in decisions about your treatment can give you more control, help you feel better through this difficult period, and may even improve your recovery.

Cancer is most often treated with surgery, radiation, or chemotherapy, or a combination of these. The goal of all three treatments is to cure the cancer—either by removing it or destroying it. The side effects of each can range from uncomfortable to debilitating.

Surgery Surgery is usually the first treatment recommended to remove a cancerous tumor and any neighboring tissue that may contain cancer cells. The success of the surgery depends on how completely the doctor is able to remove the cancerous tissue.

Radiation Radiation therapy involves the use of high-power X-rays or radioactive materials to kill cancer cells. Radiation kills cells that are dividing rapidly, as cancer cells do. Some normal cells are also destroyed during radiation treatment, but they are eventually replaced by normal cells.

Radiation is also sometimes used before surgery to shrink a tumor or after surgery to destroy any remaining cancer cells. When radiation is targeted at a woman's pelvis to treat a reproductive cancer, she will no longer be able to conceive or bear children. In some cases, to preserve a woman's ovaries for childbearing, a doctor surgically lifts them into the abdomen and out of the direction of the radiation. The ovaries continue to have at least some function and they are safe from direct exposure to radiation. Radiation therapy can be given internally or externally.

External radiation In external therapy, a machine directs a beam of high-power X-rays at the cancerous tissue. You can usually receive this type of radiation therapy 5 days a week for several weeks as an outpatient (a hospital stay is not required).

Internal radiation In internal radiation, radioactive implants are placed inside the body next to the tumor. The implants contain materials that provide a high dose of radiation to the cancerous tissue while sparing the surrounding healthy organs. This type of radiation therapy usually requires a hospital stay.

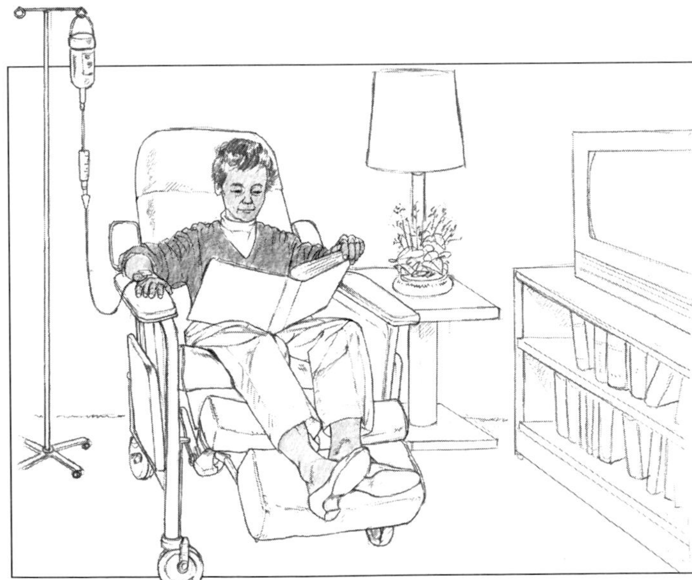

RECEIVING CHEMOTHERAPY

When using internal radiation, the radioactive material is left in place for 1 to 2 days, during which time the woman remains in bed. A screen around the woman protects other people from the radiation; her contact with other people is restricted during this time. When treatment is completed, the radioactive materials are removed from her body.

Side effects The side effects of radiation therapy depend on the part of the body being treated. Side effects can include fatigue, skin reactions, diarrhea, urinary incontinence, and loss of appetite. Radiation therapy may also lower your level of infection-fighting white blood cells, making you more susceptible to infection during this time.

When used to treat reproductive cancers, radiation therapy slows hormone production by the ovaries, stops menstruation, and causes other symptoms of menopause (see page 353). In some cases, ovarian function and menstruation resume later. Whether or not you will be fertile is more difficult to predict. Such effects often depend on your age, general state of health, number of radiation treatments, and dose of radiation you receive.

Chemotherapy Chemotherapy uses potent anticancer drugs to destroy cancer cells that are invading vital organs and cannot be removed surgically, or that have left the tumor and are circulating in the body. This treatment disrupts cancer cells' ability to grow and multiply. Many different drugs are used in chemotherapy. Some drugs are given by mouth; others work better if they are injected into the bloodstream, a muscle, or directly into the abdomen. Several drugs are often given in combination and in cycles.

Unlike surgery and radiation, which eliminate or destroy isolated cancers, chemotherapy acts throughout the body. The treatment affects all rapidly growing cells, including cells that line the digestive tract and hair cells. This is why people undergoing chemotherapy experience nausea and, sometimes, hair loss. In some cases, medications can help reduce nausea.

Chemotherapy may also affect the bone marrow, which produces all the body's blood cells. A reduction in the bone marrow's production of infection-fighting white blood cells compromises the immune system, which can temporarily increase a person's risk of infection.

Various courses of chemotherapy are recommended for different cancers, depending on the type of cancer, the degree of abnormal cell change, and the extent to which the cancer has spread. Your doctor will discuss the treatment options with you.

Hormone therapy Some types of cancer—such as cancer of the breast, endometrium, or ovary—are stimulated by hormones. For this reason, they can be treated with drugs that prevent the hormones from binding to and stimulating the cancer cells to grow. For example, some forms of breast cancer are effectively treated with the estrogen-blocking drug tamoxifen (see page 285).

Like other cancer treatments, hormone therapies can produce side effects, depending on the particular hormone used. Mild nausea, vomiting, fluid retention, or a slight weight gain are potential side effects of hormone therapy. In some cases, the synthetic hormone may interfere with the body's normal production of hormones. For example, by interfering with the production of estrogen, tamoxifen can produce symptoms of menopause, such as hot flashes. Sometimes nonhormonal drugs—such as clonidine (a blood pressure medication) or ergotamine (a mild sedative)—are prescribed to help relieve these symptoms.

COPING WITH CANCER TREATMENT

Taking care of both your physical and emotional needs can significantly improve your ability to cope with the side effects of cancer treatment. Don't hesitate to talk to your doctor about any concerns you have. It is especially important at this time to eat a nutritious diet, stay as active as possible, and get help when you need it.

Eating well Good nutrition is an especially important part of your treatment and recovery because it can significantly boost your immune system and help you withstand the effects of cancer treatments such as surgery, radiation, and chemotherapy.

Having cancer can make it difficult to get the nutrition you need. The side effects of treatment—including nausea, constipation, and a sore mouth—can make eating unenjoyable. Your basic goal is to eat a balanced diet high in fruits, vegetables, and whole grains and low in fat. It is especially important to get enough calories to fulfill your daily needs. Drink lots of liquids to avoid dehydration. If nausea is a problem, tell your doctor. Antinausea medications, taken as tablets or suppositories, are usually very effective. Here are some tips for maintaining a healthy diet while you are undergoing treatment for cancer:

- Ask a friend, relative, or neighbor to help with grocery shopping. Spend your limited energy planning and preparing meals.
- Keep it simple—choose simple menus. Complicated recipes take more time and energy, and exotic foods may not appeal to you if nausea is a problem.
- Make large batches and freeze leftovers in one-meal portions.
- Plan your meals around your treatment. Some people feel better if they eat before their treatment; others do better eating several small meals a day rather than three large ones.
- To help prevent nausea, drink liquids well before mealtime. Drink clear liquids that are free of caffeine and artificial sweeteners. Drinks that contain sugar can help reduce nausea by slowing the digestive process.
- Eat slowly and small amounts at a time, until you are sure the food will stay down. Try plain, carbohydrate-rich foods such as crackers, breads, and cereals; avoid high-fat foods such as butter, peanut butter, cheese, and ice cream.
- If the smell of cooking makes you feel nauseous, always keep cold foods on hand.
- If you are on your own and have no energy to cook, find out if Meals on Wheels is available in your area; keep a drawer full of menus from places that deliver.
- Don't suffer in silence if you are experiencing dry mouth, diarrhea, or other side effects of treatment; ask your doctor to refer you to a registered dietitian.
- Keep an open mind. It's OK to buy prepared meals or foods from the deli or frozen-food sections.
- Most importantly, eat what appeals to you. If you are not feeling well this week, eat "comfort" foods that you enjoy. Balance your diet later.

Dealing with fatigue Cancer itself, as well as the treatments, will take a toll on your energy resources. Here are some strategies for coping with fatigue:

- Set priorities. Make a list of all the things that need to be done. Sort out what you can ask others to do, what you can do by phone, and what can wait. Concentrate on the necessities.
- It's OK to feel tired. Recognize that your fatigue is caused by your illness and not by laziness.
- Make sure family and friends are aware that fatigue is a major problem for you at this time. It will reduce their expectations of you and prompt them to offer help. People like to feel needed. Ask friends who are already planning to stop by to pick up groceries or other items on their way.
- Plan rest periods throughout the day. You may need to rest only once or several times a day. Find out what works best for you. Don't count on one day being the same as the next.
- Plan mild, regular exercise for a time of day when you are likely to stick with it. Exercising may seem like the last thing you want to do when you are tired, but maintaining your muscle strength and cardiovascular fitness can help boost your energy level. Exercise can lift your mood, too.

Getting help Joining a support group of other people with cancer can make you feel less isolated and may even improve your recovery by reducing stress and making you more active in your fight against the disease. Support groups are especially valuable for gathering and sharing information and experiences. Listening to other people who have already gone through some of the things you are experiencing can help you cope better.

Support groups vary widely, depending on their structure and dynamics. Look for a group that is led by a trained professional such as a psychologist, social worker, or cancer nurse. Ask your doctor for a recommendation, check with a local hospital, or call the local branch of the American Cancer Society. If you don't like the first group you join, try another until you find one you feel comfortable with.

Surgical procedures

Disorders of the reproductive system are sometimes most effectively treated with surgery. If your doctor recommends surgery, ask him or her to explain to you why you need the surgery and if there are other treatment options. Learning as much as you can about a recommended surgical procedure can help put your mind at ease. You may want to seek a second opinion.

HYSTERECTOMY

Hysterectomy, removal of the uterus, is the second most common major surgical procedure in the US after cesarean delivery (see page 442). But the number of hysterectomies performed is declining as doctors find that, in many cases, other procedures and medications can treat some gynecologic problems as effectively.

Hysterectomies are performed for a number of reasons. One third are performed to treat fibroids (see page 221), 20 percent to treat abnormal bleeding from the uterus (see page 221), and 20 percent to treat endometriosis (see page 230). Other gynecologic problems treated with hysterectomy include uterine bleeding that does not respond to medication, prolapse of the uterus (see page 234), and cancer.

Hysterectomy may be required when fibroids cause persistent pelvic pain or anemia and severe bleeding that does not respond to treatment. But surgical removal of only the fibroids (leaving the uterus intact)—a procedure called myomectomy (see page 222)—is at times a viable alternative to hysterectomy. Myomectomy is performed most often in women who want to preserve their ability to have children.

Hysterectomies are sometimes done to treat women with endometriosis. But most doctors will remove large areas of endometriosis while doing surgery to diagnose the disorder, often making hysterectomy unnecessary. The woman then takes hormones (see page 231) to prevent the growth of the remaining

Donating your own blood before surgery

If you are faced with surgery that may require a blood transfusion, you may want to donate your own blood in advance. That way, it will be available in case you need a transfusion during or after surgery. Donation of your own blood is called an autologous blood donation.

Although the supply of blood donated from other people has been carefully screened for disease-causing organisms, there is a remote possibility that you might acquire an infection from it. You may also develop an allergic reaction to the donated blood because it is not identical to yours.

The amount of blood you donate depends on your physical condition, the time available before your scheduled surgery, and the amount of blood your doctor anticipates you may need. Usually, no more than 1 or 2 pints are required. You may be given iron supplements during this time to help replenish any iron you lose. Your blood will be drawn from 6 weeks to 3 days before your scheduled surgery and labeled and stored until it is needed.

endometriosis. If treatment with hormones does not reduce this growth, or if the doctor thinks that a particular woman may not be able to tolerate the long-term side effects of a given hormone treatment, hysterectomy may be the only option.

If you are having a hysterectomy, your doctor will recommend removing your ovaries (along with your uterus) if they are damaged or diseased, as they may be if you have had endometriosis, or if you are past menopause. Some doctors recommend removing healthy ovaries during a hysterectomy to prevent ovarian cancer in the future; women over 45 who have completed childbearing or who have a family history of ovarian cancer may choose this option. Removing your ovaries removes your source of estrogen and induces menopause, so your doctor will recommend taking estrogen in hormone replacement therapy (see page 359). Before your hysterectomy, discuss thoroughly with your doctor the advantages and disadvantages of having your ovaries removed. Remember, the final decision is yours.

Like any major surgery, hysterectomy can have complications, including infection and bleeding. Bleeding that cannot be immediately controlled during surgery may require a blood transfusion. Because of this possibility, you may wish to donate your own blood ahead of time in case you need to have a transfusion during surgery (see box at left). Ask your doctor about this option.

Another potential complication of hysterectomy is injury to the intestines, bladder, or ureter (a tube that carries urine from a kidney to the bladder). The surgeon almost always sees such an injury during the operation and repairs it immediately. Although doctors take many precautions, injuries are sometimes extremely difficult to avoid. For example, in cases of severe endometriosis or advanced cancer in the pelvis, the tissues may be so bonded together that they are nearly impossible to separate.

In rare cases, an injury to the bladder, ureter, or intestine is so small that it is not obvious at the time of the operation. Symptoms may not appear until days later. Such symptoms may include a fever and a greater degree of pain in the area of the operation than usual. Usually, your doctor will recommend an X-ray of the painful area to determine the cause.

Possible long-term complications of hysterectomy can in rare instances include the formation of a fistula, an abnormal passage between an injured organ and the vagina or rectum. Secretions then drain through the opening of the fistula. Such secretions vary, depending on the organ that was injured. For example, urine drains from a bladder fistula. A fistula usually has to be repaired in another surgical procedure.

Another complication of hysterectomy can be blood clots that form when circulation slows or the blood thickens. Blood circulation slows down during the first few days after major surgery because people are usually confined to bed. The clots most often develop in veins in the legs or pelvis. A blood clot is life threatening if it breaks away and travels to the lungs, blocking the oxygen supply to the blood and vital organs.

Doctors take precautions after surgery to prevent blood circulation from slowing and causing clots to form. For example, "compression boots" or inflatable thigh leggings are used to pump the leg muscles periodically, which stimulates circulation. Elastic support stockings may also be used to keep blood circulating in the legs. Getting out of bed and moving around as soon as possible after surgery also helps prevent the formation of blood clots.

If you are at high risk of developing a blood clot—for example, you have had one in the past or you have an abnormal or artificial heart valve—you may be given medication before surgery to help thin your blood and prevent it from clotting. Make sure you discuss your medical history thoroughly with your doctor before surgery. Something you might think is unimportant may be vital information for helping to reduce complications.

Having a hysterectomy does not in any way affect your ability to have sexual intercourse. Your sex life may even improve if the surgery relieves a painful condition. You may no longer feel pain or experience bleeding during intercourse or have to worry about becoming pregnant.

However, rare complications of hysterectomy include narrowing of the vagina from scarring, and pain with intercourse.

Hysterectomy

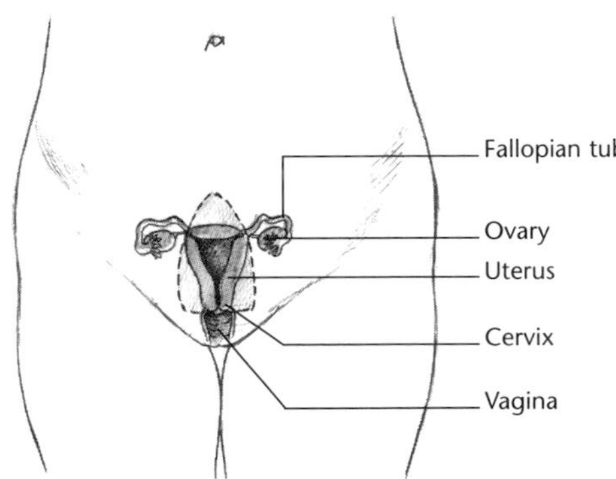

TOTAL HYSTERECTOMY
In a total hysterectomy, the entire uterus, including the cervix, is removed. The fallopian tubes and ovaries are left intact.

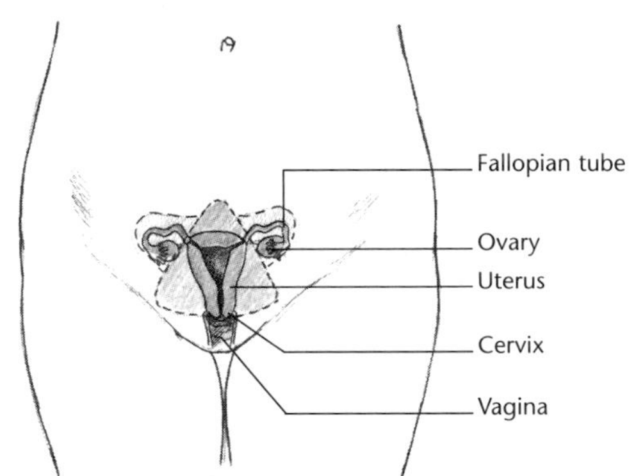

RADICAL HYSTERECTOMY
In a radical hysterectomy, the doctor removes the uterus as well as surrounding tissue, lymph nodes, part of the upper vagina, and, sometimes, the ovaries and fallopian tubes.

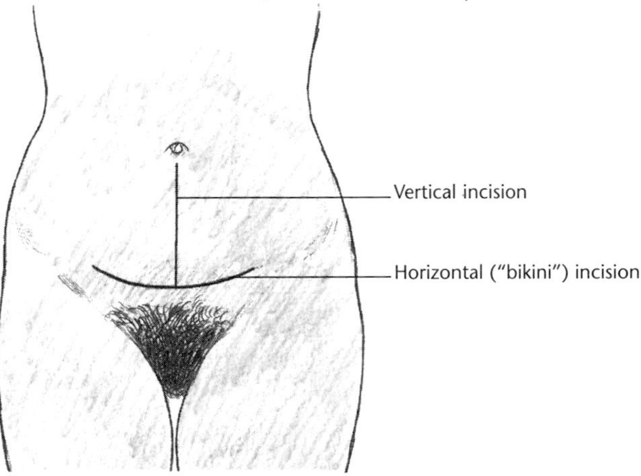

DIFFERENT INCISIONS FOR AN ABDOMINAL HYSTERECTOMY
For an abdominal hysterectomy, the doctor will make either a vertical or a horizontal incision. The scar from a horizontal ("bikini") incision is usually concealed by the pubic hairline.

These complications are more common after a vaginal hysterectomy than after an abdominal hysterectomy. If you are experiencing any of these problems, talk to your doctor. These conditions can often be corrected with medication, vaginal lubricants, or surgery.

Before your surgery, discuss your future sexual activity with your doctor. You and your doctor should decide together on the best treatment for you. Don't be embarrassed about discussing the impact of surgery on your sex life—your doctor needs to know your concerns.

If your doctor recommends hysterectomy, make sure you ask as many questions as you need to about more conservative treatments including hormone therapy (see page 223) and less extensive surgical options such as a myomectomy (see page 222). Always get a second opinion when major surgery is recommended. However, do not delay treatment too long for a serious problem such as cancer.

Vaginal hysterectomy In a vaginal hysterectomy, the uterus is removed through the vagina. The doctor makes an incision at the top of the vagina around the cervix. The uterus is cut free from its supporting ligaments and the connecting blood vessels are tied off. The cervix is cut away from the bladder and the uterus is cut away from the vagina and removed through the vagina. If necessary, the ovaries and fallopian tubes are also removed with the cervix and uterus.

Abdominal hysterectomy If the uterus is enlarged or cancerous, it is usually removed through an abdominal incision. This allows the doctor to determine the extent of the cancer's spread and remove any cancerous tissue. In an abdominal hysterectomy, the doctor makes an incision, either horizontally above the pubic hairline or vertically from the navel to the pubic bone. The uterus is cut free from its supporting ligaments and blood vessels. The cervix is separated from the bladder, and the uterus is cut away from the vaginal wall and removed through the incision in the abdomen. If necessary, the ovaries and fallopian tubes are also removed with the cervix and uterus.

Laparoscopically assisted vaginal hysterectomy (LAVH) In LAVH, the doctor

Recovering from a hysterectomy

A hysterectomy is major surgery, and you will need time to recover. Complete recovery can take several weeks or months. Prepare ahead of time for child care, help with housework, and work arrangements. Here is what you can expect:

- Your hospital stay will be about 3 to 5 days if you have an abdominal hysterectomy. If you have a vaginal hysterectomy, your hospital stay may be shorter and your recovery easier and faster.
- For several days after a hysterectomy, you will feel some pain from the incision. The incision in an abdominal hysterectomy causes more severe pain that lasts longer than that from the small incision you have in laparoscopy. Your doctor will prescribe pain medication to help make the pain manageable.
- For the first day or two after the operation, you will have a tube (urinary catheter) inserted into your bladder to help you urinate. The urine flows into a bag attached to the tube.
- If your ovaries are removed, you lose your source of estrogen and go into immediate menopause. Your doctor will probably recommend that you begin taking estrogen (see page 359) before you leave the hospital. Estrogen can relieve the symptoms of menopause, including hot flashes, and help speed your recovery.
- Expect a recovery period of 3 to 6 weeks at home before you can resume normal activities. During this time, refrain from heavy lifting or other physical exertion or from having sexual intercourse. You will need plenty of rest and should not resume a full-time work schedule until you have recovered completely. Return to your former routine gradually.
- You will have a tendency to tire easily for several weeks after the surgery.
- Don't get depressed if you do not bounce back as quickly as you thought you would. Your recovery may take a little longer if you are an older woman, your surgery was more extensive than usual, or you have cancer, diabetes, a heart condition, or arthritis. If you are concerned about how your recovery is progressing, talk to your doctor.

Preparing for Anesthesia

When you have any kind of surgery, you are given a drug called an anesthetic, which causes loss of sensation to prevent you from feeling any pain. Before your surgery, ask your surgeon and your anesthesiologist, the doctor who will administer the anesthesia, to explain thoroughly the type of anesthesia you will receive. Express any concerns you have. If you have options to choose from, make sure you understand the pros and cons of each, and ask why your doctors are recommending one method over another. The final choice of anesthesia should be made by you and your doctor together.

Local anesthesia

Local anesthesia numbs only the area that is being treated and the surrounding area.

- Local anesthesia is used for more minor procedures such as dilation and curettage (D and C; see page 262) or tooth extractions.
- Local anesthesia can be injected directly into the area to be treated. For accessible areas such as the skin, eyes, or throat, it can be applied as a spray or ointment.
- Sedatives are often used with local anesthesia to help you relax, and to blur uncomfortable sensations of touch, pulling, or pressure.

Patient-controlled analgesia

Patient-controlled analgesia is a technique in which patients themselves administer medications called narcotics, according to their need for pain relief. You receive the medication by controlling a pump attached to an intravenous line, which has been inserted into a vein to deliver fluids to prevent you from becoming dehydrated. A small but constant amount of the narcotic flows into the intravenous solution. If you are not getting enough pain relief, you can push a small button that allows the pump to increase the dose of medication. You cannot get too much of the narcotic because the maximum amount you receive in a set period is regulated.

Regional anesthesia

Regional anesthesia numbs a larger area of your body than local anesthesia but you remain conscious (unlike with general anesthesia).

- Regional anesthesia is used for moderately complicated procedures, such as a cesarean delivery (see page 442).
- A regional anesthetic can cause numbness from the waist down for surgery that is done in your abdominal or pelvic area or legs.
- The anesthesiologist injects the medication directly into your spinal column—either in one injection (called a spinal) or in a continuous injection during surgery (called an epidural). You may also receive a sedative to help you relax.

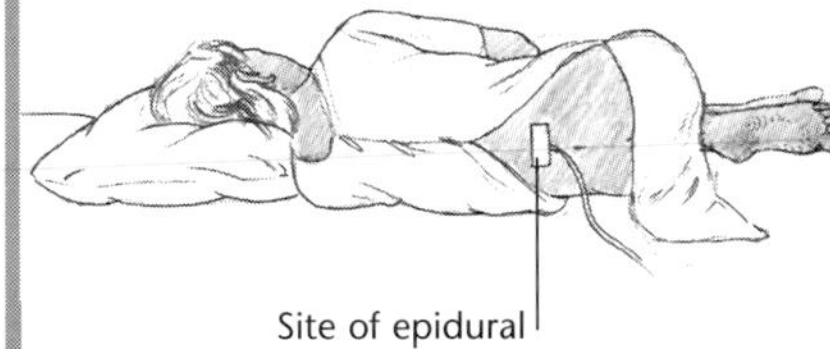

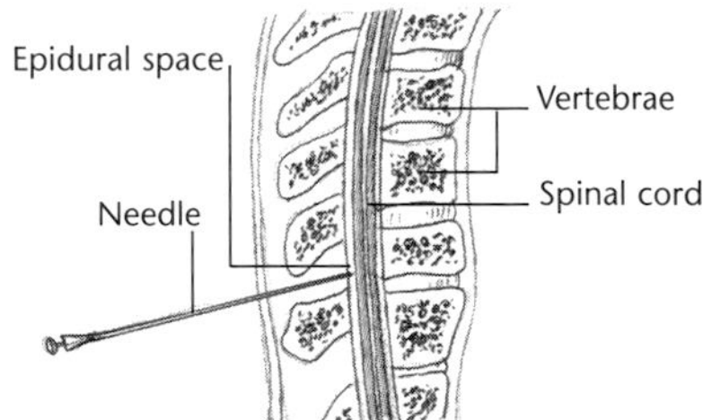

EPIDURAL ANESTHESIA
An epidural causes numbness from the waist down, but you remain fully conscious. It is often used to relieve pain during labor and delivery. For an epidural, you lie on your side (top) or sit up straight while the doctor injects the anesthetic between your vertebrae into a narrow space that surrounds the spinal cord (bottom).

General anesthesia

More extensive operations require general anesthesia, which induces loss of sensation and consciousness.

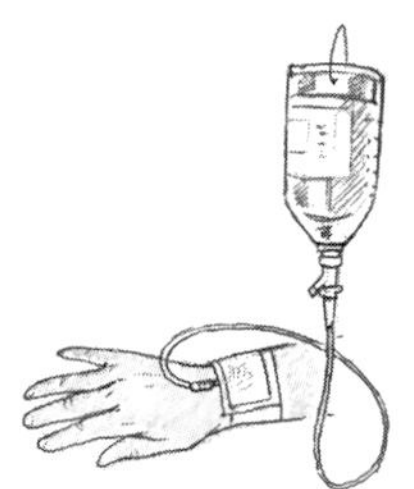

INDUCING UNCONSCIOUSNESS
After an intravenous line is inserted into a vein in your hand or arm, a medication is injected through it to help you relax. The anesthesiologist then injects a sedative through the tubing to induce unconsciousness. The tubing is left in place during the operation so that additional anesthetics or other drugs can be administered if necessary.

MONITORING VITAL SIGNS
Once you are unconscious, a tube is inserted through your mouth into your lungs and connected to a mechanical ventilator. The ventilator carefully regulates the amount of oxygen delivered to your lungs during the entire operation. You are also attached to monitors that continuously check your heart rate, breathing, blood pressure, and temperature. You remain unconscious throughout the procedure.

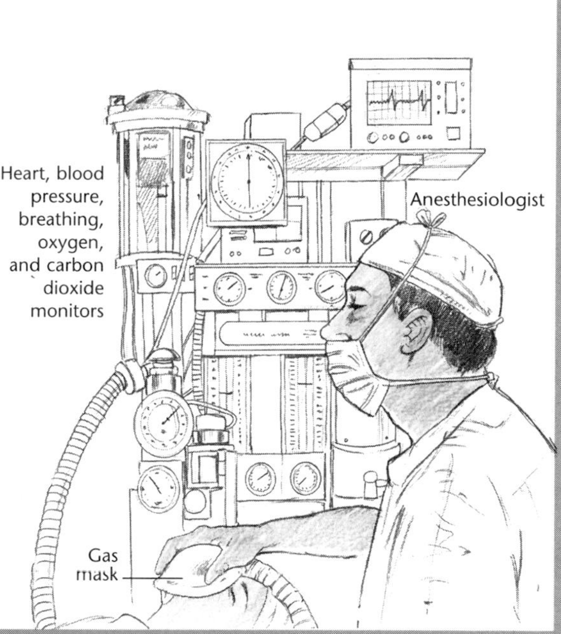

After anesthesia

Side effects are most common after general anesthesia, but can sometimes also occur after regional anesthesia. Ask your doctor the following questions:

■ **How will I feel for the first few hours after my surgery?** If you have general anesthesia, you will probably be groggy. You may also feel sleepy, dizzy, forgetful, and unable to concentrate. If you are in pain, medication is available to control it.

■ **Will the anesthesia make me feel nauseous?** Some people feel nauseous when they wake up after surgery, but new anesthetic drugs cause far less nausea and vomiting than earlier ones did. Often the expectation of nausea causes people to become queasy. Ask your doctor for medication if you feel nauseous.

■ **Can I drive myself home afterward?** Even if you feel completely normal, you should not drive for at least 1 day after having general or regional anesthesia; the drugs may affect your reflexes and coordination. If you will be leaving the hospital the same day as the procedure, arrange beforehand to have someone drive you home, or take a taxi.

■ **Can I eat or drink afterward?** This depends on the type of anesthesia you had and how long your operation took. If you had inpatient abdominal surgery performed through a large incision, you can have liquids after a few hours and gradually progress to solid food over the next few days. Before you can eat solids, your doctor will determine if your bowels are working properly. If you have had outpatient surgery, your doctor will give you instructions about what you can eat or drink as you recover at home.

■ **Does anesthesia have any long-term effects?** The aftereffects of anesthesia rarely last longer than 3 days. Some people who lose a great deal of blood during surgery feel exhausted for up to a month; this is usually caused by anemia from blood loss (see page 493), not from the anesthetic. If you have anemia, your doctor may recommend iron supplements to build up your red blood cell count.

inserts a laparoscope (a lighted viewing instrument) through a small (1/4- to 3/4-inch) incision in the abdomen, just below the navel. Using surgical instruments inserted through one or more other small incisions in the abdomen, the doctor cuts away the uterus from its supporting ligaments and blood vessels. The cervix is cut away from the bladder, and the uterus is cut away from the vaginal wall and removed through an incision in the vagina. The ovaries and fallopian tubes can also be removed during this procedure by cutting their attachments to the side wall of the pelvis and taking them out with the uterus.

Oophorectomy Sometimes the ovaries are also removed during a hysterectomy; removal of the ovaries is called an oophorectomy. Any hysterectomy results in the end of childbearing and menstruation. But the removal of the ovaries (the source of the hormone estrogen) also produces menopause in a woman who has not yet gone through menopause naturally. The symptoms of menopause, caused by the lack of estrogen, can be relieved by taking estrogen in hormone replacement therapy (see page 359).

Oophorectomy is performed without a hysterectomy in some cases of endometriosis (see page 230), or if a woman has a large, noncancerous (benign) tumor or cyst on an ovary (see page 224). If the benign tumor or cyst on the ovary is small, only it will be removed, leaving the ovary intact; this is called a partial oophorectomy or an ovarian cystectomy. When only one ovary is removed, and the other ovary is still functioning and producing eggs, a woman is still able to get pregnant.

Salpingectomy In a salpingectomy, one or both fallopian tubes are removed. A salpingectomy is usually performed to treat a pregnancy that develops in a fallopian tube (an ectopic pregnancy, see page 233) or a pelvic infection that has damaged the fallopian tube. The fallopian tube is usually removed when the adjacent ovary is removed because the tube is often damaged by the same condition that affects the ovary.

DILATION AND CURETTAGE

Dilation and curettage (D and C) is a procedure in which the endometrium (lining of the uterus) is scraped away. D and C has been used for many years to diagnose and treat a variety of disorders that affect the uterus, such as excessive bleeding during menstrual periods. Today, endometrial biopsy (see page 129) is frequently done instead of a D and C for diagnosing uterine disorders. D and C is now mostly performed after a woman has had a miscarriage or for abortions early in a pregnancy.

D and C is usually performed using local anesthesia (see page 260) to numb the cervix. You may also be given a sedative intravenously to relax you. In a D and C, the doctor first inserts a speculum into your vagina to open it. Next, using a series of progressively larger rods (inserted through the vagina into the cervix), the cervix is gradually opened (dilated). The doctor then inserts a tiny, spoon-shaped instrument called a curet into the uterus and uses it to scrape all the walls of the uterus to remove the endometrium. The scrapings are examined under a microscope to check for abnormalities such as endometrial hyperplasia (see page 221) or endometrial cancer (see page 239).

Most women experience some bleeding following a D and C or have cramps that resemble menstrual cramps for a couple of days. Complications from a D and C, which are rare, include infection, perforation of the uterus, and excessive bleeding.

If the doctor needs only a small sample of tissue to make a diagnosis, he or she can perform a procedure called endometrial biopsy right in the office. In this procedure, the doctor inserts a tiny suction device through the cervix to obtain a small portion of the endometrium for examination under a microscope.

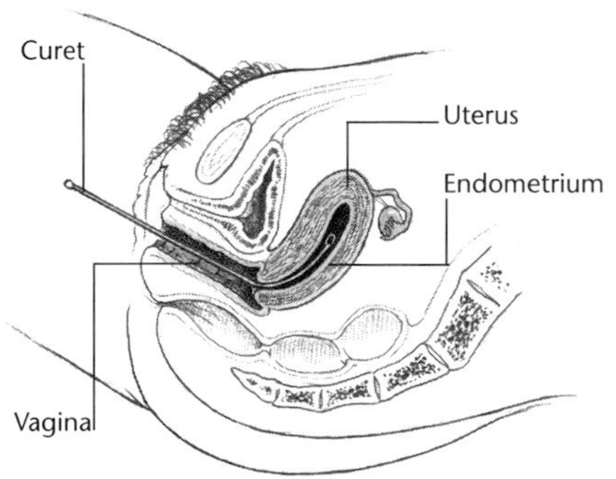

DILATION AND CURETTAGE
Dilation and curettage (D and C) is a common gynecologic procedure, performed using local anesthesia, in which the lining of the uterus (endometrium) is scraped out with a spoon-shaped instrument called a curet. D and C is used to treat a variety of disorders of the uterus, including excessive menstrual bleeding.

LAPAROSCOPY AND LAPAROTOMY

Laparoscopy and laparotomy are surgical procedures used for diagnosing and treating a variety of symptoms and disorders in the pelvic area. Laparoscopy is performed more often than laparotomy because it is a less extensive procedure. Laparoscopy requires only one to four small (½- to ¾-inch) incisions in the abdomen, while laparotomy requires a large abdominal incision. Both procedures are used to treat a variety of disorders in the pelvis or abdomen, including fibroids (see page 221), ovarian cysts (see page 224), endometriosis (see page 230), and pelvic inflammatory disease (PID; see page 232).

Laparoscopy Laparoscopy is performed in the hospital and requires general anesthesia (see page 261). However, the procedure usually does not require an overnight stay in the hospital unless it is very complicated or lengthy.

For the procedure, the doctor first inserts a hollow needle into the abdomen, usually just below the navel, to pump in a harmless gas. The gas expands the abdominal cavity and pushes the intestines back from the area to be treated. The doctor inserts a lighted viewing instrument (laparoscope) through the incision to examine the inside of the abdomen and pelvis and the reproductive organs. The doctor views an image of the organs on a nearby video screen. One to three additional small (⅛- to ¼-inch) incisions may be made in the abdomen for inserting surgical instruments.

Recovery from laparoscopy varies, depending on the extent of the surgery. You can go back to your usual routine, including your job, as soon as you feel up to it. The gas pumped into your abdomen may cause discomfort for a day or two. You will probably be able to resume exercise within 3 to 4 days. Your doctor

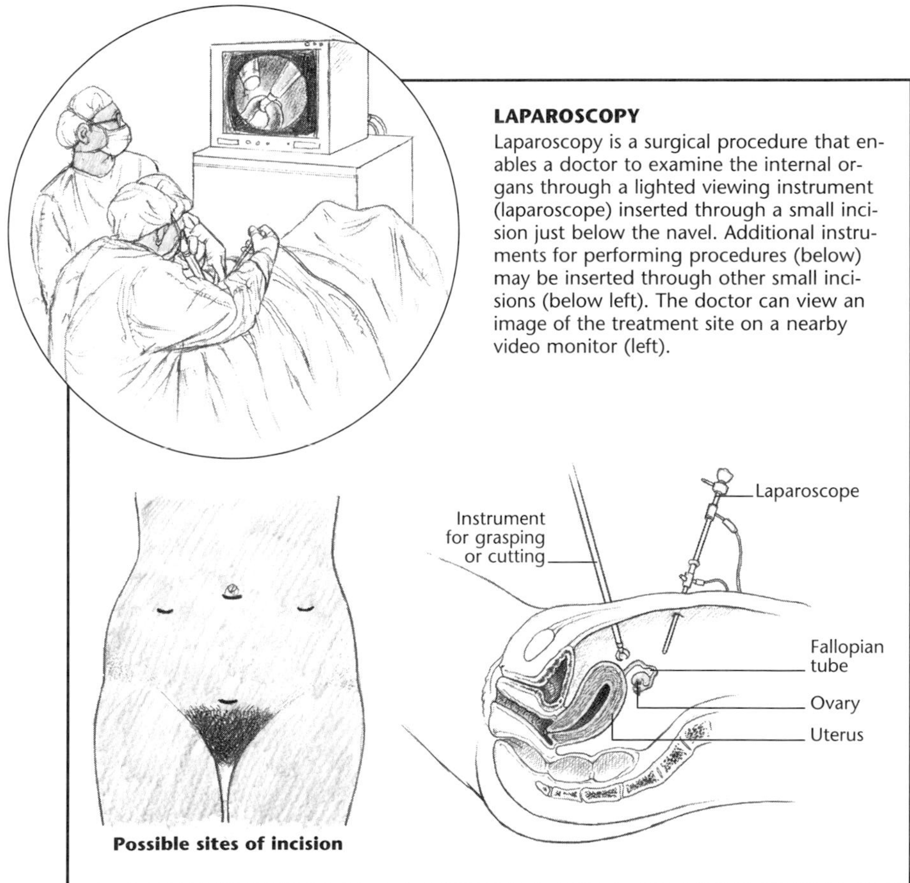

LAPAROSCOPY

Laparoscopy is a surgical procedure that enables a doctor to examine the internal organs through a lighted viewing instrument (laparoscope) inserted through a small incision just below the navel. Additional instruments for performing procedures (below) may be inserted through other small incisions (below left). The doctor can view an image of the treatment site on a nearby video monitor (left).

will discuss with you when you can resume sexual intercourse.

Laparotomy Laparotomy is a general term that refers to a variety of surgical procedures that involve opening the abdomen to diagnose or treat disorders. Laparotomy requires general anesthesia and a hospital stay. The doctor makes a horizontal or vertical incision in the abdomen and looks for signs of disease. A laparotomy is usually performed to remove part or all of a diseased organ, take a tissue sample for laboratory testing, or perform any necessary repairs.

Because laparotomy requires a much larger incision than laparoscopy, it is used less frequently. But some procedures are performed more easily and completely with laparotomy. For example, if there is a large amount of abnormal tissue to be removed, or if the work that needs to be done is in a difficult-to-reach location, laparotomy is more effective. Laparotomy is also more effective when a doctor needs to explore a large area of the abdominal cavity to investigate the cause of symptoms that other tests have failed to uncover. If you have extensive scar tissue in the abdominal area that can interfere with the insertion of surgical instruments in laparoscopy, your doctor may recommend laparotomy.

The recovery period after laparotomy varies widely depending on the disorder, the treatment, and the extent of the surgery. You may feel sore in the abdominal area (including the incision) and experience some fatigue. You should refrain from exercising strenuously, lifting heavy objects, or having sexual intercourse for 6 weeks after the operation.

HYSTEROSCOPY

For some symptoms or conditions, such as abnormal uterine bleeding (see page 221) or fibroids (see page 221), your doctor needs to look inside your uterus to make an evaluation. A procedure called hysteroscopy allows the doctor to directly view the interior of the uterus and perform some procedures there. A hysteroscopy is performed either in an operating room or in the doctor's office. Some type of anesthesia (see page 260) or sedation is usually required, depending on the extent of the procedures to be performed.

In a hysteroscopy, the doctor inserts a lighted, tubular viewing instrument (a hysteroscope) through the vagina and cervix into the uterus. The cervix is opened (dilated) slightly by introducing progressively larger rods through the vagina into the cervix to allow insertion of the hysteroscope. A liquid or gas is injected through the hysteroscope to expand the cavity of the uterus and allow a clear view of the inside. Instruments can then be passed through the hysteroscope to perform procedures.

Doctors use hysteroscopy to inspect the endometrium (the lining of the uterus); to perform biopsies (take tissue samples for laboratory testing); and to remove fibroids, adhesions (abnormal scar tissue), or polyps (tiny, usually noncancerous growths) from inside the uterus. Hysteroscopy can uncover the cause of some cases of infertility by enabling doctors to see blockages at the openings of the fallopian tubes into the uterus. Doctors can also use hysteroscopy to retrieve a lost intrauterine device (see page 324).

In women who have severe, persistent uterine bleeding that has not responded to treatment and who cannot undergo a hysterectomy because of a life-threatening medical condition such as severe heart disease, hysteroscopy can be used to perform a procedure called an endometrial ablation. In endometrial ablation, a laser is introduced through the hysteroscope into the uterus to burn off the endometrium, thereby eliminating the bleeding tissue.

Complications from hysteroscopy are not common but can include injury to the uterus, bleeding, or infection. Recovery can vary depending on the extent of the procedures performed. Doctors usually recommend refraining from exercise for 3 to 4 days and sexual intercourse for 1 to 2 weeks after a hysteroscopy.

CHAPTER 9

Your breasts

Contents

The primary biological function of the breasts is to produce milk to feed an infant. Within a day or two following childbirth, the milk ducts inside the breasts begin to produce milk to nourish the infant. Breast milk can be a baby's sole nourishment for the first 6 months of life.

The breasts also play a significant role in a woman's sexuality. Although breast sensitivity and sexual response vary greatly, most women's breasts respond to sexual stimulation by undergoing a number of physiologic changes.

The size and shape of a woman's breasts are determined mainly by her genes. Many women have breasts about the same size and shape as their mother's, or the same size as the women on their father's side of the family.

The healthy breast

The size and shape of adult women's breasts vary widely but the average breast weighs about 1/2 pound and is 4 to 5 inches in diameter. Most of the breast tissue is fat, especially the middle and lower parts, layered around milk glands and ducts and supporting fibers. Because most of the breast is composed of fat, body weight plays a role in the shape and size of your breasts.

At the center of the breast is the nipple. The nipple contains 15 to 20 tiny holes. Some of the holes are the openings of milk ducts and others are the openings of sebaceous (oil) glands. These glands produce a small amount of a white, oily substance that lubricates and protects the skin.

Surrounding the nipple is a dark area called the areola. Its size, shape, and color vary greatly from one woman to the next. The nipple and areola are covered by a membrane that is lubricated by slightly raised glands in the areola. Tiny muscles beneath the areola allow the nipple to become erect when stimulated.

Each breast contains a system of milk glands and ducts that radiate from the nipple like the spokes of a wheel. During pregnancy, a web of tiny glands called lobules begins to secrete milk into ducts that act as holding reservoirs until an infant needs the milk. The glands are divided into compartments; each compartment of glands and duct tissue is called a lobe. Between the lobes are fat and connective tissue, including ligaments that support the breasts and attach them to the chest wall.

Lymph nodes drain lymph fluids from the breast to five major areas—the armpit; the area just above the collarbone; the area under the sternum (the bone in the center of your chest); across to the opposite breast; and through passages that lead to the lymph nodes in the upper abdomen. The lymph nodes that make up the lymphatic system play an important part in the body's ability to fight infection. The lymph nodes filter out bacteria and other disease-causing organisms, and abnormal cells including cancer cells.

The breasts contain very little muscle. Their size depends not on the muscles in them or the muscles behind them but on the amount of fat they contain. That's why when you lose weight your breasts get smaller and when you gain weight, your breasts get larger. It is also why you cannot increase the size of your breasts with exercise. Nor can exercise prevent them from sagging with age. Short of surgery or a major change in weight, there is little you can do to change the size of your breasts.

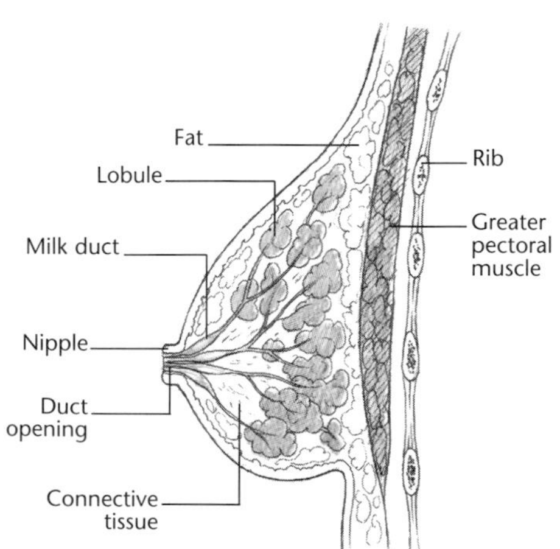

HEALTHY BREAST
Milk ducts radiate out from the nipple, leading to clusters of milk glands called lobules. After childbirth, the lobules secrete milk into the ducts. Fat and connective tissues fill the areas around the ducts and lobules. Beneath the breast is a layer of muscle covering the rib cage.

BREAST DEVELOPMENT

Girls are born with tiny breasts that consist of a nipple and an undeveloped system of ducts that empty into the nipple. At puberty, between ages 8 and 15, a girl's ovaries begin to secrete estrogen, stimulating the first changes in her breasts. The nipples begin to grow and darken, and may protrude slightly. They may itch or feel somewhat tender or painful.

The duct system begins to grow, and branches begin to form. Sometimes it feels as though a lump is forming under the nipple, which may alarm a girl or her parents. Your doctor will reassure you that this is a normal part of development. This kind of lump in breast tissue during puberty should never be surgically removed because doing so can prevent the breast from developing normally.

By the time a girl has her first period (see page 201), her breast development is well underway. The female hormone progesterone, produced by the ovaries, causes the ends of the branches of glands in the breasts to bud, forming groups of glands. The rate of breast development varies widely among girls, sometimes causing anxiety for those girls whose breasts develop earlier or later than average. But this is just the normal variation among people.

Another source of anxiety for girls is having one breast that is slightly larger than the other. This, too, is normal. Growth may begin earlier or advance more quickly in one breast than in the other. This asymmetry is not a cause for alarm—the other breast will catch up eventually. Even fully developed breasts are not always identical. In rare cases, a woman's breasts may be so asymmetrical that she may consider surgery to make them the same size. Depending on the situation, the surgery would either enlarge the smaller breast (see page 698) or reduce the size of the larger breast (see page 702).

Some women have an inverted nipple, which points in rather than out. A nipple that has been inverted since birth is normal for that woman and not a cause for concern. However, if your nipple suddenly becomes inverted, see your doctor immediately; it may be a sign of a tumor in your breast.

CHANGES DURING THE MENSTRUAL CYCLE

During your reproductive years, your breasts may go through normal changes that correspond to the phases of your menstrual cycle (see page 204). In the first part of the cycle, the breasts are usually soft and not especially tender. At midpoint in the cycle (about day 14), around the time of ovulation (release of an egg from an ovary), the breasts may begin to enlarge and feel fuller. In the last days of the cycle, before menstruation, some women feel discomfort because their breasts are swollen and sensitive to touch and motion. Once menstruation starts, the breasts usually return to feeling soft and less sensitive again.

Examining your breasts

Every woman needs to do a monthly self-examination of her breasts. The best time to do a breast self-examination is a few days after your period ends, when your breasts are most soft. (For illustrated instructions, see page 276.) You should also have an annual breast examination by your doctor. If you are over 40, you should have a mammogram (see page 127) as often as your doctor recommends; after 50, you should have a mammogram every year.

CHANGES DURING PREGNANCY AND BREAST-FEEDING

During pregnancy and breast-feeding, the breasts undergo many changes that enable them to produce milk to nourish an infant. Outwardly, the breasts grow larger, the veins become more prominent, and the pigmented areas around each nipple (areolas) grow larger and darker; some women may also develop stretch marks, which usually fade somewhat with time. Inwardly, the changes are far more complex. Milk-producing cells increase in number and the milk ducts develop further. Glands inside the breast enlarge and secrete an oily substance that softens and lubricates the skin of the nipple and areola, to protect it during breast-feeding. After a woman has weaned her child from breast-feeding, her breasts may be larger or smaller than before her pregnancy, and they may have less elasticity. (For more about breast-feeding, see page 452.)

THE BREASTS AFTER MENOPAUSE

When a woman reaches menopause, generally in her early 50s, the ovaries stop producing the hormones estrogen and progesterone. Firm breast tissue shrinks and the proportion of fat tissue increases, causing the breasts to sag. It is normal for breasts to sag with age. Taking estrogen in hormone replacement therapy (see page 359), however, may help slow this natural process.

Many older women find that their breasts are easier to examine by hand for lumps or other changes because they are softer. These changes are easier to detect because breast tissue is less dense in older women.

Noncancerous conditions of the breast

Like every other part of your body, your breasts are subject to various types of treatable problems. Not every lump or change in the breast means that you have cancer. In fact, the vast majority of breast conditions are noncancerous. But you should report any change that you notice to your doctor.

BREAST PAIN OR DISCOMFORT

Breasts are sensitive to touch, heat, and cold. Breast sensitivity often changes during the menstrual cycle. Your breasts may become noticeably painful about midway through your menstrual cycle and increasingly tender until your period. Your breasts may even become swollen or lumpy.

No single treatment for premenstrual breast pain is effective for all women. Many doctors recommend first trying to eliminate or decrease your consumption of caffeine (see page 65). For reasons that are not clear, reducing caffeine intake decreases breast discomfort in some women. Other doctors may recommend reducing salt intake or prescribe diuretics to relieve water retention. Water retention in the breasts can cause the same feeling of heaviness and bloating that it does anywhere else in the body. A doctor may also prescribe birth-control pills (see page 310), which relieve breast discomfort that results from the fluctuation in hormone levels during the menstrual cycle.

NIPPLE DISCHARGE

Many women, especially those who have been pregnant, may have a small amount of discharge from their nipples when they squeeze their nipples or breasts. Although nipple discharge is usually no cause for alarm, you should always report it to your doctor without delay. He or she can examine the discharge—which may be milky or watery or contain pus or blood—and determine its cause.

Some drugs—such as birth-control pills and some high blood pressure medications or tranquilizers—may increase nipple discharge because they increase the level of prolactin. Prolactin is a hormone, produced in the pituitary gland in the brain, that stimulates milk production normally during breast-feeding. Such milky discharge usually occurs in both breasts and is usually no cause for concern.

The level of prolactin may also be raised by a small, noncancerous hormone-producing tumor in the pituitary gland called a prolactinoma (see page 628). If your doctor determines that you have a prolactinoma, he or she is likely to recommend treatment with a medication called bromocriptine, which blocks the production of prolactin by the pituitary gland. This treatment can decrease the size of the tumor, thereby lowering the level of prolactin in your blood and stopping the production of breast milk. A large tumor may have to be removed surgically.

If the discharge appears without squeezing your nipple, if it persists, or if it comes from only one nipple, it requires immediate medical attention.

Bloody discharge, which usually occurs in only one breast, can be a warning sign of several conditions, including cancer, and should be reported to your doctor and investigated immediately. Although you should be concerned about the possibilities of cancer, in most cases bloody discharge from a nipple is caused by a noncancerous disorder such as an intraductal papilloma (see page 272).

BREAST INFECTIONS

Mastitis is the most common breast infection and occurs most often in women who are breast-feeding. Mastitis occurs when a milk duct gets blocked with milk and creates a closed area in which bacteria can accumulate. The bacteria, which usually come from the nursing infant's mouth, get trapped in this area, causing an infection.

The symptoms of mastitis include a skin infection that is red, swollen, and painful and hot to the touch. Mastitis usually causes a high fever and headache. Breast-feeding should continue unless pus begins to drain from an abscess.

Mastitis is most often treated with antibiotics taken by mouth. For severe infections, or when an abscess (a pus-filled pocket within a tissue) develops, hospitalization may be necessary. In the hospital, antibiotics are given intravenously to deliver the medication directly to the infected tissue.

In rare cases, women who are not breast-feeding develop mastitis. Women most at risk include those who have had breast surgery in which infection-fighting lymph nodes were removed or who have a suppressed immune system due to such conditions as diabetes, AIDS, or chemotherapy for cancer.

Boils—inflamed, pus-filled areas of skin that are usually caused by staphylococcal bacteria—can form on the breast just as they can on other parts of the body. Boils most often occur in people who are vulnerable to infection, such as those with diabetes. It is important to see a doctor to make sure the boil is not a symptom of another, more serious condition. Skin boils are usually treated by applying heat to the boil and by taking antibiotics.

A breast abscess is a collection of pus that may result from mastitis that is not treated or is treated inadequately. An abscess is an infection of the sebaceous glands, which produce a protective lubricant that comes out of tiny openings in the nipple. Infection results when bacteria get inside the glands and multiply, causing the tissue to swell from inflammation and eventually blocking the openings. Sometimes the blocked glands form an abscess that appears as a hot, red, sore area on the border of the areola. A breast abscess is not related to breast cancer.

A breast abscess needs to be treated surgically. A small incision is made around the areola, usually with the aid of a local anesthetic, and the abscess is drained. Antibiotics are also prescribed to fight the infection after surgery. Mastectomy (surgical removal of the breast) is not warranted as a treatment for this condition, except in severe, life-threatening conditions.

FIBROCYSTIC BREASTS

Many women have healthy breasts that are lumpy. In the past, women with lumpy breasts were sometimes diagnosed with "fibrocystic disease." However, doctors now know that lumpy (or fibrous) breasts, with or without other symptoms, do not indicate a disease. Rather, having lumpy breasts—which is very common—is now called "fibrocystic condition" or simply "fibrocystic breasts."

Although fibrocystic breasts are not a medical problem, they can make it more

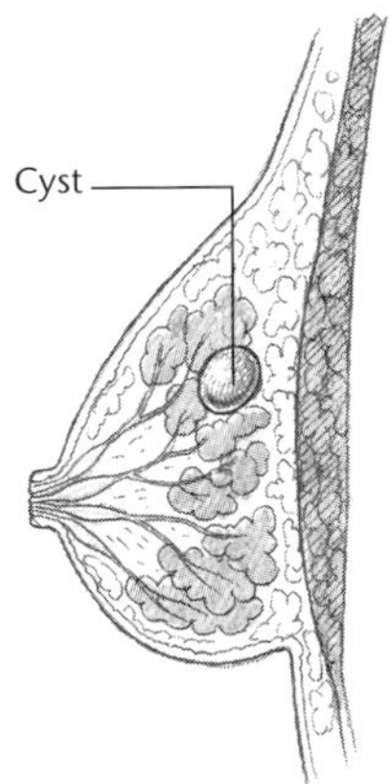

BREAST CYST
A cyst is a fluid-filled sac that may develop in the breast for unknown reasons. Cysts are not harmful. A cyst sometimes disappears by itself; if it does not, a doctor can withdraw the fluid with a needle.

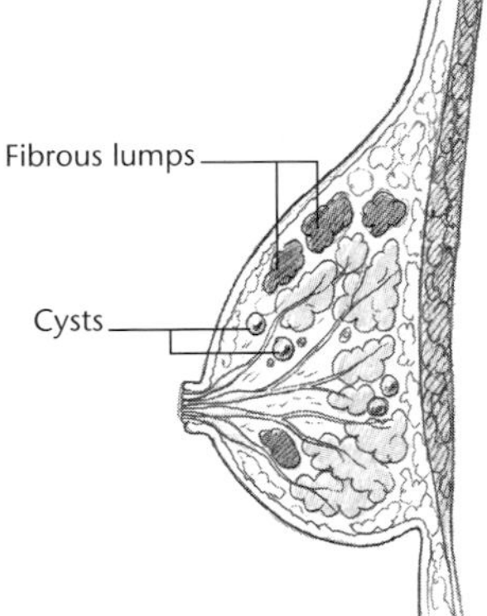

FIBROCYSTIC BREAST
A fibrocystic breast contains small, nodular lumps and cysts.

difficult to notice new cysts or to find cancerous lumps. Therefore, it is especially important for women with lumpy breasts to perform monthly breast self-examinations (see page 276). If you have lumpy breasts, you should become familiar with the shape and location of all the lumps so you can detect any changes. The lumps may become larger and sometimes feel tender just before your period; for this reason, it is best to do a breast self-examination about a week after your period begins, when the swelling has subsided. Limiting your intake of caffeine-containing foods and beverages can reduce the tenderness associated with fibrocystic breasts.

Some women with fibrocystic breasts develop cysts (noncancerous fluid-filled sacs) that can appear very suddenly. Although their cause is unknown, these cysts are not difficult to treat and are not harmful. Any woman can develop cysts, but they are more common in women who have fibrocystic breasts.

Breast cysts are treated with a procedure called needle aspiration, in which the doctor inserts a needle into the cyst and draws out the fluid. The procedure is usually performed in the doctor's office without anesthesia and is no more painful than having blood drawn. All major lumps that are detected in a woman's breast are usually aspirated in this way, especially if they feel like cysts. If the lump is a cyst, it will shrink when the fluid is withdrawn from it. Lumps that do not produce fluid when they are aspirated are tested further. These lumps may be solid tumors that could be cancerous. To make a diagnosis, a small sample of tissue (biopsy) must be removed from the lump and sent to the laboratory for testing.

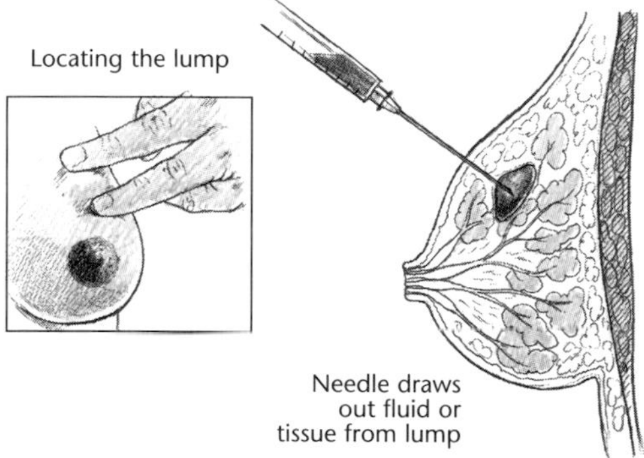

NEEDLE ASPIRATION OR BIOPSY
Fluid from a cyst is usually aspirated, or drawn out, with a needle. The doctor stabilizes the area of the lump between his or her fingers (far left), inserts the needle, and withdraws the fluid (left). If no fluid comes out, further tests may be needed to determine the nature of the lump, including whether or not it is cancerous. If the lump is solid, a needle biopsy is performed. In a needle biopsy, the doctor may use a slightly larger needle to withdraw a sample of tissue.

FIBROADENOMA

A fibroadenoma is a solid lump that does not contain fluid. It is a firm, rubbery lump that moves around easily when you feel it. A fibroadenoma can range from the size of a pea to that of a lemon. Usually the size and sensitivity of the lump do not change significantly during the menstrual cycle. Fibroadenomas cause no nipple discharge and no pain. Most women who get a fibroadenoma never develop another. Some women develop several. A fibroadenoma is likely to start developing during the teenage years and sometimes grows larger during pregnancy or breast-feeding.

Having a fibroadenoma does not increase a woman's risk of breast cancer. However, a doctor may recommend

FIBROADENOMA
A fibroadenoma is a firm lump that moves around easily. It is harmless and seldom causes pain. A fibroadenoma is often removed surgically to make sure it is not cancerous. Having a fibroadenoma does not increase your risk of breast cancer.

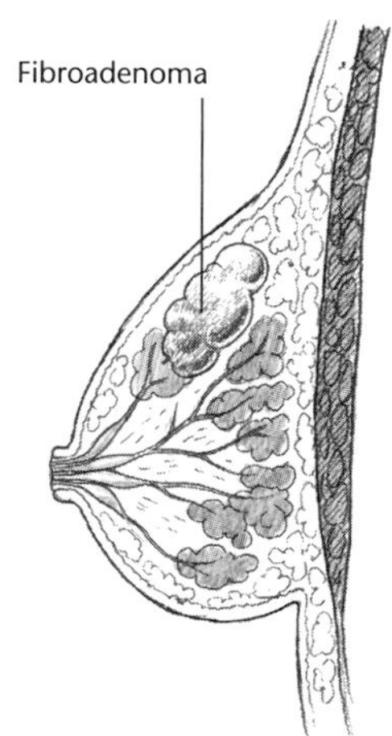

SYMPTOM CHART

Pain or lumps in your breast

Aching, pain, tenderness, or lumps in one or both breasts that you notice when you examine your breasts.

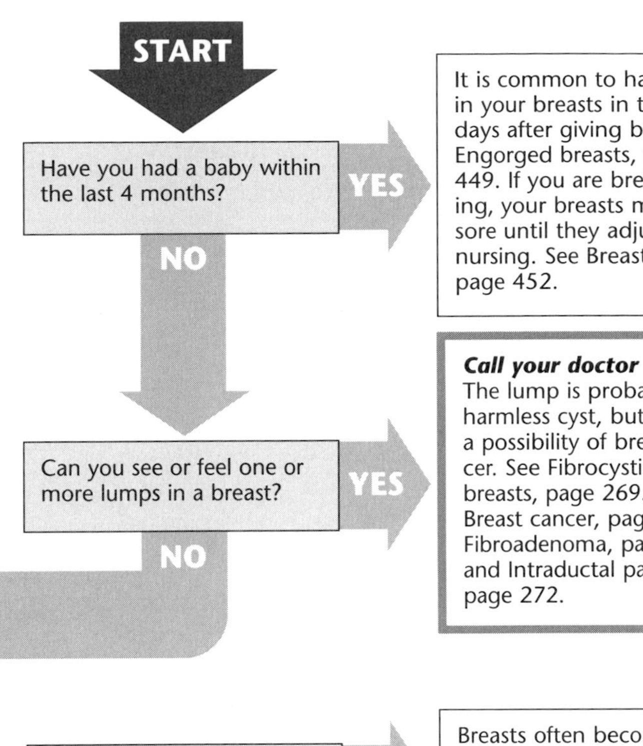

removing the fibroadenoma if it is unusually large, if the woman has a strong family history of breast cancer, or if she herself has a history of breast cancer. The surgery, which is the same as that for an excisional biopsy (see page 275), is usually performed using a local anesthetic and does not require a hospital stay.

INTRADUCTAL PAPILLOMA

An intraductal papilloma is a small, benign (noncancerous) tumor that grows in the cells lining a breast duct. After a pregnancy, many women notice some clear or milky discharge when they squeeze their nipples. This is normal. If you have not been pregnant and notice a discharge, see your doctor right away. The color of the discharge may be clear and sticky (like an egg white), greenish yellow, or bloody. The discharge often appears as a small wet spot on your clothes.

Intraductal papilloma is not a cancer, but it can mimic the symptoms of cancer. For this reason, an intraductal papilloma is usually removed surgically and sent to a laboratory for examination under a microscope to rule out cancer. In some cases, nipple discharge is a symptom of cancer. Your doctor is likely to order a mammogram (see page 127), test the discharge for the presence of blood, and send a sample of the discharge to the laboratory for examination to rule out cancer.

Breast cancer

Many women fear breast cancer more than any other disease and are alarmed by the widely reported statistic that one woman out of eight will develop breast cancer at some time in her life. But this figure is a somewhat confusing statistic that only applies to women now in their 20s, 30s, or 40s who live into their 90s. The likelihood that you will get breast cancer now or in the next few years is far lower than that. Even if you are the average 60-year-old woman (and breast cancer is primarily a disease of older women), the chance that you will get breast cancer by the time you are 70 is much lower than one in eight (see box on page 273). For most women, the risk of breast cancer is much lower than the risk of several other life-threatening diseases, including heart disease, stroke, type II diabetes, and osteoporosis.

Great progress has been made in the diagnosis and treatment of breast cancer in recent years. Breast cancer responds well to treatment and often can be cured. More than 90 percent of women whose breast cancer is detected at an early stage are free of cancer 5 years after treatment and are considered cured. Most women who are successfully treated for breast cancer live out the remainder of their life without a recurrence of the disease.

Early detection of breast cancer is vital to your chances for a cure. Monthly breast self-examinations (see page 276), regular examinations by a doctor, and regular mammograms (see page 127) can be lifesaving. If you are diagnosed with breast cancer, you and your doctor together can approach the problem with optimism to find the treatment that is best for you. By educating yourself about your options for treatment, you can feel confident about whatever decisions you make in consultation with your doctor.

RISK FACTORS

Breast cancer is believed to result from a series of alterations (mutations) in the genes of breast cells. Some women inherit genes that are more susceptible to mutations that can lead to breast cancer. The exact causes for these genetic mutations are not completely understood, but age, hormones, and family history appear to play an important role.

Regardless of your age, hormones, or family history, there is no known way to prevent breast cancer, so your best weapon against the disease is early detection. Performing monthly breast self-examinations, having annual manual breast examinations by a doctor, and having regular mammograms are lifesaving measures every woman should take.

Age Breast cancer risk increases with age (see box on page 273). The disease is far more common in older women, probably because it usually takes years for cancer-causing mutations to occur. Women in their early 60s are twice as likely to get breast cancer as women in their 40s. Therefore, the older you are, the more important it is to monitor your breasts for changes. It is easiest to detect breast cancer in the early stages in older women because the breast tissue is less dense than that of younger women; in older women, signs of cancer show up more clearly on mammograms and breast lumps are easier to feel by touch.

But young women can also get breast cancer. Breast cancer that appears in a woman before menopause is more likely to be caused by inherited genetic factors. Women who develop breast cancer at a young age often have a strong family history (mother or sister with the disease).

Hormones Exposure to the female hormone estrogen plays a role in a woman's risk of breast cancer. Women who began menstruating early (age 11 or younger) or who reach menopause late (age 55 or older) are at increased risk of breast cancer. Doctors believe this is because these women are exposed to more circulating estrogen in their body over a lifetime. For the same reason, it appears that women who have uninterrupted menstrual cycles—that is, they have never been pregnant or breast-fed a child—are exposed to estrogen over a longer time and are, therefore, at increased risk of breast cancer.

Conversely, women who have a first pregnancy before age 30 and breast-feed for longer than 6 months are at a lower risk of breast cancer. Pregnancy and breast-feeding may cause changes in breast cells that make the cells less sensitive to estrogen. Women who have their estrogen source—the ovaries—removed surgically before they go through natural menopause appear to have a lower risk of breast cancer. You are also at reduced risk of breast cancer if you started menstruating late (after age 16), have maintained a healthy weight (fat cells produce more estrogen), or go through menopause early (before age 40).

The low doses of estrogen given in hormone replacement therapy (see page 359) after menopause do not appear to cause an increased risk of breast cancer. The benefits of hormone replacement therapy—most importantly, protection against heart disease and osteoporosis—far outweigh any potential risk of breast cancer. You are ten times more likely to die of a heart attack or stroke than breast cancer, and three times more likely to die of complications from osteoporosis.

Birth-control pills, which contain low doses of estrogen, do not increase a woman's risk of breast cancer. Even if you have risk factors such as a close relative (mother or sister) with breast cancer, you can safely take birth-control pills (see page 310).

Genes Some women inherit genes that appear to protect them from breast cancer, while others inherit genes that make them highly susceptible. Scientists have already found some genes that are associated with breast cancer and are searching for others. Once they know the specific genes that increase a woman's risk, they will be able to develop tests, such as a simple blood test, to identify women who have those genes. With such forewarning, cancer can be diagnosed at earlier stages. Knowledge about the genetic mechanisms involved in breast cancer may also make it possible to find ways to prevent it.

Although family history is a factor in evaluating your risk of breast cancer, the vast majority of cases occur in women who have no family history of the disease. Still, some family patterns of breast cancer suggest a genetic vulnerability for women in those families. These family patterns are:

- Breast cancer in at least one first-degree relative (a mother, sister, or daughter)
- Breast cancer that appears before menopause in a first-degree relative
- Breast cancer that occurs in both breasts at the same time—either in a woman herself or in a first-degree relative

These family patterns are indications that the cancer may be inherited and may put a woman at increased risk. However, many women with these risk factors never get breast cancer.

For a woman who has a family history of breast cancer, particularly one whose mother or sister developed cancer before menopause, there is some encouraging news. The fact that your relative was diagnosed with breast cancer before menopause raises your risk, but that risk diminishes as you age. For example, a woman under 40 with a family history of breast cancer has a higher risk of developing the cancer than a woman with no

Your risk of getting breast cancer

This chart shows the average woman's risk of developing breast cancer at different ages. If you have a family history of breast cancer, your risk may be slightly higher.

AGE	RISK
25	1 in 19,608
30	1 in 2,525
35	1 in 622
40	1 in 217
45	1 in 93
50	1 in 50
55	1 in 33
60	1 in 24
65	1 in 17
70	1 in 14
75	1 in 11
80	1 in 10
85	1 in 9
90	1 in 8
95	1 in 8

family history of the disease. But if she does not develop the cancer by the time she is 60, her risk is the same as any other 60-year-old woman.

Even if you develop breast cancer that appears to be inherited, your chances of surviving it are just as good as those of any other woman whose cancer was diagnosed at the same stage as yours. Knowing that you have a genetic susceptibility to developing breast cancer may actually work to your advantage if it makes you more diligent about taking measures for early detection, including breast self-examinations, regular mammograms, and regular medical checkups. Nine out of 10 breast cancers that are detected early are cured.

PREVENTION

Because it is not fully understood what triggers cells in the breast to become cancerous, there are no firm guidelines for women to follow to reduce their risk. Early detection with regular mammograms and breast examinations makes early treatment possible, which is a woman's best hope for a cure.

More studies are needed to confirm possible links between the risk of breast cancer and lifestyle factors such as a high-fat diet, alcohol consumption, cigarette smoking, and other environmental factors. The best advice for now is to eat a low-fat diet that is rich in fruits and vegetables (particularly those that contain antioxidants such as vitamin A, beta carotene, and vitamin C) and whole grains, exercise regularly, drink alcohol only occasionally if at all, and don't smoke. (For more about diet and cancer, see page 63.)

DETECTION

Like many cancers, breast cancer develops slowly. It may not form a lump large enough to feel by hand or detect on a mammogram until it has been growing for several years.

The only way to know for certain if a lump is cancerous is to perform a biopsy. For a biopsy, the doctor removes a tiny piece of tissue from the lump with a needle or by cutting it out and sends it to a laboratory for examination. There is no blood or urine test that can determine if a woman has breast cancer. Regular breast self-examinations, examinations by your doctor, and mammograms are extremely important in order to find a tumor as early as possible—when treatment is most effective and a cure more likely. (For more about mammography, see page 277; for how to perform a breast self-examination, see page 276.)

If you discover a lump in your breast, don't panic. Most lumps are not cancerous. Many lumps accompany a common, harmless condition called fibrocystic breasts (see page 269). When you do find a lump, you should see your doctor for an examination. After examining your breasts, he or she may recommend further evaluation. The following techniques are used to evaluate a lump in the breast:

Manual examination In a manual examination, the doctor feels the breast and underarm tissue. A doctor can tell a lot about a lump by feeling it, but no one can know for sure if a lump is cancerous by touch alone.

Needle aspiration In needle aspiration, the doctor inserts a thin needle into the center of a breast lump and tries to withdraw fluid. If fluid can be withdrawn and the lump collapses, it is a cyst (see page 270), which is not cancerous. The fluid may be sent to the laboratory to make sure there are no abnormal cells. If no fluid can be withdrawn, it does not necessarily mean the solid lump of tissue is cancerous. The most common noncancerous solid growth in the breast is a fibroadenoma (see page 270), a firm, rubbery lump that usually begins to form during the teenage years. To confirm this, the doctor may order a mammogram or remove a sample of cells (using a slightly larger needle) to be tested in the laboratory. If you have other risk factors for breast cancer (see page 272) or the mammogram looks suspicious, your doctor may recommend a biopsy, in which the entire lump is removed for laboratory testing.

Mammogram and ultrasound If the doctor is unable to withdraw fluid from a breast lump to confirm that it is a cyst, the next step may be a mammogram (see page 127), a low-level X-ray of the breast.

A cancerous tumor usually shows up on a mammogram not as a smooth, round, defined mass, but as an irregular area with radiating arms (see illustration below right).

A cancerous tumor can also appear as an abnormal cluster of white spots, which are deposits of calcium (calcifications). Some calcifications that are tiny and isolated are noncancerous—the doctor (a radiologist) reading the X-ray can tell the difference. The image created by the mammogram is used not only for breast-cancer screening and diagnosis, but also as a guide for a surgeon during the biopsy procedure.

Another imaging technique that is sometimes used to help diagnose breast cancer is ultrasound (which forms an image with sound waves). Especially in women with thick, dense breast tissue, an ultrasound can help distinguish between a noncancerous fluid-filled cyst and a solid tumor that is more likely to be cancerous. In these cases, an ultrasound may be performed in addition to a mammogram to help a doctor determine the need for a biopsy (see below). Ultrasound is particularly helpful in younger women and in women who are pregnant or breast-feeding because their breast tissue tends to be thicker and denser.

Biopsy A biopsy, in which tissue is removed and examined under a microscope for the presence of cancer cells, is the only sure way to diagnose breast cancer. There are several different techniques for performing biopsies.

Needle biopsy A needle biopsy (see page 270) is performed in the doctor's office when he or she suspects cancer and wants to confirm the diagnosis immediately. For a needle biopsy, the doctor inserts a needle into the lump and removes a small amount of tissue. If no evidence of cancer is found from microscopic examination of the tissue sample, the doctor will recommend a more thorough biopsy in the hospital to make sure no cancerous tissue was missed.

Needle localization Needle localization, also called mammographic localization or wire localization, is sometimes used to perform a biopsy on a suspicious area that shows up on a mammogram but cannot be felt by touch. If the doctor cannot feel an abnormality, it is more difficult to withdraw a sample of tissue from it for testing.

For needle localization, you are given local anesthesia (see page 260) to numb your breast. The doctor (usually a radiologist) then introduces one or more very fine needles into your breast to the precise site of the abnormality shown on the mammogram. You are then taken to the operating room. The doctor makes an incision in the breast and, guided by the path of the needles, removes the suspicious area. This suspicious area is often a cluster of calcium deposits that can be an indication of cancer. The tissue will be examined in a laboratory under a microscope for cancer cells. You will have a tiny scar on your breast where the incision was made.

Excisional biopsy In an excisional biopsy, the doctor removes the entire lump or area that looks abnormal on a mammogram. Excisional biopsy is the most common biopsy procedure because doctors often feel safer removing a whole lump since one area of the lump may have no cancerous cells while another area may be cancerous.

For an excisional biopsy, you usually go to the hospital. You will be given local anesthesia (see page 260) to numb your

BREAST CANCER
The most common area for a cancerous lump to develop is the upper, outer portion of the breast—the area closest to the armpit. A breast tumor may develop for several years before it can be detected by touch or on a mammogram. Other than a lump, signs of breast cancer include swelling, tenderness, discharge from the nipple, indentation of the nipple, or a dimpled appearance of the skin of the breast.

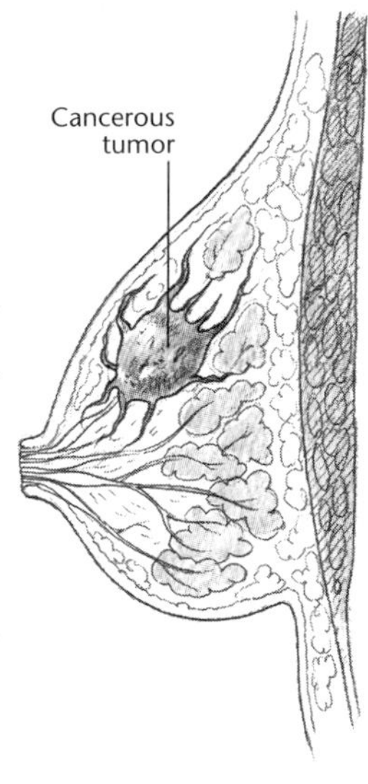

A Practical Guide to Finding Breast Cancer Early

WHEN BREAST CANCER is found at an early stage, it is easier to treat and the possibility of cure is greater. Every woman needs to examine her breasts monthly. If you are over 40, you should have mammograms as often as your doctor recommends; after 50, you should have a mammogram every year. The older you are, the greater your risk of developing breast cancer. Make these examinations a regular part of your life. (For more about breast cancer, see page 272.)

Breast self-examination

Most breast lumps are found by women themselves during regular breast self-examinations. If you menstruate, do the examination a few days after your period ends. If you use oral contraceptives, do it on the day you begin a new pill pack. If you feel any new lumps or notice anything else unusual, bring it to your doctor's attention immediately.

1 Stand in front of a mirror with your arms at your sides. Look for irregularities, puckering, dimples, changes in size or shape, or pushed-in or misshapen nipples. Look for the same changes while resting your hands on your hips and then while holding your hands behind your head.

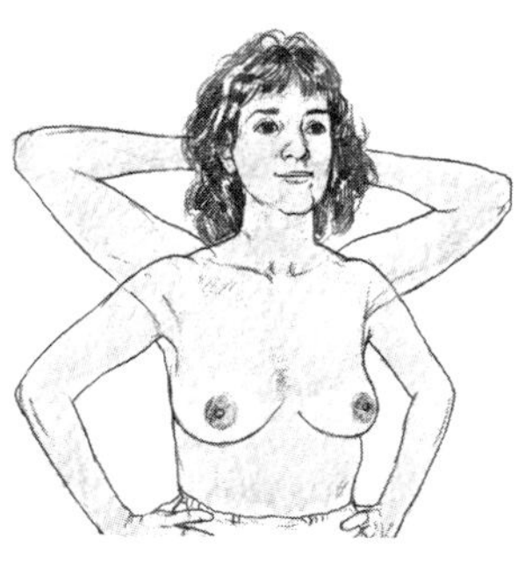

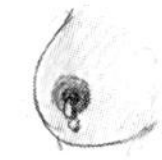

Retraction of nipple

Dimpling

Nipple discharge that is bloody or clear and sticky

2 Standing, use your left hand to examine your right breast. (Some women do this in the shower, when their skin is lubricated by soap.) Feel your breast with the pads of your index and middle fingers, moving in increasingly smaller circles, from the outside in. Compress gently, feeling for lumps. As you circle your nipple, look for discharge.

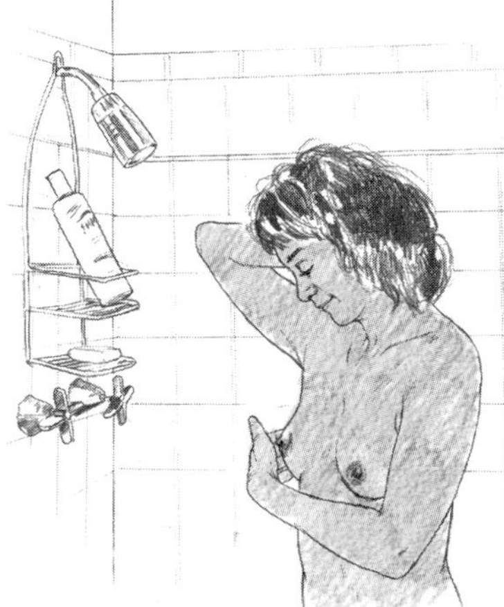

3 Continue the gentle massaging to examine the area adjacent to your breast and below your armpit. This area also contains breast tissue.

4 Repeat, using your right hand on your left breast.

5 Examine your breasts with your fingertips again while lying on your back. Put a pillow under your right shoulder and place your right hand under your head. Use your left hand to examine your right breast. Repeat on the left breast.

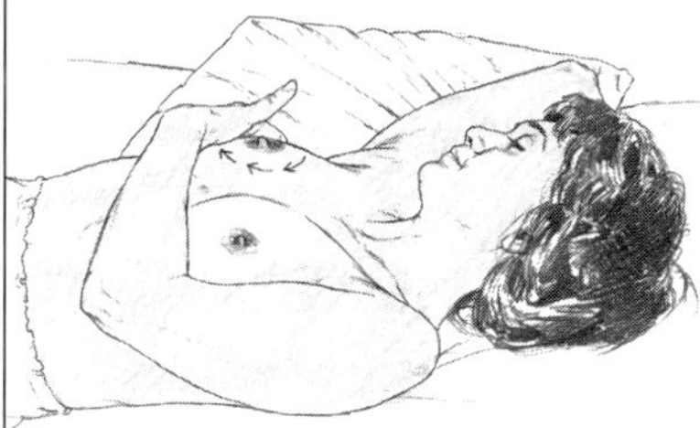

6 If your breasts are normally lumpy (see page 269), note how many separate lumps you feel and their locations. Next month, check for changes—especially an increase in size that persists after your next period.

Warning signs
Breast cancer

See your doctor immediately if you find:

- Any new lump
- Nipple discharge, particularly if it is bloody or dark or occurs without squeezing your nipple
- A nipple drawing inward or pointing in a new direction
- Any change in the shape or symmetry of your breast
- Any lump or thickening that does not shrink or lessen after your next period
- Any dimpling or dent

Examine these areas especially carefully

Cancerous tumors are more likely to be found in some parts of the breast than in others. Three out of four breast cancers occur in the upper, outer region of the breast, toward the armpit, or behind the nipple. Examine these areas especially carefully, but be sure to examine all of each breast thoroughly every month.

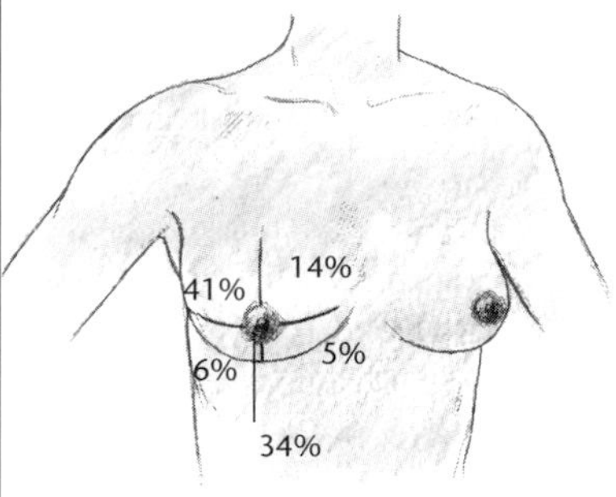

MOST COMMON TUMOR SITES
This illustration shows the percentage of cancerous tumors that are found in each quadrant of the breast and in the area behind the nipple.

The size of tumors when detected

The average size of cancerous tumors found by different methods varies dramatically. The average tumor found by chance is about 12 times larger than the average tumor that is found on a regular mammogram.

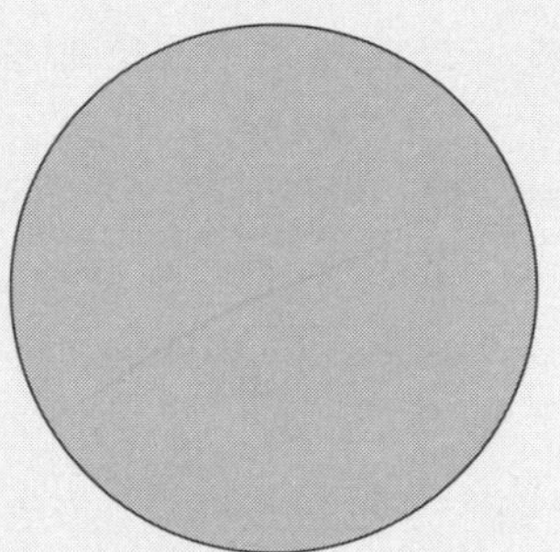

By chance ($1\frac{1}{2}$ inches; 38 mm)

With occasional breast self-examination (1 inch; 25 mm)

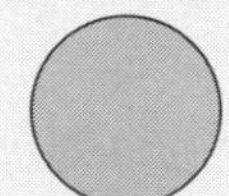

With regular breast self-examination ($\frac{1}{2}$ inch; 13 mm)

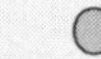

With regular mammograms ($\frac{1}{8}$ inch; 3 mm)

Mammography: Finding cancers too small to feel

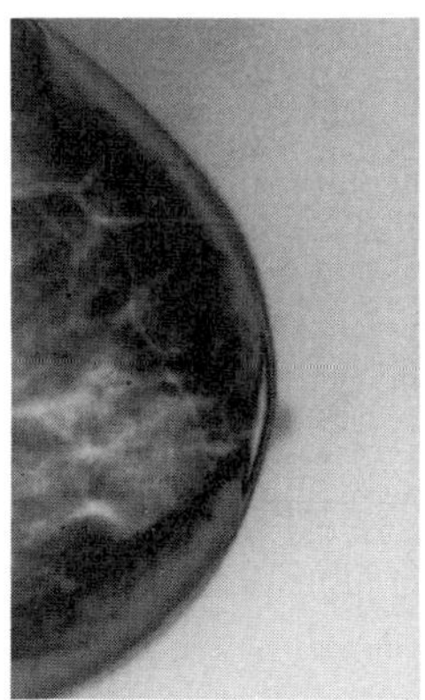

Healthy breast

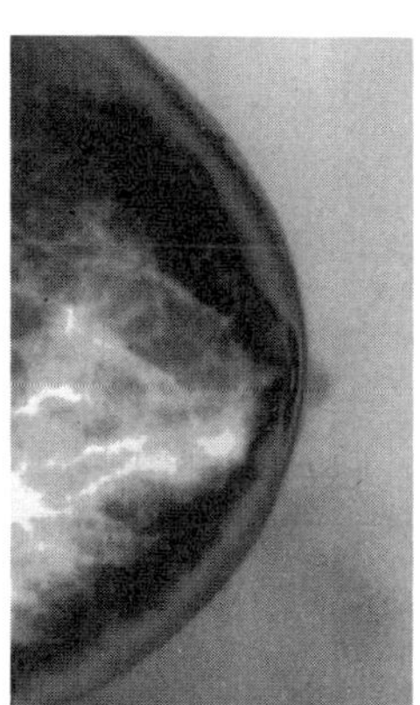

Breast with cancerous tumor

A mammogram is a low-intensity X-ray that can detect a breast tumor before it is large enough to feel by hand. When you have a mammogram, each breast is placed on an X-ray plate and gently compressed while several views are taken. If you have no family history of breast cancer or other risk factors, have a mammogram every 2 years between the ages of 40 and 49 (or as your doctor recommends) and every year after 50. For a complete description of the procedure, see page 127.

What if I feel a lump?

If you find a lump or any other change in your breast, see your doctor immediately. The vast majority of breast lumps turn out to be noncancerous (benign). Many are fluid-filled cysts that can be easily drained. You may have naturally fibrous breasts that feel lumpy—many women do. Although this is normal for you, you still need to be diligent about self-examinations. Your doctor will investigate a suspicious lump by manual examination, needle aspiration, mammography, or biopsy. (For more about diagnosing breast cancer, see page 274.)

Breast cancer responds to treatment and can often be cured, especially if it is detected early. If you are diagnosed with breast cancer, you and your doctor can work together to design the treatment program that is best for you (see page 281).

Questions to ask your doctor about a biopsy

The questions below will help you better understand the biopsy procedure. If you have any other questions that do not appear here, don't hesitate to ask them. There is no such thing as a dumb question. Take a list of questions with you to the doctor—and be sure to write down the answers so you will have the information to review later.

- What kind of biopsy will I have?
- Will it be done using local anesthesia or general anesthesia (see page 260)?
- What are the risks of the anesthesia?
- Will the tissue be examined for estrogen and progesterone receptors in a hormone receptor test (see right)?
- How visible will the scar from the biopsy be?
- What are the expected aftereffects?
- How soon after the biopsy will I find out whether or not I have cancer?
- If I have cancer, what other tests will I need to have?
- If I have cancer, how much time can I take to decide what type of treatment to have?

breast. The doctor makes an incision, cuts the lump away from the surrounding tissue, removes it, and sends it to the laboratory for examination. He or she stitches up the incision and sends you to the recovery room. You can usually go home after a couple of hours and return to work and resume your normal activities the next day. Your doctor will discuss with you when you can remove the bandage over the stitches. You will receive the diagnosis from the laboratory results within 2 days to a week. You will have a tiny scar on your breast where the incision was made.

In some cases, a doctor may recommend waiting a month or more after finding a lump before doing a biopsy. A lump that disappears during or shortly after your menstrual period and reappears again each month is usually not cancerous. However, if you feel uncomfortable about waiting, tell your doctor. You may want to have a biopsy or another diagnostic test immediately to ease your mind. Or you may want to get a second opinion to confirm that it is safe to wait.

Hormone receptor test If a breast tumor is found to be cancerous, it will be tested further to determine if the surfaces of the cancer cells have receptors for either of the female hormones estrogen or progesterone. Receptors are specific areas on cell surfaces to which hormones attach, like a key fitting a lock. If a cell has receptors for estrogen or progesterone, the hormone can attach to the receptors and stimulate the cell to grow. Not all breast cancers have cells with these receptors. A hormone receptor test is important in determining treatment (see page 284), because cancers that are influenced by hormones are treated differently than other cancers.

RECEIVING THE DIAGNOSIS

The days spent waiting to find out if you have breast cancer can seem like an eternity. "Hoping for the best" works for some women, but, if you are like most people, you are likely to fear the worst. You may feel overwhelmed by thoughts about deforming surgery, weakness and hair loss from chemotherapy, inability to continue work or maintain home responsibilities, and disrupted relationships. Remember, the vast majority of all tumors are not cancerous.

If you are diagnosed with breast cancer, you will likely experience a variety of emotions that are a normal part of the adjustment process. These emotions may include fear, feelings of helplessness, obsessive thoughts about the cancer or denial of it, difficulty concentrating, insomnia, irritability, anger, anxiety, fatigue, and depression. You may feel any or all of these things right away or later, after you have had time to consider the diagnosis. At the same time, you will probably be bombarded with facts, statistics, and information about the disease and treatment options and asked to make difficult and complicated decisions about your treatment.

Your reaction will depend on your personality and circumstances. It will be influenced by the way you have handled stress or bad news in the past, the availability of support from friends and family, the flexibility of your lifestyle and job, and your ideas about cancer.

Here are some things you can do that may be helpful during this trying time:

- Take one step at a time. Focus on what is happening now and what the immediate next step is rather than becoming absorbed with morbid possibilities.

- Ask your doctor questions. Don't be afraid to bring a list of questions or concerns to visits with your doctor. There are no "dumb" or unimportant questions. If something troubles you, have your doctor explain it until you understand it. Take notes.
- Ask your doctor to recommend books, pamphlets, or other materials for women who have been diagnosed with breast cancer. Learning more about your illness will help you be a more confident participant in decisions about your treatment. Call the National Cancer Institute or a local branch of the American Cancer Society for information.
- Consider joining a support group. Your doctor, hospital, or a local branch of the American Cancer Society may recommend a group in your area. You may find it reassuring to spend time with other women who share your experience and know what you're feeling. Learning from women who have already gone through breast cancer treatment can help you make your own decisions about treatment. Y-Me is a nationwide breast cancer support group that you may want to get involved with.
- Try to stick to your regular routine. Structure and routine help to reduce anxiety. Set reasonable daily or weekly goals for yourself and reward yourself for your accomplishments.
- Don't keep everything inside. Letting other people in can often be a tremendous relief. Friends and family can be a rich source of support and nurturing.

STAGING

Once breast cancer has been diagnosed, you and your doctor need to know its stage—how far it has progressed—before you can decide on treatment. Today most breast cancers are found in stage I or II, when they are most likely to respond to treatment. Stage III cancers sometimes respond to treatment. Stage IV cancers usually are not curable but may respond to treatment; however, a small percentage are cured.

Knowing the stage a cancer is in helps you and your doctor make decisions about your treatment. For example, the goal of surgical procedures such as mastectomy (removal of the breast) is to remove the cancer. But if the cancer has already spread (metastasized) to other parts of your body, there may be no point in removing your breast. In this case, other treatments (such as chemotherapy, which treats the whole body) are more useful.

Blood and urine tests as well as imaging procedures such as a computed tomography (CT) scan (see page 572) or a bone scan may show whether a cancer has spread to the bones, lungs, or liver. Signs that an advanced cancer has probably spread include:

- A tumor larger than 2 inches across
- Swelling, called edema, that causes a small dimple on the skin of the breast
- A tumor that is sticking to the underlying muscles or lymph nodes that you can feel above the collarbone or in the armpit
- Red, itchy, or scaly skin over a tumor

During a biopsy, some of the lymph nodes under the arm may be removed for examination under a microscope. The tumor itself will be examined for indications that the cancer has spread and will be tested for other characteristics such as hormone receptors (see page 278). The doctor will evaluate the test results to determine the stage of the cancer and the most appropriate treatment. The stages are usually described as follows:

Carcinoma in situ About 5 to 10 percent of breast cancers are detected at a very early stage called carcinoma in situ. In this stage, a cancer has not spread to nearby tissues (in situ means "in place"). A carcinoma may take different forms, such as ductal carcinoma or lobular carcinoma.

Treatment Treatment for this early form of breast cancer will depend on whether the cancer is in the milk ducts or in the lobules (bulblike glands that can produce milk). If the cancer is in the ducts, your treatment is likely to be one of the following:

- Lumpectomy and radiation
- Total mastectomy

If the cancer is in the lobules, which is less common, you are more likely to have it in both breasts. Not all doctors agree on the best treatment for this type of cancer. Your treatment is likely to be one of the following:

- Lumpectomy, followed by regular examinations and mammograms

CARCINOMA IN SITU

Ductal carcinoma is an early-stage breast cancer that occurs in the milk ducts, usually in one breast. **Lobular carcinoma** is an early-stage breast cancer that occurs in breast lobules, often in both breasts. Lobular carcinoma is less common than ductal carcinoma.

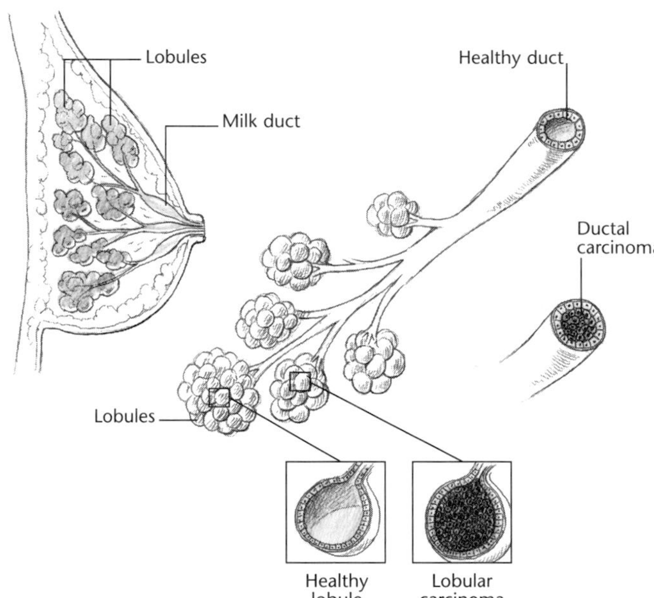

■ Total mastectomy; lymph nodes under the arm may or may not be removed

Stage I A cancer in stage I is no larger than about 1 inch (2 centimeters) across and has not spread to parts of the body other than the breast.

Treatment Treatment for stage I cancer is likely to be one or more of the following:
■ Lumpectomy, or partial mastectomy, and removal of some of the lymph nodes under the arm followed by radiation
■ Total mastectomy
■ Modified radical mastectomy
■ Chemotherapy or hormone therapy in addition to one of the above treatments

Stage II For stage II breast cancers, any of the following may be true:
■ The cancer is no larger than about 1 inch (2 centimeters) across but has spread to the lymph nodes under the arm.
■ The cancer is between about 1 to 2 inches (2 to 5 centimeters) across and may or may not have spread to the lymph nodes under the arm.
■ The cancer is larger than about 2 inches (5 centimeters) across, but has not spread to the lymph nodes under the arm.

Treatment Treatment for stage II cancer is likely to be one of the following:
■ Lumpectomy and removal of some of the lymph nodes under the arm followed by radiation
■ Total mastectomy
■ Modified radical mastectomy
■ Radical mastectomy (rarely)

Stage IIIA For stage IIIA cancers, either of the following is true:
■ The cancer is smaller than about 2 inches (5 centimeters) across and has spread to the lymph nodes under the arm. The lymph nodes have grown into each other or into other structures and are attached to them.
■ The cancer is bigger than about 2 inches (5 centimeters) across and has spread to the lymph nodes under the arm.

Treatment Treatment for stage IIIA cancer may be one or more of the following:
■ Modified radical mastectomy
■ Radical mastectomy
■ Radiation therapy before surgery to shrink the tumor or after surgery to reduce the risk of a recurrence of the cancer
■ Chemotherapy, with or without hormone therapy, after surgery

Stage IIIB In stage IIIB breast cancer, the cancer has spread to tissues near the breast such as the chest wall, ribs, or muscles.

Treatment Treatment for stage IIIB cancer may be one of the following:
■ Radiation therapy possibly followed by chemotherapy and hormone therapy
■ Radiation therapy followed by mastectomy, chemotherapy, and hormone therapy

Stage IV Stage IV is the most advanced stage of breast cancer. Either of the following is true:
■ The cancer has spread to other parts of the body, most often the lungs, liver, bones, and sometimes the brain.
■ The cancer has spread to the lymph nodes near the collarbone.

Treatment Treatment for stage IV cancer may be one of the following:
■ Radiation therapy possibly followed by chemotherapy and hormone therapy

LYMPH NODES AND BREAST CANCER
There is a concentration of lymph nodes near the breast. The cancer can enter the lymphatic system and bloodstream and circulate throughout the body—often to the lungs, liver, bones, or brain.

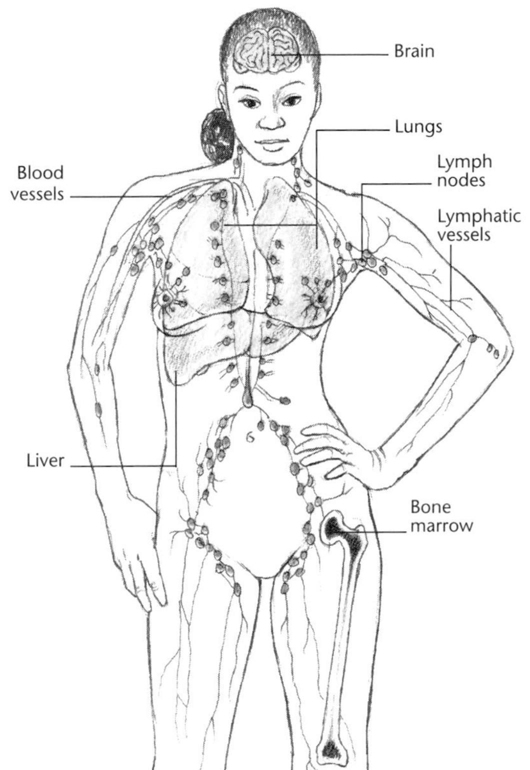

- Radiation therapy followed by mastectomy, chemotherapy, and hormone therapy

Inflammatory breast cancer Inflammatory breast cancer is a rare, fast-spreading form of cancer in which the breast looks red and feels warm and the skin may look ridged or pitted. Because of these symptoms, this type of breast cancer can be misdiagnosed as an infection of the breast or overlying skin.

Treatment Treatment is likely to be similar to that for stage IIIB or stage IV: a combination of chemotherapy, hormone therapy, and radiation therapy, possibly followed by mastectomy.

Recurrent cancer After breast cancer has been treated, it sometimes returns in the treated breast, the untreated breast, the muscles of the chest wall, or in another part of the body. This is called a recurrence of the cancer.

Treatment A recurrent breast cancer can often be treated again and sometimes cured, especially if it has not spread to other parts of the body. Treatment options for recurring breast cancer depend on the results of a hormone receptor test (see page 278), your previous treatment and how long ago you had it, where in your body the cancer has recurred, whether or not you still have periods, and other factors. Your treatment may be one of the following:

- Surgery and/or radiation therapy if your cancer has recurred in only one place
- Radiation therapy to help relieve pain resulting from the spread of cancer to the bones or other sensitive areas
- Chemotherapy or hormone therapy
- Your volunteer participation in a study involving new chemotherapy drugs, new hormonal drugs, or bone marrow transplants (see page 284). Ask your doctor for information if you are interested in participating in a study.

TREATMENTS

Once you have been diagnosed with breast cancer, and doctors have determined what stage the cancer is in, you will be faced with many decisions regarding your treatment. There are four standard treatments for breast cancer—surgery, radiation, chemotherapy, and hormone therapy—which are often used in combination. A fifth option—autologous bone marrow transplant (see page 284)—is being used increasingly in women who are at high risk of a recurrence of their cancer after the standard treatments.

Treatment for breast cancer can save your life. However, the idea of losing a breast to surgery or dealing with the side effects of chemotherapy and radiation therapy can be frightening. For this reason, it is essential to get as much information as possible from your doctor and other reliable sources, and to have the support of relatives and friends every step of the way.

Surgery Some form of surgery is involved in the treatment of almost all cases of breast cancer. Surgery removes the cancer and some or all of the surrounding tissue.

Radical mastectomy—removal of all the breast tissue and muscle of the chest

Options for breast cancer surgery

LUMPECTOMY
In a lumpectomy, doctors try to conserve as much of the basic shape and appearance of a woman's breast as possible. However, if you are small-breasted, any surgery is likely to alter the appearance of your breast. The cancerous lump and some surrounding tissue are removed. Some of the lymph nodes under the arm are usually removed as well to determine if the cancer has spread. The nipple is usually preserved. A lumpectomy is usually followed by radiation therapy to destroy any cancer cells that may remain.

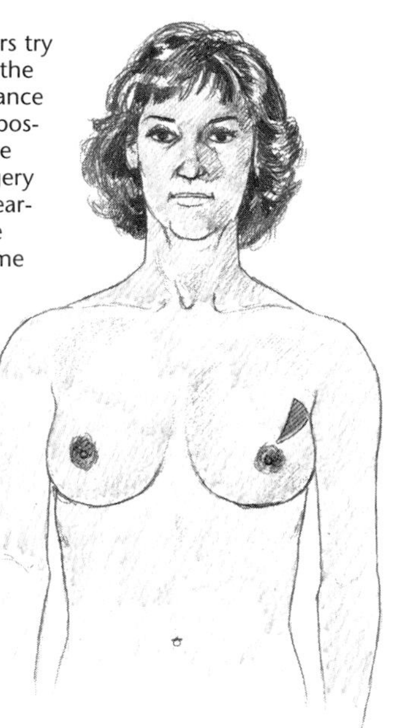

SIMPLE MASTECTOMY
In this procedure, the entire breast is removed. Radiation therapy may follow.

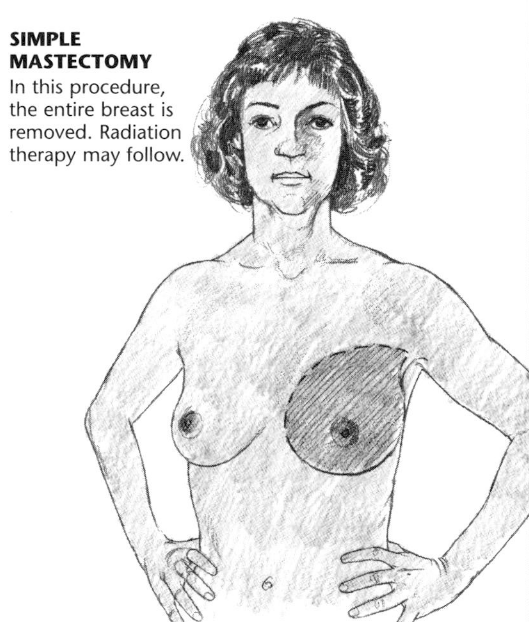

MODIFIED RADICAL MASTECTOMY
In this procedure, the entire breast and the lining over the chest muscles are removed. Lymph nodes under the arm may also be removed. Radiation therapy may follow.

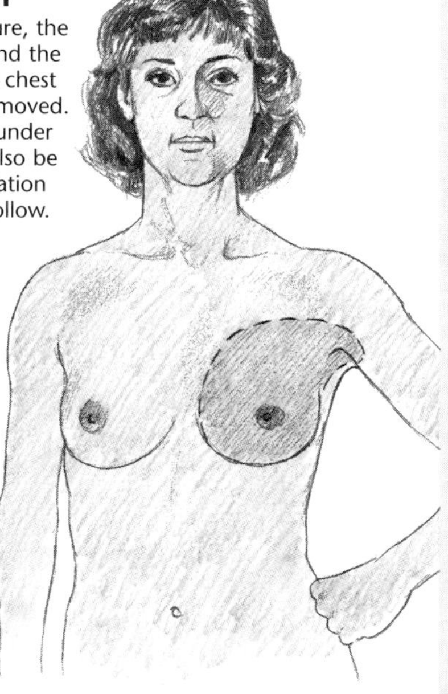

PROPHYLACTIC SUBCUTANEOUS MASTECTOMY
This procedure is not performed to treat cancer but to prevent it in women who are at high risk. Only the internal breast tissue is removed, leaving the nipple and skin intact. A breast implant replaces the tissue that has been removed. But no type of mastectomy can completely eliminate the risk of developing breast cancer because a small amount of breast tissue is always left behind.

wall—used to be the most common treatment for breast cancer. But doctors now know that lumpectomy—removal of only the cancerous tumor and surrounding tissue—can be an equally successful treatment, particularly of early-stage cancers. Radical mastectomy is rarely performed today because most breast cancers are found before they have invaded the underlying chest muscles. It is important to discuss the different surgical approaches with your doctor.

Before having surgery, you are likely to have many questions and some fears about whether the surgery will cure your cancer, whether you will be in pain after the surgery, and how your body will look after the procedure. Breast surgery has an emotional impact on women because their breasts are connected with their self-image and sexuality. Discuss your thoughts and feelings with a person close to you and talk with your spouse or partner about how the surgery will affect your relationship. Prepare in advance to get help at home from a friend, family member, or hired helper during your recovery or during the time you will be undergoing further treatment such as radiation or chemotherapy.

Before the surgery, talk to your surgeon and make sure you have a clear understanding of the procedure and your treatment plan. Find out how long you are likely to be in the hospital. Make arrangements for someone to be at the hospital after you come out of surgery.

You will be asked to not eat or drink anything after midnight the night before your surgery. You should talk with the anesthesiologist about what form of anesthesia you will have. The type of surgery will determine the type of anesthesia. Some form of general anesthesia, in which you will be asleep during the entire procedure, is usually used.

Modified radical mastectomy In a modified radical mastectomy, the entire breast and some lymph nodes under the arm and the lining over the chest muscles are removed. The lymph nodes are sent to a laboratory for examination for cancer cells. The incision is in the shape of an elongated oval (see page 282) and is usually positioned so that the scar will not show when you wear low-cut clothing. A scalpel is usually used for this procedure, although a laser is sometimes used to cut through tissues.

Mastectomies are generally performed with the idea of breast reconstruction (see page 286) in mind. If you have decided in advance that you want breast reconstruction at the time of your surgery, a plastic surgeon will be standing by to perform this procedure. Some women wait several months to decide whether or not they want breast reconstruction.

Simple mastectomy A simple mastectomy is similar to a modified radical mastectomy

Questions to ask your doctor about breast cancer

- What kind of breast cancer do I have? What stage is it in?
- What were the results of my hormone receptor test and tests investigating the aggressiveness of my cancer?
- How likely is the cancer to spread?
- What are my treatment options?
- What do you think about treating breast cancer with a lumpectomy followed by radiation therapy? Am I a good candidate for these treatments?
- What are the potential risks of the various treatments? What are the side effects?
- Will I need chemotherapy or hormone therapy? If I do, will you refer me to an oncologist (a doctor who specializes in treating cancer)?
- Would you recommend breast reconstruction in my case? If so, should I have it at the time of surgery or later?
- How long do I have to make decisions about my treatment?
- Can you recommend an oncologist from whom I can get a second opinion?
- When can I expect to be able to resume my normal routine?

RADIATION TREATMENT FOR BREAST CANCER
Radiation therapy is usually given to women with stage I or stage II breast cancer who have chosen to have a lumpectomy. This therapy, which uses X-rays to kill cancer cells, is usually administered five times a week for 5 weeks to help prevent recurrence of the cancer. For radiation therapy, you are positioned on a table under the X-ray beams, which are directed toward the cancerous area.

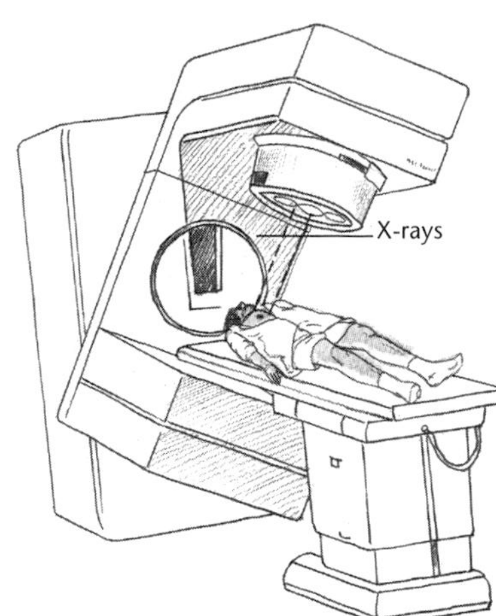

except that the chest muscle lining is not removed. This surgery is most common for some kinds of stage I and II cancers.

Lumpectomy Lumpectomy, also called a partial mastectomy or breast conservation surgery, removes the cancerous tissue and a margin of surrounding tissue from the breast. Lumpectomy has become more common as evidence mounts in favor of its success. Many women prefer this procedure because it leaves some or most of the breast intact, including the nipple. Lumpectomy is always followed by radiation therapy and sometimes by chemotherapy as well.

Make sure to discuss the procedures to be used in a lumpectomy with your surgeon. The appearance after the surgery will depend on the size of your breast and the size of the tumor. Sometimes so much of the breast must be removed that you would get better results with a mastectomy and reconstructive surgery.

Recovering from mastectomy During recovery from breast surgery, most women do not feel a great deal of pain. You will be given pain medication for any that you have; it usually subsides the first day or so after surgery. It is common to feel numb in the area of the incision; this often disappears gradually over a few weeks or months. The hospital stay is usually about 5 days for mastectomy and about 2 to 3 days for lumpectomy.

You can speed your recovery by exercising as soon as possible after surgery. Your stitches are not likely to pull apart. A physical therapist at the hospital will discuss exercises with you and help you perform them in the days following surgery. After you leave the hospital, you can expect to resume a normal schedule a few days after a lumpectomy or 2 to 3 weeks following mastectomy. You can shower after the stitches have been removed and bathe after the incision has healed.

Radiation The goal of radiation therapy after surgery for breast cancer is usually to help prevent the recurrence of cancer in the affected breast and the lymph nodes that surround it. Radiation therapy uses high-power X-rays to kill cancer cells and shrink tumors. Radiation may be administered externally from a machine positioned outside the body (usually five times a week for about 5 weeks) or internally from radioactive materials that are implanted in the affected area through thin plastic tubes. Radiation works best on small, isolated areas of cancer. (For more about radiation therapy, see page 253.)

Chemotherapy When a cancer has moved beyond the breast, powerful medications can be used to kill cancer cells that have spread throughout the body. This treatment, called chemotherapy, is often used in addition to surgery, radiation, or both to destroy any cancer cells that may remain after those treatments. Chemotherapy is sometimes used even when the cancer does not appear to have spread, but doctors suspect that it may have. Chemotherapy drugs may be taken by mouth or injected into the bloodstream or a muscle over a period of several months. (For more about chemotherapy, see page 254.)

Hormone therapy Hormone therapy is used for women whose breast cancer has been found on a hormone receptor test (see page 278) to be sensitive to the effects of estrogen. A doctor may prescribe an estrogen-blocking drug such as tamoxifen, which prevents estrogen from binding to cancer cells and stimulating them to grow. This type of hormone therapy is sometimes used after surgery or chemotherapy to help prevent a recurrence of the cancer. In some cases, the ovaries are removed to stop the body's production of estrogen.

Autologous bone marrow transplant When a breast cancer is very aggressive,

Estrogen and breast cancer

The female hormone estrogen is thought to accelerate the growth of some types of breast cancer cells. For this reason, breast cancer risk is lower for women whose levels of estrogen have been reduced over the years—for example, by late puberty, early pregnancy, or more pregnancies. Because obesity increases estrogen levels, it increases breast cancer risk.

In treatment for breast cancer, a drug called tamoxifen is sometimes used to reduce the production of estrogen and prevent it from binding with cancer cells. Tamoxifen is also being tested as a possible breast cancer–prevention drug for women who are at high risk of developing the cancer.

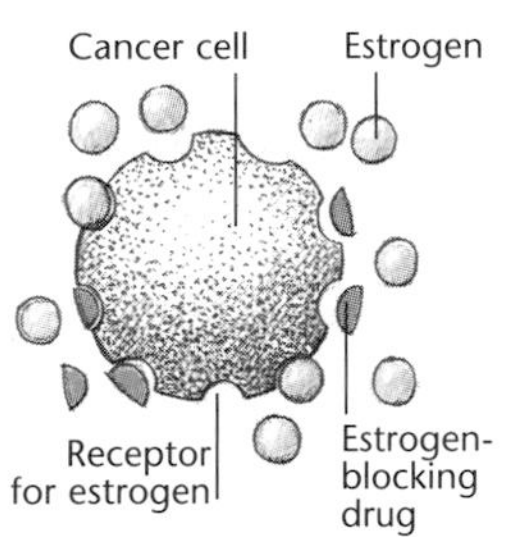

HOW ESTROGEN-BLOCKING DRUGS WORK

Estrogen-blocking drugs such as tamoxifen fit into estrogen receptors on a cancer cell, preventing estrogen from binding to the cell and stimulating it to grow.

has spread, and does not respond to standard treatments, doctors sometimes recommend an autologous bone marrow transplant. The term autologous means that it originates from a person's own body. A bone marrow transplant is often the only hope for women whose breast cancer has spread.

For an autologous bone marrow transplant, a woman's bone marrow is removed (through a needle) to allow doctors to give her extremely high doses of chemotherapy (10 to 50 times the normal dose) in an effort to kill all the cancer cells in her body. If the marrow is not removed first, such high doses of chemotherapy can be fatal—the bone marrow, which produces all the body's blood cells, would be destroyed along with the cancer.

Before the high-dose chemotherapy treatment, the removed bone marrow is examined to make sure it is free of cancer cells, and then frozen. When the chemotherapy is complete, the bone marrow is thawed and injected back into the woman's body. The marrow cells migrate back to the center of bones where they resume their job of producing new blood cells.

CHOOSING A TREATMENT

Although there are standard recommended treatments for breast cancer in each stage, the final decision is yours in consultation with your doctor. You are usually given options to choose from. For example, you may have to decide between having a lumpectomy or a mastectomy based on the stage of your cancer, your own circumstances, and your feelings about losing a breast. Discuss all of your concerns with your doctor and listen closely to his or her explanation of each treatment option and associated risks.

The results of a hormone receptor test (see page 278) are important for determining whether or not your cancer is likely to respond to hormone therapy. If you have an estrogen-dependent cancer (see box above), taking an estrogen-blocking drug such as tamoxifen or cutting off the estrogen supply by having your ovaries removed may help slow the growth of the cancer or help prevent it from recurring.

Until the 1980s, almost all women who were diagnosed with breast cancer had their breast removed. But for the earlier stages of cancer, women who undergo lumpectomy (removal of only the cancerous lump) survive just as long as those who have their entire breast removed. As a result, doctors now often recommend a breast-preserving lumpectomy rather than a mastectomy for women whose cancer is in stage I or II. Radiation therapy usually follows a lumpectomy.

The final decision about what kind of treatment to have for breast cancer is a woman's to make, usually based on some very personal considerations. If you have been diagnosed with breast cancer, give yourself enough time to learn all you can about the disease and your treatment options. Read everything you can find, ask your doctor questions, and join a support group to learn about the experiences of other women who have or have had breast cancer. Get a second or third opinion from other doctors if you are not satisfied with your doctor's recommendations. The more you know, the more comfortable you will be with your decision. Cancer takes several years, even decades, to develop. Waiting a couple of weeks while you gather information, get answers to your questions, and get another medical opinion will not make any difference in the outcome. Do not, however, delay making decisions for months; in that time your cancer can spread, reducing your treatment options.

When visiting the doctor, it is often difficult to absorb all the information and ask the right questions at the same time you are dealing with an array of emotional issues. It may help to ask a good friend or a relative to come with you when you see the doctor. That person can take notes, ask questions, and later may be able to fill in information you missed.

BREAST PROSTHESIS OR RECONSTRUCTION

Most women who have had all or part of a breast removed want to do something to recreate the appearance of two normal breasts. You can decide between wearing a prosthesis, a custom-made bralike device that includes a false breast, or undergoing one of several surgical procedures to reconstruct your breast. Some women choose to go without either, saying they feel comfortable the way they are.

Prosthesis Almost immediately after surgery to remove your breast, and before you leave the hospital, you will be offered a temporary prosthesis. Later on, you can shop for a permanent one; they are available in medical supply stores, in some lingerie stores, and at some large department stores. You can order one custom-made. Check with your insurance company to make sure your choice is covered; you may need to get a prescription from your doctor in order to be reimbursed.

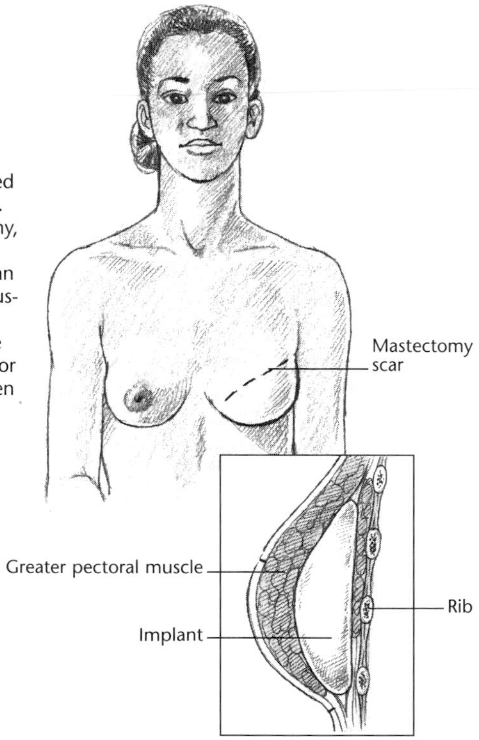

BREAST IMPLANTS
Breast implants are filled with saline (salt water). Following a mastectomy, reconstruction may include the insertion of an implant behind the muscle wall. If a woman chooses to have nipple reconstruction, tissue for the nipple may be taken from the inside of her thigh.

Reconstruction Whether or not to have breast reconstruction after surgery is entirely up to you. You need to do what will make you feel good about your body and yourself. Most health insurance plans cover breast reconstruction surgery.

Surgeons can create a new breast and nipple with varying degrees of success. The greatest challenge is to create a breast that looks the same as the natural one. Often, the results fall a little short of perfection but the breast looks normal when covered by clothing. Small breasts are somewhat easier to duplicate than large breasts. Breast reconstruction cannot create a breast that feels as natural to you as your own breast. Even if it looks and feels real to someone else, it will lack sensitivity. Most women who have undergone breast reconstruction become accustomed to this lack of feeling.

Breast reconstruction can create a new breast using either your own tissues (taken from your back or abdomen) or an artificial implant. Implants are used more often to create a large breast, sometimes in addition to the woman's own tissue, because there may not be enough tissue to make the breast the size of the remaining one. In some cases, if the surgeon thinks the remaining breast is too large to match with the reconstructed breast, he or she may recommend surgically reducing the size of the natural breast.

Some women have breast reconstruction at the same time as the mastectomy, but many wait several months to a year. Other women who do not want to go through the physical and emotional trauma of more surgery put the decision off indefinitely or decide against reconstruction altogether. You do not have to make a decision immediately. Choose whatever makes you feel most comfortable. Women who have follow-up radiation treatments may be advised to wait as long as a year before having breast reconstruction because the radiation can interfere with healing and cause scar tissue to form in the space available for the implant.

Following are brief descriptions of some breast reconstruction procedures, all of

Breast reconstruction

Many women choose to have breast reconstruction after surgery for breast cancer. Doctors may use tissue from the woman's abdomen or back to form a new breast.

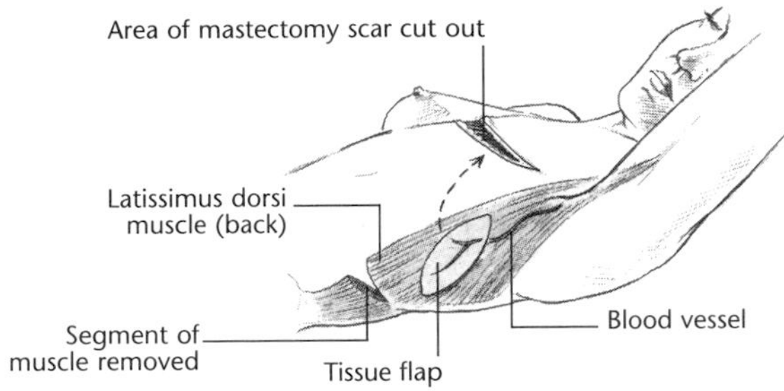

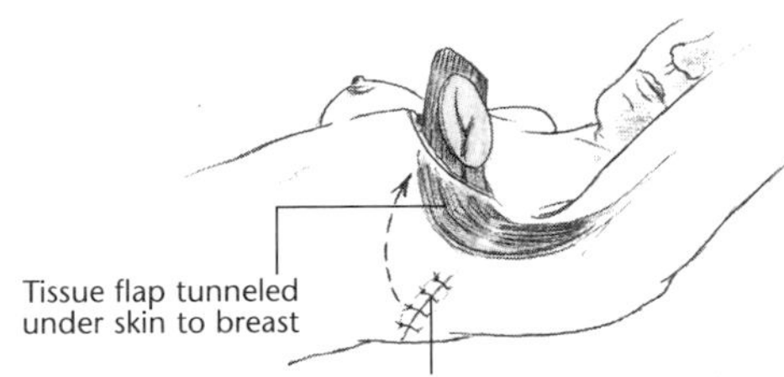

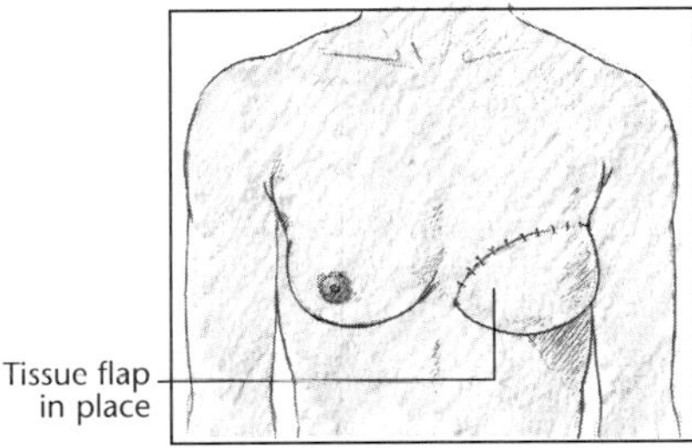

USING TISSUE FROM THE BACK

While you are under general anesthesia, the surgeon cuts out the area of the scar from the mastectomy (top). He or she cuts out a flap of tissue including skin, muscle, fat, and attached blood vessels from the back just below the armpit. The tissue flap, with its blood vessels still intact, is tunneled underneath the skin (center) and attached to the chest in the area of the breast (bottom). A nipple may be reconstructed in later surgery.

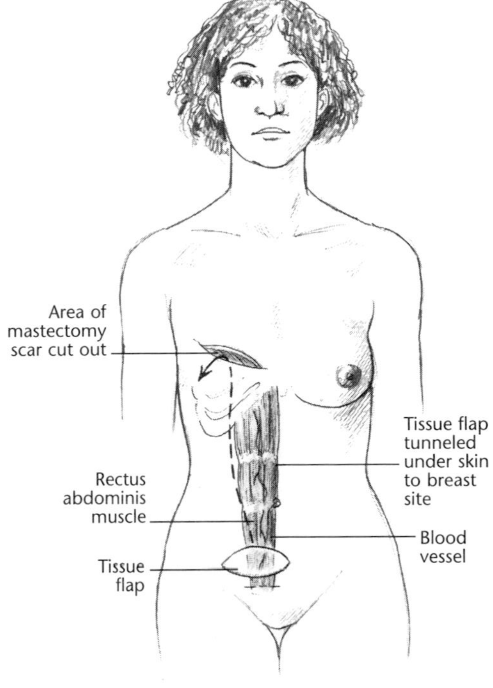

USING TISSUE FROM THE ABDOMEN

In this procedure, which is similar to the one described at left, tissue from the abdomen, rather than from the back, is used to reconstruct the breast. An advantage of using abdominal tissue is that it has a larger proportion of fat and can, therefore, produce a larger breast. A nipple may be reconstructed in later surgery.

which are performed while you are under general anesthesia (see page 261).

Reconstruction using body tissue In breast reconstruction using a woman's own tissues, the surgeon must first prepare the tissue (a flap of skin, muscle, and fat taken from either the back or abdomen) that will be used to reconstruct the breast. To keep the tissue alive, the blood vessels supplying it remain attached.

If tissue from the back is to be used, the surgeon will make an almond-shaped incision parallel to the muscle fibers that are located just under and behind the arm. Leaving the blood vessels attached, the doctor tunnels this tissue under the skin to the site from which the breast has been removed. The skin flap is secured and sewn in place. The area from which the skin flap was removed is stitched close. Sometimes an artificial breast implant is used along with a woman's own tissue to create a larger breast.

If tissue from the abdomen is used, the surgeon makes a wide, almond-shaped incision across the abdomen below the navel for the flap of skin, muscle, and fat for the new breast. With its blood vessels still attached, the tissue flap is tunneled underneath the skin to the new location, secured, and stitched in place. Because abdominal tissue has more fat than tissue from the back, it can create a larger breast. However, removing muscle from the abdominal wall can cause weakness in the abdomen and a possible hernia (in which intestines bulge through the weakened muscle wall) later in life.

Immediately after this type of breast reconstruction surgery, you will be sore in the area from which the tissue was removed. Try to limit the movement of your chest and the arm on that side for several days to avoid disrupting the stitches. Hospitalization is usually about 1 week.

Doctors can create a nipple using tissue from the inside of a woman's thigh and some of the nipple tissue from her remaining breast. A nipple gives the breast a more natural contour. The nipple is usually added to the reconstructed breast several months after the reconstruction operation in order to ensure proper healing. A woman may choose to have the reconstructed nipples tattooed to give them a more natural color.

Reconstruction using implants The Food and Drug Administration (FDA) has restricted the use of breast implants made of silicone, citing lack of information about their long-term health effects (see page 700). Saline implants, which are filled with a salt water solution, are now used almost exclusively.

The insertion of an implant behind the muscle wall in the chest is the easiest procedure to perform in breast reconstruction, requiring a hospital stay of only 2 to 3 days. The doctor makes an incision in the muscle wall, secures the implant behind the muscle, and stitches the incision close. An implant cannot create a very large breast, however, because it is flattened by the muscle wall. For this reason, implants work best in small-breasted women, or in women who have had both breasts removed and are happy with reconstructed small breasts.

To create a larger breast with implants, some women undergo a procedure in which the skin over the breast site is gradually stretched over a period of 6 months. To do so, a device called a tissue expander (a hollow, empty sack with a tube and a valve on it) is placed behind the chest muscle. Over several months, the doctor injects more and more saline through the tube into the sack, allowing the skin covering it to gradually stretch. Finally, when the breast reaches the desired size, the expander is removed and replaced with a permanent implant.

All surgery carries the risk of infection but, for breast reconstruction using implants or an expander, the risk is slightly greater. Because implants and expanders are foreign objects, they may interfere with the body's natural healing process. In the case of a serious infection, an implant will be removed.

BREAST CANCER DURING PREGNANCY

Each year, about 4,000 American women are diagnosed with breast cancer during pregnancy. If the diagnosis is made at an early, treatable stage, these women have the same chance for a cure as nonpregnant women of the same age and at the same stage of the disease. Therefore, pregnancy is not the time to let down your guard. Although the cancer risk is small, you should continue to examine your breasts regularly throughout your pregnancy and make sure your doctor examines them too.

If you or your doctor finds a lump, together you will make any decisions about diagnosis and treatment during your pregnancy. A diagnosis of cancer does not mean that your pregnancy must be terminated. Your doctor will discuss all your treatment options and you can then make an informed decision based on your own situation.

CHAPTER 10

Your sexuality

Contents

Every woman fulfills her sexual nature in her own, unique way, influenced by her circumstances, desires, choices, beliefs, fantasies, needs, and self-imposed controls. Many women today are talking more openly about their sexuality and taking a more active role in fulfilling their sexual and emotional needs and desires.

Sexuality in a mature relationship involves caring, intimacy, communication, and bonding between two people who wish to fulfill each other's needs and desires. Sexuality also involves responsibility. An important part of this responsibility is protecting yourself and your partner from unwanted pregnancy and sexually transmitted diseases.

Exploring your sexuality

Sexual pleasure is infinitely variable. Taboos and restrictions on sexual activity still exist but many have lifted in recent years, particularly for women, giving them the freedom to explore their sexuality. Learning about your sexual responsiveness and what kinds of sights, sounds, physical contact, and fantasies excite you can add new dimensions to your sexual life.

Pleasurable sexual contact between a woman and another consenting adult covers a broad spectrum that varies among cultures and individuals. A woman's rearing and values influence her attitudes about sex and her capacity to enjoy it. For example, growing up with a religious tradition or in a family that represses all discussion of sex can make it difficult for a person to learn about sex or to relax and fully enjoy sexual encounters. Your parents' attitudes about sex can have an impact on your sexuality. Experiencing sexual abuse (see page 728) as a child or adult can undermine your ability to build loving, trusting sexual relationships. If you feel that your background or experiences are harming your sex life—or your life in general—you may want to seek the help of a qualified therapist (see page 194).

As you build a relationship with your partner, you may be faced with questions and decisions about how your sexual feelings can be accommodated. When you are deciding whether or not a sexual activity is appropriate for you, ask yourself these questions: Will it bring pleasure to me or my partner? Can it be harmful or painful to me or my partner? Will I regret it later? Will I feel exploited? Will it deepen or lessen our feelings for one another? Your answers to these questions will help guide you toward a sexual experience that is enjoyable for you and your partner and at the same time respectful of your needs and values as well as those of your partner.

BUILDING A HEALTHY SEXUAL RELATIONSHIP

Like any relationship, a sexual one inevitably has periods of confusion, disagreement, or disillusionment. In heterosexual relationships, some common problems arise from differences in how men and women think about sexuality and love. For example, women's and men's attitudes and physical needs are sometimes at odds. Some men may be more oriented than some women toward performance or achieving the goal of orgasm. Some women may need more touching or foreplay to become sexually aroused, and may need longer periods of touching to achieve orgasm.

Problems may arise when partners have different expectations of their sexual relationship. For some people, sex represents love or commitment or a means of establishing emotional intimacy. For others, sex is primarily a means of achieving physical fulfillment or relaxation. A couple's sexual expectations do not need to match precisely, but huge differences can cause tension. Whether you are just starting a relationship or are in the midst of one, it is always a good idea for you and your partner to discuss your feelings about the role of sex in your relationship.

When discussing your feelings, it is important to be honest with your partner at all times. Openness and honesty will help you develop mutual trust and respect and grow together in your relationship. On the other hand, such honesty may help you learn more quickly if this person is not right for you.

SEXUAL RESPONSE

The ways in which our body responds when we are attracted to another person are as different as people themselves. But generally, both women and men experience a three-phase pattern of sexual response: (1) desire, (2) excitement, and (3) orgasm. These phases do not occur for every woman or man during every sexual encounter and do not always include orgasm. Each person can choose to express or control these responses at any time.

While sexual response in both women and men is similar, the timing is significantly different (see page 294). A couple making love may not go through the three phases at the same time. While a few couples occasionally achieve simultaneous orgasm, most do not. Sometimes, one person may have an orgasm and the other does not. Only 20 to 30 percent of women climax during intercourse but they often do so before or after. (For descriptions and illustrations of the female reproductive system, see chapter 7.)

Female sexual response Understanding the stages your body goes through during your sexual response enables you to guide your partner during lovemaking to help you achieve sexual satisfaction.

Desire The desire stage of sexual response is similar for both women and men. In the desire stage, you become interested in having sex and feel an urge to engage in sexual activity. Consciously or unconsciously, you choose either to act on that urge or suppress it. Sexual desire, which is controlled by nerve centers in your brain, can be triggered by anything you interpret as having sexual meaning. If an opportunity to have sex is available and no external circumstances influence you to suppress the desire at that particular time, you reach a state of readiness to have sex that enables you to proceed to the next stage.

Excitement The excitement stage includes both physical and emotional responses you experience when you engage in sexual activity of any kind. Sexual excitement, or arousal, is enhanced by physical and emotional stimulation—touching, fondling, rubbing, and kissing, or arousing words and fantasies.

Your body undergoes many physical changes during the excitement phase that you may not be fully aware of. When you are sexually aroused, cells in your vaginal wall secrete a lubricating fluid. With stimulation, your nipples may become erect. You may become flushed as blood circulates more rapidly closer to the surface of your skin. As your pulse rate and blood pressure increase, your breathing may become more rapid and your muscles tense. Your clitoris may elevate and enlarge slightly and the upper part of your vagina grows longer and wider and the lower part narrows. Excitement can eventually build to the next stage—orgasm.

Orgasm An orgasm is a reflexive response to high levels of sexual excitement and is usually accompanied by a variety of pleasurable sensations and physical reactions. The intensity of orgasm can differ from one person to the next and from one time to the next in the same person. Physically, orgasm is a series of contractions of the muscles of the vagina and uterus. Each contraction lasts only a few seconds, and they are less than a second apart. These vaginal contractions may be accompanied by involuntary contractions of muscles in your hands, arms, legs, feet, spine, face, or neck. Your pulse, blood pressure, and breathing rate increase. With continued stimulation, some women may experience more than one orgasm.

After orgasm, or at the end of sexual stimulation, blood flows out of your genital area; pulse, blood pressure, and breathing rate return to normal. You usually feel relaxed and sometimes sleepy. If you do not have an orgasm, the relaxation process takes longer because there are no muscle contractions to help return blood from your genital area back into the general circulation.

Changes in sexuality during the menstrual cycle

Many women experience normal changes in sexual response that correspond to hormonal fluctuations during their menstrual cycle. Some women are more sexually responsive in the days before their period, in the middle of their cycle, or during menstruation.

Male sexual response Your male partner's sexual response progresses through the same three phases as yours. Recognizing the male anatomical changes that correspond to your own sexual response helps you participate fully in your shared sexual experience.

Desire The desire stage of sexual response is approximately the same for men as it is for women, although the physical or mental cues that spark the desire may be different. Men usually require less time to reach a state of readiness to have sex.

Excitement Blood pressure, heartbeat, and breathing increase during the early stage of sexual excitement. The penis fills with blood and becomes erect. The scrotum (the sac that contains the testicles) contracts and raises the testicles closer to the body. As blood pressure, pulse, and breathing continue to increase, the man's penis continues to harden, and the testicles elevate further. In some men, the head (tip) of the penis becomes larger and darker as the erection continues. A drop of clear fluid may appear at the tip of the penis. This fluid, called pre-ejaculate, contains some sperm and therefore can cause pregnancy. If you are using a barrier method of contraception such as a condom or diaphragm, it should be in place before this fluid comes in contact with your vagina.

Orgasm In males, orgasm includes two separate events: ejaculation (the emission of semen from the penis) and involuntary muscle contractions in the pelvic area. Ejaculation occurs after fluids and stored sperm combine inside a man's body to form semen, which passes out of his body through the urethra. Once semen is produced, ejaculation is reflexive and inevitable. Muscle contractions in the penis and urethra occur a few seconds later. It is these muscle contractions that a man feels as an orgasm. For a few men, ejaculation and orgasm are distinctly separate events, but, for most, they seem simultaneous. For this reason, withdrawal of the penis from the vagina before ejaculation is not a very reliable means of birth control.

After ejaculation, a man's body returns to its pre-excitement state. Blood gradually flows out of the penis and the erection softens. Heart rate and breathing slow and blood pressure returns to normal. Unlike women, men cannot reach orgasm again immediately. The length of time necessary to achieve another orgasm varies greatly from person to person; it is much shorter in teenage boys and longer in men over 50.

THE MALE REPRODUCTIVE SYSTEM

The most visible parts of the male reproductive system are the penis and testicles. The two testicles hang suspended in a pouch of skin called the scrotum. During sexual arousal, spongy tissue inside the penis becomes engorged with blood. The testicles produce the primary male sex hormone testosterone, which is released into the circulation. Sperm are also produced in the testicles. From the testicles, sperm travel through a long duct called the vas deferens into a pair of sacs called the seminal vesicles. The seminal vesicles produce a fluid that is added to the sperm to create semen—the whitish fluid that a man ejaculates at orgasm.

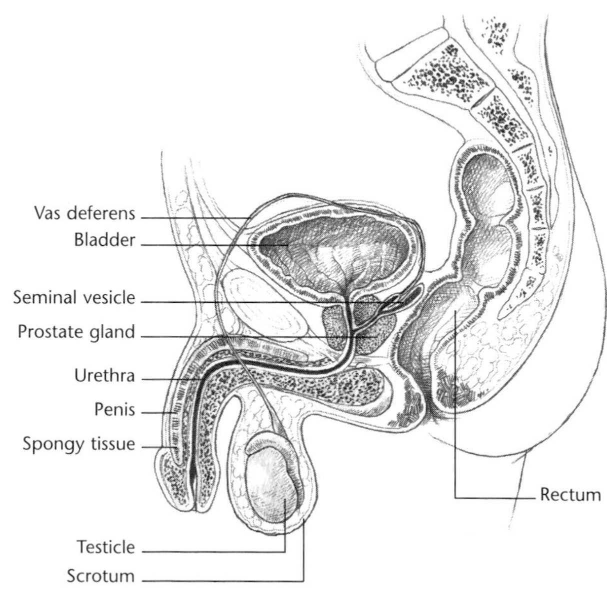

COMMUNICATION

The single most important way to improve your sexual experience with another person is to develop good communication so you can convey to each other what you like and dislike when making love. Sincere, gentle, sensitive directions from you to your partner are best. It takes time and practice to learn to communicate comfortably and well about your sexual needs and desires. You may want to try discussing your sexual relationship in a nonsexual setting in which there is less pressure to perform. Expressing what you are already enjoying in your sexual relationship is a positive way to start a conversation about making changes.

Communication does not always have to be verbal. A sigh of pleasure and body language—a touch on your partner's hand or a turn of your body—are good ways to tell your partner how and where you like to be touched during lovemaking. Guiding your partner's hand with your own can show your desire without your having to say a word.

LEARNING ABOUT EACH OTHER

There is much more to sex than intercourse. Many parts of the body are sexually responsive. Often, in the earliest stages of a relationship, any touch at all from a desired person can be wildly exciting. Later, as lovers explore and become familiar with each other's body, they discover where to touch to bring the greatest pleasure. Sharing intimate touch is an important part of making love, not only as a prelude to intercourse, but to bring sexual satisfaction to both partners.

Extended foreplay can help many women achieve orgasm (or even multiple orgasms) who would not otherwise be able to. With your partner, relax and warm up to making love with simple, nongenital body massage and progress to touching more intimate parts of each other's body. Although some parts of the body—called erogenous zones (especially

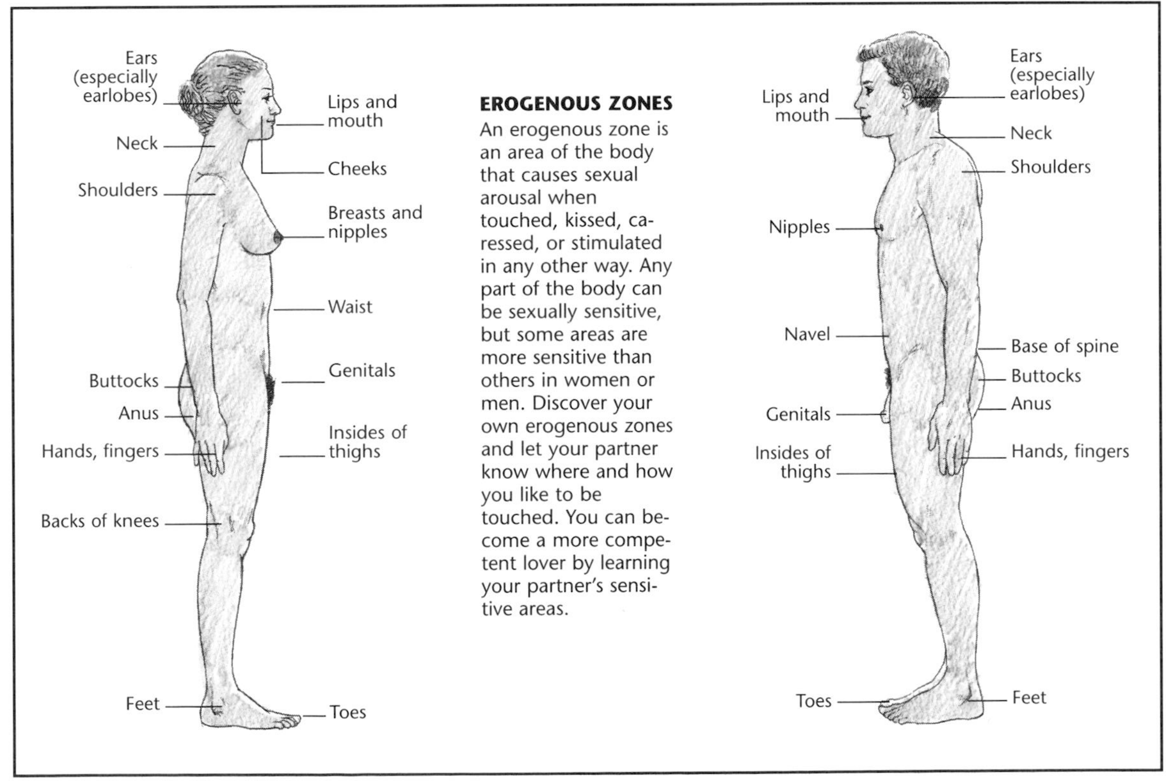

EROGENOUS ZONES
An erogenous zone is an area of the body that causes sexual arousal when touched, kissed, caressed, or stimulated in any other way. Any part of the body can be sexually sensitive, but some areas are more sensitive than others in women or men. Discover your own erogenous zones and let your partner know where and how you like to be touched. You can become a more competent lover by learning your partner's sensitive areas.

the breasts, genitals, mouth, and anus)—are especially responsive, sensual touch of virtually any part of the body can bring pleasure.

To reach intense sexual excitement and climax (orgasm), most men and women usually need direct stimulation of their genitals. Direct stimulation of the clitoris or penis often brings a person to climax. Women can get sexual pleasure from having their clitoris stimulated in a number of ways. It is a good idea to experiment with different techniques and patterns to find what is most stimulating for you. Try different lengths of time for stimulation, direct or indirect touching, and different sexual positions. Vibrators may also be a pleasurable form of stimulation for both partners.

The moments after making love can be a time of closeness for a couple—a time to share their most intimate feelings and thoughts. However, for some men and women, the intense intimacy of making love is overwhelming; they want to back away and regain some emotional distance. If their partner views this instead as a time for growing closer, disappointment and hurt feelings may result. If you are the partner who wants to maintain the intimacy, make your feelings known, so that you and your partner can gradually find a satisfying way to relate to each other after lovemaking.

ACHIEVING ORGASM

Some women achieve orgasm quickly and easily; others take longer. Some women never have an orgasm or have one only occasionally; they may be upset about it or feel inadequate. Sometimes a partner may be more concerned than the woman about her not having an orgasm during their lovemaking because he wants to please her. In fact, only about 20 to 30 percent of women have an orgasm solely as the result of intercourse; most have an orgasm only if their clitoris is directly stimulated. About 5 to 10 percent of all women never reach orgasm.

Many men do not realize that women need foreplay and stimulation of their clitoris to reach orgasm. No matter how long a man sustains his erection, the act of intercourse itself is often not sufficiently stimulating to bring a woman to climax. It may also take a woman longer to climax than a man, particularly if she has not had an extended period of foreplay. On the other hand, it is not always necessary for a woman to have an orgasm to feel sexually satisfied. Placing

Differences in timing of orgasm for men and women

On average, it takes a woman four times longer than a man to have an orgasm. A man can usually reach orgasm in less than 3 minutes; a woman usually needs about 14 minutes of stimulation before climaxing. A man can try to delay his orgasm to have one at the same time as his partner, but simultaneous orgasm is difficult to achieve and not necessary for sexual satisfaction.

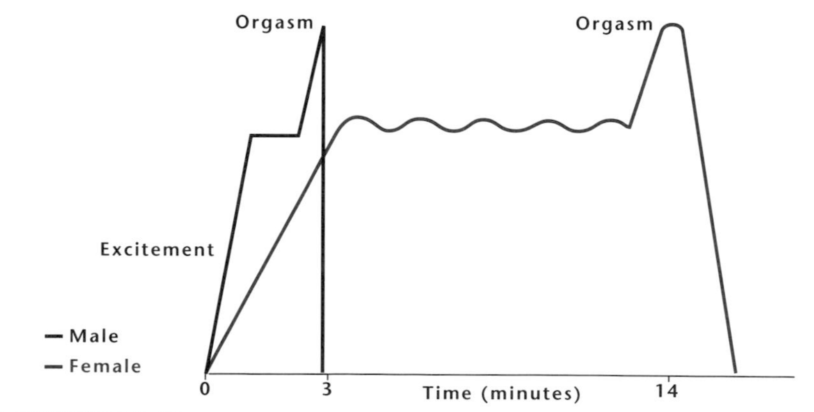

too much emphasis on achieving orgasm with every sexual encounter can lead to "performance anxiety" for both sexes. Sometimes it is enough to feel aroused, stimulated, close, and caressed. For both men and women, understanding the realities of the female orgasm can help dispel the damaging myths and reduce hurt and disappointment.

You may be able to increase your enjoyment of sex by doing pelvic-floor exercises (see page 238) to strengthen muscles in your pelvis. Some women find these exercises improve their ability to contract their vaginal muscles and give pleasure to both themselves and their partner during intercourse. Pelvic-floor exercises are especially useful in restoring muscle tone to the vagina after childbirth.

INTERCOURSE

Heterosexual intercourse usually involves penetration of the woman's vagina by the man's penis. The penis releases (ejaculates) a fluid called semen, which contains millions of sperm. Sperm can travel through the uterus into a fallopian tube, where a sperm can fertilize an egg if one is present. It is important to use contraception during sexual intercourse if you wish to prevent pregnancy. (For information about contraceptive methods, see chapter 11.)

Intercourse is the most common way for sexually transmitted diseases to be spread because disease-causing organisms may be present in vaginal fluids or semen. Therefore, if you are not in a stable, mutually monogamous relationship (see page 338), you need to practice safer sex (see page 171) by always using a latex or polyurethane male condom or a female condom with spermicide during intercourse. A male condom must be on the penis before it touches any part of your genital area because a small amount of fluid (called pre-ejaculate), which may contain disease-causing organisms, is often released before ejaculation.

A man's penis must be erect or semierect to enter the vagina. Sometimes it is necessary for you or your partner to hold his penis and guide it into your vagina as he pushes forward or you both move closer together. When you are sexually aroused, your vagina usually becomes lubricated, allowing the penis to enter comfortably. A lack of lubrication does not mean you are not aroused; all women are different and their degree of natural moisture may vary. If your vagina is not sufficiently lubricated before intercourse, you or your partner can massage your clitoris or other sexually responsive areas of your body to help stimulate you sexually. You can also use your own saliva or a water-based gel to lubricate your vagina. But keep in mind that water-based lubricants are not spermicides; if you use a barrier method of birth control, such as a diaphragm, that requires use of a spermicide, do not substitute the spermicide with a lubricant.

There are many different positions for intercourse. In some positions, partners face each other; in others, the woman's back is against her partner's chest. You can have intercourse lying down, sitting, crouching, or standing—whichever you prefer. When the woman is on top, she can control more of the motion. The woman-on-top position can be especially comfortable for women who are pregnant or for some people who are disabled. In some positions, the woman's partner can stimulate her clitoris by hand during intercourse.

ORAL SEX

Oral sex is stimulation of the genitals with the mouth and tongue. Oral stimulation of a man's penis is called fellatio; oral stimulation of a woman's genitals is called cunnilingus. A couple can perform oral sex on each other simultaneously or they can take turns. During oral sex, both partners can stimulate other parts of each other's body with their hands. For many women, having their clitoris stimulated by their partner's mouth and tongue is the most effective way to achieve orgasm.

Some sexually transmitted diseases—such as herpes (see page 342) or genital warts (see page 341)—can be transmitted during oral sex. Therefore, if you are not in a stable, mutually monogamous relationship (see page 338), you should always make sure your partner uses a latex or polyurethane condom when you are performing oral sex on your partner. You should wear a female condom to protect your partner during oral sex performed on you.

ANAL SEX

Anal sex is sexual stimulation of the rectal area, usually by penetration with a penis, finger, or vibrator. While many women have never tried anal intercourse, some engage in it regularly. Some women find anal intercourse painful and uncomfortable and do not choose to participate; their partner must respect this. Unlike the vagina, the anus and rectum produce no natural lubrication, so using saliva or a water-based lubricating gel is usually necessary to help ease penetration. (Oil-based lubricants can break down the latex in male condoms.) Letting out a long, relaxed breath as your partner's penis enters your rectum can also help reduce discomfort.

The tissues of the anus are delicate and prone to small tears, which can bleed and cause pain. Because these injuries can allow bacteria and viruses, including the AIDS virus (HIV), to enter and gain access to your bloodstream, your partner should always wear a latex condom during anal sex. Penetration and thrusting should be gentle. Your partner should wash his penis and hands thoroughly after anal intercourse and before any further contact with your vagina or mouth to avoid spreading infection.

MASTURBATION

Masturbation—touching your own genitals and other sexually responsive areas of your body for sexual pleasure and stimulation—is a healthy way to explore, enjoy, and express your natural sexual response, from arousal to orgasm. About 80 percent of women and a larger percentage of men masturbate at least occasionally. Masturbation is a safe and healthy way to explore your own erogenous zones and learn about your sexuality, which can enhance intimate sexual contact with another person.

Masturbation is a helpful way to find out what type of stimulation arouses you and what brings you to orgasm. You can then communicate this information to your partner or use it for your own pleasure. Becoming skilled at reaching orgasm through masturbation makes it easier for many women to climax during intercourse. Masturbation may also be a way of satisfying your sex drive when you have no partner, when your sex drive is greater than that of your partner, or when you choose to abstain from having sex with another person. Some people who have sexual partners masturbate as a pleasurable addition to their sexual relationship. Some people masturbate with their partners as part of lovemaking.

Learning to masturbate

If you are trying masturbation for the first time, it will be easier if you find a quiet time when you will not be interrupted. Do whatever it takes to get yourself in the mood—for example, play music or read an erotic passage in a book.

You can lie down or sit up. There is no "correct" position. Begin exploring your body with your hands to find out what feels good. Many women find that fantasizing about a person or situation is a pleasurable way to masturbate. You may want to moisten your fingers with saliva or with a water-based lubricating gel. Some women stimulate their clitoris with a vibrator, which you can buy in many drugstores. Vibrators are often sold as massagers. Other women use a stream of water from a shower or tub to stimulate their genitals. Do whatever works for you. Give yourself as much time as you need. Continue as long as it feels good and you are enjoying the sensation. It is not always necessary to reach orgasm during masturbation.

Dimensions of sexuality

Every woman's unique experience of her sexuality is influenced by factors such as her age, her physical condition, and her sexual orientation. These factors affect a woman's sexual activity as well as her feelings about her sexual self. A mutually satisfying sexual relationship with another person can enhance her enjoyment of life.

SEX AND TEENAGERS

Adolescence is a time of sexual awakening, curiosity, and exploration. The teen years bring on many emotions connected with friendship, romance, early attachments, and desires. These feelings are new and exciting, and they provide the basic structure on which to build fulfilling, mature relationships later in life.

Adolescent girls may find that fantasy and masturbation provide a safe and healthy outlet for their sexual feelings. Masturbation is extremely common for both sexes at this age and can help young people learn about their sexual responses in preparation for a mature sexual relationship with another person.

Adolescence is the time to form your own identity, or sense of who you are, including your sexual identity. This means learning about your own sexuality by reading, talking to friends, and forming relationships. You do not need to have intercourse in order to explore your sexuality. In fact, your first sexual feelings and thoughts may arise years before you first have sex. Curiosity and experimentation are normal, positive stages of growing up.

Often, a girl knows by her early teens whether she is sexually attracted to people of the opposite sex or of her own sex. Some young women may feel confused if they are attracted, in different circumstances, to members of both sexes. Having sexual feelings for members of the same sex during adolescence does not necessarily mean that a girl is or will be a lesbian.

Adolescence can also be a time of confusion, guilt, unplanned pregnancy, sexually transmitted diseases, or damaged self-esteem. Many of these problems stem from conflicting messages about sexuality that adolescent girls receive from parents, friends, boys, and the media. They are told to be popular, attractive, and sexy and, at the same time, to be "good," which usually means not having sex. Boys often assume that girls who look and act sexy want to engage in sex when, in fact, they may only be seeking approval from their peers. If you have questions or are troubled about any of these issues, talking to a trusted adult, such as a school counselor or a relative, can be helpful.

The age at which girls are ready for their first sexual relationship varies widely, and only a girl herself can judge her own level of maturity. In the US, the average age of first sexual intercourse is 16 but many young women wait until they are older. Although many teenagers think that having sex is a sign of being grown up, waiting until you are ready to have sex is, in fact, a more mature course to take. It means you are able to make an important decision for yourself without being pressured by your peers. Do not let anyone—male or female—pressure you into having sex before you feel ready. You will have a much more meaningful relationship with a person who is willing to wait until you are ready.

Learn how to set limits for yourself—to say "no" to sex when it seems dangerous or inappropriate, or simply because you are not interested or ready. It can be hard to say "no" to sexual activities, particularly if you are with someone you really like or love. Be firm. Try to avoid being in situations you might not be able to handle, such as being alone with a person to whom you are sexually attracted—especially if you have been drinking alcohol or using other drugs. Alcohol and other drugs can impair your judgment. Think ahead about what you might do or say if the situation arises.

If you make the decision to include sex in your life, do so carefully. Sex is a

Questions teenagers ask about sex

Q Is something wrong with me if I masturbate?

A Masturbation is natural and healthy. The majority of people masturbate, whether they are male or female, heterosexual or homosexual, young or old. For adolescents, masturbation is a safe, harmless way to explore sexual sensations.

Q If my boyfriend gets aroused and I don't have sex with him, will this harm his genitals?

A Men and boys frequently become aroused and have erections without having sex or climaxing. After several minutes, the erection goes down. Your boyfriend will have no permanent damage, and you are not being a tease for saying "no."

Q During intercourse, if my partner withdraws his penis from my vagina before he ejaculates, will that prevent me from getting pregnant?

A Withdrawing the penis is not an effective means of birth control. Some sperm-containing fluid often leaks from the penis before ejaculation. This fluid contains enough sperm to make you pregnant.

Q Can I get a sexually transmitted disease from someone who is a virgin?

A It is always best to protect yourself from disease by using a latex or polyurethane male condom or a female condom. A person who has never had sex before probably cannot transmit an infection. But keep in mind that people do not always tell the truth about their past sexual experiences.

special part of a mature, loving, responsible relationship between consenting partners. Before having sex, discuss with your partner how you will protect yourselves from unwanted pregnancy and sexually transmitted diseases. Ask your partner if he is willing to use a condom *every* time you have sex. If you and your partner are too embarrassed to talk about these issues, you are probably not ready to take on the responsibility of sex in your relationship.

For help with these important problems, check the phone book for a local branch of Planned Parenthood, a national organization that provides education about reproductive issues and medical care for sexually active women. Planned Parenthood is a reliable source of information, and it will keep your questions and medical history confidential. Talking with parents or a trusted adult about the emotional aspects of sexuality and a sexual relationship can be helpful.

SEX AND THE OLDER WOMAN

Our culture sometimes perpetuates the myth that older women are neither interested in sex, nor sexually desirable. In reality, most women are capable of enjoying a full range of sexual activities throughout their life. The most common reasons for not having sex are lack of a sexual partner or health problems. Among older adults who enjoy an active sex life, the majority of women and men say sex feels as good or better than when they were younger. In fact, the changes that come with age offer an opportunity for many couples to become more sexually compatible. A man who takes longer to achieve orgasm himself may give his partner more time and stimulation, which can help her reach climax. Without the constant distraction and demands of children, or worries about birth control, a couple may find themselves in a stage of life that is much more conducive to sexual intimacy. Retirement can allow a couple time for morning or afternoon lovemaking sessions.

Changes with age Orgasms continue to be part of a woman's life as she gets older, although they may take longer to achieve. After menopause, the drop in a woman's level of the female hormone estrogen causes her vagina to become lubricated more slowly and it may become smaller and less elastic. This lack of lubrication and elasticity can cause pain during intercourse (see page 303).

Vaginal dryness can be remedied in a number of ways, including the use of water-based lubricating gels or estrogen creams that you apply directly inside your vagina (see page 355). Treatment with estrogen (hormone replacement therapy, see page 359) after menopause significantly reduces dryness and thinning of vaginal tissue. Estrogen improves circulation to tissues in the vagina and helps the skin layers thicken. The increased lubrication reduces pain during intercourse, allowing you to regain your enjoyment of sex.

In older men, a decline with age in the male sex hormone testosterone can reduce sexual desire. Genital sensitivity can also decrease with age. Longer and more direct stimulation of the penis is usually necessary to produce a firmer erection. While some older men find they can maintain an erection longer than they could when they were younger, others find their erections last for shorter periods. A few men can no longer achieve or maintain an adequate erection. However, both older and younger men can have an orgasm and ejaculate without achieving a full erection.

Health considerations Poor health can hinder your sex life but, in many cases, you can do a great deal to enhance your enjoyment of sex. For example, if you have arthritis that causes pain in your joints, taking pain medication before lovemaking can help. You or your partner may be inhibited or embarrassed about making love if either of you has urinary incontinence (involuntary leaking of urine). This common problem can often be cured or treated (see page 540); talk to your doctor.

Impotence (the long-term inability to maintain an erection; see page 304) is sometimes a symptom of illnesses such as diabetes or blood circulation problems. Some older people with heart disease develop impotence from worrying about having a heart attack during intercourse. This is not a danger for most people, but check with your doctor. An active sex life may actually benefit a person with heart disease. Still, people who have chest pain from heart disease may choose to take nitroglycerin (a drug that widens the coronary arteries) as a precaution shortly before making love to prevent chest pain.

Older people are also more likely than younger people to be taking one or more medications that may affect their sex life. Many drugs that are used to control high blood pressure can reduce sex drive in both men and women and cause impotence in men. Several medications, including those used to treat disorders such as anxiety or depression (see page 594), can decrease sex drive and the ability to achieve orgasm.

Some drugs used to treat digestive disorders or some mental disorders may impair sexual functioning. If you suspect that the medication you or your partner is taking may be interfering with sex drive or sexual functioning, talk to your doctor. He or she may be able to change your prescription or reduce the dose of medication you are taking.

Adapting to change Sometimes the changes that occur in men and women as they age cause them to abandon their sex life rather than adapt it to their new circumstances. Modifying lovemaking techniques, learning to communicate better, or using alternative means to achieve sexual pleasure (such as mutual massage, masturbation, or vibrators) can often keep an older couple's sexual relationship active and fulfilling. If you are unhappy with your sex life and are unable to improve it on your own, you may want to seek help from a qualified sex therapist.

With or without sexual intercourse, the quality of your life with your partner is enhanced by physical closeness. Affection and intimacy are very beneficial stress reducers. If health problems prevent you from being able to have sexual intercourse, you and your partner can still maintain an intimate relationship through talking, kissing, and caressing.

For women, one of the major obstacles to continuing an active sex life in older age is the lack of a partner. At age 65, women outnumber men by 25 percent; at age 80, there are twice as many women as men. For older women who would like to be sexually active, finding a male partner, older or younger, may be difficult. Some women find that masturbation (see page 296) helps fulfill their sexual needs during this time. For other women, close relationships with family and friends and physical gestures of affection such as hugs can help fill some of these needs.

SEX AND THE DISABLED

Many people who are or have become disabled find their sex life less active than they would like. People who have lived with a disability all their life may find their opportunity for sexual contact limited by their circumstances and by other people's assumptions that they are uninterested in or incapable of having sex. In reality, everyone has sexual needs and desires and sexual activity can be a fulfilling part of every person's life.

Physical challenges can affect your ability to meet your sexual needs. Most sexually active people who have a disabling accident or illness experience a major decrease in their sexual activity. However, for some people this is only temporary. A woman who has had a stroke may have difficulty positioning herself for intercourse or her sexual sensitivity may be reduced. A woman with arthritis may find some sexual positions painful to her joints. Men and women who have injuries to their spinal cord often cannot experience orgasm. It is sometimes the medication that is used to treat a physical disability rather than the disability itself that interferes with a person's sex drive or ability to reach orgasm.

If you are unhappy with your sex life, you may want to discuss it with your doctor or a qualified sex therapist (see page 305). A doctor can evaluate whether any aspect of your treatment, such as medication you are taking or surgery you have had, is interfering with your sexual desire or performance. A qualified sex therapist can recommend possible alternative techniques for making love.

Fulfilling sexual needs There are many ways to fulfill your sexual needs, even if you are disabled. Remember to use birth control if you are still fertile. If you are unable to insert a diaphragm or other contraceptive device before having intercourse, have your partner insert it for you. You might try the following to increase your sexual pleasure:

- If you have pain in your joints or muscles, try taking a hot bath before lovemaking. You might also try positions for lovemaking (such as lying on your side for intercourse) that do not require you to support your partner's weight. Ask your doctor about pain-relief medications you can take before having sex.
- If lack of vaginal lubrication is a problem, use water-soluble lubricants to make intercourse more comfortable. Check with your doctor to find out if any medications you are taking may be affecting your sexual arousal or vaginal lubrication.
- If you are having difficulty achieving orgasm, try using a vibrator, which may provide more intense stimulation of your clitoris. Ask your doctor if any medications you are taking may be affecting your ability to achieve orgasm.
- If you have limited use of your hands, try using a vibrator to stimulate your clitoris. You can probably still have intercourse or oral sex.
- If you lack sensation in your pelvis resulting from an injury to your spinal cord, parts of your body above the paralyzed area may become more responsive to touch. You may prefer making love in ways other than vaginal intercourse. If your injuries require you to wear an ostomy (a bag attached to the skin to collect urine or feces), emptying your bladder and bowels before engaging in sexual activity reduces the chance of an accident and increases your confidence.

Fulfilling sexual needs if your partner is disabled If your partner is disabled, do not assume he or she has no interest in sex or ability to be aroused. Even if a man can no longer have an erection, he can have emotional erections and mental orgasms. Here are some ways you and your partner may continue to have an enjoyable sex life:

- Communicate. Find out what feels good to your partner and tell him or her what to do to help you achieve sexual satisfaction. If communication is too difficult, talking with a counselor may help. If your partner is reluctant to see a therapist, go on your own.
- Focus on your partner's erotic "hot spots." Caress and kiss the parts of his or her body that he or she can feel. If your partner is paralyzed from the waist down, kissing his or her neck or nipples can give a sensation similar to that of oral sex.
- Even if your usual role is caregiver, let your partner be in charge some of the time during lovemaking. This is a good time to let him or her feel less dependent. You can benefit from using sexual fantasies to get you into the mood for sex.
- If your partner cannot have intercourse, try different positions for sexual activity. For example, with you on top, try stimulating your clitoris with your hand or with a vibrator while moving in the same way you would during sexual intercourse. This can be visually stimulating for your partner and erotic for both of you.
- Find ways for your partner to help you achieve orgasm. Do not feel guilty if you climax when your partner cannot. You are both likely to enjoy your orgasm and your partner can feel good about participating in and contributing to your sexual pleasure.

LESBIAN SEXUALITY

A woman who is homosexual, or lesbian, is sexually attracted to other women. Sexual orientation varies so widely that many scientists question the usefulness of labels such as homosexual, heterosexual, or bisexual. Many men and women exhibit a range of sexual behavior that may include one or more sexual experiences with a person of the same sex. One of the most common fantasies among heterosexuals is to have sex with a person of the same sex, even though they may never act on it.

Estimates of the percentage of women who prefer other women as sexual partners are inexact. Most experts believe that sexual orientation is not an absolute, and includes not just sexual experience but sexual fantasies and self-identity as well. Sexual orientation may change or shift back and forth over time. For example, a woman who identifies herself as a lesbian may have had heterosexual experiences, just as a woman who considers herself to be exclusively heterosexual may have had sexual experiences with other women. Women of either orientation may have sexual fantasies that include partners of the opposite or same gender, or both, but may not act on these fantasies.

Many of the activities that heterosexual couples consider a prelude to sexual intercourse—including kissing and caressing the breasts and genital area—are central in sexual relations between women. Lesbians bring each other to climax in a variety of ways, including oral sex and the use of vibrators.

Many of the same diseases, such as genital herpes, that can be transmitted during heterosexual encounters can also be spread during lesbian lovemaking. (See page 337 for guidelines on safer sex.)

The biggest problems facing lesbians may be social ones—including dealing with the negative attitudes of parents and other family members, friends, and coworkers. Parents may assume that something they did while raising their child caused her to become homosexual. In fact, scientific evidence shows that parents have very little influence on their children's sexual orientation. Research also indicates that children raised by homosexual parents are no more likely to grow up to be homosexual than are children raised by heterosexuals.

Many women who are lesbians keep their sexual orientation confidential rather than deal with possible disapproval or maliciousness. On the other hand, a woman may choose to tell others she is a lesbian and be willing to deal with their reaction. Either course can be difficult. Developing a network of friends within the lesbian community can provide the emotional and social support you may need.

Sexual problems

More and more people, usually as a couple, are seeking help for sexual problems. The most common sexual problems are lack of desire, difference in sex drive, difficulty achieving orgasm, painful intercourse, premature ejaculation, and impotence. These conditions can have physical or emotional causes or a combination of both, and can often be successfully treated.

If you and your partner are having sexual problems, you may wish to consult your doctor, who can rule out or treat physical causes. For example, painful intercourse can result from a vaginal infection (vaginitis), insufficient vaginal lubrication, irritation of the external genitals, or other physical problems. Some sexual difficulties can arise from something as basic as fatigue from a busy lifestyle.

Some sexual problems result from one or both partner's psychological inhibitions or an earlier experience of sexual abuse. In many cases, a sexual problem is rooted in other aspects of a couple's relationship. If sexual problems arise between you and your partner, you may consider seeing a qualified sex therapist, who can help you identify the cause of the problem and regain a satisfying sex life. The goal of sex therapy is to solve a mutual problem, not to focus on either partner. The patient is the relationship itself.

LACK OF DESIRE

Low libido, or diminished sexual desire, is the most common sexual problem. Nearly half of all people who seek sex therapy have problems with low libido. Lack of sexual desire occurs in both men and women and has many causes.

Physical causes Lack of interest in sex can have physical causes. For example, illness or cancer treatment (chemotherapy or radiation) can affect a person's desire to have sex. Some medications used to treat high blood pressure, peptic ulcers, anxiety, or depression can reduce libido. Your sex drive can also be reduced when your supply of estrogen declines, which occurs when you go through menopause or have your ovaries (your source of estrogen) removed surgically. Hormone replacement therapy (HRT; see page 359) can correct this problem in most women. In some women, adding small amounts of the male hormone testosterone to HRT increases their sexual desire. Lack of desire in a person who has previously enjoyed sex may be a symptom of depression (see page 594). In many cases, the depression can be treated with medication and counseling.

During or after pregnancy or while breast-feeding, most women experience many physical, hormonal, and emotional changes that affect their sexuality. Some women may have less interest in sex at these times, while others may feel even more erotic. The physical demands of pregnancy and caring for an infant often cause fatigue, which can diminish a woman's interest in sex. It is important for both partners to integrate their new roles as parents with their feelings toward each other and the place of lovemaking in their relationship.

Psychological causes Lack of sexual desire can often have psychological causes. Some common causes of problems with sexual desire include ongoing conflict or lack of intimacy or trust between partners, low self-esteem, poor body image, unrealistic ideas about what sex should be, pressure from one partner to have sex more frequently than the other partner wants, distraction, or boredom. A hectic lifestyle with too many responsibilities can cause fatigue and contribute to or cause loss of interest in sex. Some people have difficulty readjusting from the extreme excitement of courtship to the day-to-day character of a long-term relationship and the often reduced level of passion.

The use of fantasy during sexual relations can boost a lack of sexual desire. If you find that certain erotic scenes in books or movies arouse you, or that some imaginary situations stimulate you, try using them to spark sexual desire during intimate moments with your partner.

DIFFERENCE IN SEX DRIVE

A difference in sex drive between two partners can often cause a problem in a couple's sexual relationship. One partner may feel that having sex once a week is enough while the other would like to have sex every day. The intensity of passion often cools as a relationship matures, which may disappoint one of the partners. When differences in sex drive cause trouble, it is a good idea for the couple to talk about the change and together come to a solution or compromise. If left to fester, these issues can lead to deeper problems in the relationship. For example, the partner who feels under constant pressure to have sex more often than he or she wants may lose all interest in sex.

Treatment If you and your partner cannot work out the problem together, you may want to seek help from a counselor who is trained in sex therapy. Treatment may involve evaluating each partner's feelings about the relationship and negotiating a mutually agreeable pattern of lovemaking. Treatment may also include helping the partner with lower sex drive identify sexual triggers that can increase his or her libido. The partner with higher sex drive might identify the needs that sex fulfills for him or her and may be encouraged to use masturbation to meet those needs, or to find ways other than sex to fulfill them.

Two partners may also learn to take turns pleasing each other sexually when

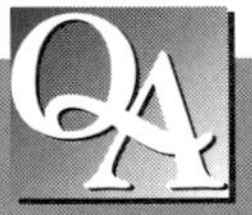

QUESTIONS WOMEN ASK
SEXUAL DESIRE

Q Is it true that men want to have sex more often than women?

A Although it is commonly believed that men have stronger sex drives than women, in fact, the desire for sex is equal in men and women.

Q Can sexual fantasies be dangerous?

A For most people, fantasies are private, safe, positive experiences that allow them to explore their sexuality and stimulate sexual desire. Some people have sexual fantasies that involve behavior that is socially unacceptable, dangerous, or even against the law. These fantasies may be healthy too, so long as you do not feel a need to act them out. If you feel a strong or growing desire to act out a fantasy that is dangerous or illegal, seek help immediately from a psychiatrist.

one of them is not in the mood. One partner sexually stimulates the other and does not necessarily expect to be stimulated to orgasm in return. Couples may also learn to view sex as a many-faceted activity rather than one activity that must go from start to finish. Engaging in less goal-oriented sexual activity than intercourse can help partners with unequal sex drives find a mutually satisfying solution. Alternatives to intercourse may include mutual, side-by-side stimulation or solo masturbation that is viewed by the other partner.

DIFFICULTY ACHIEVING ORGASM

Most women cannot reach orgasm through sexual intercourse alone; they require direct or indirect stimulation of their clitoris. Many couples use positions for intercourse in which the man or woman can stimulate the woman's clitoris directly to help her achieve orgasm. Many women find it easier to stimulate themselves to orgasm during sex using the same technique they use when they masturbate.

About 5 to 10 percent of women have never had an orgasm through any type of sexual activity; this condition is called anorgasmia. These women may benefit from counseling by a qualified sex therapist. Researchers have found that a woman's inability to reach orgasm is sometimes linked to a wide variety of psychological factors, such as low self-esteem or an inability to trust others, or to physical factors such as fatigue.

Treatment Therapists usually use a combination of counseling and masturbation therapy to treat anorgasmia. The goal is to help a woman learn what kind of stimulation can bring her to climax and how to relax and use sexual fantasy during sex. She first learns to enjoy the sensations of touching without feeling pressured to achieve orgasm or engage in intercourse. When she knows what stimulates her, she can use that knowledge to achieve sexual satisfaction.

Male difficulties A man can also experience an occasional inability to ejaculate or achieve orgasm, even though he can have an erection. This condition, called retarded ejaculation, is usually no cause for concern but, if it continues, he should see a doctor to rule out a physical problem. Retarded ejaculation is usually caused by such medical problems as overuse of alcohol or drugs, advanced diabetes (see page 620), nerve damage, or some medications. This problem is also common during fertility treatment when a couple is trying to conceive because the man is under pressure to perform at a specific time, on a specific day, following a set of instructions. He may also feel ambivalent about becoming a father. In this case, a sex therapist may be able to help him deal with his emotions after physical causes have been ruled out by his doctor.

PAINFUL INTERCOURSE

Painful intercourse for a woman can have a number of causes, but insufficient lubrication of the vagina is the most common. The lack of lubrication causes painful friction as the penis enters the vagina. In many cases, poor lubrication is caused by lack of arousal. If you are having difficulty becoming sexually aroused, your partner may need to spend more time on foreplay to stimulate you sufficiently before attempting intercourse. You may want to learn more about the sexual fantasies and types of stimulation that arouse you. Have your partner massage your clitoris with water-based lubricant, and apply it to your partner's penis and the entrance to your vagina to help reduce discomfort during intercourse. If none of these measures is effective, you may want to seek counseling from a qualified sex therapist (see page 305).

After menopause, drying of vaginal tissue and a lack of lubrication can make intercourse painful. Some women use hormone replacement therapy (HRT; see page 359) to prevent vaginal dryness. Estrogen creams (see page 360) applied directly inside the vagina replenish the lubricating cells. Using water-based lubricating gels can also help relieve discomfort during sexual intercourse.

Because a wide variety of other conditions can also cause painful intercourse, ask your gynecologist or family doctor about any pain that is not relieved by increasing lubrication of your vagina. It is important to resolve the problem of painful intercourse as soon as possible because, once intercourse is associated with pain, it can become a pattern. The anticipation of pain can inhibit sexual arousal, which reduces lubrication of the vagina, causing further pain and sometimes leading to an avoidance of sexual activity altogether.

Vaginitis (inflammation of tissues in the vagina; see page 216) is another common cause of painful intercourse. It is important for a woman with vaginitis to see her doctor for a diagnosis. Because vaginitis is often caused by infection with a fungus or with bacteria, it is easy to treat with medication. Vaginitis can also be caused by irritation from chemicals in soaps, lotions, and douches.

Vaginismus—a strong, involuntary tightening of the vaginal muscles—is another cause of painful intercourse. Muscle contractions in the outer vagina can make it extremely painful when a penis, finger, tampon, or speculum (a medical instrument used in pelvic examinations) is introduced into the vagina. Vaginismus can result from an anticipation of pain, lack of sexual knowledge, or fear of pregnancy. The condition can also be a reaction to an earlier, traumatic sexual experience, such as abuse, incest, or rape.

Treatment If a medical examination finds no physical cause of your pain during intercourse, a sex therapist may be able to help you overcome an emotional problem. Therapy usually involves desensitizing your vaginal area to touch through simple exercises you can do at home, such as inserting a finger or tampon into your vagina. If the therapist helps you find the underlying cause of the problem, he or she will work with you to design a treatment program to help you overcome it.

PREMATURE EJACULATION

Premature ejaculation is ejaculation that occurs either before the penis enters the vagina or before both partners have had an opportunity to enjoy intercourse fully. Premature ejaculation usually starts with a man's first sexual experiences and may persist for years. This condition occurs because a man has not learned to control his ejaculation reflex. The cause of premature ejaculation is usually not physical and treatment is often successful, especially when the man's partner participates. In some cases, men are so frustrated by their inability to delay ejaculation that they become impotent. For this reason, it is important to seek treatment as soon as possible.

Treatment One common treatment for premature ejaculation is the stop-start technique. In this technique, the couple begin their usual sexual activity and proceed until the man has a full erection. He lies on his back, closes his eyes, and focuses on the erotic sensations he is feeling while his partner stimulates his penis with her hand. When he feels near orgasm, he tells his partner to stop. When the urge to ejaculate goes away in a few seconds, he tells his partner to start stimulating him again, until just before ejaculation. The couple repeats this four times; on the fourth time, the man ejaculates. By focusing on his increasing excitement and learning to recognize the signs of impending ejaculation, the man learns to control ejaculation without using the stop-start technique. He then becomes more self-confident during sexual intercourse.

IMPOTENCE

Impotence is the long-term inability to maintain an erection or to keep it long enough to achieve sexual intercourse. Almost all men are occasionally unable to maintain an erection. However, when this becomes a pattern, it can harm a couple's sex life and relationship and both partners' self-esteem. The woman may feel she is not sexually attractive enough to her partner.

Impotence affects nearly 10 million men in the US and is more common among older men. However, impotence is not an inevitable consequence of aging and it is treatable. Physical causes of impotence that result from aging include changes in blood vessels and nerves of the penis. Some medications that many older men take (such as medication for high blood pressure) can cause impotence. Changing the medication or dose may help. Because impotence can often be treated, it is important to see a urologist (a doctor who specializes in treating

IMPOTENCE
The inability to maintain an erection can happen occasionally to any man, but sometimes it becomes a continuing problem. Erection occurs when two strips of spongy tissue that run the whole length of the penis fill with blood, causing the penis to become hard. If physical factors (such as illness) or psychological factors (such as stress) prevent this from happening, the penis remains soft and sexual intercourse is impossible.

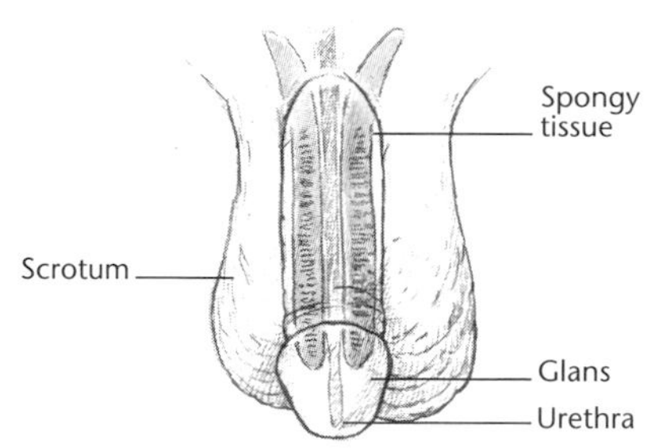

disorders of the urinary and genital tracts) for an accurate diagnosis.

Half of all cases of temporary impotence are caused by stress or anxiety. If a man cannot relax, it is difficult for him to focus on sexual stimulation and have an erection. Some men may experience impotence after using even small amounts of alcohol.

Treatment Before recommending treatment for impotence, a doctor will first rule out a physical cause. He or she will ask the man about any medications he is taking. He or she will also ask if he has erections when he wakes up in the morning, if he notices one when he awakens during the night, or if he can achieve an erection during masturbation. If he can have an erection at times other than during intercourse, the problem is probably not physical. In this case, counseling with a qualified sex therapist may be helpful.

If a man is not able to achieve orgasm at any time, a urologist will look for

Choosing a sex therapist

It is not easy to discuss your sex life with a stranger, but to professionals who are trained in the field of sexual dysfunction, sex is like any other aspect of physical or mental health that requires appropriate diagnosis and treatment. Sex therapists have information and treatments that may help you.

If you or your partner has a sexual problem, a good place to start seeking a solution is to ask your doctor to refer you to a qualified therapist. Keep in mind that some sexual problems that may appear to be psychological in origin—such as lack of sexual desire, difficulty reaching orgasm, or impotence—may have physical causes, such as a medication you are taking. A therapist will first rule out any physical causes or send you to an internist to do so.

If you are not comfortable asking your doctor for a referral to a sex therapist, or if he or she does not know a therapist to recommend, call your state medical society or the social work office of a major hospital or medical school in your area for listings of counselors who are trained in treating sexual dysfunction.

When you contact a therapist, briefly describe your problem and ask if he or she has experience treating it. Ask about his or her training, how many years he or she has been practicing, and how many cases like yours he or she has treated. You are looking for a person with a doctoral degree (PhD or PsyD), medical degree (MD), or degree in social work (MSW, MA, or MS) from an accredited university or college. Ask the therapist if he or she is licensed by the state. You should also ask about the fee for the initial visit.

At your first appointment:

- Briefly state your problem and ask what professional training the therapist has that would qualify him or her to treat your problem.
- Ask if the therapist regularly refers people to other professionals for testing when necessary.
- Ask how many cases similar to yours the therapist has treated and the outcome of those cases.
- Ask what kinds of treatment programs the therapist usually recommends for someone with a problem such as yours. He or she may not be able to give you a precise answer but should be able to provide a general idea of the treatment that may be involved.
- Ask what you can expect in the way of number of appointments, length of treatment, and fees. Go to three visits and then evaluate how you feel about the therapist and the treatment you are receiving.
- Ask what kinds of activity will take place during therapy sessions.
- If you feel uncomfortable with the therapist's training, level of expertise, or professional manner, continue your search.

physical causes. Physical causes of impotence include nerve damage caused by diabetes (see page 620), heart and blood vessel disorders that block the flow of blood to the penis, some medications, some surgical procedures such as surgery for cancer of the prostate (the gland that produces semen), radiation therapy or chemotherapy for cancer, spinal cord injuries, multiple sclerosis (a progressive disease that affects the brain and spinal cord), or alcoholism or other forms of drug abuse.

Treatment for impotence depends on the cause. Hormone replacement, use of a device called a vacuum pump to achieve erection, injections of muscle relaxants, or surgery are among the treatments available. The man's partner must be cooperative and accepting of the form of treatment; otherwise, it can cause conflict rather than improve the relationship.

CHAPTER 11

Preventing pregnancy

Contents

Contraception—controlling fertility to prevent pregnancy—is nothing new. For centuries, sexually active women have looked for ways to prevent unplanned pregnancy. Today, women and their partners have a wide variety of safe, reliable contraceptive options available to them.

Some of these choices require a doctor's prescription, while others are available over-the-counter. Some require your partner's cooperation before the act of intercourse, while others are solely the woman's responsibility. Some require a conscious effort before intercourse takes place, while others allow for more spontaneity. Such a range of choices means that, at any age and under almost any circumstances, a woman can take responsibility for avoiding an accidental pregnancy and its consequences.

Still, in the US, more than half of all pregnancies are unplanned, including most pregnancies among teenagers. For any woman, an unplanned pregnancy can derail plans for the future. It is essential to educate yourself about various contraceptive methods that can prevent you from getting pregnant when you do not want to be.

Choosing a contraceptive

All contraceptive methods have the same goal—preventing pregnancy—but each has advantages and disadvantages. Whether you are choosing a method of birth control for the first time or reevaluating your current method, the more you know about your options, the easier it will be to find a method of contraception tailored to your particular needs.

Contraception works best when both you and your sexual partner agree on the choice of method and take responsibility for its use. But when sharing the responsibility is not possible, do not let your partner's reluctance prevent you from taking charge. You are the one, after all, who will bear most of the consequences of an unplanned pregnancy.

When evaluating information about the side effects and health risks of various birth-control methods, keep in mind that your most risky choice is not to make any choice at all. At any age, pregnancy and childbirth are far more dangerous to your health than any form of contraception.

QUESTIONS TO ASK

When deciding which method of contraception is right for you, consider questions such as these:

- **Does the contraceptive provide protection against sexually transmitted diseases?** Only a latex or polyurethane male condom or a female condom provides effective—although not complete—protection against sexually transmitted diseases (STDs). Diaphragms, cervical caps, and spermicides provide some protection against STDs, but each must be combined with a condom to be most effective. Natural family planning methods and contraceptives that use hormones, such as the birth-control pill, provide no protection against STDs. If there is any possibility that you are not in a stable, mutually monogamous relationship (you and your partner are having sex only with each other; see page 338), you should always use a latex or polyurethane male condom or a female condom with spermicide in addition to your usual method of birth control *every time you have sex.*
- **How reliable is the method in preventing pregnancy?** Along with surgical sterilization (vasectomy in men and tubal ligation in women, see pages 328 and 327, respectively), methods that use hormones, such as the birth-control pill and hormone implants, provide the most reliable contraception when used correctly. If you cannot take the pill for a medical reason (see page 312), so-called barrier contraceptives such as the diaphragm and condom are reliable if you use them correctly and consistently with spermicide every time you have sexual intercourse. Other methods, such as spermicides used alone, are much less effective in preventing pregnancy. Natural family planning methods (see page 329) can be fairly effective, but only when practiced with a great degree of diligence and accuracy. The effectiveness of the withdrawal method of birth control

depends on the man's ability to withdraw his penis from the vagina before he ejaculates. In addition, a fluid (called pre-ejaculate) that is released before ejaculation contains sperm.

■ **Is the birth-control method convenient?** Convenience often depends on your circumstances. For example, the birth-control pill or another method that uses hormones may be most convenient if you prefer not to interrupt lovemaking to use a contraceptive. But if you have sex infrequently, you may feel that taking a pill every day is not as easy as using a condom and spermicide, or a diaphragm, when needed.

■ **Is the contraceptive easy for you to use?** There are many reasons why contraception fails. You may forget to take your birth-control pills as prescribed or to reinsert spermicide into your vagina before having intercourse again if you are using a diaphragm. You may not have the contraceptive with you when you need it. Consider any potential drawbacks to using a particular type of contraceptive. For example, if you know you are likely to forget to take a pill now and then, you may find hormone implants more practical and reliable.

■ **How comfortable are you with your chosen method?** If you and your partner find a particular method of contraception so awkward or inconvenient that you do not use it every time you have intercourse, switch to a different method. It only takes one act of sexual intercourse without contraception to get pregnant.

■ **How much does the method cost?** Some birth-control methods, such as the intrauterine device (IUD) or hormone implants, have a relatively large up-front cost but are less expensive than many other methods in the long run because they provide continuous protection that lasts from months to years. Condoms and spermicides are the least expensive initially but may be less reliable than the long-lasting contraceptives—especially when you are using them for the first time and are unfamiliar with their correct use.

■ **Is the method a good choice for a woman with your health history?** Thoroughly discuss your medical history with your doctor when you are deciding on a contraceptive method. For example, if you have a family history of ovarian cancer or endometrial cancer, your doctor may recommend the birth-control pill because it can significantly reduce your risk of these cancers.

■ **Is there any reason you absolutely should not use a particular contraceptive?** If you are a smoker and you are over 35, you should not take the regular, combined birth-control pill because it increases your risk of heart attack and stroke. However, if you smoke very few cigarettes—less than one pack per week—you may be able to use a birth-control pill that has a very low dose of the female hormone estrogen. If you have a history of pelvic inflammatory disease (PID), an infection of the upper reproductive tract, you should not use an intrauterine device (IUD) because it can increase your risk of infection.

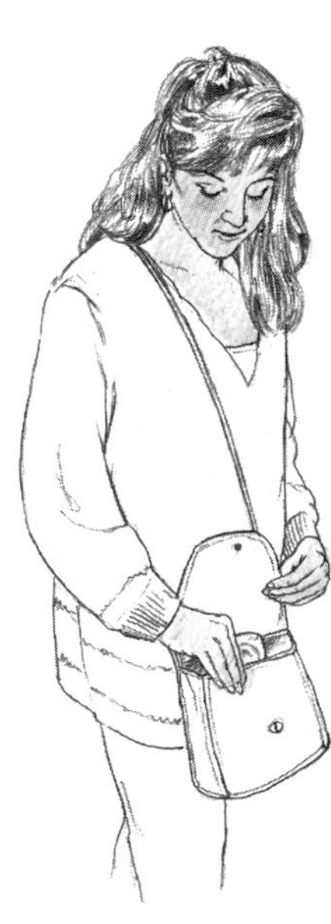

BE PREPARED
If you use a condom, diaphragm, or spermicide for birth control, you need to have it with you when you have intercourse.

How reliable is your method of birth control?

This table shows the effectiveness of various methods of contraception in the first year of average use by women between the ages of 18 and 44. Effectiveness is based on the percentage of women using a particular method of contraception who did not have an unintended pregnancy during the first year of use.

CONTRACEPTIVE METHOD	EFFECTIVENESS (%)
Hormone implants	99.9
Vasectomy	99.8
Hormone injections	99.6
Tubal ligation	99.5
Intrauterine device (IUD)	98.0
Combined pill	97.0
Minipill	96.0
Male condom	88.0
Diaphragm	82.0
Natural family planning	81.0
Female condom	79.0
Cervical cap	73.0
Spermicides	70.0
No contraception	15.0

Hormonal contraceptives

Contraceptives that use hormones—in pills, implants, or injections—to block ovulation (the release of an egg from an ovary) are among the most effective and convenient methods of birth control. More women use hormonal methods to control their fertility than any other method except surgical sterilization (tubal ligation).

Some hormonal contraceptives provide health benefits as well. The birth-control pill significantly reduces your risk of endometrial cancer (see page 239) and ovarian cancer (see page 249). This protection against cancer lasts at least 15 years after you stop taking the pill. The birth-control pill can also increase your bone density in the years preceding menopause. Hormone injections and implants reduce your risk of endometrial cancer.

The biggest drawback to hormonal contraceptives is that they provide no protection against sexually transmitted diseases (STDs). If you are not in a stable, mutually monogamous relationship (see page 338), always use a latex or polyurethane male condom or a female condom with spermicide each time you have sex (vaginal, oral, or anal).

COMBINED BIRTH-CONTROL PILLS

The most widely used birth-control pills contain both of the key female hormones—estrogen and a synthetic form of progesterone (progestin). The combined pill prevents ovulation by interfering with the cyclical hormonal changes that cause ovulation to take place. Also, progestin causes the cervical mucus to remain thick and scanty throughout the menstrual cycle, which helps block sperm from entering the uterus. (During ovulation, cervical mucus becomes thinner and more abundant, which enables sperm to reach the uterus more easily.)

Combined birth-control pills deliver estrogen and progestin into your system in varying amounts and according to different schedules. The pills are packaged so that you can take one clearly marked pill each day without worrying about the formula of hormones the pills contain. Some pills are packaged so that you take one pill each day for 21 days, and then stop taking the pill for 7 days. During the 7 pill-free days, you will usually have a period. After those 7 days, whether or not your period is over, you start a new 21-day course of pills.

Other combined birth-control pills are packaged so that you take one hormone-containing pill each day for 21 days and then one pill containing no hormones each day for 7 days. Doctors call these pills without hormones "reminder" pills because they keep you in the habit of taking a pill every day. Reminder pills are always a different color than the 21 hormone-containing pills. You will usually get your period at some point during the 7-day, reminder-pill period. Whether or not your period is over, you will begin a new package of pills the day after your old package runs out.

There are three kinds of combined birth-control pills—monophasic (one phase), biphasic (two phase), and triphasic (three phase). One-phase pills provide the same steady dose of estrogen and progestin throughout your cycle. Two-phase and three-phase pills are designed to mimic your natural hormone cycle and limit the total amount of hormones you take in the pills. Two-phase pills increase the amount of progestin in the middle of the cycle of pills, while the dose of estrogen remains constant. Three-phase pills vary the amount of progestin at different times in the cycle. In some three-phase pills, the dose of estrogen remains constant throughout the cycle; in others it varies. Ask your doctor to explain these different types of pills; together you can decide which is best for you.

Birth-control pills are 99.9-percent effective in preventing pregnancy when they are taken as prescribed. Even for women who occasionally forget to take a pill, their effectiveness is about 97 percent. Still, the two most common reasons for contraceptive failure with the pill are forgetting to take a pill or two during the cycle or forgetting to start a new cycle of pills on the right day.

If you forget to take one pill, take it as soon as you remember, even if it means taking 2 pills on the same day (the one you missed and the one for that day). If you miss more than one pill or take more than one pill late during a cycle, you lose your contraceptive protection and must use another form of birth control, such as a condom with spermicide. Call your doctor; he or she can tell you the best way to get back on the correct pill cycle and for how long you need to use alternative birth control. If you repeatedly forget to take your pills, consider using a different form of hormonal contraception such as implants (see page 314).

If you start taking birth-control pills exactly as recommended—that is, starting within 7 days of the first day of your period—you are immediately protected against pregnancy because the pill will prevent you from ovulating that month (and every month thereafter for as long as you stay on the pill). You can take birth-control pills for as many years as you want.

Taking the pill does not affect your future fertility. When you decide you want to get pregnant, finish the cycle of pills you are on. You do not have to stop taking the pill for any length of time before trying to conceive. If you change your mind and decide to go back on the pill, wait until you have a period before resuming the pills. Waiting for a period ensures that you have not gotten pregnant while you were off the pill.

You should not take the combined pill when you are breast-feeding because the hormone levels may slow the production of breast milk. While breast-feeding, you can take a different type of birth-control pill (the minipill, see page 313), which contains smaller doses of hormones.

Side effects Some women experience light bleeding or spotting (called breakthrough bleeding) between periods when they first start taking the birth-control pill. This bleeding usually occurs when you miss a pill or take one or more pills late.

If breakthrough bleeding continues after the first or second cycle you are on the pill, talk to your doctor about trying a pill with a different dose of hormones. You should also have a physical examination to rule out other possible causes of breakthrough bleeding, such as a sexually transmitted disease.

To reduce your risk of sexually transmitted diseases while you are on the pill, always use a latex or polyurethane male condom or a female condom with spermicide every time you have sex (vaginal, oral, or anal).

Sometimes, women taking birth-control pills for the first time feel nauseous during the first month. You may be able to prevent nausea by taking the pill at bedtime or with a meal or snack. The nausea usually goes away by the second or third month you are on the pill. If it does not go away, talk to your doctor; he or she may recommend a different pill formulation.

Many women experience a slight increase in the size of their breasts and breast swelling and tenderness when they begin taking birth-control pills. Breast tenderness usually goes away after the first few cycles of pills but, in some women, breast enlargement persists for as long as they are on the pill. Most of these side effects can be reduced by switching

Tips for helping you remember to take your pill

Forgetting to take birth-control pills is a major cause of unwanted pregnancies among women who use oral contraceptives. Here are some tips for helping you remember:

- Take a pill at the same time every day so that it becomes a habit.
- Do not keep your pills in a drawer you rarely open; leave them out where you will see them every day, such as next to your toothbrush.
- If your routine changes, such as when you take a trip, write a note to remind yourself and put it where you will see it (taped to the inside of your purse or on your cosmetic bag).
- Some women keep their pills with them at all times in their purse so if they realize they have forgotten to take a pill, they can take one immediately instead of waiting until they get home.

to a birth-control pill that contains less estrogen. Discuss this with your doctor.

Many women with acne notice an improvement in the condition of their skin when they begin taking birth-control pills and further improvement the longer they are on the pill. Rarely, a woman may get acne for the first time when she starts taking birth-control pills, especially pills that contain more progestin than usual. Switching to a pill with either more estrogen or a milder form of progestin usually eliminates this problem.

Headaches are another possible side effect of the pill. Some women may notice they get more headaches when they first start taking the pill. Mild, so-called tension headaches usually decrease in frequency after the first or second month on the pill. Some women who are prone to migraine headaches find they increase in frequency while they are on the pill; other women have fewer migraines. If your headaches become more frequent or severe, your doctor may recommend trying a pill with a lower dose of estrogen or no estrogen at all, or switching to a different form of birth control.

Some women may retain fluids, which can cause puffy ankles, while they are taking birth-control pills. Reducing salt intake may help. Your doctor may also prescribe a mild diuretic, a medication that reduces water retention. Most women do not gain weight from taking birth-control pills. If a woman does gain weight while on the pill, it is usually because of a change in lifestyle—she is eating more and exercising less.

Most women taking birth-control pills lose less blood during menstruation. The pill often relieves painful menstrual cramps and pain during the middle of the cycle that some women experience during ovulation. Occasionally, the pill stops menstrual bleeding completely. If you skip a period, take a pregnancy test just to be safe. It is extremely unlikely that you are pregnant if you have not missed taking any pills or taken any late. However, if you would find it more reassuring to have regular periods, talk to your doctor about trying a different pill formulation.

Combined birth-control pill

Advantages

- Is very effective in preventing pregnancy when taken as prescribed
- Decreases your risk of cancers of the ovary and endometrium, a benefit that continues for at least 15 years after you stop taking the pill
- Decreases your risk of pelvic inflammatory disease (PID; see page 232) by reducing the risk of infection in your fallopian tubes
- Decreases your risk of osteoporosis (see page 552) by providing a steady supply of estrogen, which maintains bone density
- Makes menstrual flow lighter and periods shorter and reduces menstrual cramps, irregular periods, and pain during the middle of your cycle
- May help prevent iron-deficiency anemia (see page 493) by reducing blood loss
- May help reduce fibrocystic changes in the breast
- Does not require cooperation of partner or interruption of lovemaking

Disadvantages

- Provides no protection against sexually transmitted diseases
- Must be taken every day whether or not you are sexually active
- Requires a prescription

Health effects The first birth-control pills that were developed had high doses of estrogen and progestin, which sometimes caused blood clots, increasing a woman's risk of heart attack and stroke. Today's birth-control pills have very low doses of these hormones and do not present this risk except for women 35 and older who smoke cigarettes. Women over 35 who smoke should not use birth-control pills. They need to use another reliable method of birth control. There are many excellent reasons to quit smoking; being able to use birth-control pills safely is just one of them.

Because women with advanced diabetes (see page 619) are at increased risk of heart disease, stroke, and the formation of blood clots, many doctors recommend that they not use birth-control pills. There is no overall increased risk of breast cancer in women who take birth-control pills.

Who should not take birth-control pills?

Although most women can safely take birth-control pills, for some women the pill is not a good choice. You should not take birth-control pills if you:

- Smoke cigarettes and are over 35
- Suspect you might be pregnant
- Have had blood clots in the veins of your legs, eyes, or lungs during pregnancy or while taking birth-control pills
- Have some types of heart disease, such as a previous heart attack or atrial fibrillation
- Have breast cancer
- Are experiencing vaginal bleeding of unknown cause
- Have active liver disease
- Have advanced diabetes

If you have high blood pressure, your doctor will want to monitor it closely while you are taking birth-control pills, because the pill sometimes increases already elevated blood pressure. If you are taking medication for high blood pressure, your medication may have to be increased while you are using birth-control pills. As long as your blood pressure is under control, you can safely use birth-control pills. Your doctor may need to find the best formulation for you.

If you have active liver disease, such as a hepatitis B infection (see page 534), or liver damage, you should not take birth-control pills. Hormones in the pill are broken down by the liver. If your liver is not functioning normally, the hormones can build up in your bloodstream. Blood tests to measure levels of particular proteins (enzymes) can determine if your liver is healthy and functioning properly. If your enzyme levels are normal, you can safely take the pill.

Drug interactions Most medications can safely be taken with birth-control pills. Some drugs that may affect the pill's effectiveness include antibiotics such as griseofulvin and rifampin. Be sure to tell your doctor that you are using the birth-control pill if he or she prescribes another medication.

Drugs used for controlling seizures (see page 578)—such as phenobarbital, phenytoin, and primidone—are broken down in the liver, as are birth-control pills. If you have been taking antiseizure medication for a long time, enzymes in your liver have become more efficient at breaking down the drug and, therefore, may also break down the birth-control pill at an increased rate. For this reason, you have to take a birth-control pill with a higher dose of estrogen (50 micrograms compared with the usual dose of 20 to 35 micrograms) to effectively prevent pregnancy. Discuss this with your doctor.

Health benefits Birth-control pills have a number of health benefits besides preventing pregnancy. Birth-control pills can reduce your risk of a number of medical conditions, including ovarian cancer (see page 249), endometrial cancer (see page 239), ectopic pregnancy (see page 233), pelvic inflammatory disease (PID; see page 232), iron deficiency anemia (see page 493), functional ovarian cysts (see page 224), fibrocystic breasts (see page 269), irregular menstrual periods, painful periods, and pain during the middle of the menstrual cycle.

If you are over 35 and do not smoke cigarettes, it can be beneficial for you to take low-dose birth-control pills. In addition to protecting against ovarian and endometrial cancers, taking the pill provides a steady supply of estrogen to replace your own, which naturally declines in the years preceding menopause (see page 352). The pill can also prevent symptoms of early menopause, such as painful, heavy, or irregular periods. A steady supply of estrogen also reduces your risk of osteoporosis (page 552) because estrogen helps maintain the strength and density of your bones.

MINIPILLS

The minipill contains small amounts of the synthetic form of the female hormone progesterone (progestin) without estrogen. The minipill is very effective when taken exactly as prescribed. However, there is less room for error than with the regular, combined birth-control pill (which contains both estrogen and progestin). For this reason, the minipill is recommended only for women who cannot take estrogen or who are breast-feeding. The minipill prevents sperm from entering the uterus by thickening the mucus that covers the cervix (the opening into the uterus). The minipill also prevents the endometrium

Minipill

Advantages
- Highly effective when taken as prescribed
- May be used by smokers over 35 (unlike the combined birth-control pill)
- May be used by women who are breast-feeding (unlike the combined birth-control pill)
- Does not require cooperation of partner or interruption of lovemaking

Disadvantages
- Provides no protection against sexually transmitted diseases
- Requires a prescription
- May cause side effects such as irregular periods

(the lining of the uterus) from growing, making it more difficult for a fertilized egg to implant itself in the wall. The low dose of progestin in the minipill also prevents ovulation (release of a mature egg from an ovary), but not as consistently as the combined birth-control pill.

You take the minipill every day throughout the month instead of stopping toward the end of the cycle as you would with the combined birth-control pill. You do not have regular periods while taking the minipill but you may have irregular bleeding.

Because the minipill contains only progestin and no estrogen, it may be used by women who smoke and women who cannot take estrogen because they have a history of blood clots in their legs during a pregnancy or while taking birth-control pills. The minipill is also recommended for women who are breast-feeding because it does not interfere with milk production, as the combined birth-control pill does. You can start taking the minipill right after delivery.

The minipill is sufficiently effective when you are breast-feeding because an elevated level of prolactin, the hormone that stimulates milk production, also inhibits ovulation. However, prolactin prevents you from ovulating only as long as breast milk is your baby's sole source of nourishment. As soon as you start to reduce the number of feedings per day, your prolactin level decreases along with your production of milk, and so does the effectiveness of the minipill. At this time, you should switch to the combined birth-control pill.

When using minipills, you must take a pill at the same time every day and never skip a day. During the first 28-day cycle of pills, you do not have the pill's full contraceptive protection and must use a backup method of birth control. If you are more than 3 hours late taking a pill after the first cycle, take one immediately and use a backup method of birth control for the next 48 hours. If you miss more than one minipill in a row, take two pills at the usual time for 2 days and use another form of birth control for the remainder of the cycle. If you do not have a period or any bleeding at all within 4 weeks, take a home pregnancy test and call your doctor.

Side effects Irregular periods are the most common side effect of the minipill. Some women do not menstruate at all while others experience bleeding between periods. Your periods may be longer than usual or occur more closely together. These changes can be annoying but they are not health problem.

The minipill sometimes produces the same side effects as the combination pill, including headaches, water retention, and nausea. These side effects usually go away after 2 or 3 months.

HORMONE IMPLANTS

Hormone implants are soft capsules made of a synthetic material that are placed just beneath the skin in your upper arm. They release a small, steady dose of the hormone progestin to block ovulation (release of an egg from an ovary) over a period of 5 years.

Hormone implants are a very effective and convenient form of birth control, but they provide no protection against sexually transmitted diseases. Implants are more effective (greater than 99.9 percent) than any other form of contraception, including surgical sterilization (tubal ligation or vasectomy). The effectiveness is due in part to their convenience; you do not have to remember to use them since they are implanted in your body.

The main contraceptive effect of hormone implants is to suppress ovulation. Like other hormonal contraceptives that contain only progestin (without estrogen), implants also prevent pregnancy by thickening the mucus that covers the cervix (the opening into the uterus), which helps block sperm from entering the uterus.

The capsules must be inserted and removed by a doctor who has been trained in performing the procedure. The capsules must be replaced every 5 years. But it is important to continue having a yearly pelvic examination, Pap smear, and breast examination.

The implants are safe for most women. You should not use them if you are breast-feeding or have serious health conditions such as liver disease, breast cancer, unexplained vaginal bleeding, or a history of blood clots in the veins of your legs, eyes, or lungs.

The major disadvantage of the implants is that they provide no protection against sexually transmitted diseases. If you are not in a stable, mutually monogamous relationship (see page 338) or you have any doubt that you are, continue to use a latex or polyurethane male condom or a female condom with spermicide every time you have sex (vaginal, oral, or anal).

Many women who have implants experience changes in their menstrual cycles, such as irregular bleeding or absent periods. The most common pattern is spotting that precedes and follows a normal menstrual period. This bleeding is not heavy enough to cause a medical problem such as anemia (see page 493) but you have to wear tampons or pads for more days than usual each month. Many of these changes decrease after the first year of using the implants.

Inserting hormone implants If you have decided to use hormone implants, see a doctor who has experience inserting them. The implants are usually inserted within 7 days after the first day of your period because of the small chance of your being pregnant at this time. The procedure takes about 10 minutes. A local anesthetic is injected into your upper arm to numb the area. The doctor makes a tiny incision and inserts the capsules one at a time in a fan-shaped arrangement just beneath your skin.

The area around the incision may feel sore or look bruised for a day or two; you can relieve the pain with ice packs or over-the-counter painkillers such as aspirin or ibuprofen. If you change your mind about having the implants or if you decide later that you want to become pregnant, talk to your doctor. He or she can remove them.

The implants are fully effective against pregnancy 24 hours after insertion. Use another form of birth control until then. The capsules are usually not visible under the skin but you can feel them if you touch them with your fingers. In a few women, the skin over the implants darkens; this discoloration disappears when the implants are removed. If you notice any pain, pus, or bleeding in the arm with the implants, call your doctor; you could have an infection.

Hormone implants must be replaced every 5 years because they lose their contraceptive effectiveness. New implants can be inserted right away if you wish to continue using this form of birth control. The procedure for removing the capsules is similar to that of implanting them but it takes a little longer—about 20 to 30 minutes. Removal is more difficult than insertion because some scar tissue forms around the capsules. The original incision can be used for inserting the replacement capsules but the capsules are fanned out

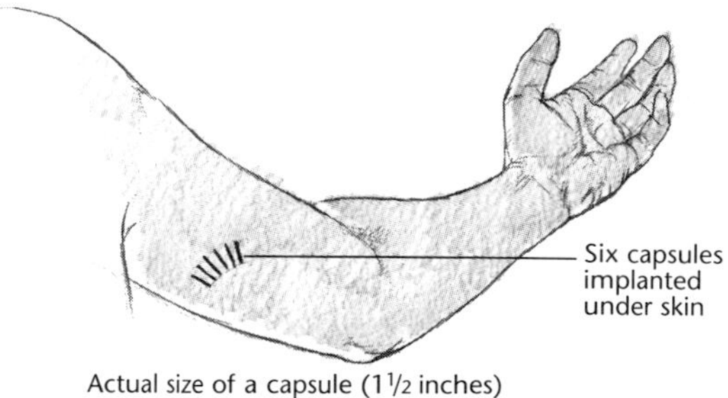

HORMONE IMPLANTS

Hormone implants are six small, matchstick-sized hormone-containing capsules placed just beneath the surface of the skin on the inside of your upper arm. The implants, which release a small, steady dose of the hormone progestin, provide contraceptive protection for 5 years.

Hormone implants

Advantages

- Are highly effective in preventing pregnancy
- Are effective for 5 years
- Are safe for women who cannot take estrogen (see page 361)
- Do not require you to remember to use birth control each time you have sex
- Do not require cooperation of partner or interruption of lovemaking

Disadvantages

- Provide no protection against sexually transmitted diseases
- Require a visit to the doctor for insertion
- Removal may be difficult and cause discomfort

in a different direction. It is sometimes necessary to make a new incision.

Side effects The most common side effects of hormone implants, especially during the first year, are irregular periods and spotting between periods. See your doctor if you experience heavy vaginal bleeding. Irregular bleeding can sometimes be treated with small doses of estrogen taken in pills.

Some women with implants have no periods at all. This is usually no cause for concern, but if you are sexually active, you may want to do a home pregnancy test every 1 to 2 months to reassure yourself. If you skip a period after having many regular periods while you have implants, take a pregnancy test and call your doctor.

Although less common, other side effects of hormone implants include weight gain, hair loss, acne, and mood changes. Not all women experience these side effects and those who do find that they usually subside after a few months. The only way to know if you are likely to experience these progestin-related side effects is to try another progestin-only birth-control method first, such as the minipill (see page 313) or hormone injections (see below). If you have any side effects using these methods and find them intolerable, hormone implants are probably not a good choice of birth control for you. It is easier to discontinue using the minipill or hormone injections than to have the implants removed.

HORMONE INJECTIONS

Injectable contraceptives have been used for many years outside the US. One type now available in this country—medroxyprogesterone acetate—has long been used here to treat gynecologic problems such as endometriosis (see page 230) and endometrial cancer (see page 239). A doctor injects the contraceptive deep into your buttocks muscle at regular intervals, usually every 3 months.

Like the minipill and hormone implants, the injectable contraceptive contains progestin (a synthetic form of the female hormone progesterone) and no estrogen. It is a highly effective (more than 99 percent) form of birth control. The injectable contraceptive prevents pregnancy by thickening the mucus that covers the cervix (the opening into the uterus), which helps prevent sperm from reaching the uterus. The contraceptive also makes the endometrium (the lining of the uterus) less receptive to implantation by a fertilized egg.

Women who are breast-feeding should not use this form of contraception because it may decrease their production of breast milk. A disadvantage of this method for women who plan to become pregnant in the future is that, after the injections are stopped, fertility may not return for several months.

Side effects The most common side effect of injectable contraceptives is

Hormone injections

Advantages

- Are highly effective in preventing pregnancy
- Do not require cooperation of partner or interruption of lovemaking
- May stop periods after 1 year or more of use
- Reduce the frequency of seizures in women with epilepsy
- Do not require you to remember to use birth control

Disadvantages

- May cause irregular periods or spotting, especially during the first year
- Do not protect against sexually transmitted diseases
- Require an injection in a doctor's office every 3 months

irregular periods. Some doctors give the first several injections closer together than every 3 months to try to prevent this. Usually, after a woman uses the contraceptive for 1 year or more, her periods gradually stop altogether. Some women see this absence of menstruation as an advantage. Others find it disconcerting because they worry that they might become pregnant and not know it.

Other side effects of the injectable contraceptive are weight gain or mood changes. Rare side effects include acne, growth of unwanted hair, or hair loss. These problems usually go away after a few months. However, if they do not subside and you find them intolerable, discuss with your doctor whether a different form of birth control might be better for you.

For women who have epilepsy (see page 578) and are taking medication to control seizures, the injectable contraceptive offers an advantage—it decreases the frequency of seizures. You may want to consider this form of birth control if you are taking antiseizure medication. Ask your doctor about this option.

MORNING-AFTER PILLS

Morning-after pills are a series of birth-control pills containing estrogen and progestin that are taken as soon as possible after intercourse without a contraceptive. This treatment prevents pregnancy by inhibiting the growth of the lining of the uterus (endometrium). The endometrium is then less able to sustain the circulation necessary for a fertilized egg.

The pills are available only by prescription. You take two pills immediately and two more 12 hours later. The treatment is effective only when the first dose is taken within 72 hours of the unprotected intercourse.

Mifepristone (see page 331), another drug used as a morning-after pill when taken within 72 hours of unprotected intercourse, is a hormone that prevents pregnancy by preventing implantation of a fertilized egg in the wall of the uterus. Mifepristone works by blocking the effect of progesterone, the hormone that nourishes the lining of the uterus in preparation for a fertilized egg.

You should not consider morning-after pills a regular form of contraception; they are not 100-percent effective and there may be a slight risk that the hormones will harm the fetus if you are already pregnant. Morning-after pills are an appropriate method of preventing pregnancy in some situations, such as after sexual assault. They can also be a good solution in an emergency when your usual form of birth control has failed—for example, a condom has ripped. Morning-after pills are a better way to deal with an unwanted pregnancy than a later surgical abortion. Call your doctor immediately if you have had sexual intercourse without a contraceptive and you want to avoid pregnancy.

Like other hormonal methods of contraception, morning-after pills are highly effective (97 to more than 99 percent). However, this effectiveness is reduced considerably 72 hours after the unprotected intercourse.

Side effects Because the composition of the pills is similar to that of combined birth-control pills, the side effects are similar (see page 311). These side effects include nausea, breast tenderness, and light vaginal bleeding, or spotting.

Seeking morning-after treatment Call your doctor to get an evaluation of your situation and, if necessary, set up an immediate appointment. Your doctor will ask the date of your last period to determine if there is any possibility you were already pregnant when you had intercourse without contraception. Your doctor may ask the date and time of the intercourse and whether you had unprotected intercourse at any other time since your last period.

Your doctor will perform a physical examination and pelvic examination and may also want to do a blood test or urine test to make sure you are not pregnant. If you were a victim of sexual assault, you will also be tested for sexually transmitted diseases.

Along with the hormone pills, your doctor may give you medication to reduce the possible side effect of nausea or vomiting. Taking the pills with a snack or a glass of milk can help you avoid nausea. Your periods should resume within a few weeks after taking the pills. If you do not have a period within 3 weeks, take a pregnancy test and call your doctor right away.

Barrier methods of contraception

Barrier methods of contraception prevent pregnancy by physically blocking sperm from the uterus. Male and female condoms, spermicides, the diaphragm, and the cervical cap are barrier methods of contraception. Each barrier contraceptive is designed to be used with a spermicide, which kills sperm on contact. Barrier methods are not as effective as hormonal methods in preventing pregnancy.

MALE CONDOMS

The male condom is a thin sheath of latex or polyurethane that is placed on a man's erect penis before intercourse to prevent semen, which contains sperm, from entering a woman's vagina. Condoms come in a variety of types and are available in most drugstores. Some condoms are already lubricated or coated with spermicide.

The average effectiveness of condoms in preventing pregnancy in a 1-year period is 88 percent, mainly because people do not use them correctly or consistently. However, when you use a condom correctly every time you have intercourse, it is 98-percent effective in preventing pregnancy; used with a spermicide, the condom can be 99-percent effective—better than any other barrier contraceptive. A latex or polyurethane male condom provides the fullest possible protection against sexually transmitted diseases because it prevents the exchange of body fluids that may contain bacteria or other disease-causing organisms. Do not use condoms made of natural materials such as lambskin, which are porous and do not block viruses (such as HIV, the virus that causes AIDS) and other disease-causing organisms.

Because the male condom must be put on an erect penis before the penis has any contact at all with your genitals, it is best to put the condom on your partner's penis as an early part of lovemaking. The tip at the end of a condom is designed to leave room (about 1/2 inch) for ejaculated semen to collect. After intercourse, you or your partner must hold the base of the condom around his penis while your partner withdraws to prevent semen from leaking into your vagina.

If you experience any discomfort while using a condom, try using a lubricant in your vagina or on the condom. Use only water-based lubricants with a latex condom; oil-based lubricants such as petroleum jelly can weaken latex. Remember, however, that lubricants are not spermicides; they do not provide any protection against pregnancy or sexually transmitted diseases.

Because condoms offer the best protection against AIDS and other sexually transmitted diseases, always use a condom in addition to another method of birth control if you have any doubt about whether you are in a stable, mutually monogamous relationship (see page 338).

Male condom

Advantages

- Provides fullest possible protection against sexually transmitted diseases
- Reduces your risk of cervical dysplasia (see page 218) and cervical cancer (see page 250)
- Provides effective protection against pregnancy
- Does not require a prescription and is widely available
- Is easy to use

Disadvantages

- Requires cooperation of male partner
- May not completely protect either partner against HIV, the virus that causes AIDS, or against herpes or genital warts, two sexually transmitted diseases that infect the external genitals
- Requires interruption of lovemaking
- May decrease sexual sensitivity in some men and women

FEMALE CONDOMS

The female condom is a soft, thin prelubricated polyurethane sheath that, when in use, lines the inside of the vagina and covers most of the outer part of the vagina. It has a soft, flexible ring at each end. The smaller ring, which is not attached to the sheath, lies inside the closed end and is used primarily for insertion and to hold the condom in place against the cervix. A larger, thinner ring forms the open end of the sheath and remains outside the vagina, allowing entry of the

Female condom

Advantages

- You control its use
- Provides effective protection against sexually transmitted diseases
- May provide more protection than the male condom against sexually transmitted diseases that infect the external genital area, such as genital herpes and genital warts

Disadvantages

- May be awkward to use at first
- May require cooperation of partner or interruption of lovemaking
- Aesthetics are not pleasing to some people
- May require use of lubricant

penis. You insert the female condom before having sex.

A major advantage of the female condom is that you control its use. It also can help protect you and your partner from sexually transmitted diseases. Unlike the male condom, the female condom provides some protection against genital herpes (see page 342) and genital warts (see page 341), two sexually transmitted diseases that infect the external genitals. In addition, using the female condom does not disrupt lovemaking because you put it in place before sexual activity begins and you do not have to remove it while your partner still has an erection. On the negative side, some couples find using the female condom awkward at first.

Be sure to read the instructions carefully before you insert the condom. It is a good idea to practice inserting it before you use it with your partner. You and your partner must be careful to use enough of the extra lubricant provided with the condom to prevent it from slipping inside your vagina. You also must be sure that your partner's penis enters inside the condom rather than to the side of it. You may want to guide your partner's penis into the condom with your hand.

Studies show an effectiveness rate of about 79 percent for average use of the female condom, compared with 88 percent for the male condom. However, the effectiveness rates for both male and female condoms are much higher than these if you use them correctly every time you have sex.

INSERTING A FEMALE CONDOM

1. With the open end of the condom hanging down, squeeze the smaller, inner ring on the closed end with your fingers.
2. Insert the condom into your vagina. With your index finger, push it as far as you can up against your cervix.
3. Check to make sure the inner ring is up just past your pubic bone. About 1 inch of the open end remains outside your vagina and lies against your external genitals.

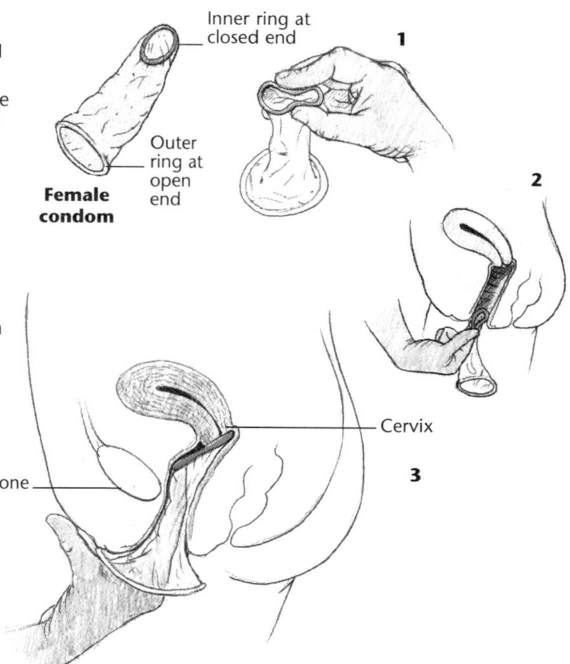

SPERMICIDES

Spermicides prevent conception by killing sperm before they can reach an egg to fertilize it. Spermicides are often combined with barrier methods of contraception such as a condom or a diaphragm.

Spermicides can be effective if they are used correctly and consistently. But nearly one out of three women who uses a spermicide alone, without combining it with a barrier method of birth control, becomes pregnant during the first year of use. This failure rate makes a spermicide alone a poor form of birth control for most women. Spermicides may provide some protection against such sexually transmitted diseases as chlamydia and gonorrhea, but not enough to rely on them alone to protect you. Spermicides do not affect your future ability to become pregnant and do not harm a fetus that results from an accidental pregnancy.

Occasionally, a particular spermicide may cause irritation in the vagina or on the penis. These problems may include mild burning or a watery discharge. Most spermicides contain the same active ingredient—nonoxynol 9—but may have different added substances. If you have a reaction to one kind of spermicide, try another brand.

Spermicides come in many forms—including gels, foams, suppositories, and squares of film that dissolve inside your vagina before you have intercourse. They require no prescription and you can buy them in most drugstores.

Creams and gels Some spermicidal creams and gels are made to be used with a barrier contraceptive such as a diaphragm or cervical cap. Some come with an applicator to insert the spermicide directly into your vagina before having intercourse. Carefully follow the directions on the package insert.

Creams and gels are effective for 1 hour. If you have intercourse after that time, you must insert more spermicide. If you have intercourse more than once, you need to insert more spermicide before each session.

Foams Contraceptive foams come in aerosol containers. You remove a specific amount of the spermicidal foam from the container using a special applicator. You then insert the applicatorful of foam into your vagina, in a similar way to using a tampon. Carefully follow the directions on the package insert.

Foams are effective for 1 hour. If you are going to have intercourse after that time, you must insert more foam before penetration occurs.

Suppositories Suppositories are bullet-shaped tablets of spermicide that you insert into your vagina with your finger. The suppository must be in position high in your vagina next to your cervix. You must insert the suppository 10 to 15 minutes before intercourse to allow time for it to melt inside your vagina. Carefully follow the directions on the package insert.

Most suppositories are effective for 1 hour; you must insert another one if you wait longer than an hour before having intercourse. You need to use a new suppository for each act of intercourse.

Contraceptive films Contraceptive films are thin, 2-inch-square films of spermicide that you insert with your finger high into your vagina next to your cervix. The film melts in about 5 to 10 minutes and is then effective for about 2 hours. You must insert another film each time you have intercourse again. Carefully follow the directions on the package insert.

Spermicides

Advantages

- May provide some protection against some sexually transmitted diseases, including chlamydia and gonorrhea
- Are easy to use
- Increase the effectiveness of barrier methods
- Do not require a prescription and are widely available in stores
- Do not need to be removed from the vagina after use

Disadvantages

- Contraceptive effectiveness is relatively low (about 70 percent), so they must be used with other barrier methods
- Provide little protection against sexually transmitted diseases
- Must be reapplied for each act of intercourse
- Are effective for only 1 hour, so accurate timing is essential
- Can be messy
- May require cooperation of partner and interruption of lovemaking

DIAPHRAGMS

A diaphragm is a thin rubber dome that covers your cervix, blocking sperm from your uterus. You use the diaphragm with spermicidal jelly or cream, either of which will kill most if not all of the sperm that might get past the diaphragm. To use the diaphragm, you must feel comfortable enough with your body to insert it into your vagina and remove it. The diaphragm can be inserted several hours before lovemaking, so it is more convenient than some other barrier methods.

The diaphragm is not quite as reliable as the male condom for contraception; its average effectiveness is about 82 percent. Most failures occur because of inconsistent or incorrect use or because the diaphragm does not fit properly or has not been replaced at the recommended time and has holes in it. If you have had at least one child, the diaphragm is more effective than the cervical cap (see page 323) because the effects of labor change the shape of your cervix—it becomes larger and less circular. This change makes the cervix more difficult to cover completely with a cervical cap, which is smaller than a diaphragm.

Few women have side effects from using a diaphragm. In rare cases, a woman may have more frequent urinary tract infections because the diaphragm puts pressure on the urethra (the small tube that carries urine from the bladder), which may block the flow of urine and allow bacteria to grow.

Diaphragm

Advantages

- May reduce your risk of cervical dysplasia (abnormal changes in cells in the cervix) and some sexually transmitted diseases
- Does not require interrupting lovemaking because it can be inserted an hour or two before having intercourse
- Can be used when having intercourse during your period to temporarily block the flow of blood

Disadvantages

- May be difficult to use for some women
- May require interrupting lovemaking if not inserted in advance
- Requires a prescription and fitting by a doctor
- Provides little protection against sexually transmitted diseases

On the other hand, women who use a diaphragm for a long time may have a reduced risk of cervical dysplasia (abnormal changes in cells of the cervix that can lead to cancer; see page 218). The diaphragm may help prevent viruses, such as the human papillomavirus, from entering the cervix. The human papillomavirus (see page 341) causes genital warts, a sexually transmitted disease that is linked to an increased risk of cervical dysplasia.

Sometimes a woman or her partner is allergic to the spermicide or the rubber of the diaphragm. If this occurs, try a different brand of spermicide or, if the rubber of the diaphragm is causing the problem, switch to a different form of contraception.

Being fitted for a diaphragm Diaphragms are available only through a doctor. Diaphragms come in sizes measured in millimeters—from 50 to 95 millimeters (about 2 to 4 inches) in diameter. Your doctor will fit you for size during a pelvic examination. In this examination the doctor can also detect any abnormalities in the shape of your vagina, cervix, or uterus that would prevent you from using a diaphragm successfully. Your doctor may have you practice inserting and removing your diaphragm in his or her office to make sure you understand how to use it and to help you feel more confident about it. Carefully follow the directions on the package insert.

You should replace your diaphragm and be refitted for a new one every year. Tiny holes can form in the rubber that are too small to see but large enough to allow sperm or disease-causing organisms through. The size of your diaphragm should also be checked if you lose or gain 20 pounds or more, if you have a miscarriage or abortion or carry a pregnancy to term, if you have any surgery involving your reproductive organs, if you experience discomfort while using the diaphragm, if you have recurring urinary tract infections (see page 542), or if you have difficulty inserting your diaphragm correctly.

For some women, particularly those whose pelvic muscles or tissues were stretched during childbirth, the diaphragm may not be the best choice. Weakened pelvic muscles and tissues may not be strong enough to hold the diaphragm securely in place. Your doctor can tell if your diaphragm fits properly; it should be snug but comfortable.

Using a diaphragm Before inserting your diaphragm, wash your hands. Put about a tablespoon of spermicidal jelly or cream in the bowl of the diaphragm. Apply the spermicide around the outer rim of the diaphragm; this will help form a seal between the diaphragm and your cervix. Insert the diaphragm into your vagina as shown below.

If more than 2 hours elapse before you have intercourse, you must insert more spermicide into your vagina, using the applicator that comes with your diaphragm. This is important because spermicides lose their effectiveness over several hours. Each time you have intercourse, you have to add more. Do not remove your diaphragm after intercourse because, if there is semen (which contains sperm) in your vagina, reinserting the diaphragm could push it up into your uterus.

Leave the diaphragm in place for at least 6 hours after intercourse, but make sure you remove it within 8 hours of intercourse to avoid the slight risk of developing a potentially serious bacterial infection called toxic shock syndrome (see page 214). If 6 hours or more have passed since you had intercourse and you expect to have sex again, remove your diaphragm, wash it, apply more spermicide, and reinsert it.

Before removing your diaphragm, always wash your hands. Hook your finger under the rim that rests behind your pubic bone and firmly pull forward and down. Wash the diaphragm on both sides with water and a mild, unscented soap; allow the diaphragm to air and store it in its case away from extreme heat or cold. Do not clean your diaphragm in boiling water (heat can weaken the rubber) or use talcum powder on it (the tiny particles can cause irritation in your genital area). If you have trouble inserting or removing your diaphragm, ask your doctor for a prescription for a diaphragm introducer, a device that may make it easier to insert.

Every few weeks, check your diaphragm for holes by holding it up to the light. Do not use the same diaphragm for more than 1 year even if it appears to be in good condition; holes that are too small to see can allow sperm through and, over time, a diaphragm can become brittle and crack.

INSERTING A DIAPHRAGM

1. Place about a tablespoon of spermicidal jelly or cream inside the bowl of the diaphragm and apply some around the entire rim.
2. Pinch the edges of the diaphragm together with your thumb and index finger.
3. Insert the diaphragm into your vagina and push it with your index or middle finger up as far as it goes. When you release the diaphragm, it will spring open and cover your cervix. Push the lower rim of the diaphragm up behind your pubic bone. Feel with your finger to make sure the diaphragm is covering your cervix, which feels like a small, firm mound. To remove the diaphragm, hook your index finger gently around the rim and pull it out.

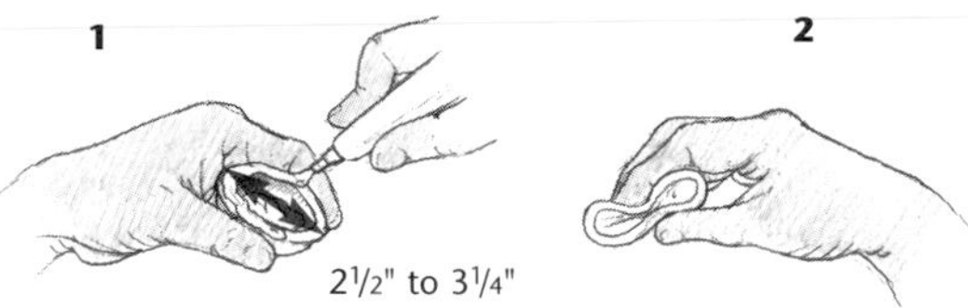

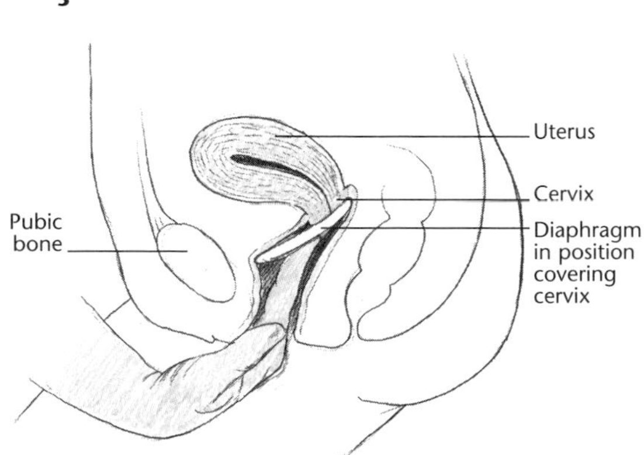

CERVICAL CAPS

The cervical cap is a small, rubber, dome-shaped cap that is filled with a spermicide and fits snugly over the cervix. The cap is held in place by suction. Because of its smaller size, some women find it more difficult to insert than the diaphragm. However, the cap can be left in place for up to 48 hours (the diaphragm must be left in for 6 hours after intercourse but for no more than 8 hours).

It is more difficult to accurately fit a cervical cap than a diaphragm because of its small size. The cap may also be more difficult for some women to insert because it has to be pushed up higher in the vagina. You must put spermicide into the cap before inserting it and insert more spermicide into your vagina each time you have intercourse.

The cervical cap is not quite as effective as a diaphragm in preventing pregnancy. Some women cannot use a cervical cap because of the shape of their cervix. The cervical cap is less effective in women who have had children, because the effects of labor change the shape of the cervix. Women who have an especially long vaginal canal or short fingers may not be able to use a cap because they cannot reach their cervix with their finger to insert the cap correctly.

As with other barrier contraceptives that are used with spermicide, the cervical cap helps protect against some sexually transmitted diseases (see page 318). However, if you develop a greenish or yellow vaginal discharge, stop using the cap and see your doctor—you may have an infection.

A doctor must fit you for a cervical cap to determine the right size to cover your cervix. Your doctor will give you detailed instructions about how to insert the device and may have you practice inserting and removing it in the office. Carefully follow the directions on the package insert. Make sure you know how to use the cap before you have intercourse.

Cervical cap

Advantages

- May be left in place for up to 48 hours
- Does not require interruption of lovemaking
- May reduce your risk of some sexually transmitted diseases

Disadvantages

- Provides less protection against sexually transmitted diseases than condoms
- Does not fit all women
- May not be an effective contraceptive for women who have had a child
- Is more difficult to insert and remove than a diaphragm
- May cause an unpleasant odor or infection if left in place for longer than 48 hours

Using a cervical cap Before inserting the cervical cap, wash your hands. You must insert the cap at least 20 to 30 minutes before intercourse to allow time for suction to form a seal between your cervix and the rubber of the cap.

Fill one third of the inside bowl of the cap with spermicidal jelly or cream. Spread some spermicide around the outer rim of the cap. If you need a lubricant to help make insertion easier, use only a water-based product. Oil-based lubricants, such as petroleum jelly, can weaken the rubber of the cap.

Before inserting the cap, make sure you know where your cervix is by feeling for it with your fingers; it will feel like a firm mound. Insert the cap into your vagina as shown on page 324. When the cap is in position correctly, it completely and snugly covers your cervix. A well-fitted cap is difficult to dislodge accidentally. However, a cap can sometimes be displaced by the penis. After intercourse, feel with your finger to make sure the cap is still in place. If the cap has been dislodged, quickly push it back into position and insert an application of spermicide into your vagina. If you plan to have intercourse again, insert another application of spermicide and do so each time you have intercourse.

Leave the cap in place for at least 8 hours after intercourse. Do not leave it in longer than 48 hours; the risk of infection increases after that time and the spermicide may begin to develop an unpleasant odor.

Do not douche while using a cervical cap. Douching may dilute the spermicide or force sperm under the cap and into the cervix. Do not use a cap while you are menstruating; it may increase your risk of infection.

To remove the cap, hook your finger gently over the back rim and pull. Or

INSERTING A CERVICAL CAP

1. Locate your cervix by inserting a finger inside your vagina and feeling for it at the top of the vagina. Squeeze the edges of the cap together with your thumb and index finger and insert it into your vagina.
2. Push the cap with your index finger as far as you can up into your vagina, until the open end of the cap reaches your cervix. Check that the cap is snugly in place over your cervix by nudging it with your finger. To remove the cap, tilt it to the side with your finger to break the suction and pull it down from your cervix and out.

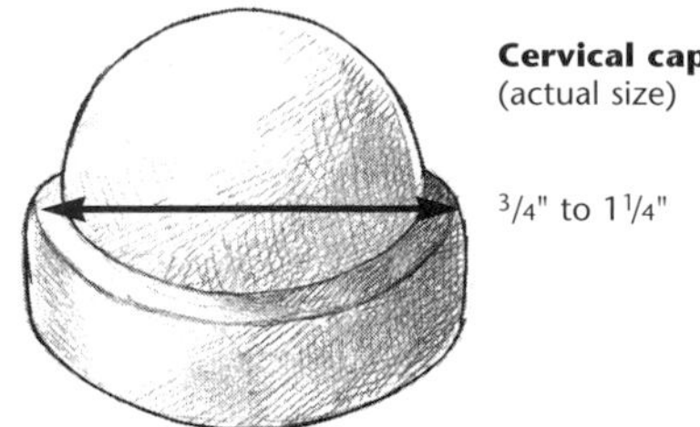

Cervical cap
(actual size)

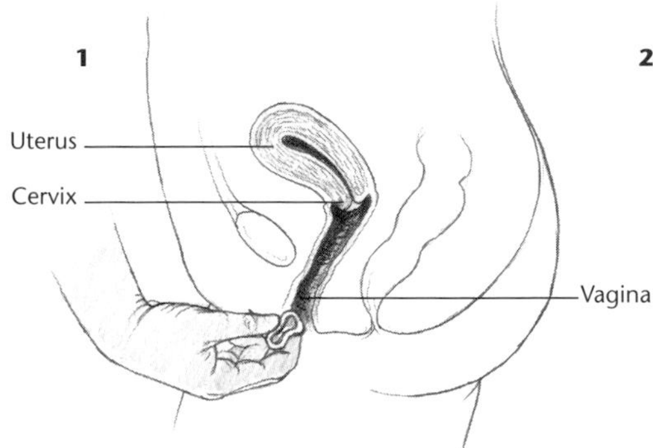

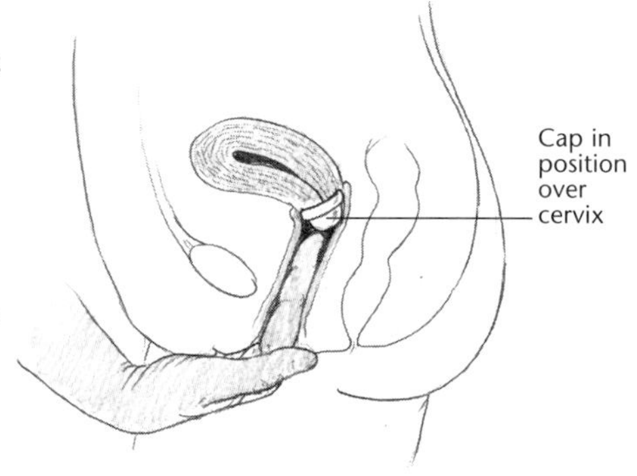

push the dome of the cap forward with your index finger while your middle finger hooks over the back and pulls it down.

After removing the cap, wash it with a mild, unscented soap, turning it inside out to clean the bowl. Do not clean your cap in boiling water (heat can weaken the rubber) or use talcum powder on it (the tiny particles can cause irritation in your genital area).

Each time you use your cervical cap, hold it up to the light to check for holes or any signs of deterioration, such as brittleness or cracking. You should be refitted for a new cap every year.

Other methods of contraception

Other contraceptive methods you may wish to consider are the intrauterine device (IUD), surgical sterilization (of you or your partner), and natural family planning. The IUD (used by relatively few women today) or male or female sterilization (used by many couples) may be a good choice if you have completed your family. Natural family planning is less reliable than all other forms of birth control and takes considerable planning and effort. None of these methods provides protection against sexually transmitted diseases.

INTRAUTERINE DEVICES

An intrauterine device (IUD) is a small (1/2 inch across and 1 inch long), T-shaped plastic device that is inserted into your uterus by a doctor. It is a highly effective method of birth control. Depending on the type of IUD you have, it can remain inside your uterus for up to 10 years before having to be replaced.

Doctors used to think that the IUD worked by preventing a fertilized egg from implanting itself in the wall of the uterus. It is now believed that the IUD causes the cervical mucus to change in such a way that sperm are unable to reach a fallopian tube to fertilize an egg.

Types of IUDs There are two kinds of IUDs—one covered with copper wire and one containing the female hormone progesterone. The copper IUD can be worn continuously for 10 years before it needs to be replaced and is more effective in preventing pregnancy than the one containing progesterone. The effectiveness of the copper IUD is 99.2 percent; the progesterone-containing IUD is 98-percent effective.

The copper IUD is more convenient than the progesterone IUD for most women because it does not need to be replaced as often. Less frequent replacement also reduces the risk of two rare but possible complications of IUD insertion: infection and injury to the wall of the uterus. Because the cervix must be dilated (opened) in order to insert the IUD, infection can occur if the bacteria that are normally present and harmless in the vagina get inside the uterus and multiply there. Injury to the wall of the uterus during the insertion process can allow the IUD to penetrate the wall and, possibly, work its way into the abdominal cavity.

The progesterone IUD slowly releases a small amount of the hormone into the uterus for 1 year and then must be replaced with a new one. The progesterone in the IUD helps prevent pregnancy by making the cervical mucus thicker and the lining of the uterus thinner. As a result, sperm are much less likely to get into the uterus and a fertilized egg is less able to implant itself in the wall.

Potential problems Contraceptive failures occur when women forget to check for the strings of their IUD regularly and do not realize that the IUD has become dislodged and has been expelled from their uterus, or has penetrated the wall.

Check for the strings of your IUD every month, right after your period. This timing is important because contractions of the uterus during menstruation can expel the IUD. Insert your finger into your vagina and feel for the soft, plastic strings at the top of the vagina. If you cannot feel the strings, call your doctor immediately. An ultrasound of your pelvis can show if the strings of the IUD have moved up inside your uterus. You may need to have surgery to remove the IUD if it has penetrated the wall of your uterus.

When contractions of the uterus during menstruation expel an IUD, which is not common, it is most likely to occur during the first 3 months of use. You may find the IUD on a sanitary pad or in the toilet if it has been expelled in this way. If your partner can feel the IUD with his penis during intercourse, or if the strings extend far down or even out of your vagina, have your doctor check to see if your IUD is being expelled. If you cannot feel the strings of your IUD, it may have already been expelled.

The most common side effects of an IUD are bleeding problems, such as spotting between periods or longer and heavier periods. These problems generally lessen over time, but in some women they are so severe that the IUD must be removed.

Who can use an IUD An IUD is usually recommended for women who have had at least one child or for women who do not plan to have children because an IUD may increase the risk of pelvic inflammatory disease (PID; see page 232). PID can cause ectopic pregnancy (see page 233) and infertility (see page 382). Because sexually transmitted diseases (primarily chlamydia and gonorrhea) are the major causes of PID, you should not use the IUD unless you are at low risk of sexually transmitted diseases—that is, you are in a stable, mutually monogamous relationship (you and your partner are having sex only with each other; see page 338).

Using an IUD An IUD must be carefully fitted and inserted by a doctor, usually during a woman's period. At this time, the possibility of pregnancy is lowest and

Intrauterine device

Advantages

- Is highly effective in preventing pregnancy
- Does not require interrupting lovemaking
- Is effective for 10 years when made of copper
- Does not require cooperation of partner

Disadvantages

- Provides no protection against sexually transmitted diseases
- Increases the risk of pelvic inflammatory disease (PID; see page 232) so it is not a good choice if you are not in a mutually monogamous relationship (see page 338) and are, therefore, at risk of sexually transmitted diseases (which cause PID)
- Can cause mild discomfort and cramping on insertion
- Carries a small risk of side effects such as heavier periods

your cervix is already slightly open to allow for menstrual flow, making insertion easier. (If you want to use an IUD after a pregnancy, doctors recommend waiting until at least 6 weeks after delivery because the IUD is more likely to be expelled as your uterus returns to its pre-pregnancy size.)

Your doctor may prescribe an antibiotic that you take by mouth about an hour before the IUD is inserted. This medication may help prevent a bacterial infection. Your doctor may also recommend a mild painkiller such as ibuprofen for uterine cramps that may occur during or right after insertion.

To insert the IUD, the doctor opens your vagina with an instrument called a speculum (the same instrument that is used to open your vagina during a Pap smear) and grasps your cervix with another instrument, which may cause mild discomfort or cramping. Next, he or she measures the length of your uterus. The IUD is introduced in a slim, plastic tube up inside your uterus as close to the top as possible. The plastic tube is withdrawn slowly, allowing the IUD to unfold into its characteristic T shape. The two strings that hang from the bottom of the IUD remain outside of your cervix and are cut to the appropriate length. During a follow-up visit a month later, your doctor will examine you to make sure your IUD is in the proper position.

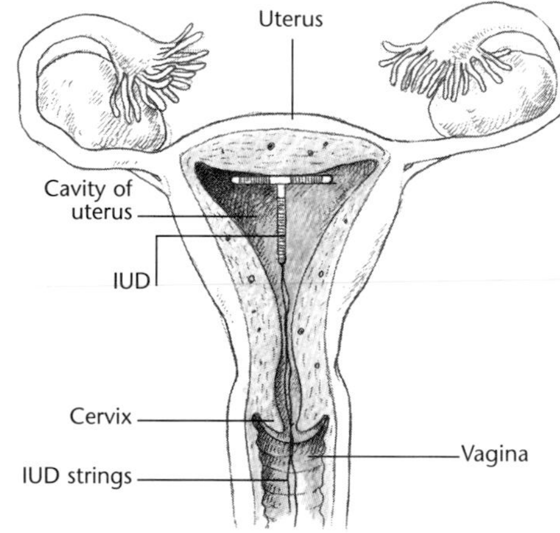

THE IUD
Only a doctor can insert or remove an IUD. When an IUD is correctly positioned inside the uterus, the strings hang slightly outside the cervix (but not outside the vagina).

Have your doctor show you how to check for the strings; checking for them monthly is the best way to make sure your IUD is in place. The first few weeks after you have an IUD inserted, check for the strings once or twice a week. If the strings feel longer than usual, if you cannot feel them at all, or if you feel the IUD itself inside your vagina, call your doctor immediately.

Some women who have a copper IUD experience heavier periods, menstrual cramps, and some spotting between periods. These symptoms usually subside or go away completely after a few months.

You can have intercourse as soon as you wish after your IUD is inserted. However, during the first month until your follow-up visit, you should use condoms and spermicide to make sure you are protected from pregnancy. Because the IUD provides no protection against sexually transmitted diseases, you should always use a condom when having sex (vaginal, oral, or anal) if you are not in a stable, mutually monogamous relationship (see page 338). An IUD can only be removed by a doctor. Do not try to remove an IUD yourself or pull on the strings—you can harm your cervix.

SURGICAL STERILIZATION

Sterilization—in either a woman or a man—is a surgical procedure that prevents reproduction. Surgical sterilization is the most common method of contraception among Americans. One out of four women of childbearing age has been sterilized using a procedure called tubal ligation in which the fallopian tubes are sealed or cut to prevent sperm from reaching an egg. A man can also be sterilized using a procedure called vasectomy, which blocks the passage of sperm from the testicles into the penis. The man still ejaculates, but his semen does not contain sperm.

In both men and women, surgical sterilization is considered permanent. Although both vasectomy and tubal ligation can sometimes be surgically reversed, reversal procedures are complicated and expensive, and usually unsuccessful. For this reason, people who do not want to have children in the future are most likely to choose sterilization as a method of birth control.

Both vasectomy and tubal ligation are nearly 100-percent effective in preventing pregnancy. However, neither procedure provides any protection against sexually transmitted diseases. You must

Surgical sterilization

Advantages
- Is considered permanent and is highly effective against pregnancy
- Does not require interruption of lovemaking
- Does not usually require an overnight stay in the hospital

Disadvantages
- Does not provide protection against sexually transmitted diseases
- Is usually not reversible
- Carries the risk of general anesthesia and surgery in the case of tubal ligation

still use a latex or polyurethane male condom or a female condom with spermicide every time you have sex (vaginal, oral, or anal) if you are not in a stable, mutually monogamous relationship (see page 338).

Vasectomy is a simpler and much less expensive operation than tubal ligation and has fewer complications. A vasectomy can be performed in 20 minutes in a doctor's office using local anesthesia (see page 260). In contrast, tubal ligation is done in an operating room and usually requires general anesthesia (see page 261). In spite of its greater difficulty and expense, tubal ligation is performed more often than vasectomy.

Tubal ligation In a tubal ligation, the fallopian tubes are either looped and banded close with rubber rings, pinched close with metal or plastic clips, cut and tied off, or burned (cauterized) with an electric current and cut. If you decide to have a tubal ligation, make sure you choose a surgeon or gynecologist who does the procedure often.

Many women who choose a tubal ligation have the operation immediately after childbirth when their uterus and fallopian tubes are still high in their abdomen and, therefore, easier to reach through a small incision under their navel. The procedure is often performed at the time of a cesarean delivery (see page 442), through the same incision. Having the procedure done at this time eliminates the need for another visit to the hospital and several extra days of rest.

Tubal ligation with laparoscopy Tubal ligation is usually performed through a small incision in the abdomen using a surgical technique called laparoscopy (see page 263). General anesthesia (see page 261) is usually used. The surgeon inserts a hollow needle into your abdomen and injects a harmless gas to expand your abdominal cavity and push the intestines out of the way. He or she then makes a tiny incision in your abdomen to insert a

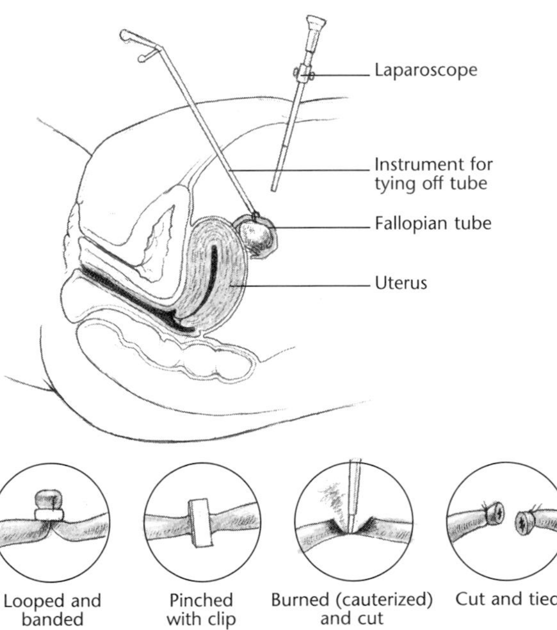

TUBAL LIGATION
In a tubal ligation, the fallopian tubes are closed off to prevent passage of an egg. The procedure is usually done through a small abdominal incision while you are under general anesthesia. The tubes are either looped and banded with rubber rings, pinched close with metal or plastic clips, burned (cauterized) with an electric current and cut, or cut and tied off with stitches.

lighted viewing instrument (laparoscope). While looking through the laparoscope, the doctor uses a second instrument to grasp and close off each fallopian tube. The tubes are then closed off using rubber rings, plastic clips, stitches, or an electrical current that burns and seals them.

During the next few days, you may have some abdominal discomfort caused by a little remaining gas, but this gradually goes away. You can return to work as soon as you wish, but you may want to take it easy for a couple of days.

Tubal ligation with laparotomy A tubal ligation can also be performed in a surgical procedure called laparotomy (see page 264). This procedure is more extensive than laparoscopy because it requires a larger incision in the abdomen. A laparotomy may be done when a woman has extensive adhesions (abnormal scar tissue) in her pelvic area that make it difficult to reach the fallopian tubes using a laparoscope. General or regional (spinal or epidural) anesthesia (see page 260) is used for laparotomy. In this procedure, the doctor makes an incision about 2 to 3 inches long in the abdomen just above the pubic hairline. Each fallopian tube is lifted out and closed off, either using stitches, rubber rings, or clips.

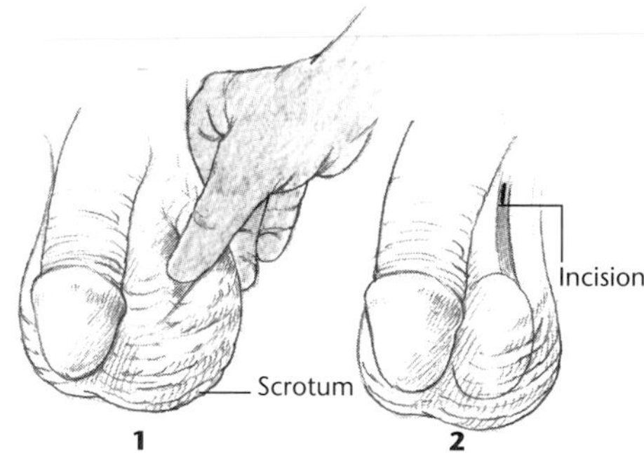

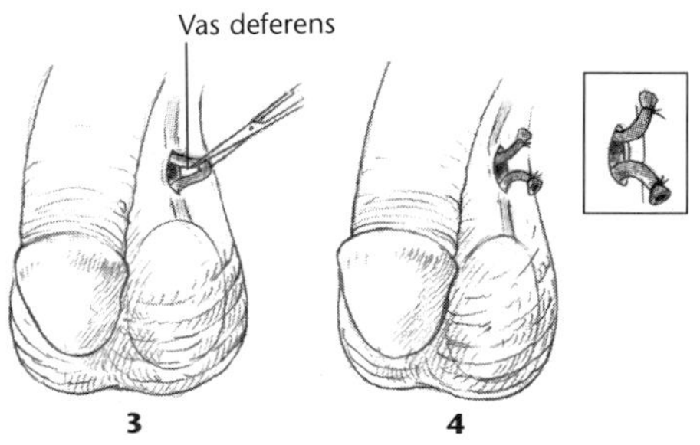

VASECTOMY

1. The doctor feels for the location of the vas deferens inside the scrotum.
2. An incision (1/4 to 1/2 inch) is made in the scrotum.
3. A loop of the vas deferens is pulled through the incision and cut.
4. The cut ends of the vas deferens are cauterized (burned) to seal them or closed with stitches. A second incision may be made on the other side of the scrotum for the second vas deferens or the same incision may be used for both. Each incision is stitched close.

Complications of tubal ligation Although rare, complications from tubal ligation may include infection, internal bleeding, or injury to adjacent organs. A possible complication of using electrocautery (burning) to close off the tubes is accidentally burning a tiny hole in a nearby abdominal organ such as the intestine or bladder.

Sterilization has a small failure rate. If a woman does become pregnant after a tubal ligation, her risk of having an ectopic pregnancy (see page 233) is greater than usual.

Vasectomy Vasectomy is a sterilization procedure for men in which the two vas deferens (the tubes that carry sperm from the testicles to the penis) are cut to prevent sperm from mixing with semen (the fluid produced at ejaculation). The sperm are instead reabsorbed into the testicles. A vasectomy does not affect a man's ability to achieve erection, have an orgasm, or ejaculate. In fact, the amount of semen ejaculated remains unchanged because the other fluids that make up most of the semen are still secreted by the prostate gland and other glands.

A vasectomy is done in the doctor's office. Vasectomy is a safer and less complicated procedure than tubal ligation because the male organs are more easily accessible and it is performed using local anesthesia. The procedure does not involve abdominal surgery so there is no risk of damaging other organs.

It is sometimes possible to reverse a vasectomy, but the reversal procedure is difficult and its success rate is less than 50 percent. A vasectomy should be considered permanent.

Standard vasectomy Before the procedure, some doctors give the man a sedative to relieve pain and relax him. The doctor locates each vas deferens by feeling it under the skin of the scrotum. Holding the skin over one of the vas deferens, he or she injects an local anesthetic to numb the area and makes a small incision. A small loop of the vas deferens is exposed and cut, and each end is sealed with electrocautery (burning) to prevent bleeding. The doctor may make another incision over the second vas deferens and repeat the procedure or use the same incision for both. Each incision is then stitched close.

No-scalpel vasectomy Another vasectomy procedure is done through a tiny puncture in the scrotum, eliminating the need for an incision. The puncture technique reduces pain, recovery time, and the risk of infection. The whole procedure takes only about 10 minutes.

After injecting a local anesthetic into the scrotum to numb it, the doctor pierces it with a sharp instrument at a place where the vas deferens is most accessible. Each vas deferens is pulled through the opening, severed, closed off, and returned to the scrotum through the same opening. No stitches are required to close the puncture, which heals on its own.

Although rare, complications may result from vasectomy. The most common problem is a hematoma, a blood clot that occurs when a blood vessel leaks. This leaking may cause painful swelling for a day or two, but then goes away on its own. A man can reduce his risk of hematoma by spending the first 24 hours after the procedure off his feet to relieve any pressure on the blood vessels in the scrotum. Any skin infection that develops near the site of the vasectomy can be treated with antibiotics taken by mouth.

A man can resume intercourse after surgery whenever it feels comfortable, which can take from a few days to a week. He will have follow-up tests to check his sperm count. Until two consecutive tests a month apart show no sperm in his semen, he and his partner should use another form of birth control.

NATURAL FAMILY PLANNING

Natural family planning methods of birth control are based on a woman's knowledge of male and female reproduction and her awareness of the signs that occur naturally during her menstrual cycle. These methods require abstaining from sexual intercourse during the time in the cycle when a woman is most likely to become pregnant. Natural family planning methods are not always reliable in preventing pregnancy because most women do not have regular menstrual cycles, many women find the close monitoring of body processes impractical, and many couples take chances and have intercourse at unsafe times in the cycle. Also, natural family planning methods alone provide no protection against sexually transmitted diseases. You or your partner must use a latex or polyurethane male condom or a female condom in order to achieve this protection.

To use natural family planning to avoid pregnancy, you must determine when you are ovulating (one of your ovaries is releasing an egg) so you can abstain from intercourse during this fertile time in your menstrual cycle. An egg survives for 12 to 24 hours after the ovary releases it, but sperm can live for 2 to 7 days in the fallopian tube. Therefore, to avoid pregnancy, you must abstain from intercourse for at least 7 days before ovulation and 3 days after.

You can use three methods to determine when you are ovulating: the calendar method, the temperature method, and/or the cervical mucus method. If you use all three methods simultaneously and refrain from intercourse during your fertile time, you can avoid pregnancy as effectively as with some other contraceptive methods, such as the diaphragm (see page 321). The calendar method alone is the least precise and effective unless you have very regular menstrual cycles. For many women, a combination of the temperature and cervical mucus methods is the most successful "natural" contraceptive technique.

Calendar method The calendar method involves tracking days between periods to estimate time of ovulation. Before starting to use the calendar method for contraception, monitor your menstrual cycles for a few months to find your longest and shortest cycle. Count the first day of menstrual bleeding as day 1 of each cycle. Subtract 20 days from your shortest menstrual cycle to determine the first day of your fertile time and 10 days from your longest menstrual cycle to determine the last day of your fertile time each month. For example, if your shortest cycle is 22 days, your first fertile day is day 2; if your longest cycle is 28 days, your last fertile day is day 18. Therefore, to avoid becoming pregnant, you have to abstain from sexual intercourse or use a backup method of birth control from the second day of your period through the 18th day of your cycle.

Temperature method The temperature method, also called basal body temperature method, involves recording your temperature daily to watch for fluctuations that indicate ovulation. You must take your temperature at the same time each day—first thing in the morning, before you get out of bed. You should use an extra-sensitive thermometer designed for this purpose. The thermometer can be used orally, rectally, or vaginally as long as you take your temperature the same way every time. Your temperature rises slightly (0.4° to 0.8°F) before, during, or right after ovulation and remains at this elevated level until your next period begins. These temperature changes are very small (less than 1°F), so to be accurate you should record your temperature each day on a chart.

You should assume you are fertile and refrain from intercourse or use a backup method of birth control from the beginning of your cycle (no later than day 4) until after your temperature has remained elevated for 3 days in a row. One disadvantage of this method is that fever, stress, or other disruptions can affect your temperature and thus the accuracy of your chart.

Cervical mucus method The cervical mucus method requires that you check your vaginal discharge every day (for example, when you use the toilet) for changes that signal ovulation. You can collect the mucus directly from your vagina either with your finger or with toilet paper. You probably will not have any mucus for a few days after your period. Then you will notice mucus that is thick, cloudy, whitish or yellowish, and sticky. As you approach ovulation, the mucus becomes more abundant and feels increasingly wet. A clear, abundant, stretchy mucus that resembles raw egg white is a sign of ovulation. After ovulation, the mucus becomes thick, cloudy, and sticky again or disappears. Consider the presence of any mucus at all to mean you are fertile. Refrain from intercourse or use a backup method of birth control during the first part of your cycle up through the fourth day after your mucus becomes noticeably most abundant. You should not use barrier methods, except for condoms, as backup birth control during fertile times while you are using the cervical mucus method; contraceptive jelly, such as that used with diaphragms, and foam may change the consistency of your cervical mucus.

The cervical mucus method may not give you enough advance warning of ovulation to prevent unplanned pregnancy. Some women do not secrete sufficient amounts of mucus to reliably evaluate changes during the menstrual cycle.

Abortion

Abortion is the termination of pregnancy. When performed by a qualified doctor, it is a safe medical procedure for a woman with an unwanted pregnancy or a fetus with a severe birth defect.

The decision about whether or not to have an abortion is a personal one. If you need to make such a decision, ask your doctor about any aspect of the procedure—medical or emotional—that concerns you. If you are under 18, call the local office of Planned Parenthood to find out if the law in your state requires that one or both of your parents be notified before you can have an abortion.

Sometimes abortions are performed not because the pregnancy is unwanted, but because the life of the woman or fetus is, or will be, in danger if the pregnancy progresses. When serious medical problems are involved, whether or not to continue a pregnancy is a decision a woman must make in consultation with her doctor. For example, a woman with severe heart disease may not be able to tolerate the stress that a pregnancy places on her heart. In a woman with advanced or uncontrolled diabetes (see page 418), pregnancy can cause serious complications for the woman and fetus, including birth defects. A woman may also choose abortion if the fetus has an abnormality that will prevent it from surviving outside the uterus or a serious genetic disorder (see page 373).

If you are considering abortion and are looking for a clinic, ask for referrals from your primary care doctor or gynecologist, the obstetrics and gynecology department of a local hospital, or a local Planned Parenthood office. If you are a student, talk to a school nurse or guidance counselor or another adult you trust.

If you are faced with an unplanned pregnancy, as soon as possible after you learn you are pregnant, think about whether you will have an abortion or continue the pregnancy. An abortion is much more easily and safely performed early in pregnancy. Up to the 12th week of pregnancy, an abortion is a private matter between a woman and her doctor. After the 12th week, state law may regulate abortion. Some states require a 24-hour waiting period before a woman can have an abortion. Check the laws in your state by talking to your doctor or ask for information from a local Planned Parenthood office.

AT AN ABORTION CLINIC

At your first visit to an abortion clinic, a medical assistant or counselor will review consent forms with you in detail. He or she will tell you that this is your decision to make and you can change your mind at any time before the abortion is performed. The counselor is there to help you; take the opportunity to talk about how you feel about your decision and to learn all you can about the procedure.

If you decide to have an abortion, you will undergo several tests beforehand, including a pregnancy test. You will have blood tests to determine if you are Rh negative (see page 371). If you are Rh negative, you will be given Rh immune globulin to avoid the risk of becoming sensitized to Rh, which can harm both you and the fetus in any future pregnancy. You may also be tested for sexually transmitted diseases (STDs). If you have an STD such as chlamydia or gonorrhea, which can spread to your upper reproductive tract, you will be treated for it before you have the abortion. The clinic may perform an ultrasound examination (see page 405) to determine the age of the fetus. (It may be dangerous to terminate a pregnancy that is too far along.)

You will be given instructions about how long before the procedure you should stop eating or drinking fluids, depending on the type of anesthesia (see page 260) you will receive for the procedure. On the day of the abortion, you may want to arrange to have a close friend or relative come along for emotional support and to drive you home. Having an abortion does not require an overnight stay in the hospital or clinic.

ABORTION PROCEDURES

The vast majority of abortions are performed during the first 12 weeks of pregnancy. The earlier in pregnancy an abortion is performed, the safer it is for the woman and the lower the risk of complications, such as bleeding.

Vacuum aspiration Vacuum aspiration, also called vacuum curettage or suction curettage, is the most common abortion procedure during the first 12 weeks of pregnancy. The doctor first performs a pelvic examination to determine the size and position of your uterus and opens your vagina with a speculum (the same instrument that is used during a Pap smear). After injecting a local anesthetic into your cervix to numb it (you may feel a slight pinching, cramping, or pressure), the doctor dilates (opens) your cervix with slender, tapered metal rods of increasingly larger sizes. This process may cause some cramping.

Once the cervix is open wide enough, the doctor inserts a suction tube, which is attached to a vacuum pump, and moves the tube around inside your uterus to loosen and remove the contents. A spoon-shaped instrument (curet) is used to scoop out any remaining tissue. The procedure takes about 10 to 15 minutes.

You may experience cramps and some nausea and vaginal bleeding afterward. The clinic will provide a place for you to rest after the procedure and will monitor your recovery. You usually can go home within an hour or two. You will have mild cramping for 2 or 3 days and bleeding that should be no heavier than a regular period. The bleeding will taper off and stop within 2 to 7 days after the abortion. Using a mild painkiller such as ibuprofen or acetaminophen can relieve any discomfort you might feel. Your doctor will tell you to refrain from sexual intercourse for 2 to 3 weeks.

Mifepristone Mifepristone, a synthetic hormone, is often referred to as an "abortion pill" because it can end pregnancy by causing the lining of the uterus to shed. The drug has been available in Europe for several years and is currently being tested in the US. When used for an abortion, mifepristone must be taken within 9 weeks of your last period. Its success rate is highest for pregnancies of less than 6 weeks. The drug blocks the action of the hormone progesterone, which is essential for pregnancy.

To induce an abortion, you take one dose of mifepristone in a pill. Two days later you take a combination of pills that stimulate uterine contractions, which expel the embryo. The effectiveness of mifepristone is 96 percent—nearly the same as that of a surgical abortion—but the drug does not carry the risks of surgery.

It may take several days to complete the termination of pregnancy using mifepristone. You will experience cramps for 2 to 3 days and bleeding similar to that of a heavy period, usually lasting about 7 to 10 days. In the meantime, you can take a mild painkiller such as ibuprofen or acetaminophen to help relieve the pain and discomfort. Other side effects of mifepristone may include nausea, vomiting, and diarrhea. Because the dose of the drug is very small, these symptoms are usually mild.

In a small number of women who take mifepristone, the pregnancy is not terminated. For this reason, your doctor will tell you when you should return for a follow-up visit to make sure the pregnancy was successfully terminated. If the pregnancy was not terminated with mifepristone, you can choose to have a surgical abortion or continue with the pregnancy. Most doctors recommend a surgical abortion if mifepristone has failed to terminate a pregnancy.

Dilation and evacuation Dilation and evacuation is the most common abortion procedure performed between weeks 13 and 16 of a pregnancy. The procedure is similar to vacuum aspiration except that the cervix must be opened wider because larger instruments are required to remove larger pieces of tissue. To open your cervix, tiny devices called osmotic dilating agents, which resemble small tampons, may be placed inside your cervical canal the day before the scheduled abortion. Osmotic dilating agents absorb water and swell, pushing open the cervical canal. You will be told not to eat or drink anything for about 12 hours before the procedure.

Dilation and evacuation is performed in an operating room in a clinic or hospital. You may be given intravenous fluids and a pain medication or sedative. The doctor injects a local anesthetic into your cervix to numb it. After removing the dilating agents (if they are used), the doctor inserts a vacuum pump and grasping instruments through your cervix into the uterus to remove tissue. A curet is used to scrape the walls of the uterus to make sure no tissue is left behind. In pregnancies beyond 14 weeks, a medication called oxytocin often is given intravenously to stimulate the uterus to contract and shrink.

After the procedure, your pulse and blood pressure will be checked and you will be examined periodically for signs of bleeding. After a few hours, if you can keep fluids down, you will be able to go home. You will be asked to return for a checkup about 1 or 2 weeks later.

Bleeding after a dilation and evacuation should be no heavier than your usual period and should decrease over the next 1 to 10 days. If bleeding is heavier than a period or does not stop within 10 days, call your doctor. You should also call your doctor if you have a temperature higher than 100°F or pelvic pain worse than menstrual cramps. These may be signs that some tissue from the pregnancy is still inside your uterus or that you have an infection.

Late second trimester abortions Although a highly skilled surgeon can perform a surgical abortion up to the 20th week of pregnancy, many abortions performed during the 16th to 24th week use nonsurgical methods. These procedures are done in hospitals or surgery centers and usually take several hours. During any of these procedures, most women are given a drug called oxytocin intravenously to stimulate the uterus to contract and shrink, which reduces bleeding.

Abortion using saline In a saline abortion, a concentrated salt solution is injected into the uterus through a needle inserted through the abdomen to end a pregnancy and induce contractions of the uterus. Over several hours, the contractions cause the cervix to dilate (open) and the contents of the uterus to be expelled.

Abortion using urea and prostaglandins Urea is a nitrogen-based solution that can be injected into the uterus to end a pregnancy. Drugs called prostaglandins are then given to induce contractions of the uterus strong enough to expel its contents.

Abortion using prostaglandins only Prostaglandins, which are drugs that stimulate powerful contractions of the uterus, are used for late pregnancies in which the fetus has died of natural causes. Prostaglandins, given in suppositories, are introduced into the vagina to induce labor and expel the fetus. Prostaglandins may also stimulate muscle contractions elsewhere in the body and cause such side effects as nausea, vomiting, diarrhea, fever, and high blood pressure. A woman is given medication before the procedure to prevent these side effects.

After all of these procedures, there is a small possibility that a dilation and curettage (D and C; see page 262) will be required to remove the placenta (the organ that connects the fetus's circulation to that of the woman) if it is not expelled during the abortion. After the procedure, you will be monitored for several hours or overnight to make sure you do not have bleeding heavier than a period. When your heart rate and blood pressure are stable, you can go home. Your doctor will recommend that you rest for a couple of days before resuming your normal activities. It is extremely important to have followup visits to your doctor as he or she recommends.

Complications of abortion The risk of complications from an abortion is extremely small—much smaller than the potential risks involved in carrying a pregnancy to term. However, the later in pregnancy you have an abortion—particularly after the 12th week—the greater the chance of problems. When they do occur, these complications usually begin within a few days of the abortion. One possible complication of any abortion is that some tissue may remain in the uterus after the procedure. Because there is more tissue to remove later in a pregnancy, it is more likely for some to be left behind after a late abortion. You may continue to expel tiny pieces of tissue for a few days. This process is normal as long as it is not accompanied by bleeding that is heavier than a period, a temperature over 100°F, or cramps worse than you experience during a regular period.

If your uterus does not expel the tissue on its own and you have signs of an infection, such as a fever, you may have to have additional surgery, such as dilation and curettage (D and C). Other symptoms of infection include cramps, abnormal vaginal discharge, and discomfort in your pelvis. An infection can sometimes be cleared up with antibiotics.

Another complication of abortion occurs when a pregnancy is not successfully terminated. A woman may continue to have such signs of pregnancy as a lack of periods, breast swelling, nausea, and a feeling of fullness in the lower abdomen. After a second trimester abortion, it is especially important to have followup checkups with your doctor to make sure the pregnancy was successfully terminated. If the pregnancy was not terminated and you wait too long to see your doctor, you may not be able to have another abortion.

Potential complications of abortion using saline—including high salt levels in the blood, abnormal bleeding, convulsions, and, in rare cases, coma—can occur if the salt is absorbed into the woman's bloodstream.

After your abortion Plan to take 1 or 2 days off from your usual activities after an abortion. You may have a sense of pelvic pressure or mild, aching discomfort. If you feel severe pain, call your doctor. After a few days, your breasts will return to their normal size and morning sickness (if you had it) will go away. You should have a period within 4 to 6 weeks after the abortion. Schedule a follow-up visit with your doctor a month after the abortion to make sure the pregnancy was successfully terminated and there are no complications, such as infection. You may feel mildly depressed or even regretful after your abortion; many women do. These feelings usually pass in a few days or weeks; if they do not, talking with a qualified therapist (see page 194) may be helpful.

If you did not discuss contraception with your doctor before your abortion, it is especially important to ask about it before you resume intercourse so that you can find a reliable method of birth control that you can use successfully to prevent another unplanned pregnancy. Having one or two abortions does not in any way affect your ability to have children in the future. However, having three or more abortions may weaken your cervix, making it difficult for you to carry a pregnancy to term and increasing your risk of having a miscarriage (see page 422) in a later pregnancy.

CHAPTER 12

Sexually transmitted diseases

Contents

Sexually transmitted diseases are infections that are spread primarily, although not exclusively, by sexual intercourse. These serious diseases, many of which have long-term health consequences (such as infertility) affect people of every age, racial, ethnic, and socioeconomic group.

The increasing risk of STDs

Although the incidence of sexually transmitted diseases (STDs) has escalated dramatically in the last several decades, many women do not think they are personally at risk. Fewer than one third of sexually active women report using condoms to help protect themselves against STDs.

Not only are women at risk of STDs, they are at greater risk than men. The warm, moist environment of the vagina may be conducive to the growth of disease-causing organisms. These organisms may be present in semen, which enters the vagina during intercourse. In a single act of unprotected intercourse with an

What is your risk of acquiring an STD?

Women are at greater risk than men of acquiring some sexually transmitted diseases—even after just one sexual encounter with an infected person. For example, half of all women exposed to gonorrhea during a single sexual encounter become infected while only one fourth of men do. The exceptions are herpes and genital warts, which pose an equal risk to both sexes.

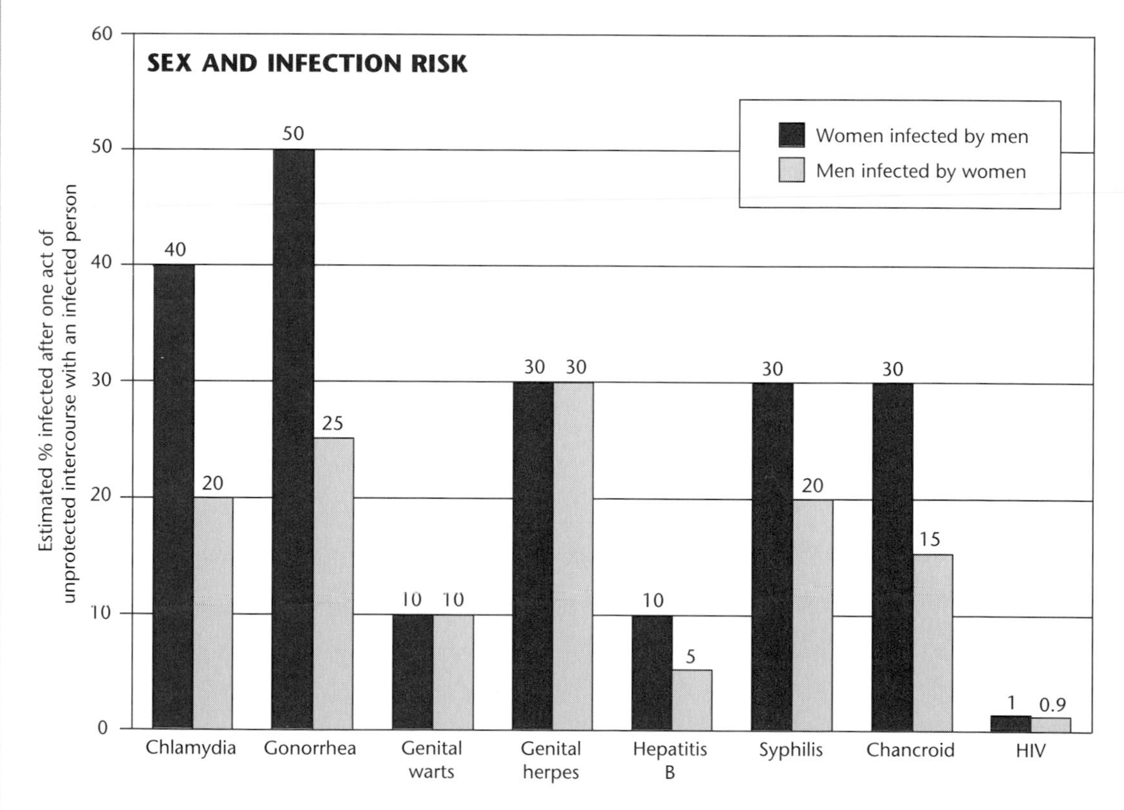

infected partner, a woman is twice as likely as a man to contract such common STDs as chlamydia and gonorrhea. It may also be easier for a woman to contract HIV, the virus that causes AIDS, from a man than vice versa because the delicate tissue of the vagina is more prone than the penis to tiny tears through which the virus can enter the bloodstream.

In women, the symptoms of an STD are often not apparent because they occur inside the vagina. For this reason, STDs can be difficult to diagnose in women. Sometimes, a woman can be infected with an STD for several months or years before she or her doctor discovers it. By that time, the infection may have spread up through her uterus and into the fallopian tubes, causing pelvic inflammatory disease (PID; see page 232). PID is an extremely serious condition—it can produce scarring in a fallopian tube, which can block the tube and lead to ectopic pregnancy (see page 233), infertility (see page 382), or persistent pelvic pain.

In addition to the dangers to her own health, a pregnant woman can transmit an STD to the fetus during pregnancy or childbirth. Some STDs can cause miscarriage or premature delivery. The viruses that cause AIDS and hepatitis B, which are present in the body fluids of an infected woman, can be transmitted to a nursing child through breast milk. Children born to women who have hepatitis B are at increased risk of cirrhosis of the liver and liver cancer. Most children infected with HIV, the virus that causes AIDS, die by age 8. A child born to a woman infected with gonorrhea or syphilis may have a low birth weight or respiratory problems or such severe birth defects as blindness and mental retardation.

Some STDs—such as chlamydia, gonorrhea, and syphilis—are caused by bacteria and therefore can be cured with antibiotics. Others, such as herpes, are caused by viruses and can be treated but not cured. AIDS is incurable and fatal.

STDs: A growing problem

It is estimated that more than 12 million new cases of STDs occur each year in the US. This table shows the estimated annual incidences of some of the most common STDs:

STDs	NEW CASES
Chlamydia	4,000,000
Trichomoniasis	3,000,000
Genital warts	1,000,000
Gonorrhea	800,000
Genital herpes	500,000
HIV/AIDS	141,000
Syphilis	101,000
Hepatitis B	53,000

PREVENTING STDs

The only sure way to protect yourself from STDs is to abstain from sexual activities, including vaginal and anal intercourse and oral sex, during which infections can be transmitted. After abstinence, your best protection against STDs is using a latex or polyurethane male condom or a female condom correctly every time you have sex.

The most popular forms of contraception—surgical sterilization (tubal ligation in women and vasectomy in men) and birth-control pills—give no protection against STDs because they do not provide a barrier between the infecting organism and the delicate mucous membranes lining the vagina and cervix. However, birth-control pills and tubal ligation may protect against the development of pelvic inflammatory disease (PID; see page 232), a serious infection that can cause infertility.

You need to use a latex or polyurethane male condom or a female condom with spermicide every time you have sex because even one act of vaginal, anal, or oral sex without a condom is all it takes to become infected. Unless you are involved in a stable, mutually monogamous relationship, there is no way to know for sure if your partner has an STD. You can ask, but your partner may have an infection and not know it, or not tell you the truth. Your partner may have contracted an undetected infection before your relationship began. Looking at your partner's genitals for sores or a discharge is a good idea, but a lack of these signs is no reassurance that the person does not have an STD.

WARNING SIGNS STDs

If you notice any of the following symptoms, see your doctor immediately:

- Any open sores, red or white bumps or rashes, or liquid-filled blisters, no matter how small, in your genital area
- Redness or swelling in your genital area
- Any unusual change in the amount, color, smell, or consistency of your vaginal discharge
- Pain in your pelvis or abdomen, with or without nausea or vomiting
- Pain, soreness, irritation, or other discomfort during intercourse, or bleeding after intercourse
- Fever, loss of appetite, fatigue, or swollen lymph nodes (infection-fighting glands) in your groin or neck
- Unusually severe menstrual cramps
- Recurring yeast infections and other infections

What is a mutually monogamous relationship?

A mutually monogamous relationship is one in which neither partner is having sex with anyone else. If either you or your partner has had sex with someone else within the last 6 months, there is a risk of exposure to an STD. If you are beginning a new sexual relationship, always use a latex or polyurethane male condom or a female condom with spermicide to protect yourself from STDs. Before you think about having sex without using a condom, make sure that the following guidelines apply to your relationship:

- You and your partner are having sex only with each other.
- You and your partner have both tested negative for HIV (the virus that causes AIDS) and other STDs (such as chlamydia and gonorrhea) 6 months after your last sexual encounter with another person.
- Neither you nor your partner is injecting illegal drugs.

Most STDs are caused by bacteria or viruses—microorganisms that enter the body through the warm, moist tissues that line the external genitals, vagina, urethra (the tube that carries urine from the bladder), mouth, or anus. If your partner has more than one STD, you can be infected with any or all of them during one sexual encounter. For example, gonorrhea and chlamydia are often transmitted together. It is unlikely that you will get an STD from a toilet seat, doorknob, or other object because the microorganisms cannot live for long on these surfaces.

Prevention is the best defense you have against STDs. Using a latex or polyurethane male condom or a female condom (see page 318) with spermicide consistently and correctly can help you avoid infection. If you get an STD, report any symptoms to your doctor immediately to ensure that you get prompt treatment and to help prevent you from passing it on to another person. Inform any sex partners if you are diagnosed with an STD so that they can also be treated. If your partner is diagnosed with an STD or has symptoms of one, see your doctor immediately for an examination even if you do not have any symptoms yourself. For more about protecting yourself from STDs, see page 171.

TESTING FOR STDs

Because the symptoms of an STD are not always apparent, it is important to have a yearly gynecologic examination (see page 124). You should have an examination more frequently if you have more than one sexual partner or if you have changed partners. During your regular examination, tell your doctor if you are sexually active so that he or she will check for signs of STDs. If you are age 25 or younger, your doctor may recommend tests for chlamydia and gonorrhea, the most common STDs, which often have no symptoms in women.

Report any unusual symptoms you have noticed, including sores in your genital area, unusual vaginal discharge or odor, or swelling, redness, or tenderness in your genital area. Pain during intercourse may also indicate an STD.

The long-term effects of STDs

If left untreated, some STDs—especially chlamydia and gonorrhea—may lead to pelvic inflammatory disease (PID), an infection of the uterus, fallopian tubes, or ovaries. PID may have few, if any, symptoms. But it can have serious consequences, including persistent pelvic pain, infertility, ectopic pregnancy, or even death. For more about the diagnosis and treatment of PID, see page 232.

Depending on your symptoms, your doctor will perform tests to identify specific infections. For example, your doctor will take a sample of cells from your cervix to be examined in a laboratory for the organisms that cause chlamydia and gonorrhea. It is especially important to detect these STDs at an early stage, because they can spread through your reproductive system and cause pelvic inflammatory disease (PID), a serious infection that can block your fallopian tubes and cause infertility.

For the most part, your doctor must rely on your sexual history, the symptoms you report, and the signs he or she sees to determine whether or not to test you for STDs. See your doctor immediately if you notice any of the symptoms described in the following pages. If you are diagnosed with an STD, notify all of your sexual partners so that they can seek treatment too. This may not be easy, but it is extremely important to help protect their health and to keep yourself from getting reinfected.

Teens and STDs

One out of four people who acquires an STD is a teenager. Sexually active girls between 10 and 19 have the highest incidence of chlamydia and gonorrhea of any group. Teenagers are the least likely to seek medical help or tell their sexual partner that they have been diagnosed with an STD. As a result, many young women who acquire STDs experience the long-term effects of these diseases—including infertility (see page 232)—many years later.

If you are a sexually active teenager, annual pelvic examinations, including a Pap smear (see page 127) to test for cervical cancer and tests for STDs, are vitally important to protect your health and your ability to have children. Your teen years are an excellent time to get into the habit of having annual examinations—a habit that you should follow throughout your adult life. If you are not comfortable talking to your parents or family doctor, talk to the school nurse or another adult you trust about helping you get the basic medical care you need. You can also receive helpful information, counseling, and other services from the local office of Planned Parenthood.

Symptoms, diagnosis, and treatment

More than 50 disease-causing organisms are transmitted sexually—through vaginal or anal intercourse or oral sex. The infections that result have varying symptoms and degrees of seriousness; the methods of diagnosis and treatment differ as well. If you do acquire an STD, being able to recognize the symptoms enables you to get immediate treatment. Prompt treatment reduces your risk of long-term consequences that can result from an untreated STD, such as pelvic inflammatory disease (PID), which can lead to infertility. Prompt treatment of an STD also decreases the likelihood that you transmit the infection to another person.

On the following pages, you will find descriptions of the symptoms of some of the most common STDs and how they are spread, and explanations of their diagnosis and treatment.

CHLAMYDIA

Chlamydia is a bacterial infection that can be acquired through vaginal or anal intercourse and, sometimes, through oral sex. Chlamydia is the most common STD—4 million new cases occur each year in the US. It is also the most frequent cause of pelvic inflammatory disease (PID; see page 232).

If a woman with chlamydia becomes pregnant, the infection can cause the amniotic sac (the fluid-filled sac surrounding the fetus) to break, resulting in premature birth. The infection can also be transmitted to an infant in the birth canal during vaginal delivery. Chlamydia can cause life-threatening pneumonia in infants, which can result in long-term respiratory problems. It is also a major cause of eye infections in newborns. For these reasons, if you are planning to become pregnant, it is a good idea to be tested for chlamydia.

Symptoms Most women who have chlamydia do not have any symptoms. Most infected men, on the other hand, do experience symptoms, which include a burning sensation during urination, a clear discharge from the penis, and swelling or pain in the testicles. In women who have symptoms (which usually appear within 1 to 3 weeks of exposure to the disease-causing bacteria), the symptoms may include abnormal vaginal discharge, a burning sensation during urination, pain or pressure in the pelvic area, pain during intercourse, or vaginal bleeding after intercourse.

Diagnosis Because people who are infected with chlamydia may not have symptoms, the infection can be difficult to diagnose. The most accurate way to diagnose chlamydia in a woman is through laboratory testing of a sample of vaginal discharge. Several laboratory tests are available, some of which provide results in 24 hours. Because chlamydia is so common, many doctors test for the infection during a regular annual pelvic examination in sexually active women who may be at risk. Ask your doctor if he or she thinks you need to be tested.

Treatment Chlamydia is usually treated with antibiotics taken by mouth. In severe cases, the medication is given by injection into a vein. Both you and your partner must be treated at the same time; you should refrain from having sex until treatment is completed. Even if you do not have symptoms, you need to be treated if your partner is infected.

If the infection has progressed to your fallopian tubes (pelvic inflammatory disease, see page 232), you may have to be hospitalized and given antibiotics intravenously to eliminate the infection. An infection in the fallopian tubes can cause scarring, which can block them and make you infertile and at increased risk of having an ectopic pregnancy (see page 233).

If you are diagnosed with chlamydia and there is a possibility you might be pregnant, tell your doctor. He or she must rule out an ectopic pregnancy and make sure you receive an antibiotic that is safe to use during pregnancy.

If the infection returns after treatment, it may indicate that you or your partner did not take the medication as prescribed, or that one of you is having sex outside the relationship with an infected person. You and your partner should discuss the situation and determine the cause. You both will have to undergo a repeat course of treatment.

GONORRHEA

Gonorrhea is a highly contagious bacterial infection that can be transmitted through vaginal, anal, or oral sex. More than 800,000 new cases of gonorrhea are reported each year in the US. The incidence of gonorrhea is highest among sexually active teenage girls. The infection can occur in the cervix, vagina, urethra (the small tube that carries urine from the bladder), rectum, or throat.

Because 80 percent of early gonorrhea infections produce few symptoms in women, the infection often goes undetected. An undetected and untreated infection of the cervix can spread to your fallopian tubes and produce abscesses (pus-filled areas) in the tubes and ovaries (pelvic inflammatory disease, see page 232). This process causes scarring in the fallopian tubes that can result in a life-threatening ectopic pregnancy (a pregnancy that occurs outside the uterus, usually in a fallopian tube; see page 233), infertility (see page 382), and persistent pelvic pain. In men, gonorrhea can lead to infertility.

A pregnant woman who is infected with gonorrhea can pass it to her baby during childbirth, causing blindness and such serious infections as meningitis (an infection of the lining covering the brain and spinal cord). To prevent gonorrhea-related blindness in infants, all states require that the eyes of newborns be treated with silver nitrate drops or an antibiotic ointment. Most pregnant women are tested for gonorrhea during their initial prenatal visit (see page 403) to their doctor. If you are pregnant or you have a new sex partner or more than one partner, you should be tested and, if necessary, treated for gonorrhea during the last trimester of pregnancy to avoid infecting your baby during delivery.

Symptoms Symptoms of gonorrhea, if any, usually appear within 2 to 10 days of exposure to the disease-causing bacteria. In women, symptoms are often mild or nonexistent. When they occur, early symptoms of gonorrhea include a green or yellow-green discharge from the vagina or rectum and burning or itching during urination. The most common symptoms in men are a slow dripping of pus from the penis and burning or itching during urination.

If you notice that your partner has a thick, milky discharge from his penis at times other than during ejaculation, do not have sexual contact (vaginal, oral, or anal) with him and see your doctor immediately. Your partner must also see his doctor for treatment. You must notify any other sex partners you have had.

Untreated gonorrhea can spread to your bloodstream and other organs of your body, infecting the joints, heart valves, or brain and causing severe arthritis, heart disease, or brain damage. In these cases, symptoms can include a fever, severe pelvic pain, abdominal pain, lower back pain, the urge to urinate more frequently than usual, swelling and tenderness in glands in the groin area, a rash anywhere on the body, a sore throat, or sharp pains in the upper abdomen or shoulders. If you have a fever, shaking chills, rash, or joint pains, seek medical attention immediately.

Diagnosis In women, gonorrhea is usually diagnosed from laboratory testing of a sample of cells from cervical secretions. The testing procedure is similar to a Pap smear (see page 127). The results of the test are usually available in a couple of days. In men, the same laboratory test is used to diagnose the infection from a sample of discharge from the penis. Sometimes, a doctor can make a diagnosis by examining a sample of discharge from the penis under a microscope in his or her office.

Treatment Gonorrhea can be cured with antibiotics taken by mouth. Several different types are effective. You and your sexual partner must be treated at the same time to avoid reinfecting each other. If the infection returns after you have been treated, it may mean that you or your partner did not take the medication as prescribed, that the antibiotic is not effective against the strain of gonorrhea you are infected with, or that one of you is having sex with an infected person outside the relationship. You and your partner should discuss this and determine the cause. You both will have to be treated again.

To make sure the antibiotic has cured the infection, your doctor may recommend a follow-up test about 2 weeks after the first one. If the infection has spread to your fallopian tubes or ovaries or if the bacteria have entered into your bloodstream, you may have to be hospitalized and given antibiotics injected into a vein.

GENITAL WARTS

Genital warts are an extremely common STD caused by strains of the human papillomavirus (HPV). HPV can be transmitted through vaginal, anal, or oral sex. The infection can produce painless, fleshy, cauliflowerlike warts on and inside the genitals, anus, or throat. An estimated 24 to 40 million people in the US are infected, and as many as 1 million new cases occur each year.

Like other STDs caused by viruses, genital warts cannot be cured. However, the warts can be treated. The virus can remain in your system and cause recurrences of the warts at any time. About half of all people infected with HPV have recurrences after treatment. You can transmit the virus to a sexual partner even if you do not have signs of warts. Male condoms do not necessarily block transmission of HPV because invisible warts may be present on the base of the penis, which is not protected by a male condom. The female condom (see page 318) may provide more protection against HPV because it covers a woman's external genitals.

Some strains of HPV appear to increase the risk of cancer of the cervix, vulva (the external genitals), vagina, anus, or penis. If you have HPV, having a Pap smear (see page 127) to test for cancer of the cervix every year—or more frequently if your doctor recommends it—is especially important. The Pap smear can detect early abnormal changes in cells of the cervix (cervical dysplasia, see page 218) caused by exposure to the virus. These abnormal cell changes can lead to cancer if not treated.

You are at increased risk of an HPV infection if you have a condition that weakens your immune system (such as AIDS or diabetes), if you are undergoing chemotherapy for cancer, or if you are pregnant.

In rare cases, a baby exposed to HPV in the vagina during delivery can develop warts in his or her throat. These warts can be removed using laser surgery. Warts may also appear on the baby's genitals. These warts can be removed using laser surgery or by applying strong chemicals, in the form of liquid or cream, to freeze or burn them. Once treated, HPV causes no permanent harm to the child and rarely recurs. A woman with HPV does not need to have a cesarean section (surgical delivery through the abdomen) because the risk of transmission during vaginal delivery is extremely low.

Symptoms Genital warts are flat or raised, pink, white, or brown areas on the genitals or anus. The warts, which are painless, can occur as one or two tiny bumps or as large clusters. They are usually visible, but sometimes are so small (in both men and women) that they are difficult to see with the naked eye. In women, genital warts can go undetected when they occur inside the vagina or on the cervix. In men, they may appear on the penis, scrotum (the pouch of skin containing the testicles), or anus. Rarely, warts appear inside the mouth on the gums.

Diagnosis A doctor can usually recognize genital warts by sight. He or she may coat the area with a diluted vinegar solution that makes the warts more visible. (The vinegar solution makes them appear white.) The doctor may also use a magnifying lens to detect very small warts.

Treatment HPV cannot be cured and recurrences are common. However, a variety of treatments—freezing, laser surgery, medication applied directly to the warts, or traditional surgery—can remove or destroy the warts. A medication called interferon can be injected into the warts. The type of treatment used in any one case depends on the extent of the infection and, in the case of a recurrence, on the way in which the warts were previously treated.

It is important to eliminate as many of the warts as possible to reduce the risk of a recurrence. Almost all the treatments cause some degree of pain (burning, soreness, or skin irritation) at the time of the procedure and for a day or two after. Before undergoing treatment, ask your doctor to describe the procedure you will have so you know what to expect.

You and your sexual partner must be treated at the same time. Either of you may still have invisible warts. If you carry the virus, you can continue to pass the infection back and forth to each other. Although condoms do not guarantee protection, you can reduce your risk of a recurrence by using a latex or polyurethane male condom or a female condom with spermicide every time you have sexual intercourse. You can also use a lubricant that is water-based (not oil-based like petroleum jelly) with either type of condom to help reduce friction during intercourse; friction can cause small tears in the skin of the genital area, making it more vulnerable to infection.

GENITAL HERPES

Herpes is a highly contagious infection caused by the herpes simplex virus. There is no cure for herpes. As many as 500,000 new cases occur each year in the US; more than 40 million Americans are already infected with the virus.

A herpes infection can cause repeated outbreaks of painful sores that look like blisters on the genitals. Most cases of genital herpes are caused by a strain of the virus called herpes simplex virus 2. Another strain (herpes simplex virus 1) usually causes cold sores (also called fever blisters or sun blisters) around the mouth. However, both viruses can cause infections on the genitals or in the mouth.

The herpes virus can be transmitted by direct skin-to-skin contact with the affected area, even when the infected person has no obvious signs or symptoms. In some women, a sample of vaginal secretions examined in the laboratory shows evidence of the virus even though the women have no visible sores. When sores are present, the infection is extremely contagious. A person with cold sores can transmit the virus to his or her partner's genitals during oral sex.

If you notice symptoms of herpes for the first time while you are pregnant, see your doctor immediately. Women who acquire herpes during a pregnancy have an increased risk of transmitting the infection to the child during labor and delivery. Although rare, a herpes infection in a newborn can cause serious eye problems, severe brain damage, and death within the first year of life.

If you were already infected with genital herpes when you became pregnant, make sure your doctor knows you have herpes. He or she will probably want you to come to the hospital early in your labor so you can be examined to rule out an outbreak. If you have an outbreak of genital herpes at the time of labor, you might be advised to have a cesarean section (surgical delivery through an incision in your abdomen) because the baby can become infected in the vagina during delivery. However, if you do not have an outbreak of herpes at the time of delivery, it is safe for you to deliver vaginally.

The herpes virus can hide in the body inside nerve cells where the immune system cannot find it. In many people, the virus periodically becomes active, causing recurring outbreaks of sores in the same area of the genitals. These outbreaks are often triggered by stress, illness, or injury to the affected area.

A herpes infection puts you at increased risk of cervical cancer (see page 250). Sores that form on the cervix make the tissue more vulnerable to infection with the human papillomavirus (HPV; see page 341), a sexually transmitted virus that can cause abnormal cell changes in the cervix, which in turn can lead to cancer.

An active genital herpes infection (with sores present) also increases your risk of becoming infected with HIV, the virus that causes AIDS, if you are exposed to it. The open sores provide HIV an entry point into the bloodstream. If you or your partner has a cold sore around the mouth, or if it feels like you may be getting one, do not have oral sex until the blister is gone. If you transfer the virus to your partner during oral sex, he may spread it to your genital area during intercourse. This sequence can be the same for either partner.

Avoid kissing people who have cold sores or fever blisters or sharing their towels, eating utensils, or drinking containers. Do not share towels with a person who has genital herpes. Avoid vaginal, oral, and anal sex completely when you or your partner has any symptoms of herpes, including sores on your genitals or tingling or itchiness in the genital area. Have sex only when you have no symptoms, and even then always use a latex or polyurethane male condom or a female condom with spermicide. However, using a condom during an outbreak does not guarantee protection against herpes because the sores can occur in an area a condom does not cover.

Relieving the symptoms of genital herpes

Although herpes cannot be cured, there are several things you can do to relieve pain and discomfort during an outbreak.

- Ask your doctor about using the drug acyclovir in pills or in an ointment that you apply to the affected area to kill the virus. The medication can also help speed healing and reduce pain. Acyclovir is available only by prescription.
- Take an over-the-counter pain medication such as aspirin, acetaminophen, or ibuprofen to relieve pain and reduce fever.
- Keep your genital area clean and dry to avoid a bacterial infection. (Open sores are susceptible to bacterial infection.) After showering, pat the area dry with a clean towel; do not rub. Use a different towel for the affected area to avoid spreading the infection to another part of your body.
- Wear loose, cotton underwear so that air can get to the affected area and help keep it dry. Avoid wearing excess layers of clothing; moisture from perspiration can slow the healing process.
- Take a sitz bath—sitting in a tub of shallow, lukewarm water—for about 10 to 15 minutes three times a day.
- Avoid stress; stress may make an outbreak worse or slow healing.

Symptoms You may have no symptoms when you are first infected with genital herpes. If you do have symptoms, they usually appear within 2 to 10 days after your exposure to the herpes virus. The symptoms, which can be very mild, may include itching, burning, or pain in your genital area or buttocks, or an unusual vaginal discharge.

Small, painful blisters appear, usually in the genital area, buttocks, or anus. Sores can also develop inside the vagina or on the cervix; you may be unaware of these. The lymph nodes (infection-fighting glands) in your groin may become swollen and tender. You may also have a mild fever and feel like you are getting the flu.

The symptoms of the initial infection, including the blisters, usually heal in 2 to 3 weeks. The virus then becomes dormant and may reappear periodically. In most people, recurrences gradually decrease in severity and frequency over time.

Diagnosis A doctor may recognize herpes sores on the genitals during a pelvic examination. But laboratory testing of a sample of fluid from a blister is the only way to confirm the diagnosis.

Treatment There is no cure for herpes. However, the antiviral drug acyclovir taken in pill form or applied to the affected area in an ointment for about 10 days during the initial infection or during an outbreak may help relieve the symptoms and speed healing of the blisters or cold sores. If you have frequent recurring outbreaks, your doctor may recommend that you take acyclovir pills two to three times a day for several months or more to help reduce the frequency and severity.

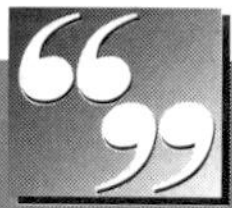

One woman's story
Herpes

I started having sex with boys fairly early. The first time was when I was 15. Before I was out of high school, I had gotten herpes. It was very painful at first. I was too embarrassed to go to a doctor, but when I had a recurrence a few months later, I decided to go. My doctor told me about genital herpes—that it cannot be cured and I would have it for the rest of my life. She told me some ways to deal with outbreaks and prescribed the drug acyclovir for me to take whenever I had an outbreak. The medication seemed to make the outbreaks less severe and go away more quickly.

"Fifteen years later, I still have to say I have herpes."

I'm 31 now and single. The outbreaks have become far less frequent, maybe only a couple of times a year, and they are very mild. The biggest problem now is that each time I start a new relationship with a man, I have to tell him I have herpes. I'm not supposed to have sex when I have an outbreak, and the rest of the time I'm supposed to use a condom whenever I have sex—even though I feel perfectly fine. Some men lose interest when I tell them I have herpes. It's very hard to tell anyone this. I find myself delaying and avoiding situations where someone I'm dating might start trying to make love to me. It's very stressful. And when I do tell someone, I never know how he'll react.

The fact is that you can have a normal sex life even if you have herpes. The best situation is to be in a monogamous relationship with a person who understands the disease and knows that there are steps to take to avoid getting it. I have to be careful to watch for any symptoms and to avoid having sex at that time, including oral sex. It's hard to believe that a mistake I made when I was a teenager is affecting my life today. Fifteen years later, I still have to say I have herpes. I hope teenagers now are better informed than I was about how important it is to use condoms to avoid STDs.

HIV AND AIDS

Acquired immune deficiency syndrome (AIDS) is a serious disease because it is almost always fatal. The virus that causes AIDS is called the human immunodeficiency virus (HIV). AIDS is now the leading cause of death of American women and men ages 25 to 44.

The disease is relatively new—the first cases were recognized in the US in 1981. In the early 1980s, most cases occurred in either homosexual men or drug users who shared contaminated needles. However, women are now one of the fastest-growing groups affected by HIV infection and AIDS. The primary route of infection is sexual contact with an infected partner.

HIV infection progressively destroys your immune system, weakening its ability to fight infections and some cancers. The virus interferes with the immune system by destroying infection-fighting white blood calls called CD4 cells.

HIV is present in an infected person's blood, semen (sperm-carrying fluid), and vaginal secretions. The virus is primarily transmitted through contact with these fluids. During sexual contact with a person infected with HIV, the virus can enter the body through the vagina, the external female genitals, penis, rectum, or mouth. As with many other STDs, women may be more susceptible to infection than men during heterosexual intercourse.

HIV can also be transmitted through blood, most often among injection drug users who share needles contaminated with infected blood. Before the development of an effective test to detect HIV antibodies in blood, the virus was transmitted through blood transfusions and some blood products. Today, potential donors are carefully screened and their blood is tested for the presence of HIV and other disease-causing organisms. As a result, donated blood, organs, or tissues for transfusions or transplants are almost always safe.

Another means of HIV transmission is from an infected pregnant woman to the fetus. About one out of four babies born to HIV-infected women is infected. The average time from HIV infection to development of AIDS in these children is 3 years. Although some infected children die by age 4, many live more than 8 years. One medication—zidovudine (AZT)—given to infected pregnant women can significantly decrease the risk of transmission of the virus to the fetus. HIV can also be transmitted to a nursing child via breast milk.

Symptoms Some people who are infected with HIV develop a flulike illness characterized by fever, muscle aches, tiredness, and swollen lymph nodes (infection-fighting glands). Some people do not have any symptoms when they are first infected. In fact, a person may have no symptoms even though he or she has been infected for 10 years or more.

But even without symptoms, infected people can transmit the virus. You can unknowingly transfer the virus to a sex partner or child. You can acquire the virus from someone who appears to be

How is HIV transmitted?

HIV *can* be transmitted through:

- **Sexual contact** You can become infected with HIV from vaginal, anal, or oral sex. If you have other STDs, especially those that cause sores in the genital area, your risk of becoming infected with HIV increases.
- **Pregnancy or breast-feeding** During pregnancy, a woman infected with HIV can transmit it to the fetus. A woman can transmit HIV to a nursing child through breast milk.
- **Sharing needles** Sharing needles to inject drugs can expose you to blood that contains the AIDS virus.

HIV is *not* transmitted through:

- **Nonsexual contact** You do not get AIDS from casual contact: sitting next to or touching an infected person (hugging or shaking hands) or having a meal together, even if you share glasses, plates, and silverware. Nor do you become infected from eating food handled, prepared, or served by an infected person.
- **Sharing water fountains, toilets, or swimming pools with an infected person** The virus that causes AIDS does not survive outside of the body.
- **Being bitten by an insect or animal** HIV is not transmitted by bites from mosquitoes or any other insect, or from animals.
- **Donating blood or having a blood test** Each time blood is taken, a new sterile needle is used so there is no risk of passing HIV from one person to another.

perfectly healthy. Most women who acquire HIV from a sex partner did not know their partner was infected.

HIV's ability to hide inside cells in the body, producing no symptoms, underscores the importance of always practicing safer sex (see page 337). You should use a latex or polyurethane male condom or a female condom with spermicide every time you have sex, unless you are in a stable, mutually monogamous relationship (both you and your partner are having sex only with each other; see page 338). It only takes one exposure to the virus to become infected.

The progression from HIV infection to the development of the array of symptoms called AIDS varies from person to person, but nearly always ends in death. As an infected person's immune system breaks down, his or her body becomes defenseless against normally harmless organisms, such as the fungus that causes yeast infections (see page 217), and other serious infections and cancers that are usually controlled by a healthy immune system. HIV infection generally follows the course described here:

Acute retroviral syndrome Some people experience flulike symptoms—loss of appetite, fatigue, enlarged lymph nodes in the neck, armpits, and groin—1 to 2 months after exposure to the virus. These symptoms usually go away even without treatment in a week to a month.

HIV infection without symptoms HIV infection can last from 2 to 10 years or more. During this time, the virus is slowly replicating inside body cells, producing no visible signs or symptoms but continuing to weaken your immune system, lowering your resistance to infections.

HIV infection with symptoms You may experience a variety of symptoms and recurring infections long before the onset of AIDS. Symptoms can include enlargement of lymph nodes in the neck, armpits, or groin that may last for 3 months or longer; weight loss; fatigue; frequent fevers or sweats; recurring yeast infections in the vagina, mouth, and esophagus; frequent, severe recurrences of genital herpes (see page 342); and susceptibility to many other infections.

AIDS As HIV infection advances, most people succumb to a succession of infections or diseases that are called "opportunistic" because they take advantage of a weakened immune system to cause illness. These conditions include a recurring form of pneumonia caused by bacteria; another type of pneumonia called *Pneumocystis carinii*; and some cancers, such as cervical cancer (see page 250), that advance more rapidly than usual in HIV-infected women. These illnesses indicate AIDS. Symptoms such as extreme weight loss and mental confusion may precede death.

Diagnosis A blood test can detect the presence of antibodies your body produces in response to HIV infection, even when you do not have any symptoms. It usually takes from 6 weeks to 3 months after exposure for your body to produce antibodies to HIV, but in a few people the process may take up to 6 months. If you think you may have been exposed to the virus, see your doctor to discuss when or if you should have a blood test. If the blood test is negative (meaning you do not have HIV antibodies), you may need another test 6 months later to make sure you are not infected. In the meantime, abstain from sex or practice safer sex to protect yourself and your partner, and do not share needles for injecting drugs.

Treatment There is no cure for HIV infection or for AIDS. Some medications, including zidovudine (AZT), may slow the disease in many people, but these drugs have limited benefits. Drugs called anti-infectives are used to prevent such common and severe opportunistic infections as *Pneumocystis carinii* pneumonia. Antibiotics can help combat the frequent infections that affect people whose immune system has been weakened by HIV. Researchers are attempting to develop a vaccine to protect against the virus and more effective drugs to treat the infection.

HEPATITIS B

Hepatitis B is an infection caused by the hepatitis B virus, which attacks the liver. The virus can be deadly; it kills about 6,000 people in the US each year. About 1.5 million people carry the virus. Carriers have no symptoms of illness, but their blood contains the virus. Carriers can transmit hepatitis B to other people. If you are a carrier of hepatitis B, you should always use a latex or polyurethane male condom or a female condom with spermicide whenever you have vaginal, anal, or oral sex. In later life, carriers are at risk of cirrhosis of the liver (a progressive disease that destroys the liver), liver cancer, and reduced immunity to other infections and illnesses.

In addition to sexual contact, hepatitis B can be spread through contaminated needles used for injecting drugs or, rarely, through contaminated medical or dental instruments that pierce the skin.

There is a safe and effective vaccine to protect against hepatitis B. Vaccination is recommended for people at high risk of exposure to the virus—including medical and dental workers, drug users who inject drugs, homosexual men, people undergoing kidney dialysis (see page 549), and people who are sexually active with a person who has any of these risk factors. All newborns in the US are vaccinated against hepatitis B because the vaccination is very safe and the consequences of a hepatitis B infection can be severe. If you have had any STDs recently or more than one sex partner during the past 6 months, ask your doctor if you should be vaccinated against hepatitis B.

During pregnancy, an infected woman can transmit the virus to the fetus. This risk is especially high (80 to 90 percent) if the woman is infected during the last trimester of pregnancy. In addition to being vaccinated, newborns whose mothers have been identified as carriers of hepatitis B are given antibodies (immune globulin) to fight the virus. This treatment prevents hepatitis B infections in more than 90 percent of these children. Of the fewer than 10 percent of the treated children who still get infected, the vast majority become lifelong carriers of the virus; they are at risk of liver disease and liver cancer and they can transmit the virus to other people.

Symptoms About one third of people with the hepatitis B virus have no symptoms. When symptoms occur, they can be mild or severe and may include fever, headaches, muscle aches, fatigue, loss of appetite, vomiting, and diarrhea.

In advanced stages of infection, symptoms may include abdominal pain and signs of jaundice—dark urine and yellowing of the skin and whites of the eyes. Jaundice results from a buildup in the blood of bilirubin, a yellow-brown pigment that is usually filtered out by the liver.

Diagnosis Hepatitis B can be diagnosed from either a blood test that detects the virus itself or one that detects specific antibodies to the virus that your body produces to fight the infection.

Treatment Most hepatitis B infections clear up on their own within 4 to 8 weeks, but some persist and can lead to permanent liver damage. There is no effective treatment or cure for hepatitis B but some symptoms of the infection, such as pain or diarrhea, can be treated or controlled with medication. Research is focused on development of new medications to treat people who are hepatitis B carriers.

SYPHILIS

Syphilis is a potentially life-threatening disease caused by bacteria. The infection is most often transmitted through vaginal, anal, or oral sex. However, the bacteria can also be transmitted through contact with a syphilis sore on an infected person's body.

With the development of antibiotics in the 1950s, the incidence of syphilis dropped sharply. But an increase in the number of reported cases of syphilis has caused doctors to return to regular testing of pregnant women to screen for the bacteria.

Syphilis can be transmitted during pregnancy; one out of four infected babies is stillborn or dies shortly after birth. More than half of pregnant women who have untreated syphilis give birth to babies with syphilis. If the infection is not detected in these children, it can damage their heart, brain, and eyes. All pregnant women should be tested for syphilis at least once during their pregnancy because, if it is detected early, it is curable with antibiotic shots administered over a period of 3 weeks.

Symptoms The first symptom of syphilis is usually a small (about ½ inch across), raised, smooth, painless sore that most often appears on the genitals but can appear anywhere on the body. The sores develop between 10 days and 3 months after exposure to the bacteria. In women, the sores sometimes develop inside the vagina or on the cervix and, because they are painless, go unnoticed. Without treatment, the sores go away on their own within a few weeks.

However, if the infection is not treated, the disease-causing bacteria can remain in the body indefinitely. In some people, the disease becomes completely dormant and never again causes symptoms. But, in most untreated cases, the infection progresses to a second, more serious stage. The second stage of syphilis begins with a rash that appears 3 weeks to 6 months after the initial sores developed. The rash may cover your body or appear only in a few areas such as the palms of your hands or soles of your feet. On the external genitals, the infection can produce large, flat, raised, grayish-white patches that may grow together and form open sores. This stage may also cause widespread symptoms including mild fever, fatigue, sore throat, hair loss, and swollen glands throughout your body.

As in the first stage of syphilis, the symptoms that occur in the second stage also disappear without treatment, but may come and go for 1 to 2 years. If not treated during this stage, the disease moves into a latent (inactive) stage, during which it is not contagious and does not cause any symptoms.

About one out of three infected people moves into the third and final stage of syphilis, which can result in irreversible damage to the heart, brain, eyes, nervous system, bones, and joints. This stage of the infection can lead to dementia, blindness, heart disease, and death.

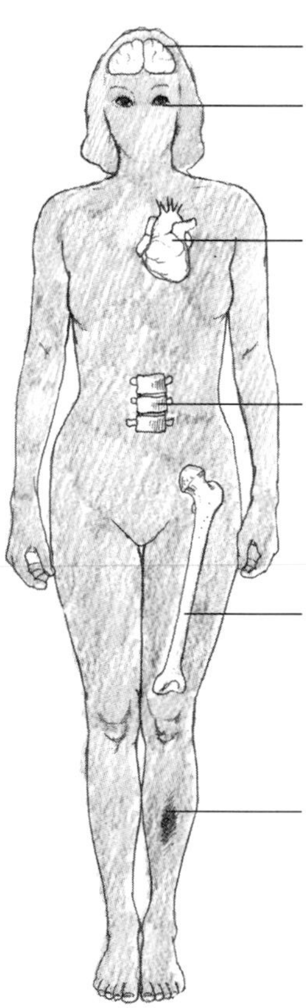

Brain damage—leading to dementia

Damage to eyes—leading to blindness

Damage to heart—leading to heart disease

Damage to spinal cord—causing paralysis

Damage to bones—causing bone deformities

Damage to skin—causing sores

LONG-TERM EFFECTS OF SYPHILIS

Syphilis can be treated with antibiotics, but it sometimes is not detected and, therefore, not treated. An untreated syphilis infection may be inactive for a long period and then become active and begin to attack organs in the body, particularly the brain, heart, spinal cord, bones, eyes, and skin. Once this damage occurs, it cannot be reversed.

Diagnosis Syphilis is usually diagnosed through a physical examination, blood test, and microscopic examination of a sample taken from a sore. A blood test done 6 weeks after the initial infection can show whether or not your body has developed antibodies to fight the disease-causing bacteria. If the results of the blood test are negative (normal), but the doctor still suspects you may have syphilis, he or she will recommend another test in 6 weeks to give your body time to develop the antibodies.

Treatment Syphilis can be cured with antibiotics given by injection, even in the later stages. However, organ damage that occurs during the third stage cannot be reversed. Both sexual partners must be treated at the same time.

CHANCROID

Chancroid—a relatively rare infection in the US—is caused by a highly contagious bacterium that produces painful, pus-filled sores on the genitals. The infection is transmitted through vaginal or anal intercourse. Sometimes people who have no symptoms carry the disease-causing bacterium and can transfer it to others. An open sore in the genital area, such as that produced by chancroid, increases your risk of contracting other STDs, especially AIDS (see page 344).

Symptoms Symptoms of chancroid appear within a week of exposure to the disease-causing bacterium. In women, the symptoms may be limited to painful urination or bowel movements, painful intercourse, or vaginal discharge. Chancroid can also cause sores that resemble pimples that do not heal. They usually occur on the external genitals and around the anus. These sores may be accompanied by swollen, tender lymph nodes (infection-fighting glands) in the groin. Unlike the sores of syphilis, which are painless, the sores of chancroid are painful. Obvious symptoms of the infection, such as sores, are more common in men.

Diagnosis Because chancroid can cause sores that resemble those of syphilis, a test to rule out syphilis is usually done first. The laboratory test to diagnose chancroid (from a sample of fluid taken from a sore) is more complicated than the test for syphilis and not all laboratories are equipped to do it.

Treatment Chancroid can be cured with antibiotics taken by mouth.

TRICHOMONIASIS

Trichomoniasis is an extremely common STD caused by a single-celled organism. The infection is usually transmitted through sexual intercourse. About 3 million new cases occur each year in the US. The infection usually occurs in the vagina in women and in the urethra (the tube that carries urine from the bladder) in men. Having trichomoniasis puts you at greater risk of contracting HIV, the virus that causes AIDS, if you are exposed to it.

During pregnancy, an untreated infection may cause such complications as premature delivery and a baby with a low birth weight.

Symptoms Trichomoniasis often causes no symptoms. When symptoms do occur, they usually appear within 4 to 20 days after exposure to the disease-causing organism.

In women, symptoms include a yellow-green vaginal discharge with an unpleasant odor, itching and irritation in the genital area, discomfort during intercourse, and pain during urination. You may also feel the need to urinate more frequently than usual. Lymph nodes (infection-fighting glands) in your groin area may become swollen and tender. When men have symptoms, they usually include a clear discharge from the penis and pain during urination.

Diagnosis The infection is often discovered by a doctor during a regular Pap smear (see page 127), even when a woman has no symptoms. An accurate diagnosis is made after examination of a sample of vaginal discharge under a microscope. In men, diagnosis is made by laboratory testing of a sample of discharge from the penis.

Treatment Trichomoniasis can be cured with antibiotics taken by mouth. Both sexual partners must be treated at the same time to avoid reinfecting each other.

If the infection returns after you have been treated, it may mean that you or your partner did not take the medication as prescribed, or that one of you is having sex with an infected person outside the relationship. You and your partner should discuss it and determine the cause. You both will have to be treated again.

NONGONOCOCCAL URETHRITIS

Nongonococcal urethritis is a bacterial infection of the urethra, the short tube through which urine passes from the bladder. This infection is more common in men than in women. Several different types of bacteria may cause the infection, but the same type of bacteria that causes chlamydia (see page 339) is responsible for most cases. Some doctors use the terms nongonococcal urethritis and chlamydia urethritis interchangeably.

The bacteria may enter the urethra during any sexual activity that involves genital-to-genital contact. Because nongonococcal urethritis may produce no symptoms or only mild symptoms in women, many delay seeking treatment. If the infection is not treated, it can spread to the uterus, fallopian tubes, or ovaries, causing pelvic inflammatory disease (PID; see page 232), which can lead to infertility. Urinating after intercourse can help flush out any bacteria that may have been pushed up into the urethra during intercourse.

Symptoms Symptoms of nongonococcal urethritis are more obvious in men. When symptoms do occur (in both men and women), they include pain during urination and a discharge of mucus from the urethra.

Diagnosis In both men and women, nongonococcal urethritis is diagnosed from laboratory testing of a sample of discharge from the urethra to detect and identify the disease-causing bacterium.

Treatment If you are diagnosed with nongonococcal urethritis, your doctor may ask for a urine specimen or he or she may take a sample of the discharge from your urethra to determine which bacterium caused the infection. You will be given a prescription for antibiotics to be taken by mouth. Drinking plenty of fluids dilutes your urine and helps reduce pain during urination. You and your sexual partner must be treated at the same time; during treatment, you should avoid sexual activities involving genital-to-genital contact.

MOLLUSCUM CONTAGIOSUM

Molluscum contagiosum is a virus that infects the skin. The virus can be spread not only by sexual contact but by any close or intimate body contact with an infected person.

Symptoms When transmitted through sexual contact, infection with molluscum contagiosum appears as small, pinkish-white, waxy-looking growths on the genitals or thighs. These growths are shaped like small domes with a depression in the center. The growths can appear from 3 weeks to 3 months after contact with an infected person. The infection does not cause any other symptoms.

Diagnosis Your doctor can diagnose molluscum contagiosum by examining a sample of cells from a growth under a microscope.

Treatment Your doctor will treat each growth by destroying it with heat (electrocautery) or cold (cryosurgery) or with chemicals that kill the virus inside the growth. These procedures are performed in the doctor's office. You may feel a stinging sensation during the procedure but it is not painful enough to require an anesthetic. Two to 3 weeks after treatment, some growths may reappear and have to be treated again.

CRAB LICE

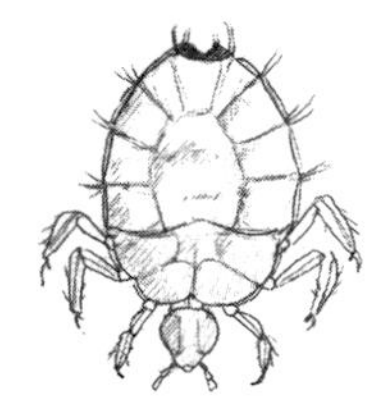

CRAB LOUSE
A crab louse (shown here about 12 times its normal size) can be seen on the skin, often at the base of hairs.

Crab lice, also known as pubic lice or crabs, are tiny insects (about the size of the head of a pin) that can be transferred from one person to another, usually through sexual contact. They can also be acquired through contact with infested clothing, bedding, or toilet seats.

Crab lice live in pubic hair and bite the skin to feed on blood. Although tiny, the lice and their egg clusters, which cling to hair shafts, can be seen with the naked eye. Crab lice may be transmitted from parents to children through physical contact. In children, the lice often attach themselves to eyelashes.

Symptoms The bites of crab lice usually cause itching and irritation. You also may be able to see the lice on hair.

Diagnosis Because crab lice are visible, a doctor can make a diagnosis from a physical examination.

Treatment Because crab lice cling to shafts of hair, they cannot be removed by scratching or washing. The only way to eliminate the lice is to use an insecticidal lotion that kills both the lice and their eggs. The medication is applied in a shampoo or skin lotion, left in place for 12 hours, and then washed off. If you still have symptoms, you may have to repeat the treatment a second time. The lotion contains a powerful chemical agent, so you should not use it more often than your doctor prescribes.

All members of the household of an infected person must be treated at the same time. All clothing (including underwear) and bedding must be washed in very hot water (exceeding 140°F) or dry-cleaned to kill the lice.

Your doctor may prescribe an antihistamine (a drug that blocks the effects of an allergic reaction) to help relieve itching caused by the insect bites.

CHAPTER 13

Menopause

Contents

The term menopause specifically refers to a woman's final menstrual period. Physically, however, menopause is a transition period in a woman's life that begins years before her last period when her body begins to slow its production of estrogen and other important hormones. The process is gradual and usually lasts several years, occurring some time between ages 40 and 55. The average age at which women stop menstruating is 51, but can vary widely.

Menopause causes many significant changes in your body, but it is a normal, healthy stage of your life—not a disease. Because the average age of the American population is rising, increasing numbers of women are approaching and going through menopause. Many are educating themselves thoroughly about the physical changes menopause brings and making informed decisions about their health, such as whether to undergo hormone replacement therapy (HRT) to maintain their body's level of estrogen.

Estrogen is a powerful hormone that affects many tissues throughout your body—the reproductive tract (vagina, external genitals, and uterus), urinary tract (bladder and urethra), heart and blood vessels, bones, breasts, skin, hair, mucous membranes, pelvic muscles, and brain. As you approach menopause, your ovaries begin to release eggs less regularly and, at menopause, stop releasing eggs completely. Your ovaries also reduce their production of estrogen. This reduction of estrogen in your body can have wide-ranging effects—from the symptoms of menopause, such as hot flashes, to increased risk of heart disease and osteoporosis, which can be life threatening.

Your changing hormones

Hormones—which are produced in your ovaries, brain, and other organs—are essential substances that control a variety of important functions in your body. A carefully orchestrated interplay of the hormones estrogen and progesterone precisely regulates your menstrual cycle.

At about age 40, your ovaries begin to gradually reduce their production of progesterone. Progesterone is produced during ovulation (when one of the ovaries releases a mature egg) to prepare the lining of the uterus (endometrium) for implantation of a fertilized egg. (For a description of ovulation, see page 204.) Because your ovaries continue to produce adequate, though decreasing, amounts of estrogen during this time, you are not yet in menopause. Estrogen is still stimulating some growth of your endometrium, which is why you continue to have menstrual cycles. However, menstrual bleeding may become irregular during this time.

As menopause progresses, other hormonal changes also occur. As you reach your late 40s and early 50s, the pituitary gland in your brain senses the decreased levels of progesterone and estrogen. The gland then produces more luteinizing hormone (LH) and follicle-stimulating hormone (FSH), which regulate the functioning of the ovaries. This increase in LH and FSH is your body's response to the drop in hormone production by your ovaries and is the cause of hot flashes.

The most important and dramatic hormonal change during menopause is an enormous drop in your body's production of estrogen—about 75 percent. The lack of estrogen causes the common physical symptoms of menopause.

MENSTRUAL CHANGES BEFORE MENOPAUSE

In the years before you have your final period, your menstrual cycle may begin to change. Women experience these changes in different ways—in the length of their cycle, amount of blood flow, or both. You should see your doctor if you have irregular bleeding between periods, if you have excessive or prolonged bleeding, or if you have gone more than 2 months without a period.

Your doctor may perform an endometrial biopsy (see page 129) to see if you have endometrial hyperplasia, which is excessive growth of cells in the endometrium (the lining of the uterus). This condition can lead to endometrial cancer if not treated. Although endometrial hyperplasia can occur at any age, it is more common in the years before menopause because a woman may not be producing the hormone progesterone in sufficient amounts to suppress excessive growth of the endometrium.

If you have endometrial hyperplasia, you may be given progestin (a synthetic form of progesterone), which stops the excessive growth of endometrial cells. Progestin is taken in pills for 7 to 21 days each month or by injection. The injections are given in the doctor's office every 1 to 3 months. If you do not have endometrial hyperplasia but you have heavy, irregular periods, your doctor may recommend the same treatment or prescribe birth-control pills. Birth-control pills regulate your cycle and make your periods lighter.

Once you have stopped having periods for a full year, you can assume you have gone through menopause. A blood test to determine your level of follicle-stimulating hormone (FSH) can confirm menopause, because FSH increases in response to a decrease in estrogen. Estrogen levels are not used to confirm whether or not a woman has gone through menopause because they vary greatly during a woman's menstrual cycle.

However, you should not wait a full year after your periods stop before seeing your doctor. If you are having severe hot flashes or other symptoms caused by a deficiency of estrogen, your doctor may recommend that you begin taking estrogen in hormone replacement therapy (HRT; see page 359) even before your periods stop. In addition to relieving your symptoms, starting HRT before your last period, or within a few months of your last period, also provides long-term health benefits, such as protection against osteoporosis and heart disease. For this reason, it is important to continue having regular gynecologic checkups (see page 124) in the years before menopause.

Contraception in your 40s Although you may ovulate less regularly as you approach menopause, you can still get pregnant well into your 40s. Unless you are planning a pregnancy, using reliable contraception is just as important as ever. Natural family planning methods (see page 329), which require extremely accurate understanding of your cycle to be effective, are much less reliable at this stage of life. The length of your menstrual cycle is changing, and "safe" times to have intercourse are even more difficult to predict.

For most women, birth-control pills and other hormonal methods (see page 310) of contraception are safe to use right up to their last period. However, a woman who smokes and uses birth-control pills after 35 is at a significantly increased risk of heart attack and stroke. If you smoke and use birth-control pills, your doctor will recommend switching to another contraceptive method as you approach the age of 35. Alternatively, your doctor may recommend birth-control pills called minipills (see page 313), which do not contain estrogen. These pills contain only progestin (a synthetic form of the female hormone progesterone) and are safe to take by women over 35 who smoke cigarettes.

An important benefit of using birth-control pills in your 40s is the protection they provide against ovarian cancer and endometrial cancer, which are more common in women over 50. This cancer protection lasts for at least 15 years after you stop taking the pill. If you are at high risk of these cancers, your doctor may recommend birth-control pills. Other hormonal methods of birth control—such as hormone implants and injections—are also thought to reduce a woman's risk of developing endometrial cancer.

Coping with the symptoms of menopause

Menopause is a new stage in your life and you can expect to experience some changes. Most women have at least some symptoms, ranging from mild to severe and lasting for months or years. If the symptoms become troublesome to you, some of the approaches described here can help make you more comfortable. If you are uncertain about whether or not the physical or emotional changes you are experiencing result from menopause, see your doctor. He or she can rule out other causes and, together, you can find solutions to your particular problems.

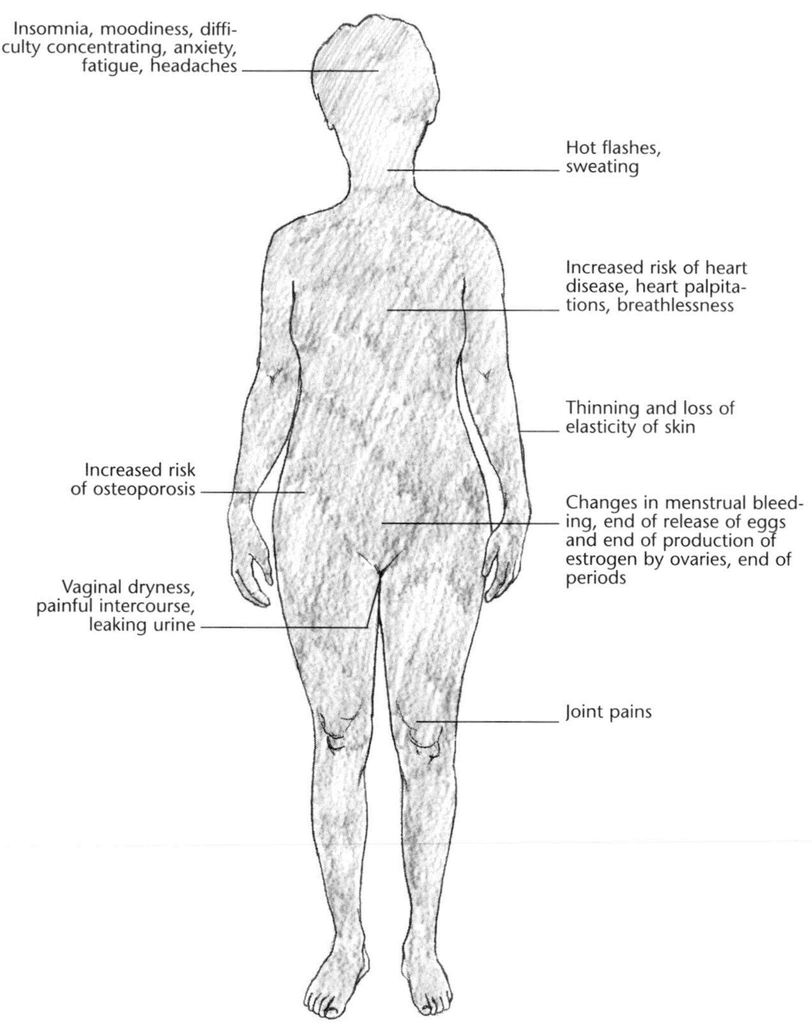

SYMPTOMS AND CHANGES IN YOUR BODY AT MENOPAUSE AND AFTER

Each woman experiences menopause in a different way. The loss of estrogen at menopause can have a variety of effects on a woman's body—including short-term symptoms such as hot flashes and long-term health risks such as heart disease, stroke, and osteoporosis.

HOT FLASHES

About 75 percent of women who are going through menopause experience hot flashes—sudden, brief increases in their body temperature. A woman may have hot flashes for only a month or for 5 years or more. They usually start before a woman's last period and continue after it. Hot flashes vary greatly in intensity and frequency from woman to woman.

In addition to an increase in the temperature of your skin—particularly of your head, neck, and upper chest—a hot flash causes an increase in your heart rate. You may flush as you experience a shock of intense heat that rises from your neck to your face and then spreads outward over your scalp and upper chest. You suddenly perspire, sometimes heavily, as your body tries to reduce its temperature. Heart palpitations and dizziness may also accompany a hot flash.

A hot flash usually lasts about 1 to 3 minutes. Some women have a less intense sensation, but are aware of an increased feeling of warmth. At the beginning of menopause, hot flashes may occur only at night or at times of stress.

Hot flashes that occur at night are called night sweats. You may wake up drenched in sweat, and you may have to change your night clothes and bedding. In many women, the frequent disruptions of sleep cause fatigue, irritability, and even depression.

Coping with hot flashes Taking estrogen is the most effective treatment for relieving the symptoms of menopause, including hot flashes and night sweats. If you cannot take estrogen for a medical reason (see page 361), a drug called clonidine, a medication for high blood pressure, may help reduce your hot flashes. But clonidine may produce side effects such as dizziness and fatigue. A mild, combined sedative preparation of belladonna, ergotamine, and phenobarbital is also sometimes used to treat symptoms of menopause—including hot flashes, sweating, restlessness, and insomnia. This combination of medications is effective in about half of the women who take it.

Hot flashes occur more frequently during the summer. Keeping cool and dressing in layers of natural fabrics such as cotton can help reduce the discomfort of a hot flash. It is a good idea to wear layers that can be easily removed and replaced. Keep a change of clothes at work in case you perspire heavily, and take advantage of air-conditioning at home, at work, and in your car. If you are perspiring heavily, drink extra fluids to keep from becoming dehydrated.

Some women find that eliminating alcohol or caffeinated beverages—including coffee, cola, tea, and hot chocolate—reduces the frequency or intensity of hot flashes. (Many over-the-counter cold preparations and pain relievers also contain caffeine; check the label.) Some women experience more hot flashes when they are under stress. If your hot flashes are triggered by stress, try the stress reduction techniques on page 190.

VAGINAL DRYNESS OR IRRITATION

The loss of estrogen at menopause may cause the lining of your vagina to thin. This thinning can cause the vagina to gradually become shorter, narrower, drier, and more prone to irritation and infection. These changes can cause pain during intercourse.

Extending the period of foreplay when making love and applying a water-based vaginal lubricant to all irritated areas can help reduce the discomfort. Ask your doctor about using a vaginal cream containing estrogen, which can relieve the dryness. You apply estrogen cream directly to the affected tissue inside your vagina (see page 363). The cream will relieve the dryness in a few weeks. Estrogen taken in pills or skin patches is also effective in relieving vaginal dryness but, in these forms, it may take several months or more to have an effect.

Maintaining the muscle tone in your pelvic area can help you continue a pleasurable sex life. Performing daily pelvic-floor (Kegel) exercises (see page 238) is especially important at this time.

URINARY PROBLEMS

The decline in your body's production of estrogen at menopause can cause the cells that line your urinary tract to deteriorate and thin and the muscle tone in your urinary tract to diminish. You may experience some loss of bladder control. In many women, the urethra (the tube that carries urine from the bladder) can no longer maintain the necessary pressure and strength to prevent urine from leaking out of the body. This condition is called incontinence.

Some women experience stress incontinence (see page 540), a sudden leaking of urine when they cough, sneeze, or exercise. Other women have urge incontinence (see page 541), in which specific triggers—such as laughing or moving suddenly—can produce the sensation of needing to urinate, followed by leaking of urine.

Losing bladder control is distressing for any woman. Doing pelvic-floor exercises (see page 238) every day can help build muscle strength and tone in your vaginal area, which can help reduce mild incontinence. Taking estrogen in hormone replacement therapy (HRT; see page 359) can significantly reduce a woman's risk of incontinence and improve the condition in women who have it. Estrogen increases circulation to all the tissues of your pelvis, including the urethra and bladder, boosting their muscle tone and strength. If your incontinence does not improve with HRT and you have to wear a pad frequently, talk to your doctor about surgery and other treatment options.

CHANGES IN YOUR BREASTS

As you age, glandular tissue in your breasts is replaced by fat tissue, which causes your breasts to sag. Larger breasts tend to sag more than smaller breasts because their heavier weight stretches the ligaments that support them. No amount of exercise can prevent this process because you do not have muscles in your breasts. Taking estrogen in hormone replacement therapy can help maintain some firmness in your breasts by preserving more of the glandular tissue.

Because your risk of breast cancer increases with age, it is especially important after menopause to continue performing breast self-examinations (see page 276) every month. Having physical examinations and mammograms (see page 127) every year is essential to detect breast cancer in its earliest, most curable stage.

CHANGES IN HAIR GROWTH

A change in the balance between your body's production of female hormones and male hormones (androgens) may affect your pattern of hair growth. A relative increase in the level of male hormones in your body after menopause and decrease in estrogen may cause some of the normally fine, light hairs that cover your face and body to darken and thicken. Taking estrogen in hormone replacement therapy can help reduce this excessive hair growth. You can remove the hairs by plucking them or using hair-removal creams. You may want to consider electrolysis, a procedure to remove hair permanently.

As they go through menopause, some women notice that their hair begins to thin, especially on their scalp and in their pubic area. Taking estrogen in hormone replacement therapy can also help reduce hair thinning.

SKIN CHANGES

Although most skin aging is caused by the damaging effects of exposure to the sun, your body's decreasing estrogen production during menopause can make your skin thinner and less elastic. This thinning and loss of elasticity can cause wrinkling and sagging.

Your body is also producing less collagen, one of the main supporting proteins of the skin. Collagen cannot be restored through lotions or creams, and injections of collagen have only temporary effects. Taking estrogen in hormone replacement therapy helps maintain collagen levels and skin thickness.

As you age, your skin becomes more delicate, making it more susceptible to damage from the sun. It is more important than ever to shield your skin from exposure to the sun by using a sunscreen with a sun protection factor (SPF) of at least 15, wearing protective clothing, and staying out of the sun when its rays are the strongest (between 10:00 AM and 3:00 PM).

EMOTIONAL SYMPTOMS

Some women experience sudden mood changes or depression as they go through menopause. Declining levels of estrogen may be part of the reason, but it is important to recognize that these feelings may be a response to the overall aging process or to changing circumstances. Many women take on new roles at this time in their life—such as becoming a mother-in-law, grandmother, widow, or caregiver for an aging parent. Some women are starting new careers. It is natural to feel some new, perhaps complicated emotions in response to these changes.

Many emotional changes associated with menopause have a physical basis. For example, hot flashes that wake you up each night can deprive you of sleep and make you irritable the next day. Eating healthfully, exercising regularly, and getting sufficient sleep can help keep your body strong and your mind better able to cope with the symptoms of menopause. Remaining active through work, interaction with family and friends, volunteering, and hobbies also helps focus your energies away from emotional highs and lows.

As at any other time of life, it is important to recognize when you need help. If your emotional symptoms are severe, if they persist for long periods of time, or if they impair your ability to function at home or at work, discuss your situation with your doctor. He or she may be able to help you or refer you to a qualified therapist who can help you ease through this period of adjustment. For many women, a short-term course of therapy is all it takes.

Long-term health risks

The hormonal changes your body undergoes during menopause not only cause short-term symptoms, but also increase your long-term risk of two life-threatening disorders—heart disease and osteoporosis. As knowledge about these major disorders increases, it becomes critically important for you to know how they can be prevented and treated. Understanding the complex biological changes that are associated with menopause gives you the basic facts you can use to ask questions, learn about your personal risk factors, and take measures that can help you reduce those risks and improve the quality of your life.

INCREASED RISK OF HEART DISEASE

More American women die of heart disease than any other disease—including all cancers combined. For much of your life, because your body produces more estrogen than a man's, you are at lower risk than a man of having a heart attack. But by the time you reach 65, your risk of a heart attack equals that of a man because your body is no longer producing estrogen.

Estrogen protects against heart disease in several ways. It reduces your total cholesterol level, raises your "good" high-density lipoprotein (HDL) cholesterol level, and lowers your "bad" low-density lipoprotein (LDL) cholesterol level. LDL is a type of cholesterol that can build up inside your arteries, narrowing them and increasing your risk of a heart attack. In contrast, HDL cholesterol clears out potentially damaging LDL cholesterol from your arteries, helping to keep them open.

There are a number of ways you can improve the health of your heart and blood vessels and avoid a heart attack. Taking the following steps not only reduces your risk of heart disease, but improves your overall health:

- Consider hormone replacement therapy (HRT). Discuss with your doctor your risk factors for heart disease (see page 461) and the benefits of HRT for you. Women using HRT after menopause cut their risk of heart disease in half. This protection lasts for as long as they are taking estrogen.
- Eat a low-fat, high-fiber diet rich in fruits and vegetables and whole grains. Reduce your consumption of saturated fat—the kind found in meats and dairy products and hydrogenated oils used in many prepared and packaged foods. Read food labels carefully for fat content (see page 67).
- Do not smoke. Cigarette smoking is a major risk factor for heart disease. If you smoke, quitting (see page 156) is the single most important thing you can do for your health.
- Exercise regularly. Regular exercise (see page 74) lowers your blood pressure and cholesterol level and your risk of developing type II diabetes (see page 621). High blood pressure, high cholesterol level, and diabetes are major risk factors for heart disease. Even moderate exercise, such as walking half an hour three times a week, significantly benefits your heart.
- Maintain a healthy weight (see page 98). By maintaining a healthy weight, you can reduce your blood pressure and cholesterol level, and your risk of developing type II diabetes.
- Take medication for high blood pressure if your doctor prescribes it. High blood pressure occurs more frequently in women after menopause.
- Reduce stress in your life. Relaxation techniques (see page 190) and exercise may help keep stress at a manageable level.

INCREASED RISK OF OSTEOPOROSIS

One of the most debilitating effects of menopause is the gradual loss of bone density that occurs when your supply of estrogen, which keeps bones strong, begins to decline. This loss of bone strength and density significantly increases your risk of developing osteoporosis (see page 552). This bone-thinning disorder can lead to disabling and potentially life-threatening fractures in the spine and hip.

Once considered an inevitable part of aging, osteoporosis is now known to be a serious disorder that is preventable and often treatable. Osteoporosis can progress without symptoms for many years; the first sign of the disorder is often a fracture. One half of all women over 50 will at some time have a fracture caused by osteoporosis.

Bone density In the process of bone formation and growth, calcium—the major component of bones—is continuously being added and removed. This process gradually builds up bone until it reaches peak density at about age 20. After age 35, both men and women begin to gradually lose more bone than their body builds. The effect of this imbalance is far more harmful in women. Their bones are already smaller than those of men so they cannot afford to lose as much.

In addition, estrogen production declines at menopause and a woman begins to lose bone at an accelerated rate. Estrogen stimulates bones to absorb calcium from the blood and slows the rate at which bones naturally lose calcium. When estrogen levels fall and the calcium supply is inadequate, bones gradually become more porous—like sponges with tiny holes that grow larger and larger. Bones become brittle and easily broken, especially in the wrist, hip, and spine. When a vertebra (one of the bones in the spine) fractures, it collapses on itself, severely weakening the spine and leading to a loss in height and the curved upper spinal column that you see in many older women.

The greatest decline in the density of your bone occurs between the ages of 45 and 70, particularly in the 5 to 7 years after your last menstrual period. During these critical years, you can lose from 1 to 3 percent of your total bone density each year. After that, the decline is more gradual—about 1 percent every year. At that rate, you can lose as much as 40 percent of your total bone tissue by the time you are 80 years old—dangerously increasing your risk of fractures.

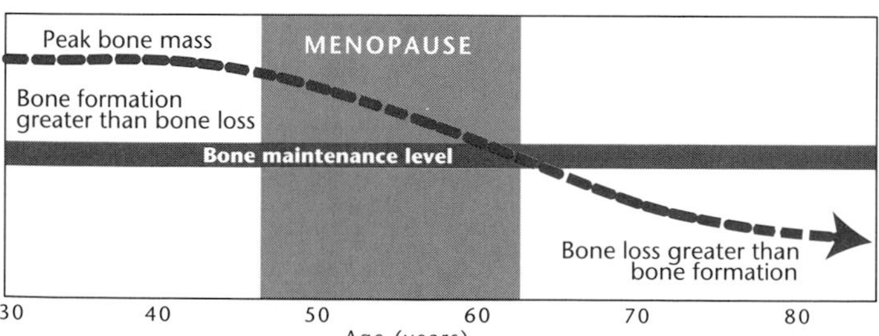

Effects of menopause on bone density

Prevention With osteoporosis, prevention is the key. Building strong bones during childhood and adolescence and maintaining the strength of your bones throughout your life with weight-bearing exercise (see page 84) and adequate intake of calcium (see page 58) are critical factors in protecting against osteoporosis. However, none of these measures can completely compensate for the deficiency of estrogen that triggers rapid bone loss in the 5 to 7 years immediately after menopause.

Not all women are at risk of osteoporosis. The following factors increase your risk of osteoporosis:

- Being white or Asian
- Having a small, thin body frame
- Having a family history of osteoporosis
- Going through menopause at an early age (before 45)
- Experiencing an absence of menstrual periods (amenorrhea, see page 210) at any time during your life, especially if brought on by excessive exercise, eating disorders such as anorexia nervosa (see page 610), or stress
- Smoking cigarettes
- Getting too little calcium
- Getting too little weight-bearing exercise
- Drinking alcohol excessively
- Using some medications (corticosteroids used to treat asthma, arthritis, or cancer; antiseizure medications; or high doses of thyroid hormone)

Treatment If you have any of the above risk factors, you should seriously consider taking estrogen in hormone replacement therapy (HRT) after menopause. If you are in any doubt about your risk of osteoporosis or are reluctant to take hormones, talk to your doctor about having tests to measure your bone density (see page 558). These tests, which are safe and painless, evaluate bone density at various sites in the body. Your doctor can use the information from these tests to predict the likelihood of future fractures and determine an appropriate course of treatment for you.

The earlier you seek treatment for osteoporosis, the more effective it is likely to be. However, the effectiveness of any treatment for osteoporosis depends on the severity of bone loss. In women with

ONE WOMAN'S STORY
HORMONE REPLACEMENT THERAPY AND OSTEOPOROSIS

I was 57 and I had gone through menopause when I was 49. I had very few symptoms during menopause—only an occasional, mild hot flash. One day, while my husband and I were out taking a walk, my foot missed the curb and I slipped. I reached out with my hand to break my fall and broke my wrist.

My doctor recommended testing my bone density to see if I had osteoporosis. The test showed that my bones had already thinned so much that I was at serious risk of breaking more bones. I found out that I have many of the risk factors for osteoporosis. I am fair-skinned, thin, and I smoke. I realize now that my mother must have had it too. She broke her hip when she was 75 and could never again walk without help.

"I found out after I broke my wrist that I have many of the risk factors for osteoporosis."

My doctor prescribed estrogen to prevent any more bone loss and maybe even help strengthen some of the bone. I quit smoking, I'm eating more foods that are rich in calcium, and I'm taking calcium supplements to make sure I get at least 1,000 milligrams a day. My doctor told me that, since I'm taking estrogen, I don't need 1,500 milligrams of calcium like women who aren't taking estrogen do. I've always hated exercising but I'm making an effort to walk as much as I can—to and from work, up and down stairs, wherever I can go without a car.

I have been taking estrogen for 5 years and I haven't had any more bone fractures. I feel better and I sleep well. I only wish I had started taking estrogen years earlier, when I first went through menopause.

osteoporosis, treatment can slow, stop, or sometimes reverse bone loss. Women who take estrogen have half as many bone fractures in their spine caused by osteoporosis as women who do not take the hormone. Estrogen is the only treatment for osteoporosis that also offers other important health benefits such as protection against heart disease.

The effects of HRT on slowing or eliminating bone loss appear to be greatest when you start treatment soon after menopause and continue therapy for at least 5 to 10 years. As soon as you stop taking estrogen, your bones lose density as rapidly as they normally would after menopause. For this reason, many doctors now recommend that women continue HRT for the rest of their lives. Even in women who do not start HRT until many years past menopause or when they already have osteoporosis, HRT can often increase bone density in their spine enough to reduce their risk of debilitating fractures.

If you are at high risk of osteoporosis or already have it but cannot take estrogen, ask your doctor about alternative treatments (see page 555), such as a newer nonhormonal medication called alendronate sodium or a thyroid hormone called calcitonin.

Hormone replacement therapy

Hormone replacement therapy (HRT) is treatment to replace vital hormones your body no longer produces in adequate amounts. HRT is used to alleviate the short-term symptoms of menopause such as hot flashes and the long-term, potentially life-threatening health effects of menopause, such as an increased risk of heart disease and osteoporosis.

For many women, HRT consists of replacement estrogen combined with progestin, a synthetic form of the other important female hormone progesterone. You can take HRT either in pills or in a patch applied to your abdomen or buttocks. (When estrogen is used alone, without progestin, it is sometimes called estrogen replacement therapy, or ERT.)

Progestin is added in HRT to protect against endometrial hyperplasia (increased cell growth in the lining of the uterus; see page 221) and endometrial cancer (see page 239). Taking estrogen alone may increase your risk of endometrial hyperplasia because estrogen stimulates the endometrium to grow. Progestin, on the other hand, prevents uncontrolled growth of the endometrium. If you have had a hysterectomy and, therefore, have no uterus, you can take estrogen alone.

Women often take HRT to relieve symptoms of menopause—primarily hot flashes and vaginal dryness. Doctors prescribe HRT mostly to prevent heart disease and osteoporosis. The only women for whom HRT may not be recommended are those who have had breast cancer or who developed blood clots in their legs, lungs, or eyes during pregnancy or when taking birth-control pills. Estrogen may increase the risk of a recurrence of these conditions. You and your doctor can evaluate your personal and family health histories and decide whether or not the benefits of HRT outweigh the potential risks in your case.

MAKING THE DECISION

Many women are unnecessarily reluctant to take HRT because they underestimate their risk of heart disease and overestimate their risk of breast cancer and endometrial cancer. If you are a woman between ages 50 and 94, you are 10 times more likely to die of heart disease than breast cancer. You are 30 times more likely to die of heart disease than of endometrial cancer.

Some women reject HRT because they feel it is not "natural." But, in fact, it may not be natural for a woman's body to be without estrogen. Until very recently most women did not grow old enough to reach menopause. At the beginning of the 20th century, the average life expectancy was only 47 years. Today, a woman can expect to live to about 80. Women now outlive their ovaries' ability to produce estrogen by about 30 years.

Some women reject HRT because they remember the problems, such as blood clots, some women experienced using the early birth-control pills. The first birth-control pills had high doses of hormones and many of the affected women were heavy smokers. Cigarette smoking is now known to be a significant risk factor for circulatory problems and even more so in women who are over 35 and also take birth-control pills. HRT provides much smaller doses of estrogen that, in most women, produce a level of the hormone that is lower than their level before menopause, when their ovaries were producing estrogen.

Educate yourself about the benefits and risks of HRT for you, based on your family health history as well as your own health history. Find a doctor who is willing to help you evaluate the benefits and risks objectively and work out a solution that is right for you. If you are not comfortable with your doctor's recommendation, get a second opinion.

TAKING HRT

Before you begin HRT, your doctor will perform a medical evaluation that includes taking your health history and measuring your blood pressure and cholesterol levels. He or she will also perform a physical examination, breast examination, pelvic examination, and Pap smear and will recommend that you have a mammogram. You should continue to have regular medical checkups while taking any kind of HRT.

Estrogen can be taken in pills or in patches applied to the skin on your abdomen or buttocks; both forms provide the same health benefits. If you tend to forget to take pills, you may want to use the patches, which you change twice a week. But if you have not had a hysterectomy, you need to take progestin along with the estrogen to reduce your risk of endometrial hyperplasia (excessive growth of the endometrium; see page 221) and endometrial cancer (see page 239). Progestin is available only in pills.

If your primary goal is treating the specific problems of vaginal dryness and pain during intercourse, you can use an estrogen cream to restore vaginal lubrication. You insert the cream with a special applicator directly into your vagina. The dose of estrogen in the cream is much lower than that in the pill or patch and is not effective for preventing heart disease or osteoporosis. Vaginal estrogen creams are usually used in addition to the estrogen you are getting from HRT in pills or patches.

When to start HRT If you are at high risk of osteoporosis or heart disease, the sooner after menopause you start HRT, the better the protection it gives to your heart and bones. Some women who develop hot flashes before their periods stop may benefit from starting HRT shortly before menopause. But starting HRT even 20 years after menopause can help slow the rate of bone loss in women with osteoporosis and reduce their risk of heart disease.

If menopausal symptoms, such as hot flashes and vaginal dryness, are your main concern, you can start HRT whenever you want. If you have had a hysterectomy that included the removal of your ovaries (your source of estrogen), your doctor is likely to recommend that you start estrogen replacement therapy (estrogen alone) immediately after the surgery to maintain your body's supply of estrogen.

SIDE EFFECTS OF HRT

Some women experience side effects from HRT, which are usually mild and can be controlled. Many of the side effects of HRT resemble those of birth-control pills (see page 311), which contain similar hormones. As with birth-control pills, many of the side effects subside within the first few months of taking the hormones. Tell your doctor about any side effects that are bothering you.

Side effects such as breast swelling and tenderness are usually caused by the estrogen. Most women become accustomed to the increased fullness of their breasts and it does not bother them. However, if you find these symptoms bothersome, they can sometimes be reduced by switching to a different form of estrogen or reducing the dose temporarily to allow your body time to adjust to the hormone. Water retention is usually caused by the progestin, which is added to HRT to reduce the risk of endometrial cancer (see page 239) in women who have not had a hysterectomy (surgical removal of the uterus). Progestin prevents cells in the endometrium from growing excessively (a condition called endometrial hyperplasia, see page 221), which can lead to endometrial cancer if it is not treated.

Women who take a steady dose of both progestin and estrogen throughout the month may experience irregular bleeding for the first few months they are taking HRT. Most women, especially if they are several years past menopause, will eventually stop bleeding altogether. If you are following a cycle of HRT in which you take progestin for only 10 to 12 days each month, you may begin having periods again. These periods, often called withdrawal bleeding, usually occur right after you finish the cycle of progestin pills.

If bleeding or spotting occurs at other times in your cycle, see your doctor. He or she may want to examine you to determine if you should have an endometrial biopsy (see page 129) or an ultrasound scan (see page 405) to rule out a problem such as endometrial hyperplasia. Like cell changes in your cervix (cervical dysplasia, see page 218), which can be detected at an early stage on a Pap smear and treated successfully, endometrial hyperplasia and endometrial cancer can also be detected at early stages and cured. After ruling out any abnormalities inside your uterus, the doctor can usually correct the irregular bleeding by adjusting your hormone dose or cycle of pills, or both.

RISKS OF OF HRT

As with any medication, the benefits of taking HRT must be weighed against the potential risks. For now, the best evidence shows that HRT is beneficial for most women and that HRT is the best treatment available to prevent some of the most serious health problems—primarily heart disease (see page 464) and osteoporosis (see page 552)—that women face in the years after menopause. However, HRT may not be for every woman, especially if you have any of the following risk factors:

Breast cancer Most studies show that HRT does not increase a woman's risk of breast cancer, or increases it only slightly. There may be a link between how long a woman takes estrogen and her risk of breast cancer, but this risk also appears to be small. Still, the current recommendation is that women should not take HRT

HORMONE REPLACEMENT

AT MENOPAUSE, YOUR BODY stops producing the essential hormone estrogen, causing short-term symptoms such as hot flashes and long-term health risks such as heart disease, stroke, and osteoporosis. Taking estrogen in hormone replacement therapy (HRT) at menopause can alleviate the immediate symptoms. Continuing to take it for the rest of your life can reduce your risk of chronic, debilitating illnesses. When making a decision about whether or not to take HRT, you and your doctor should thoroughly discuss the benefits and risks of HRT for you personally.

You may benefit from HRT if you have:

- Symptoms of menopause such as hot flashes, night sweats, or vaginal dryness
- Osteoporosis or a family history of the disease or other risk factors (see page 555)
- A high total cholesterol level or low HDL level (see page 131)
- A family history of heart disease
- Gone through menopause or had a hysterectomy that involved removal of your ovaries (your primary source of estrogen)
- A family history of colon cancer

You may not be a good candidate for HRT if you have:

- Had breast cancer
- Had a blood clot in a vein in your legs, lungs, or eyes during pregnancy or while taking birth-control pills
- Active liver disease or severely impaired liver function

Choosing a form of HRT

Hormones in HRT can be taken in various forms. If you decide to take HRT, you and your doctor can determine which form is best for you.

Pills

You take one estrogen pill every day of the month or for 25 days in a row (usually the first 25 days of the calendar month). Because estrogen taken by itself for long periods may increase your risk of cancer of the endometrium (lining of the uterus), doctors recommend taking progestin, a synthetic form of the hormone progesterone, along with the estrogen to reduce that risk. If you have had a hysterectomy, you take only the estrogen because you are not at risk of endometrial cancer.

You usually take progestin for 10 to 14 days of the pill cycle. Toward the end of the cycle of progestin pills, many women experience withdrawal bleeding, which is usually much lighter than a menstrual period and does not cause cramps. If you take a continuous daily dose of both estrogen and progestin, you do not have withdrawal bleeding but you may experience irregular bleeding for the first few months.

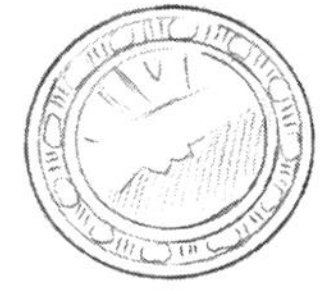

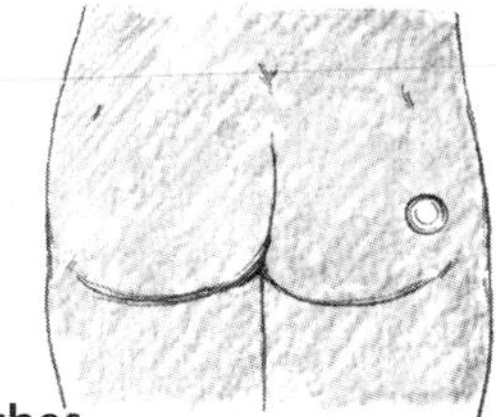

Patches

Estrogen (not progestin) can be administered through a skin patch impregnated with estrogen in gel form and attached with adhesive to the skin of your abdomen or buttocks. The patch, which is about 2 to 3 inches wide, releases a steady dose of estrogen into your body. You wear a patch every day of the month, replacing it with a new one every 3 to 7 days. You can shower, bathe, and swim while wearing a patch. Estrogen that enters your body through the skin provides the same health benefits as estrogen taken in pills. If you have not had a hysterectomy and your

Evaluating the benefits and risks

You are probably reading and hearing a great deal about HRT—both pro and con. HRT significantly reduces your long-term risk of heart disease, stroke, and osteoporosis. The question has been raised about a possible link between HRT and a slightly increased risk of breast cancer. Most studies find no association between HRT and breast cancer. The average American woman is 10 times more likely to die of heart disease or stroke than breast cancer and many times more likely to develop osteoporosis than breast cancer. When making a decision about taking HRT, you and your doctor will carefully evaluate your risk of heart disease, osteoporosis, and breast cancer.

Other benefits of HRT are now emerging. Taking estrogen may delay symptoms of Alzheimer's disease. HRT may also reduce your risk of colon cancer, which can be an important deciding factor if you have a family history of the cancer. Before you make your decision about HRT, learn as much as you can about it, keeping an open mind about all of your options. If you have any concerns about anything you have heard or read, talk to your doctor.

HAVING A BONE DENSITY TEST
If you are not sure about whether or not to take HRT, your doctor may recommend having a test to measure the density of your bones and determine your risk of osteoporosis. If the results of a bone density test show that you are at increased risk of osteoporosis, taking HRT would be beneficial for you.

Possible side effects of HRT

Few women experience side effects from HRT, and many who do are not bothered by them. However, if you have any of the following side effects and find them troublesome, your doctor may be able to change your dose or prescribe a different form of hormone therapy. Do not stop HRT without talking to your doctor.

- Breast tenderness or swelling (caused by estrogen)
- Water retention (caused by estrogen or progestin)
- Monthly periods, which usually stop after a few years (if you are taking progestin several days in the pill cycle instead of every day)
- Irregular bleeding, which usually stops after several months (if you are taking progestin every day in the pill cycle)

uterus is intact, you also take progestin pills for 10 to 14 days each month or every day. If you take progestin for 10 to 14 days, you may have a period toward the end of the progestin cycle.

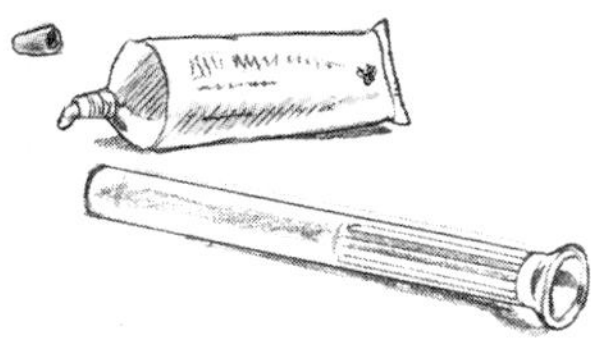

Creams

Estrogen creams are applied directly inside the vagina to alleviate vaginal dryness, which often follows menopause and can cause pain during intercourse. Estrogen creams deliver a lower, more erratic dose of estrogen than pills or patches, so creams do not provide the same health benefits as those forms.

Get regular checkups

If you are taking HRT, your doctor will recommend an annual examination to watch for any signs of problems that occur in a small number of women who are on HRT. Your doctor will examine your breasts for lumps and do a pelvic examination for signs of abnormalities in your ovaries, uterus, cervix, or vagina. Your blood pressure will also be measured, because hormones can increase blood pressure in some women. Tell your doctor about any side effects that are bothering you.

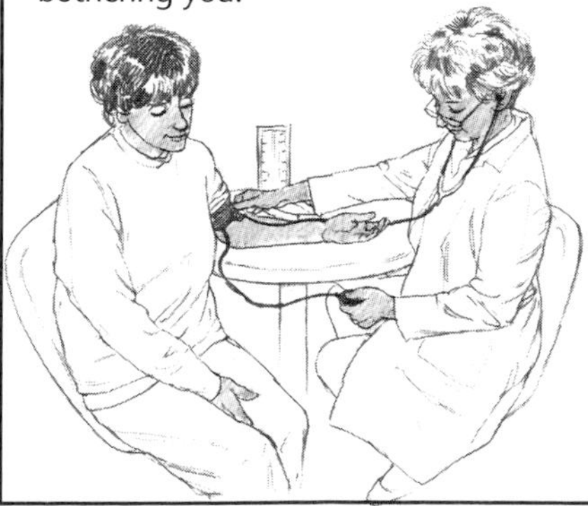

if they have or have had breast cancer. Because some breast cancers are stimulated by estrogen, the hormone may make some undetected cancers grow more quickly or increase the risk of a recurrence of a cancer.

As more becomes known about breast cancer and its relationship to estrogen, it is possible that this recommendation will change. Some doctors believe that 10 years after a diagnosis of breast cancer, a woman with no evidence of a recurrence can consider taking HRT. Even if you have breast cancer, whether or not to take HRT is an individual decision for you to make in consultation with your doctor. Women with a family history of breast cancer (a close relative with the cancer) can safely take HRT.

Endometrial cancer Taking estrogen alone for several years can increase a woman's risk of endometrial cancer (see page 239). For this reason, HRT is usually given as estrogen in combination with progestin, which counteracts the effect of estrogen on the endometrium. Estrogen stimulates growth of the endometrium while progestin limits its growth. This protection against endometrial cancer is the only reason progestin is added to estrogen in HRT. If you have had a hysterectomy, you can take estrogen alone because you no longer have a risk of endometrial cancer. Both endometrial hyperplasia (abnormal cell changes inside the uterus) and endometrial cancer can be detected at an early stage and cured.

Blood clots HRT does not appear to increase your risk of developing blood clots if you have no history of this kind of problem. But if you have had blood clots in the past, you may be more susceptible to developing them again. High levels of estrogen have been associated with an increased susceptibility to blood clots. However, even if you developed a blood clot while taking birth-control pills or during pregnancy, both of which increase the level of estrogen circulating in the body, your doctor may still recommend HRT. The dose of estrogen in HRT is much lower than the dose of the hormone that is provided in birth-control pills or the level your body produces during pregnancy. Your doctor may recommend tests to evaluate the circulation in your veins before you begin HRT.

If you had a blood clot in a deep vein in your leg after an injury such as a bone fracture, you can safely take estrogen because this type of blood clot is not related to your level of circulating estrogen. If you have had a heart attack or stroke, your doctor will probably not recommend HRT.

Liver disease Women with active liver disease or severely impaired liver function should not use HRT. A healthy liver breaks down estrogen and prevents it from building up in the bloodstream. If you have had hepatitis (an infection of the liver; see page 534) in the past and your liver is functioning normally now, you can safely take HRT.

Sexuality at menopause

You can continue to have a satisfying sex life well into old age. How you viewed your sexuality in the past and as you approach and go through menopause has a great deal to do with the quality of your sex life after menopause. Taking estrogen, which preserves the health of vaginal tissues, can help you maintain your enjoyment of sex and may even enhance it at this stage of your life.

CHANGES IN THE VAGINA

Women who have regular sexual intercourse (about once a week) have fewer problems with vaginal dryness than women who are less sexually active. The drop in estrogen production at menopause reduces the vagina's secretion of a lubricating fluid when you become sexually aroused. The thrusting of the penis inside the vagina during intercourse may stimulate vaginal cells to continue multiplying and producing this lubricating fluid.

If it takes longer for your vagina to become lubricated after you are sexually aroused, try extending foreplay a few minutes before having intercourse. If this does not work, try using a water-based lubricant. Many women of all ages (and their partners) benefit from using a lubricant during foreplay and intercourse. You can apply the lubricant to yourself or your partner, or have your partner apply it.

Hormone replacement therapy (HRT) is the best way to maintain the functioning of your reproductive system. Even 10 years or more after menopause in women who have experienced severe changes in their vagina, HRT can restore and thicken the vaginal lining. HRT can also renew the vagina's ability to produce the lubricating secretions that enhance sexual pleasure.

CHANGES IN SEXUAL DESIRE

Many women report a loss of sexual desire as they reach menopause. Some women experience no change in their desire for sex and others find their sex life becomes even more satisfying as they are freed from the concerns of pregnancy and birth control.

The ovaries produce some male hormones, called androgens, as well as female hormones. Androgens, which include the male hormone testosterone, affect sex drive (libido) in both women and men. In some women, the production of androgens by the ovaries decreases at menopause. This drop in androgens may reduce a woman's sexual desire.

If you have experienced a significant drop in sexual desire during menopause, you may want to talk with your doctor about the possibility of adding the male sex hormone testosterone to your HRT. Some forms of HRT contain small doses of testosterone to help increase libido in women who are concerned about their loss of sexual desire. In rare cases, long-term use of testosterone may produce such side effects as a slight increase in facial hair or acne. These effects will disappear when treatment stops.

Some women choose to let sex become less important. For the growing number of older women who are alone, the lack of a partner limits their opportunities for a regular sex life and may decrease their interest. This is not uncommon. If you have chosen to eliminate sex from your life and you are happy with your decision, you have made the right choice for you. On the other hand, if you do not have a partner but you want to experience sexual stimulation, you might consider alternatives. Masturbating (see page 296) can help relieve tension and maintain vaginal tissues. Keep an open mind.

CHANGING SEXUAL RELATIONSHIPS

As you and your partner get older, communication is just as important as ever for maintaining a healthy relationship. Expressing your feelings openly to your partner whenever something bothers you can prevent a problem from festering and compromising your relationship. Letting your partner know what gives you pleasure sexually can help both of you continue to have a mutually satisfying sex life.

Keep in mind that pleasure can take many forms. Closeness, companionship, caring, and laughter are as necessary as sex for a fulfilling life with another person—no matter how old you are. For many couples, retirement brings new opportunities to enjoy life together and nurture their relationship without the constraints of time, a job, and other commitments.

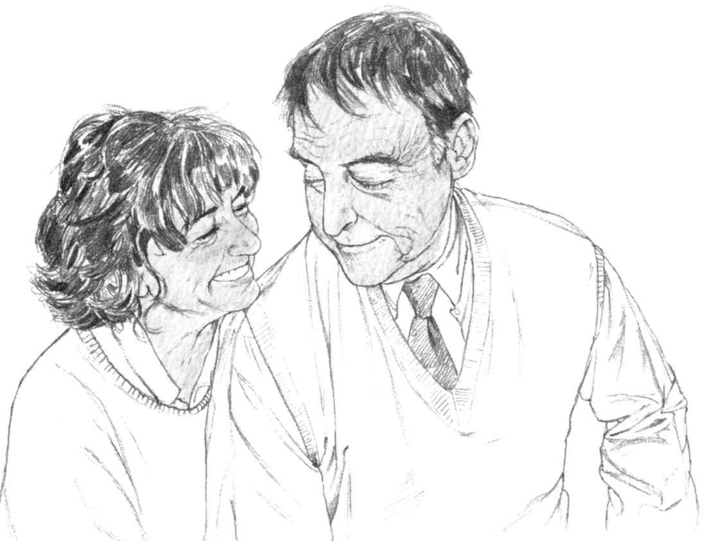

KEEPING YOUR RELATIONSHIP VITAL
Although your body may undergo changes as you age, these changes need not prevent you from having a satisfying sex life. You and your partner can continue to enjoy an affectionate, caring, rewarding relationship well into old age.

On the other hand, some couples find that retirement and their increased time together brings new challenges to their relationship. The many distractions of their formerly busy life may have prevented them from seeing and dealing with underlying problems in their relationship.

Unresolved difficulties can cause a growing distance between two people that may extend into the bedroom. Either partner's attitude can influence the other's self-image and sexuality. A negative self-image can make a person feel less sexually desirable and cause the relationship to deteriorate further. Counseling is often the best solution in this case. It is important to begin counseling while you and your partner are still willing to work constructively toward a shared goal.

If the problem is rooted in the relationship itself, a marriage counselor or a therapist who specializes in counseling couples is a good choice. If the problem is sexual, a qualified sex therapist may be able to help you. For information about finding a qualified sex therapist, see page 305. For sexual difficulties that result from medical conditions, you need to work with a medical doctor; many of these problems are treatable.

·3·

Pregnancy

CHAPTER 14

Planning a pregnancy

Contents

The best time to prepare for a healthy pregnancy is long before you decide to become pregnant. Let your doctor know that you are planning to become pregnant and make an appointment to see him or her. During the months before pregnancy, your doctor can help you build a strong foundation for a healthy pregnancy and healthy baby. If you are concerned about any inherited disorders or birth defects that have occurred in your family—or any health conditions you have that could affect your pregnancy—this is the time to ask about any tests or treatments you should have. Most couples who are actively trying to conceive do so within a year. If you have been trying to become pregnant for a year or more without success, you and your partner may want to consider having a doctor evaluate your fertility.

Before you get pregnant

Like any major event in your life, pregnancy requires planning. Prepare your body for pregnancy by establishing healthful habits—including eating a nutritious diet and exercising regularly—and eliminating unhealthy habits, such as smoking or drinking. If you have a family history of a genetic disorder or birth defects, or if you are adopted and don't know your family health history, ask your doctor to refer you to a genetic counselor (see page 373), who can help you evaluate your risk of having a child with a birth defect.

PRECONCEPTION CHECKUP

If you are thinking about getting pregnant, make an appointment with your doctor to discuss your plans and to have a physical examination. Your doctor will ask about your health history and that of your family. He or she will probably ask about any harmful habits you should stop or lifestyle factors you should change before getting pregnant.

Your preconception checkup will probably include:

- Gathering information about your personal and family health histories and previous pregnancies and deliveries, including any problems or complications you have had.
- A physical examination that includes measurement of your blood pressure, a pelvic examination to check for abnormalities in your cervix or uterus, a Pap smear, and a breast examination.
- Testing to determine if you are immune to rubella and hepatitis B, if you do not know for sure. These infections can harm the fetus if you acquire them while you are pregnant. If you are not immune to rubella or hepatitis B, your doctor may recommend a vaccination, especially for rubella, at least 3 months before you conceive. If given during pregnancy, a rubella vaccination can cause complications, such as cataracts (clouding of the lenses of the eyes), in the fetus. Although it is safe to have a hepatitis B vaccination during pregnancy, it is a good idea to have it before you get pregnant in order to minimize the risk of an active infection during pregnancy.
- Testing to see if you have an active syphilis infection, which can cause birth defects. There is no vaccination against syphilis but, because it is a bacterial infection, it can be treated with antibiotics.
- Testing for Rh factor (see page 371).
- Evaluating your family health history to see if you should have testing to determine if you carry a gene for a serious inherited disorder such as cystic fibrosis (see page 512) or sickle-cell anemia (see page 493).

PREPARING FOR PREGNANCY

The healthier you are before you get pregnant, the easier your pregnancy will be and the healthier your baby is likely to be. Several months before you start trying to conceive, evaluate your lifestyle to determine if you have any habits—such as smoking or drinking or using drugs—that can pose a risk to your fetus. The first weeks of pregnancy, often before you even know you are pregnant, are a crucial period in a fetus's development. Nearly all of a fetus's major organs—including the heart, brain, and lungs—are formed in the first 3 months of pregnancy.

Rh factor incompatibility

If you are thinking about getting pregnant or are already pregnant, you should have a blood test to determine if you have Rh factor, a protein found on the surface of red blood cells, the blood cells that carry oxygen. If you have the Rh factor, as most people do, your blood is Rh positive. If you do not have the Rh factor, your blood is Rh negative.

If you have Rh-negative blood and your partner has Rh-positive blood, you could become pregnant with a fetus whose blood is Rh positive. Because the fetus's Rh factor differs from yours, if the baby's blood enters your bloodstream during delivery, your body's immune system may recognize the fetus's red blood cells as foreign and produce antibodies to eliminate them. In a first pregnancy, the number of antibodies produced usually is not enough to harm the fetus. However, the antibodies remain in your body and, during a second pregnancy in which the fetus also has Rh-positive blood, the level of the antibodies could rise sharply and attack the fetus's red blood cells, potentially causing anemia (insufficient oxygen in the blood), organ damage in the fetus, or death.

You should be tested for Rh factor before you get pregnant for the first time, or early in your first pregnancy. If you have Rh-negative blood, your doctor will prescribe a type of vaccine called Rh immune globulin that prevents your immune system from producing antibodies to Rh-positive blood.

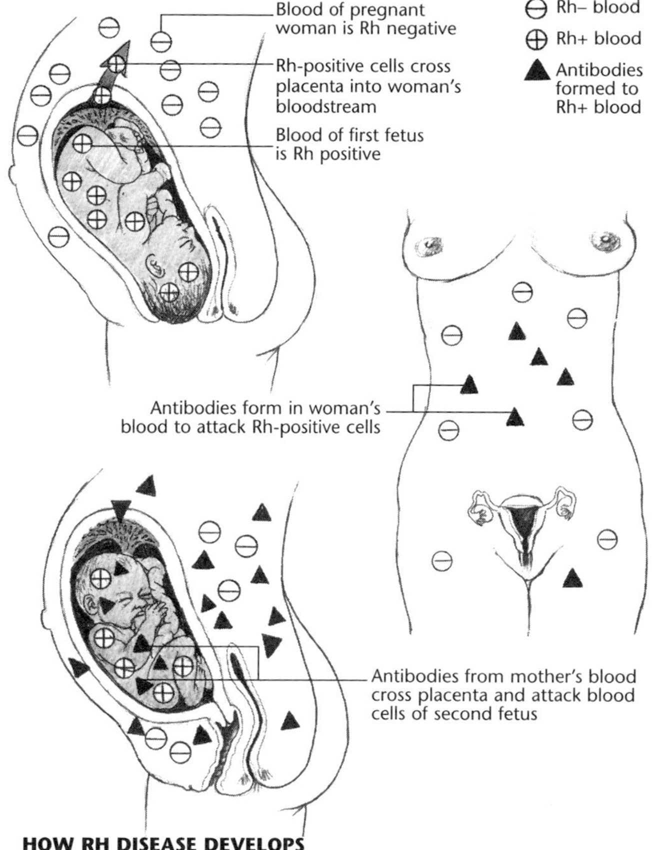

HOW RH DISEASE DEVELOPS
During delivery, some blood from the fetus can enter the mother's bloodstream (top). If a woman's blood is Rh negative and her first child's blood is Rh positive, her body will develop antibodies (center) that can recognize and destroy the Rh-positive blood (though usually not enough to harm the first fetus). The woman must be vaccinated within 48 hours of this first birth. If she is not vaccinated and she has a subsequent pregnancy with an Rh-positive fetus, her antibodies may go through the placenta and destroy the fetus's red blood cells (bottom).

Eat well and maintain a healthy weight
Eating a nutritious diet (see page 44) will help prepare your body for the demands of pregnancy. A healthful diet is low in fat and rich in fruits, vegetables, and whole grains.

It is especially important—at least 2 months before you become pregnant—to begin taking a vitamin/mineral supplement that contains 400 micrograms (0.4 milligrams) of folic acid. Folic acid, a B vitamin, reduces the risk that your child will be born with a birth defect, such as a neural tube defect. Neural tube defects, which can range from mild to life threatening, are abnormalities that result when the spine fails to develop completely. Because many pregnancies are unplanned, and many women do not know they are pregnant until 4 to 6 weeks after conception, it is recommended that all women who may become pregnant take this supplement every day in a vitamin supplement or as part of a multivitamin supplement.

Limit your daily consumption of caffeine to less than the equivalent of two cups of coffee (see page 65). Although doctors do not fully understand how caffeine affects a developing fetus, it may increase the risk of miscarriage or low birth weight.

Exercise Moderate exercise, such as brisk walking for half an hour three to four times a week, will make you feel better and more comfortable throughout your pregnancy and may make your pregnancy and delivery easier. If you have not been exercising regularly, begin an exercise program (see page 78) before you get pregnant. If you have always been a regular exerciser, keep it up throughout your pregnancy. Pregnancy is not a good time to start a strenuous or new exercise program because pregnancy makes extra demands on your body. If you have a history of miscarriage (see page 422) or preterm labor (see page 427), it is essential that you check with your doctor before starting any exercise routine.

Quit smoking Each cigarette you smoke during pregnancy deprives the fetus of oxygen it needs to develop and grow. Smoking increases the risk of miscarriage, stillbirth, and having a baby with a low birth weight. It is best to quit smoking before you get pregnant, but quitting at any time during pregnancy is beneficial. (For more about the effects of smoking during pregnancy, see page 413; for information about how to quit smoking, see page 157.)

Eliminate alcohol and other drugs Heavy drinking, particularly during the early weeks and months of pregnancy, can cause fetal alcohol syndrome. Fetal alcohol syndrome is the major preventable cause of mental retardation in the US. Because no safe level of alcohol consumption during pregnancy has been established, doctors recommend that you do not drink at all if you are pregnant, think you may be pregnant, or are trying to become pregnant.

If you use any illegal drugs, stop doing so several months before you conceive and refrain throughout your pregnancy. Increasing numbers of women are using cocaine during pregnancy, which is linked to miscarriage (see page 422), preterm labor (see page 427), premature detachment of the placenta (placental abruption, see page 426), fetal brain hemorrhage, and birth defects. If you are using alcohol or other drugs to relieve stress, you may need help learning more positive ways of coping with problems (see page 186). If you think you may be addicted to alcohol or another drug, see page 164.

Some prescription and over-the-counter medications can also harm the developing fetus. Tell your doctor about any medications, including vitamins and health food store preparations, you take regularly. You should not use any drug without your doctor's knowledge.

Avoid harmful substances Make sure you are not exposed to chemicals, such as paint thinners, that are known to be potentially harmful to a developing fetus. For information about environmental hazards at work and at home during pregnancy, see page 414.

Engage only in safe sex If you are not in a stable, mutually monogamous relationship (see page 338), having sex without a latex or polyurethane male condom or female condom with spermicide puts you at risk of contracting sexually transmitted diseases (STDs). Some of these infections, especially genital herpes (see page 342) and HIV (the virus that causes AIDS; see page 344), can be transmitted to the fetus or put the pregnancy at risk. Because many STDs do not cause symptoms, women often have an STD and do not know it. Some STDs, such as chlamydia (see page 339), can lead to infertility. Your doctor will ask you about your risk of exposure to STDs and determine whether or not you should be tested.

IF YOU ARE OVER 35

If you are over 35, getting pregnant may take longer for you than for a younger woman because fertility begins to decline at 30 and drops significantly after 35. Your risk of having a child with a chromosome abnormality (see page 375) such as Down syndrome increases significantly with age. The risk of other birth defects also increases slightly as a woman ages. Depending on your age and family history, your doctor may recommend that you have a prenatal test—such as amniocentesis (see page 406) or chorionic villus sampling (CVS; see page 407)—

early in your pregnancy to detect chromosome abnormalities and some other birth defects.

Women over 35 are also more likely to have health conditions that can increase their risk of complications during pregnancy. For example, older women are more likely than younger women to have high blood pressure, which can cause premature birth or miscarriage. They are also more likely to have diabetes (see page 617) or to develop a type of diabetes called gestational diabetes (see page 418) that is brought on by the added physical stress of pregnancy. If you have diabetes, your doctor will recommend a special diet, more frequent checkups during your pregnancy, and, sometimes, early delivery to ensure the health of the baby. An older woman is also more likely to have a cesarean delivery (see page 442) or a delivery using forceps (see page 441).

If you are over 35 and planning a pregnancy, your doctor will closely monitor any existing health problems you have and will take steps to manage any risks to your pregnancy. Most women over 35 have uncomplicated pregnancies and give birth to healthy babies.

GENETIC COUNSELING

If you are concerned about birth defects or genetic diseases in your family, you should talk to your doctor about genetic counseling. A genetic counselor can translate complex scientific knowledge about genetic inheritance into practical information you can use when planning your family. For example, a genetic counselor can evaluate your risk of transmitting a particular genetic disease or birth defect to your child and the effect that a particular disorder can have on your family in terms of care, treatment, and long-term prognosis. How much knowledge you and your partner pursue and how that knowledge affects your plans for pregnancy is your choice. The information that a genetic counselor provides can mean completely different things to different couples.

For many genetic disorders, blood tests can show whether or not a person with a family history of the disorder has the gene. If you consider the risk of transmitting a genetic disorder to a child too great, you may want to consider adoption rather than take the chance of conceiving a child with a life-threatening condition. If you do get pregnant, in some cases prenatal diagnostic tests such as amniocentesis (see page 406) or chorionic villus sampling (CVS; see page 407) can tell you at an early stage in the pregnancy whether or not the fetus has the disorder. You can then decide with your partner whether or not to continue the pregnancy. If the fetus is affected and you decide to continue the pregnancy, you can begin to plan for the care of a child with special needs. Some couples choose to use assisted reproductive technology (see page 392) to substitute the egg or sperm of the partner who carries the disease-causing gene with an egg or sperm from a donor.

Who should consider genetic counseling?

If you have questions about genetic diseases or birth defects that have occurred in your family, consider genetic testing and counseling. A genetic counselor can help you understand your risk of passing a genetic disorder to your children, or help you find treatment for an inherited disorder that you have. Consider genetic counseling if:

- You have or think you may have an inherited disorder or birth defect.
- You are pregnant or planning to be pregnant after age 35.
- You already have a child with mental retardation, an inherited disorder, or a birth defect.
- You have had two or more miscarriages (see page 422) or babies who died in infancy.
- You would like to be tested for a genetic disease or want more information about birth defects that occur frequently in your ethnic group.
- You and your partner are first cousins or other close blood relatives, which increases your risk of carrying the same defective recessive gene.
- You are already pregnant and prenatal tests, such as ultrasound imaging (see page 405) or blood tests for alpha-fetoprotein (AFP; see page 404), have shown that your fetus may be at increased risk of a birth defect.

Recessive disorders For disorders that follow a recessive pattern of inheritance (see page 377), a child must inherit two copies of the faulty gene (one from each parent) to have the disorder. When parents are carriers of a recessive disease gene, they are not affected by the disease themselves, but, if they each transmit the defective copy of the gene to offspring, the child will be affected. Every child of this couple has a 25-percent chance of inheriting both defective copies of the recessive gene and having the disorder, a 50-percent chance of inheriting one defective copy of the gene and being a carrier like his or her parents, and a 25-percent chance of inheriting both healthy copies of the gene and being neither affected nor a carrier.

If a test is available to detect a particular recessive disease gene, a woman who may be at risk of carrying the gene can be tested, usually before she becomes pregnant. If the test shows she does not carry the faulty recessive gene, her partner does not have to be tested because there is no risk of their transmitting the disease to offspring. However, their children may want to be tested before they have children themselves to see if they carry the faulty gene. Diseases that follow a recessive pattern of inheritance include cystic fibrosis (most common among whites; see page 512), sickle-cell anemia (most common among blacks; see page 493), Tay-Sachs disease (most common among people of eastern European Jewish descent), and beta-thalassemia (most common among people of Mediterranean descent, such as Italians or Greeks).

Some recessive genetic disorders, such as Duchenne's muscular dystrophy or hemophilia, are carried on the X sex chromosome. Women are usually not affected by a so-called X-linked disorder because they have two X chromosomes. If a gene on one X chromosome is defective, the healthy copy of the gene on their other X chromosome compensates, for the most part, for the harmful effects of the defective gene. Each child of these women has a 50-percent chance of inheriting the X chromosome with the faulty gene. A son who inherits the gene will be affected by the disorder because he does not have a healthy copy of the gene to override the effects of the disease gene; a daughter who inherits the gene will be an unaffected carrier like her mother. The daughter may be tested for the disease-causing gene (if a test is available) before she has children to find out if she is at risk of transmitting the disease to a son.

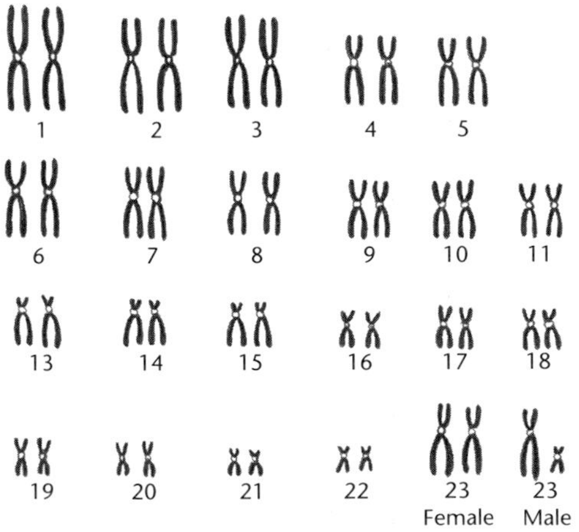

Dominant disorders For genetic disorders that follow a dominant pattern of inheritance (see page 377)—such as achondroplasia (a form of dwarfism) and familial hypercholesterolemia (a disorder that causes cholesterol to build up in the blood)—a person need inherit only one defective copy of the gene to be affected. When one member of a couple has a gene for a dominant disorder, each of their children has a 50-percent chance of inheriting the gene and having the disorder. For some dominant disorders, testing is available that may be useful in prenatal diagnosis or diagnosis before a person has symptoms. A genetic counselor can tell you if testing is available for a particular dominant genetic disorder that may run in your family.

Chromosome abnormalities Other genetic disorders are caused by mistakes that can occur when eggs or sperm are formed. When an egg and sperm combine at conception, they each contribute 23 chromosomes to make a total of 46 in the new cell, which has a unique mix of genes. If an error occurred when the egg or sperm was formed or when they combine at conception, the fertilized egg may contain extra or missing chromosomes, or the chromosomes may have an abnormal structure or arrangement. Such an error is repeated in the millions of cells that form the growing embryo and affects a number of body structures or functions.

Down syndrome, which results from an extra copy of chromosome 21, is a

1 2 3 4 5
6 7 8 9 10 11 12
13 14 15 16 17 18
19 20 21 22 23 Female 23 Male

CHANGE IN CHROMOSOMES
A chromosome disorder results from a change in the number or structure of the chromosomes, which usually occurs during the formation of an egg or sperm. In the most common chromosome disorder, Down syndrome, the fetus has three copies of chromosome 21 instead of the usual two.

Your risk of having a child with a chromosome abnormality

As you age, your risk of giving birth to a child with a chromosome abnormality, such as Down syndrome, increases. However, not all cases of chromosome abnormalities occur in children born to women over 35. Many babies with chromosome abnormalities are born to women under 35 because more women in this age group are having babies. Chromosome disorders can range from very mild to life threatening.

MOTHER'S AGE	RISK OF HAVING A CHILD WITH DOWN SYNDROME	RISK OF HAVING A CHILD WITH ANY CHROMOSOME ABNORMALITY
20	1 in 1,667	1 in 526
30	1 in 952	1 in 385
33	1 in 602	1 in 286
35	1 in 378	1 in 192
38	1 in 173	1 in 102
40	1 in 106	1 in 66
42	1 in 63	1 in 42
45	1 in 30	1 in 21

good example of how a single change in chromosome number can affect many parts of the body. People with Down syndrome usually have a characteristic facial appearance, short limbs, defects of the heart and other internal organs, and varying degrees of mental retardation. Testing for Down syndrome and other chromosome abnormalities is routinely offered to all women over 35, who are at significantly higher risk of having a child with this type of disorder.

DISEASES THAT CAN AFFECT PREGNANCY

A number of disorders that a pregnant woman may have—including high blood pressure, diabetes, epilepsy, and obesity—can increase the risk of complications during pregnancy, both for the woman and the fetus. Before you get pregnant, tell your doctor about any medical condition you have. Your condition may require an adjustment in treatment or more frequent monitoring by your doctor during your pregnancy.

Diabetes A pregnant woman who has diabetes has an increased risk of having a child with birth defects that affect the nervous system, heart, skeleton, or urinary tract. This risk can be reduced if the woman begins a treatment program to get her diabetes under control before she becomes pregnant. Because the physical stress of pregnancy can make diabetes worse, she may need to take more insulin or eat a special diet to keep it under control. (For more about controlling diabetes, see page 418.)

High blood pressure Blood pressure increases to some degree during most pregnancies, so, if you already have high blood pressure, the extra stress of pregnancy may cause it to reach dangerous levels. It is important to lower your blood pressure—with weight loss, exercise, and a diet low in sodium—before you become pregnant. If these measures do not lower your blood pressure, your doctor may prescribe medication. Make sure your doctor knows you are trying to get pregnant, so he or she can prescribe a medication that is safe for you to take during pregnancy.

Epilepsy Some medications used to control seizures in women with epilepsy (see page 578) can cause birth defects if taken during pregnancy. However, doctors recommend that pregnant women who have epilepsy continue taking their medication during pregnancy. If a woman has a seizure during pregnancy, she may stop breathing temporarily, which can

A Practical Guide to Genetic Inheritance

An understanding of genetic inheritance gives you a clearer picture of how some of your traits were passed on to you from your parents and how you could pass on traits to children of your own. If you are planning to become pregnant, or already are, an understanding of how genes are inherited can help you make decisions about having genetic counseling and prenatal testing.

What are genes?

Genes are the chemical units of heredity. You have between 50,000 and 100,000 genes in every cell of your body. You receive half of your genes from each parent—packaged in structures called chromosomes. Each parent contributes 23 chromosomes to make a total of 46. Your unique mix of genes is responsible for your physical characteristics, regulates all the functions of your body, and contributes to traits, such as your height, that are influenced by environmental factors (such as diet) as well.

Genes can be either recessive or dominant. Recessive genes usually have no outward effects unless you have two copies of the same recessive gene. Dominant genes always have an effect, even if you have only one copy, because they are the working gene in a pair.

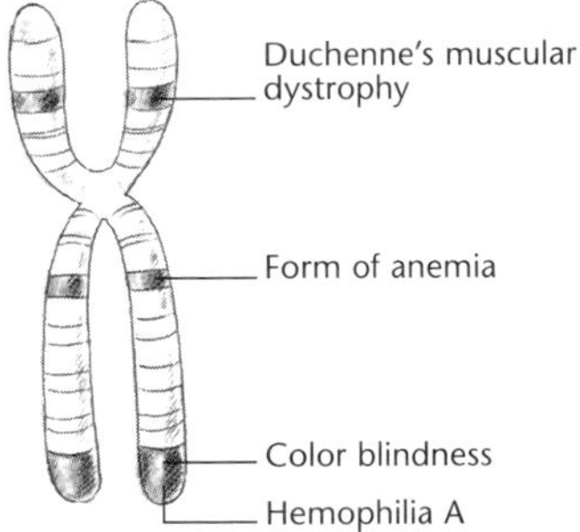

GENE MAPPING

The illustration above shows the general location on the X sex chromosome of some genes that cause disease. Scientists are working to identify and map the location on chromosomes of all the genes in the human body. They have found many of the genes that cause serious disorders such as cystic fibrosis (see page 512). This new knowledge has led to the development of diagnostic tests and new treatments for some genetic disorders and may lead to ways to prevent or cure them.

Chromosome abnormalities

Chromosome abnormalities usually occur spontaneously during the formation of an egg or a sperm or during the first few cell divisions after fertilization. In most cases, if an embryo has abnormal chromosomes, the pregnancy will end in miscarriage. In a child born with a chromosome abnormality, the effects can vary from minor to life threatening. The most common chromosome abnormality, Down syndrome (see page 374), causes multiple birth defects and mental retardation.

As a woman ages, her risk of having a baby with a chromosome abnormality gradually increases. Most pregnant women over age 35 have a prenatal test—amniocentesis or chorionic villus sampling (CVS)—that can detect chromosome abnormalities and some inherited genetic disorders in the fetus.

Genetic counseling

If either you or your partner has a family history of a genetic disorder, you may choose to see a genetic counselor before you become pregnant or early in the pregnancy. Ask your doctor for a referral to a genetic counselor. Most genetic counseling is performed by a team of experts—usually a doctor who specializes in genetics, a counselor who is trained in the scientific and practical aspects of genetics, and scientists who perform laboratory tests.

Genetic counseling before pregnancy evaluates your risk of transmitting a genetic disorder to a child. A blood test can show whether you or your partner carries a specific disease-causing gene that may run in your families. Once you are pregnant, tests such as amniocentesis or chorionic villus sampling (CVS) can determine if the fetus has a chromosome abnormality or some other genetic disorder.

Recessive disorders

- Recessive genetic disorders, the most common inherited disorders, occur when both parents pass on an abnormal (mutated) copy of the same recessive gene to a child.
- A person who has only one abnormal copy of a recessive gene is a carrier of the disease-causing gene but is not affected by the disease. The healthy copy of the gene on the paired chromosome overrides the effects of the abnormal gene. A carrier can, however, pass on the abnormal gene to a child.
- When one parent has one abnormal and one healthy copy of a recessive gene and the other has two healthy copies of the gene, they cannot transmit two of the abnormal genes to a child. Therefore, none of their children will be affected by the disease.

RECESSIVE INHERITANCE

Each of these parents carries one abnormal copy of a recessive gene but are not affected by the disease; they are called carriers. Each of their children has a one-in-four chance of inheriting an abnormal copy of the gene from both of them and having the disorder; a one-in-two chance of inheriting the abnormal copy of the gene from one parent and being a carrier like the parents; and a one-in-four chance of inheriting two healthy copies of the gene and being neither affected nor a carrier.

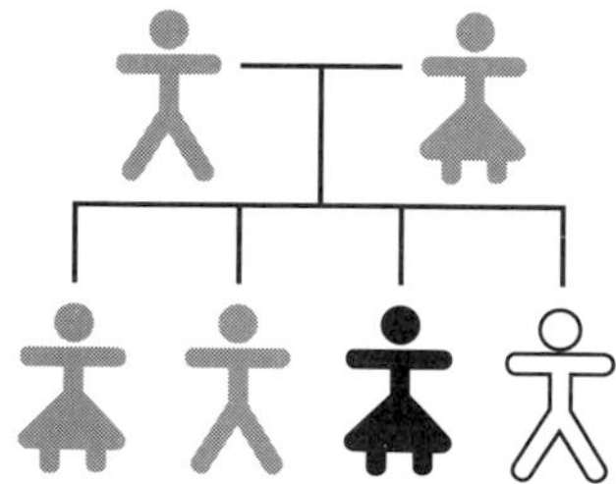

DOMINANT INHERITANCE

A person who inherits only one copy of a disease-causing dominant gene will be affected by the disease. Each of his or her children has a one-in-two chance of inheriting the abnormal gene and having the disorder. Each child also has a one-in-two chance of inheriting the parent's healthy copy of the gene and being unaffected.

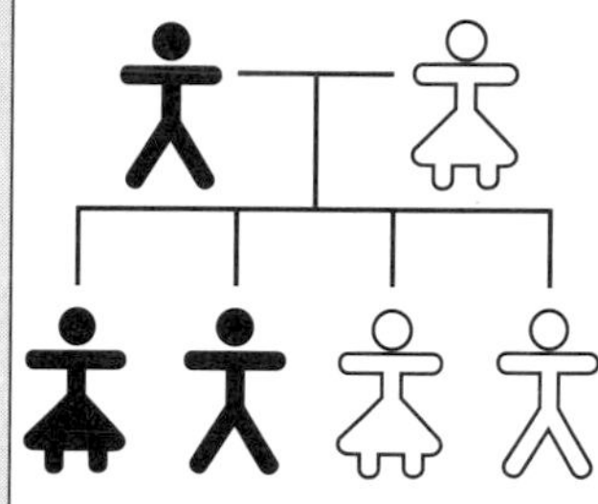

Dominant disorders

- A dominant genetic disorder occurs when a person inherits one copy of an abnormal dominant gene. A child who inherits a disease-causing dominant gene will be affected by the disease.
- If one parent has a disease-causing dominant gene, each of his or her children has a one-in-two chance of inheriting the gene and also having the disease. Each child also has a one-in-two chance of not inheriting the gene and, therefore, being unaffected by the disorder and not at risk of passing the gene on to his or her own children.

X-LINKED INHERITANCE

Each son of a woman who carries an X-linked disease gene has a one-in-two chance of inheriting the gene and having the disease. Each daughter also has a one-in-two chance of inheriting the gene, but she will be an unaffected carrier.

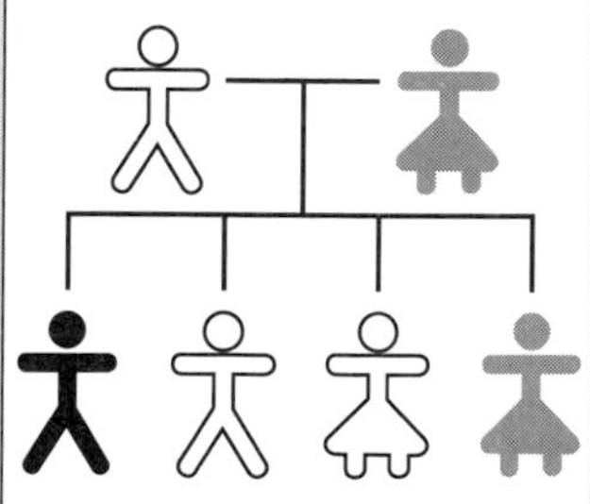

X-linked recessive disorders

- Of the 23 pairs of chromosomes, one pair—the X and Y sex chromosomes—determines whether a child will be male or female. Females have two X chromosomes, one from each parent. Males have an X and a Y chromosome—the X from their mother, the Y from their father. A disorder caused by an abnormal gene on the X chromosome is called an X-linked disorder.
- Only males are affected by X-linked disorders.
- A woman with an abnormal gene on an X chromosome is an unaffected carrier of the gene. If she passes the gene on to a son, he will have the disease. If she passes the gene to a daughter, the daughter will be an unaffected carrier like her.

Key: ■ Affected ■ Unaffected carrier □ Healthy

cut off the oxygen supply to the developing fetus. Before you get pregnant, talk to your doctor about the seizure medication you are taking. He or she may recommend a different medication that is safer to take during pregnancy but effective enough to prevent seizures.

Gynecologic disorders Some gynecologic conditions—such as endometriosis (see page 230), pelvic inflammatory disease (PID; see page 232), and fibroids (see page 221)—can cause infertility. Some of these conditions can worsen with age, so it is advisable for women with one of these disorders to try to get pregnant before age 30. If one of these disorders is preventing you from conceiving, you may be able to have surgery to enable you to get pregnant. Discuss the treatment options with your doctor.

Phenylketonuria Women with a rare disorder called phenylketonuria (PKU)—which results from a deficiency of an essential liver enzyme—have excessive levels of a protein component called phenylalanine in their blood. Phenylalanine can pass through the placenta to the fetus, causing mental retardation, low birth weight, and microcephaly (an abnormally small head). However, if the woman follows a diet low in protein before she gets pregnant and throughout her pregnancy, the risk of abnormalities in the fetus is substantially reduced. Because of the importance of starting a low-protein diet before you get pregnant, talk to your doctor if you have PKU and you are planning a pregnancy.

Other disorders that can affect pregnancy Some other disorders can affect your pregnancy and require more diligent monitoring. Ask your doctor how you can work together to manage your condition. If you have asthma (see page 635), pregnancy may trigger worse attacks, sometimes so severe that they require emergency treatment. Crohn's disease (see page 527) may hinder the absorption of enough nutrients from a pregnant woman's intestinal tract to provide nourishment for the fetus to grow. In this case, your doctor will monitor the growth of the fetus throughout your pregnancy to ensure that it is getting adequate nutrition, and recommend appropriate treatment when necessary. A woman with a thyroid disorder (see page 624) may have to have the dose of her medication changed during pregnancy. For any of these disorders, careful planning with your doctor will increase the likelihood of a healthy outcome for you and your baby.

Childhood diseases If you have not had the common childhood diseases measles, mumps, or rubella (German measles) or been vaccinated against them, you should be immunized before you become pregnant. Having any of these infections during pregnancy can cause birth defects in the fetus. If you are not sure whether or not you are immune to any of these infections, your doctor can test your blood to see if you need a vaccination.

Fifth disease, which is caused by a virus called parvovirus, is a mild childhood infection for which there is no vaccination. Most adults are immune to the virus. However, if a pregnant woman who is not immune is exposed to a child with fifth disease, she may pass the infection to her fetus, potentially causing anemia, swelling, or death in the fetus. If you have been exposed during pregnancy to a child with fifth disease, your doctor can test your immunity to see if your fetus is at risk.

Becoming pregnant

Many couples who want to have a child simply have sexual intercourse without contraception. For other couples—such as those who want to have a child as soon as possible or those who have been having regular intercourse without contraception for several months and have not conceived—more concerted effort may be required. You can choose from several methods that can help increase your chances of becoming pregnant. These methods are based on your ability to understand your menstrual cycle and determine when during your cycle you are most fertile and, therefore, most likely to conceive.

If you have had intercourse at least once a week without contraception for a year and have not gotten pregnant, talk to your doctor about having an evaluation of your fertility. He or she can often determine whether or not you and your partner have a fertility problem and recommend appropriate treatment.

KNOWING YOUR FERTILE DAYS

To increase your chances of becoming pregnant, it is important to know when during each month you ovulate—one of your ovaries releases an egg into one of your fallopian tubes. This is the optimal time to have intercourse. Ovulation occurs in the middle of your menstrual cycle—on or around day 14 of the average 28-day cycle, counting the first day of your period as day 1. If your cycle is longer than 28 days, you can estimate the day of ovulation by counting back 14 days from the expected first day of your period. This so-called calendar method is a general indication of when you ovulate.

There are several ways to pinpoint ovulation more precisely so that you know the best time to have intercourse. You can use an at-home ovulation test, which measures a hormone in your urine that signals ovulation; you can take your temperature every day to see when it increases, which occurs right after ovulation; or you can monitor mucus secretions from your cervix for changes that signal ovulation.

At-home ovulation tests You can purchase an ovulation predictor kit, sold over the counter, to help pinpoint when you are ovulating. These tests measure your level of luteinizing hormone (LH; see page 205), which rises just before you ovulate. You have to perform the test each day for several days around ovulation (days 12 to 16 of a 28-day cycle). The test must be done at the same time every day. The tests vary, so read the instructions on the package carefully to find the best time to test your urine. In most of the tests, you dip a chemically treated strip of paper into a sample of your urine and, if the paper changes color, you know that you will ovulate soon. You and your partner should have sexual intercourse at least once a day for 2 days after a positive test. Although home ovulation tests are easy and reliable, they can be expensive because you must buy a new kit each month.

Basal temperature method Charting your body temperature every day can be an inexpensive and relatively easy way to determine when you are ovulating. Using a basal body thermometer, a very precise thermometer that you can buy in most drugstores, take your temperature when you first wake up each morning before you get out of bed. (Any activity at all, including having a conversation, can change your body temperature.) Make sure you take your temperature at the same time every day. For 3 to 4 months in a row, chart your daily temperature on a sheet of graph paper (see below), using a new graph each month. Some women have a slight drop in their temperature right before or during

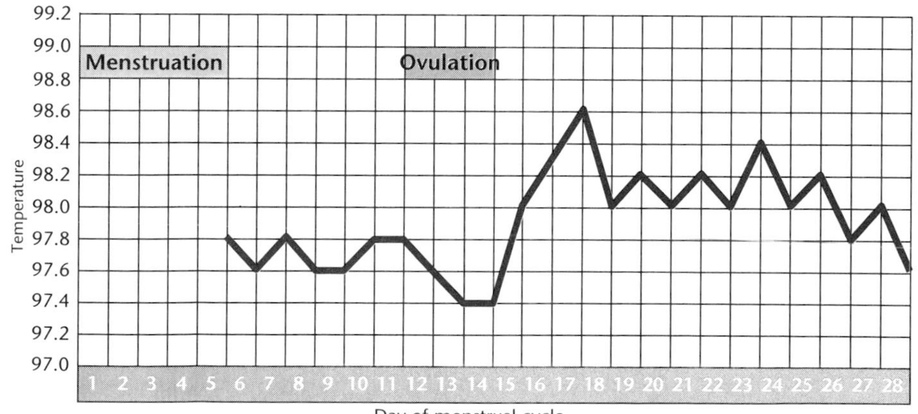

FINDING YOUR FERTILE DAYS
You can identify the days you are most likely to be fertile by charting your temperature each day and checking your normal vaginal discharge (note on the chart when it becomes clear, stretchy, and abundant). According to this chart, this woman probably ovulated around day 14 (right before a steep rise in her temperature) and noticed a change in her discharge on days 12 to 14.

How conception takes place

Reproduction is a complex process in which cells from two different people combine to form an offspring. Here are the basic steps in fertilization:

1. A developing follicle in one of a woman's ovaries releases an egg into her fallopian tube.
2. Millions of sperm ejaculated in fluid (semen) from her partner's penis during intercourse travel up through the uterus and into a fallopian tube.
3. One of the sperm penetrates the egg in a process called fertilization.
4. The fertilized egg begins dividing from one cell into many as it travels through the fallopian tube toward the uterus.
5. About 5 days after fertilization, the egg (which is now a mass of cells) implants itself in the wall of the uterus, where it will develop into a fetus and continue to grow for the next 9 months.

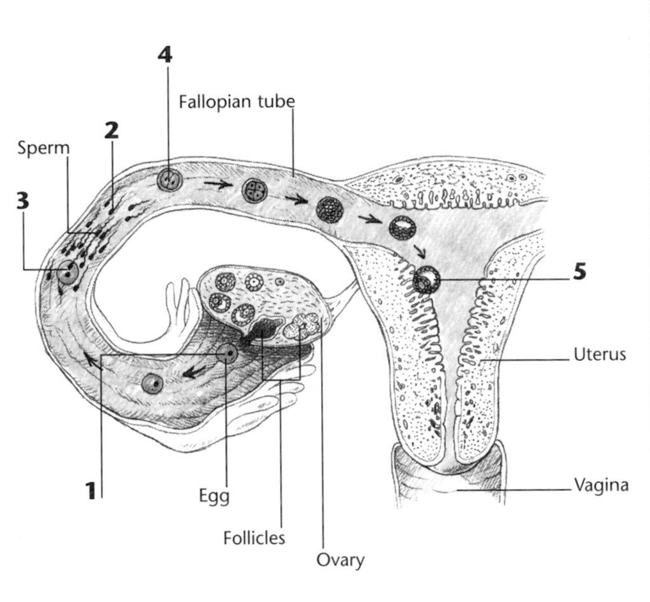

ovulation. Your temperature rises immediately after ovulation; this temperature rise indicates the end of your most fertile time. Do not wait until you see a sustained increase in temperature before having intercourse because your fertile period may already be over by then.

Once you recognize a pattern in your cycle, you can use the graph to predict the day you will ovulate. Have intercourse every day around this time of the month, starting 5 days *before* the expected temperature rise. Illness or stress may affect your body temperature, so note these on your chart.

Cervical mucus method The look and feel of the discharge from your vagina change throughout your menstrual cycle. If you monitor your vaginal discharge every day, you will notice that you have very little discharge in the days right after your period. Most women are not fertile at this time. After several days, a small amount of sticky mucus may appear that is white, cloudy, or yellow; it may be possible for some women to become pregnant at this time. However, it is not until a few days later that most women are most fertile, when a more abundant, clear, thin, slippery mucus appears, signaling ovulation. This mucus is stretchy and looks and feels like egg white. If you can stretch the mucus between your thumb and index finger into a thin strand 2 to 3 inches long, you are about to ovulate and, therefore, are fertile. A few days later, your mucus becomes sticky again and less abundant, and you are less fertile.

Understanding the variation in your mucus takes a lot of practice. This method is more effective for some women than for others because some women secrete greater amounts of cervical mucus and can recognize the differences more easily.

AM I PREGNANT?

After an egg is fertilized by a sperm, it may implant itself in the lining of the uterus. If it does implant, you are pregnant. But how do you know for sure? The sign that women most often associate with pregnancy is a missed period. But some women have irregular menstrual cycles and the length of their cycles can be affected by factors such as stress or illness. You can also miss a period for reasons other than pregnancy. So it is a good idea to be aware of other

Girl or boy?

Eggs and sperm each have 23 chromosomes that carry genes, the hereditary units that provide instructions for building and maintaining a living organism. When an egg and a sperm unite at conception, their chromosomes combine in the fertilized egg, making a total of 46. Of these 46 chromosomes, two are called sex chromosomes—one contributed by the mother and one by the father. Females have two X sex chromosomes; males have an X and a Y. Therefore, an egg from the mother can provide only an X sex chromosome; the father's sperm can provide either an X or a Y chromosome. If the sperm carries a Y chromosome, the fetus develops into a male; if the sperm carries an X chromosome, the fetus remains female.

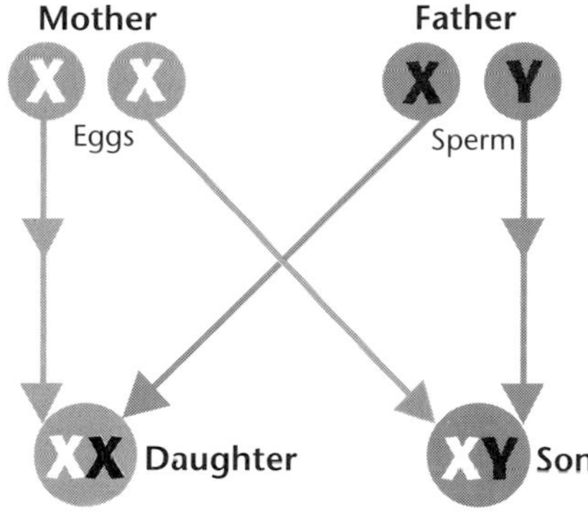

possible early signs of pregnancy such as the following:

- Nausea (morning sickness)
- Breast tenderness or swelling
- Flulike symptoms such as fatigue or loss of appetite
- Increased sensitivity to odors
- Spotting, or very light bleeding, from the vagina

Even before you miss a period, you can have a blood test in your doctor's office to see if you are pregnant. The test detects a hormone called human chorionic gonadotropin (HCG), which the fertilized egg begins secreting into your bloodstream as soon as the egg implants in your uterus. The blood test can give accurate results 11 to 12 days after conception. If you have missed a period, HCG can be detected in your urine. You can bring a urine sample to your doctor's office or test it yourself at home with a home pregnancy test that you can buy over the counter. If you follow the directions carefully, the home test is 95-percent accurate. If your home test shows you are pregnant, make an appointment with your doctor to confirm your pregnancy and begin prenatal care. If the home test is negative (shows you are not pregnant) but you continue to have signs of early pregnancy and you do not get your period at the expected time, see your doctor for a pregnancy blood test or to explore other possible causes of your symptoms.

Do not wait too long to see your doctor—the earlier in pregnancy you begin prenatal care, the better for you and the fetus. You may have an ultrasound scan (see page 405) performed to determine the date you conceived if you are unsure of when you had your last period or if you have irregular menstrual cycles. An ultrasound scan can date your pregnancy more accurately if it is done early in pregnancy. Because many prenatal tests, such as the alpha-fetoprotein test (AFP; see page 404), must be performed at a specific time during pregnancy, accurate dating of conception is extremely important.

Similarly, some treatments, such as control of diabetes, should begin as early as possible in your pregnancy. If you have a history of diabetes (see page 418), making sure your sugar levels are under control before you conceive and during the first trimester of pregnancy can decrease the risk of birth defects in your fetus. Getting enough folic acid (see page 371) before you conceive and throughout the first trimester decreases the risk of neural tube defects (spine abnormalities) and other birth defects.

Infertility

Most couples who actively try to conceive do so within 1 year. Actively trying to conceive means you are monitoring your menstrual cycle to know when you are ovulating (your most fertile time) and then having intercourse on those days (see page 379). But one out of five couples does not conceive after a year of actively trying. Doctors recommend that couples consider fertility counseling after

1 year of trying without success. In some situations, such as when a woman is over 35 or has a known ovulation problem, it may make sense to begin the evaluation after 6 months of trying to conceive.

Infertility is a problem shared by a couple. There is often more than one cause—it may be a problem in either the woman or man, or both may have borderline infertility problems that, when combined, make it difficult for them to conceive. Many infertility problems are treatable and curable; some are not. About 15 percent of the time, no clear cause is ever found. For these couples, infertility testing and treatment can be especially difficult because there is no focus for treatment and no clear explanation of their problem. However, even in cases of infertility in which the cause remains unclear, there are techniques that doctors can use to help couples bear a child.

Fertility treatment is not a guarantee of pregnancy. Because the treatment can be emotionally difficult, time-consuming, and expensive, make sure you have a clear idea of the entire process before you begin so you know what to expect. Discuss it thoroughly with your doctor and read as much as you can about the various diagnostic tests and treatment options so you and your partner can decide what procedures may be appropriate for you. Check with your health insurance provider when you are first considering infertility treatment to find out what, if any, part of the evaluation and treatment is covered.

Preventing infertility

In many cases, infertility can be prevented. Pelvic inflammatory disease (PID; see page 232), an infection of the upper reproductive tract that results from untreated sexually transmitted diseases (STDs), is the most common cause of preventable infertility in American women. Some causes of male infertility, including STDs and injury to the testicles, are also preventable. Taking the following steps can improve your and your partner's chances of being able to conceive when you decide to:

- When you are not in a stable, mutually monogamous relationship (see page 338), use a latex or polyurethane male condom or a female condom with spermicide to avoid STDs; some very common STDs, such as chlamydia and gonorrhea, can cause infertility in both men and women.
- Watch for symptoms of infection—including vaginal discharge; irritation, warts, or sores in the genital area; pain during urination; or tenderness in your pelvic area—and see a doctor immediately if any symptoms develop. Have an annual pelvic examination and Pap smear; remember that many STDs cause no symptoms.
- If possible, get pregnant before you are 35. Fertility decreases with age.
- Boys should be immunized against the childhood infection mumps long before puberty to avoid orchitis (inflammation of the testicles), a complication of mumps that can lead to infertility.
- Men should wear protective gear such as athletic supporters while playing sports, including football or soccer, in which their testicles might be injured.

INFERTILITY IN WOMEN

Infertility in women is increasing, probably for several reasons. One possible explanation for this increase is the escalation in the incidence of STDs, such as gonorrhea and chlamydia, that can lead to pelvic inflammatory disease (PID; see page 232), a common cause of infertility. In addition, more and more women are postponing childbearing until their late 30s and early 40s, when they are less fertile. In women over 35, a condition called endometriosis (see page 230) is a common cause of infertility.

Infertility can develop in several ways in women. The most common problems are blockage of the fallopian tubes or failure of an ovary to release an egg at the appropriate time (called failure to ovulate). Less frequently, infertility results from abnormalities in the lining of the uterus (endometrium) or the shape of the cavity of the uterus, or from a narrowing of the cervix.

Before recommending a treatment, a doctor must first determine the cause of infertility. He or she usually performs a series of tests to determine if your reproductive system is functioning normally. Some causes of infertility can be treated with surgery; others with medication. In some cases, a simple change in lifestyle, such as losing weight or quitting smoking, is the first treatment to try.

The doctor visit The first part of your appointment with a doctor for an evaluation of infertility will include questions about your medical, reproductive, and menstrual histories. Have you been pregnant or had any children? If so, how long did it take for you to conceive? Do you have regular periods? Have you always had regular periods? If you have been pregnant in the past and you have always had regular periods, you are probably not infertile. Your doctor also will ask if you have had any vaginal infections, STDs, or other conditions, such as fibroids (see page 221) or endometriosis (see page 230), that can interfere with fertility.

Your doctor will do a pelvic examination to evaluate the shape and position of your reproductive organs. He or she may recommend a variety of fertility tests to diagnose your specific problem.

Ovulation tests If your ovaries do not release eggs (a condition called anovulation), you cannot become pregnant. Your doctor may recommend tests or methods you can use at home—such as an ovulation predictor kit (see page 379) or monitoring your cervical mucus (see page 380)—to see if you are ovulating. If these indicators show that you are ovulating, your doctor may recommend a blood test to measure how much of the hormone progesterone your body produces after ovulation and how long the progesterone level stays elevated. Progesterone prepares the lining of the uterus (endometrium) to receive a fertilized egg; the hormone is essential for nurturing a pregnancy. The progesterone blood test is performed 5 to 10 days before your next period is due. An endometrial biopsy (see page 129) can be performed just before your period to determine if you have ovulated and if your endometrium has responded sufficiently to the effects of progesterone.

Tests for cervical mucus Around the time of ovulation, mucus secreted from the cervix is normally clear, slippery, watery, abundant, and stretchy. These qualities help sperm pass through the cervix and into the uterus. A test called a postcoital test performed in your doctor's office 2 to 12 hours after you and your partner have had sexual intercourse can determine if your cervical mucus is of the right consistency and can confirm that your partner's sperm are present in your mucus and are active. In a procedure similar to a Pap smear, the doctor takes a sample of mucus with sperm from your vagina and examines it under a microscope to determine the number of sperm and evaluate their activity.

If your doctor sees signs that your immune system is producing antibodies in your cervical mucus that are blocking the sperm, he or she may recommend that you and your partner have blood tests to detect these antibodies. Because this type of response is very rare, an antibody test is one of the last to be performed to evaluate infertility.

Tests of the uterus and fallopian tubes Abnormalities of the uterus—such as fibroids (noncancerous tumors in or on the uterus), polyps (small, projecting growths), an abnormally shaped uterus, or scar tissue resulting from previous infections—can prevent a fertilized egg from implanting in the wall of the uterus. Your doctor can use a number of methods to diagnose and, in some cases, treat infertility that results from an abnormality in the uterus or fallopian tubes.

Ultrasound Ultrasound (see page 405), an imaging method that produces pictures using sound waves, can detect abnormalities in your internal pelvic organs. Ultrasound can reveal the size and shape of your uterus and ovaries, as well as the thickness of the endometrium (the lining of the uterus). If you are trying assisted reproductive technology (see page 392), you may have an ultrasound to monitor the growth of egg follicles in your ovaries to determine the best time for the doctor to retrieve eggs for the procedure.

Hysterosalpingography Your doctor can also look for abnormalities in your uterus or fallopian tubes using an X-ray imaging procedure called hysterosalpingography (HSG), which is performed in a radiologist's office or the X-ray department of a hospital. For HSG, a small amount of dye is injected through a tube that has been inserted through your vagina into your cervix. The dye flows

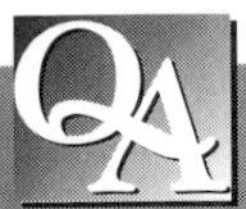

Questions Women Ask
Infertility

Q I'm 38 years old and married for the second time. My husband and I have been trying to have a child for almost a year and I am still not pregnant. I had been putting off having children until my career was established. In all my years of being sexually active, I have never had an accidental pregnancy. What could be our problem?

A There are several possible explanations for your situation. The most likely reason you never had an unplanned pregnancy is that you were using reliable contraception correctly and consistently. You and your husband simply may not have had intercourse during the times you were most fertile (see page 379) over the last year. Because of your age, you also may wish to have an evaluation by a doctor. You may have a condition called endometriosis (see page 230), which is a common cause of infertility in women over 35. Endometriosis can be treated. Your husband's semen also should be analyzed to make sure his sperm are healthy.

Q I have become a running fanatic over the last few years. I just don't feel right unless I run at least 50 miles a week. Although my body weight is normal, my periods have gradually decreased from every 4 weeks to every 7 weeks. Can this affect my chances of becoming pregnant?

A The change in your menstrual cycle is a sign that you are not ovulating regularly. Although you may not feel that you are exercising excessively, your longer menstrual cycles may indicate that this amount of exercise is straining your system. Another reason you are not ovulating regularly may be that your percentage of body fat is so low that you are not producing an adequate amount of estrogen (fat cells produce estrogen). Talk to your doctor about having tests to determine if you are ovulating (see page 383). You may need to cut back on your running and exercise at a more moderate level, or you may need to take medication to induce ovulation (see page 386).

Q A doctor once told me that I have a "tipped" uterus. Could that affect my ability to get pregnant?

A A tipped uterus is a common and normal variation and does not affect a woman's chances of conceiving. Your uterus is tilted backward, toward the base of your spine, rather than forward, toward your bladder.

into your uterus and out your fallopian tubes, if they are open. The image shows the interior of the uterus and the dye outlines anything that is taking up space inside the uterus, such as a fibroid (see page 221). The image can also highlight narrowed areas or blockages in the fallopian tubes.

Hysteroscopy Your doctor can directly view the interior of your uterus using a procedure called hysteroscopy (see page 264), which can be performed with either local or general anesthesia (see page 261). Using a magnified viewing tube (hysteroscope) inserted through your vagina and cervix into your uterus, the doctor can see the inside of your uterus and look for any abnormal tissue, such as fibroids, polyps, or scar tissue. In many cases, if there is abnormal tissue, it can be cut out and removed using tiny scissors inserted through the hysteroscope. The doctor can also examine the fallopian tubes at the point where they open into the uterus. If the tubes are found to be blocked, they can sometimes be opened using surgical instruments inserted through the hysteroscope.

Laparoscopy The doctor can directly examine the exterior of your uterus, fallopian tubes, and ovaries in a procedure called laparoscopy (see page 263) in which a long, narrow, viewing tube (laparoscope) is inserted through a tiny incision in your abdomen. Laparoscopy, which is usually performed using general anesthesia, is used to diagnose a number of gynecologic problems, including endometriosis (abnormal growth of tissue on organs in the pelvic area), and to detect the presence of scar tissue resulting from other causes, such as pelvic inflammatory disease (PID; see page 232). The laparoscope also enables the doctor to find ovarian cysts, fibroids, abnormally shaped organs, or other abnormalities that may be affecting your fertility. For example, to determine whether your fallopian tubes are open, the doctor injects a liquid dye through a tube inserted into your vagina and cervix and watches (through the laparoscope) to see if the dye flows out the ends of the tubes.

Treating endometriosis If endometriosis is suspected to be the cause of a woman's infertility, surgery is often performed through a laparoscope to burn or remove as much of the abnormal tissue as possible (see page 231). After the surgery, you may be given medication (to take by mouth, injection, or nasal spray) to shrink any remaining abnormal tissue and suppress the growth of more. The success of this procedure depends on the extent of the condition. If a pregnancy is going to occur, it usually does so within a year. After this time, some couples choose to improve their chances of conceiving by using an assisted reproductive technology method such as in vitro fertilization (see page 393).

Treating fibroids Fibroids (noncancerous tumors in or on the uterus) can sometimes interfere with a woman's fertility. When fibroids are very large or numerous, hysterectomy (surgical removal of the uterus; see page 256) is usually recommended, ending a woman's ability to conceive. In some cases, it is possible to remove only the fibroids, leaving the uterus intact and preserving the woman's ability to have a child. For more about this procedure, called myomectomy, see page 222.

Treating a blocked fallopian tube Surgery can sometimes be performed to open a fallopian tube that is blocked by scar tissue. This tissue usually has formed from infection, including pelvic inflammatory disease (PID; see page 232). In some cases, fallopian tubes that have been closed by surgical sterilization (tubal ligation, see page 327) can be surgically reopened. Your ability to become pregnant after having surgery on a fallopian tube depends on many factors, including the length of the remaining tube and your age. The procedure a doctor uses to reopen a blocked fallopian tube is determined by the location and extent of the blockage.

Tubal cannulation Tubal cannulation is a procedure in which a thin, flexible tube (cannula) is inserted into a blocked fallopian tube to open it. Tubal cannulation is used to open a fallopian tube that is blocked near its opening into the uterus. The procedure may be performed using laparoscopy (see page 263) or hysteroscopy (see illustration). When performed using hysteroscopy, a hollow, flexible tube called a hysteroscope is inserted through the vagina into the uterus. A balloon-tipped tube or wire is then manipulated through the hysteroscope and into the

Ovary
Fallopian tube
Uterus
Cervix
Vagina
Cannula
Hysteroscope

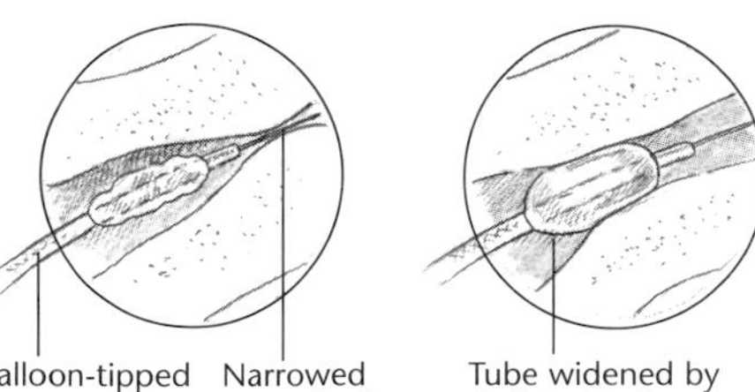

TUBAL CANNULATION: OPENING A BLOCKED FALLOPIAN TUBE

To open a blocked fallopian tube using a procedure called tubal cannulation, a thin, balloon-tipped tube (cannula) is guided through a hollow, flexible tube (hysteroscope) inserted through your vagina into your uterus and up to the site of scarring or narrowing inside the blocked tube. The balloon is then inflated to open up the tube. When the fallopian tube is opened, the balloon is deflated and withdrawn through the vagina.

narrowed fallopian tube to open the tube and allow passage of eggs in the future.

Tubal reanastomosis Tubal reanastomosis is the surgical rejoining of two parts of a fallopian tube, which is performed after a blockage has been removed or to reverse a tubal ligation (see page 327). Before you have this procedure, your doctor will make sure that you are ovulating and that your partner's semen is healthy, and rule out any other problems that could prevent fertilization. This procedure is performed in the hospital using general anesthesia (see page 261) and may take several hours. Through an incision in your abdomen, the blocked area of the fallopian tube is cut out and the severed ends are tested to make sure they are open. These ends are then stitched together using very delicate instruments that decrease the risk of scarring. Before having the procedure, ask your doctor about his or her experience and success rate (the percentage of women who have had pregnancies after having the surgery). You may want to ask several medical centers their record of success.

Surgery for an abnormally shaped uterus Some women are born with an abnormally shaped uterus. In some cases, a uterus with an unusual shape, such as a double uterus, may not be able to support the full growth of a fetus or carry a pregnancy to term. Surgery can sometimes be performed to create a uterus of sufficient size and shape to support a pregnancy. This type of surgery is usually performed only when other causes of infertility have been ruled out.

Drugs to induce ovulation If you are having difficulty conceiving because you ovulate irregularly or not at all, your doctor may recommend medication—often called fertility drugs—to make you ovulate more frequently. These medications usually do not improve fertility in women who ovulate regularly. The doctor will evaluate your ovulation problem, primarily with blood tests, before selecting the appropriate drug and dosage to induce ovulation. While you are taking any of these medications, you may have periodic blood tests and monitoring procedures to make sure the drugs are safe and effective for you. During treatment, you should keep a calendar documenting your menstrual periods, days of ovulation, and days you have intercourse.

Ovulation-inducing drugs may also be used to precisely control the time of ovulation in a woman who is undergoing artificial insemination (see page 392) or other assisted reproductive technology.

Causes of infertility in women

Infertility can result from a number of factors, including sexually transmitted diseases (STDs) and medical conditions such as diabetes. The following are among the most common causes of infertility in women:

- Lack of ovulation—failure to release an egg from an ovary—can result from a number of factors, including obesity, extreme underweight, or excessive exercise.
- Infections caused by STDs or other conditions such as appendicitis can lead to scarring of organs in the pelvis. Scarring in a fallopian tube can block the passage of an egg.
- Endometriosis can cause scarring and the formation of abnormal scar tissue (adhesions), which may block the fallopian tubes. Endometriosis can also cause scar tissue to form on the ovaries, which can prevent an egg from reaching the fallopian tube.
- Surgery performed in the pelvic area can cause the formation of abnormal scar tissue (adhesions). Adhesions can block or bind together tissues in the pelvic area, preventing sperm and egg from coming together in the fallopian tube or blocking the passage of a fertilized egg into the uterus.
- Scarring, tumors such as fibroids (see page 221), or other abnormalities inside the uterus can prevent a fertilized egg from implanting in the wall of the uterus.
- Cervical mucus that is too scanty or too thick can prevent sperm from entering the uterus.
- Medical conditions that alter metabolism, such as hypothyroidism (see page 624) or diabetes (see page 617), can affect the frequency of ovulation and the production of certain hormones at ovulation. These hormones prepare the lining of the uterus to receive a fertilized egg and are necessary for nurturing a pregnancy.

These drugs are sometimes used to produce more than one egg during a woman's cycle to increase the chances for successful fertilization when using assisted reproductive technology, but they also can increase the likelihood of a multiple birth such as twins.

Clomiphene citrate Clomiphene citrate is a drug used to stimulate ovulation in some women who have infrequent periods and long menstrual cycles. You take the medication once a day, usually for 5 days in a row beginning on the fifth day of your cycle, counting the first day of your period as day 1. Clomiphene citrate works by preventing estrogen from binding to receptor sites in the brain, fooling the hypothalamus in the brain into thinking that estrogen levels are lower than they really are. In response, the hypothalamus signals the pituitary gland to secrete more follicle-stimulating hormone (FSH) and luteinizing hormone (LH) into the bloodstream, which encourages the growth of an egg-containing follicle in the ovary and the release of an egg.

If the drug is successful, ovulation will usually occur about a week after you take the last pill. If you do not ovulate, the dose of the drug may have to be increased during your next cycle. Because most women for whom treatment with clomiphene citrate is effective become pregnant within the first four to six cycles of therapy, it is recommended that the drug be used no longer than six cycles. Side effects of clomiphene citrate may

One Woman's Story
Infertility Treatment

I always knew I wanted children, but, when my husband and I got married in our early 30s, we decided to give ourselves a couple of years together before having a child. When we did decide to conceive, I was 35. Nothing happened after a year of trying, so we started to get worried and decided to go in for fertility testing. It turned out to be a long and difficult process. It was strange to think that one of us might be infertile, and I think we each hoped it was the other.

One of the first things the doctors wanted to do was analyze Mike's semen. That meant Mike had to produce a sample of semen by masturbating into a jar in a little room at the infertility clinic. I know he was embarrassed and anxious about it but he went along with it. He was relieved when it turned out his sperm count was normal.

I had to have all kinds of tests. They checked my hormone levels with blood tests and asked me to test my urine at home to find out if and when I was ovulating. But the color change on the home tests was sometimes hard for me to detect. It was confusing. We had to have intercourse and then go to the clinic right away so they could take a sample of my cervical mucus with Mike's sperm in it to see if his sperm were moving in my mucus. The doctor told me that the consistency of a woman's mucus can prevent sperm from entering her uterus.

Finally, the doctors determined that my irregular periods were a sign of infrequent ovulation. When they told me that the best chance for getting pregnant at that point meant taking a drug to make me ovulate, I was worried about having a multiple birth. The doctors reassured me that the drug clomiphene citrate has a much lower rate of multiple births than other ovulation drugs. I decided to do it and took clomiphene for 5 days every menstrual cycle to induce ovulation. I took it for 5 months and was nervous about it the entire time. Mike began to say maybe we should forget the whole thing and get on with our lives.

I felt my life was on hold. I couldn't plan for anything—my career, buying a house, even our relationship—until I knew if we were going to have children. Finally it happened, just when we were considering quitting the treatment. I'm now 39 and we feel very lucky to have a wonderful 2-year-old boy. Although the whole experience was difficult emotionally and at times I wondered whether we should be going through it all, we are grateful that we were able to get the kind of help we needed to have a family.

"It was strange to think that one of us might be infertile, and I think we each hoped it was the other."

SYMPTOM CHART

Failure to conceive

Failure to get pregnant after more than 12 months of trying without contraception.

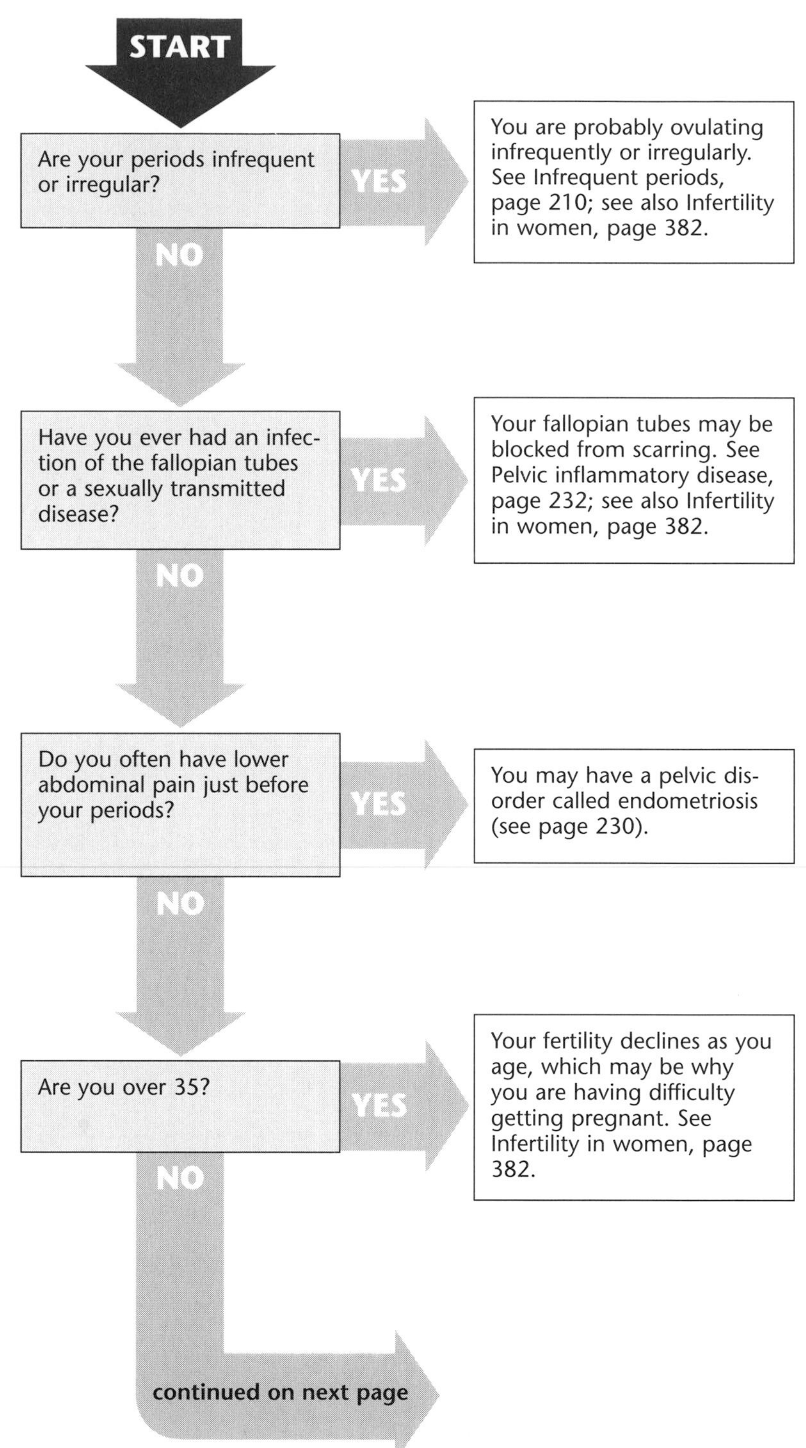

Evaluating infertility

If you are having difficulty conceiving, it is important to talk to your doctor. Infertility can result from some gynecologic conditions that are easier to treat when they are detected early.

continued from previous page

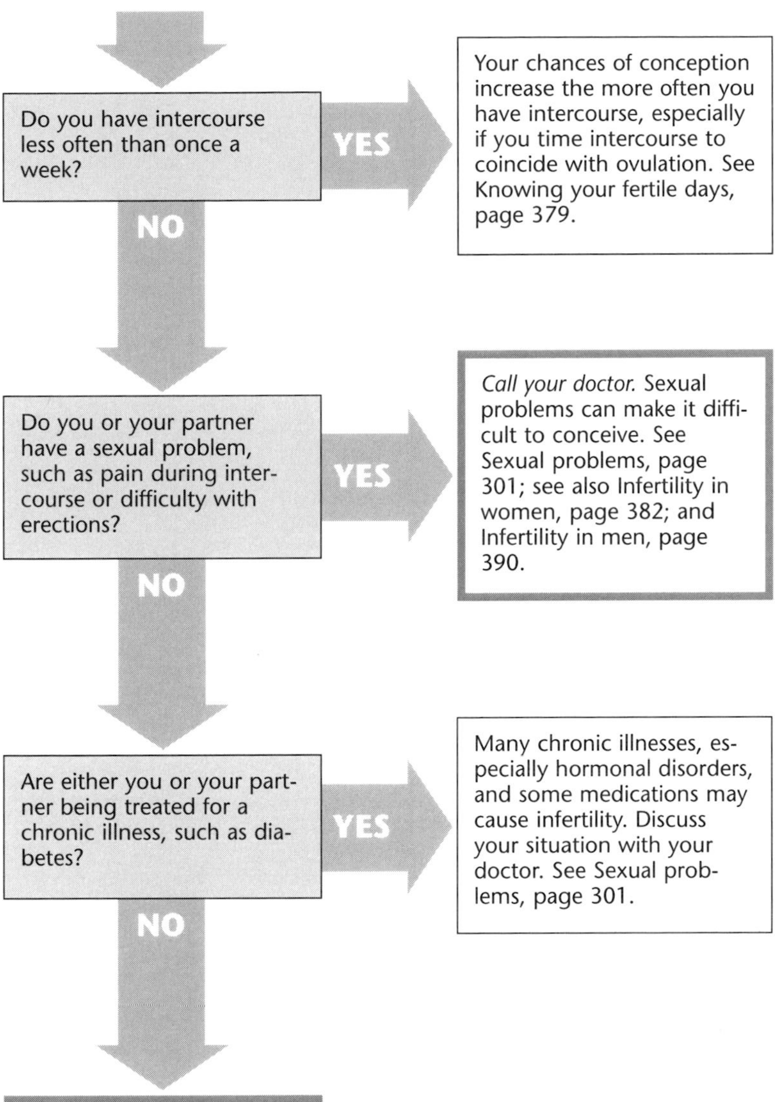

Causes of infertility in women

- Lack of ovulation
- Scarring of fallopian tubes from infection
- Endometriosis
- Scarring or fibroids inside the uterus
- Scarring in pelvic area resulting from surgery
- Cervical mucus that is too thick or too scanty
- A medical condition that affects hormone levels

include hot flashes, headaches, nausea, mood swings, or breast tenderness. Although the evidence is not yet clear, the drug may slightly increase a woman's risk of ovarian cancer if it is taken for more than a year.

Human menopausal gonadotropin The most potent fertility drug, called human menopausal gonadotropin, may contain both follicle-stimulating hormone (FSH) and luteinizing hormone (LH), or FSH alone. This drug is prescribed for women who are not ovulating and have not responded to treatment with clomiphene citrate. You take human menopausal gonadotropin in injections once a day for several days in a row. The drug is also used to stimulate the growth of multiple egg-containing follicles when a woman is undergoing an assisted reproductive technology (see page 392). As more follicles develop, there are potentially more eggs to remove for artificial fertilization. Not all of the removed eggs are successfully fertilized, so removing more eggs than you need increases the likelihood of successfully fertilizing at least one or two. Multiple pregnancies occur in 10 to 20 percent of the women using this drug; of these pregnancies, most are twins. Triplets and multiple births of a higher number are rare.

Side effects of human menopausal gonadotropin include breast tenderness, swelling or rash at the site of injection, bloating, mood swings, and abdominal pain. The most serious side effect of the drug is hyperstimulation syndrome, a condition in which multiple follicle cysts develop in the ovaries, causing swelling and pain. This condition may require hospitalization. In rare cases, these cysts rupture and may require surgery.

Bromocriptine Bromocriptine is a medication prescribed for women who ovulate irregularly because their pituitary gland, located in the brain, secretes too much prolactin, the hormone that stimulates milk production for breast-feeding. If your prolactin levels are high, you are likely to have X-rays taken of your head to see if you have a tumor in your pituitary gland (prolactinoma, see page 628). Bromocriptine reduces the amount of prolactin released by the pituitary and can sometimes shrink any small prolactinomas that are present. You usually take this medication one to three times a day until your prolactin level is normal. Most women treated with this drug become pregnant if they do not have any other fertility problem. Taking this drug does not increase the likelihood of multiple births. Possible side effects of bromocriptine include nasal stuffiness, headaches, nausea, and dizziness.

INFERTILITY IN MEN

About 40 percent of the time, a couple's inability to conceive results from a problem in the male partner. Most of these problems are related to the inability of sperm to fertilize an egg. For example, a man may not be producing enough sperm, his sperm may not be active enough to reach an egg and fertilize it, or a vas deferens (one of the tubes that carry sperm from the testicles to the urethra) may be blocked from scarring or infection. When a couple seeks fertility treatment, a semen analysis is one of the first tests performed. Evaluating the male partner also includes a health history, physical examination, and laboratory tests.

The doctor visit If your partner's semen analysis shows abnormalities, the doctor usually refers him to a urologist, a doctor who specializes in treating disorders of the male reproductive system. At your partner's first appointment with the urologist, he will be asked about his reproductive history, such as whether or not he has fathered any children, and about his health history. The doctor will give your partner a physical examination to look for evidence of past or present infections or other conditions that can affect sperm production.

Semen analysis Because most male fertility problems involve the production of sperm, a semen analysis is the first test. Before the test, the man is asked to refrain from ejaculating for 2 to 3 days and then produce a sample of semen by ejaculating into a container. Some men find it difficult or embarrassing to produce "sperm on demand" in a doctor's office. If so, a man may be able to produce the sample at home as long as he can bring it to the clinic within an hour. To keep the sperm alive, he must maintain the semen

Causes of infertility in men

Most of the advances in the diagnosis and treatment of infertility have been developed to treat infertility in women. However, many conception problems result from abnormalities in the male partner's sperm. Infertility in men can result from a number of causes.

- Some sexually transmitted diseases, including chlamydia and gonorrhea, can cause scarring that may block a vas deferens, one of the tubes that carry sperm from the testicles to the urethra.
- Some infections (such as mumps), if they occur after puberty, can cause inflammation of the testicles, where sperm are produced. In some cases, infection destroys sperm-producing tissues.
- Some types of surgery performed on the male reproductive tract can harm various tissues, which can result in the formation of scar tissue, blockages, or nerve damage. For example, surgery to repair a hernia (an abnormal opening in supporting tissues in the groin) may result in injury to a vas deferens. Surgery to remove the prostate gland may damage the surrounding nerves and disrupt the passage of semen through the ducts. Vasectomy (surgical sterilization; see page 328) or surgery performed to reverse a vasectomy may also injure a vas deferens.
- Varicose veins in the testicles, called varicoceles, can affect sperm production and movement.
- Some prescription medications that are used to treat depression or high blood pressure can cause impotence.
- Exposure of the testicles to high temperatures—which can result from wearing tight clothing, using hot tubs, or some workplace conditions—can reduce sperm count.
- Use of drugs such as tobacco, marijuana, cocaine, or alcohol can temporarily reduce sperm count and increase the number of abnormally formed sperm.
- Some medical conditions such as diabetes can cause impotence.
- Injury to the testicles can produce scar tissue that blocks the passage of sperm.

near body temperature by placing it inside the waistband of his clothing until he gives it to the doctor. The doctor analyzes the semen for:

- Sperm count—the number of sperm per milliliter of semen. Normal semen contains a minimum of 20 million sperm per milliliter of semen.
- Sperm motility—determining whether enough of the sperm are sufficiently active to swim up into the uterus and fallopian tubes to fertilize an egg. Sperm motility is considered normal if at least half of the sperm are moving vigorously.
- Sperm morphology—determining whether enough sperm are of normal shape. All men have some sperm that are shaped abnormally and cannot fertilize an egg. A man's fertility is considered normal if at least half of his sperm are of normal shape.

Other sperm tests In some cases, more sophisticated tests are required to find the cause of a man's infertility. One test, performed from 2 to 12 hours after a couple has intercourse during the most fertile day in the woman's cycle, determines if her partner's sperm are able to live and move about in the mucus secreted by her cervix. In this test, the doctor takes a sample of cervical mucus during a pelvic examination similar to a Pap smear and sends it to the laboratory for examination under a microscope. A sperm antibody test determines if a man's immune system produces substances (antibodies) that make his sperm clump together or become immobile or incapable of fertilizing an egg. A test called a sperm penetration assay can determine whether sperm are capable of attaching to and penetrating an egg.

Treatment Treatment of male infertility depends on the cause. Varicose veins in a testicle, called varicoceles, may be treated with surgery to tie off the affected veins. This procedure often improves the results of a semen analysis, especially the percentage of sperm that are of normal shape. Low sperm count or insufficient sperm motility (movement) occasionally can be improved by treatment with hormones or other medications taken for several months. If infertility is the result of an active bacterial infection, such as gonorrhea or chlamydia, it is treated with antibiotics. Surgery can often correct a blockage in the ducts that carry sperm from the testicles to the penis.

ASSISTED REPRODUCTIVE TECHNOLOGY

If traditional fertility treatments with drugs or surgery have not helped you and your partner conceive, you may want to explore other fertilization techniques that are referred to collectively as assisted reproductive technology. While this technology has helped many couples conceive, the rate of successful pregnancies is only about 10 to 30 percent per attempt. Some of these procedures, which are very expensive, are not covered by many health insurance plans and you must undergo numerous tests. Your partner may have to produce sperm on demand many times. You will have to take ovulation drugs, which sometimes have side effects.

Nevertheless, some couples so strongly want to conceive that they are willing to pursue every option. Other couples choose adoption. Still others decide that their lives are fulfilling and happy without children. Learning about the different types of assisted reproductive technology can help you and your partner make a decision that is right for you.

Intrauterine insemination For intrauterine insemination, sperm (from a partner or donor) is placed inside a woman's uterus around the time she ovulates. The sperm is inserted through a slim tube into the woman's vagina, through the cervix, and into her uterus. The goal is to make it easier for the sperm to reach the fallopian tube and fertilize the egg as the egg travels from the ovary through the fallopian tube. Intrauterine insemination is used when a couple has a problem with cervical mucus or when the cause of their infertility is not known. The procedure may also be used if the male partner is physically disabled and unable to achieve intercourse. The woman must have at least one functioning fallopian tube and she must be able to ovulate. Sometimes, drugs such as clomiphene citrate (see page 387) are used to induce the release of extra eggs from an ovary. Ultrasound imaging (see page 405) may also be used to determine if and when a woman will be ovulating in order to know when to perform the insemination procedure.

Going through intrauterine insemination can be emotionally and physically stressful. The man may have to produce semen in the doctor's office on short notice. The woman must be tested frequently for the time of ovulation, and often she must take ovulation-inducing drugs, which can cause unpleasant side effects. The procedure may have to be repeated several times before fertilization is successful.

If the male partner cannot produce enough normal sperm, the couple may choose to have the woman's egg fertilized with donor sperm from a sperm bank. Single women who choose to become pregnant without a male partner may use intrauterine insemination with donor sperm. Fertilization techniques using donor sperm can raise some emotional issues (see page 395). Donor insemination also raises legal questions about paternity, so you should talk to an attorney before undergoing this procedure. However, the procedure is extremely safe when it is performed at a reliable

Could you benefit from artificial fertilization?

Before recommending any type of assisted reproductive technology, a doctor will evaluate your infertility problem to find the cause and determine whether or not you are likely to benefit from such treatment. Assisted reproductive technologies are not recommended for everyone. They may be appropriate for you if you have one of the following fertility problems:

- A blockage in a fallopian tube that cannot be corrected with surgery
- Endometriosis that does not respond to surgery or medication
- Cervical mucus problems that have not been circumvented using intrauterine insemination
- Infertility that is traced to sperm antibodies (see page 391)
- Some kinds of male fertility problems such as low sperm count or poor sperm motility (see page 391)
- Long-standing, unexplained infertility

infertility center by a doctor who is board certified in the subspecialty of reproductive endocrinology and has experience with the procedure. Sperm donors are carefully tested for medical problems and sexually transmitted diseases. All donors are registered by age, race, hair and eye color, and body build so that a couple can choose a donor who has a genetic background that is similar to theirs.

In vitro fertilization In vitro fertilization means that a woman's egg is fertilized outside her body. To have this procedure, the woman usually takes ovulation drugs (see page 386) to stimulate the development of multiple eggs. Just before she ovulates, these eggs are removed from her ovary, usually by withdrawing them through a needle inserted through her vaginal wall (see illustration below). The collected eggs are fertilized in a plastic dish with sperm from her partner or with donor sperm. One to four of the fertilized eggs are then placed in the woman's uterus, using a thin plastic tube inserted through her vagina. Fertilized eggs that are not used may be frozen and stored for possible use later. The rate of successful pregnancies from in vitro fertilization ranges from 10 to 30 percent; ask the staff at your fertility clinic what their success rate is.

Gamete intrafallopian transfer Gamete intrafallopian transfer (GIFT) is the transfer of a gamete (egg or sperm) into a fallopian tube. The most important difference between GIFT and in vitro fertilization is that, with GIFT, fertilization takes place inside the woman's fallopian tube instead of outside her body. The woman must have at least one healthy fallopian tube. After the eggs are removed from her ovaries through her vagina using needle aspiration (see illustration below), the eggs and sperm (from her partner or a donor) are placed together in her fallopian tube, where fertilization can occur. Placement of the eggs in the fallopian tube is usually done through a small incision in the abdomen (see page 394).

Zygote intrafallopian transfer and tubal embryo transfer Zygote intrafallopian transfer (ZIFT) and tubal embryo transfer (TET) are similar to GIFT except that, in these procedures, eggs that are already fertilized (zygotes) are placed in the fallopian tube instead of separate eggs and sperm (gametes). Eggs are removed from the woman's ovary, fertilized in the laboratory with her partner's sperm or with donor sperm, and placed in an incubator for 1 or 2 days. The doctor inserts up to four of the fertilized eggs into the woman's

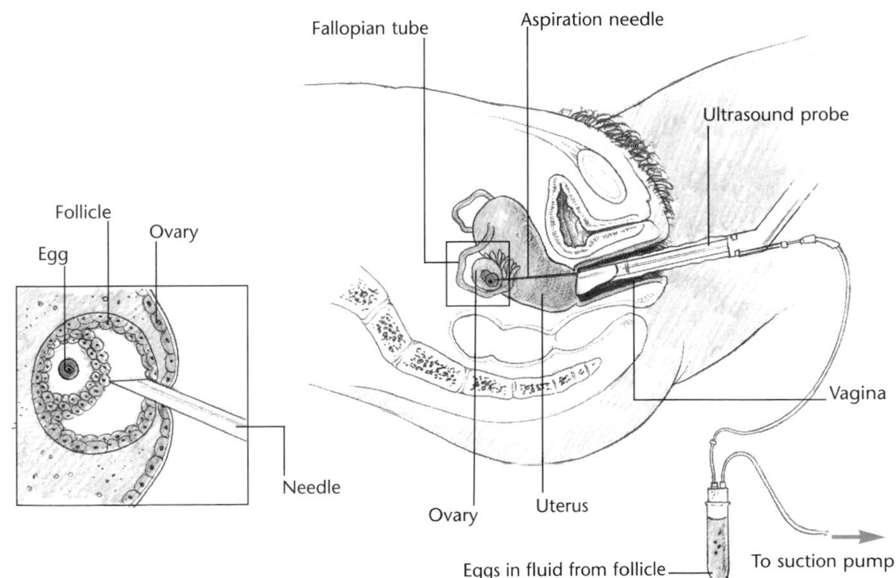

VAGINAL EGG RETRIEVAL

To remove eggs from a woman's ovary for artificial insemination, the doctor inserts a hollow needle into her vagina, through the vaginal wall and along the outer wall of the uterus to the ovary. An ultrasound probe is also inserted into the vagina to produce an image that guides the doctor. Several eggs, along with fluid from the follicles, are extracted through the needle using gentle suction.

fallopian tube through a laparoscope. ZIFT and TET procedures are used in cases in which there is a problem with the partner's sperm, the woman's cervical mucus is not of the right consistency to help sperm enter her uterus, or the cause of a couple's infertility is unknown.

Frozen embryo transfer Of the embryos produced during in vitro fertilization, some can be frozen and saved in case the procedure, such as ZIFT or TET, is unsuccessful and the couple wants to try again at a later time. The frozen embryos can be transferred into the woman during another menstrual cycle. Some doctors recommend that the woman take the hormones estrogen and progesterone before the procedure to prepare her uterus to receive a fertilized egg.

Fertilization using a donated egg The use of an egg donated by another woman is possible for women who want to have children but are unable to produce viable eggs because of their advanced age or because their ovaries have stopped functioning prematurely or have been damaged by radiation therapy or chemotherapy for cancer. Eggs from another woman are fertilized by the partner's sperm and transferred to the infertile woman's uterus or fallopian tube. In some cases, a woman's sister or another close relative or friend provides the eggs. Eggs from anonymous donors are sometimes available through the fertility clinic or hospital in which the woman is undergoing infertility treatment.

A woman who is an egg donor must undergo the same testing, use of ovulation drugs to increase the number of eggs she produces, and extraction of her eggs by needle aspiration that all women do who are having in vitro fertilization. Both the infertile woman and the woman donating the egg have to sign legal agreements, so they should each discuss the situation thoroughly with a lawyer.

Surrogate motherhood Some women are unable to carry a fetus to term because they have had a hysterectomy (surgical removal of the uterus) or repeated miscarriages, or because they were born without a uterus (but have functioning ovaries). A surrogate mother is a woman who makes a legal agreement with an infertile couple to have an egg from the infertile woman, which has been fertilized by her partner's sperm, implanted into her uterus. She then carries the pregnancy to term. This approach is very controversial and is illegal in some states. If you are considering it, discuss all the ramifications thoroughly with your doctor and a lawyer.

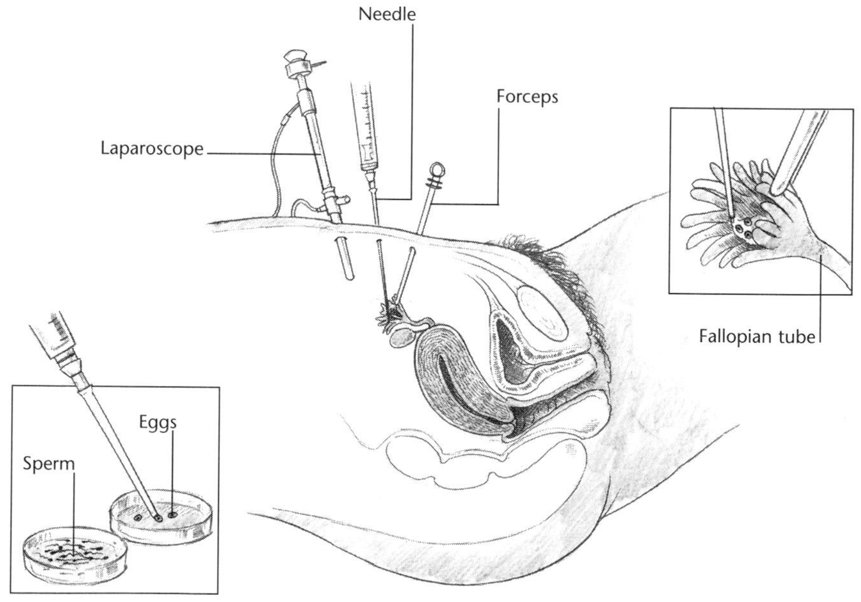

GAMETE INTRAFALLOPIAN TRANSFER

In gamete intrafallopian transfer (GIFT), eggs and sperm that have been removed from the partners are placed together inside one of the woman's fallopian tubes, with the intent that fertilization will occur there. Using a lighted viewing instrument called a laparoscope inserted through a small incision in the woman's abdomen, the doctor views the pelvic organs. Forceps are used to hold the fallopian tube in place during the procedure, and the doctor inserts a hollow needle through the laparoscope and injects the eggs and sperm into the fallopian tube.

Is donor insemination for you?

Choosing to use donor sperm from a sperm bank raises a number of questions. There are no right answers to these questions—you and your partner have to evaluate your feelings before making a choice. Joining a support group for infertile couples who are considering these same questions or seeking counseling may help you decide whether or not donor insemination is right for you.

- Have you and your partner come to terms with the feelings of loss about not being able to have your own biological child?
- Does your partner feel obligated to agree to the procedure to please you?
- Do you fear that your partner will not be able to feel close to a child who is not his biological offspring?
- Will there be an imbalance of power in the family because the child will be biologically related to you but not your partner?
- Will you tell friends and family? Or will you choose to retain your privacy and let people assume the child is biologically yours and your partner's?
- Will you tell your child?
- If you are a single woman or a lesbian couple, will you have emotional support from family and friends during the pregnancy and after the birth of your child?

ADOPTION

If you are having difficulty conceiving, you may want to consider adoption. It is a good idea to explore this option while you are undergoing testing and treatment for infertility because about 30 to 50 percent of couples who undergo such treatment never conceive. Many adoption agencies do not accept couples over a certain age, so begin the application process as early as possible.

Closed adoptions, in which the birth parents and adoptive parents are unknown to each other, were once the norm. In a closed adoption, adoptive parents receive little information about the child's origins and the adoption agency makes every effort to keep the records closed to all parties involved, including the child.

Open adoption, which has become more common, allows some exchange of information and contact between birth parents and adoptive parents. Some agencies allow the birth mother to choose the adoptive parents. The adoption process may even involve a face-to-face meeting between the adoptive parents and birth mother. Adoptive parents can learn about their child's background, and the birth mother gains the security of knowing about her child's new family.

To begin the adoption process, most couples apply to an agency. On the application, you will be asked to state your preference about the child's age, sex, race, or national heritage, and the degree of openness you want in the adoption proceedings. A representative from the agency will come to your home to determine your suitability as parents. If you are approved, the agency will at some point identify a child who is available to you for adoption. You must then decide whether to accept the child. Once you accept the child, there will be a supervisory period during which the child lives with you. After this period has expired (the length of time varies with the laws in each state), you can legally adopt the child.

Private adoption is an alternative in which couples independently seek out a woman who is pregnant and considering giving her baby up for adoption when it is born. Seek the advice of a lawyer before pursuing a private adoption.

Fees vary widely, but any type of adoption can be expensive. Ask an agency for a fee schedule well in advance. In private adoption, the cost can be even higher because you must pay a lawyer as well as hospital costs and doctors' fees for the birth mother and baby. There may also be travel expenses and other costs, depending on your arrangement with the birth mother. For a list of adoption agencies in your area, contact the department in your state government that is responsible for licensing adoption agencies. You also may be able to find a support group of adoptive parents in your area who can share information with you. Some people choose to adopt a child from another country. If you are interested in this option, discuss it with a lawyer.

CHAPTER 15

Pregnancy

Contents

Pregnancy can be a wondrous time in your life. You may find it fascinating to understand how your body is changing and follow the development of your fetus through each stage of growth. Being aware of these astonishing changes as they occur can help make your pregnancy a more rewarding and comfortable experience. You should take especially good care of yourself throughout your pregnancy—avoiding hazards to yourself and the fetus and managing any complications—to help ensure that your pregnancy is a healthy one.

Choosing your doctor

Even if you are a healthy woman experiencing an uncomplicated pregnancy, you need to have medical care to monitor your own health and that of your developing fetus. There are many things to consider before choosing the doctor who will care for you during your pregnancy and delivery. Begin by checking your health insurance plan to see what options are available to you. With many plans, you must choose from a selected list of doctors or midwives. Health maintenance organizations (HMOs) offer a limited choice of doctors and hospitals, but they usually cover all aspects of pregnancy and childbirth.

Many doctors or health plans coordinate a group of health care professionals who provide various types of care to pregnant women. Such a group might include one or more obstetricians, a nurse-midwife, a nurse practitioner, and childbirth educators who provide or direct you to classes on conception, pregnancy, nutrition, and childbirth.

Even after you have carefully chosen your doctor, another member of the group may actually deliver your baby. Because women go into labor and give birth at all times of the day and night, doctors and nurse-midwives work on a rotating schedule to make sure someone is always available. If your doctor is part of a group practice, you should schedule appointments with several members of the group during your series of prenatal appointments. This way you are more likely to know the person who delivers

Questions to ask a doctor

Before you get pregnant, find a doctor in whom you have confidence to help you through pregnancy and delivery. Many women interview more than one doctor before making a decision. Here are some questions to consider when choosing a doctor:

- What kind of training does the doctor have? Is he or she board certified in obstetrics and gynecology?
- Do you have any health problems or conditions that might require the care of a specialist?
- How does the doctor answer questions about issues that may concern you, such as ultrasound (see page 405), prenatal testing (see page 404), methods of preparing for childbirth, cesarean delivery (see page 442), fetal monitoring (see page 440), pain relief during labor and delivery, episiotomy (see page 441), birthing rooms (see page 399), induced labor (see page 439), or breast-feeding (see page 452)?
- Does he or she answer all your questions thoroughly, or do you feel rushed?
- With what hospital is the doctor affiliated? What facilities does the hospital have (birthing rooms, a pediatrician on call 24 hours, or a neonatal intensive care unit)?
- Is the office or clinic convenient to your home or work? (You will have regular checkups there throughout your pregnancy.)
- What are the arrangements for emergency care outside of office hours?
- What are the fees for the doctor and hospital? Are they covered by your health plan?

your child and to be comfortable with him or her.

An obstetrician-gynecologist is a doctor who specializes in the reproductive health of women. In addition to medical school, most obstetrician-gynecologists have completed 4 years of residency training in their specialty. The doctor may also be board certified in obstetrics and gynecology, which means that he or she has passed a rigorous examination in the specialty. Some obstetrician-gynecologists are further specialized and certified in an area called maternal-fetal medicine, or high-risk obstetrics. These doctors have had extra years of training in treating pregnancies that carry a risk of complications in either the woman or fetus, or both.

A family physician has 3 to 4 years of training in all aspects of primary care or internal medicine, including obstetrics. A family physician may serve as your obstetrician, gynecologist, and internist, as well as your child's pediatrician. If complications occur during your pregnancy or delivery, your family physician may refer you to a specialist, while remaining your primary doctor.

A certified nurse-midwife is a registered nurse who has additional certification in the care of healthy pregnant women and newborns. A nurse-midwife has had supervised training in a maternity hospital and is qualified to give care to women who have uncomplicated pregnancies and deliveries as well as to provide regular gynecological care (such as Pap smears) to healthy women throughout their reproductive years. Some nurse-midwives are in group practices with doctors. Others have ongoing professional relationships with doctors to whom they refer patients with special needs.

If you choose a nurse-midwife, you should know the obstetrician with whom the midwife is working. The nurse-midwife arranges for the obstetrician to be available to take care of you in a hospital in the event of an emergency, which can arise even in the healthiest of pregnancies. You will want to know the hospital with which the midwife and doctor are affiliated and where you will deliver your baby. You will also want to know their approach to childbirth and how it corresponds with your own and how comfortable you are with the doctor and the nurse-midwife.

The role of a birth partner

Throughout your pregnancy and the delivery of your baby, a reliable and caring partner can be an important source of support. This person—the baby's father or a close, reliable friend or relative—should attend childbirth classes with you and learn techniques to help make your labor more comfortable. If the baby's father is not involved in your life, choose someone early in your pregnancy. He or she should try to be available when delivery is imminent to bring you to the hospital or birthing center and stay with you throughout your labor and delivery.

A partner who feels squeamish about being present during the delivery often can overcome this feeling by attending childbirth classes and becoming familiar with the process. Fathers or other partners are welcome in the delivery room except in the case of an emergency cesarean delivery.

Some nurse-midwives are associated with birthing centers where women receive prenatal care throughout their pregnancy and go through labor and delivery. "Natural" childbirth, which generally means childbirth without the use of pain-relieving drugs, is usually emphasized at birthing centers. These centers are not equipped to handle complications of childbirth. For example, if a cesarean delivery (see page 442) becomes necessary, you will be transferred to a hospital immediately. If you have a medical condition such as high blood pressure (see page 480), diabetes (see page 418), or heart disease (see page 421)—which can complicate pregnancy and delivery—you should plan to deliver your baby in a hospital that is well-equipped to handle complications. If you choose to receive your care during pregnancy and childbirth at a birthing center, make sure it is licensed by the state and has arrangements with consulting obstetricians and with a nearby hospital for your transfer in case of an emergency.

The stages of pregnancy

Pregnancy is divided into three stages called trimesters, each about 13 weeks long. A normal, healthy pregnancy lasts an average of 40 weeks. Your doctor will calculate how many weeks along you are, counting from the first day of your last menstrual period—not the estimated time of conception. Each stage of pregnancy brings dramatic changes in your body as the fetus develops and grows. While many of these changes follow a predictable pattern, each woman is unique and experiences pregnancy in a different way.

FIRST TRIMESTER

The first trimester of pregnancy is the most critical time in the development of a fetus. By the end of the first trimester, all the fetus's major organs and arms and legs are fully formed. During this early stage, the fetus is especially vulnerable to damage from exposure to agents such as bacteria and viruses, environmental hazards, or alcohol and other drugs, all of which can cause birth defects.

The developing fetus As soon as the fertilized egg implants itself in the wall of the uterus, the lining of the uterus (endometrium) thickens further and covers the egg. The placenta, the organ that links the blood supplies of the mother and fetus, begins to develop inside the uterus and is completely formed by the end of the third month. The fetus is linked to the placenta by the umbilical cord. Blood flowing through the placenta carries oxygen and nutrients to the fetus and removes carbon dioxide and other wastes. Inside the uterus, the fetus is contained in a thin membrane called the amniotic sac, which is filled with amniotic fluid. This watery fluid surrounds the fetus, providing cushioning that protects it from external pressure or movement.

The embryo grows rapidly. By the end of the first month, the head and trunk are formed. The heart begins to beat around the 25th day. By the end of the second month, all the major organs have begun to develop. Fingers and toes develop. By the third month, hair begins to grow and buds for teeth appear. At the end of the third month, the fetus is about 4 inches long and weighs about 1 ounce.

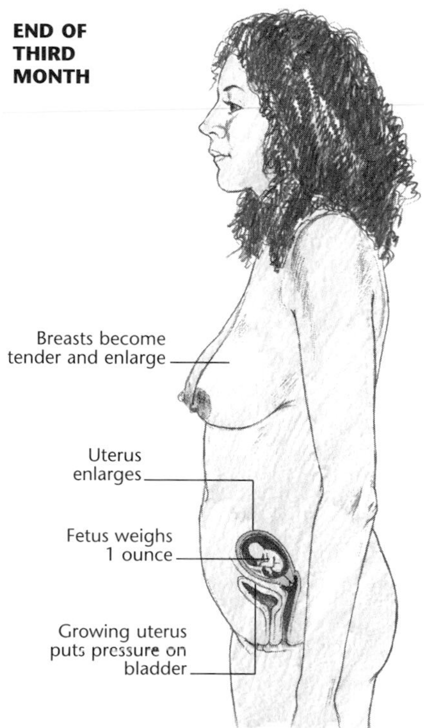

Your changing body Your body undergoes many changes during the first months of pregnancy. You will not have a menstrual period, but you may have some spotting around the time you would have had a period. You may feel tired and sleepy during these early months. Try to get extra rest and don't push yourself too hard.

Your breasts may begin to enlarge and become tender. The areola, the dark area around each nipple, may become even darker. These changes are caused by increased levels of the hormones estrogen and progesterone, which are preparing your breasts for breast-feeding. Breast tenderness usually subsides by the end of the first trimester. By this time, you may have gained enough weight to make your clothes feel tighter around your waist.

Many women feel nauseous during the first trimester (see page 415). Some also experience aversions to foods, drinks, or odors; cravings for certain foods or drinks; and heartburn, indigestion, flatulence, or bloating.

You may feel the urge to urinate frequently. This is your body's response to a higher volume of fluids and increased efficiency of your kidneys, which are producing more urine. The higher volume of fluids during pregnancy is necessary to circulate blood sufficiently through the placenta and fetus. Your enlarging uterus also puts pressure on your bladder. Make sure you drink at least eight glasses of water or other non-alcoholic, noncaffeinated fluids each day.

Because the first trimester is a critical time in the fetus's development, do not use any potentially harmful drugs, including alcohol or tobacco, and be especially diligent about eating a well-balanced, nutritious diet (see page 44). Check with your doctor before you take any prescription drugs or over-the-counter medications, including aspirin. Avoid exposure to environmental hazards (see page 414) such as pesticides and lead paint. Make sure you take the daily prenatal multivitamin supplement your doctor recommends.

Many miscarriages (see page 422) occur in the first weeks of pregnancy, often before a woman knows she is pregnant. An early miscarriage is usually the body's way of rejecting a fetus that would not have developed normally.

SECOND TRIMESTER

For many women, the second trimester of pregnancy is the easiest and most comfortable. The most rewarding time of this trimester may be when you first feel the fetus moving inside you. Morning sickness has usually subsided, your risk of miscarriage is reduced, and your energy level returns. Although you will begin wearing maternity clothes during this trimester, you are not so large that exercise and sexual intercourse are uncomfortable.

END OF SIXTH MONTH

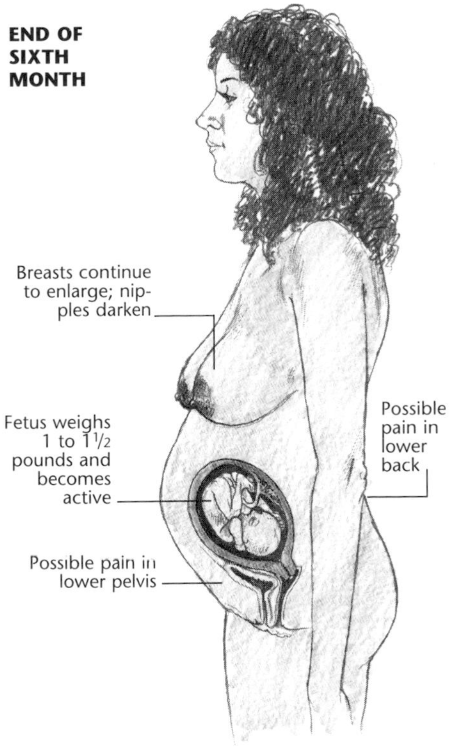

Breasts continue to enlarge; nipples darken

Fetus weighs 1 to 1½ pounds and becomes active

Possible pain in lower pelvis

Possible pain in lower back

The developing fetus Usually by about the 16th week (from the first day of your last period), you will begin to feel the fetus moving and kicking. Tell your doctor or nurse-midwife when you first begin to feel this movement because it helps to more accurately predict your due date.

The fetus now sleeps and wakes, passes urine into the surrounding amniotic fluid, and can hear sounds. It even has hair on its head. Around the fifth month, the fetus has a growth spurt. The internal organs are maturing and the fetus is more physically active. By the end of the sixth month, the fetus will be about 11 to 14 inches long and weigh about 1 to 1½ pounds. Because the fetus is still tiny and its lungs are not fully developed, it cannot live outside the uterus without highly specialized medical care.

Your changing body The middle 3 months of pregnancy are often the easiest because many of the discomforts of the first trimester have subsided and you are not yet large enough to be uncomfortable. You may feel as energetic and be as interested in sex as you were before you got pregnant. The size of your abdomen will increase significantly as your uterus expands to accommodate the growing fetus. Supporting tissues (called round ligaments) that stretch from the sides of your uterus to your groin may cause a sensation of pulling or tugging in your lower pelvis. You may have uncomfortable symptoms such as heartburn, indigestion, flatulence, and constipation. Your breasts continue to enlarge, but the tenderness may subside. Elevated hormone levels may cause your nipples to darken and a dark line (called the linea nigra) to form on your skin, running from your navel to your pubic hair. Your appetite will probably increase and you will continue to gain about a pound a week.

You may begin to experience lower back pain as your back adjusts to supporting the increased weight of your abdomen. You may have difficulty sleeping as you struggle to find a comfortable position.

THIRD TRIMESTER

During the last 3 months of pregnancy, you begin anticipating and preparing for labor and delivery. You may feel more uncomfortable as the fetus reaches its birth weight and your uterus expands even more. You may be less interested in sex during this time.

The developing fetus During the last 3 months of pregnancy, the fetus grows from about 3 pounds to its final birth weight of about 6 to 9 pounds or more. It exercises by kicking and stretching, sucks its thumb, and opens and closes its eyes. You may even feel it hiccuping inside you. The fetus's bones are hardening as they absorb calcium from your body, so it is essential for you to take in 1,200 milligrams of calcium every day (see page 58) to avoid losing calcium from your own bones.

The fetus shifts into position for birth, which is usually head down and facing toward your back with its arms and legs curled.

THE NINTH MONTH

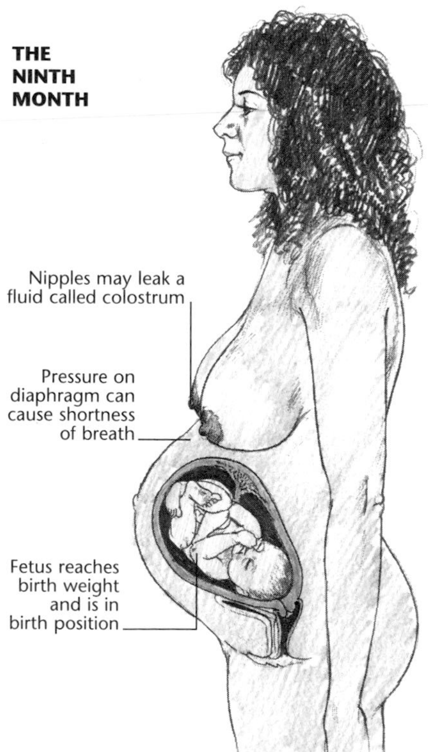

Your changing body During the third trimester, the increased size of the fetus may make moving about, exercising, and sleeping more difficult. Stretch marks may appear on your abdomen and breasts. Toward the end of your pregnancy, your nipples may begin to leak a small amount of colostrum, a fluid that is secreted as the breasts prepare for milk production. Your navel may protrude slightly. You may feel more tired and need to rest more frequently. Your ankles and other parts of your body may retain fluid and become puffy.

By the end of the ninth month, the upper part of your uterus reaches the lower part of your diaphragm and you may feel short of breath; large meals may make you feel uncomfortable. The shortness of breath usually goes away when the fetus "drops," or descends into the pelvic cavity; this usually occurs 1 to 2 weeks before delivery but may not occur until labor begins if you have already had a child. You may also feel an increasing sensation of pressure or cramps in your lower pelvis, especially if this is a second or later pregnancy.

In the ninth month, you may feel mild contractions of your uterus, called Braxton Hicks contractions, that can last from 30 seconds to 2 minutes. These are not true labor contractions (see page 432) but are sometimes mistaken for them. Braxton Hicks contractions are sometimes called false labor pains because they often increase in intensity and frequency a few days before true labor begins. True labor usually begins during the 37th to 42nd week.

Prenatal care

As soon as you think you may be pregnant, see a doctor to confirm the pregnancy and begin prenatal care. Even if you have already had one or more healthy pregnancies, it is always important to see a doctor as early as possible. Each pregnancy is different, and problems that cause few symptoms can arise suddenly. Throughout pregnancy, you will see your doctor or nurse-midwife regularly to monitor your health and that of the fetus.

THE FIRST PRENATAL VISIT

The first appointment with your doctor after your pregnancy is confirmed will be longer than usual. After this initial visit, you and your doctor will arrange a schedule for subsequent appointments and tests throughout your pregnancy. During your first visit, your doctor will probably take your medical history, do a physical examination, establish a due date, and perform some tests.

Medical history Your doctor will ask you questions about any previous pregnancies and your personal health history and that of your family. Tell your doctor about any past pregnancies and your family and personal health histories. Some conditions recur in future pregnancies or tend to run in families. You will be asked whether you smoke cigarettes, drink alcohol, or use any other drugs. Your doctor will also want to know if there is a possibility that you have a sexually transmitted disease (STD) such as genital herpes or another health condition that could affect your pregnancy or delivery. All pregnant women are tested for the STDs gonorrhea and syphilis.

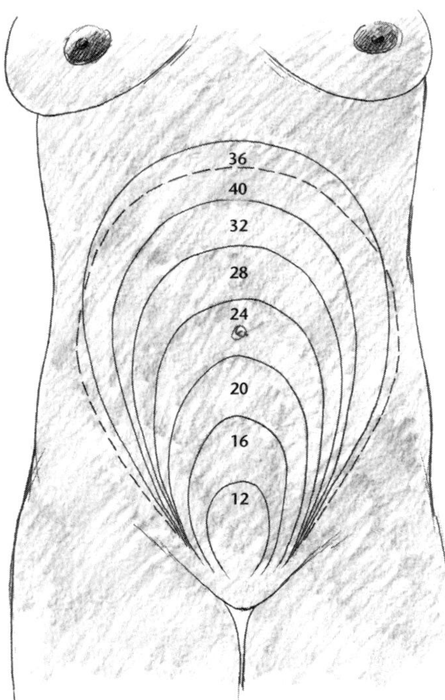

MEASURING THE GROWING UTERUS

The size of your expanding uterus helps the doctor determine how many weeks along your pregnancy is. At each prenatal visit after the 12th week of pregnancy, your doctor will feel the top of your uterus and measure the distance from there to your pubic bone using a measuring tape. By the 36th week, the top of your uterus will be just below your rib cage. By the 40th week (dotted line), this measurement is sometimes smaller because the fetus has begun to descend into the pelvic cavity in preparation for birth.

Physical examination Your height, weight, and blood pressure will be measured. You will have a regular physical examination as well as a pelvic examination to determine the size of your uterus, which helps calculate your due date. Your doctor will look for changes in your cervix that may indicate an incompetent cervix (see page 423), a condition in which the cervix cannot support the weight of a pregnancy. You will have a Pap smear during this visit if you are due for one.

Establishing your due date A healthy, full-term pregnancy lasts from 37 to 42 weeks, but the due date is usually set at 40 weeks from the first day of a woman's last menstrual period. If you are not sure of the date of your last period, or if your uterus appears larger or smaller than expected, your doctor may recommend an ultrasound scan (see page 405) to estimate your due date and determine the size of the fetus.

Routine tests You will have several tests during your first visit to the doctor; some of these tests, such as measurement of your blood pressure and weight, will be repeated throughout your pregnancy. You will have blood tests for blood type, Rh factor (see page 371), anemia (see page 493), some sexually transmitted diseases, and immunity to German measles (rubella) and hepatitis B. Urine tests show the approximate levels of protein and sugar in your urine. Excessive levels of protein (albumin) in your urine can indicate a life-threatening condition of pregnancy called preeclampsia (see page 428); excessive levels of sugar in your blood may indicate diabetes (see page 418), which can also cause complications during pregnancy. Urine tests can also detect some infections, such as kidney infections, that can cause preterm labor or other complications during pregnancy.

REGULAR PRENATAL VISITS

Your prenatal doctor appointments are likely to be scheduled on a monthly basis up to the 28th week of pregnancy, every 2 to 3 weeks up to the 36th week, and weekly thereafter. You will have many questions for your doctor throughout your pregnancy. Plan for each visit by writing down your questions and bringing them with you. At most appointments, the doctor or nurse-midwife will measure the growth of your uterus, listen to the fetus's heartbeat—and let you listen too—and ask about any symptoms you may be having. You will also have blood and urine tests and your weight and blood pressure will be measured. All women are tested for diabetes in the sixth month, but you will be tested for it earlier in pregnancy if you developed diabetes during your last pregnancy or if you have a strong family history of the disease.

PRENATAL TESTING

As your pregnancy continues, tests can be done to help determine the health of the fetus. Discuss with your doctor whether you should have any of these tests and when you should have them. Although prenatal tests cannot cure a problem, they can alert you and your doctor to it and help determine if special care is necessary. Prenatal tests can also detect some birth defects or genetic disorders in the fetus.

Fetal heart rate monitoring Doctors can monitor the health of the fetus by listening to its heartbeat with an ultrasound transducer (see page 405) or with a stethoscope held against your abdomen. You will be able to listen to the heartbeat too. Sometimes more sophisticated heart-rate monitoring is required to make sure there is no problem with the fetus. This extended monitoring is most often done in pregnancies that are considered to be high risk because the woman has a medical condition such as high blood pressure or diabetes or in pregnancies that have passed the due date.

The most common test to evaluate fetal heart rate is the nonstress test in which the doctor uses a fetal monitor (see page 440) to make sure the heart rate increases when the fetus moves, indicating it is healthy. A decrease in the fetus's heart rate would be an unhealthy response to stress.

If the doctor needs more information after doing the nonstress test, he or she may recommend a test called a biophysical profile. This test, which uses ultrasound, provides information about the fetus's breathing, movement, muscle tone, and the amount of amniotic fluid surrounding the fetus. The results of the biophysical profile are combined with the results of the nonstress test to help determine if an early delivery is necessary, if the woman should be hospitalized for more testing, or if the pregnancy can continue for the time being with further monitoring.

An alternative to a biophysical profile is a contraction stress test, also called an oxytocin challenge test. The same fetal monitoring equipment used in the nonstress test is used in a contraction stress test but, in addition, you are given an intravenous solution of oxytocin, a drug that stimulates mild contractions of your uterus. The doctor observes the fetus's response to the stress of the contractions for signs of difficulties, such as decreased heart rate. A fetus that does not respond normally may already be having problems that could worsen before the onset of labor. In such a case, it might be necessary to deliver. A normal response to the contractions suggests that the fetus is healthy, receiving sufficient oxygen, and will be able to withstand the stress of labor.

Alpha-fetoprotein test A blood test offered to all pregnant women between the 15th and 18th weeks of pregnancy measures the level of alpha-fetoprotein (AFP), a protein produced by the growing fetus. AFP is present in amniotic fluid and, in smaller amounts, in the pregnant woman's blood. An elevated level of AFP can indicate that the fetus has a neural tube defect, a type of birth defect that occurs when the brain or spinal cord fails to develop properly and is not covered by normal bone and skin. Increased amounts of AFP leak through the abnormal opening in the fetus's spine and cross the placenta into the woman's bloodstream. The AFP test cannot detect neural tube defects in which the spinal cord is covered by normal skin.

You may have an elevated level of AFP in your blood even if the fetus does not have a neural tube defect. If the test shows a high AFP level in your blood, you are likely to have further testing to get more accurate information about the health of the fetus. You may have an ultrasound examination, which can detect larger neural tube defects. If the ultrasound appears normal and there is no error in dating the pregnancy, a test called amniocentesis (see page 406) may be performed. Because amniocentesis provides a more direct measurement of the AFP level, the test can detect the presence of a small neural tube defect that may have been missed by ultrasound. If amniocentesis confirms a neural tube defect in the fetus, your doctor will recommend genetic counseling (see page 373) to evaluate the severity of the abnormality and help you make a decision about whether or not to terminate the pregnancy, or to prepare for special care of the child at delivery and after.

The AFP test can detect some cases of Down syndrome in fetuses of women under age 35, which otherwise would be missed because women this age are not routinely offered testing for Down syndrome and other chromosome abnormalities. Women over 35 are routinely offered such testing—amniocentesis or chorionic villus sampling (CVS; see page 407)—because they are at much higher risk of having a child with a chromosome abnormality (see page 374). If an AFP test on a woman under 35 shows a lower-than-normal level of AFP, she will have another blood test, called a PAN-AFP test or triple screen, that detects two other hormones—estriol (a form of estrogen) and human chorionic gonadotropin (HCG)—in addition to AFP to more accurately predict the risk of Down syndrome in the fetus. If the result of the PAN-AFP test is abnormal, the woman will have amniocentesis or CVS to confirm the diagnosis.

Ultrasound Ultrasound is a painless and safe imaging procedure that uses sound waves to create a picture on a video screen. Doctors use ultrasound during pregnancy to help determine the age of the fetus, its rate of growth, and its position in the uterus. They can also tell if there is more than one fetus or any visible birth defect, such as a missing limb. Ultrasound shows the position of the placenta and the amount of amniotic fluid. Most pregnant women in the US have an ultrasound examination at least once during their pregnancy. During the last months of a pregnancy, it is sometimes possible to determine the sex of the fetus. However, ultrasound is not a precise method of determining the sex of a fetus and is never recommended for this reason alone.

Although ultrasound can identify a variety of fetal abnormalities, including structural defects such as missing limbs, it cannot detect minor structural abnormalities such as an extra finger or toe; genetic disorders such as cystic fibrosis, sickle cell anemia, or Tay-Sachs disease; or chromosome abnormalities such as Down syndrome.

Before the ultrasound examination, you may be asked to drink several glasses of water; your full bladder pushes the uterus up out of the pelvic area, allowing the doctor to get a better view. Fluids in the bladder also improve the transmission

HAVING AN ULTRASOUND

Ultrasound is a painless imaging procedure that produces a picture of the fetus on a nearby video screen. For an ultrasound, a medical technician moves a device called a transducer over your abdomen. The transducer transmits sound waves into your abdomen that reflect back off the fetus and are electronically converted into an image on a screen.

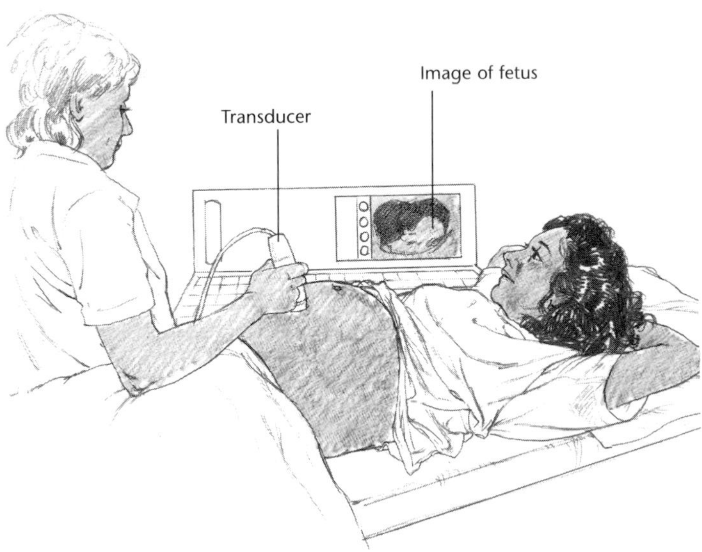

of sound waves. During the procedure, you lie on an examining table and the doctor rubs a gel over your abdomen to improve contact between your skin and the ultrasound transducer, a wand that transmits sound waves as it is moved over your abdomen. The sound waves are converted into an image on a video screen, which is examined by a doctor who is trained in radiology. If the doctor wants a clearer view of a small fetus early in pregnancy, he or she may recommend a vaginal ultrasound. In a vaginal ultrasound, the transducer is narrower and is inserted into the vagina.

Amniocentesis Amniocentesis is a test performed between the 14th and 18th weeks of pregnancy to analyze the liquid that surrounds the fetus throughout pregnancy (amniotic fluid, which contains fetal cells) to detect abnormalities in the genetic material inside the fetus's cells. Amniocentesis can detect chromosome abnormalities (see page 374)—such as Down syndrome—or genetic disorders—such as cystic fibrosis (see page 512), sickle-cell anemia (see page 493), Tay-Sachs disease, or hemophilia in the fetus. You and your doctor will decide which of these diseases to test for based on your family health history, your own health history, your ethnic or racial background, or whether or not you carry a gene for a particular disorder. Some genetic disorders, such as sickle cell anemia, are more likely to occur in some ethnic or racial groups than in others. If you are a carrier of an X-linked genetic disorder such as hemophilia, which affects only males, the fetus would not be tested for it unless amniocentesis shows that the fetus is male.

Amniocentesis is usually performed by a specialist in a hospital or a doctor's office. For the procedure, the doctor uses ultrasound to locate the position of the fetus and determine the best place to insert the needle without harming the fetus, placenta, or umbilical cord. The doctor injects a local anesthetic just beneath the skin of your abdomen and, using the ultrasound image as a guide, carefully inserts a needle through your abdomen into your uterus and withdraws about an ounce of amniotic fluid. The fetal cells in the fluid are grown in a laboratory for 2 to 3 weeks. Then the chromosomes are analyzed to detect genetic defects and to make an exact diagnosis.

Amniocentesis is not painful. After the procedure, some women may have mild cramps, light vaginal bleeding, or leaking of amniotic fluid. Injury to the fetus is rare, but there is a slightly increased risk of miscarriage (1 in 200) in women who have the procedure. For this reason, amniocentesis is performed only in women

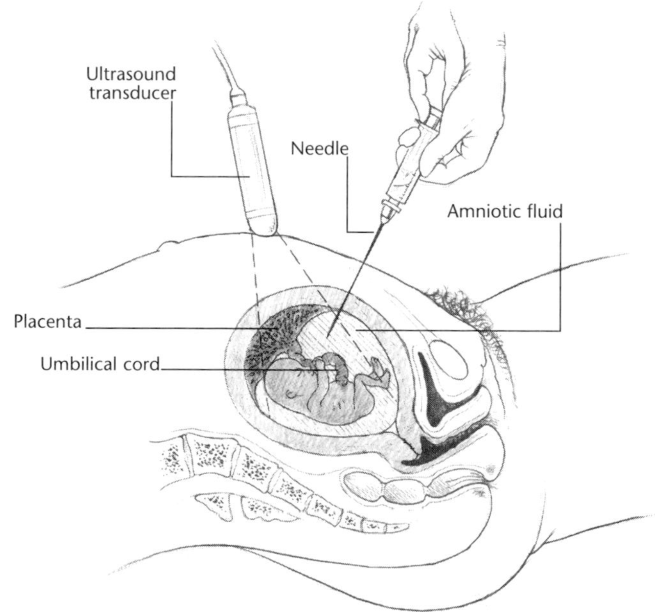

AMNIOCENTESIS
Amniocentesis is performed between the 14th and 18th weeks of pregnancy to test for a variety of chromosome abnormalities such as Down syndrome and genetic disorders such as cystic fibrosis. Guided by an ultrasound image showing the position of the fetus, the doctor inserts a needle into the pregnant woman's abdomen to withdraw a sample of amniotic fluid, which surrounds the fetus. The fetal cells present in the amniotic fluid are grown in a laboratory and studied for genetic abnormalities.

If prenatal test results are abnormal

If prenatal testing shows that the fetus may have a genetic disorder, chromosome abnormality, or serious birth defect, you will be faced with difficult decisions. Read everything you can find about the abnormality and get in touch with a support group to find out from other parents what it is like to care for a child with the disorder. Your decisions include whether or not to terminate the pregnancy or how to make special preparations for the birth and care of the infant.

When making your decision, consider your situation. Will you have sufficient support from your partner, family members, or friends to help you raise a child who needs special care? Will the child require so much specialized care that he or she will have to live in an institution? Will the child need special equipment for eating, sleeping, or moving around? If one parent must be available at all times to care for the child, can your family survive financially on one income? In case of your death, what financial and custodial arrangements should be made for the care of the child? If you already have children, what effect will having a seriously handicapped child in the family have on them? If you are single, where will you get support? Whatever your decision, seeking counseling, participating in support groups, and relying on relatives and friends can help you cope.

who may be at risk of having a fetus with a birth defect, such as women over 35 or who have a family history of a genetic disorder. Your doctor or a trained genetic counselor (see page 373) will evaluate your personal risk factors and your family health history before recommending amniocentesis. You may or may not choose to have the test; the decision is yours.

Chorionic villus sampling Like amniocentesis, chorionic villus sampling (CVS) is a prenatal diagnostic test that can detect genetic abnormalities in a fetus. Chorionic villi are microscopic threadlike projections that form part of the developing placenta and contain the same genetic material as cells of the fetus. In CVS, a small sample of chorionic villi is taken from the placenta without disrupting the development of the fetus or placenta. The major advantage of CVS over amniocentesis is that it can be done earlier in pregnancy, between the 10th and 12th weeks, and results are available faster—in 10 to 14 days. The disadvantage of CVS is that it has a higher rate of complications than amniocentesis and a higher risk of miscarriage (1 in 100 compared with 1 in 200 for amniocentesis).

CVS is performed between the 10th and 12th weeks of pregnancy (counting from the first day of your last period) because the risk of miscarriage from the procedure is higher before and after this time. In some cases, such as to rule out a neural tube defect, amniocentesis must be used instead of CVS because amniotic fluid rather than tissue from the placenta must be tested.

During CVS, the doctor inserts a speculum into your vagina to open it and, guided by ultrasound, inserts a thin catheter through your vagina and cervix and withdraws a tiny sample of tissue from the placenta. The tissue sample is sent to a laboratory where the cells are grown and studied for genetic abnormalities. CVS can also be done through the abdomen. In this procedure, the tissue sample is withdrawn through a needle inserted through the abdomen and uterus. The insertion of the needle is also guided by ultrasound. CVS done through the abdomen may have fewer complications than CVS done through the vagina because inserting the needle through the abdomen is often an easier way to obtain a tissue sample from the placenta.

Percutaneous umbilical cord blood sampling Percutaneous umbilical cord blood sampling (PUBS) is a prenatal diagnostic test for genetic abnormalities that is performed after the 17th week of pregnancy and is used only when other diagnostic procedures cannot provide a definite diagnosis. In PUBS, a sample of blood is drawn through a needle from the umbilical cord (guided by ultrasound) and studied in the laboratory for various abnormalities, including infections. Because PUBS is a complicated and difficult procedure, it is performed only by doctors who are highly trained and experienced in the procedure. Complication rates are higher with PUBS than with amniocentesis or CVS because there is a risk of injuring the umbilical cord.

Because PUBS is performed late in pregnancy, it cannot be used for early testing for genetic diseases or chromosome abnormalities. However, if your doctor does not suspect a genetic abnormality until later in pregnancy, PUBS can be used to make a diagnosis. PUBS can also be used to determine if the pregnant woman has transmitted a potentially harmful infection to the fetus and to evaluate the fetus's health. PUBS can detect life-threatening anemia in the fetus caused by Rh incompatibility (see page 371). If anemia is detected, PUBS can be used to treat the condition by giving the fetus a blood transfusion directly into the umbilical cord.

Toward a healthy pregnancy

It is extremely important to take care of yourself throughout your pregnancy—both physically and emotionally. Eating a balanced, nutritious diet, gaining the right amount of weight, and exercising moderately can make you healthier during pregnancy, which is the best thing you can do for the health of your fetus. Avoiding excess stress can also make you feel better and help you withstand the physical and emotional demands that pregnancy places on you.

NUTRITION AND WEIGHT GAIN

"Eating for two" means you are filling the nutritional needs of two people, *not* that you should eat twice as much food. You do not need to consume additional calories during the first 3 months of pregnancy, but you should eat about 300 extra calories a day during the remainder of your pregnancy to support the growth of the fetus and placenta. Most women get hungrier at this time and do not need to consciously increase their calorie intake.

What is a healthy weight gain? Although you need to take in additional nutrients and calories during pregnancy, gaining too much weight can cause the fetus to grow too large, potentially leading to complications in late pregnancy and during childbirth. Excess pounds you gain during pregnancy can be hard to take off after pregnancy and can set the stage for an unhealthy weight in the long term.

Your target weight gain during pregnancy depends on your weight before you got pregnant. For women who are at a healthy weight before pregnancy, doctors recommend a weight gain of 25 to 35 pounds. For overweight women who are otherwise healthy, 15 to 25 pounds is the recommended weight gain; for obese women (those who are more than 20 percent over their ideal weight; see page 98), 15 pounds is the recommended gain. A thin woman can safely gain up to 40 pounds. If you are carrying twins, you need to take in more nutrients and gain more weight—between 35 and 45 pounds.

During the second and third trimesters you should take in from 2,000 to 2,600 calories each day, depending on your height and body frame (see page 99); those calories should come from healthy foods. Be careful. Most women tend to gain too much weight during pregnancy; 300 extra calories a day is not much.

Most women do not gain much weight during their first trimester. After this time, it is best to gain weight gradually, about the same amount each week. Underweight women should not gain more than 2 pounds per week; women of average weight should gain about 1 pound per week; overweight women should gain no more than about two thirds of a pound each week. If you are obese, ask your doctor about how much weight you can gain safely during pregnancy.

Do not try to lose weight during pregnancy, even if you are overweight, because doing so can deprive the fetus of essential nutrients. At delivery you will lose about 12 to 14 pounds and in the 6 weeks after delivery you will lose weight as your uterus shrinks to its normal size and you lose excess body fat and fluids. You will lose weight faster if you breastfeed because your body burns calories producing milk.

Nutrients for a healthy pregnancy Your diet should include plenty of fresh fruits and vegetables, whole grains, and protein sources such as lean meats, fish, and nonfat dairy products. Your doctor will prescribe a prenatal vitamin supplement to ensure that you get adequate amounts of vitamins and minerals. It is a good idea to start taking these vitamin supplements 3 months before you plan to become pregnant so that your body has sufficient levels of essential vitamins and minerals before conception.

Folic acid Folic acid is a type of B vitamin that is important for fetal development, especially during the first month of pregnancy. A developing fetus needs folic acid to form a healthy brain and spinal cord, the bundle of nerves running from the base of the brain down the spinal column. A deficiency of folic acid increases the risk of birth defects such as neural tube defects, in which the tube of nerve tissue that forms the brain and spinal column does not close properly. Some of these defects can be life threatening. Because many birth defects occur early in fetal development, often before a woman knows she is pregnant, doctors now recommend that all women of childbearing age get 400 micrograms (0.4 milligrams) of folic acid every day in a supplement.

Nutrients for women who are pregnant or breast-feeding

When you get the essential nutrients your body needs during pregnancy, you also enhance the healthy development of your fetus. If you are breast-feeding, it is important to take in the nutrients your body requires for producing milk to feed your infant. It is recommended that you get the following amounts of vitamins and minerals every day when you are pregnant or breast-feeding.

NUTRIENT	PREGNANT	BREAST-FEEDING	
		FIRST 6 MONTHS	SECOND 6 MONTHS
VITAMINS			
Vitamin A	800 mcg*	1,300 mcg	1,300 mcg
Vitamin C	70 mg†	96 mg	90 mg
Vitamin D	10 mg	10 mg	10 mg
Vitamin E	10 mg	12 mg	11 mg
Vitamin K	65 mcg	65 mcg	65 mcg
Vitamin B_1 (thiamine)	1.5 mg	1.6 mg	1.6 mg
Vitamin B_2 (riboflavin)	1.6 mg	1.8 mg	1.7 mg
Niacin	17 mg	20 mg	20 mg
Vitamin B_6	2.2 mg	2.1 mg	2.1 mg
Vitamin B_{12}	2.2 mg	2.6 mg	2.6 mg
Folic acid	400 mcg	280 mcg	260 mcg
MINERALS			
Calcium	1,200 mg	1,200 mg	1,200 mg
Phosphorus	1,200 mg	1,200 mg	1,200 mg
Magnesium	320 mg	355 mg	340 mg
Iron	30 mg	15 mg	15 mg
Zinc	15 mcg	19 mcg	16 mcg
Iodine	175 mcg	200 mcg	200 mcg
Selenium	65 mcg	75 mcg	75 mcg

* Microgram
† Milligram

Foods to avoid when you are pregnant

Some foods that might normally cause only a brief illness or not affect you at all can severely harm a fetus. Avoid the following foods during pregnancy:

- Raw meat may contain the microorganism that causes an infection called toxoplasmosis (see page 420). Although this infection may cause few or no symptoms in a pregnant woman, it can affect a fetus severely.
- Raw fish, freshwater fish, many ocean fish (including salmon and swordfish), and shellfish (such as clams, mussels, and oysters) are often contaminated with a variety of microorganisms or chemical pollutants. The safest varieties of fish are those that live deep in the ocean, such as cod, red snapper, pollack, halibut, yellowfin tuna, and haddock.
- Unwashed fruits and vegetables may have residual amounts of pesticides on the surface. Peel or wash all produce thoroughly before cooking or eating.
- Unpasteurized soft cheeses, such as Brie or Camembert, may contain bacteria that can infect you and your fetus.

Protein Proteins are the building blocks of cells and are especially important during pregnancy. Lean meats, poultry, egg whites, fish, low-fat or nonfat dairy products, and legumes (such as dried beans and peas) are good sources of protein. Try to get 60 grams of protein each day—the equivalent of three glasses of skim milk, a cup of low-fat yogurt, and 3 ounces of turkey. Because protein is abundant in many foods, there is no need to take high-protein powders or drinks.

Calcium The fetus needs calcium to build strong bones and teeth as well as to develop muscle, heart, and nerve tissue. Four 8-ounce glasses of skim milk will provide the minimum recommended daily intake of 1,200 milligrams of calcium without adding excess fat. Nonfat yogurt and cottage cheese are also good sources of calcium. (For more about good sources of calcium, see chart on page 58.) If you do not get sufficient calcium in your diet, take calcium supplements to reach the recommended level. Some antacid tablets also contain calcium in the form of calcium carbonate, which your body absorbs easily.

Iron During pregnancy, you have to take in twice as much iron as usual—30 to 60 milligrams each day. Most prenatal multivitamin/mineral supplements contain this amount. Your body absorbs iron more efficiently from animal foods such as red meat, chicken, and tuna than from plant foods such as dried beans and whole grains. The fetus needs iron to build blood cells. If you are not getting enough iron, the fetus will take it from your blood supply, which can cause anemia (see page 493) in you. Nearly one out of five pregnant women experiences anemia, usually beginning around the 20th week of pregnancy. If you have anemia, your doctor will prescribe a supplement that contains more iron.

EXERCISE

If you exercised regularly before pregnancy, exercise will continue to help you control your blood pressure, reduce stress, tone your muscles, and improve your mental and physical well-being. Exercise can also help curb excessive weight gain and reduce constipation, which often accompanies pregnancy. If you did not exercise before becoming pregnant, you can begin a moderate walking program, but nothing more strenuous. Starting an intensive exercise program during pregnancy may increase your risk of injuries such as sprains. Whether or not you exercised previously, talk with your doctor about exercising during pregnancy, especially if you have an incompetent cervix (see page 423) or you have had any preterm deliveries. Some complications that can arise during pregnancy, such as preterm labor (see page 427), require bed rest and therefore preclude any exercise at all.

The best exercise program during pregnancy is a moderate aerobic workout three to five times a week for 30 minutes at a time. Walking is ideal. Doing pelvic floor exercises (see page 238), also called Kegel exercises, can help prevent the leaking of urine that sometimes follows childbirth if these muscles are damaged.

As healthy as exercise can be during pregnancy for both you and your fetus, it is important not to overdo it. Here are some guidelines:

- Exercise at the same level of intensity you did before you were pregnant—no more.
- If you did not exercise regularly before you got pregnant, start a moderate program now; try walking for half an hour at least three times a week.
- Do not exercise beyond a level at which you can carry on a conversation; your heart rate should not exceed 140 beats per minute.
- Expect to have less energy, especially in the last trimester.
- Swimming is an excellent exercise during pregnancy because the water helps support the increased weight of your body.
- Stretch gently to avoid straining your joints. Do not engage in sports that require quick changes in direction, such as tennis and racquetball. Extra weight on your joints can cause injury to the ligaments. Bouncing exercises, such as high-impact aerobics, may put excessive pressure on your cervix, especially if you have a weakened cervix (incompetent cervix, see page 423).
- Do not participate in sports that can result in a blow or other injury to your abdomen and uterus, such as springboard diving, horseback riding, downhill skiing, or fencing. Do not scuba dive because it can change the pressure in your uterus. Sudden pressure changes inside the uterus can cause the placenta to separate from the wall of the uterus prematurely (see page 426).
- Do not exercise at high altitudes; doing so can deprive the fetus of oxygen. However, if you live at a high altitude and have been exercising regularly, you can continue doing so during pregnancy.
- Avoid saunas and hot tubs, which can raise your body temperature to levels that can be harmful to a fetus.
- Stop all exercising and see your doctor immediately if you have pain in your pelvis or abdomen, vaginal bleeding, or a watery vaginal discharge that may indicate the amniotic membrane has ruptured, or if you do not feel the fetus moving.

A LOWER-BACK EXERCISE
Stretching your lower back can help relieve backache throughout pregnancy and even during labor. To do this exercise, sometimes referred to as the cat stretch, get on your hands and knees, keeping your head straight and in line with your spine. Do not let your spine sag or your back arch. Hump your back, tightening the muscles of your abdomen and buttocks and letting your head drop down. Gradually raise your head and relax your back, returning to the starting position. Repeat several times.

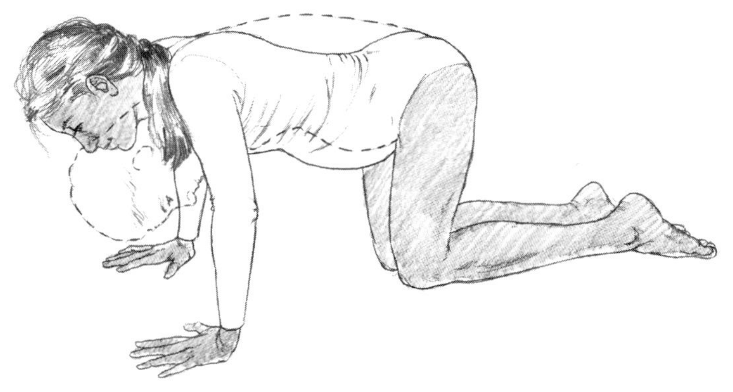

SEX

Having sexual intercourse during pregnancy will not harm the fetus. Most couples can continue to have intercourse right up to the onset of labor. As your uterus enlarges, you may find intercourse more comfortable in positions that place less pressure on your abdomen, such as side by side, you on top, or your partner entering you from behind. Couples who find intercourse more difficult or less enjoyable during this time may want to try other ways to give each other sexual pleasure.

Many women have less sexual desire during pregnancy. Neither partner should feel guilty about being less interested in sex during this time. As your body undergoes dramatic changes, so may your feelings about your sexuality. At the same time, you may be focusing on becoming a mother, a role that may conflict with your sexual image. Your partner must also change his perception of you to include your role as mother in addition to sex partner, and redefine himself as an expectant father. You both may need some time to reconcile these different concepts.

If you have placenta previa (see page 426), vaginal bleeding, preterm labor (see page 427), premature rupture of the membranes (see page 444), or an incompetent cervix (see page 423), your doctor may recommend limiting or avoiding intercourse and nipple stimulation. In women with any of these conditions, intercourse and nipple stimulation can trigger contractions of the uterus that may bring on labor. As at any other time, monogamy is important during pregnancy. Having multiple sexual partners increases your risk of infections such as AIDS or genital herpes, which can be transmitted to the fetus during pregnancy or childbirth, or genital warts, which can complicate delivery.

TRAVEL

It is usually safe to travel during pregnancy. If you are planning a trip, weeks 14 to 28 are probably the best time because you are not likely to have morning sickness and you will not be so large that you have trouble getting around comfortably. In the eighth and ninth months, try to avoid travel in case labor begins.

Travel by commercial airline is considered safe for pregnant women, but avoid unpressurized private planes. Sudden or extreme changes in pressure can cause premature separation of the placenta (see page 426). Here are some things you can do to make travel during pregnancy more comfortable:

- Plan your trip to allow you to get up and walk around every hour or two; this maintains blood circulation and prevents swelling in your feet and legs.
- Request a bulkhead seat on the airplane to give yourself more room.
- Take a copy of your prenatal medical records with you; ask your doctor for a copy.
- Wear comfortable, nonbinding clothes.
- Drink plenty of water and other fluids to avoid dehydration.
- Do not take medication for motion sickness, insomnia, or any other travel-related condition unless your doctor says it is OK.
- If you are considering foreign travel, talk with your doctor about the safety of any vaccinations you may need. To avoid traveler's diarrhea, drink only bottled water and avoid eating raw vegetables and fruits.
- If you want to travel late in your pregnancy, check with your doctor first. Ask about your risk of preterm labor (see page 427) or your need to avoid delivery in a hospital that is not equipped to take care of a difficult delivery or a newborn with problems.
- Bring crackers with you to help prevent nausea.
- If you are traveling by automobile, always wear your seat belt.

CORRECT POSITION OF SEAT BELT DURING PREGNANCY

Wear a lap and shoulder belt whenever you travel in a car. The lap belt should be placed under your abdomen and against your upper thighs. Position the upper part of the belt between your breasts. The belt should cross your shoulder without rubbing against your neck. Adjust both lap and shoulder belt as snugly as is comfortable. Don't slip the shoulder part of the seat belt off your shoulder and place it under your arm; it will not work as effectively that way.

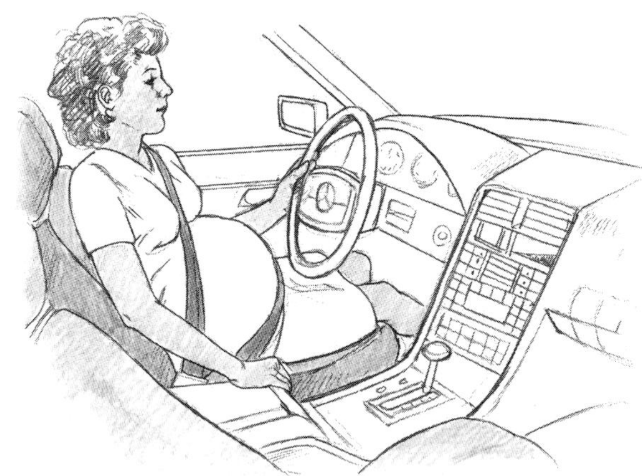

PSYCHOLOGICAL ASPECTS OF PREGNANCY

For some women, pregnancy is a period of peaceful anticipation. For other women, pregnancy is a time of crisis and upheaval. Most women fall somewhere in the middle, looking forward to bringing new life into the world but feeling ambivalent about the many changes that are involved and concerned about their baby's welfare as well as their own. Some of the factors that play a role in a woman's adjustment to pregnancy are her life circumstances; the amount of emotional support she has from her partner, family, and friends; her prior emotional stability; and her attitudes toward femininity and motherhood. Although changes in body image, lifestyle, and focus are common and expected parts of pregnancy, they can be sources of tension and stress.

Letting people know how you feel and what you are worried about is an important first step in getting the extra support and reassurance you need during pregnancy. Your obstetrician can be a great source of information and comfort, as can friends and relatives who have been through a pregnancy themselves. Classes that prepare you for childbirth and parenting are valuable learning and social experiences. You and the other women and couples in these classes can commiserate and share advice. The knowledge you gain also can help diminish the fear of the unknown associated with pregnancy and childbirth.

Hazards in pregnancy

Substances in the environment—some of which you can control and some of which you may never have given a thought to before—can harm a fetus. It is not always possible to avoid exposure to every potentially damaging substance around you but there are many things you can do to limit your exposure and help protect your fetus. For example, you can avoid drinking alcohol or taking other drugs or smoking cigarettes while you are pregnant.

SMOKING

Each cigarette you smoke exposes the fetus to harmful chemicals. For example, carbon monoxide produced by the cigarette lowers the amount of vital oxygen delivered to the fetus, which can reduce its ability to thrive and withstand stress, such as the stress of labor. Women who smoke during pregnancy are more likely to have a miscarriage, stillbirth, or premature delivery than women who do not smoke. Babies born to smokers have a lower birth weight and are more susceptible to medical problems than are babies of nonsmoking women. They are also more likely to die of sudden infant death syndrome. Your exposure to secondhand smoke during pregnancy can also harm the fetus.

Quitting smoking before you get pregnant is best. However, even quitting during pregnancy, especially in the early months, can reduce your chances of giving birth to a baby with a low birth weight or other health problems. For more about smoking and how to quit, see page 152.

DRINKING

Heavy drinking by pregnant women often causes a serious birth defect called fetal alcohol syndrome, which is the most common preventable cause of mental retardation in the US. Fetal alcohol syndrome has a wide range of symptoms, including facial and limb deformities, heart defects, slow growth, mental retardation, impaired motor coordination, and abnormal speech. Because alcohol can disrupt cell growth during early fetal development when the major organs are being formed, it can cause permanent abnormalities in organ systems throughout the body.

No safe level of drinking during pregnancy has been established. Because it is not known whether or not moderate drinking (no more than one drink a day) can cause problems during pregnancy, doctors recommend that women not drink any alcohol at all during pregnancy. You also should avoid alcohol if you are trying to get pregnant or if there is any possibility that you may be pregnant or become pregnant.

TAKING DRUGS

Eliminating the use of all illegal drugs is an important step to take during pregnancy. The earlier in pregnancy you stop using drugs, the better. Many drugs pass through the placenta and can harm the health of the fetus. For example, cocaine and a form of cocaine called crack can cause a sudden increase or change in blood pressure, leading to placental abruption (see page 426), in which the placenta separates from the wall of the uterus, cutting off the fetus's circulation and sometimes causing death. Having only a single "hit" of cocaine during pregnancy can cause a brain-damaging stroke and sometimes permanent paralysis in a fetus because of cocaine's ability to rapidly elevate blood pressure. Cocaine use during pregnancy can also prevent a woman from getting adequate nutrition and gaining a sufficient amount of weight.

Many other illegal drugs can also harm a fetus (see page 168). For more information about drugs and pregnancy, see page 169.

Check with your doctor before taking any prescription or over-the-counter medication, even aspirin. As soon as you find out you are pregnant, ask your doctor about any medication you have been taking regularly.

CAFFEINE

The effects of caffeine during pregnancy are not known for sure. An intake of caffeine that is the equivalent of more than two cups of coffee a day may increase the risk of miscarriage. Your best bet is to eliminate caffeine during pregnancy or reduce your consumption to one or two cups of coffee a day. Tea and soft drinks have about half as much caffeine per serving as coffee (see page 65).

ENVIRONMENTAL THREATS

Exposure to some environmental substances, such as those mentioned here, can make it more difficult for a woman to become pregnant or for a fetus to develop normally. Although the effects of some of these chemicals are not fully understood, they are known to be potentially harmful to a developing fetus. Try to avoid exposure to them at home or at work. If you are regularly exposed to any known harmful substances at work, make arrangements with your employer to protect yourself. Most employers are willing to do what is necessary to protect the health of their employees. Put your request in writing and save a copy. Job discrimination because of pregnancy is illegal.

Lead and mercury If you work in a factory or laboratory, ask your employer if you are being exposed to lead or mercury. These metals are known to cause delay in development and mental retardation in a fetus. People who work near heavy traffic, such as toll collectors, are exposed to both lead and mercury. At home, do not scrape or sand old paint when you are pregnant because it contains lead. Varnish also contains lead, so do not breathe its fumes.

Radiation Large doses of ionizing radiation, the kind of radiation used in medical X-rays and in many industries, can harm a developing fetus. Find out from your employer if you are being exposed to any radiation in your workplace. Normal exposure to nonionizing radiation, the kind emitted from computer and television screens, does not cause problems. If you need to have any diagnostic tests, ask your doctor to see if another medical procedure, such as ultrasound (see page 405), can be used instead of X-rays.

Pesticides and solvents Halogenated hydrocarbons—a group of chemicals used in agriculture and industry—are considered harmful to a fetus. This group of chemicals includes polychlorinated biphenyls (PCBs; used in plastics, insulation, and flame retardants), dioxin (a manufacturing impurity found in many industrial products including wood preservatives, sealants, and bleached paper products), and some pesticides. Ask your employer whether you are being exposed to any of these chemicals. At home, stay away from pesticides and lawn and garden fertilizers. Paints available today are safe because they no longer contain lead. However, you should avoid exposure to solvents, such as paint thinners used for cleaning up oil-based paint and deck sealers and other wood preservatives.

Health concerns during pregnancy

Most of the changes your body undergoes during pregnancy are normal, healthy, and expected. Some effects of pregnancy may cause you temporary discomfort, but many of these common discomforts can be prevented or relieved by simple measures. However, you should be aware of symptoms that are not usual and may indicate a serious problem that requires careful monitoring or special treatment during your pregnancy. Make sure your doctor knows about any health condition you have, such as high blood pressure or diabetes, that can pose a risk to you or the fetus. Tell your doctor about any discomfort, pain, or symptoms you are experiencing, no matter how minor they may seem to you.

COMMON DISCOMFORTS

Most common discomforts of pregnancy are no cause for concern but it is a good idea to ask your doctor about them. There are usually simple things you can do to prevent or relieve many of these symptoms.

Tender breasts Your breasts will grow throughout your pregnancy and may become tender or swollen. A properly fitting bra with good support may help relieve the discomfort. If you are planning to breast-feed, you may want to purchase several nursing bras and wear them during the last trimester. Breast tenderness often subsides as pregnancy progresses.

Nausea and vomiting A rapidly rising level of the hormone estrogen in the first few months of pregnancy often causes nausea. Although nausea is most common in the first trimester, in some women it lasts into the second trimester. Because these symptoms most often occur in the morning, they are referred to as "morning sickness," but nausea can occur at any time, especially when your stomach is empty. The following steps may help you avoid nausea:

- Get out of bed slowly in the morning, first sitting on the edge of the bed for a few minutes. Have crackers available on your nightstand and eat one or two as soon as you wake up.
- Eat dry toast, crackers, or a peeled apple every few hours during the day.
- Between meals, drink plenty of beverages or soups but avoid those that are either very hot or very cold.
- Avoid foods that are greasy, fried, or highly seasoned, especially those containing pepper, chilies, or garlic.
- Do not take medication without your doctor's approval.
- Contact your doctor if your nausea or vomiting become severe.

Indigestion Indigestion occurs when food and acids in your stomach back up into your esophagus, the tube leading from your mouth to your stomach. This often occurs during pregnancy because an increased level of the hormone progesterone relaxes the muscles that usually prevent this backup. Your enlarging abdomen can also cause indigestion by pressing on your stomach and esophagus. Signs of indigestion include heartburn; a feeling of discomfort, fullness, or burning in your upper abdomen; or nausea.

To avoid indigestion, you should eat several small meals during the day instead of three large ones. Avoid foods that cause gas or irritate your stomach, including spicy foods or acidic foods such as citrus fruits. Wait an hour after eating before you lie down and 2 hours before you exercise.

Constipation and hemorrhoids About half of all pregnant women have some degree of constipation. Hormones released during pregnancy slow the movement of food through the digestive tract. Constipation is often most severe during the last trimester, when your enlarged uterus puts pressure on your rectum, making it difficult to pass stool. The best way to avoid constipation is to eat a high-fiber diet and drink plenty of liquids. Eat a bowl of high-fiber cereal for breakfast and lots of fruits and vegetables throughout the day. Drink at least eight glasses (8 ounces each) of water each day. If you have severe constipation, talk to your doctor about using a natural fiber laxative.

Constipation can put increased pressure on veins in the rectum, causing hemorrhoids (see page 522). Hemorrhoids are swollen veins in the rectum that may protrude and bleed. Eating plenty of fiber and drinking fluids may help relieve hemorrhoids as well as constipation. Do not take over-the-counter hemorrhoid medications without consulting your doctor.

Cravings At some time during your pregnancy you may crave a particular food. Food cravings may signify a need for a particular nutrient or mineral. For example, many women crave salty foods. It is fine to respond to your cravings, but watch out for high-fat foods that might cause you to gain too much weight or high-sodium foods that can make you retain water.

Fatigue Most women feel more tired than usual during pregnancy. Fatigue is most common during the first and third trimesters. It is important to get enough sleep throughout your pregnancy, and rest whenever you can.

Leg cramps For unknown reasons, leg cramps sometimes occur during the last 3 months of pregnancy, usually while you are lying down. Stretching your calf muscles before going to bed and first thing in the morning (see page 87) may help prevent cramps. If you get a cramp in the middle of the night, get up and walk around slowly until it subsides.

Swollen ankles Many women find that their ankles and feet swell as their pregnancy progresses. This swelling is caused by the increasing pressure an enlarging uterus puts on the veins that carry blood from the legs to the heart. To help improve the circulation in your legs, try to lie down and put your feet on a raised pillow several times throughout the day, or sit with your feet elevated as often as possible. Limiting salt in your diet and wearing support stockings may also be helpful.

Skin changes Your skin may change in a number of ways during pregnancy. Patches of darker skin may appear on your face. This condition, called chloasma or, sometimes, "mask of pregnancy," will fade when your hormone levels return to normal. In some women, a dark line appears that runs from the navel to the pubic hair. This dark line is also caused by hormones and will fade after delivery. As your skin expands over your growing abdomen and breasts, stretch marks may appear. Although stretch marks may be permanent, on most women they fade with time.

Dental problems Hormonal changes during pregnancy sometimes cause sore, swollen gums. In extreme cases, eating becomes painful. Therefore, it is important to see your dentist at least once during your pregnancy for a checkup and cleaning. To prevent gum inflammation and pain, brush and floss your teeth at least twice a day. Try to limit sweets and avoid snacking throughout the day to help reduce the buildup of a bacteria-containing substance called plaque. If your gums become painful or bleed when you brush your teeth, see your dentist. You may need a special type of cleaning or gum treatment. If not treated, some forms of gum disease—gingivitis (see page 662) or periodontitis (see page 663)—may lead to unnecessary loss of teeth.

Dental X-rays are considered safe during pregnancy but are only done when required for a specific purpose, such as to

Warning signs During pregnancy

Although most of the symptoms you experience during pregnancy are normal, some may indicate problems. Call your doctor immediately if you experience any of the following:

- **Pain** Any prolonged pain you have in your pelvis or abdomen during pregnancy may be a sign of trouble. Pain may also be related to a condition other than pregnancy, such as appendicitis.
- **Vaginal bleeding** Bleeding and cramps in early pregnancy can be signs of miscarriage. Bleeding can also be a sign of an ectopic pregnancy (see page 233).
- **Sudden, rapid weight gain** Gaining more than 2 pounds a week during pregnancy and sudden swelling of your feet, hands, and face can be signs of high blood pressure. If not treated, high blood pressure can worsen and cause seizures in a pregnant woman (eclampsia, see page 428) and stillbirth (see page 430).
- **Headaches, blurred vision, pain in the upper right abdomen** These may be signs of high blood pressure.

Lower back pain during pregnancy

Lower back pain is a common problem during pregnancy as the growing uterus puts strain on the lower back. Lifting objects the proper way (see illustration on page 557) is especially important during pregnancy for helping to prevent back pain. You can help relieve lower back pain by applying ice or a heating pad to the sore area. Here are some other ways to prevent or relieve backache:

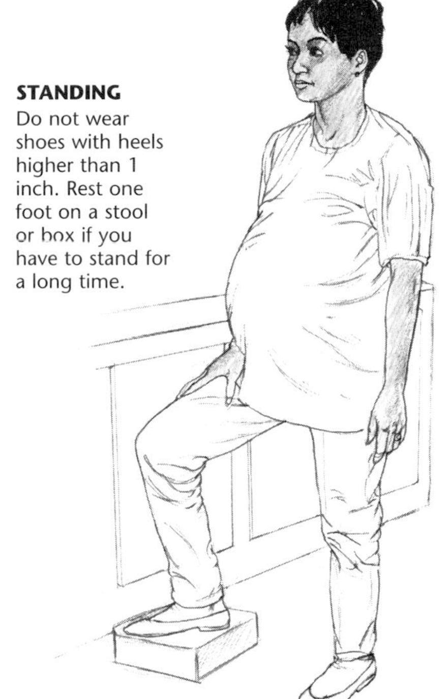

STANDING
Do not wear shoes with heels higher than 1 inch. Rest one foot on a stool or box if you have to stand for a long time.

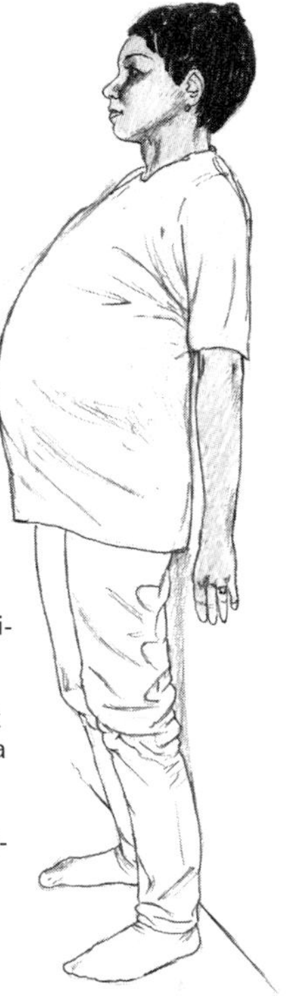

STRETCHING
Doing stretches called pelvic tilts can help strengthen your abdominal muscles and relieve lower back pain. For a pelvic tilt, stand straight with your back against a wall. Press your lower back into the wall by tightening your abdominal muscles.

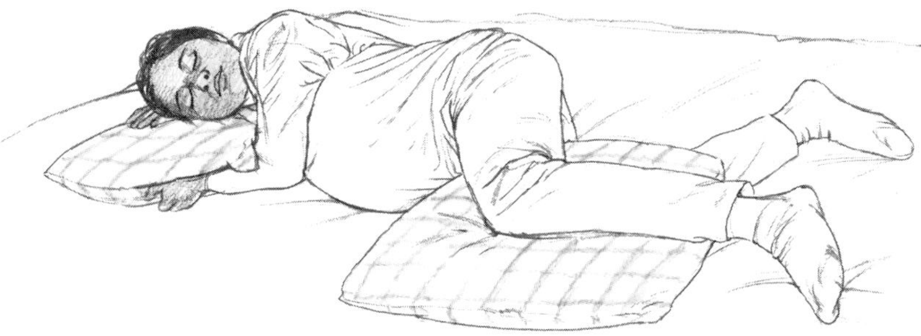

SLEEPING
Sleep on your side with your upper knee bent and supported by a pillow.

rule out a serious medical problem, such as an abscess (an infected, pus-filled sac) in the gums. If you need to have an X-ray, your abdomen will be shielded with a lead apron to protect the fetus from exposure to radiation. Your dentist will delay routine X-rays until after your pregnancy.

HIGH BLOOD PRESSURE

If you had high blood pressure before you became pregnant, you can safely carry a pregnancy to term as long as you have frequent checkups to monitor your blood pressure closely. Make sure your doctor knows if you have a history of high blood pressure. Mild high blood pressure that is controlled with exercise, diet, or low doses of medication may cause no complications at all during pregnancy. However, extremely high blood pressure that is not under control during pregnancy can cause such complications as delayed growth of the fetus, preeclampsia (see page 428), preterm labor (see page 427), placental abruption (see page 426), and low birth weight.

In addition to having more frequent checkups to measure your blood pressure, you may also have ultrasound examinations (see page 405) to monitor the growth of the fetus. The physical stress of pregnancy may raise already elevated blood pressure in women who have reduced kidney function that has resulted from high blood pressure. In this case, your doctor will recommend more frequent blood and urine tests during pregnancy to monitor the functioning of your kidneys.

DIABETES

Diabetes (see page 617) occurs when the body cannot make or use insulin, a hormone that converts sugar (glucose) from food into energy. If you have diabetes that is not controlled before you get pregnant, there is a greater risk of birth defects in the fetus. During pregnancy, uncontrolled diabetes increases the risk of miscarriage, high blood pressure (preeclampsia, page 428), hydramnios (excess fluid in the amniotic sac), postpartum hemorrhage, and a larger-than-average baby. A larger fetus is less likely to fit through the birth canal, increasing the likelihood of a cesarean delivery (see page 442). Pregnant women with diabetes are also more likely to have infections and these infections are likely to be more severe than usual.

Gestational diabetes Some women develop high sugar levels in their blood only while they are pregnant. Their pancreas is unable to produce enough insulin to counteract a hormone produced during pregnancy that increases sugar levels. This condition, called gestational diabetes, is more common in women who are over 30, obese, have a family history of diabetes, or had problems in a previous pregnancy such as a stillbirth or an unusually large baby. If you have any of these risk factors, you may be asked to have a test for diabetes in the first trimester of pregnancy. If the results of this first test are normal, you will have another test later in pregnancy—between weeks 24 and 28—as all pregnant women do. It is at this time in pregnancy that gestational diabetes usually develops.

For a glucose tolerance test, you drink a sugar solution and, 1 hour later, the sugar level in your blood is tested. If the level is high, you will have a 3-hour glucose tolerance test. This more extensive test measures your sugar level after 3 days of eating a special diet high in carbohydrates, which is designed to stimulate your pancreas to produce as much insulin as it can. After you have followed the diet for 3 days, your doctor will ask you to fast overnight. The next morning, your blood sugar level is measured. Then you are given another sugar solution to drink and your blood sugar level is tested 1, 2, and 3 hours later. If two out of the four tests are abnormal, you have gestational diabetes. If you are diagnosed with this form of diabetes, your doctor will recommend a diet and eating pattern to follow throughout your pregnancy to help control the condition. Most women with gestational diabetes can control it with diet.

Controlling diabetes during pregnancy If you have diabetes and are pregnant, your doctor will prescribe a diet that consists of eating recommended meals and snacks throughout the day. The number of calories you should eat depends on your weight and the stage of your pregnancy. Your intake of carbohydrates (starches and sugars) must be timed carefully so that your body does not take in too much or too little sugar in any one period. Your diet may need to be adjusted periodically to improve control of your sugar level or to meet the needs of the growing fetus. Regular exercise is also important in controlling diabetes. Your doctor will help you design an exercise program that is right for you, depending on your blood sugar levels and the stage of your pregnancy.

Some women with diabetes must take injections of insulin, sometimes four times a day, to control their diabetes. Insulin does not affect the fetus because the hormone does not cross the placenta. Your doctor will adjust the dose of insulin from time to time, depending on your blood sugar level. If you are taking insulin, you must monitor your sugar levels closely throughout the day. Many women use a blood glucose meter or chemically treated strips of paper to measure their sugar level.

If you have diabetes, you may need to have more frequent testing during pregnancy. For example, you may have tests for a type of hemoglobin (the oxygen-carrying protein in red blood cells) that has a sugar molecule attached to it. The level of this hemoglobin in your blood shows how well your glucose has been controlled over a period of several weeks. An increased level of this type of hemoglobin indicates inadequate control of your glucose level over the previous 4 to 8 weeks. This information can be useful in estimating the risk of birth defects in early pregnancy. You might also have other tests—such as an ultrasound (page 405), amniocentesis (page 406), or fetal monitoring (page 440)—to monitor the health of the fetus. If your glucose levels are not under control, you may have to be hospitalized to stabilize them. Your doctor may determine that you need additional treatment—including insulin shots and a regulated diet—to maintain your glucose level in a healthy range.

INFECTIONS

Although many infections, such as the common cold, cause no problems during pregnancy, some infections can result in serious complications, including birth defects, growth retardation, miscarriage, premature delivery, and stillbirth. Call your doctor immediately if you think you have an infection; do not try to treat it yourself.

Colds and influenza The symptoms of a cold and influenza are the same during pregnancy as at any other time—including fatigue, fever, pain in muscles and joints, and a runny nose. If you get a cold or the flu during pregnancy, do not treat yourself with over-the-counter medications—they may harm the fetus. Instead, ask your doctor what you can do to relieve the symptoms. During pregnancy, influenza is more likely to lead to pneumonia, which can be life threatening. It is a good idea to get a flu shot when you are pregnant, especially during an epidemic or if you are at increased risk of infection or complications that can result from infections—for example, if you have tested positive for HIV, the virus that causes AIDS (see page 344) or if you have sickle-cell anemia (see page 493). Because the influenza vaccine is made of killed viruses, flu shots are very safe.

Childhood diseases The childhood diseases chickenpox, rubella (German measles), and fifth disease can harm a fetus if a woman acquires them during pregnancy. If you have not had these infections or have not been vaccinated against rubella (see page 138) and you are planning a pregnancy, talk to your doctor. If you are already pregnant and you are not immune to these infections, avoid people who have these very contagious diseases. In general, do not visit households with sick children, especially if they have a rash.

Cytomegalovirus Cytomegalovirus is a virus that causes few, if any, symptoms. About 60 to 70 percent of all people have been previously infected with the virus, often without knowing it. The virus is spread through saliva, urine, or sexual contact. Cytomegalovirus rarely causes serious illness in adults, but, when transmitted to a fetus, it can cause severe illness, birth defects including blindness and mental retardation, or death—especially if the woman has the infection for the first time. The virus can be transmitted to the fetus through the placenta or through the vagina at birth, or to a nursing infant through breast milk. The risk of harming the fetus is greatest if the woman becomes infected during the first trimester of pregnancy. Still, only a small percentage of children who are born with the infection have severe adverse effects from it.

You should be tested for cytomegalovirus if you think you have been exposed to an infected person or if you have a flu-like illness. If a cytomegalovirus infection occurs early in pregnancy, especially if it is your first infection, talk to your doctor about the risk to your fetus.

Pneumonia Pneumonia, an infection of the lungs, can be more serious during pregnancy than at other times because it can reduce the oxygen supply of both the woman and fetus. It is important to diagnose and treat pneumonia as early as possible. The infection is diagnosed from a chest X-ray—a lead apron over the pregnant woman's abdomen shields the fetus from radiation.

Treatment often includes antibiotics that are safe to take during pregnancy. In some cases, a hospital stay is necessary.

Sexually transmitted diseases Some sexually transmitted diseases (STDs)—HIV (the virus that causes AIDS), genital herpes, hepatitis B, and genital warts—can be transmitted to the fetus during pregnancy or childbirth, with serious consequences. If you suspect you have an STD, tell your doctor. He or she can test you and take steps to protect the fetus. (For more about STDs, see chapter 12.)

Toxoplasmosis Toxoplasmosis is an infection caused by a parasite that lives in raw meat and in some mammals, including cats. In adults, the infection can cause mild flulike symptoms, including fatigue and muscle pain. If a pregnant woman becomes infected, there is a one in three chance that her fetus will become infected. Most infants born with toxoplasmosis have only minor symptoms, but some children eventually develop neurological problems and even blindness. In rare cases, the infection is fatal.

If you have a cat, your doctor can test you to see if you are immune to toxoplasmosis. If you are immune, your fetus cannot become infected. If you are not immune, you need to take precautions to avoid infection. Do not eat uncooked or rare meat and avoid contact with cat feces in litter boxes, garden soil, and sandboxes. Wash your hands frequently. If you suspect you may have been infected during pregnancy, your doctor can test you and, if necessary, the fetus. You can be treated with antibiotics, which decreases, but does not totally eliminate, the risk of infection in the fetus.

Urinary tract infections Infections of the urinary tract are common during pregnancy. Hormonal changes cause the smooth muscles of the bladder to relax, which may allow more bacteria to enter. When the enlarging uterus presses on the bladder, it can slow the flow of urine, making the bladder more susceptible to infection. Most urinary tract infections clear up quickly with treatment but, when not treated, can cause problems for both pregnant woman and fetus, including preterm labor (see page 427).

Cystitis (infection of the bladder; see page 543) is the most common urinary tract infection. Symptoms of cystitis include more frequent urination, burning pain during urination, and blood in the urine. Treatment with antibiotics is usually effective. Another urinary tract infection, pyelonephritis (infection of the kidney; see page 544), has symptoms similar to those of cystitis, but they are usually accompanied by fever and back pain. Pyelonephritis is more serious than cystitis and, if untreated, can lead to preterm labor. In rare cases, pyelonephritis progresses to chronic kidney disease. The infection is usually treated in the hospital with antibiotics administered intravenously. See page 542 for more about urinary tract infections.

KIDNEY DISEASE

During pregnancy, your kidneys filter your waste products and those of the fetus. If your doctor suspects from your health history or a physical examination that you have kidney disease, he or she will prescribe blood and urine tests to make an accurate diagnosis. For example, protein in the urine is one sign of kidney disease. Treatment depends on the cause of the problem. If kidney disease is not treated during pregnancy, it can worsen and lead to growth retardation in the fetus and preterm labor (see page 427). Some kidney problems are caused by high blood pressure and subside once the blood pressure is under control. Urinary tract infections can also contribute to kidney disorders. (See page 546 for more about kidney disorders.) Urinary tract infections are more common during pregnancy. See your doctor if you experience pain during urination.

EPILEPSY

Most women with epilepsy have normal pregnancies. However, some medications used to control seizures increase the risk of birth defects. Medications such as valproic acid and trimethadione should not be used during pregnancy. Although the reason is unclear, these drugs substantially increase the risk of birth defects such as neural tube defects (which affect the spine or brain), heart defects, or cleft lip and palate. Many other common drugs used to control seizures, including phenytoin and phenobarbital, carry a lower risk of birth defects. Discuss your medication with your doctor.

You may have to take higher doses of your medication because of the physical stress of pregnancy and the increased blood circulation through your uterus to the placenta and fetus. Because you have more blood in your circulatory system, which continues to increase as the pregnancy progresses, your usual dose of medication may no longer be sufficient to control your seizures. If your seizures are poorly controlled, they may increase in frequency as your pregnancy advances. If you have a seizure during pregnancy, the oxygen supply to the fetus can be cut off, potentially causing great harm or even death. For this reason, doctors recommend that pregnant women with epilepsy continue taking their usual medication or a safe alternative. The level of the medication in your blood will be measured periodically throughout your pregnancy to make sure that you are receiving an adequate dose.

HEART DISEASE

Women who have heart disease during their reproductive years usually have either rheumatic heart disease (which results from a childhood infection called rheumatic fever) or congenital heart disease (a heart defect that was present at birth). These conditions are usually diagnosed before pregnancy. A woman with heart disease must be carefully monitored throughout her pregnancy because pregnancy increases the workload of the heart, and labor and delivery place added stress on the heart. Your doctor may prescribe extra rest and medications.

If your heart condition does not cause any symptoms or limit your activity before pregnancy, you can probably withstand the stress of pregnancy with no difficulty. However, if your condition already limits your activities, you will be monitored especially carefully throughout your pregnancy for signs of declining heart function or an inadequate blood supply to the placenta and fetus.

Women with heart disease are more likely to give birth prematurely and their babies tend to be smaller because blood circulation through the placenta to the fetus is often less than normal. Women who have congenital heart disease have an estimated 4- to 5-percent risk of giving birth to a baby with the same disorder. Sophisticated ultrasound tests done after the 20th week of pregnancy can diagnose most heart defects in the fetus and make it possible to plan in advance for an infant who may need special care after delivery.

Complications during pregnancy

While most women have a normal, uncomplicated pregnancy and delivery, a number of serious complications can occur that can endanger the health of the fetus and the pregnant woman. Being aware of the signs and symptoms of potential problems during pregnancy helps you recognize them if they occur and enables you to bring them to your doctor's attention. You can learn about the signs of possible complications by attending childbirth education classes offered by hospitals and local groups. Ask your doctor about these classes. The earlier in pregnancy a problem is recognized, the more likely treatment is to be successful.

MISCARRIAGE

A miscarriage is the spontaneous termination of pregnancy before the fetus is developed enough to survive outside the uterus. Miscarriage is very common—it occurs in 15 to 20 percent of all pregnancies. The most common causes of miscarriage are abnormalities of the chromosomes (genetic structures) of the developing embryo or fetus. Most chromosome abnormalities (see page 374) are detected by a woman's body and rejected, usually before the eighth week of pregnancy.

Vaginal bleeding and cramps in the pelvic area are the major signs of impending miscarriage. In many cases, the fetus has died days or weeks before the miscarriage occurs. Some women discover that the usual symptoms of pregnancy, such as nausea and breast tenderness, begin to subside even before their miscarriage is diagnosed. Blood tests that show decreasing levels of human chorionic gonadotropin (HCG), a hormone released by the developing embryo, and an ultrasound examination that shows no fetal heartbeat can confirm that the fetus has died.

A small percentage of miscarriages result when a woman's uterus has an

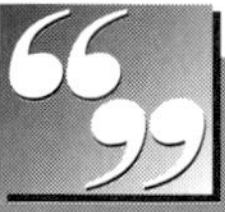

ONE WOMAN'S STORY
MISCARRIAGE

We had been married 3 years when my husband and I decided to start our family. We wanted to have two or three children. I stopped taking the pill and, after 4 months of trying, I became pregnant. We were elated and told our family and friends right away. We even started shopping for baby furniture and clothes.

In about the sixth week of pregnancy (8 weeks after my last period), I began to have some vaginal bleeding. I went to the doctor right away. She examined me and did an ultrasound. She told me she could not detect a fetal heartbeat on the ultrasound. She said it may just be too early in the pregnancy to see a heartbeat or I may not be as far along in the pregnancy as I thought. The other possibility was that I was about to have a miscarriage. She described what would happen if I had a miscarriage and what I should do if it occurred at home. She told me to go home and take it easy until the bleeding stopped or until she reexamined me the next week.

A few days later I had a miscarriage at home. It was like having an especially heavy period. Even though I was very upset I did exactly what the doctor had told me to do—I collected as much of the tissue as I could and put it into a jar to bring to the doctor's office so she could send it to a laboratory for examination. She told me that the laboratory could confirm that I had had a miscarriage. She said that most miscarriages during the first trimester of pregnancy are caused by errors that occur in the genetic material of the embryo and are the body's natural way of ending a pregnancy that isn't normal.

My husband and I were devastated. My doctor reassured us that a single miscarriage didn't reduce our chances of having a healthy pregnancy the next time. In fact, she said my chances of giving birth to a healthy, full-term baby were just as good as anyone else's.

"My doctor reassured us that a single miscarriage didn't reduce our chances of having a healthy pregnancy the next time."

The doctor told me some things I could do to help reduce my risk of having another miscarriage. I'm making these changes now—before I get pregnant again. I'm eating a much healthier diet and I'm taking a prenatal multivitamin/mineral supplement that has the right amount of the nutrients, including the vitamin folic acid, that are essential for a healthy pregnancy. My doctor told me that folic acid is especially important because it helps prevent many birth defects that can occur in the first 3 months of pregnancy. I'm avoiding alcohol, caffeine, and all drugs except those my doctor says are OK to take during pregnancy. I'm walking every day so that I'll be in good shape when I get pregnant. I plan to continue exercising throughout my pregnancy.

abnormal shape. In many cases, the abnormality can be corrected surgically to allow the woman to carry a future pregnancy to term. Daughters of women who took a medication called DES (diethylstilbestrol) when they were pregnant often have this problem.

Other causes of miscarriage include scar tissue on the lining of the uterus (endometrium) that has resulted from a complicated dilation and curettage (D and C; see page 262) or fibroids (see page 221) that take up space inside the uterus. Both of these conditions interfere with a fertilized egg's ability to implant itself in the endometrium.

There is nothing you can do to prevent a miscarriage that is about to occur. If you have a miscarriage at home, it is important to save all of the tissue that passes out of your body and bring it to your doctor in a clean glass jar. The tissue will be examined to make sure you have eliminated all of it. If there is any tissue remaining behind, you may have to have a D and C or vacuum aspiration (see page 331) to remove it.

The tissue from the miscarriage can be analyzed in a laboratory to help determine the cause. This information can be useful if you plan to become pregnant again. After a miscarriage, you can try to conceive again once you have had one normal period.

Your risk of having another miscarriage depends on the cause of the first one. A single miscarriage does not reduce your chances of having a healthy pregnancy the next time. However, a series of several miscarriages in a row may indicate a more serious problem such as an abnormally shaped uterus or a chromosome abnormality in you or your partner that does not affect you but can affect an egg or a sperm. Genetic testing (see page 373) and treatment may be available that can help you have a successful pregnancy in the future.

INCOMPETENT CERVIX

During normal labor, the cervix opens (dilates) to allow the fetus to pass through the vagina during delivery. In some women, the cervix is too weak to hold the increasing weight of the fetus during the entire pregnancy. This condition is called incompetent cervix. If the cervix opens too soon (during the second trimester), the result may be extremely premature birth—before the fetus can survive outside the uterus.

There are many things that can cause an incompetent cervix. Occasionally, a woman is born with insufficient connective tissue to hold her cervix closed. An abnormality of the cervix may also occur in women whose mother took a medication called DES (diethylstilbestrol) during pregnancy to prevent morning sickness. Often, incompetent cervix results from previous injury to the cervix. For example, surgery performed on the cervix, including a cone biopsy (see page 220) to rule out cervical cancer after an abnormal Pap smear, can weaken the cervix.

An incompetent cervix is difficult to diagnose in first pregnancies and in many women who have no symptoms. Frequently, a diagnosis is not made until a woman has a miscarriage. If your doctor suspects you may have a weak cervix or if you have previously been diagnosed as having an incompetent cervix, he or she will ask you to report immediately during your pregnancy any feeling of pressure or cramps in your pelvic area, or any bloody or watery discharge from your vagina. Your cervix will be examined frequently during your pregnancy for signs of dilation.

Treatment of an incompetent cervix depends on the stage of pregnancy and the certainty of the diagnosis. The most common treatment is to stitch the cervix close after the 12th week of pregnancy to prevent it from opening too early or from opening any further. If the diagnosis is uncertain, your doctor may continue to examine your cervix once a week for signs of dilation. He or she may also recommend bed rest and abstinence from sexual intercourse during this time. The stitch is removed when you go into labor or when your pregnancy reaches full term, whichever comes first.

BLEEDING IN THIRD TRIMESTER

Some women experience vaginal bleeding during the third trimester. Abnormalities of the placenta, the organ that grows inside the uterus to nourish and sustain the fetus, are responsible for most of this bleeding. The placenta allows nutrients and oxygen in the pregnant woman's blood to flow to the fetus and

SYMPTOM CHART

Vaginal bleeding during pregnancy

Any vaginal bleeding at all during pregnancy.

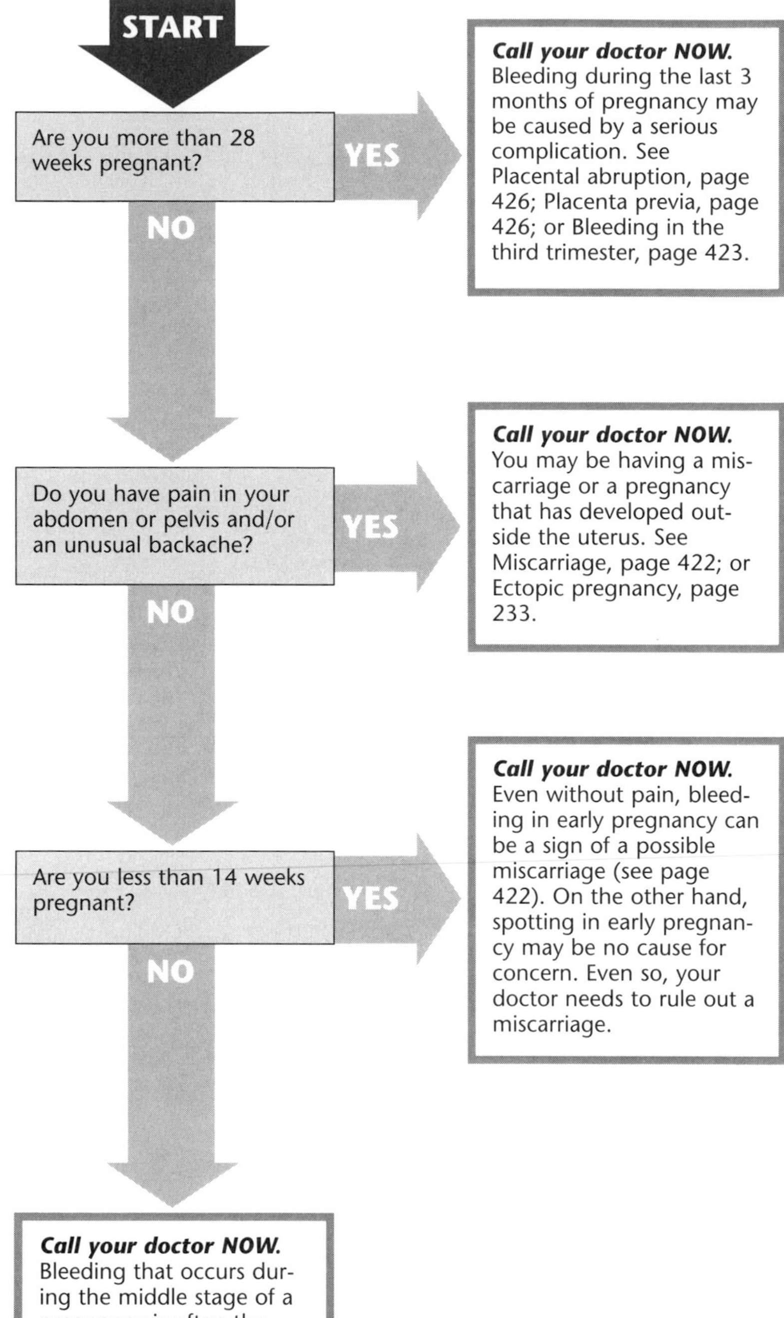

Bleeding

If you experience bleeding at any time during your pregnancy, call your doctor immediately. Bleeding can be an indication of a miscarriage; a pregnancy that has developed outside the uterus, usually in a fallopian tube; or another serious complication.

SYMPTOM CHART

Back pain during pregnancy

Dull pain and stiffness in your middle and lower back that make it difficult for you to get up from a sitting or lying position; the pain is likely to worsen as your pregnancy progresses.

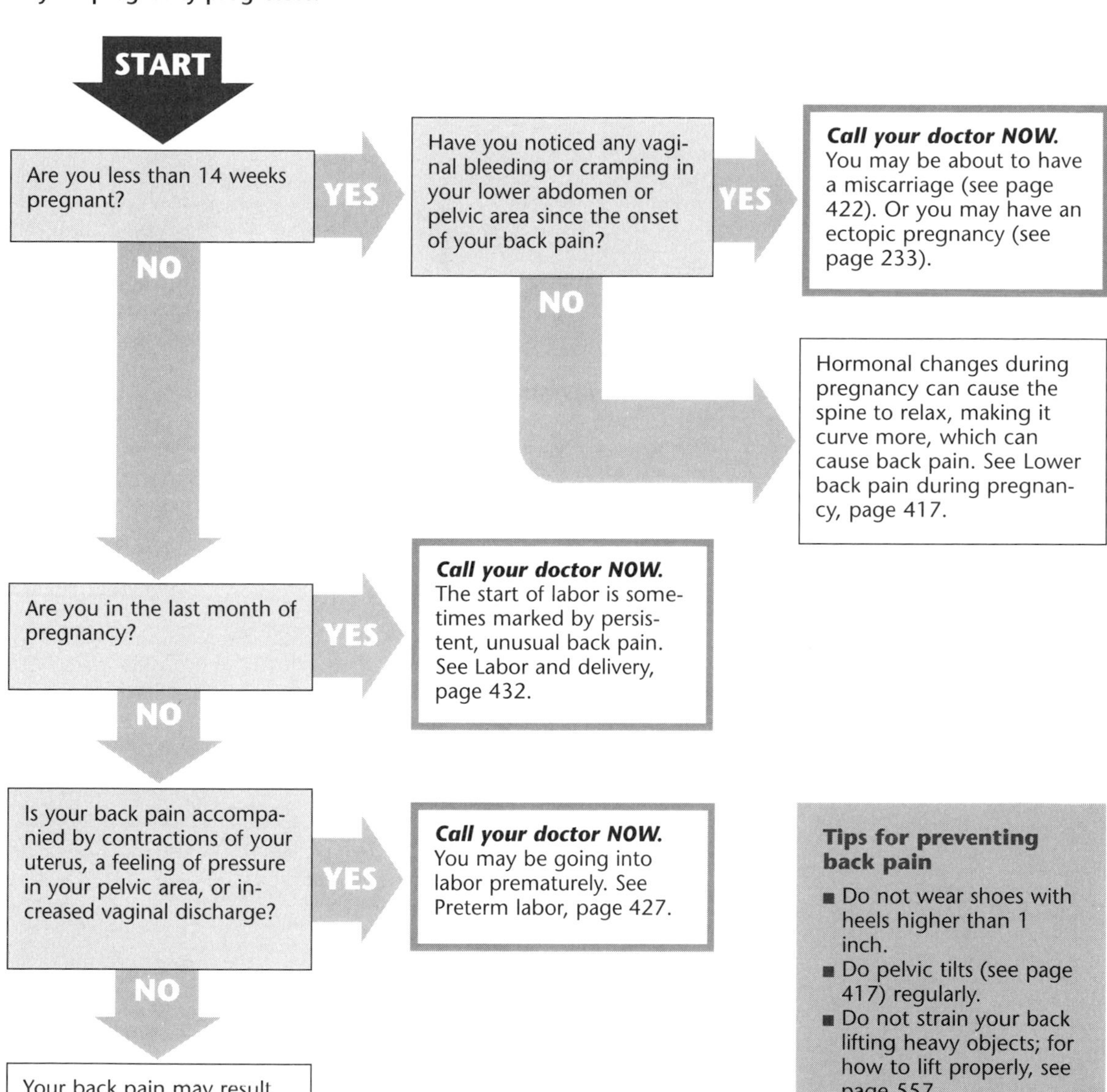

Tips for preventing back pain

- Do not wear shoes with heels higher than 1 inch.
- Do pelvic tilts (see page 417) regularly.
- Do not strain your back lifting heavy objects; for how to lift properly, see page 557.

If you have lower back pain that persists, see your doctor.

waste products from the fetus to be passed into the woman's blood for elimination. Call your doctor immediately if you notice any bleeding at any time during your pregnancy.

Placenta previa In a condition called placenta previa, the placenta covers the cervix to some degree, partially or completely blocking the entry into the vagina. Normally, the placenta is attached to the top portion of the uterus—at the part farthest away from the cervix. Although you will not experience any pain with placenta previa, you may have bleeding, usually during the last trimester of pregnancy. Call your doctor immediately.

The severity of placenta previa can be determined by an ultrasound examination (see page 405). Your doctor can evaluate the health of the fetus with the ultrasound, as well as with fetal heart rate monitoring (see page 404). Because the position of the placenta can change as the uterus grows, your doctor may recommend another ultrasound at a later time to watch for these changes. If the placenta is only marginally blocking your cervix, it may not affect your pregnancy in any way. If the placenta moves away from the cervix as your uterus grows larger, and no longer blocks the vagina, you can have a normal delivery.

In cases in which the placenta is partially blocking the cervix, a doctor may recommend limiting physical activity or abstaining from sexual intercourse. If the placenta completely blocks the cervix and birth canal, precautions such as bed rest may be necessary. Walking around can cause the weight of the fetus to put pressure on the portion of the placenta that covers the cervix, sometimes causing bleeding. Vaginal bleeding that is severe or recurrent may require hospitalization. If you are in labor, your cervix begins to dilate (open) and the lower part of your uterus expands. Portions of the placenta that are attached to these areas may tear away and begin to bleed. Very heavy bleeding may indicate that the placenta has detached, thereby cutting off the blood supply to the fetus. Immediate delivery may be necessary, usually by cesarean section (see page 442); although severe bleeding is rarely fatal to the pregnant woman, it can cause the death of the fetus.

If bleeding is light or stops on its own and the fetus is not in any danger, your doctor may want to monitor your condition with more frequent checkups. If you have experienced more than one episode of bleeding, you may be hospitalized for closer observation.

Placental abruption Placental abruption, or abruptio placentae as it is sometimes called, occurs when a placenta that is implanted normally inside the uterus separates prematurely from the wall of the uterus, usually during the third

PLACENTA PREVIA

In placenta previa, the placenta is attached to the uterus at the wrong place—near the bottom instead of at the uppermost portion. In complete placenta previa (right), the placenta covers the entire cervix, blocking entrance to the vagina. In partial placenta previa (center), the placenta blocks part of the cervix. In marginal placenta previa (far right), the placenta does not cover the cervix, but reaches to its edge.

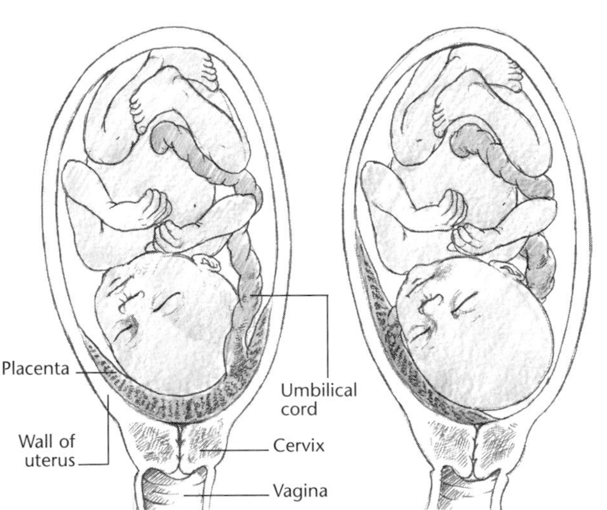

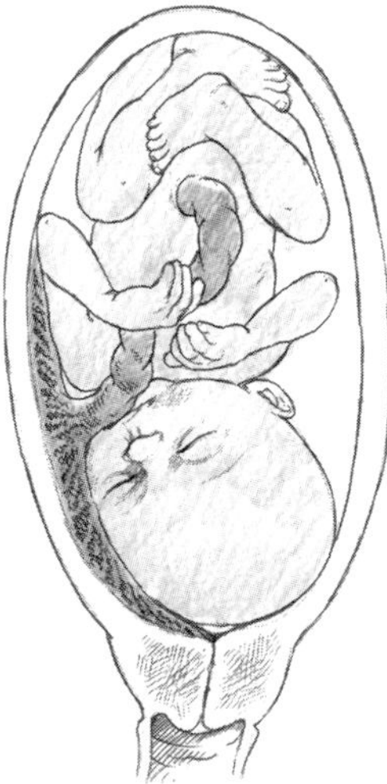

trimester of pregnancy. This detachment severs the blood vessels that attach the placenta to the wall of the uterus, cutting off the fetus's circulation, which can be life threatening. Placental abruption often causes vaginal bleeding.

In most cases, the cause of placental abruption is unknown, but it occurs most often in pregnancies of women who have high blood pressure, either long-term or related to pregnancy (preeclampsia, see page 428). Because the separation of the placenta from the wall of the uterus may be rapid and complete or slow and partial, the signs and symptoms of placental abruption vary greatly. The condition frequently causes vaginal bleeding and pain during the third trimester of pregnancy.

In some cases, the blood stays between the placenta and the wall of the uterus and does not escape through the cervix and vagina. The irritation caused by blood collecting beneath the placenta may trigger contractions of the uterus, initiating preterm labor (see page 427). If the degree of separation of the placenta is high enough to interfere with blood circulation to the fetus, fetal monitoring will detect an abnormal heart rate pattern in the fetus. In a complete placental abruption, all of the placenta detaches from the wall of the uterus and the fetus's heart rate shows signs of severe difficulties. At this point, immediate delivery, usually by cesarean section, is required to save the life of the fetus.

PRETERM LABOR

Preterm labor is labor that occurs before the 37th week of pregnancy and can threaten the life of the fetus. About 10 percent of all infants are born preterm. Because their lungs have not had time to develop fully, many infants who are born before the 36th week die of a condition called respiratory distress syndrome.

Women at greatest risk of going into labor early are those who:

- Are carrying more than one fetus.
- Had a previous premature delivery or preterm labor.
- Have an abnormality of the uterus, such as an abnormal shape, or cervix, such as an incompetent cervix.
- Have a condition (hydramnios) in which there is too much amniotic fluid around the fetus.
- Have an infection, especially a kidney infection, during pregnancy.
- Use cocaine (see page 414).
- Have had previous surgery on their cervix, such as a cone biopsy (see page 220).
- Have bleeding after the first trimester (see page 423).
- Have had two or more abortions during the second trimester of pregnancy (see page 332).
- Have been exposed to DES (see page 252).

After you report your symptoms to your doctor, he or she will examine you to see whether your cervix has begun to open (dilate) or shorten. You may have an ultrasound (see page 405) to estimate the size and age of the fetus and determine its position in your uterus. Your doctor will ask you to monitor your contractions over the next several days and report any increase in their frequency or severity. Your cervix will be examined more frequently to watch for changes, such as dilation or thinning (effacement, see page 432), that may indicate you are in labor. These changes in your cervix are the most accurate indication that you are in labor.

Treatment of preterm labor depends on the stage of the pregnancy. If there are no signs that the fetus is in danger from infection, bleeding, or other complications, doctors usually recommend bed rest to decrease pressure on the cervix. Your doctor may also tell you to drink more fluids to avoid dehydration, which can sometimes cause mild contractions of the uterus. In some cases, medication can stop or lessen contractions.

WARNING SIGNS
PRETERM LABOR

The signs that you are going into labor prematurely may be obvious or subtle. Call your doctor immediately if you have any of the following symptoms at any time during your pregnancy:

- Vaginal discharge that is bloody or watery, or contains more mucus than usual
- Pressure in your pelvis or lower abdomen
- Abdominal cramps, especially if accompanied by diarrhea and a fever
- Regular contractions or tightening of the uterus

You should refrain from intercourse during this time; do not insert anything (such as a tampon or medicated cream) into your vagina.

If your contractions stop, your doctor may tell you to go home and feel the surface of your abdomen regularly for tightening, which might indicate contractions. If you feel contractions, count them for an hour. If you feel more than six per hour, call your doctor. You may be hospitalized until the contractions stop or, possibly, you deliver. In some cases, labor is too far along to be stopped. In other cases, delivery is allowed to proceed because there are signs of an infection or bleeding or indications that the fetus may be having problems—all of which can make it riskier to prolong the pregnancy than to deliver the baby early.

PREECLAMPSIA

In some women, pregnancy causes high blood pressure. When high blood pressure is accompanied by fluid retention and leaking of protein into the woman's urine, it is a condition called preeclampsia (or toxemia or pregnancy-induced hypertension). In cases of preeclampsia, high blood pressure can cause severe complications for both the woman and fetus. Extremely high blood pressure (higher than 160/110) can damage the woman's kidneys, brain, eyes, and liver by causing bleeding in these organs.

If preeclampsia causes seizures, which can be fatal for both the woman and fetus, it moves into a stage called eclampsia. High blood pressure may lead to seizures by decreasing the amount of oxygen delivered to the woman's brain. Seizures caused by eclampsia may also be linked to brain hemorrhage (stroke). Stroke is the most common cause of maternal death from eclampsia. Even mildly high blood pressure can decrease the flow of blood and oxygen to the placenta, causing malnourishment and retarded growth of the fetus. Premature delivery sometimes results.

Frequent visits to your doctor throughout your pregnancy, beginning early in pregnancy, are the best way to detect early signs of high blood pressure. The earlier you begin treatment for high blood pressure, the better the chances for successful treatment and the less likely that your blood pressure will reach dangerously high levels. Although all pregnant women are monitored for high blood pressure, those at greatest risk are women under 20 or over 30, or who have a history of high blood pressure or are overweight.

You are considered to have high blood pressure during pregnancy if the reading shows an increase over your level before pregnancy of 30 points in the systolic pressure (the top number of your reading) or 15 points in the diastolic pressure (the bottom number); any diastolic pressure over 100 indicates high blood pressure. If you have high blood pressure, your doctor will probably ask you to come in for more frequent visits so your blood pressure can be monitored.

Many medications that are usually prescribed for high blood pressure are not safe to take during pregnancy. Your doctor will prescribe a medication that is safe. He or she will also prescribe bed rest and ask you to log the fetus's movements on a "kick chart" throughout the day. If you feel eight or more kicks in your abdomen within 1 hour, it usually indicates that the fetus is healthy.

When preeclampsia is mild, the doctor will prescribe bed rest and allow the pregnancy to continue if there are no signs of difficulties for the fetus. You will have ultrasound (see page 405) to monitor the fetus's growth and the amount of amniotic fluid inside the uterus. Lack of growth of a fetus and a low level of amniotic fluid indicate that the placenta is unhealthy and not delivering adequate nutrients to the fetus. In this case, early delivery may be necessary. If the pregnancy is not yet full term, various tests are used to help determine whether or not early delivery is required. For example, a doctor may perform a nonstress test (see page 404) to evaluate the health of the fetus. If the pregnancy is already full term, most doctors will forego further testing and deliver the baby.

In severe cases, eclampsia threatens the woman's life, and the only choice is to deliver the baby by induced labor (see page 439) or cesarean delivery (see page 442), regardless of how far along the pregnancy is. After delivery, the woman's blood pressure usually returns to normal and she has no adverse long-term effects. However, she may have an increased risk of high blood pressure later in life.

MULTIPLE BIRTHS

Twins occur once in every 90 births; two out of three are fraternal twins. Fraternal twins result when two different eggs are fertilized by two different sperm; identical twins result when a single egg fertilized by one sperm divides at an early stage into two identical embryos. The incidence of identical twins is nearly the same throughout the world. However, the incidence of fraternal twins varies between races and within countries and is affected by factors such as the pregnant woman's age and the number of pregnancies she has had. Black women and women between 35 and 40 are more likely to have twins than other women. The more pregnancies a woman has had, the more likely she is to have twins.

The incidence of fraternal twins and other multiple births has been increasing in recent decades because more women are taking fertility drugs (see page 386). A suspected multiple birth can be confirmed by an ultrasound examination (see page 405). In some cases, a multiple birth is discovered during an ultrasound done for another purpose.

If you are carrying more than one fetus, there is a greater risk of complications during your pregnancy. You will have more frequent prenatal checkups so that any problems are found as early as possible. Because your nutritional needs are greater, you should gain about 35 to 45 pounds during your pregnancy—about 1½ pounds per week during the second and third trimesters.

High blood pressure is more common in women with multiple births. If you have high blood pressure, your doctor may recommend bed rest; in severe cases, an early delivery may be necessary. See page 418 for more about high blood pressure during pregnancy.

Preterm labor (see page 427) is common in multiple births. About half of all multiple births occur before the 37th week of pregnancy because the fetuses grow too large for the uterus, triggering contractions. If early delivery seems likely, your doctor may recommend bed rest, which can increase blood flow to the uterus by helping muscles in the uterus relax. Your doctor may also recommend abstinence from sexual intercourse because intercourse can stimulate the cervix and cause the uterus to contract.

Labor may be slower and more difficult for a woman with a multiple birth. Depending on the number of fetuses and their position inside the uterus, a cesarean delivery (see page 442) may be necessary.

Multiple births are more likely to be of lower-than-average birth weight because of decreased space to grow inside the uterus and increased demands on the placenta for nutrients and oxygen. You will have more frequent ultrasound examinations to monitor the growth of the fetuses and to watch for changes in their positions. Nonstress tests (see page 404) may also be necessary, especially if one fetus or both are not growing at the normal rate.

Signs of multiple births

Although it is sometimes difficult to tell if there is more than one fetus in the uterus, your doctor will look for signs of a multiple birth if any of the following conditions exist:

- Your uterus is larger than expected or growing at an unusually rapid pace.
- You used fertility drugs.
- You have a family history of twins.
- The doctor detects more than one fetal heartbeat.
- You feel more fetal movement than in previous pregnancies.

POSTTERM PREGNANCY

Most women give birth at some time between the 37th and 42nd week of pregnancy. Ten percent of pregnancies last longer. If a pregnancy goes beyond 42 weeks, it is called postterm, or postdate. Most doctors recommend inducing labor (see page 439) at this point, or even before the 42nd week. Before making a decision about inducing labor, your doctor will perform tests to make sure that your expected due date was calculated correctly and the fetus is healthy. He or she will also examine your cervix to see if it is dilated and ready for delivery.

Although more than 90 percent of babies born between weeks 42 and 44 are completely healthy, a fetus is considered to be at increased risk when a pregnancy continues beyond the 42nd week. In some postterm pregnancies, a fetus may have an abnormal heart rate in response to labor because the blood vessels in the placenta are less healthy and do not transport oxygen as efficiently to the fetus. Another potential problem in postterm pregnancies is that the fetus may be so large (9 pounds or more) that it is difficult to deliver vaginally. It is common in postterm pregnancies for a fetus to have a first bowel movement (called meconium) into the amniotic fluid; this can be dangerous if the fetus inhales the meconium, which can block its air passages.

At this late stage, there is also a risk that the placenta will stop functioning normally, which can reduce the amount of oxygen and nutrients to the fetus or cause the fetus to secrete less urine, thereby reducing the volume of amniotic fluid. Amniotic fluid provides cushioning between the fetus and the wall of the uterus. A deficiency of amniotic fluid decreases this cushioning during labor contractions, which can cause the umbilical cord to be compressed, cutting off the fetus's life support.

An accurate due date is the most important factor in helping doctors diagnose postterm pregnancy. However, it is not always possible to calculate an exact due date, especially in women who have irregular periods. The health and well-being of the fetus are also evaluated using fetal monitoring such as nonstress tests (see page 404). If the fetus appears to be healthy, the doctor may continue monitoring its health while waiting for labor to begin naturally. If the fetus appears to be at risk, the doctor may induce labor with the drug oxytocin, which stimulates contractions of the uterus, or recommend a cesarean delivery (see page 442). Whether or not to deliver the baby surgically depends on the condition of the fetus, including its size, and how dilated the woman's cervix is.

STILLBIRTH

A stillbirth is the birth of a dead baby after the 28th week of pregnancy. There are many possible causes of stillbirth but about 20 percent result when the fetus has severe birth defects. Stillbirth can also be caused by hemorrhage (see page 423), high blood pressure, diabetes or another condition that affects the placenta, or Rh factor incompatibility (see page 371). About one third of stillbirths have no known cause. If not treated, some infections (see page 378)—including measles, chickenpox, influenza, toxoplasmosis, rubella, cytomegalovirus, genital herpes, syphilis, and malaria—may cause stillbirth. If you acquire an infection during pregnancy, call your doctor immediately.

Coping with loss in pregnancy

Many women experience profound distress and sadness after losing a fetus. Most miscarriages occur in early pregnancy but they can also occur late, or the pregnancy can end with a stillbirth. Some women are able to "put on a happy face," minimize their emotional distress, and look forward to future pregnancies. But it is natural to have feelings of inadequacy, anger, sadness, guilt over something that may have contributed to the loss (real or imagined), embarrassment, or a feeling of hopelessness. You may be reluctant to talk about your loss or not know what to say. Advice and attempts at consolation from family and friends are sometimes more upsetting than comforting.

Your response to the loss of a fetus depends on your personality, ability to cope, and the meaning the pregnancy has for you personally and in your relationship with your partner. Support from loved ones and the opportunity to grieve are extremely important in the process of accepting your loss and moving on with your life. Some women find that holding a funeral or memorial service helps resolve this painful experience. If you become unable to function at home or at work for a prolonged period, or if you feel the need for help, you may benefit from counseling or joining a support group of other women who have had a similar experience. Talk to your doctor; he or she may be able to help you or refer you to a counselor or support group.

CHAPTER 16

Childbirth and new motherhood

Contents

For many women, giving birth is one of the most joyful experiences of their life. But childbirth can also involve intense pain and anxiety. Your experience can be influenced by your level of understanding of the process of labor and delivery and your expectations after delivery. Understanding what is going on inside your body enables you to work more effectively with your doctor to make the choices that are appropriate for you.

Labor and delivery

The experience of childbirth is different for every woman. In fact, the same woman goes through the process in a different way each time she has a baby. But for the majority of women, the stages of labor and delivery follow a general pattern that can give you a good idea of what to expect.

THE STAGES OF LABOR

Labor is divided into three main stages—dilation and effacement (opening and thinning of the cervix), delivery of the baby, and delivery of the placenta. The duration of labor can vary greatly—from an hour or less to more than a day. In a woman giving birth for the first time, labor usually lasts about 18 to 24 hours from the time the uterus begins to contract to the time of delivery. The length of labor is often, but not always, shorter for subsequent births.

Stage 1: Dilation and effacement The first stage of labor varies the most among women and is usually the longest. This stage begins when your cervix starts to thin (efface) and open (dilate) to allow the baby to pass through. The extent of effacement is expressed in percentages, with 100 percent as the goal. The extent of dilation is expressed in centimeters, with 10 centimeters as the goal. Effacement and dilation can occur independently of one another. For example, as your labor progresses, you may be told, "You are 4 centimeters dilated and 80 percent effaced." The first stage ends when your cervix is fully dilated.

The muscles of your uterus contract in a regular pattern to open the cervix and push the baby out of the uterus and down the vagina. Contractions feel different to every woman but in early labor they often feel like menstrual cramps with a mild backache. As labor progresses, the intensity of contractions gradually increases, although contractions can vary in intensity from one to the next.

This first stage of labor has three phases—early, active, and transition. In the early phase of labor, your cervix dilates to 4 centimeters. Contractions are generally mild, occurring every 15 to 20 minutes and lasting 60 to 90 seconds. (You time the spacing of contractions from the beginning of one contraction to the beginning of the next.) They gradually become stronger and more frequent until they occur about every 5 minutes. During the active phase, your cervix dilates from 4 to 8 centimeters. Contractions become stronger, occurring about every 3 minutes and lasting about 45 seconds.

In the transition phase, your cervix dilates fully to 10 centimeters (about 4 inches in diameter). Contractions, which are now 2 to 3 minutes apart and last about a minute, seem to come one right after the other, almost in waves, and are usually the most intense of labor. This phase can be the most difficult, but it seldom lasts longer than 1 or 2 hours. It is during transition that many women feel most tense, irritable, or out of control. At the end of this stage, the baby has usually begun to descend into the vagina and you may be feeling a strong urge to push.

Stage 2: Delivery In the second stage of labor, contractions help push the baby through the vagina. After your doctor confirms that your cervix is fully dilated, you will be told to push or bear down when you feel a contraction. If your cervix is not fully dilated, you will be asked not to push, even though you may have a strong urge to do so because of the pressure of the baby's head low in your pelvis. Pushing before full dilation may press the baby's head against your cervix, causing the cervix to swell, which would be counterproductive.

The length of the pushing stage

DILATION OF THE CERVIX
In the first stage of labor, the cervix gradually dilates, or opens. When the cervix is open 10 centimeters, it is fully dilated, and the baby's head will begin to press through the cervix and enter the vagina.

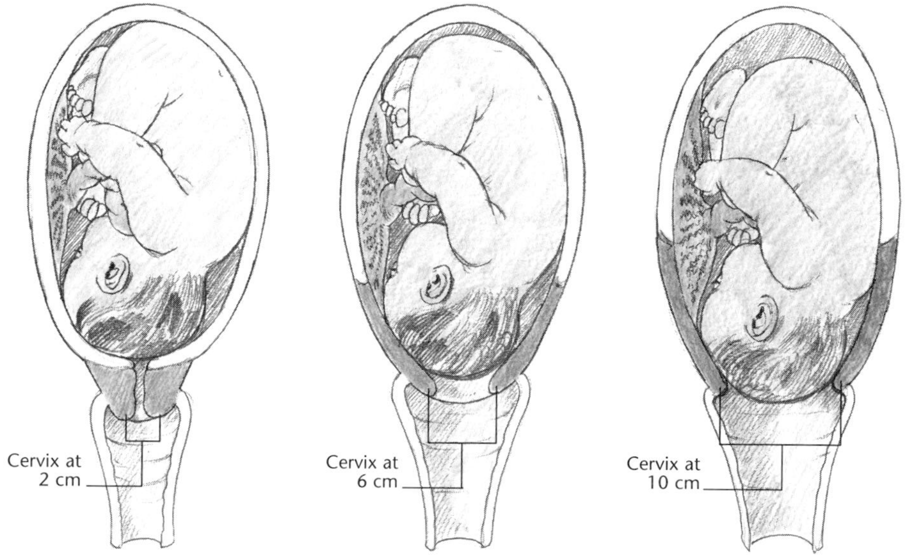

Actual size of the cervix during dilation, in centimeters

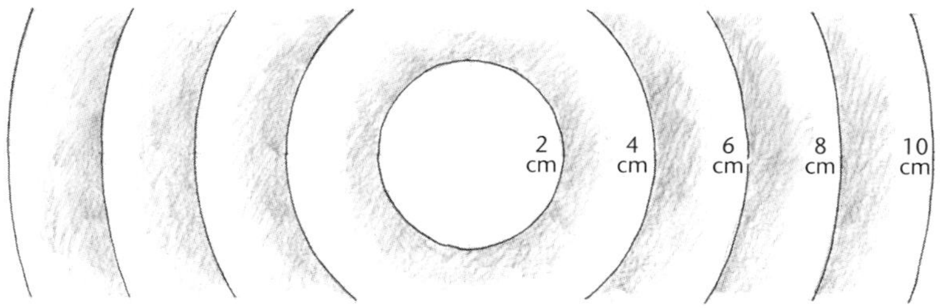

depends on the frequency and intensity of the contractions and the woman's ability to bear down. Contractions may slow down, separated by 2 to 5 minutes and lasting 60 to 90 seconds. This stage can be 2 hours or longer if it is a woman's first delivery or 1 to 2 hours in a second or later delivery. This stage ends when the baby is born.

Stage 3: Expulsion of the placenta (afterbirth) In the third stage, which occurs shortly after delivery, the placenta, or afterbirth, detaches from the wall of the uterus and passes from your body. Contractions that are less painful than those of delivery help to expel this tissue from your uterus. This stage usually lasts from a few minutes to half an hour.

HAS LABOR BEGUN?

Because you cannot predict when labor may begin, find out where you can reach your doctor if you should go into labor at night or on a weekend. Make arrangements ahead of time for someone to take you to the hospital at any time of the day or night. If no one is available, call a taxi. If you have other children, make arrangements in advance for someone to take care of them on short notice.

In the days or weeks before labor starts, you may feel some mild, irregular contractions, called false labor or Braxton Hicks contractions. These pains do not indicate the start of labor but are a sign that your body is preparing for it. These contractions may increase in frequency and intensity right before true labor begins. Call your doctor if you experience any of the following signs of true labor:

Vaginal delivery

Most vaginal deliveries follow this pattern:

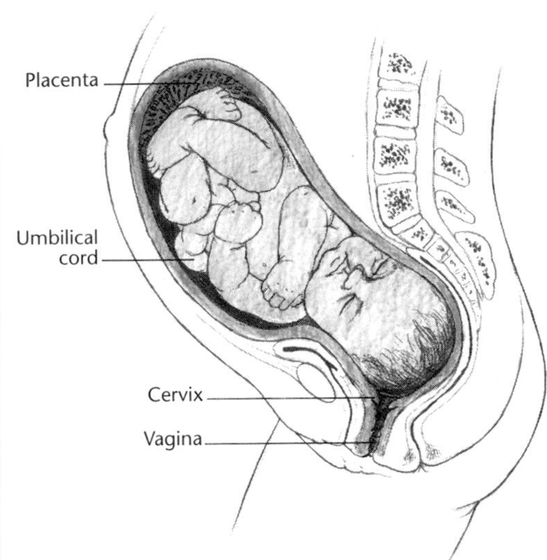

1. The baby's head rests against the cervix, which has thinned and started to dilate.

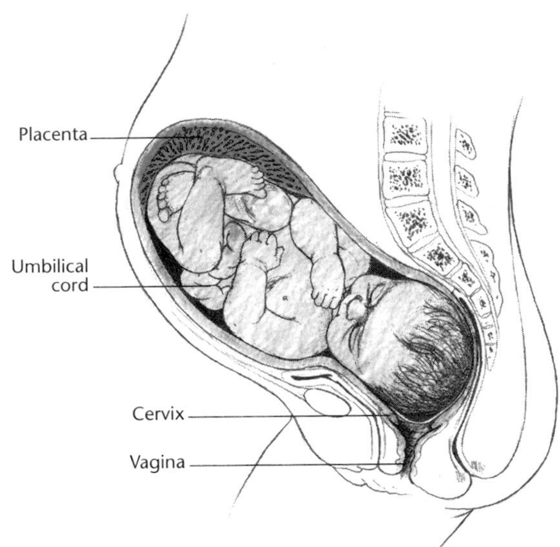

2. As the cervix dilates, the baby's head begins to press into the vagina.

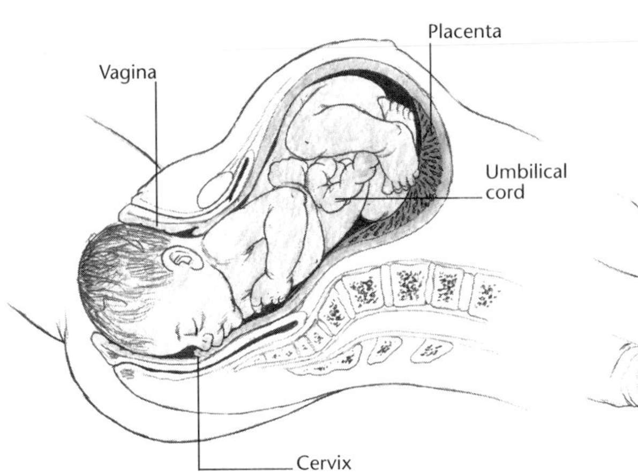

3. The baby makes a quarter turn so the narrowest part of its head can slide through the vagina first. The top of the baby's head becomes visible outside the vagina.

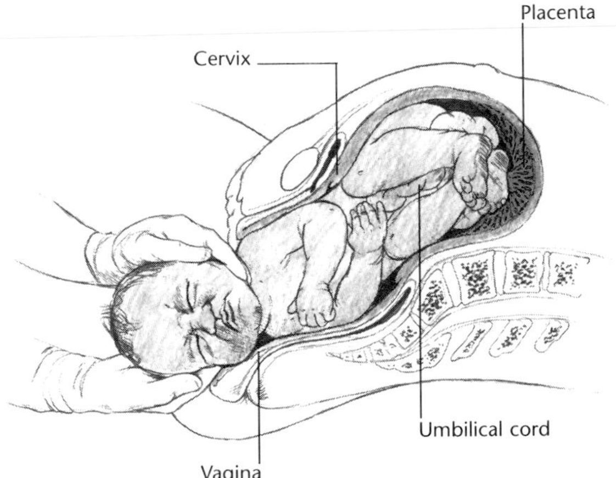

4. Once the baby's head is out of the vagina, the doctor assists the delivery of the baby's shoulders and the rest of the body while you continue to push.

WARNING SIGNS
LABOR

Call your doctor if you experience:

- Regular contractions that do not go away when you walk around; ask your doctor how long and how frequent they should be before you go to the hospital
- A trickle or gush of fluid from your vagina
- Bloody discharge from your vagina
- Persistent, severe pain with no relief between contractions

Strong, regular contractions When labor begins, the contractions of your uterus, which may feel mild and irregular at first, will progressively become stronger and regular. These contractions are more painful than the false labor pains you may have experienced days or weeks earlier. It is a good idea to begin timing the spacing and duration of the contractions and jotting the numbers down on paper so you will have a sense of how your labor is progressing. Check in with your doctor when you think you are in labor (it is not always easy to tell, especially if it is your first baby), and ask him or her how frequent and how long your contractions should be before you call again. Many doctors ask that women call them again when the contractions have been spaced 4 or 5 minutes apart for an hour or so. If you are having regular contractions, your doctor may want to examine you to see whether your cervix is dilating (opening), which is the only way to know for certain that you are in labor. If your cervix is not dilated, your doctor may recommend that you go home and wait until your contractions are stronger and more frequent.

Bloody discharge When your cervix begins to dilate, the mucus plug that has sealed it off during pregnancy passes out of your vagina. The mucus plug forms early in pregnancy to prevent bacteria and other organisms from entering the uterus from the vagina. You may see some mucus tinged or streaked pink or brown with blood (called bloody show). The birth process may begin at any time after the bloody show—in an hour or several days. Although the passing of the mucus plug is a normal part of labor, you should report it to your doctor, especially if it is accompanied by bleeding. Bleeding from the vagina can be a sign of serious complications, such as premature separation of the placenta from the wall of the uterus (placental abruption, see page 426). It is important for your doctor to be able to make an accurate diagnosis as early as possible.

Rupture of the membranes The membranes of the amniotic sac that surrounds the fetus can rupture, or break, before labor begins or at any time during labor. When your "bag of water breaks," as this process is often called, a clear fluid (amniotic fluid) trickles or gushes from your vagina. Usually, but not always, labor begins within 12 hours after the membranes rupture. If labor has not yet begun, most doctors induce it within 24 hours after rupture to avoid the possibility of infection or other complications. When the membranes rupture, bacteria that are usually harmless in the vagina can enter the uterus, causing an infection around the fetus. In addition, if the membranes rupture and fluid leaks quickly, the umbilical cord may be squeezed between the fetus and the wall of the uterus. (The fluid acts as a protective cushion around the fetus.) The umbilical cord is the fetus's lifeline; any compression may reduce the amount of oxygen it receives.

Call your doctor as soon as your water breaks. He or she will determine when you should come to the hospital. Depending on your condition and that of the baby, your doctor may recommend inducing labor (see page 439). If you have not had any contractions before the rupture of the membranes, they are likely to begin. If you are already having contractions, they are likely to increase in frequency and intensity after the membranes rupture.

Dark amniotic fluid When your water breaks, the fluid should be clear. If the fluid is dark green or brown, report it to

Timing your contractions

Have a stopwatch or a watch or clock with a second hand, a pen, and a piece of paper ready for timing your contractions when they begin. Start timing as soon as you feel a pain, which indicates the beginning of a contraction. When the pain subsides, write down the number of seconds from when it started to when it stopped. To find how often your contractions occur, write down the number of minutes that pass from the beginning of one contraction to the beginning of the next. Time several contractions in a row and take the average. You do not have to time every contraction, but check periodically, especially as labor progresses and your contractions become stronger and more frequent.

your doctor immediately. This dark substance, called meconium, is the baby's first bowel movement. Meconium may be expelled from the baby before birth if the pregnancy goes beyond the due date or if the baby is not getting enough oxygen. This can be dangerous; if the baby inhales the meconium, it can block its airway. A baby that is not getting enough oxygen may have heart rate abnormalities, which can be detected through fetal monitoring (see page 440).

Reddish amniotic fluid may indicate bleeding inside the amniotic sac, usually resulting from premature separation of the placenta from the wall of the uterus (placental abruption, see page 426). Notify your doctor immediately.

AT THE HOSPITAL OR BIRTHING CENTER

When you arrive at the hospital or birthing center, you will go through a brief admitting procedure. If your labor is active (your contractions are strong and regular), your birth partner may be able to take care of the paperwork for you. You may be asked to sign hospital consent forms. Many hospitals and birthing centers allow pregnant women to fill out all the necessary routine forms ahead of time. Ask your doctor if you can get this paperwork done in the weeks before delivery.

In the birthing or delivery room, you will be asked to change into a hospital gown and produce a sample of urine. A nurse will check your pulse, blood pressure, temperature, and breathing rate, and the baby's heart rate. A nurse or doctor will examine your cervix to see if it has dilated and look for signs of leaking amniotic fluid or bleeding. Tell the doctor or nurse of anything unusual you have noticed, such as vaginal bleeding or a lack of movement by the fetus.

Your doctor may stay with you throughout labor and delivery or may keep in touch with your progress through reports from the nurses in the hospital. If the nurses report that labor is proceeding normally, your doctor will probably arrive close to the time of delivery.

What to bring to the hospital

As your due date approaches, pack a bag to have ready to take to the hospital or birthing center. If you take a birth preparation class or get a chance to tour the delivery facility, ask what you should bring. Here are some suggestions:

Things to bring to help make labor more comfortable:

- A watch or clock with a second hand to time your contractions
- Heavy, absorbent socks in case your feet get cold
- Extra pillows in case the hospital runs short; make sure your pillows have colored pillowcases so they are not confused with hospital pillows
- Small tape player and tapes if music helps you relax
- Lotion that your partner can use to massage your back during contractions
- Hard candies or lollipops to keep your mouth moist
- Change for vending machines and phone
- A camera

Things to bring for after delivery:

- A loose, comfortable gown; a robe; slippers; nursing bras; extra underwear
- Toiletries including shampoo, lotions, or soaps
- Going-home clothes for you (you will still need to wear your maternity clothes)
- Going-home clothes for your baby, including a heavy blanket or bunting if it is cold
- Child car seat; make sure your partner or whoever picks you up from the hospital remembers to bring the car seat
- Phone numbers of people you want to call with the news after delivery

Relieving the discomfort of labor and delivery

You and your partner can learn what to expect during labor by taking a childbirth class and asking your doctor questions. You can also learn various ways to cope with the pain of contractions. Some women choose so-called natural childbirth that minimizes the use of pain-relieving drugs. Other women, in consultation with their doctor, may choose medication to help keep the pain under control. Many women decide to start labor without pain-relieving drugs but use pain medication when it becomes necessary. There is no "right" or "wrong" choice; you must decide what works best for you.

SELF-HELP FOR EASING LABOR

There are many things you can do on your own to make yourself more comfortable during labor—at home or in the hospital. Here are some tips:

- When a contraction begins, breathe deeply and slowly.
- Practice positions that will help you relax during a contraction.

Positions for labor

As you prepare for delivery, try a variety of positions and find several that are comfortable. For example, try sitting up or lying down, leaning against a wall or your partner, or lying on one side or the other. Do not lie flat on your back because this position can reduce blood flow to the baby if your uterus puts pressure on veins returning blood to your heart. Positions in which you are upright, either standing or sitting, take advantage of gravity to speed up dilation of your cervix and help the baby descend. Practice relaxing every muscle of your body, from the muscles in your face to those in your toes.

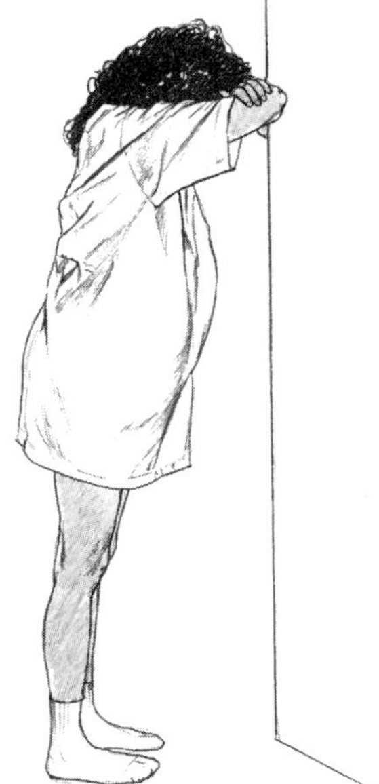

STANDING DURING A CONTRACTION
While standing, lean forward against a wall. Try this position during a contraction if the pain is not severe enough to keep you from walking around.

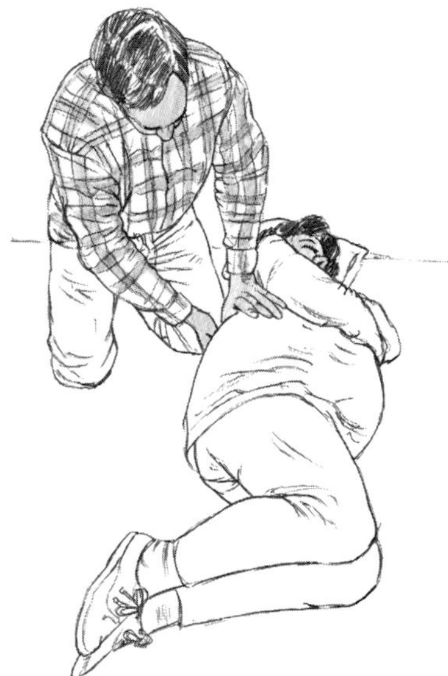

BACK RUB
If you feel pain in your lower back, ask your partner to give you a back rub. During contractions, your partner can press firmly on the point where you feel discomfort.

■ Stay active as long as possible as your labor progresses. Walking can help your cervix dilate during the early stage of labor.

■ Relax between contractions. Take a few slow, deep breaths and exhale completely. Focusing on your breathing can help distract you from the pain. Breathing exercises are the basis for many childbirth preparation courses.

■ Drink plenty of clear fluids (such as water, tea, or ginger ale) during early labor to maintain your energy level; suck on ice chips throughout labor. Ask your doctor if you can have a light snack such as toast or soup before you leave for the hospital. If there is a chance you might have a cesarean delivery (see page 442), your doctor will probably recommend against eating or drinking anything.

■ Focus positively on how much each strong contraction is accomplishing, and how you have one more contraction behind you. Try to picture your cervix opening up—your body is doing the work for you.

■ If you feel the urge to push before your doctor tells you your cervix is sufficiently dilated, doing quick pants, blowing, or shallow breathing may help make you feel more comfortable and able to resist the urge until it subsides.

■ Once you have the go-ahead to start pushing, you may want to try different positions, such as sitting or squatting, in which gravity works with you.

PAIN-RELIEF MEDICATION

Many medications are available to relieve pain during labor. Because it is impossible to predict the amount of pain you will experience during labor or the level of pain you can tolerate, you may not make your final decision about whether or not to use pain medications until your labor is under way. Still, it is a good idea for you and your partner to learn about the available pain-relief options ahead of time, so you can make decisions about which methods you prefer.

Analgesics Pain medications called analgesics can be given in an intravenous line or injected into a muscle to reduce pain during labor. These medications have an effect on your entire body and often on the baby as well. Possible side effects in the pregnant woman include drowsiness and decreased ability to concentrate. If the drug is given too close to the time of delivery, the newborn may be drowsier than usual and may not cry immediately. Small doses of narcotics that last an hour or two when given intravenously are usually safe, as long as the baby's heart rate is being monitored.

Epidural anesthesia An epidural (see page 260), also called an epidural block, numbs the body below the waist. While you are sitting or lying down, the anesthetic is injected through a tiny tube (catheter) threaded into the epidural space—the region around the spinal cord—at the lower part of your spine. An epidural is very effective in relieving pain, but it may make it more difficult for you to know when to push with contractions, potentially lengthening your labor. Sometimes, an epidural causes the walls of the woman's blood vessels to relax, which can cause her blood pressure to drop. A significant drop in blood pressure may slow the baby's heart rate. To help prevent this problem, you will be given intravenous fluids before and during administration of the epidural. Serious complications are unusual. After receiving an epidural, you will not be able to get up or walk because the catheter stays in place in your lower spine in case more medication is needed as your labor progresses.

Spinal anesthesia A spinal (see page 260) is similar to an epidural except that you are paralyzed, not just numb, from the waist down. For this reason, this type of anesthesia is not useful during a vaginal delivery because a woman's muscle power is essential to help push the baby out. Spinals are usually used only for cesarean deliveries.

Pudendal block In a procedure called a pudendal block, performed shortly before delivery, an anesthetic is injected into tissues surrounding one of the pudendal nerves on either side of the vagina. The anesthetic blocks pain in the tissues between the vagina and anus so it is especially helpful when an episiotomy (see page 441) is performed. A pudendal block is one of the safest forms of pain relief during delivery and rarely causes side effects.

General anesthesia General anesthesia (see page 261) causes loss of consciousness and is rarely used during delivery unless complications arise and there is not enough time to give an epidural or a spinal. General anesthesia is used for emergency cesarean deliveries because it causes numbness quickly. It is not used simply to relieve the pain of labor contractions or vaginal delivery. If there is any chance you may need to have an emergency cesarean delivery, you will be told not to eat any solid food once labor has started. (General anesthesia increases the risk of vomiting and suppresses the reflex that prevents vomit or acid from entering your windpipe and lungs and obstructing the passage of air.)

Procedures to assist labor and birth

A doctor may recommend one or more techniques that can help the birth process go smoothly and improve the chances of a healthy outcome for mother and baby. These techniques range from monitoring the status of the baby to assisting the birth with the use of instruments, such as forceps, or surgery.

INDUCED LABOR

In some cases, your doctor may decide to start, or induce, labor medically before it occurs naturally. Labor is induced when the health risks of speeding up delivery are less than the risk of continuing the pregnancy. For example, labor may be induced if your pregnancy has gone 1 to 2 weeks beyond the due date, your blood pressure is dangerously high (see page 428), the amniotic fluid around the baby is low, the baby is unusually small and not growing, or there is an infection in the amniotic fluid surrounding the baby (chorioamnionitis, see page 447).

Before inducing labor, your doctor will check the condition of the baby and examine your cervix to see if it has already started to dilate in preparation for labor. One technique doctors use to start or speed up labor is to break the membranes of the amniotic sac surrounding the baby and release the amniotic fluid. This procedure, called amniotomy, is painless—you feel only a gush of warm liquid. The major advantage of amniotomy is that it allows your doctor to see if there is any meconium (the baby's first bowel movement) present in the amniotic fluid. Amniotomy also makes it possible for the doctor to use internal monitoring (see page 440) in order to closely monitor the health of the baby.

Use of medications The synthetic hormone oxytocin can also be used to speed up labor that is not progressing. This process, called augmentation of labor, is sometimes used when the membranes of the amniotic sac have ruptured and labor has not started after 12 to 24 hours, or labor is taking so long that the health of the woman or baby is at risk.

Oxytocin is also used to induce labor. The hormone is administered intravenously using a pump that precisely dispenses the required doses. The baby is continuously monitored for the remainder of labor to make sure that he or she receives sufficient oxygen between contractions, especially if the contractions are very close together. If the baby's heart rate is abnormal, you may be given oxygen to breathe (to increase the oxygen supply to the baby) and more intravenous fluids (to increase blood flow to the baby). The administration of oxytocin may be reduced or discontinued.

If your due date has passed, your doctor may try to help labor begin by separating the amniotic membranes from their attachments in the cervix and lower wall of your uterus. This procedure, called stripping the membranes, is done in the doctor's office. The doctor inserts a finger through your vagina and cervix and peels the amniotic membrane away from the cervix. This activity triggers the release of prostaglandins, hormones that stimulate contractions of the uterus. There is little risk involved in the procedure but you may feel some mild cramps or contractions during or immediately after the procedure.

Risks Forcing labor to begin before the pregnancy has come to term and the cervix is ready can cause a variety of complications for the pregnant woman

Fetal monitoring

Doctors use fetal monitoring techniques to evaluate the baby's heart rate during labor to determine if he or she is getting enough oxygen. There are various methods a doctor can use to evaluate the status of the baby. For example, your doctor can listen to the baby's heartbeat by pressing a stethoscope or hand-held ultrasound device (see page 405) to your abdomen periodically. Other methods provide precise and continuous electronic monitoring if necessary.

One such method is external monitoring, which is done from outside your body. Some doctors or hospitals routinely perform external monitoring when a woman first arrives at the hospital. While you are resting in a hospital bed, two belts are placed around your abdomen to hold instruments that measure the baby's heart rate and the length, frequency, and relative intensity of your contractions. The instruments are connected to a monitor that prints out the information. If everything is normal, the monitoring is discontinued and the belts are removed. You can then move about freely. Some women find external monitoring reassuring; others find it intrusive. Discuss your doctor's monitoring policies in the weeks before you go to the hospital.

If a complication such as bleeding develops that increases the risk to you or the baby, your doctor may recommend internal fetal monitoring. Internal monitoring can be done only after the membranes of the amniotic sac have been broken (see page 439). Internal monitoring gives the doctor a much clearer idea of the baby's heart rate and the strength of your contractions. An electrode that measures the baby's heart rate is inserted through your vagina and cervix and attached to the baby's scalp. A thin tube called a pressure catheter may also be inserted into your uterus to precisely measure the intensity, length, and frequency of your contractions. The instruments are connected to a monitor that prints out the information. You usually have to stay in bed during this type of monitoring procedure. Internal monitoring usually continues until delivery.

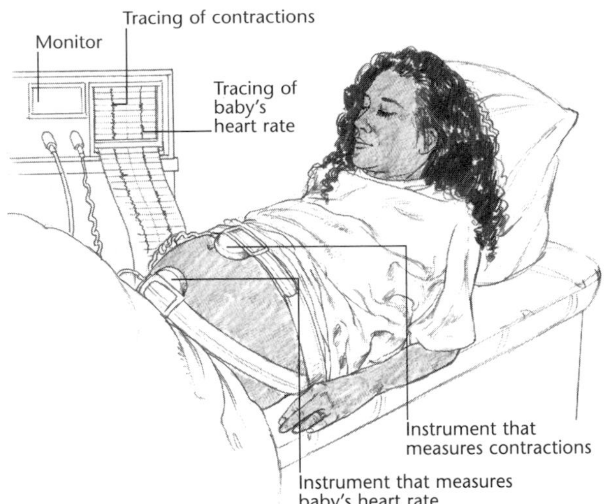

EXTERNAL MONITORING
In external monitoring during labor, instruments attached to belts wrapped around your abdomen measure the baby's heartbeat and the length, frequency, and relative intensity of your contractions. (Only an internal monitor can measure the actual intensity of contractions.) These devices are attached to a monitor that prints out the information.

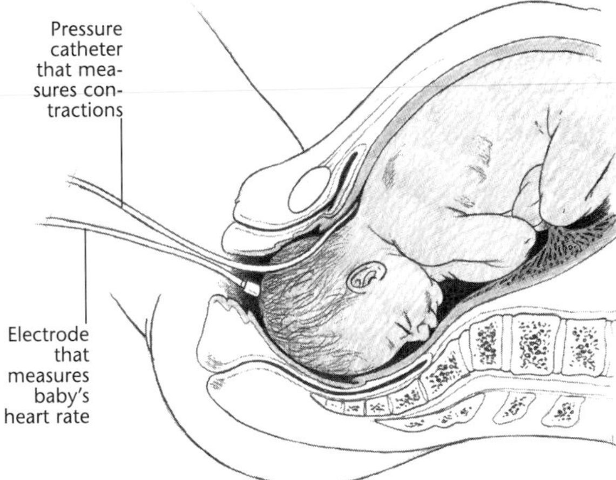

INTERNAL MONITORING
An electrode inserted through your vagina and cervix into your uterus and attached to the baby's scalp measures the baby's heart rate. A long thin tube called a pressure catheter may be inserted through the vagina into the uterus to measure the intensity, length, and frequency of contractions. These devices are attached to a monitor that prints out the information.

and baby. Therefore, labor is not induced for nonmedical reasons, such as convenience. Labor is seldom induced before 39 weeks because the baby's lungs may not be fully developed. If the exact due date is not known and there is a chance that the pregnancy is less than 39 weeks along, the amniotic fluid may be evaluated by amniocentesis (see page 406) to determine if the baby's lungs are mature enough to function outside the uterus. Inducing labor too early in a pregnancy—before the cervix has softened—may also result in a failure of labor to progress, which increases the risk of a cesarean delivery (see page 442).

EPISIOTOMY

An episiotomy is a procedure in which a small cut is made in the perineum, the area of skin between the opening of the vagina and the anus, to allow the baby to pass through more easily. An episiotomy is usually done when the head of the baby is just beginning to emerge from the vagina. The most common reason for performing an episiotomy is to avoid excessive tearing of the perineum during childbirth, which can permanently weaken the tissues that surround the vagina and anus. Episiotomy is also done to ease the delivery of a large baby during a difficult, prolonged labor or a forceps delivery. Episiotomies are more common in the delivery of first babies than in subsequent deliveries.

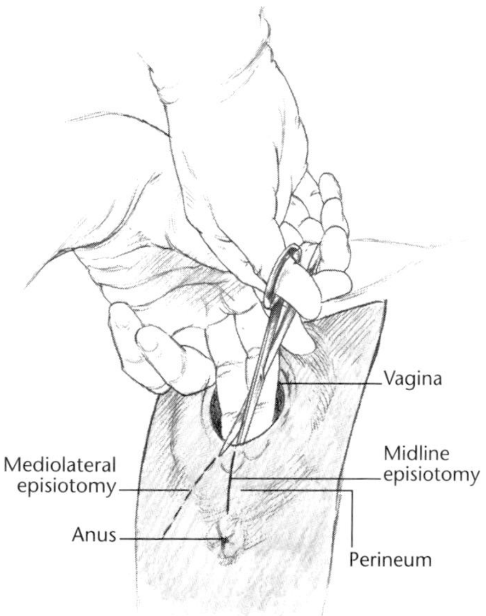

EPISIOTOMY
For an episiotomy, the doctor administers a local anesthetic to numb the perineum (the area of skin between your vagina and anus) and cuts the tissue with sterile scissors or a knife. In a midline episiotomy (solid line), the incision is a straight line from the vaginal opening toward the anus. In a mediolateral episiotomy (broken line), the incision is diagonal from the vaginal opening to one side of the anus. After delivery, the incision is closed with dissolvable stitches.

Although episiotomy is one of the most common surgical procedures in the US, fewer doctors are now doing it routinely. Most doctors do an episiotomy only when they think it is necessary to prevent vaginal tissue from tearing, such as when the baby is unusually large.

There are two types of episiotomy—midline (or median) or mediolateral. In a midline episiotomy, which is the most common type, the incision is made straight down from the vagina toward the anus. In a mediolateral episiotomy, the incision is made at an angle from the vagina to the side of the anus. A midline episiotomy cuts through fewer layers of tissue, usually causes less discomfort after delivery, and heals more easily. A mediolateral episiotomy may be necessary in some cases, such as when the baby is very large or when forceps have to be used during delivery. In these cases, a mediolateral incision may be less likely than a midline episiotomy to extend and tear into the rectum during delivery. Talk to your doctor ahead of time to find out if he or she plans to do an episiotomy and, if so, under what circumstances. Episiotomy can be beneficial in the following situations:

- If the baby is larger than the woman's vaginal opening is able to stretch.
- If labor is prolonged and the woman is exhausted and unable to push the baby out.
- If forceps are going to be used for the delivery.
- If there are signs that the baby's heart rate is abnormal during the second (pushing) stage of labor, and delivery must occur immediately.

FORCEPS DELIVERY AND VACUUM EXTRACTION

If labor contractions have been successful in helping push the baby to the vaginal opening but the woman cannot push the baby out completely, the doctor may use forceps, a pair of metal instruments shaped to fit around the baby's head, to pull it out of the vagina. Before using forceps, a doctor administers a local anesthetic, a pudendal block (see page 438), or an epidural (see page 438) to numb the area around the vaginal opening. Forceps are sometimes used when a woman is unable to push the baby out after prolonged effort, such as when the pushing stage of a woman's first delivery lasts longer than 3 hours. Forceps may also be used when signs of heart rate abnormalities in the baby make an immediate delivery necessary. In some cases, a doctor using forceps can deliver a baby more quickly than he or she could by performing a cesarean delivery. An episiotomy is usually performed before a forceps delivery.

A procedure called vacuum extraction is sometimes used instead of, or in addition to, forceps in a difficult or prolonged delivery. In vacuum extraction, a metal or plastic cup is attached to the baby's scalp and suction is applied to gradually pull the baby down the vagina. The baby's scalp may be swollen from the procedure but this swelling subsides within a few days. An episiotomy is usually required before vacuum extraction to expand the opening of the vagina.

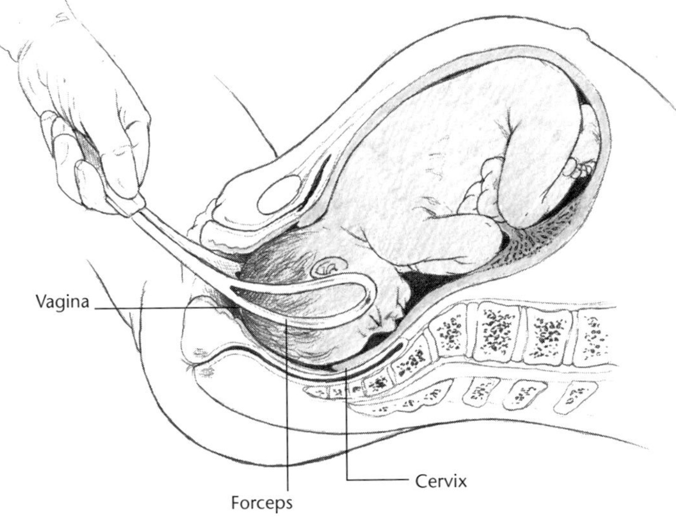

FORCEPS DELIVERY
To perform a forceps delivery, the doctor inserts the blades into your vagina along either side of the baby's head. He or she helps the baby's head descend by pulling gently while you continue to push with your contractions.

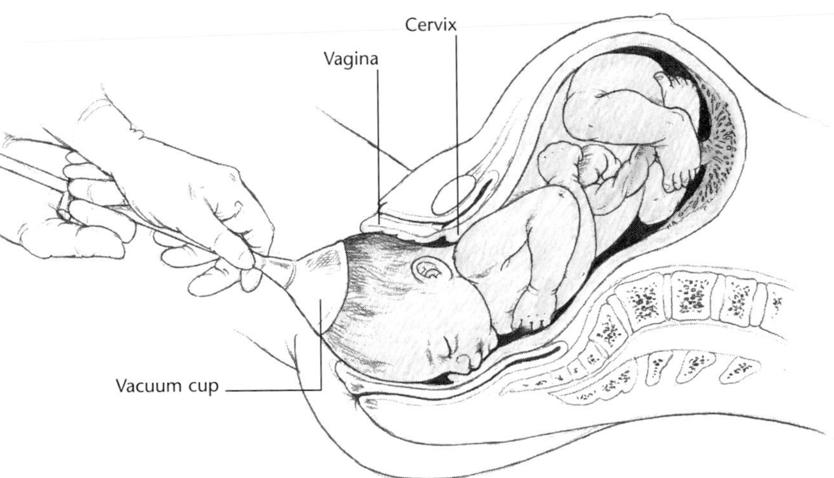

VACUUM EXTRACTION
In vacuum extraction, a plastic cup attached to a vacuum tube is placed on the baby's head inside the vagina. The vacuum pump is turned on to secure the cup to the baby's head. Using a handle attached to the cup, the doctor gently pulls the baby through the vagina in time with each contraction. After the baby's head appears, the vacuum is turned off and the doctor assists the delivery of the rest of the baby's body while you continue to push with your contractions.

CESAREAN DELIVERY

Cesarean delivery is the surgical delivery of a baby through an incision in the wall of the uterus and an incision in the abdomen. A cesarean delivery, sometimes called a cesarean section or C-section, is major surgery and requires regional anesthesia, such as an epidural (see page 438) or a spinal (see page 438), or, in an emergency, general anesthesia (see page 261). A cesarean delivery lengthens a woman's hospital stay and recovery. Cesarean deliveries are being done less frequently than in the past. Many women prefer to deliver vaginally whenever possible so they can be more directly involved in the birth and recover more quickly. However, if you and your doctor decide a cesarean delivery is necessary, you should not feel that you have failed in any way.

A cesarean delivery may be planned well in advance because of a condition such as placenta previa (see page 426) or may be done at the last moment if complications occur, such as an abnormal heart rate in the baby or failure of labor to progress. Unless the cesarean is an emergency procedure, your birth partner can probably be in the operating room and will be able to hold the baby after the delivery.

Following are the most common reasons cesarean deliveries are performed, and some possible alternatives:

■ **Prolonged labor** About one third of cesarean deliveries are done because labor is prolonged and contractions are not effective in dilating the cervix. Doctors usually try methods that may help labor along before deciding to do a cesarean. For example, the drug oxytocin can be used to speed up labor (see page 439). Walking around sometimes helps stimulate contractions. In some women, the cervix may stop dilating at some point during labor and then start up again. For this reason, doctors often wait a few hours after dilation stops before performing a cesarean delivery in order to see if dilation begins again. During this time, the baby is monitored to make sure it is tolerating the stresses of labor.

■ **A large baby** Improved nutrition has led to a greater number of large babies and, as a result, more cesarean deliveries. Many women can vaginally deliver a baby weighing more than 10 pounds, but a cesarean delivery may be performed if a woman's pelvic cavity is too small for a very large baby to pass through.

■ **The baby is affected by the stress of labor** Some cesarean deliveries are performed when there are indications (such as an abnormal heart rate) that the baby is not tolerating the stresses of labor. If a baby has an abnormal heart rate, further testing can be done of the level of oxygen in the baby's blood. If the baby's heart rate or blood oxygen level is worrisome, a cesarean delivery is usually done.

■ **Breech presentation** Most babies in the breech position (buttocks or feet first; see page 445) are delivered by cesarean. As an alternative in some cases, the doctor may perform a procedure called external version, in which the baby is manually turned before labor begins. To perform external version, the doctor presses his or her hands on the woman's abdomen and slowly and firmly turns the baby; the baby's heart rate is being monitored at the same time. This procedure is not tried in all cases because there is not always enough extra room inside the uterus to turn the baby in this way. It is also possible that the baby will go right back to its original position after the external version.

■ **Previous cesarean delivery** If you had a cesarean delivery in a previous pregnancy, talk to your doctor about whether there is any reason why you should not have a vaginal delivery in this pregnancy. Although rare, the major risk of having a vaginal delivery if you have previously had a cesarean delivery is possible rupture of the scar on your uterus left by the cesarean delivery. The risk of rupture is greatest if you had a vertical incision on your uterus. (The scar on your uterus does not necessarily match the scar on your abdomen.) However, because most cesarean deliveries in the US are performed using a horizontal incision low on the uterus, most women can safely have a vaginal delivery after having had a cesarean.

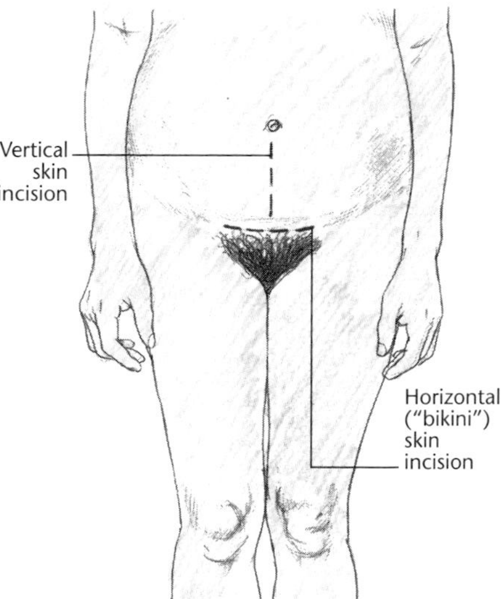

CESAREAN INCISION

The most common skin incision for cesarean delivery is a horizontal cut made across the abdomen just above the pubic hairline. In some cases, a vertical incision may be made from just below the navel to the top of the pubic hairline. The incision made into the uterus (not shown) is usually horizontal.

The procedure In preparation for a cesarean delivery, the nurse will wash your abdomen with an antiseptic solution. A catheter will be inserted through your urethral opening to drain urine from your bladder. The catheter remains in place during the delivery and until the next morning. You will be given fluids intravenously through a vein in your arm or hand.

You will receive anesthesia. If you have an epidural or a spinal (see page 438), you will be numb from the waist down. If you have general anesthesia, you will be unconscious. A cloth drape will probably be placed below your chest to shield your view of the procedure. Your doctor will make a horizontal or vertical incision in your abdomen and another incision in the wall of your uterus. The baby will be pulled out through the incisions, the umbilical cord will be cut, and the placenta will be removed. The incision on your uterus is closed with dissolvable stitches; the incision on your abdomen is closed with stitches or staples that are usually removed before you leave the hospital.

Like any major surgery, a cesarean delivery carries risks, such as infection, excessive blood loss and anemia, and the development of blood clots in the legs, pelvic organs, or lungs. In rare cases, injury may occur to nearby organs, such as the bladder, which is immediately repaired. Most cesarean deliveries are uncomplicated and cause no problems for the woman or baby. You can probably hold your baby shortly after the delivery, as you would after a vaginal delivery.

Problems during labor and delivery

Although labor and delivery usually proceed smoothly, unanticipated problems sometimes develop. Hospitals are well equipped to deal with these complications. It is important to be aware of the warning signs of possible complications so you can alert your doctor immediately of any problems.

PREMATURE RUPTURE OF MEMBRANES

For most women, if the amniotic membranes rupture ("the water breaks") early, labor follows within a few hours. But the earlier in pregnancy this rupture occurs, the longer it may take for labor to begin afterward. Conditions that most often cause the premature rupture of membranes include infection of the uterus or cervix, multiple births (see page 429), incompetent cervix (see page 423), or premature separation of the placenta (placental abruption, see page 426).

If your membranes rupture, you are likely to feel a gush or trickle of fluid out of your vagina. (Sometimes, a woman thinks her membranes have broken when, in fact, urine has been pushed out by the weight of the baby on her bladder.) Your doctor can tell in a pelvic examination if your membranes have ruptured and if your cervix has started to thin (efface) or open (dilate). He or she may also take samples of amniotic fluid to evaluate the maturity of the baby's lungs and to check for infection.

If the membranes rupture after the 36th week of pregnancy, labor usually begins in 24 to 48 hours. If it does not, labor will probably be induced. The risk of infection begins to increase 24 hours after the membranes rupture. Because of the risk of infection, you should not have intercourse or put anything into your vagina, including tampons.

Although rare, the membranes can rupture before the 25th week of pregnancy. When the membranes rupture this early in pregnancy, a doctor will try to delay the onset of labor for as long as it is safe for the baby. The woman is usually admitted to the hospital so that her temperature and the baby's heart rate can be monitored continuously; an increase in either may be an indication that an infection is developing inside the uterus. Exposure to infection inside the uterus can significantly reduce a baby's chances of survival.

Only one fourth of babies born before the 25th week of pregnancy survive outside the uterus. Because they are not fully developed at birth, those that do survive may have permanent disabilities, including slow development, mental retardation, inadequate development of their lungs, or blindness.

BREECH PRESENTATION

During birth, the baby is usually positioned head down and facing back. In 3 to 4 percent of deliveries, the baby is in the breech position with its buttocks against the cervix. When a baby is in this position, a vaginal delivery may be possible, but a doctor is likely to discuss with the woman the possibility of cesarean delivery as an alternative. Breech presentation is more common when a baby is smaller than average, the uterus is an abnormal shape, there is more than one baby, or the woman has already had children and her uterus is relaxed.

In some cases, a baby in the breech position can be delivered vaginally; when the legs and lower half of the body are out, the doctor then completes the delivery of the shoulders and head, sometimes using forceps. Because of the potential risk of complications in a vaginal delivery of a baby in a breech position, many doctors now regularly deliver such babies by cesarean. If a vaginal delivery is done, electronic fetal monitoring (see page 440) and episiotomy (see page 441) are usually used. A vaginal delivery may be attempted for a baby in the breech position if:

- The baby is in a frank breech position—its hips are bent and its legs extend up.
- The baby is small enough (usually under 8 pounds) to pass easily through the vagina.
- The pregnant woman has no obstetrical problems, such as placenta previa (see page 426), that might complicate the delivery.
- The pregnant woman's pelvis is a normal or above average size.
- The baby has already descended well into the pelvis as labor begins.
- The baby's head is tucked down toward its chest—not extended.

In some cases of breech presentation, a doctor can try to reposition the baby (called external version) late in pregnancy. Usually guided by ultrasound (see page 405), the doctor uses his or her hands on the outside of the woman's abdomen to try to manipulate the baby inside the uterus into the normal birth position, with head down. Although this procedure can be uncomfortable for the woman, it is sometimes a viable alternative to cesarean delivery. Because of the slight possibility of rupturing the membranes or causing labor to begin, external version is attempted only when the baby is mature enough for delivery.

PROLONGED LABOR

In a normal labor, the cervix gradually opens, or dilates, and the head of the baby descends into the pelvis and through the vagina. Labor is considered prolonged if it lasts more than 20 hours in a woman's first delivery and 14 hours in a subsequent delivery. Labor can slow down at any stage. Causes of prolonged labor include a thick cervix, which takes longer to dilate, or poorly synchronized contractions. A common remedy for prolonged labor in the early stage is to induce labor by administering the hormone oxytocin (see page 439) intravenously to stimulate contractions of the uterus.

Labor can also slow down during the active phase (see page 432), when the cervix is dilated from 3 to 7 centimeters. In this phase, labor can be prolonged if the baby is too large for the woman's pelvis, if an epidural (see page 438) was administered too early, if contractions are not strong enough to open the cervix, or if the baby is in an abnormal position. Because two thirds of women with prolonged active labor eventually deliver vaginally, doctors usually allow labor to proceed on its own during this phase.

However, one third of these women stop dilating, usually because the baby's head is too large to pass through their pelvis, a condition known as cephalopelvic disproportion. In this case, a cesarean delivery may be necessary. If the baby is not considered too large for the woman's pelvis, the hormone oxytocin may be administered to stimulate contractions of the uterus and help the labor continue. If oxytocin fails to cause the cervix to dilate after 2 to 3 hours of adequate contractions, a cesarean delivery is usually performed.

Labor may also fail to progress during the final stage, when the cervix has already dilated 8 to 10 centimeters. This slowdown usually occurs because the baby is too large for the woman's pelvis. A doctor may consider this a possibility if the baby's head has not descended, even though the cervix is fully dilated. Cesarean delivery may be necessary, especially if oxytocin has been given and has not helped labor progress.

Breech presentation

The usual position for a baby at the time of birth is head down. The head is the largest part of the baby. During delivery, the head emerges first, which causes the cervix to dilate fully and allows the rest of the body to follow easily. In a breech presentation, the baby's buttocks emerge first, which may not cause the cervix to dilate fully. Insufficient dilation of the cervix may make the remainder of the delivery more difficult because the largest part of the body is still to come.

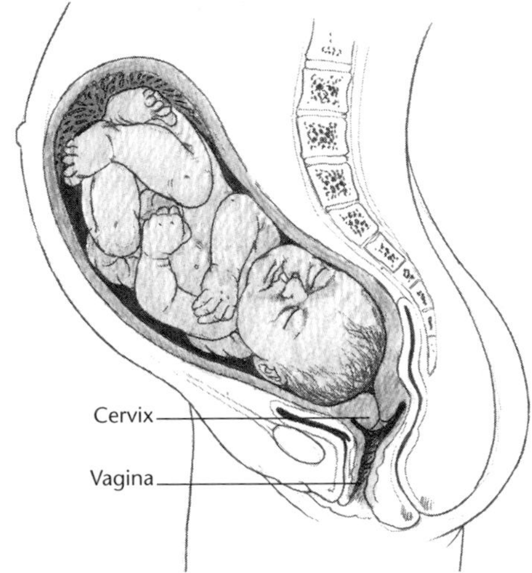

NORMAL POSITION
The normal position of a baby for birth is head down with arms and legs curled in front of his or her body.

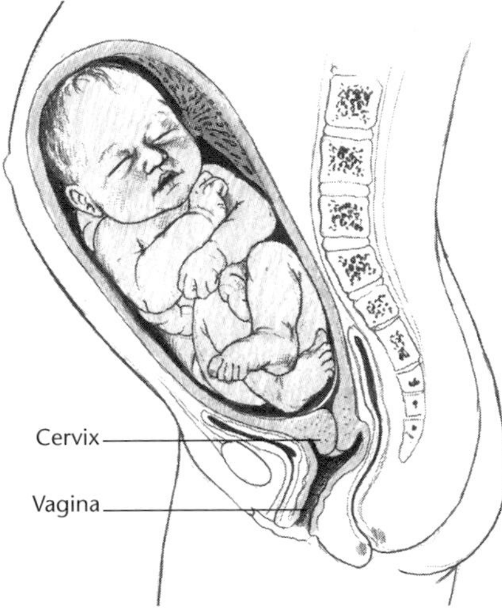

COMPLETE BREECH
If a baby is in a complete breech position, the hips and knees are bent. A baby in this position can sometimes be delivered vaginally if all other factors are favorable.

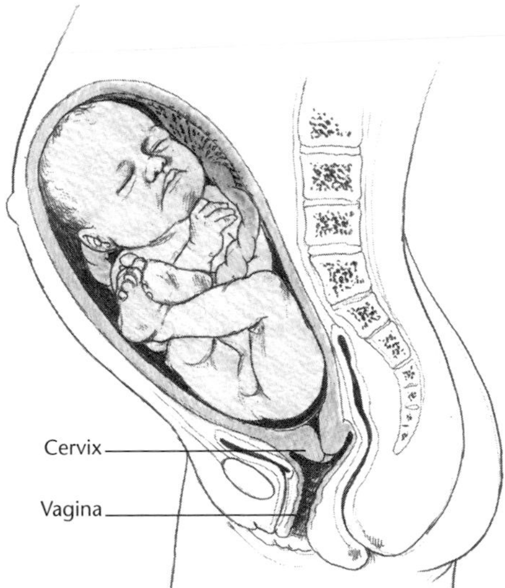

FRANK BREECH
If a baby is in a frank breech position, the hips are bent but the legs extend up toward its head. A vaginal birth is usually possible when the baby is in this position.

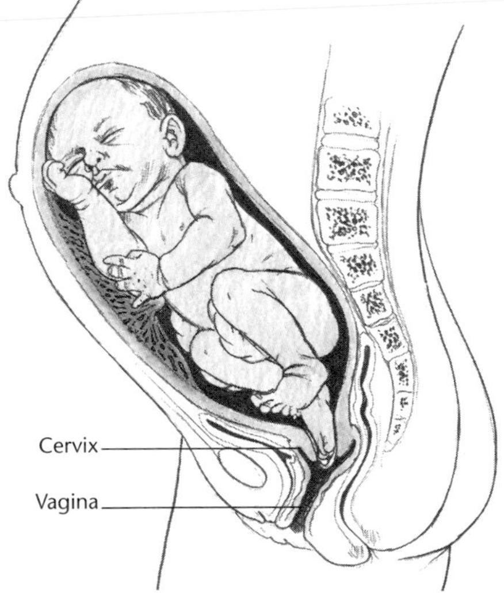

INCOMPLETE BREECH
If a baby is in an incomplete breech position, such as a footling position (in which the feet protrude through or cover the cervix), delivery is usually by cesarean.

CHORIO-AMNIONITIS

Chorioamnionitis is an infection of two membranes of the placenta (the chorion and the amnion) and the amniotic fluid that surrounds the baby. The infection, which occurs in about 2 percent of all pregnancies, is caused by bacteria that reach the uterus through the vagina. Chorioamnionitis usually occurs at the end of a pregnancy when more than 24 hours elapse between the time that the membranes rupture (see page 435) and delivery. This time lapse allows the bacteria to multiply, increasing the risk of infection.

In rare cases, chorioamnionitis occurs when there is no obvious rupture of the membranes. The infection may be the cause of some cases of preterm labor (labor that begins before the 37th week of pregnancy; see page 427). For this reason, doctors check first for infection in women who have preterm labor. The infection occasionally occurs early in pregnancy in women who have a type of bacteria called beta streptococcus in their vagina. Because this bacteria can cause severe infections, such as pneumonia, in the newborn, a doctor tests a woman's vaginal secretions to determine if beta streptococcus is present. If it is, the infection is treated immediately.

Symptoms of chorioamnionitis include fever and tenderness in the uterus. The baby may show signs of infection, such as a fever or a higher-than-normal heart rate. The infection is treated with antibiotics, usually given intravenously in the hospital. Because antibiotics given to the woman do not reach the baby in quantities sufficient to treat its infection, immediate delivery is recommended. If the baby is born with a severe infection, he or she is given antibiotics intravenously to prevent or treat other infections—such as pneumonia or meningitis (an infection of the membranes covering the brain)—that can be caused by the same bacteria.

After delivery

The first moments after giving birth are very special for most women. You will probably be able to hold your baby right away and may want to try to breast-feed. If, for some reason, you are not able to hold your baby right after delivery (for example, because you have had a cesarean, your baby requires immediate medical attention, or you are simply too exhausted), do not be overly concerned. The first few minutes after delivery are not critical; you will have the time you need in the weeks and years ahead to get to know and bond with your child.

THE FIRST MOMENTS

You may not feel about your baby the way you expected. Along with the joy of having brought a new life into the world, you may feel overwhelmed, scared, or even distant. For many women, it can take time for deep feelings and a sense of connection to develop.

Your baby may not look the way you expected. A newborn is often covered with a greasy white coating called vernix, which protected his or her skin inside the uterus. Your baby's head may be narrowed from passage through the cervix and vagina and his or her eyes may be swollen shut. His or her skin may be blotchy and red, blue, or gray. Most, but not all, babies cry at birth.

Immediately after delivery, the staff at the hospital goes into action to help ensure your baby's health. Using a suction device, they remove any mucus that may be inside the baby's nose and mouth. An antibiotic ointment or solution is placed in the baby's eyes to help protect against infection. The doctor will check the baby's heart rate, observe to make sure the baby is breathing normally, and measure the baby's length and weight. Your baby will demonstrate some early reflexes such as grasping, reacting to light and noise, and sucking.

While most babies are healthy at birth, a variety of unexpected complications can occur. Breathing difficulty is the most common problem in newborns. Symptoms include increased breathing rate, labored chest movements, or bluish skin. If your baby is having difficulty breathing, he or she will probably be placed in the neonatal intensive care unit (see page 450) of the hospital for treatment until his or her condition improves.

Your baby's Apgar score

One minute after birth and again in 5 minutes, all newborns are given a score, called an Apgar score, that reflects their heart rate, respiration, muscle tone, reflexes, and color. The Apgar score is one of many ways a doctor evaluates your baby's general health. However, a low score is not necessarily a cause for concern. The score does not measure a baby's long-term potential or development. A baby who has been through an unusually long labor or stressful delivery may have a low initial Apgar score. But, like most babies, he or she is likely to develop normally.

To get an Apgar score, the doctor adds up the scores given on five signs of a baby's condition. The total score can range from 0 to 10.

	APGAR SCORE		
SIGN	**0**	**1**	**2**
Heart rate	None	Under 100 beats a minute	Over 100 beats a minute
Breathing and crying	None	Cry weak, breathing irregular	Cry strong, breathing regular
Skin color*	Blue or pale	Body pink, hands and feet blue	All pink
Muscle tone	Limp	Arms and legs bending some	Arms and legs bending actively
Reflex response	None	Grimaces	Cries

* For nonwhite infants, skin color is assessed by examining the inside of the mouth and the lips, the whites of the eyes, the palms, and the soles of the feet.

ADJUSTING AFTER CHILDBIRTH

In the first days after delivery and at home with your baby, while you are learning how to take care of your infant, your body will be readjusting from the demands of pregnancy and childbirth. Whether you have had a vaginal delivery or cesarean, you will have to cope with a number of discomforts during this challenging time.

Contractions after delivery Although regular labor contractions stop when the placenta (afterbirth) is delivered, you will continue to feel some less painful contractions (called "afterpains") for several days. These contractions help your uterus return to its normal size. A nurse will massage your abdomen several times the first day after delivery to help stimulate your uterus to contract. If the contractions are painful, ask your doctor for pain-relief medication. Breast-feeding also stimulates contractions that can help the uterus return to its normal size more quickly. Over a period of about 6 weeks, your uterus gradually shrinks from 1½ pounds to about 2 ounces. Your abdomen will feel soft and flabby for several weeks and you will probably have to wear your maternity clothes for a while after delivery.

Soreness If you had a vaginal delivery, your perineum, the area of skin between your vagina and anus, was stretched and may have torn on its own or been cut during an episiotomy (see page 441). For this reason, the area around your vagina may be sore and swollen for several days; urination may be a little painful. Applying cold packs for the first hours after delivery can help reduce the discomfort and swelling. Later, a warm sitz bath (sitting in warm water for a short time) may help make you more comfortable. You might want to try a pillow shaped like a doughnut, which you can purchase in a drugstore, to help make sitting more comfortable. Follow the instructions you were given about how to clean your vaginal area to prevent infection. As soon as you want, you can begin doing pelvic floor exercises (Kegel exercises; see page 238) to restore strength to the muscles in your vaginal area.

WARNING SIGNS
POSTPARTUM DEPRESSION

Many women experience emotional highs and lows after giving birth. If the emotional lows substantially interfere with your ability to function, you should get help. Talk with your doctor about the need for counseling if you experience any of the following symptoms of severe depression:

- Feelings of anxiety or hopelessness that do not go away after 2 weeks
- Inability to sleep even when you feel tired
- Sleeping too much, even when your baby is awake
- Anxiety or panic attacks
- Lack of interest in your baby or other members of the family
- Fear of harming the baby or yourself

Vaginal discharge For the first few days after delivery you will probably have a bloody discharge from your vagina called lochia, which consists of blood and the remains of the placenta. This discharge can be quite plentiful; you may need to change your sanitary napkin every few hours or so at first. Over the next 2 to 6 weeks, this discharge will become pink, then clear, and gradually stop. Use sanitary napkins only; do not use tampons until your doctor has examined you at the postpartum visit. Refrain from vaginal intercourse for as long as your doctor recommends, usually 4 to 6 weeks after delivery.

Engorged breasts Your breasts may swell painfully as your milk comes in 2 to 4 days after delivery. A properly fitted support bra and hot showers will help relieve some of the discomfort, especially if you are breast-feeding. Ask your doctor if you can take a painkiller if you are nursing. Nursing your baby frequently helps relieve the pressure in your breasts caused by the buildup of milk. Do not be discouraged—the discomfort will go away in a few days as you and your baby adjust to breast-feeding.

If you are not breast-feeding, a support bra is just as essential. Ice packs (frozen bags of vegetables work nicely) may help relieve the pain of engorgement. Because you want your breasts to stop producing milk, do not pump them because doing so stimulates the production of more milk, which causes further engorgement. This engorgement subsides after about 3 days, when the lack of stimulation causes your breasts to stop producing milk. If the pain is severe, talk to your doctor about pain-relief medication.

Hemorrhoids and constipation Many women experience hemorrhoids (see page 522) and constipation after childbirth. You can relieve both problems with a diet high in fiber and liquids. Over-the-counter ointments or sitz baths may help relieve the discomfort of hemorrhoids. Do not use laxatives, suppositories, or enemas without checking with your doctor, especially if your episiotomy extended to your anus or you had stitches in that area.

Postpartum depression Most women become somewhat moody and depressed in the first few days after giving birth. This is normal. These "blues" may make you feel lonely, overwhelmed by your new responsibilities, anxious, or angry. For most women, these feelings go away within several days or weeks.

Some women develop a longer-lasting condition called postpartum depression. They feel intense anxiety or despair that makes it difficult for them to function. The cause of severe postpartum depression may result from a sudden reduction in a woman's hormone levels combined with other factors, such as lack of sleep, pain from an episiotomy, or breast engorgement. Some women may have a difficult time adjusting to caring for a new infant at home and all the emotional challenges that entails.

Getting emotional support to help you cope with these new circumstances is a key to resolving the minor depression that can occur after delivery. Share your feelings with your partner and other relatives and friends who have children. Make some time for yourself whenever you have a chance by letting friends or relatives provide help with meals, cleaning, and child care. If your depression does not lift or becomes overwhelming, talk to your doctor. He or she can help you or refer you to a psychiatrist or counselor.

Menstruation and contraception If you are not breast-feeding, your period will return 6 to 8 weeks after delivery. You can use tampons if you want for this first period. If you are breast-feeding, you

Neonatal intensive care

If your baby is born preterm (before the 37th week of pregnancy or weighing less than 5 pounds) or with a serious infection, respiratory problem, or birth defect, he or she will be taken immediately to the neonatal intensive care unit of the hospital, or transferred to another hospital that has such a unit. If you are at risk for a preterm birth, your doctor will plan ahead of time for your baby's transfer to a neonatal intensive care unit after birth, if necessary. Immediate care improves the baby's chance of survival and long-term health,

In general, babies born after the 26th week have a good chance of survival. Their development may be delayed, but most preterm babies catch up to full-term babies before the end of their first year. Preterm birth can result as a complication of pregnancy-related conditions such as preeclampsia (see page 428) or placenta previa (see page 426), or a chronic illness the mother has, such as diabetes (see page 418). However, in many cases, the cause of preterm birth cannot be determined.

If your baby is preterm, he or she will not look like the plump infant you envisioned. He or she will be tiny and thin, with reddish skin. In the neonatal unit, a baby will be kept warm in an incubator and attached to electronic monitors that check his or her vital signs. Oxygen may be supplied if the baby's lungs are undeveloped.

At first, the baby will be fed through a tube inserted into the stomach through the nose, or intravenously. Later, he or she will be fed with a bottle. You will be able to breast-feed your baby as soon as he or she gains strength and develops the sucking reflex. To provide breast milk for your baby during this time, and to keep your breasts producing milk for when you can nurse him or her, you should regularly express milk from your breasts. Any extra breast milk can be frozen for later use. Breast milk can be beneficial for a preterm infant because, along with providing nutritional benefits, breast milk contains antibodies that help protect the baby from infections.

Because preterm birth can be caused by an infection, a preterm infant is usually treated with antibiotics for the first 2 days, until the doctor is certain there is no infection. Blood samples are taken regularly from the infant's umbilical cord or from a tube in the arm to make sure the kidneys and liver are functioning properly. Your baby will probably stay in the hospital until his or her weight reaches 4 to 5 pounds and any life-threatening conditions have been treated successfully.

One of the hardest parts of having a preterm or ill baby is being separated at a time when you would normally be holding, cuddling, and breastfeeding your baby. It is essential for you and your partner to spend time touching, stroking, and talking to the baby while he or she lies in the incubator. This kind of stimulation can dramatically improve your baby's breathing and physical development. The contact will also help you both form emotional bonds with your baby.

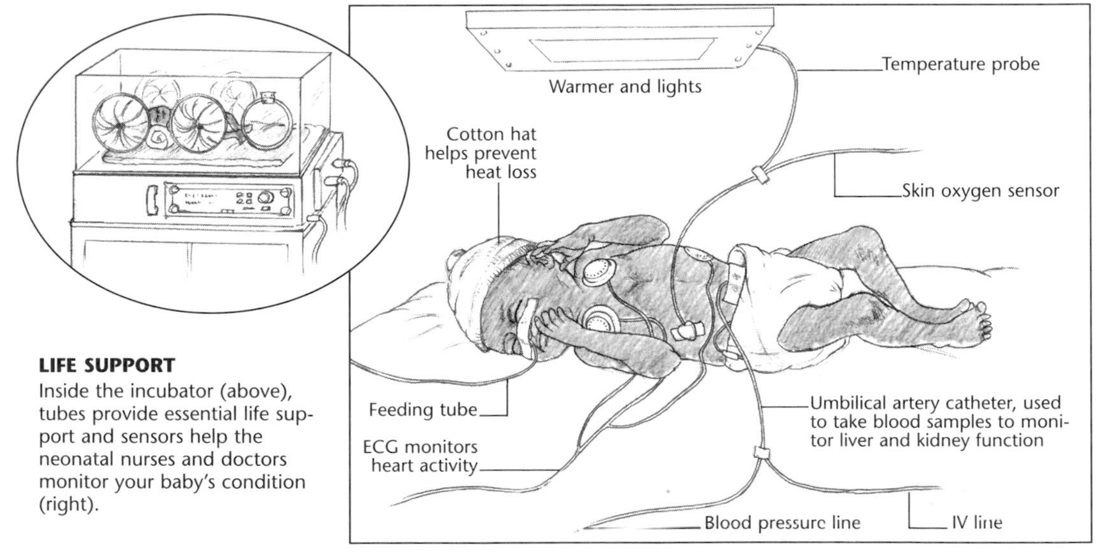

LIFE SUPPORT
Inside the incubator (above), tubes provide essential life support and sensors help the neonatal nurses and doctors monitor your baby's condition (right).

may not have a period for as long as you nurse your baby. However, breast-feeding by itself is *not* a reliable form of contraception. Even if you do not have a period, you may ovulate (release an egg from an ovary) and, therefore, you can become pregnant. If you are having sex, you need to use some form of contraception. If you are breast-feeding, do not use hormonal methods of contraception (see page 310), such as birth-control pills, for the first 6 weeks after delivery because the hormones may lessen the amount of breast milk you produce. Use a barrier method of birth control (see page 318), such as a condom, diaphragm, or spermicide. If you have decided you do not want to have any more children, you or your spouse may consider surgical sterilization (see page 326).

Sexual intercourse You can resume sexual intercourse as soon as the tissue of your vagina and surrounding area is completely healed. It usually takes about 6 weeks for a tear in the tissue or an episiotomy to heal. Although you are physically capable of having intercourse, you may find that you are less interested than usual in sex during the first months after delivery. A major cause of this lack of interest is fatigue caused by interrupted sleep. You may experience pain during intercourse for up to 3 months after delivery, especially if you are breast-feeding. This is because breast-feeding lowers the level of the hormone estrogen, which may cause your vagina to be dry. A water-based vaginal lubricant may help relieve this discomfort. If you have had an episiotomy, you may feel some tenderness for weeks or months during intercourse.

Exercising after delivery After about 6 weeks you can begin to do exercises, such as sit-ups, to strengthen your abdominal muscles, and start a program of regular aerobic exercise. Do not swim for the first 3 weeks after delivery because bacteria from the water may enter the healing tissue of your vagina, possibly causing infection. If you have had a cesarean delivery, avoid strenuous activity for at least 3 weeks; do not do any abdominal exercises for at least 6 weeks.

Questions women ask
New motherhood

Q I'm home with my healthy new baby but I find I'm crying all the time and reacting emotionally to things that never would have phased me before. Is this postpartum depression?

A What you are experiencing is not unusual. More than half of new mothers experience mood swings, including crying episodes, during the first week after childbirth. Most women recover within a few days. But a small percentage of women experience severe depression that can last longer than 2 weeks and require professional help. Postpartum depression is a serious illness that can be treated. Call your doctor immediately if your crying and emotional highs and lows continue for 2 weeks or longer. He or she can help you or refer you to a psychiatrist or other mental health professional.

Q I've always been a perfectionist. I like things neat, organized, and running smoothly. Now, with the baby waking up for feedings around the clock, everything is disorganized. How can I make our lives more sane?

A It is important to accept the idea that things are going to be disorganized for the first few weeks or months after childbirth. Don't expect the house to look perfect or meals to be much more than frozen foods or take-out dishes for a while. Rely on your partner, friends, and relatives to help with meals, chores, and housework so you can concentrate your energies on the baby. Try to get some time for yourself.

WARNING SIGNS
COMPLICATIONS AFTER CHILDBIRTH

Call your doctor immediately if you experience any of the following symptoms in the days or weeks after delivery:

- Heavy vaginal bleeding
- Fever over 100.4°F
- Hot, tender breasts
- Pain or a burning sensation while urinating, or a sudden urge to urinate
- Swelling or tenderness in your legs
- Chest pain or cough
- Increasing or persistent pain in the vaginal area

Recovering from a cesarean delivery If you have had a cesarean delivery, your hospital stay and recovery period will be longer. The catheter used to empty your bladder during the delivery will be left in place for about 24 hours. You may find bowel movements difficult. Drinking liquids and eating a high-fiber diet (lots of fruits, vegetables, and whole grains) can help. If necessary, your doctor may recommend a stool softener.

If you require pain medication and you are breast-feeding, be sure that your doctor knows you are breast-feeding so that he or she can prescribe a pain medication that is safe to take. Walk around as much as possible to get your body systems working normally again. You may feel some gas pains as your bowel function returns to normal. You will have bleeding from the vagina resembling a period (called lochia) for 2 to 6 weeks, just as you would after a vaginal delivery. This bleeding may taper to a pinkish discharge.

After a cesarean delivery, you are likely to remain in the hospital for 3 to 4 days. Once you are home, you will probably need extra help with the baby, housework, and meal preparation. In addition to your partner, ask a relative or friend to help. Avoid lifting anything over 15 pounds for the first 2 weeks.

Breast-feeding

Breast-feeding a child is a unique and rewarding time in a woman's life. The interdependence between mother and child created by the act of nursing helps create a special bond between them. In addition, breast milk is the most nutritious and beneficial form of nourishment a newborn can have.

BENEFITS OF BREAST-FEEDING

Breast-feeding is good for both you and your baby in many ways. If you are unsure about whether or not to breast-feed, consider the advantages:

For you:

- Helps your uterus return to its normal size more rapidly.
- Helps you lose weight faster; your body burns calories producing milk.
- Helps reduce your risk of breast cancer if you nurse for at least 3 months because breast-feeding may cause changes in breast cells that have a protective effect (see page 273). Your risk of breast cancer is reduced further each time you nurse another baby for at least 3 months.
- Helps form an emotional bond between you and your child because it is a regular time for being close and sharing a warm, pleasant experience.
- Eliminates the inconvenience of preparing formula and washing bottles; your milk is immediately available whenever your baby is hungry.

For your baby:

- Provides a unique mixture of nutrients and hormones and other essential proteins, making it the healthiest food available for an infant.
- Reduces the incidence of ear infections and infections of the digestive and respiratory tracts during the first years of life.
- Causes fewer food allergies.
- Causes fewer digestive problems; babies are less likely to be constipated.

If you cannot breast-feed or choose not to breast-feed, a variety of nutritious commercially prepared formulas are available. Ask your pediatrician which formula he or she recommends. In some cases, it may not be appropriate for a woman to breast-feed. It is currently recommended that women not breast-feed if they are undergoing chemotherapy for cancer or if they are infected with HIV (the virus that causes AIDS) or hepatitis B. These viruses can be passed to a nursing baby in breast milk. You can continue breast-feeding if you have the breast infection mastitis (see page 454), even if you are taking antibiotics.

GETTING STARTED

Even though breast-feeding may not seem simple or natural at first, almost every woman can breast-feed. The size of your breasts before you became pregnant has nothing to do with your ability to breast-feed. Some infants are naturally adept at nursing from the start, but many need to learn how. Breast-feeding is a learning experience for you as well. Be confident; you and your baby are likely to become skilled breast-feeding partners within a few weeks.

The first few days after delivery, your breasts produce and secrete a small amount of colostrum, a thick, creamy substance that supplies your baby with essential nutrients and antibodies (to fight infection) until your milk begins to flow. Usually, milk "comes in" between the second and fourth days after delivery but it can take longer for some women.

Some mothers worry that their baby is not getting enough milk. You will not know exactly how many ounces your baby is drinking at each feeding, as you do with bottle-feeding. However, you can tell that your baby is getting enough milk from your breasts if he or she is gaining weight regularly, wetting six or more diapers a day, and is sleeping well. The more frequently and longer you nurse, the more milk your breasts produce.

Breast-feeding can benefit you and your baby whether you continue for a

Tips for breast-feeding

Here are some ideas to help you get started breast-feeding your infant:

- Be patient with yourself and your baby. Few nursing "partners" hit it off from the start; it takes time and practice to perfect a nursing routine.
- Feed your baby whenever he or she is hungry; you will eventually establish a pattern. A newborn may need to nurse as often as every 2 hours or perhaps even more frequently. As your baby grows, he or she can hold more and more milk and go for a longer time between feedings. Don't worry; your baby will eventually sleep through the night.
- Sit or lie down in a comfortable position. Vary the position from feeding to feeding, especially at first, to prevent breast soreness.
- Use both breasts at every feeding and try to alternate the breast you start with. It is important to alternate breasts because the composition of the milk in one breast differs from the beginning of the nursing session to the end; it is a good idea to let your baby empty one breast completely before starting on the other.
- Hold your baby so that his or her whole body is facing you.
- Use your thumb and index finger to point your nipple outward and brush it against the baby's cheek to stimulate the rooting reflex, which makes the baby turn toward the touch. Repeat if necessary but do not force it; your baby will respond eventually.
- Be sure your whole nipple and part of the areola, the dark circular area around it, are in the baby's mouth.
- If your baby's sucking is strong, steady, and rhythmic, you can be sure he or she is receiving nourishment.
- When the baby is finished nursing and before you remove the baby from your breast, it helps to break the suction by gently pressing your fingers into your breast near his or her mouth.
- Expect to feel some soreness for the first week or two as the baby clamps onto your nipples at the beginning of each nursing session. This soreness will subside as your nipples begin to toughen. You can aid in the process by keeping your nipples exposed to the open air after nursing, scrubbing them with a washcloth as you bathe or shower, and cleaning them with water alone—soap can be drying.
- Contact your doctor if you have a fever, if a breast becomes red and warm to the touch, or if you feel a hard lump in a breast. You may have a clogged or infected milk duct (see page 454). Your doctor can show you how to apply heat to your breast or massage it to unclog the duct. If you have a breast infection, your doctor will prescribe medication.

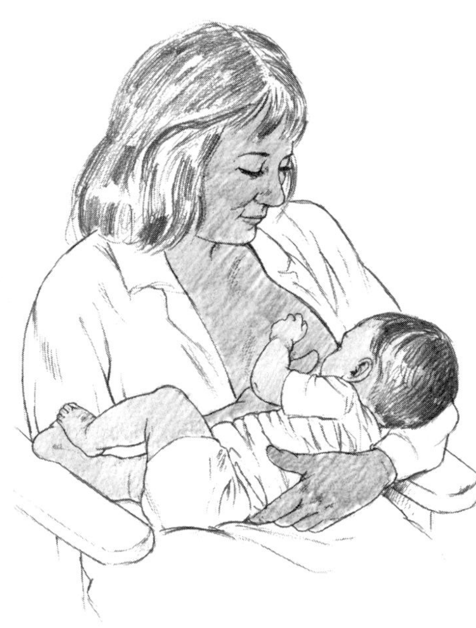

BREAST-FEEDING
Position your infant so that he or she is facing you. Support the baby's head in the bend of your arm, using an armrest or pillows to support your arm if necessary. Make sure you are comfortable because you will be sitting in this position for 15 to 30 minutes. Check to be sure your whole nipple and part of the dark circular area around it are in the baby's mouth.

few weeks or several months or more. Some working mothers breast-feed for as long as they are on maternity leave and then wean their infant to a bottle before they return to work. They may continue to nurse the baby in the morning, evening, and night. Some working mothers continue providing breast milk to their baby by expressing milk from their breasts at work using a breast pump, refrigerating the milk, and bringing it home for the baby's caregiver to feed to the baby the next day. Whichever route you choose, your milk production will automatically adjust to your baby's demand for it.

As you and your baby learn how to breast-feed, some problems may arise and you may have questions. Ask your doctor or hospital for a referral to a nurse who specializes in breast-feeding. Another resource for helpful advice is a local chapter of La Leche League, a volunteer organization that provides information and encouragement to women who are breast-feeding.

DIET, EXERCISE, AND WEIGHT

When you are breast-feeding, you need to take in about 600 more calories each day than you did before you became pregnant. You also need extra fluids and calcium. You should take in about the same amount of calcium each day that you did during pregnancy—1,200 milligrams. If you do not take in enough calcium, your body will take the calcium it needs from your bones. Drinking several glasses of skim milk each day helps fulfill this requirement and also provides extra fluid. Do not restrict calories to try to lose weight while you are breast-feeding. Many women find that breast-feeding helps them lose weight more quickly.

Regular aerobic exercise is healthy for you and does not affect the quality of your milk in any way. You may find it more comfortable to nurse right before exercising so your breasts will be less heavy with milk. Avoid alcohol, tobacco, caffeine, prescription drugs, and over-the-counter drugs; these substances can pass into your milk supply and to a nursing baby.

PROBLEMS

Most women do not have serious difficulties once they and their baby establish a breast-feeding pattern. However, it is common to have sore nipples when you begin breast-feeding. Gradually, the skin will toughen. In the meantime, there are some things you can do to reduce the discomfort. Wash your nipples with water only—soap can be drying. Vary your nursing position so that the baby is not always sucking on the same spot. Make sure that the whole nipple and areola, not just the nipple, are in the baby's mouth. Do not use lotions or lubricants around your nipples that your baby may swallow while nursing.

It is possible for an infection to develop while you are breast-feeding. Call your doctor if you or your baby experience any symptoms of the following infections:

Mastitis Mastitis, an infection of the milk ducts in the breasts, is the most common problem in women who breast-feed. It occurs when bacteria enter the breast through the nipple, usually from a nursing baby's mouth. Symptoms, which can be very painful, include soreness, hardness, redness, and swelling of the breast. You may also have chills and a fever. Call your doctor if you have any of these symptoms. He or she will prescribe an antibiotic and, if necessary, a pain reliever that is safe to take while breast-feeding. Continue to breast-feed; emptying the breast of milk helps relieve the symptoms. Have the baby nurse first on the infected breast so that the hardest sucking is on this side, when the baby is hungriest. If the baby does not empty the breast completely, empty it with a breast pump. Some women have recurring mastitis.

Breast abscess A breast abscess, caused by infection, is a collection of pus in breast tissue that forms a red, hot, firm lump in the breast that is extremely tender. A breast abscess occurs when bacteria from the baby's mouth enter the breast through a cracked or sore nipple. Report this problem to your doctor immediately. An abscess can usually be treated with antibiotics that you take by mouth. In more severe cases, a doctor may also recommend draining the abscess with a needle or a tiny incision. This procedure can be performed in the doctor's office using a local anesthetic. You can continue to nurse during treatment.

Thrush Some women develop a yeast infection called thrush when they are nursing. Thrush causes the nipples to become sore and cracked. The nursing baby will also have the infection, which appears on his or her tongue as white patches. Your doctor will prescribe medicated cream that you apply several times a day to your nipples and another medication to give by drops into the baby's mouth. Thrush may also spread through the baby's digestive tract and cause a form of diaper rash, which can be treated with a medicated cream. Thrush often requires several weeks of treatment and can be recurring. Continue to breast-feed during treatment.

Medical care for your child

As your child grows and develops, he or she will require routine medical care, such as immunizations. Your child's doctor can be either a pediatrician or a family physician. A pediatrician is trained in caring for infants and children, and should be board certified by the American Board of Pediatrics. A family physician, whose medical training includes all aspects of family medicine, should be board certified by the American Board of Family Practice.

To find a doctor for your child, ask for recommendations from your obstetrician or friends or family members who live in your area. Your health insurance plan may supply a list of doctors from which you must choose. It is a good idea to have an initial interview with the doctor before making a final decision. Here are some things to consider when choosing a pediatrician:

- Ask the doctor about his or her philosophy and attitudes about things that are important to you, such as breast-feeding.
- Find out if the doctor's office hours—and the location of the office—accommodate your schedule. A doctor who has some evening or weekend time may be better for working parents.
- How long is the average waiting time in the doctor's office?
- Find out the system that is used for phone inquiries. Frequently, you may have questions that do not require an office visit. Will the doctor take phone calls and, if so, when is he or she available for calls?
- What is the doctor's hospital affiliation? To what hospital will your child go in case of serious illness or injury?
- Find out how billing and financial matters are handled. Make sure the doctor is covered by your insurance plan.

HAVING YOUR CHILD IMMUNIZED

It is essential that you have your child immunized. The recommended vaccinations protect your child against potentially life-threatening infections, including polio, measles, and hepatitis B. The federal government recommends that all American children be vaccinated against the following nine serious infectious diseases: diphtheria, pertussis (whooping cough), and tetanus (together in one shot called DPT); measles, mumps, and rubella (in one shot called MMR); poliomyelitis; *Haemophilus influenzae* type b (Hib); and hepatitis B.

When should your child be immunized?

Your pediatrician can guide you as to the exact timing of each of the following vaccinations. If you have any questions about immunizations, ask your doctor to discuss them with you. Most public school districts require proof of immunization for enrollment.

CHILD'S AGE	VACCINE
At birth	Hepatitis B
1-2 months	Hepatitis B
2 months	DPT; OPV; Hib
4 months	DPT; OPV; Hib
6 months	DPT
6-18 months	Hepatitis B
12-15 months	MMR
15-18 months	DPT; OPV
4-6 years	DPT; OPV
11-12 years	MMR
14-16 years	Diphtheria, tetanus

KEY	
DPT	Diphtheria, pertussis, tetanus
OPV	Oral polio vaccine
Hib	*Haemophilus influenzae* type b
MMR	Measles, mumps, rubella

·4·

Health concerns of women

CHAPTER 17

Your heart, blood, and circulation

Contents

Heart disease is the number-one killer of American women. If you are a woman, you are at risk of developing heart disease at some time in your life, particularly after menopause. Your risk of heart disease is three times greater at age 65 than at 45. Educating yourself about the symptoms of heart disease and ways to prevent it—through diet, exercise, and lifestyle changes—can be especially beneficial because the condition is more likely to go undetected in women than in men.

The subject of heart and blood vessel disorders is vast and complex. This chapter focuses on the disorders that affect the greatest number of women or are more common among women than men.

Your heart

Your heart is a muscular organ that is about the size and shape of a fist. It consists of two side-by-side pumps. Your veins carry used, oxygen-depleted blood to the right side of your heart, which pumps it to the lungs to receive a fresh supply of oxygen. This newly oxygenated blood returns to the left side of your heart and is pumped through the aorta, a large blood vessel that directs blood to a system of arteries. Your arteries carry fresh blood to tissues throughout your body. The veins return the used blood to the heart and the process starts again, about 100,000 times every day.

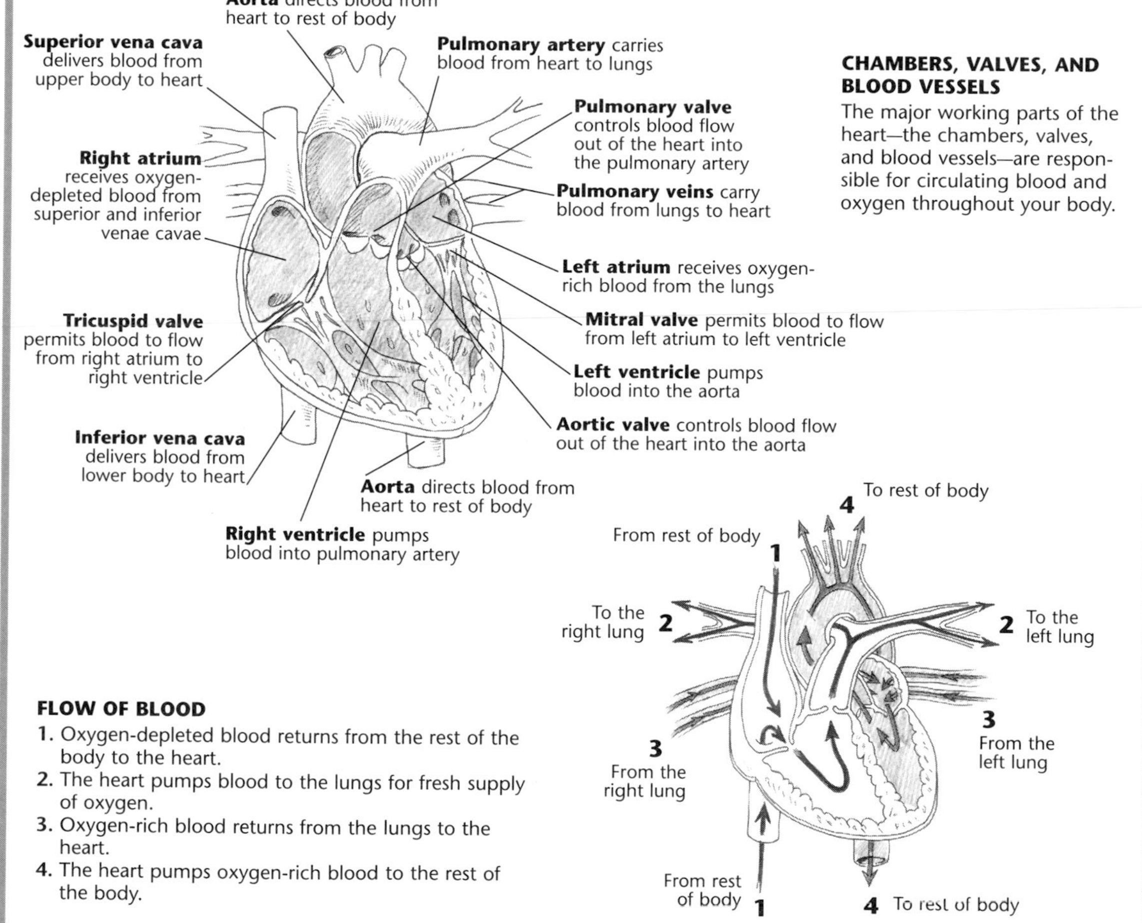

CHAMBERS, VALVES, AND BLOOD VESSELS

The major working parts of the heart—the chambers, valves, and blood vessels—are responsible for circulating blood and oxygen throughout your body.

FLOW OF BLOOD

1. Oxygen-depleted blood returns from the rest of the body to the heart.
2. The heart pumps blood to the lungs for fresh supply of oxygen.
3. Oxygen-rich blood returns from the lungs to the heart.
4. The heart pumps oxygen-rich blood to the rest of the body.

Coronary artery disease

The coronary arteries are branching blood vessels on the surface of the heart that supply the heart muscle with the nutrient-rich blood it needs to function. If these arteries become narrowed or blocked by the buildup of fatty deposits (plaque) in a process called atherosclerosis (see page 468), the heart muscle does not get a sufficient amount of oxygen and may be damaged. This condition, called coronary artery disease, can lead to a heart attack.

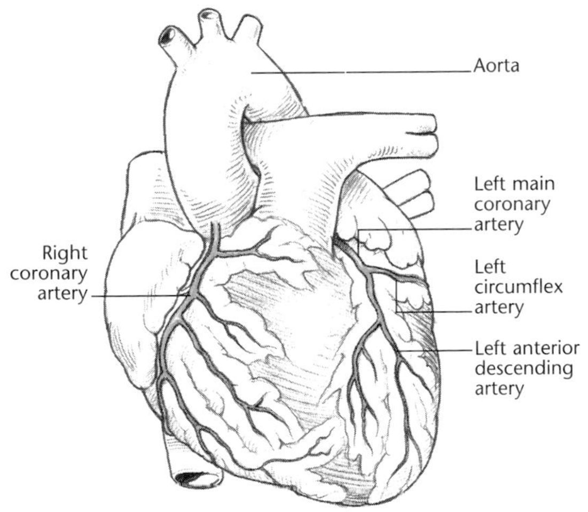

CORONARY ARTERIES
The coronary arteries supply oxygen-rich blood to the heart muscle itself. Both the right and left coronary arteries branch off the aorta. The left main coronary artery immediately branches into two major arteries—the left anterior descending artery and the circumflex artery. The left anterior descending artery supplies the front portion of the heart muscle; the circumflex artery circles around to the side and back of the heart. The right coronary artery delivers oxygen to the right ventricle and the lower surface of the heart. A narrowing or blockage in a coronary artery can cut off the supply of blood to the heart, causing a heart attack. A heart attack causes damage to the heart muscle itself.

RISKS YOU CAN CONTROL

There are several factors that can increase your risk of having a heart attack, some of which you can control. You cannot control factors such as age or a family history of heart disease. The four biggest risk factors for heart disease in women—high cholesterol level, smoking, high blood pressure, and diabetes—are controllable. You can do many relatively simple things to reduce your risk of heart disease, including eating a low-fat diet, exercising regularly, not smoking, maintaining a healthy weight, and getting treatment for high blood pressure or diabetes if necessary. A gradual decline in the number of deaths from heart disease in the US over the last several years is the result of an increased understanding of these risk factors and the corresponding changes in lifestyle that many people have made.

High cholesterol level High levels of cholesterol in the blood increase the likelihood that the coronary arteries will become narrowed, which can lead to a heart attack. Before menopause, the presence of the female hormone estrogen in the blood gives most women lower total cholesterol levels than men and higher levels of the good, heart-protecting cholesterol called high-density lipoprotein (HDL). However, estrogen's heart-protecting advantage is lost after menopause, when the ovaries reduce their production of the hormone. The presence of estrogen in women's blood is one reason they tend to develop heart disease later in life than men.

At age 20, you should have a cholesterol test that evaluates your total cholesterol level and your level of HDL cholesterol; if these levels are normal, have your cholesterol tested every 5 years (or as often as your doctor recommends) until menopause. After you go through menopause, have a cholesterol test every year. For more about

What is your risk of heart disease?

For each of the following characteristics that apply to you, write down the corresponding number. Then add up the points to determine your risk of coronary artery disease.

YOUR AGE

Although heart attack and stroke affect women of all ages, your risk increases as you age, especially after menopause.

Over 50 and past menopause 10
Between 35 and 50 and past menopause 8
Past menopause but taking estrogen 4
Over 34 and not menopausal 4
Age 34 or under 1

YOUR FAMILY HEALTH HISTORY

If a member of your immediate family has had a heart attack or stroke, your risk of heart disease is increased.

Family member had a heart attack or stroke before age 55 5
Family member had a heart attack or stroke after age 55 3
No immediate family history of heart attack or stroke .1

SMOKING

The more you smoke, the greater your risk of heart disease.

Smoke 11 or more cigarettes a day 5
Smoke 1 to 10 cigarettes a day 3
Never smoke 1

WEIGHT

Determine your body mass index (BMI): Multiply your weight in pounds by 705. Divide the result by your height in inches. Divide this result by your height in inches again.

BMI of 27 or more 5
BMI between 22 and 26 3
BMI below 22 1

BODY SHAPE

If you carry most of your weight around your hips and thighs, your risk of heart disease is lower than if you carry your weight around your waist and upper body. Calculate your waist-to-hip ratio by dividing your waist measurement by your hip measurement.

Waist-to-hip ratio of .80 or more 5
Waist-to-hip ratio of less than .80 1

DRINKING

Moderate drinking—the equivalent of one glass of wine each day—can reduce your risk of heart disease, but heavy drinking can raise your cholesterol level and blood pressure, increasing your risk of heart disease.

Binge drinking 5
More than two drinks a day 3
One drink a day 1

STRESS

If your job is demanding but allows you little or no control over your working conditions, your risk of heart disease is increased.

High job pressure 5
Any other job situation 1

EXERCISE

Lack of regular aerobic exercise is a major risk factor for heart disease.

Exercise rarely 5
Exercise occasionally .3
Exercise at least three times a week 1

BLOOD PRESSURE

If your blood pressure is usually above 140/90, your risk of heart disease is increased.

Above 160/95 5
140/90 to 160/95 3
Below 140/90 1

DIETARY FAT

Reducing your intake of saturated and hydrogenated fats (see page 51) can help keep your cholesterol at a healthy level. How often do you eat red meat, butter, margarine, or cheese?

Eat them almost every day 5
Eat them several days a week 3
Eat little or none 1

IF YOUR SCORE IS:

13 or fewer points: You have little or no risk of heart attack or stroke. Keep doing what you're doing.

14-30 points: You have a moderate risk of heart attack or stroke. Keep an eye on your diet and exercise regularly. If you smoke, quit now.

31 or more points: You have a high risk of heart attack or stroke. See your doctor.

the different types of cholesterol and cholesterol testing, see page 131.

You can help maintain your cholesterol level in a healthy range by eating a low-fat diet (see page 51) and getting regular exercise (see page 78). If you have a high cholesterol level and you already have heart disease, or you have other risk factors for heart disease (such as high blood pressure), your doctor may recommend a medication to lower your cholesterol level. You may have to take cholesterol-lowering drugs for many years. While you are taking the medication, your doctor will ask you to watch for possible side effects such as constipation and he or she will examine you regularly for changes in liver function or other potential problems.

There are a variety of cholesterol-lowering drugs from which doctors can choose; your doctor will recommend a particular drug for you, depending on your cholesterol profile. For example, some drugs are effective in lowering the level of harmful, low-density lipoprotein (LDL) cholesterol, while other drugs increase the level of good HDL cholesterol or modify levels of other fats in the blood called triglycerides. Following are descriptions of the most commonly used cholesterol-lowering medications:

Bile acid binding resins Bile acid binding resins are drugs that make bile acids (body chemicals that aid digestion) and cholesterol combine in the small intestine. This combination, or binding, lowers cholesterol level by preventing cholesterol from being absorbed into the blood and by stimulating the liver to remove cholesterol from the blood. Resins come in a powder form that can be mixed with water or orange juice, or with food during meals. These medications are safe because they are not absorbed into the body. However, they have some irritating side effects. Most people do not like the taste of these drugs because they have a gritty texture.

Genetic susceptibility to high cholesterol

Some people have genetic abnormalities that can have an adverse effect on their cholesterol profile (see page 131). For example, some people inherit a gene that puts them at high risk of having a very high total cholesterol level. This condition is called familial hypercholesterolemia. Other people may inherit a susceptibility to having a low level of the good, heart-protecting cholesterol called high-density lipoprotein (HDL). In women, a low level of HDL (below 35 milligrams per deciliter) may be an even more powerful risk factor for heart disease than a high total cholesterol level. If you have a family history of high cholesterol or another cholesterol abnormality, have your cholesterol tested beginning at age 20. Your doctor will analyze your cholesterol profile and determine what kind of treatment you need. You are likely to have to take medication throughout your life to maintain your cholesterol profile in a healthy range.

A heart-healthy lifestyle

A healthy lifestyle can greatly reduce your risk of heart disease. Here are the most important things you can do to keep your heart strong and working efficiently:

- Eat a low-fat, low-cholesterol diet. Saturated fats and cholesterol in foods can raise your cholesterol level—a strong risk factor for heart disease. For information about how to limit fat and cholesterol in your diet, see page 107.
- Get regular exercise. You are twice as likely to develop heart disease if you are inactive than if you exercise regularly. Exercise that increases your heart rate—such as brisk walking, swimming, or weight lifting—lowers your blood pressure and cholesterol level, and strengthens your heart so that it can pump more blood with less effort.
- Maintain a healthy weight (see page 99). Being overweight increases your risk of high blood pressure and diabetes—two important risk factors for heart disease. If you are 20 percent or more over your ideal weight, you are putting your health in danger. This is particularly true if your body shape is such that you carry excess weight around your waist (see page 97).
- Do not smoke cigarettes. If you smoke, quit. Smoking dramatically increases your risk of heart disease (see page 464).

Resins can also cause bloating and constipation.

Fibrates Fibrates are drugs that lower the level of potentially harmful fats in the blood called triglycerides. Fibrates can also lower the level of harmful LDL cholesterol and slightly increase the level of good HDL cholesterol. Side effects include a slightly increased risk of gallstones (see page 532) and gallbladder disease.

HMG CoA reductase inhibitors Human menopausal gonadotropin coenzyme A (HMG CoA) reductase inhibitors are drugs that block an enzyme in the liver called HMG CoA reductase. Blocking the action of this enzyme significantly decreases the production of cholesterol in the liver. These drugs are very effective in lowering the level of harmful LDL cholesterol. Most people tolerate these drugs very well but, in rare cases, they may cause some liver damage. For this reason, you will be given a blood test periodically to make sure the medication is not harming your liver.

Niacin The vitamin niacin, or nicotinic acid, decreases the production of harmful LDL cholesterol in the liver. In order to lower your total cholesterol level significantly, you have to take relatively large doses of the drug. At high doses, niacin can also increase good HDL cholesterol. The dose must be built up gradually to avoid side effects such as flushing of the skin. In some cases, the side effects can be controlled by taking the drug along with aspirin. In rare cases, niacin can cause liver damage.

Probucol Probucol is a drug that lowers the level of harmful LDL cholesterol. The drug may also work as an antioxidant, a chemical that helps prevent fatty deposits from building up in artery walls. However, probucol can also lower the level of good HDL cholesterol. The most common side effect of the medication is diarrhea.

Smoking For women who smoke cigarettes, quitting is the most important way to reduce the risk of heart disease. Smoking decreases the levels of two substances in the blood that help protect against heart disease—HDL cholesterol and the female hormone estrogen. Smoking as few as one to four cigarettes a day doubles your risk of heart disease; smoking more than a pack a day increases your risk up to 15 times. Heart attacks are more severe and deadly in people who smoke.

Smoking puts strain on your heart because it causes blood vessels to constrict, which reduces the flow of blood to your heart and makes the heart work harder to pump blood to other parts of the body. In addition, toxic substances in cigarette smoke may directly damage artery walls and cause atherosclerosis (see page 468), a process in which fatty deposits accumulate on the inside of artery walls, potentially narrowing or blocking the blood vessels. When you stop smoking, your risk of heart disease drops rapidly. For information about how to quit smoking, see page 157.

High blood pressure Blood pressure is the force of blood against the walls of arteries. High blood pressure, also called hypertension, dramatically increases your chances of developing coronary artery disease and stroke. In a woman who is not pregnant, blood pressure is considered high when the reading stays over 140/90 for an extended period. Your risk of having high blood pressure increases after menopause. More than half of all women over 65 have high blood pressure. Black women are more likely to have high blood pressure than women in any other racial group.

Estrogen and heart disease

Estrogen helps protect your heart and circulatory system by reducing your total cholesterol level and increasing your level of the heart-protecting type of cholesterol called high-density lipoprotein (HDL). Estrogen may also help protect you from heart disease by making the inside lining of your arteries less susceptible to the buildup of fatty deposits (atherosclerosis). When your ovaries reduce their production of estrogen at menopause, your blood pressure and cholesterol level go up and your level of good HDL cholesterol goes down, increasing your risk of heart disease. Women who take estrogen in hormone replacement therapy (HRT; see page 359) after menopause are half as likely to die of heart disease as women who do not take the hormone. If your risk of heart disease is high, or you have been diagnosed with heart disease, talk with your doctor about whether taking estrogen will reduce your risk.

If you have high blood pressure, talk to your doctor about the possible need for treatment, including taking medication to lower your blood pressure and making changes in your lifestyle, such as losing weight, exercising more, and limiting your intake of salt. For more about high blood pressure and treatment, see page 480.

Diabetes People with diabetes (see page 617) have an increased risk of heart disease and stroke. In the most common form of diabetes, called type II diabetes, an elevated level of insulin (a hormone the body uses to regulate sugar), raises blood pressure and adversely affects cholesterol levels and causes cholesterol to be deposited in artery walls. For most people with type II diabetes, weight reduction and exercise can increase the burning of excess sugar in their blood and reduce their risk of heart disease and stroke.

People with type II diabetes have high levels of insulin in their blood because their body is resistant to the effects of the insulin they do have; in response, their body produces more and more insulin. However, this is often not enough to lower their blood sugar levels to normal. These people may have to take medication that improves insulin's efficiency in regulating sugar, or injections of insulin. For more about controlling diabetes, see page 622.

ANGINA: AN IMPORTANT WARNING SIGN

Even at an advanced stage, coronary artery disease often has no symptoms. This is especially true for men, whose first sign of trouble is often a sudden heart attack. But many women are given a warning—they may first experience angina, chest pain caused by a reduced supply of oxygen to the heart muscle, which indicates heart disease. You may feel a tight, heavy, or squeezing sensation deep beneath your breastbone or in a band across your chest. The pain may radiate to your left arm, shoulder, neck, jaw, or down your back. You may also experience nausea, sweating, or shortness of breath. The pain of angina is similar to the pain of a heart attack (see page 471). Angina often occurs during physical exertion or emotional stress and may last only a few moments. You may have this recurring chest pain on and off for several years before you actually have a heart attack. As your arteries become narrower, the pain becomes more severe and may occur at any time, not just during exercise or stress; this is called unstable angina.

Because the symptoms of heart disease can be subtle, in some people the condition is not diagnosed for years. You may not have any warning chest pains at all. It is possible to have coronary artery disease and even a heart attack without knowing it. As many as a third of heart attacks in women are not recognized and the symptoms are sometimes misdiagnosed as indigestion. Being aware of the warning signs of heart disease (chest pain in particular), and bringing them to your doctor's attention immediately, may save your life.

WARNING SIGNS
HEART DISEASE

The major symptom of heart disease is chest pain called angina. See your doctor immediately if you have:

- Mild or severe chest pain or pressure
- Chest pain or shortness of breath during physical activity (such as climbing stairs)
- Relief of chest pain after a short rest
- Nausea, sweating, dizziness, or difficulty breathing

DIAGNOSING HEART DISEASE

If you experience angina or are at high risk of heart disease, your primary care doctor may refer you to a cardiologist, a doctor who specializes in disorders of the heart. To determine the health of your heart, you may have one or more of the following tests. These tests are listed in the order in which you are likely to have them, starting with the test that is easiest to perform and the least invasive (does not require entering your body or cutting into it).

Electrocardiogram An electrocardiogram (ECG but sometimes called an EKG) is a painless test that records the flow of electricity through your heart. Electrodes attached to your skin transmit this electrical activity to a machine that prints it out on a recording that your

SYMPTOM CHART

Chest pain

Pain anywhere between your neck and the bottom of your rib cage, which may be dull and pressing or stabbing, burning, or crushing.

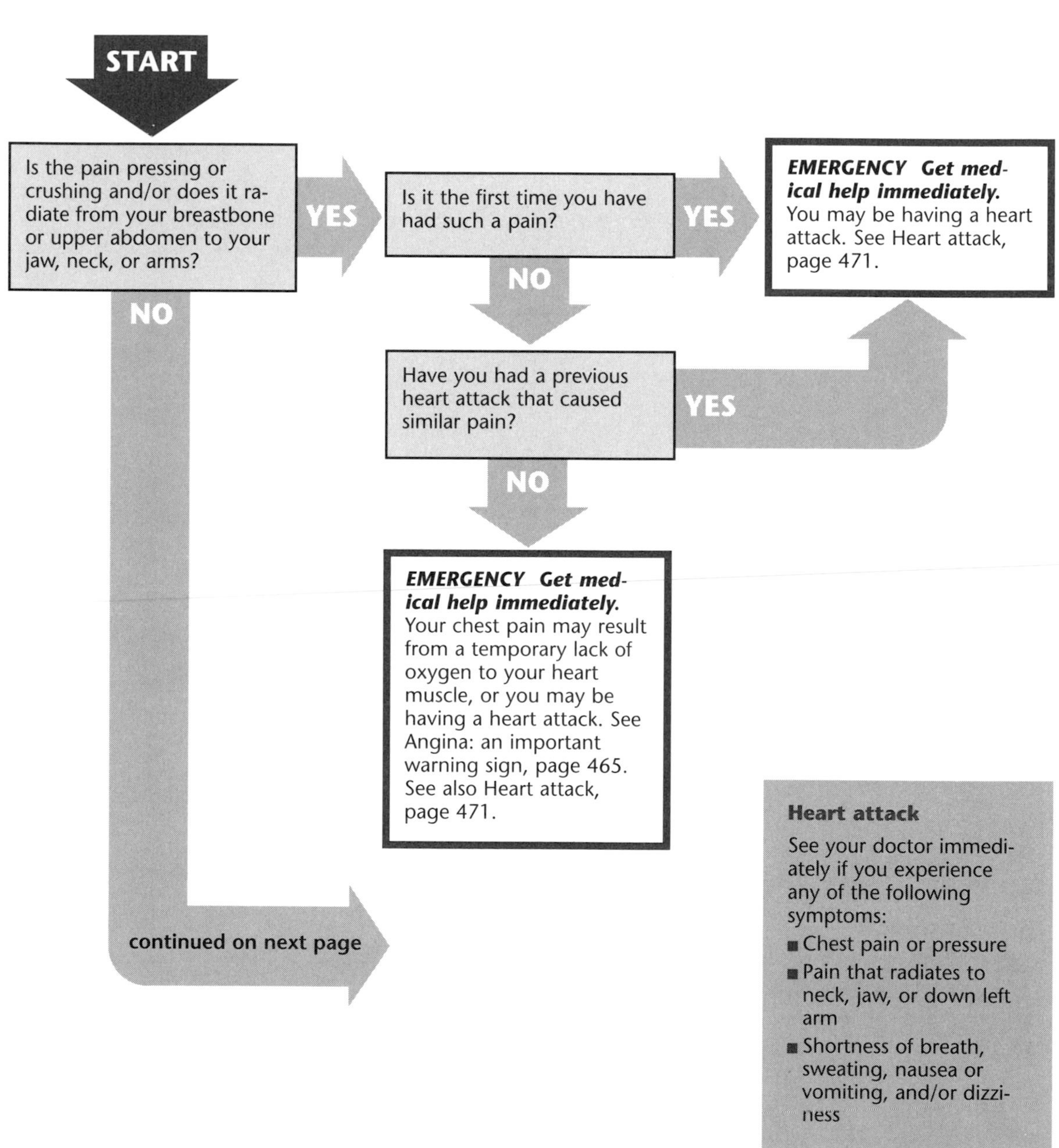

Heart attack

See your doctor immediately if you experience any of the following symptoms:

- Chest pain or pressure
- Pain that radiates to neck, jaw, or down left arm
- Shortness of breath, sweating, nausea or vomiting, and/or dizziness

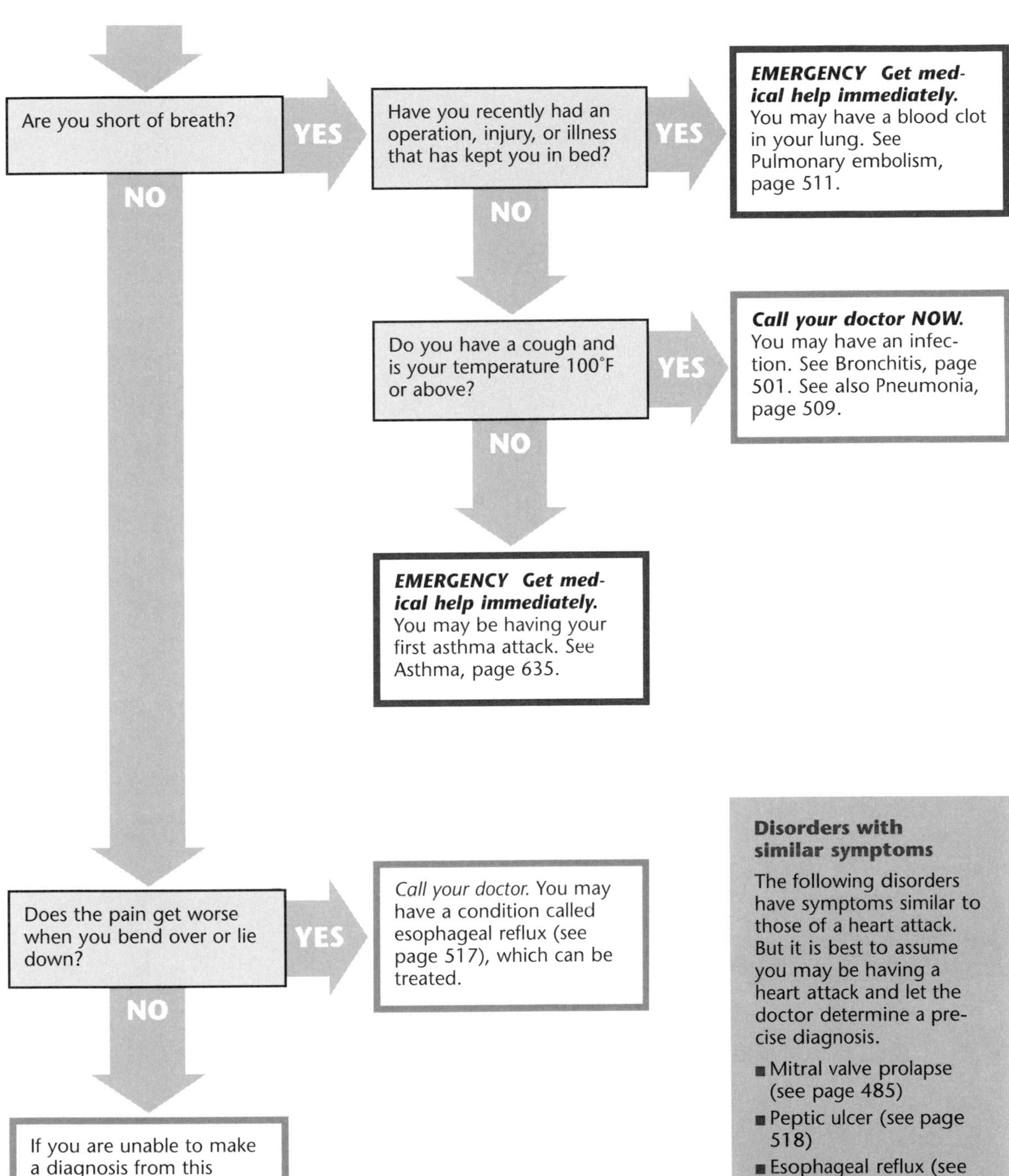

Disorders with similar symptoms

The following disorders have symptoms similar to those of a heart attack. But it is best to assume you may be having a heart attack and let the doctor determine a precise diagnosis.

- Mitral valve prolapse (see page 485)
- Peptic ulcer (see page 518)
- Esophageal reflux (see page 517)
- Asthma (see page 635)
- Pulmonary embolism (see page 511)

What is atherosclerosis?

Atherosclerosis is the buildup of fatty material called plaque on the inside walls of arteries. The formation of plaque begins when a fatty substance called lipoprotein—made of cholesterol and other fatty materials and protein—deposits itself on the inside walls of arteries. This process stimulates abnormal growth of cells in the lining of the arteries, which causes scarring and inflammation. The scarring and inflammation damage the artery walls, leading to the formation of plaque. Over a lifetime, as more and more fatty deposits accumulate, the size of the plaque grows, potentially narrowing the artery or even blocking it completely. Blocking of an artery can cut off the flow of blood to vital organs, destroying those tissues. If the blockage occurs in the arteries that nourish the heart, the result is chest pain (angina, see page 465) or a heart attack (see page 471). If the blockage cuts off the flow of blood to the brain, the result is a stroke (see page 569). Blockages in blood vessels in the legs can make walking painful.

Atherosclerosis can lead to blocking of an artery in other ways as well. Plaque is susceptible to cracking. Your body interprets these cracks as injuries and forms blood clots around them to seal them (see illustration below). If these blood clots grow large enough, they can block an artery, causing a heart attack. An accumulation of plaque can also trigger blood clotting by creating a turbulent flow of blood around it. This abnormal agitation of the blood stimulates the formation of blood clots, which can block an artery.

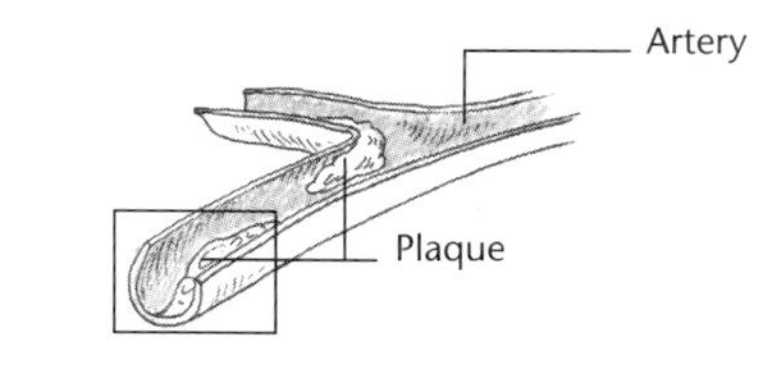

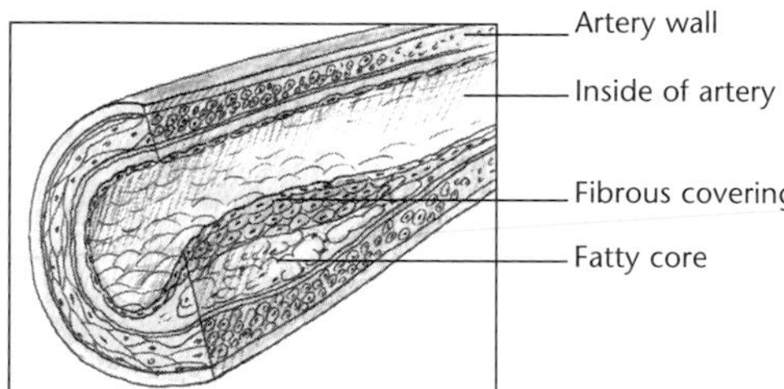

ATHEROSCLEROSIS
Atherosclerosis is the buildup of a cholesterol-containing substance called plaque inside arteries. Plaque often has a fatty core with a fibrous covering. Areas where arteries branch (top) are common sites for plaque formation and buildup. The buildup of plaque can impede or cut off the flow of blood to vital organs.

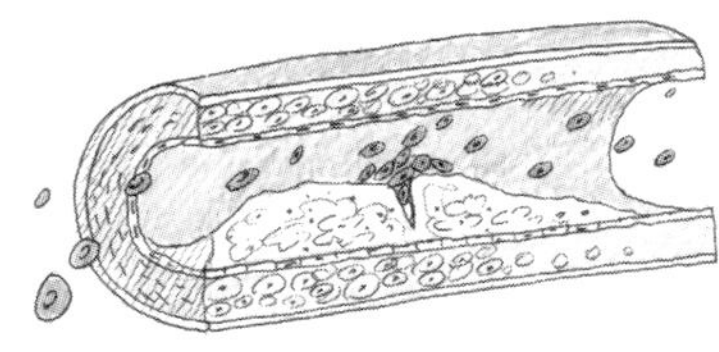

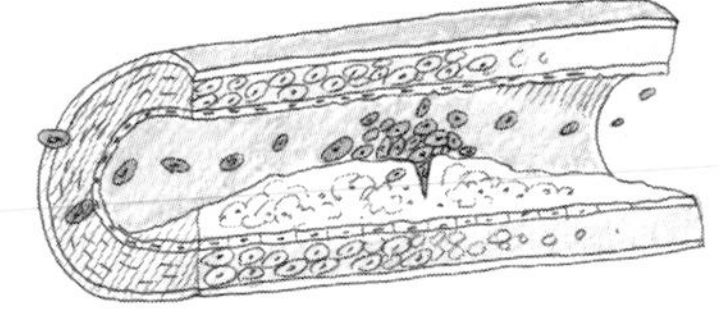

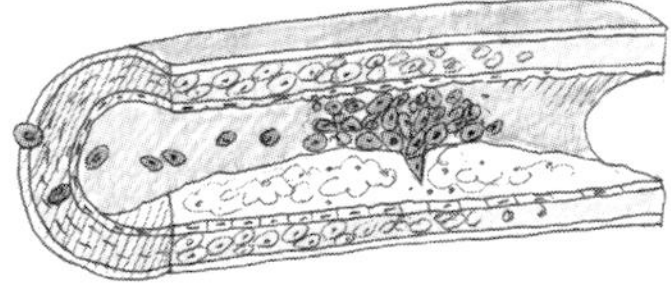

HOW PLAQUE CAN LEAD TO A BLOOD CLOT
A buildup of plaque can be the start of a clot. Plaque is prone to cracking (top). Your body interprets these cracks as injuries and forms blood clots around them to seal them (center). If a clot inside a coronary artery grows large enough (bottom), it can block the artery and cause a heart attack.

doctor can read. Each beat of your heart starts with an electrical impulse. When there is an abnormality in your heart, the flow of electricity through your heart changes. An ECG can help detect such a change. Your doctor can also use an ECG to help diagnose a wide range of heart problems—including abnormal heart rhythms, abnormal thickening of the heart muscle, defects in electrical impulses through the heart, and damage to heart tissue resulting from heart disease. However, this test sometimes fails to detect the presence of heart disease, especially if it has not caused any damage to the heart muscle. For a more thorough description of how an ECG is performed, see page 132.

If the ECG reveals irregular heart rhythms, your doctor may want to monitor your heart rate over a 24-hour period using a portable ECG machine called a Holter monitor. The Holter monitor is a device that is about the size of a portable cassette tape player. The monitor is attached to a shoulder strap. Electrodes attached to the skin of your chest transmit your heartbeat to a cassette tape inside the monitor, which is later interpreted by your doctor. You wear the monitor continuously for 1 day while you follow your usual routine. Your doctor may also recommend using the Holter monitor for 24 hours if you have been experiencing chest pain, dizziness, fainting episodes, or heart palpitations (sudden, rapid heartbeats).

The monitor can detect periods of ischemia, which occur when the oxygen supply to the heart is temporarily decreased. These episodes of ischemia may cause no symptoms and are then called "silent" episodes because you are unaware of them. However, with or without symptoms, these periods of ischemia may put you at increased risk of having a heart attack. Ischemia usually indicates that your heart needs more oxygen than your arteries are able to supply, usually because of a blockage caused by atherosclerosis (see page 468). If you are experiencing episodes of ischemia, your doctor may prescribe medication to reduce their occurrence or recommend further testing to evaluate the severity of your condition and help determine treatment.

WEARING A HOLTER MONITOR

A Holter monitor is a portable ECG machine that monitors your heart over a 24-hour period.

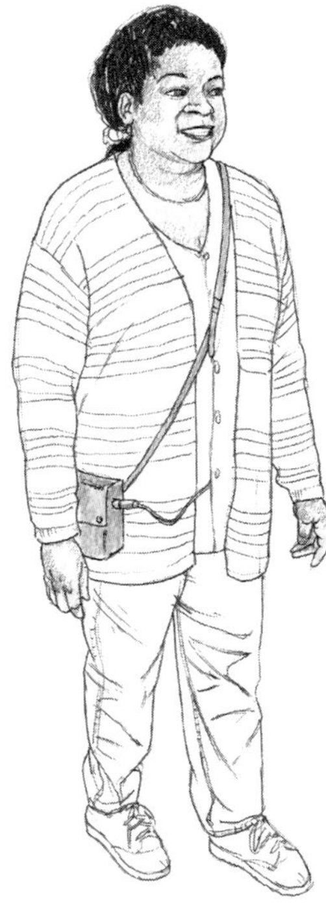

Exercise stress test An exercise stress test is an ECG that is taken while you walk on a treadmill or ride a stationary bicycle. The purpose of this test is to determine whether your heart is getting enough oxygen during exertion, when it requires more oxygen than usual. Electronic sensors are attached to your body and connected to an ECG machine. You begin exercising, slowly at first and then more quickly, until you reach a target heart rate.

Your target heart rate is expressed in a number of beats per minute that is determined by your age and physical condition. Your doctor will monitor your blood pressure at the same time. An exercise stress test does not usually detect a problem unless one or more coronary arteries are more than 50-percent blocked. The signs of significant narrowing in a coronary artery include intolerable fatigue or chest pain while exercising or an irregular heart rhythm detected on the ECG. In this case, further testing, such as angiography (see page 470), is necessary to determine the location and extent of the blockage.

Thallium exercise stress test A thallium exercise stress test is similar to an exercise stress test but is more accurate at measuring the flow of blood to the heart. Toward the end of the exercise session, your doctor injects a low dose of a radioactive substance called thallium into one of your veins. After exercising, you lie down on the examining table and the doctor uses a large scanning machine to detect the movement of thallium from your bloodstream into your heart cells. If there are areas in your heart in which little or no thallium shows up on the scan, your heart is not getting enough blood, probably because a coronary artery is narrowed or blocked.

A few hours later, while you are resting, another scan is performed. This second test may show that it is only during exercise that blood is not reaching that area of your heart. This is a sign that there is significant narrowing in a coronary artery but not permanent damage or scar tissue in the heart. A test result that shows that blood is not reaching an area of your heart while you are resting indicates permanent damage to that part of your heart, usually as the result of a heart attack.

Although the thallium exercise stress test is more accurate than the exercise stress test, it is not performed as frequently because it is more expensive and takes more time. In addition, in some women, breast tissue may interfere with the camera's ability to get a good picture of the heart.

Echocardiogram An echocardiogram is a painless test that uses ultrasound (see page 405) to produce a picture of the structure of the heart. In this test, an ultrasound transducer (a hand-held device that sends out sound waves that are translated into an image on a monitor) is placed on your chest, under your left ribs, and directed toward your heart. The image on the monitor shows the size and shape of the heart chambers and the activity of the chambers and valves.

An echocardiogram can also detect a blood clot in the heart chambers and sometimes shows evidence of scarring in the heart, which usually indicates a previous heart attack. Although a doctor cannot directly view the coronary arteries and see blockages on an echocardiogram, evidence of damage from a previous heart attack is a good indicator of the presence of heart disease. To make an accurate diagnosis of heart disease, the doctor will perform more definitive tests, such as an angiogram.

Angiogram An angiogram is a test in which a dye is injected through a thin, flexible tube (catheter) into the coronary arteries to make them visible on an X-ray. An angiogram is used to diagnose narrowing of arteries or damage to tissues of the heart. An angiogram is considered the definitive test for diagnosing heart disease in people who are experiencing chest pain (angina, see page 465) or who have abnormal results on a stress test or echocardiogram. A doctor always performs an angiogram before making a decision to treat heart disease surgically—either by opening a narrowed artery (angioplasty, see page 476) or by redirecting blood away from obstructed vessels and through healthy ones (coronary bypass surgery, see page 477).

To perform an angiogram, a specially trained cardiologist inserts a wide, hollow needle into an artery in your upper thigh (femoral artery) or arm (brachial artery). Before the needle is inserted, you will be given a local anesthetic to numb the area but you will be conscious throughout the procedure. The doctor inserts the catheter through the needle and threads it through the artery up to the coronary arteries. You may feel a small amount of pressure but usually no pain. Once the catheter is in place in a coronary artery, dye is injected through it. During this injection, you may feel hot or nauseous or have the urge to urinate, but all of these symptoms will pass quickly. You may be asked to cough or take deep breaths during the procedure, which may last 30 to 60 minutes.

If the catheter was inserted through your thigh, a special bandage called a pressure dressing is put over the area and it is immobilized for up to 6 hours to prevent it from bleeding, often by placing a weight (usually a 10-pound bag of sand) on it. If the catheter was put in your arm, bleeding from the site of the needle insertion is prevented using a pressure dressing or, possibly, a stitch. You can eat as soon as you like after having an angiogram. If you are in pain, ask your doctor for medication.

An angiogram sometimes requires an overnight stay in the hospital. Serious complications from angiography are uncommon but can include bleeding or the formation of blood clots. The artery in which the catheter was inserted may be damaged and bleed, or may become infected. If a blood clot forms, it usually occurs around the site in the groin where the catheter was inserted. This is not dangerous unless the clot breaks off and travels to the heart or lungs. Sudden arrhythmia (abnormal heartbeat), stroke (see page 569), or allergic reaction to the dye occurs in extremely rare cases.

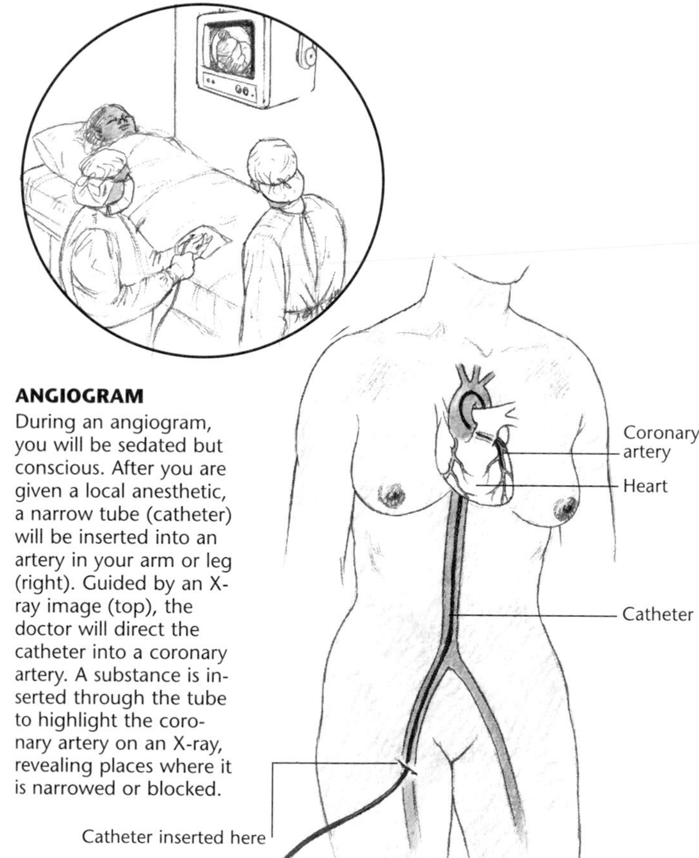

ANGIOGRAM
During an angiogram, you will be sedated but conscious. After you are given a local anesthetic, a narrow tube (catheter) will be inserted into an artery in your arm or leg (right). Guided by an X-ray image (top), the doctor will direct the catheter into a coronary artery. A substance is inserted through the tube to highlight the coronary artery on an X-ray, revealing places where it is narrowed or blocked.

HEART ATTACK

When a blood clot blocks a coronary artery, the heart muscle is deprived of oxygen. The result is a heart attack. Part of the heart muscle may die or become damaged; sometimes the heart fails altogether, causing death. A heart attack can be sudden, painful, and easy to identify, or it can cause few or no symptoms and go entirely undetected. A heart attack can feel different to different people. You may have crushing pain, dull pain, or a squeezing sensation in your chest that may spread to your neck, jaw, arms, or down your back; or you may feel pain only in your arms, jaw, or back. Women are less likely than men to call for help when they are having a heart attack, possibly because they have not been diagnosed with heart disease or they think that heart attacks only happen to men. Heart attacks in women are often mistaken for indigestion.

Learn how to perform CPR—you could save a life

Everyone should learn how to perform cardiopulmonary resuscitation (CPR). It is especially important to know CPR if you live with a person who has heart disease or is at high risk of heart disease. CPR is required when a person's breathing or pulse has stopped after a heart attack. When giving CPR, you breathe for the person by blowing air into his or her mouth and compressing his or her chest wall to squeeze blood out to vital organs. Courses on CPR are widely available through local chapters of the Red Cross and the American Heart Association.

Severe and moderate heart attacks

A heart attack is caused by a blockage in a coronary artery, one of the blood vessels that supply blood to the heart muscle. The portion of heart muscle that does not receive oxygen-rich blood is damaged. The severity of a heart attack depends on the amount of muscle that is affected. In many cases, the surrounding healthy muscle keeps working, allowing the heart to continue pumping while the damaged area of heart muscle heals and recovers its strength.

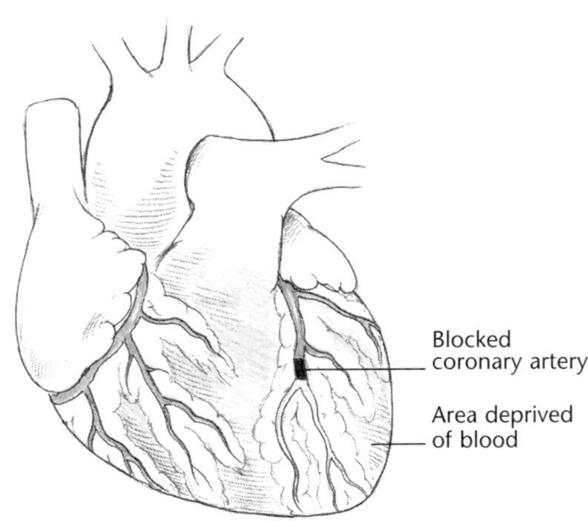

CARDIAC ARREST
In rare cases, a heart attack causes the heart to stop beating completely (cardiac arrest or asystole) or to beat in an ineffective, fluttering pattern (called ventricular fibrillation).

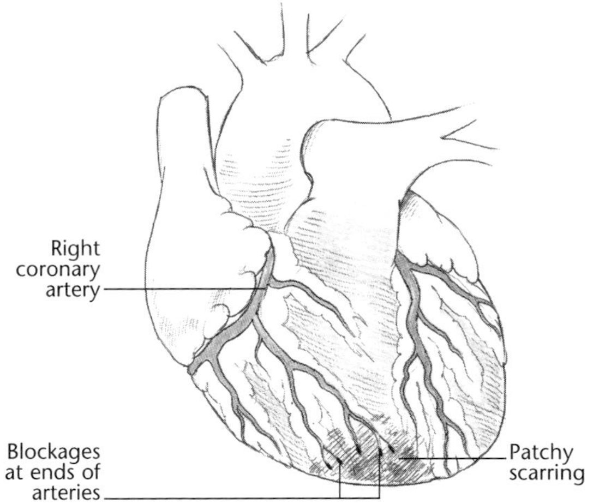

MODERATE HEART ATTACK
When a blockage occurs at the small end of a coronary artery, only a small portion of the heart muscle dies. If similar blockages occur in several arteries, scar tissue may form that can weaken the heart's ability to pump.

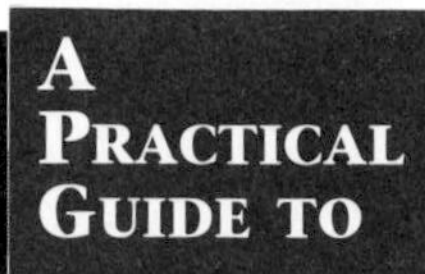

Recognizing a Heart Attack

THE SIGNS OF A HEART ATTACK can be subtle and hard to identify. Many women don't recognize the symptoms even when they are in the middle of a major heart attack. The amount of time that passes before you receive treatment can mean the difference between life and death. Learn about the symptoms of heart disease and your own risk factors (see page 461). Get help immediately even if you are not sure you are having a heart attack.

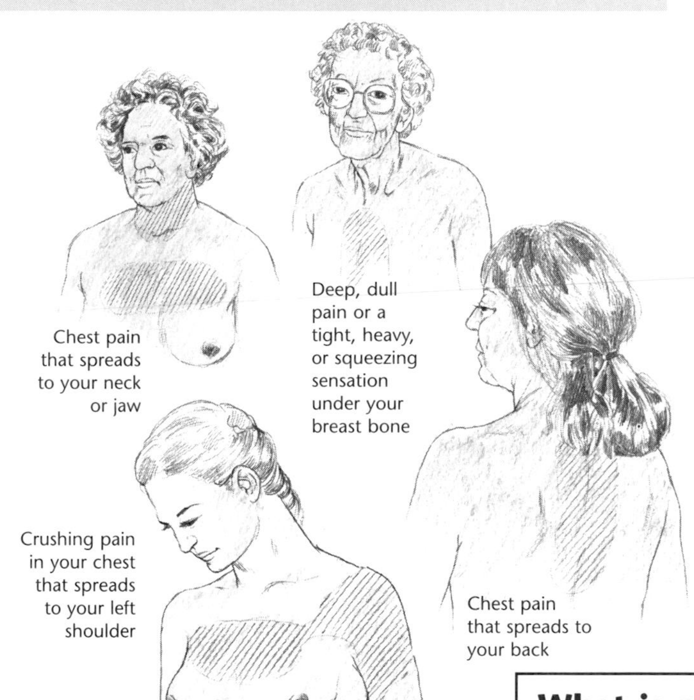

Chest pain that spreads to your neck or jaw

Deep, dull pain or a tight, heavy, or squeezing sensation under your breast bone

Crushing pain in your chest that spreads to your left shoulder

Chest pain that spreads to your back

HEART ATTACKS: NO TWO ARE THE SAME

A heart attack feels different to different people. Even if you have already had a heart attack, a second one may not feel the same. You may feel pain in any of the areas of the body shown above. Or you may feel pain only in your arms, jaw, or back. Other warning signs of a heart attack include dizziness, fainting, sweating, nausea, or weakness.

Don't ignore angina

Angina—a feeling of pain, heaviness, tightness, burning, or squeezing in your chest—is an indication that you have heart disease and are at risk of having a heart attack. Angina occurs when the heart muscle does not receive enough oxygen because of a temporary narrowing of one of the coronary arteries that supply it with oxygen-rich blood. Angina usually occurs during physical exertion or emotional stress.

Tell your doctor immediately if you have any symptoms of angina, which are similar to those of an actual heart attack (see page 471). Prompt treatment for angina can prevent you from having a heart attack. Many women experience angina for years, but do not seek treatment and eventually have a heart attack.

What is a heart attack?

A heart attack occurs when a coronary artery, one of the blood vessels that supply oxygen-rich blood to the heart muscle, becomes blocked. The area of heart muscle that does not receive blood begins to die. The seriousness of a heart attack depends on how much of the heart is affected. Often the surrounding healthy muscle keeps working, allowing the heart to keep pumping while the injured muscle heals and recovers some of its strength.

What is nitroglycerin?

Nitroglycerin is a drug that reduces the pain of angina by widening blood vessels to allow more blood to reach the heart muscle. You place nitroglycerin tablets under your tongue whenever you feel the pain of angina or anticipate it coming on. Women who have angina should have nitroglycerin with them at all times and should take it immediately if they feel pain in their chest.

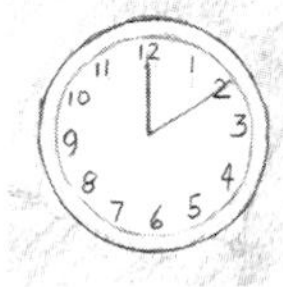

Don't delay

A heart attack does the most damage in the first 2 hours. The longer you delay seeking treatment, the more damage your heart is likely to sustain. Responding promptly to signs of a heart attack can dramatically increase your chances of recovery. If your symptoms last more than 2 minutes, call 911. Here are some common reasons why people delay calling for help, and the facts in each situation:

Reason for delay: You think that only men have heart attacks.
Reality: Heart disease is the most common cause of death in women as well as men. If you have symptoms, call for help.

Reason for delay: You are not sure it is a heart attack.
Reality: Call anyway—heart attack symptoms can be vague.

Reason for delay: It feels like heartburn.
Reality: If you have a history of heart disease, angina, or high blood pressure, the heartburn you feel may actually be a heart attack. Call for help immediately.

Reason for delay: You'd feel embarrassed if it turned out you didn't need medical help after all.
Reality: Never feel embarrassed about calling for help. A little embarrassment might save your life.

Reason for delay: You're hoping that it is not a heart attack.
Reality: Wishful thinking can be deadly. You can't wish a heart attack away, and getting treatment quickly can save your life. Most people who survive a heart attack can return to their normal life, including work, within 3 months.

At the hospital

Much can be done to help you recover from a heart attack, but you must take the first and most important step—getting medical help immediately. At the hospital, the emergency room staff will determine if you have had a heart attack by doing a test called an electrocardiogram (ECG; see page 132) and by taking a blood sample to test for chemicals that are secreted by damaged heart muscle. You may be given drugs immediately to help dissolve a clot that may be causing the blockage. If your heartbeat is abnormal, the doctor may need to restore a normal rhythm with a defibrillator, which delivers an electric current to your heart. If your heart has stopped, doctors will compress your chest rhythmically to try to maintain normal pumping action until your heartbeat has been reestablished. Later, you may be given blood-thinning medications to help prevent a clot from forming again or to prevent new clots from forming. Your care will continue in the coronary care unit until you are out of danger. For more about treatment of heart attacks, see page 474.

Take action

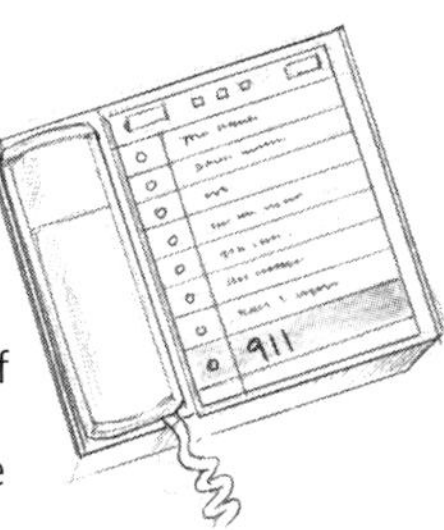

Getting prompt treatment for a heart attack can be lifesaving. If you experience one or more symptoms of a heart attack, act quickly and take the following steps:

- Sit down or lie down.
- If symptoms persist for 2 minutes, call 911 or your local emergency number and say you may be having a heart attack. Leave the phone off the hook so that medical personnel can locate your address if you should become unconscious.
- If you have nitroglycerin tablets, take up to three pills, one at a time every 5 minutes.
- Ambulances are well equipped to provide emergency care for people who are having heart attacks. It is usually better to have medical personnel come to you than for you to start off for the hospital.
- If you can get to the hospital faster by car than by ambulance, have someone drive you. Do not drive yourself—it could be dangerous.
- Do not delay getting medical treatment, even if you are not sure you are having a heart attack. A delay can cause permanent damage to your heart muscle or even death. Let the doctor determine whether or not you are having a heart attack.
- If your breathing or pulse stops, any person who is trained in cardiopulmonary resuscitation (CPR; see page 471) should immediately begin the procedure. Call 911 first.
- When you arrive at the emergency room, you or the person who brought you should announce clearly that you may be having a heart attack. Make sure you are seen at once.

Women tend to have their first heart attack 10 years later than men—at an average age of 69 compared with 59 for men. Women also tend to have smaller heart attacks that cause less damage to the heart muscle. Still, heart attack is the single largest killer of both women and men. Nearly 250,000 women die of heart attacks each year—about the same as the number of men.

A heart attack—or, in medical terms, myocardial infarction—occurs when the blood supply to an area of the heart is severely reduced or cut off. The process begins when one of the coronary arteries (the blood vessels that supply blood to the heart) becomes narrowed by deposits of a fatty substance called plaque. The buildup of plaque inside arteries is a process called atherosclerosis (see page 468). A narrowed coronary artery is then blocked further, sometimes completely, by an obstruction, usually a blood clot that sticks to the plaque. The formation of a blood clot in an area of an artery in which plaque has built up is called a coronary thrombosis. If the supply of oxygen-rich blood to the heart is severely blocked and remains blocked for too long, the lack of oxygen causes irreversible damage to the heart muscle. Extensive damage to the heart muscle is often fatal because the heart can no longer continue to pump blood to the rest of the body.

If you are having a heart attack, the faster you get help, the greater are your chances of surviving it. Eighty percent of people who do survive a heart attack can return to their normal life, including work, within 3 months. The following facts show how acting quickly can help save your life if you think you are having a heart attack.

- The longer you delay treatment for a heart attack, the more severely your heart is likely to be damaged.
- Most people who die of a heart attack do so within 2 hours of the onset of symptoms.

Warning signs
Heart attack

Call your doctor immediately if you are experiencing any of the following symptoms:

- Uncomfortable tightness or pressure, fullness, or squeezing deep in your chest or across your chest
- Chest pain that spreads to your neck, jaws, or down your back
- Pain in your jaw, arms, or back
- Unusual shortness of breath
- Dizziness, fainting, sweating, nausea, or weakness
- Indigestion that does not respond to antacids
- Chest pain (angina) that does not respond to the prescription heart drug nitroglycerin (see page 472)

TREATING CORONARY ARTERY DISEASE

A woman who has a heart attack is more likely than a man to die of it. This is partly because women tend to be older than men when they have their first heart attack. Women are also less likely to receive aggressive treatments, such as medication to dissolve blood clots during a heart attack or surgery to open blocked arteries (angioplasty, see page 476) or to redirect blood flow from narrowed arteries (coronary bypass surgery, see page 477). Knowing the many effective treatments that are available for heart disease can help you get the treatment you may need.

Medication The array of drugs for treating heart disease continues to grow. It often takes some adjusting to determine the right combination of medications for a particular person. Your doctor may prescribe different drugs alone or in combination to find what works best for you and causes the fewest side effects. It is important to tell your doctor about any side effects you are experiencing while you are taking any medication. Heart disease medications fall into the following major categories:

Alpha blockers Alpha blockers are drugs that help lower blood pressure by preventing the blood vessels from constricting. These drugs also prevent hormones your body releases in response to stress (such as adrenaline) from raising your blood pressure. Alpha blockers are often combined with other drugs to lower blood pressure. Alpha blockers sometimes cause dizziness.

ACE inhibitors ACE inhibitors (ACE stands for angiotensin-converting enzyme) help lower blood pressure by blocking production of a hormone produced by the kidneys called angiotensin II, which causes blood vessels to constrict. These drugs are often used to control blood pressure in people with diabetes (see page 617) or congestive heart failure (see page 492). ACE inhibitors can cause a dry cough in some people.

Antiarrhythmic drugs Antiarrhythmic drugs are used to correct an irregular heartbeat, called arrhythmia. Because these drugs control the heart rate, it is extremely important to take them exactly as prescribed. Although most people have no side effects from these drugs, possible problems include liver inflammation, muscle weakness, loss of balance, slow heart rate, increased susceptibility to sunburn, or lung inflammation.

Anticoagulants, antiplatelet agents, and thrombolytics Anticoagulants, antiplatelet agents, and thrombolytics are groups of drugs used to "thin" the blood, making it less likely that blood clots will form that can block the coronary arteries or the lungs. Aspirin is an antiplatelet drug—it prevents blood cells called platelets from sticking together and forming clots. Aspirin is frequently prescribed to prevent clots from forming in the arteries of people who are recovering from a heart attack. Thrombolytic drugs—such as streptokinase or tissue plasminogen activator (TPA)—are often given intravenously during a heart attack to help dissolve a clot that is blocking a coronary artery. These drugs can cause bleeding in some people.

Beta blockers Beta blockers slow the heart rate and reduce blood pressure. These drugs can effectively treat angina, which is chest pain caused by a reduced oxygen supply to the heart muscle during physical exertion. Your doctor may prescribe beta blockers alone or with a diuretic (a drug that increases the output of urine) or other blood-pressure medication. Because beta blockers slow the circulation, they can cause your hands and feet to be cold. Other possible side effects include nausea or, in men, impotence.

Calcium channel blockers Calcium channel blockers reduce constriction of blood vessels, allowing blood to flow more freely, thereby reducing blood pressure. These drugs occasionally cause headache, nausea, tiredness, ankle swelling, dizziness, or skin rash.

Centrally acting drugs Drugs called centrally acting drugs lower blood pressure by acting on the brain to reduce the nerve impulses that can cause blood vessels to constrict. These drugs, which are not used widely, may also slow the heartbeat. Centrally acting drugs are sometimes used to enhance the effects of a diuretic or other blood-pressure medication. Possible side effects include drowsiness, constipation, dry mouth, headache, dizziness, skin rash, depression, ankle swelling, or cold hands.

Digitalis drugs Digitalis, an extract of the foxglove plant, has been used for more than 200 years to treat heart disease. It strengthens the force of the heart's contractions by increasing its supply of calcium, which is necessary for all muscles to contract. Digitalis is used primarily to treat congestive heart failure (see page 492) and often improves symptoms of heart failure, such as breathlessness, that result from fluid congestion in the lungs. The drug also increases a person's capacity to exercise. Digitalis can be used to treat disturbances in the heartbeat, called arrhythmias. Possible side effects include fatigue, nausea, loss of appetite, or disturbed vision.

Diuretics Diuretics are drugs that reduce blood pressure by increasing the kidney's output of water and sodium, which reduces the volume of blood that the heart has to pump through the circulation. With a reduced workload, the heart has less need for oxygen. Diuretics are among the oldest and most effective blood-pressure medications. Side effects are uncommon but may include lethargy, cramps, or skin rash.

Nitrates Nitrates are drugs that dilate (widen) blood vessels—both arteries and veins. When veins widen, more blood collects, or pools, in the system of veins, reducing the amount of blood returned to the heart and decreasing the workload of the left ventricle of the heart. Widening of the arteries reduces blood pressure because blood pumped from the heart can flow more easily through them. Nitrates are often used to relieve chest pain (angina, see page 465) in heart disease by allowing more blood to flow through the widened coronary arteries. Possible side effects of nitrates include headaches, flushing, or dizziness.

Peripheral adrenergic antagonists Drugs called peripheral adrenergic antagonists widen blood vessels and reduce blood pressure by blocking the effects of adrenaline, a hormone released during stress that can cause blood vessels to constrict. These drugs are sometimes combined with a diuretic. In high doses, these drugs may cause drowsiness.

Angioplasty and other procedures to open arteries A variety of procedures can be used to open a narrowed or blocked artery. In some of these procedures, a tiny balloon (for angioplasty) or cutting device (for atherectomy) attached to the end of a long, thin tube (catheter) is inserted into the blocked artery to open it. In many cases, these procedures to open an artery can replace coronary bypass surgery (see page 477), which carries higher risks and has a longer recovery time. You may be a good candidate for this type of procedure if you have a significant blockage in only one or two of your arteries or if you have angina (chest pain) that cannot be controlled with medication.

Before any of these procedures to reopen blocked arteries you will be given a sedative to relax you and a local anesthetic at the site at which the catheter enters your body—usually the skin over the femoral artery in your groin or upper thigh. The cardiologist threads a thin, flexible wire called a guide wire through this artery into your coronary artery to a point just beyond the blockage. A catheter is then placed in the coronary artery, and the size and location of the blockage is confirmed by injecting dye through the catheter into the blocked artery to show its outline on an X-ray (angiogram, see page 470).

In balloon angioplasty, a catheter with a balloon at its tip is threaded into the artery, over the guide wire, to the site of the blockage. A tiny balloon at the end of the catheter is inflated at the blockage site, sometimes several times for 30 to 120 seconds each time. The pressure of the balloon pushes the fatty buildup (plaque) back against the artery walls and opens the artery to allow blood to flow more freely. Balloon angioplasty is virtually painless, but you may feel some pressure in your chest when the balloon is inflated. When the procedure is finished, the doctor removes the catheter and balloon and performs another angiogram to see if the artery has been opened successfully.

Possible complications of balloon angioplasty are spasm of the artery, which causes it to close abruptly (constrict), or tearing of the artery, which causes it to collapse. You may be given medication after the procedure to prevent spasm. If a spasm or tearing occurs, emergency coronary bypass surgery may have to be done. In about 3 percent of cases, a person experiences a heart attack during balloon angioplasty, which also may require emergency bypass surgery.

The technology is developing rapidly for alternatives to balloon angioplasty to open blocked coronary arteries and restore the normal flow of blood to the heart. Your doctor may not be able to determine which technique will work best in your case until the procedure is under way. In one type of an artery-opening procedure called atherectomy (see illustration on page 477), a cutting device at the tip of the catheter shaves through

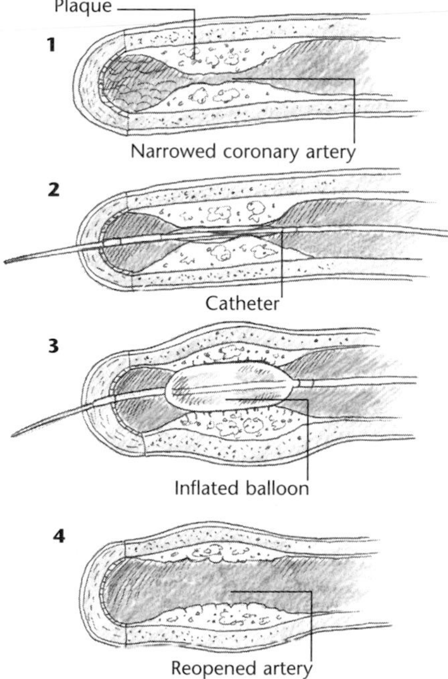

BALLOON ANGIOPLASTY

Balloon angioplasty is a procedure used to reopen an artery that has become blocked by a buildup of fatty deposits called plaque (1). A long, thin, flexible tube (catheter) is inserted into an artery in your groin and threaded through the artery to the site of blockage in the coronary artery (2). A tiny balloon on the tip of the catheter is then inflated with liquid, splitting the plaque and pressing it into the walls of the artery (3). This reopens the artery (4), allowing blood to flow freely to the heart.

ATHERECTOMY

In a procedure called atherectomy, a tiny cutting device is threaded through a catheter to the site of the blockage inside a coronary artery. The cutting device shaves the buildup of plaque off the sides of the artery walls, reopening the blood vessel. The shaved fatty debris is removed with the catheter.

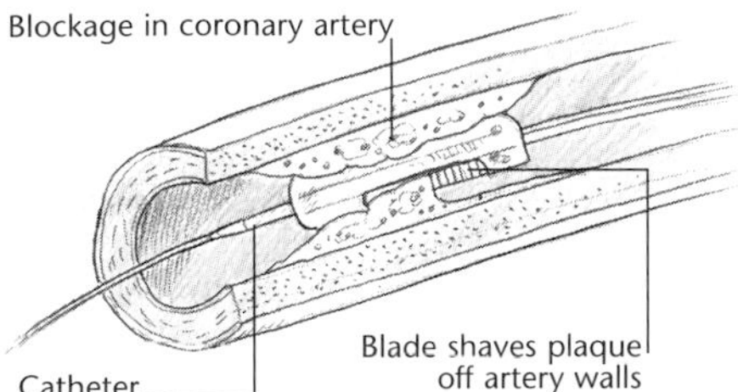

the plaque; the shaved fatty debris is removed with the catheter. Laser angioplasty uses precisely focused heat to vaporize a blockage. Another procedure that is being used increasingly to open arteries is the insertion (through a catheter) of a spiral spring called a stent; a stent serves as a brace to prevent the artery wall from narrowing again. A drawback of balloon angioplasty and all artery-opening procedures is that, one third of the time, the fatty buildup recurs within 6 months. If the artery stays open longer than 6 months, it is less likely to close again.

Coronary bypass surgery Coronary bypass surgery is performed to redirect blood around a blocked coronary artery using a healthy piece of blood vessel taken from another part of your body. Bypass surgery is done to relieve chest pain (angina, see page 465) that has not responded to intense drug therapy and to prevent a heart attack. Your doctor may recommend bypass surgery if an artery recloses after one or more angioplasty procedures to open it, or if all three of your coronary arteries are significantly blocked. Sometimes a bypass graft, a healthy replacement blood vessel used in a previous bypass, becomes blocked over the years, necessitating another bypass operation.

Women are twice as likely as men to die after coronary bypass surgery. For years doctors thought the procedure was more difficult to perform and less effective in women because women's blood vessels are smaller than men's. In fact, women are usually older and have more advanced heart disease than men when they have bypass surgery and, therefore, are likely to have a more difficult time recovering. In addition, most people, including many doctors, wrongly consider women to be at less risk of heart disease than men. As a result, women are less likely to receive an angiogram (see page 470), a test used to determine the need

What to expect after angioplasty or atherectomy

After a procedure to open a blocked artery, such as balloon angioplasty or atherectomy, you will probably stay in the hospital for a day or less. Here is what to expect during your recovery in the hospital and at home:

- You may feel tenderness or see a bruise at the site where the catheter entered your body. The bruise may extend as far down as your knee but will fade gradually over the next 4 to 6 weeks. Call your doctor if the area around the catheter insertion site becomes swollen; this may indicate an enlarging blood clot or bleeding that requires attention.
- For the first 24 hours, whenever you cough or sneeze, press down on the insertion site lightly with your hand to prevent bleeding.
- If the insertion site was in your groin, do not bend over or strain for the first 48 hours after the procedure. Do not lift heavy objects for the first week.
- You can bathe or shower as usual, but do not use a hot tub or whirlpool.
- You can take over-the-counter painkillers.
- You can resume sexual activity after 48 hours.
- If you notice any numbness, tingling, or coolness in your toes, foot, or leg, call your doctor immediately.
- If you notice bright red bleeding from the insertion site, lie down and apply firm pressure to the area around the site for 20 minutes and then release gently. This is easier if you have someone else do it. If you cannot stop the bleeding, call 911 and notify your doctor immediately.

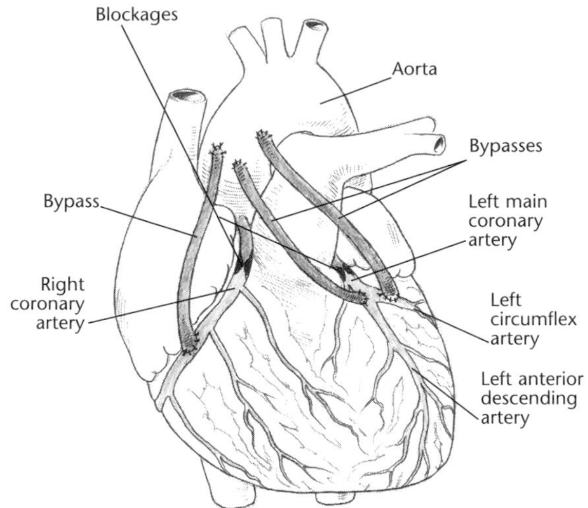

CORONARY BYPASS
In this example, three bypasses using replacement blood vessels from other parts of the body have been created to reroute blood around blockages in the left and right coronary arteries.

for potentially lifesaving procedures such as angioplasty (see page 476) or coronary bypass surgery.

Bypass surgery is open heart surgery. You are placed on a heart-lung machine during the surgery so that your heart can be stopped long enough to stitch the healthy replacement blood vessel in place. The heart-lung machine mimics the functioning of your lungs and heart by supplying fresh oxygen to used blood and pumping it throughout your body during the time your heart is stopped. The replacement blood vessel used for the bypass graft can be taken from a vein in your leg (the saphenous vein) or from an artery that runs along your inner chest wall (the internal mammary artery). Both of these blood vessels are often used in the same procedure if more than one bypass is required.

Following are the general steps in a coronary bypass operation:

- An anesthesiologist administers general anesthesia (see page 261) to make you unconscious. The surgeon makes an incision down the center of your sternum (breastbone) and opens your chest to expose the heart.
- The surgeon makes an incision in one of your legs to obtain a blood vessel or cuts a vessel off the inner surface of your chest wall. This blood vessel is used to form the bypass around your blocked artery.
- A heart-lung machine is connected to your heart and your heart is stopped. The surgeon stitches one end of the section of blood vessel to the aorta and the other end to an area of the coronary artery beyond the obstruction.
- If necessary, several bypasses are performed in the same operation.
- The doctor restarts your heart, disconnects the heart-lung machine, and closes your chest with stitches.

Cardiac rehabilitation Cardiac rehabilitation is a program of regular exercise, low-fat diet, and lifestyle counseling designed to recondition your heart, lungs, and muscles and keep your cholesterol level low to prevent plaque from building up in your arteries again. A cardiac rehabilitation program can benefit anyone who has heart disease, whether or not he or she has had a heart attack or any kind of heart surgery or procedure. Before you leave the hospital, you will be referred to a cardiac rehabilitation program near your home. If not, ask your cardiologist for a recommendation at your first follow-up office visit.

Although you can maintain an exercise program and healthful diet on your own, it is far better to join an organized program because you receive support from an experienced staff. Also, you are with other people who are going through the same experience. The usual rehabilitation process starts in the hospital a day or two after surgery with simple activities such as moving to a bedside chair while an attendant makes the bed. You are encouraged to gradually engage in more activity.

What to expect before and after bypass surgery

Before you have bypass surgery, you will meet with the cardiac surgeon who will perform the procedure. This is the time to ask questions and express any fears you may have. The surgeon can tell you, based on the results of your tests, which procedures he or she recommends and why. You may want to bring a family member with you to take notes and discuss the care you will need while you are recovering after surgery.

You will check into the hospital a day or several hours in advance of the surgery and undergo a variety of tests. You will be asked about your use of medications and alcohol, cigarettes, and other drugs. Your honest answers to these questions are important because they can affect your healing and recovery. The anesthesiologist who will administer general anesthesia will visit you before your operation to discuss the procedures that he or she will use. You will be asked to shower the night before or the morning of your surgery to reduce the amount of bacteria on your skin and thereby reduce your risk of infection. You will not be able to eat or drink after midnight the night before surgery (general anesthesia is much safer to have on an empty stomach).

Before the operation, intravenous lines will be placed in your arms or neck to administer fluids and a sedative to relax you. You will be connected to machines that check your vital signs (such as your heart rate) continuously throughout the procedure. A catheter will be inserted into your bladder to collect urine and another catheter will be inserted into an artery in your wrist to monitor your blood pressure. You will be given general anesthesia to make you unconscious.

After surgery, you will be taken to the intensive care unit of the hospital where your condition will be monitored continuously. Although your family will be allowed to visit, you will be groggy and unable to talk because a tube will have been placed down your throat to connect your lungs to a ventilator, a machine that helps you breathe until the effects of the anesthetic wear off. You may find your inability to speak frustrating, particularly if the ventilator has to be used for more than a day. However, nurses are specially trained to communicate with you by touch and with signboards and you may be able to communicate by writing on a note pad. Most people are taken off the ventilator the morning after surgery; the catheters and intravenous lines are removed within 2 days.

You will be instructed about healthful lifestyle factors—such as quitting smoking, eating a nutritious diet, and exercising regularly—that can help keep your arteries open. A nutritionist will describe an eating program you should follow at home. Many programs have counselors available to help you learn how to reduce stress and deal with any anxiety or depression (see page 594) you may be experiencing, as many people do after having a heart attack or undergoing heart surgery. If you do have anxiety or depression, make sure you tell your doctor about it. He or she may refer you to a qualified counselor or support group.

Questions to ask about a cardiac rehabilitation program Joining a good cardiac rehabilitation program greatly increases the chances that you will succeed in making the changes in your lifestyle that are necessary to keep your heart healthy. You need not do it alone. You will get support and positive feedback from participating in an organized program. Consider the following questions when choosing a cardiac rehabilitation program:

- Is the program directed by a qualified doctor?
- Is the program covered by your health insurance?
- Is the program tailored to each person's needs?
- What provisions are there for handling emergencies? For example, is there a defibrillator (see page 491) on hand and a person trained to use it in case you develop an abnormal heart rhythm?
- How are the conditions of participants monitored during exercise? Are pulses checked regularly?

Sex during your recovery from heart surgery

If you had angioplasty or atherectomy, you will probably be able to resume sexual activity after 48 hours. If you have had a heart attack or bypass surgery, you may need to wait about 4 weeks before resuming sexual activity. Discuss the timing with your doctor. Some people worry that having sex will cause them to have a heart attack, but your heart rate rarely rises above 130 beats per minute during intercourse, a safe level for most people with heart disease. Your blood pressure may also rise slightly during sexual activity. If your doctor has prescribed the medication nitroglycerin, ask him or her if you should take it before you have sex to help prevent chest pain (angina).

Some medications used to treat angina or high blood pressure can reduce your sexual desire or affect your ability to have an orgasm. If you notice any change in your sexual response, ask your doctor whether your medication may be causing this change and, if so, if there is an alternative medication you can take. Talk to your doctor if you experience any of the following symptoms during sexual activity:

- Rapid heartbeat and breathlessness that continue 10 minutes after sexual activity
- Heart palpitations (sudden, rapid heartbeats) that continue 10 minutes after sexual activity
- Chest pain during sexual activity
- Extreme fatigue the day after you have sex

- What are the requirements for being accepted into the program? Do you need a physical examination or referral from a doctor?
- Is the program convenient to your home?
- Does the program have equipment such as a track and exercise bicycles?
- In addition to exercise, does the program address diet, weight control, smoking, and drinking? Is counseling part of the program?

High blood pressure

High blood pressure, or hypertension, is excessive pressure of the blood against the walls of the blood vessels and heart. High blood pressure is the most common chronic illness in the US, the most common cause of stroke (see page 569), and a major risk factor for heart disease. In the vast majority of people who have high blood pressure, the cause is unknown. High blood pressure is called the silent killer because it seldom causes symptoms but can gradually damage tissues and organs, eventually leading to heart failure, stroke, or kidney failure. In young adulthood, high blood pressure is more common in men than women. Later in life, women with high blood pressure outnumber men and more women die of its effects. More than half of all women 65 and over have high blood pressure. The disease is more common among black and Hispanic women than any other group. High blood pressure is relatively easy to treat but millions of Americans who have high blood pressure do not know they have it.

High blood pressure makes your heart work harder than usual. At first, this extra effort makes your heart muscles stronger and larger. But, over time, your heart becomes stiff and weak, which sometimes leads to congestive heart failure (see page 492). High blood pressure can harm other parts of the body as well. In the brain, stroke is more likely to occur because high blood pressure weakens arteries, making them susceptible to rupture. High blood pressure can also lead to stroke by promoting the formation of blood clots in arteries in the brain.

High blood pressure can damage tiny blood vessels in the kidneys, reducing the amount of blood the kidneys can filter. Protein that is normally returned to the bloodstream may be excreted into the urine, and waste products that should be eliminated from the bloodstream may build up in the blood, eventually leading to kidney failure (see page 548).

Treating high blood pressure early can be lifesaving because of its severe long-term effects, which you may be unaware of until you have heart failure, a stroke, or kidney failure. Make sure you have your blood pressure measured regularly and, if you have high blood pressure, carefully follow your doctor's recommendation for treatment.

MEASURING BLOOD PRESSURE

Your blood pressure fluctuates from moment to moment. It is usually highest right after you get up in the morning and lowest while you are sleeping. Throughout the day, physical activity or stress can cause it to rise suddenly. These brief, temporary increases in blood pressure are normal. Blood pressure that is consistently high is not normal.

To measure your blood pressure, a nurse or doctor wraps a cuff around your upper arm and pumps air into it until it restricts your circulation. You will feel moderate squeezing but no pain. When the doctor or nurse first places a stethoscope over the artery inside your elbow, he or she hears nothing. But, as air is slowly released from the cuff, the sound of circulating blood can be heard through the stethoscope. This first sound is the point of greatest pressure. The reading taken at this point is called the systolic pressure.

Systolic blood pressure is the first, or top, number on your reading. Normal systolic blood pressure in a young woman who is not pregnant is less than 130. Blood pressure is expressed in millimeters of mercury (mm Hg). Older women have higher systolic blood pressure; up to 160 mm Hg may be considered normal. As air continues to be released from the cuff, the sound of blood pulsing in the arteries drops off. At this point, a second reading is taken—diastolic pressure. A normal diastolic pressure is less than 85 mm Hg. A sustained level of 140/90 mm Hg or higher is classified as high blood pressure.

A diagnosis of high blood pressure should not be based on a single reading except when it is extremely high—above 180/110 mm Hg. Usually, several readings are taken over a period of time. The circumstances under which a blood pressure reading is taken can influence the outcome. For example, blood pressure measured at a time of severe stress may be higher than it would be otherwise. Blood pressure rises if a person is nervous about being in a doctor's office. If this is a problem for you, talk to your doctor. You may be able to take your blood pressure several times at home.

If your blood pressure reading is consistently elevated, your doctor may look for signs of organ damage. For example, the doctor may shine a light into your eyes to inspect the blood vessels for thickening or narrowing or for signs of tiny hemorrhages. He or she will listen to your heart for unusual sounds and may take an electrocardiogram (ECG; see page 132). Your pulse may be taken at several points in your body, including your wrists, neck, and ankles.

TREATING HIGH BLOOD PRESSURE

High blood pressure is usually treated with a combination of lifestyle changes, such as weight loss and exercise, and medication. If your blood pressure is only mildly elevated (see page 482), you and your doctor can discuss the possibility of trying to treat it without medication. In many cases, weight loss and exercise alone are effective in reducing mildly elevated blood pressure.

Losing excess weight Losing excess weight is probably the single most effective way to reduce your blood pressure. People who are 20 percent or more over their desirable weight are more likely to have high blood pressure. Eating a low-fat diet that is rich in fruits, vegetables, and whole grains can help you lose weight and keep it off. For information about determining your healthy weight and losing excess pounds, see chapter 3.

Exercise Moderate, regular aerobic exercise (such as brisk walking) can also help lower your blood pressure, especially

A Practical Guide to Controlling Blood Pressure

HIGH BLOOD PRESSURE, or hypertension, has been called "the silent killer" because it often causes no symptoms, but can lead to a heart attack, stroke, or kidney failure. In many cases, the cause of high blood pressure is unknown.

Many people can control their blood pressure by exercising regularly, maintaining a healthy weight, and not smoking. Some people need to take medication to keep their blood pressure in a healthy range. Other measures to help control blood pressure include eating a diet that is low in fat and salt and drinking alcohol moderately, if at all. Ask your doctor if there are other steps you can take to keep your blood pressure in the normal range.

How high is your blood pressure?

Every woman should have her blood pressure checked regularly. A blood pressure test is simple, painless, and fast.

Ask your doctor to explain your blood pressure reading. The chart below shows different blood pressure ranges and how they are classified. Find your systolic pressure (the first or top number in your reading) in the first column of numbers and your diastolic pressure (the second or bottom number in your reading) in the second column. Look in the left column to find what the numbers mean. For example, if your blood pressure is 120/80, it is considered normal.

Blood pressure classifications for people over 18

Category	Systolic (mm Hg)	Diastolic (mm Hg)
Normal	Under 130	Under 85
High normal	130-139	85-89
Mild hypertension	140-159	90-99
Moderate hypertension	160-179	100-109
Severe hypertension	180-209	110-119
Very severe hypertension	Over 209	Over 119

Take your medication

If your doctor prescribes blood pressure medication, it is extremely important that you take it as prescribed. Because high blood pressure seldom causes symptoms, some people don't understand the need for medication. But, even though you may feel fine, uncontrolled high blood pressure can lead to life-threatening conditions, including heart attack and stroke.

Here are the major types of blood pressure medications and descriptions of how they lower blood pressure. Your doctor may prescribe one of these drugs or a combination of them.

Diuretics These drugs increase the kidneys' excretion of water and sodium, reducing the volume of blood the heart has to pump.

Beta blockers These drugs reduce the workload of the heart.

Calcium channel blockers These drugs reduce narrowing of blood vessels, letting blood flow more freely.

ACE inhibitors ACE stands for angiotensin-converting enzyme. These drugs block production of a hormone (angiotensin II) that causes blood vessels to narrow (constrict).

Alpha blockers These drugs block the effects of the stress hormone adrenaline (which can increase blood pressure) and cause the muscles in artery walls to relax.

Centrally acting drugs These drugs act on the brain to reduce the nerve impulses that can cause blood vessels to narrow (constrict).

All blood pressure medications have potential side effects, such as swelling, headache, or dizziness. If you experience any, talk to your doctor. Do not stop taking your medication. Suddenly discontinuing your medication can cause your blood pressure to increase to a dangerously high level.

Effects of high blood pressure

High blood pressure seldom causes symptoms but it can cause severe damage to major organs over time.

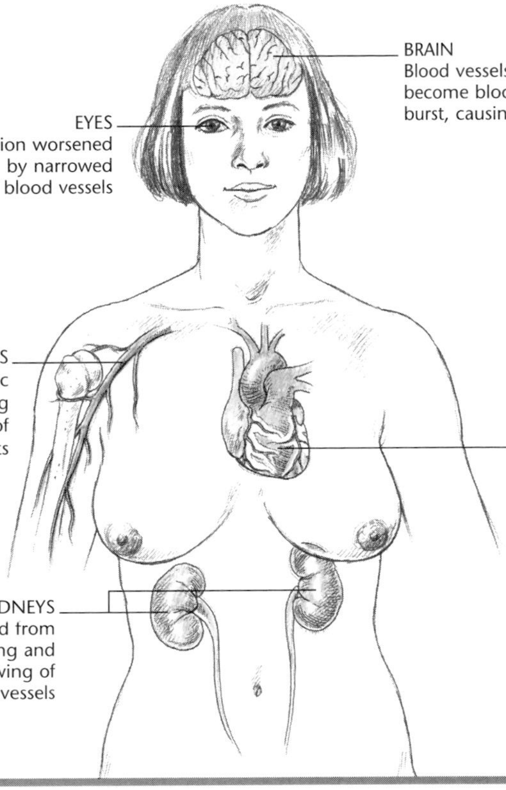

BRAIN
Blood vessels can become blocked or can burst, causing a stroke
EYES
Vision worsened by narrowed blood vessels
BLOOD VESSELS
Become less elastic and prone to narrowing from a buildup of fatty deposits
HEART
Increased pressure in blood vessels causes the heart to strain and grow larger, increasing the risk of angina, heart attack, or heart failure
KIDNEYS
Damaged from hardening and narrowing of blood vessels

Change in blood pressure (mm Hg)
40
20
0
-20
-40
-60
Diastolic
Systolic
-20
-10
Original Weight
10
20
Change in body weight (pounds)

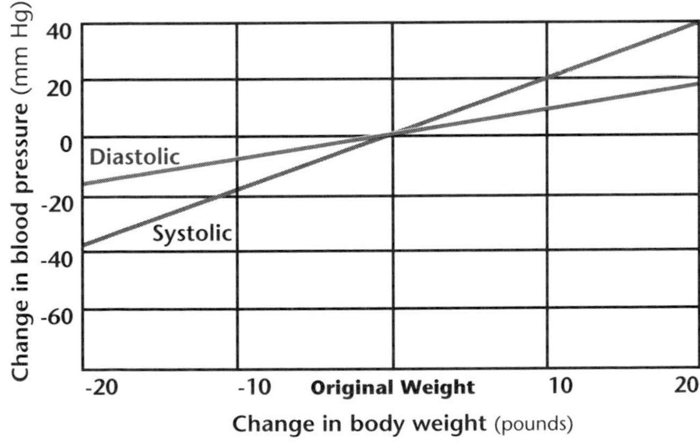

BODY WEIGHT AND BLOOD PRESSURE

If you are overweight, losing weight is the most important way to reduce your blood pressure. Even a moderate weight loss can significantly decrease your blood pressure. Conversely, a weight gain can increase your blood pressure.

Cutting back on salt

In a small percentage of people, eating salt (sodium) causes their blood pressure to rise. Because it is difficult to know who is sensitive to salt and who is not, most doctors recommend that all people who have high blood pressure reduce the salt in their diet to no more than 4 to 6 grams (1 to 1½ teaspoons) a day. The average American eats more than twice that amount.

When cutting back on salt, try to eliminate prepared foods, or substitute reduced-salt versions. One bowl of some canned soups can contain more salt than anyone should eat in a whole day. Once you get used to eating less salt, your craving for it will diminish and you'll enjoy the true flavors of the foods you eat.

Drug interactions

Some medications, including some over-the-counter painkillers, can make your blood pressure medication less effective. For example, some nonsteroidal anti-inflammatory drugs used to treat the pain and inflammation of arthritis, such as ibuprofen, may reduce the effectiveness of drugs that lower blood pressure. Be sure to tell your doctor about any medications you are taking. If your doctor prescribes blood pressure medication, ask him or her what other drugs you should avoid.

when it is combined with weight loss. In order to achieve this effect, you have to increase your heart rate for 20 to 30 minutes several times a week.

Relieving stress Practicing techniques to reduce stress (see page 186) in your everyday life may also help lower your blood pressure.

Reducing salt intake For most people, eating salt does not affect their blood pressure. But, in a small percentage of people, the amount of salt they eat causes their blood pressure to go either up or down. Blacks are more often sensitive to salt than people of other racial groups. If you have high blood pressure or a strong family history of high blood pressure, you should limit your salt intake to about 4 to 6 grams (1 to 1½ teaspoons) a day, including the salt you eat in prepared foods. The average American consumes more than twice that amount. Read package labels carefully for sodium content. (Six grams of salt is equal to 2,400 milligrams of sodium.)

Medications Many different types of medications are available that can help lower blood pressure. You may have to try several before you and your doctor find the one that works best for you and has the fewest side effects. You may have to take a combination of several blood pressure drugs to get your blood pressure under control. Because high blood pressure has no symptoms and some of the medications have unpleasant side effects, some people stop taking their medication against their doctor's recommendation. However, it is extremely important to

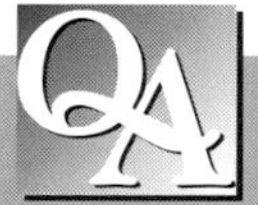

Questions Women Ask
High blood pressure

Q Why do I have high blood pressure?

A In most cases, the cause of high blood pressure is never found. High blood pressure is known to run in families and is more common in blacks than in other groups. People who have diabetes or are overweight are also more likely to have high blood pressure.

Q My high blood pressure is not causing any problems. I don't have any symptoms, so why do I have to take medication?

A High blood pressure is called the silent killer because it often has no symptoms until it reaches an advanced, life-threatening stage. Long before high blood pressure causes any noticeable symptoms, it is damaging vital organs throughout your body. Your first "symptom" may be a stroke or heart attack, which can be fatal. For this reason, it is extremely important to keep your blood pressure under control by taking the medication your doctor prescribes, exercising regularly, and maintaining a healthy weight.

Q My blood pressure medication causes some side effects I don't like. Do I have to keep taking it?

A A number of different medications are available for treating high blood pressure. If the medication you are taking is causing side effects, your doctor may be able to prescribe a different drug that you will tolerate better.

continue taking your blood pressure medication even when you are feeling healthy and see no obvious need for it. If the side effects of the medication you are taking are bothering you, your doctor can prescribe a different medication that you may tolerate better. For descriptions of the major groups of blood pressure medications, see Controlling blood pressure, page 482.

Heart valve disorders

When one or more heart valves do not function correctly, the result is a condition called valvular heart disease. Just as a faucet opens to allow water to flow through and closes to cut off the flow, the valves of your heart open to allow blood to flow through and close to prevent it from backing up. The heart has four chambers—a right and left ventricle and a right and left atrium. Each chamber is closed by a one-way valve. When something goes wrong with a heart valve, the normal flow of blood through the heart may be obstructed and blood is not pumped efficiently to the rest of the body.

The mitral valve, which allows blood to flow into the left ventricle (the main pumping chamber of the heart), and the aortic valve, which allows blood to flow from the left ventricle into the aorta, are the most common sites of disease. These valves are under the greatest strain from the powerful contractions of the left ventricle, which pumps blood throughout the body.

Damaged heart valves or replacement valves are susceptible to infection. Dental treatments and some surgical procedures may release bacteria into the bloodstream. To reduce the risk of infection if you have a heart valve disorder, you may be required to take antibiotics before going to the dentist or having surgery. Make sure all of your dentists and doctors know of your condition.

MITRAL VALVE PROLAPSE

Mitral valve prolapse, the most common valve disorder, is a usually inherited structural defect of the mitral valve, a valve that permits blood to flow from the left atrium into the left ventricle. About 5 percent of adult Americans have mitral valve prolapse, which is twice as common in women as in men. Although it may sound alarming, the condition is rarely serious. In a person with a normal valve, oxygen-rich blood returning from the lungs enters the left atrium and flows from the atrium through the mitral valve into the left ventricle, which pumps the blood throughout the body. In a person with mitral valve prolapse, the two parts of the valve, called leaflets, thicken and elongate, which can prevent them from coming together properly. One or both leaflets may fall back into the left atrium. When the valve does not close, blood may leak backward into the left atrium. Mitral valve prolapse is usually diagnosed by chance when a woman is in her 30s or 40s.

Symptoms Most people who have mitral valve prolapse have no symptoms. If symptoms appear, they usually begin in a person's 30s or 40s. The disorder may cause chest pain, palpitations (sudden, rapid heartbeats), shortness of breath, fatigue, or dizziness. These symptoms may occur during exercise but more frequently occur during rest. Severity of symptoms does not necessarily correspond to the degree of abnormality or the severity of leaking from the valve.

Diagnosis A doctor can identify mitral valve prolapse by listening through a stethoscope for the characteristic sounds of clicks and murmurs made by the abnormal activity of the valve. The diagnosis is usually confirmed with an echocardiogram (see page 132), which can show the severity of the abnormality. Depending on the severity of the prolapse, your cardiologist may recommend regular checkups.

Treatment Mitral valve prolapse is usually mild and seldom requires treatment of any kind. In a small number of people with the disorder, extra heartbeats and tachycardia (abnormally rapid heartbeat) may become bothersome enough to require medication. In rare cases, the leaking of blood back through the valve becomes severe enough to require treatment, such as open heart surgery, to repair or replace the valve (see page 488). People with mitral valve prolapse may also be at risk of endocarditis, an infection of the valve that can lead to serious damage that may require surgery. Although women with mitral valve prolapse are not as susceptible to endocarditis as are men with the disorder, you should tell all your doctors and dentists that you have it. You will need to take antibiotics before any kind of surgical or dental procedure to avoid infection.

MITRAL VALVE PROLAPSE

A healthy mitral valve (right) allows oxygen-rich blood to flow from the left atrium into the left ventricle, the heart's main pumping chamber. In mitral valve prolapse (far right); parts of the valve leaflets thicken and elongate, which can prevent them from coming together and may cause blood to leak backward into the left atrium.

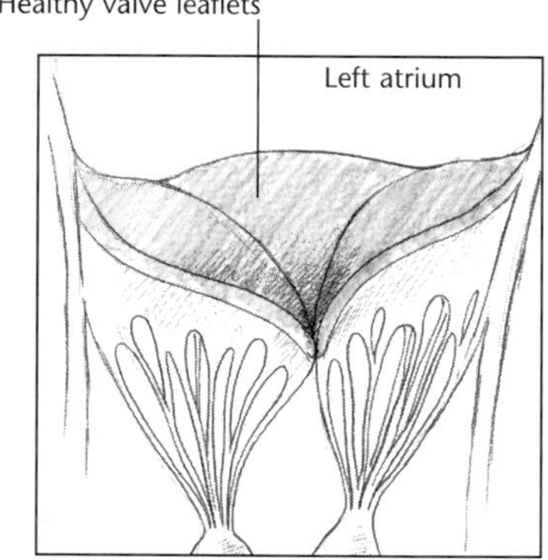

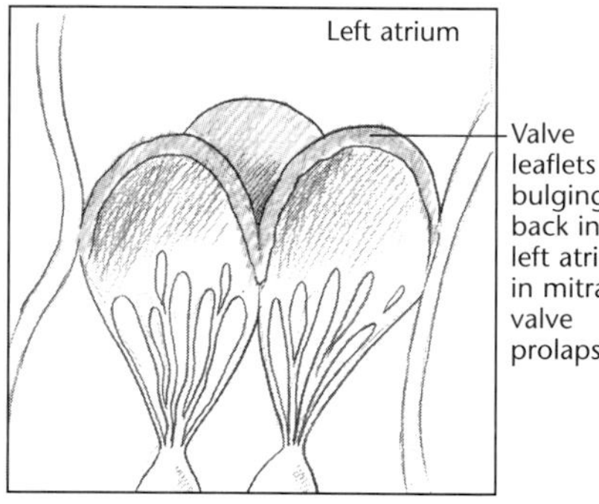

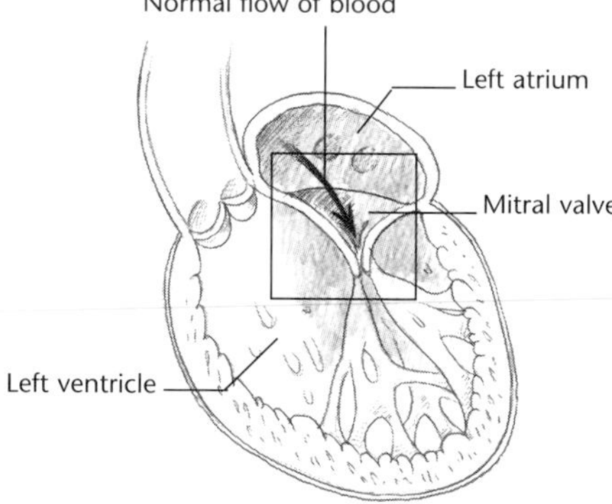

Healthy mitral valve

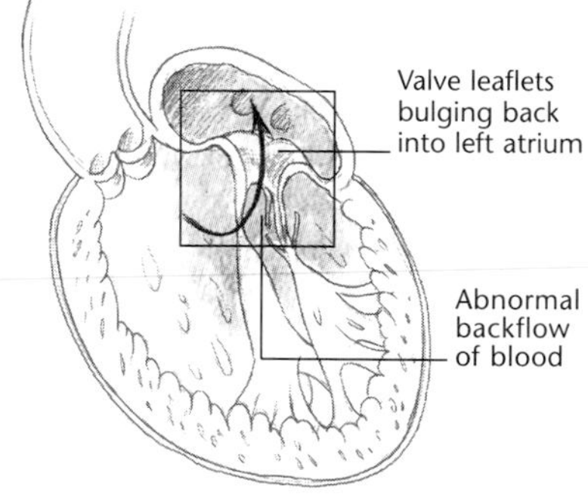

Mitral valve prolapse

MITRAL VALVE STENOSIS

Mitral valve stenosis, which is less common than mitral valve prolapse, is narrowing of the mitral valve, usually as a result of rheumatic fever. Rheumatic fever, a condition that can follow a throat infection caused by streptococcal bacteria, causes inflammation in tissues throughout the body, including the heart. The damage may occur over a long period of time and symptoms may not appear until 20 to 30 years after a childhood episode of rheumatic fever.

When the mitral valve narrows, less blood is able to flow from the left atrium into the left ventricle (the main pumping chamber of the heart), causing pressure to build up in the atrium. This pressure then backs up through the veins into the lungs, causing increased pressure and congestion in the lungs. The buildup of pressure and fluid in the lungs often causes shortness of breath and can eventually lead to congestive heart failure (see page 492).

If you develop symptoms from mitral valve stenosis, surgical treatment is usually necessary. In severe cases, the valve may have to be widened in a procedure called balloon valvuloplasty or it may have to be surgically opened and replaced (see page 488). Balloon valvuloplasty is a procedure in which a thin, flexible tube (catheter) with a balloon at its tip is placed across the abnormal mitral valve and the balloon is inflated to open up the narrowed valve.

AORTIC STENOSIS

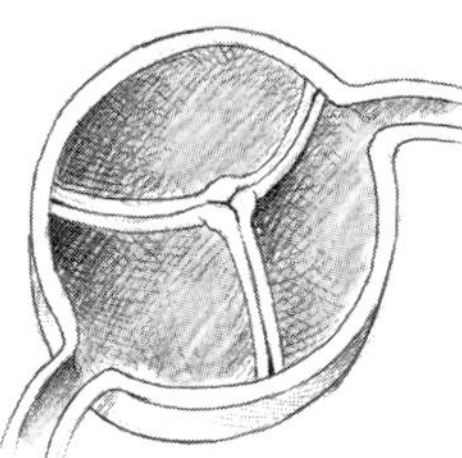

Healthy aortic valve

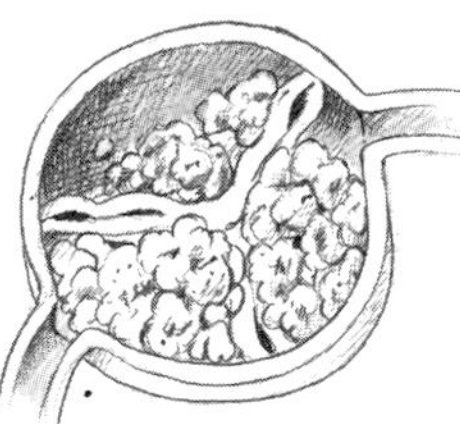

Aortic valve in stenosis

AORTIC STENOSIS
In aortic stenosis, the aortic valve becomes abnormally thickened and narrow from a buildup of calcium deposits.

Aortic stenosis is an abnormal narrowing or stiffening of the aortic valve, the valve that controls the flow of blood from the left ventricle (the main pumping chamber of the heart) into the aorta. Blood is pumped from the aorta throughout the body. When the aortic valve narrows, the left ventricle has to work harder with each beat to push blood into the aorta and out to the rest of the body. Over time, the muscle wall of the left ventricle thickens and the ventricle may enlarge, which can eventually lead to congestive heart failure.

The most common cause of aortic stenosis is the gradual buildup of deposits of calcium on the aortic valve. Because this buildup is a natural consequence of aging, the condition is most common in older people. Aortic stenosis may also be the result of an abnormality that was present at birth. Another condition, called aortic insufficiency, may occur if the valve does not close properly. If the valve does not close, blood may leak back into the left ventricle, which can lead to congestive heart failure.

Eventually, the stress on the valve may cause it to enlarge or thicken and weaken. Even in a person with aortic stenosis, the heart can usually maintain adequate pumping of blood to the rest of the body. However, during exercise or physical exertion, the heart may not be able to pump hard enough to supply sufficient blood to the brain, which may cause the person to faint. A narrowed aortic valve may also reduce the delivery of blood to the coronary arteries, which supply blood to the heart muscle itself. This reduced supply of oxygen-rich blood to the heart muscle can cause the chest pain of angina (see page 465).

Symptoms Aortic stenosis usually causes no symptoms for many years. Eventually, you may have chest pain during exercise, fainting spells during exercise or at rest, or shortness of breath during exercise.

Diagnosis A doctor can usually detect aortic stenosis by listening to the heart through a stethoscope for a characteristic loud murmur and the absence of the sound of the valve closing. He or she may also recognize a characteristic feel to the pulse. An echocardiogram (see page 132) can confirm the diagnosis and determine the severity of the condition.

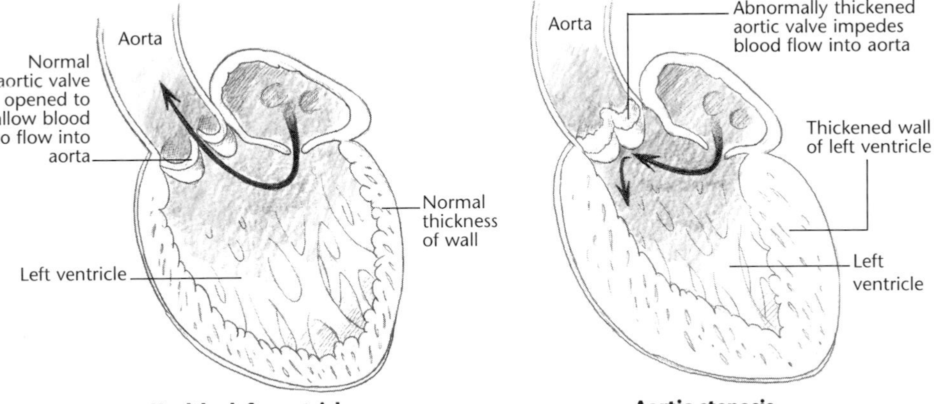

HOW AORTIC STENOSIS AFFECTS THE LEFT VENTRICLE
The left ventricle pumps blood into the aorta, which directs it to the rest of the body. The aortic valve controls the flow of blood from the left ventricle into the aorta (left). But, in aortic stenosis, the thickened valve impedes the normal flow of blood (right), making the left ventricle work harder to pump blood to the rest of the body and causing the ventricle to enlarge and thicken.

Treatment If you have aortic stenosis, your doctor will tell you not to engage in intense physical activity, although moderate exercise, such as walking, usually causes no problem. Your doctor may prescribe medication to help reduce the severity of your symptoms. Medications called vasodilators relax the blood vessels, which helps reduce the pressure against which the heart must pump. Medications called diuretics (see page 475) can reduce the amount of salt and water in the bloodstream, which in turn reduces the workload on the heart. In severe cases of aortic stenosis, surgery may be required (see below).

Valve replacement surgery

Surgery is performed only for severe cases of heart valve disease, usually when there are signs of congestive heart failure (see page 492). Surgery is done for mitral valve stenosis when the opening of the valve is less than a quarter of its normal size. For aortic stenosis, surgery is done when the valve opening is less than a third of its normal size. Although a diseased or damaged valve can sometimes be repaired, it usually has to be replaced.

Mechanical replacement valves are made of metal and plastic. Biologic replacement valves are made of human tissue or animal tissue (usually taken from pigs). Mechanical valves are more durable than biologic ones and can last 20 years or more before they have to be replaced. But mechanical valves tend to promote the formation of blood clots and, therefore, require long-term use of anticoagulants (see page 475), drugs that prevent clotting. Surgery to replace a heart valve involves open heart surgery. The general steps in valve replacement surgery are as follows:

- You are given general anesthesia (see page 261) to make you unconscious. The surgeon makes an incision in your sternum (breastbone) and opens your chest to gain access to the heart.
- You are hooked up to a heart-lung machine, which functions for your heart and lungs to pump oxygen-rich blood to the rest of the body while your heart is stopped during the surgery.
- The diseased valve is carefully cut out, leaving enough tissue to which to attach the replacement valve.
- The replacement valve is positioned and stitched in place.
- Your heart is started again, the heart-lung machine is disconnected, and your chest is closed with stitches.

Weak or abnormal heartbeat

Some heart conditions result from an irregular heartbeat. For example, the heart may beat too quickly, too slowly, or erratically. Abnormal heartbeats are more common in people who have an underlying heart condition, such as congestive heart failure, but they can occur in otherwise healthy people as well.

ARRHYTHMIA

An arrhythmia is an abnormally fast or slow heartbeat. It is normal for your heart to beat faster or slower at certain times. For example, when you exercise or when something startles you, your heart temporarily speeds up and then gradually slows down to its normal pumping rate. But some people feel their heart beating irregularly at unusual times.

An irregular heartbeat is caused by a malfunction in the heart's electrical system. An electrical impulse triggers each beat of your heart. The sinus node (a cluster of specialized muscle cells) located at the top of the right atrium is the heart's natural pacemaker—it sends out electrical impulses that normally range between 60 to 100 beats a minute. When something interferes with the transmission of these electrical signals, an irregular heartbeat, or arrhythmia, may result. Coronary artery disease (see page 461) is the most common underlying cause of arrhythmia. An arrhythmia may also result from a heart abnormality that was present at birth.

A heart rate that is too fast most of the time (more than 100 beats per minute) is called tachycardia. A heart rate that is too slow most of the time (fewer than 60 beats per minute) is called bradycardia. These two types of irregular heartbeat are divided further according to the rhythm of the beat and the place of origin of the electrical impulses that trigger each beat.

Atrial (of the atrium) flutter and atrial fibrillation are common forms of an abnormally fast heartbeat (tachycardia). The fast, erratic beating of the heart caused by these arrhythmias reduces the efficiency of the heart as a pump, decreasing its ability to supply a sufficient amount of blood to the rest of the body. The increased pumping of the ventricles can have serious effects on an already diseased heart and can significantly worsen heart failure. Treatment is designed to slow the heart rate and return the irregular rhythm to normal.

Atrial flutter and atrial fibrillation occur most often when the heart is enlarged as a result of heart disease. But sometimes these conditions occur in a heart that is otherwise healthy. Lack of sleep, excessive intake of caffeine, some drugs, or excessive alcohol consumption can increase the risk of atrial flutter or atrial fibrillation.

Symptoms The most common symptoms of arrhythmia include heart palpitations (sudden, rapid heartbeats) or a fluttering sensation in the chest, as well as dizziness, fainting, chest pain, or shortness of breath. Sometimes, even with a serious arrhythmia, a person has none of these symptoms. Some people become more aware of the symptoms just before they go to sleep at night, particularly when they lie on their left side, because the heart moves closer to the chest wall when you lie on that side.

Diagnosis If your doctor suspects you have an arrhythmia, he or she takes your pulse and listens through a stethoscope to evaluate the rate and rhythm of your heart. A more exact diagnosis of the particular type of arrhythmia you have can be made from an electrocardiogram (ECG; see page 132), a test that shows the rate and pattern of electrical activity in your heart. If the arrhythmia occurs sporadically, it may be necessary to do an ECG using a portable monitor called a Holter monitor (see page 469) that you wear continuously for 24 hours. Your blood may be tested to evaluate the

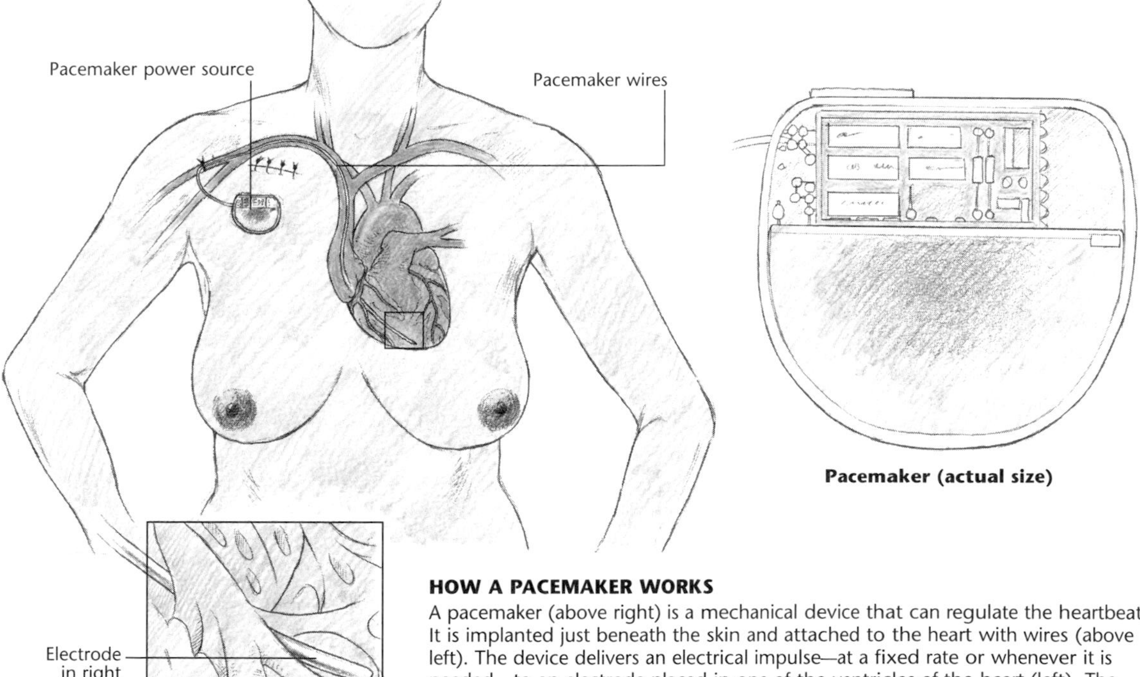

Pacemaker (actual size)

HOW A PACEMAKER WORKS

A pacemaker (above right) is a mechanical device that can regulate the heartbeat. It is implanted just beneath the skin and attached to the heart with wires (above left). The device delivers an electrical impulse—at a fixed rate or whenever it is needed—to an electrode placed in one of the ventricles of the heart (left). The pacemaker switches on whenever the heart slows down or misses a beat. A pacemaker can run for several years until the battery wears down and must be replaced.

functioning of your thyroid gland or to detect a chemical imbalance. A thyroid disorder or an imbalance of body chemicals can cause some types of arrhythmias.

Treatment Many arrhythmias are mild enough that they do not require treatment. More serious arrhythmias can be treated with medication or by installing a pacemaker (a device that regulates the heartbeat) or a defibrillator (a device that corrects an abnormal heartbeat).

Medication The medication used to treat an arrhythmia depends on the type of arrhythmia. Heart disease medications (see page 474), such as beta blockers, calcium channel blockers, and digitalis, are sometimes used. You may be given drugs designed specifically to control or prevent an irregular heartbeat by slowing the transmission of electrical impulses in the heart. Because of the wide variety of medications available to treat arrhythmias and because some of the drugs have unpleasant side effects, you may have to try different medications until you and your doctor find what works best for you and, at the same time, produces the fewest side effects.

Pacemaker A pacemaker is a small, battery-powered device that provides electrical impulses to the heart to keep it beating regularly. Pacemakers are usually used to regulate a very slow heart rate, but, occasionally, they are used to control a heart rate that is too fast. The device is implanted just beneath your skin and attached to the heart muscle with delicate wires. A pacemaker can produce an electrical impulse at a fixed rate or it can work on demand—switching off when the heart is beating normally and switching on when the heart slows down or misses a beat. A pacemaker can run for many years before the battery wears down and must be replaced. Your doctor can insert a replacement battery in a minor operation that is usually performed in the hospital using local anesthesia. Your doctor will recommend regular checkups to make sure your pacemaker is working properly.

A pacemaker is inserted in the following way:

- After administering a local anesthetic to numb your chest, a thin tube (catheter) is inserted, usually through the subclavian vein, a large vein just beneath the skin in your upper chest.
- One or more electrodes that supply the electrical impulse to your heart are threaded through the catheter to one of the chambers of the heart.
- The surgeon makes a small pocket in the pad of flesh under the skin of your

Living with a pacemaker

For the first several weeks after you get your pacemaker, refrain from any strenuous activity or movement that may dislodge one of the wires. In particular, you should limit the motion of your arm on the side the pacemaker was implanted. Do not raise your arm above your head except to wash or dress, and avoid sudden, jerking movements. Do not engage in any strenuous activities that involve your arms, including swimming, bowling, tennis, vacuum cleaning, carrying heavy laundry or trash, raking, or mowing the lawn. After 8 weeks, the wires will become set and less likely to become dislodged. You can then resume all of your normal activities.

Although it is not necessary, you may want to check your pulse at rest for 1 full minute and again for 1 minute after you exercise. Your doctor will tell you the normal ranges for your pulse at rest and after exercise. You should have your pacemaker checked by your doctor about 2 weeks after it is implanted, again at 3 and 6 months, and then at least once a year. You may be able to monitor the functioning of your pacemaker by phone; a call-in service can provide you with a special transmitter that relays a signal over the phone. Ask your doctor about this service.

In unusual situations, external sources of electrical signals such as antennas, high-voltage equipment, and high-powered electrical machinery can disrupt the functioning of a pacemaker. Old microwave ovens with leaky seals may also cause disruption. At airports, ask to be checked by an attendant instead of going through the metal detector. Ask your doctor for a list of situations you should avoid because of your pacemaker. For example, you cannot have any medical tests that use magnetic resonance imaging (MRI; see page 572). If you have any concerns about your pacemaker's functioning, see your doctor immediately.

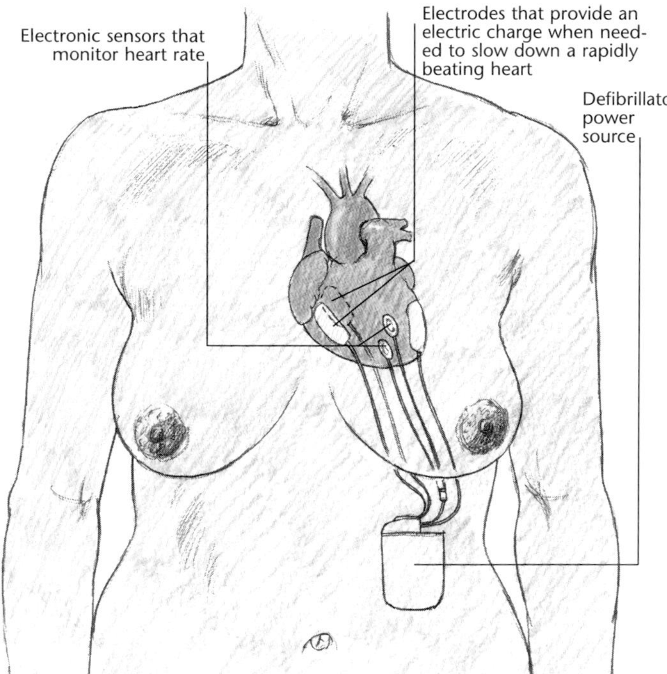

HOW A DEFIBRILLATOR WORKS

An implantable cardiac defibrillator slows down or stops a potentially dangerous rapid heart rate that arises in the ventricles—the pumping chambers of the heart. The power source of the defibrillator is implanted in a pocket underneath the skin of your abdomen. Two electronic sensors attached to the heart and connected to the power source monitor the electrical activity of your heart. When this activity becomes erratic, the defibrillator sends a charge of electricity through two other electrodes connected to the heart. This electric charge delivered to the heart restores its normal beating.

chest wall below the collarbone to hold the power source, which is about the size of a tiny beeper. After inserting the power source, the surgeon stitches the skin flap close. (You will have a small scar.)

You will remain in the hospital 1 to 2 days after the procedure. Complications are rare but include the same complications that are possible in all procedures in which a catheter is threaded through a blood vessel—including bleeding, a punctured vein, an infection, or a collapsed lung.

Implantable defibrillator A defibrillator is a device that is surgically implanted inside your body to slow down or stop potentially dangerous rapid heartbeats that arise in the ventricles, the pumping chambers of your heart. A cardiac defibrillator prevents ventricular fibrillation—a very rapid, quivering, uncoordinated rhythm in the ventricle that prevents the ventricle from pumping sufficient amounts of blood. Uncontrolled ventricular fibrillation is the major cause of sudden death.

Implanting a defibrillator is a more complicated and difficult procedure than implanting a pacemaker and requires a longer hospital stay. For this reason, the procedure for implanting a defibrillator is usually performed only on people who are in danger of sudden death from ventricular fibrillation. The procedure, which uses general anesthesia (see page 261), is done through an incision in the chest wall (called a thoracotomy) in the following general way:

- An incision is made either in your chest or along your left side, to expose your heart.
- Two 2 x 3-inch electronic sensors are attached to the surface of the heart to monitor its electrical activity. Two other electrodes are attached to the surface of the heart to give an electric charge when necessary to slow a potentially dangerous rapid heartbeat.
- Wires connected to the four electrodes are tunneled underneath the skin to the abdomen.
- A battery-operated power source is implanted in a pocket created under the skin of the abdomen.
- In some cases, corrective heart surgery, such as coronary bypass surgery (see page 477), may be performed at this time. Many people who require an implantable defibrillator also have coronary artery disease (see page 461).
- After surgery is completed, you are taken to the intensive care unit for a day or two so that your condition can be monitored for potential complications.

You will have to stay in the hospital for about a week for recovery after the procedure. You may have to wear a portable ECG monitor (see page 469) for 24 hours after the procedure to monitor the electrical activity of your heart. Your recovery at home will take another 6 to 8 weeks. You must take the same precautions and restrictions with an implantable defibrillator that you would with a pacemaker (see page 490). In addition, there is always a risk that you may lose consciousness briefly when the defibrillator provides an electric charge to your heart. For this reason, if you have an implantable defibrillator, you cannot drive a car.

CONGESTIVE HEART FAILURE

Congestive heart failure is a condition in which the heart pumps inefficiently and may not pump an adequate amount of blood to the lungs and the rest of the body. Congestive heart failure is a life-threatening condition, but it can be treated with medications that can stop the progression of the disease and control it. A person who has experienced heart failure can lead a productive life for many years. However, if not treated, congestive heart failure can cause irreversible damage to the heart and, ultimately, death.

Congestive heart failure can result from damage to a heart muscle caused by a heart attack, a heart valve disorder (see page 485), high blood pressure (see page 480), or a buildup of pressure in the lungs caused by lung disease. Because the heart is not pumping a sufficient amount of blood, pressure backs up into the veins, causing fluid buildup and swelling in tissues of the lungs, liver, and ankles. The heart's inability to pump a sufficient amount of blood to the rest of the body can also lead to fatigue, dizziness, and low blood pressure. In extreme cases, the rhythm of the heartbeat becomes dangerously abnormal and causes death.

Many people who have congestive heart failure have abnormal heart rhythms. These abnormal rhythms, which may occur at any time (even when the person is feeling fine) may instantly worsen symptoms or cause sudden death. Abnormal heart rhythms are responsible for half of all deaths of people with heart failure.

Symptoms Symptoms of congestive heart failure include unusual tiredness or shortness of breath, wheezing caused by fluid in the lungs, swelling of the ankles and lower legs, frequent urination at night, and a sudden, unexplained large weight gain of 20 to 30 pounds (caused by an accumulation of excess fluid). You may also experience a feeling of being unable to breathe when you lie down. This difficulty breathing is caused by pooling of fluid inside your lungs. Blood pools in the lungs because the heart has insufficient strength to push it forward to the rest of the body.

Diagnosis To diagnose congestive heart failure, your doctor may do an echocardiogram (see page 132) to evaluate the size and thickness of your heart and its ability to contract and relax, and the health of the valves and pericardium (the tissue lining the outside of the heart). An exercise stress test (see page 469) can determine how much work your heart is able to do. A stress test is safe for people with congestive heart failure as long as it is carefully administered.

Other tests may also be done to diagnose congestive heart failure. For example, your doctor may test your lungs to differentiate between congestive heart failure and some types of lung disease. A test called a radioisotope study, which evaluates blood flow through the heart, can help determine how the left ventricle of the heart is pumping. A test result showing a lower rate of pumping efficiency indicates a greater severity of heart failure.

Treatment If you are diagnosed with congestive heart failure, the first advice your doctor will give is to decrease your physical activity, at least until your condition stabilizes. Your heart cannot meet the demands of extra physical exertion, which forces the heart to work harder to supply more oxygen. You will also be told to cut back on salt (which causes water retention), avoid caffeine (which can worsen an irregular heartbeat), and eat more frequent but smaller meals (which require less effort to digest).

Congestive heart failure is treated with a combination of three kinds of drugs—digitalis drugs (see page 475), vasodilators such as ACE inhibitors (see page 474) or alpha blockers (see page 474), and diuretics (see page 475). Together, these medications increase your heart's pumping action and lower blood pressure by widening (dilating) blood vessels and helping your body eliminate excess fluid. In cases in which medication fails to improve the condition, heart failure may be treated with surgery.

In some people who are severely ill with congestive heart failure, a heart transplant may be done. More and more people are having heart transplants every year and about 85 percent of those who have a transplant are alive at least 5 years after the surgery. However, donor hearts are scarce and not everyone is a good candidate for this major surgery. Your doctor can tell you whether or not you might benefit from a heart transplant.

Disorders of the blood and small blood vessels

Some disorders of the blood, such as anemia, are more common among women than men. These disorders may result when the body's production of red blood cells cannot keep up with the demand, when the composition of the blood changes, or when a disease affects the condition of the blood vessels.

ANEMIA

Anemia is a blood disorder caused by a reduction in the amount of oxygen delivered to tissues by red blood cells. Anemia may occur when a person has fewer red blood cells than normal or less hemoglobin, the oxygen-carrying protein in red blood cells. A deficiency of red blood cells or hemoglobin can result from bleeding or, occasionally, an insufficient amount of iron in the diet. Iron is necessary for the normal growth of blood cells. Women sometimes develop anemia from heavy menstrual bleeding. If you have heavy periods, particularly if they have recently become heavier, see your doctor to be tested for anemia.

Anemia sometimes occurs in women who are pregnant or breast-feeding because the developing fetus or nursing infant increases the woman's need for iron. For this reason, doctors prescribe a multivitamin/mineral supplement that contains iron for women who are pregnant or breast-feeding; 30 milligrams of iron a day is sufficient in many cases.

Persistent bleeding, the most common cause of severe anemia, often occurs in the intestines from an abnormal growth such as a polyp or tumor. Internal bleeding can also result from regular use of aspirin, ibuprofen, or other nonsteroidal anti-inflammatory drugs.

Symptoms Mild iron deficiency anemia may cause vague symptoms, including listlessness and fatigue. If the anemia becomes more severe, the inability of the blood to supply oxygen to tissues can result in shortness of breath, rapid pulse, and the sensation that your heart is working harder or faster. The linings of your eyelids and the skin underneath your nails sometimes become pale. See your doctor if you experience any of these symptoms.

Diagnosis To diagnose anemia, your doctor can perform a simple blood test to measure your level of red blood cells. Your doctor may also measure the level of iron in your blood to determine whether or not you need to take iron supplements.

Treatment If the blood test shows your level of red blood cells is low, your doctor will prescribe an iron supplement. You can try to increase the amount of iron in your diet by eating iron-rich foods (see page 66), but it is difficult to treat anemia with diet alone. Treatment for other causes of anemia, such as bleeding from the intestines, depends on the cause. You should never try to treat anemia yourself by taking iron supplements. The amount of iron necessary to correct iron deficiency anemia is much more than is found in most over-the-counter supplements.

You should not take an iron supplement at any time unless your doctor has prescribed it. Your body stores iron and an excess can build up over time. A high level of stored iron in your body can interfere with your body's ability to use other nutrients and can damage organs.

SICKLE-CELL ANEMIA

Sickle-cell anemia is an inherited deformity in red blood cells that reduces their ability to carry oxygen to tissues. The disease results from an abnormal type of hemoglobin (the oxygen-carrying protein in red blood cells) that causes red blood cells to form in the shape of a sickle. This abnormal shape makes the oxygen-carrying red blood cells fragile and less able to pass through tiny blood vessels called capillaries, from which tissues get most of their oxygen. A lack of oxygen can result in damage to tissues and organs. Until recently, most children born with sickle-cell anemia died in early childhood. Now, many people with the

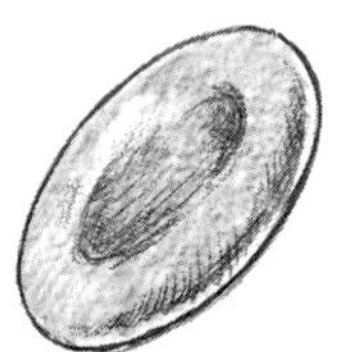

Shape of normal red blood cell

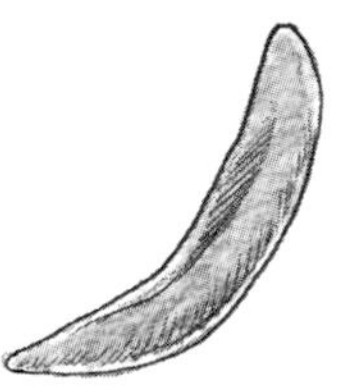

Shape of sickled red blood cell

disease are reaching adulthood and living relatively normal lives.

Because sickle-cell anemia is a recessive genetic disorder (see page 377), a child must receive a copy of the defective gene from both parents to have the disease. A person who inherits only one copy of the sickle-cell gene will not have the disease but will be a carrier and, therefore, can transmit the disease to children if his or her partner is also a carrier. Sickle-cell anemia is most common among blacks and people of Mediterranean origin, although it can affect people of any race or ethnic group. About 1 in every 12 blacks carries the sickle-cell gene. If you are planning a pregnancy and are black or have a relative with the disease, consider being tested (see page 373) to find out if you are a carrier of the gene. If you are a carrier, your partner should also be tested. If you are not a carrier, there is no risk of transmitting the disease to your children because a child has to receive a copy of the sickle-cell gene from both you and your partner. A test performed in early pregnancy can determine whether a fetus is carrying two copies of the sickle-cell gene.

Symptoms The first symptoms of sickle-cell anemia usually appear around 6 months of age. In some children, the spleen becomes enlarged and traps damaged red blood cells, causing a severe form of anemia that can be life threatening. Persistent anemia causes fatigue, headaches, shortness of breath on exertion, and jaundice (a condition characterized by yellowing of the skin and whites of the eyes). Damaged or dead red blood cells can collect in joints or elsewhere in the body, causing extreme pain. Episodes of severe pain are called sickle-cell crises. A crisis can be brought on by infection, cold weather, or dehydration from prolonged vomiting and diarrhea. Children with sickle-cell anemia are at increased risk of pneumonia and gallstones.

Diagnosis Sickle-cell anemia is diagnosed by a blood test. The abnormally shaped red blood cells can be seen under a microscope, and the amount of hemoglobin (the oxygen-carrying protein in red blood cells) can be measured.

Treatment There is no cure for sickle-cell anemia, but immunization against infectious diseases and the use of antibiotics to fight infection have increased the life span of many people with the disease. Affected people usually take supplements of folic acid (a B vitamin) throughout their life; this vitamin helps the body regenerate new red blood cells to replace damaged and dead cells.

In a sickle-cell crisis, immediate treatment is essential. Painkillers are usually required to relieve the severe pain of a crisis. You may receive intravenous infusion of fluids to prevent dehydration, and antibiotics to prevent infection. You may have to breathe concentrated oxygen to increase the supply of oxygen to tissues. A blood transfusion may be required to increase the amount of normal hemoglobin in your blood.

IDIOPATHIC THROMBOCYTOPENIC PURPURA

Idiopathic thrombocytopenic purpura (ITP) is an autoimmune disease in which an antibody mistakenly produced by the immune system binds with and damages blood cells called platelets, the cells that are necessary for clotting. In most cases, this failure of blood to clot normally causes little more than bruising of the skin. ITP is most common between ages 20 and 50 and affects twice as many women as men. The condition is often long-term and usually does not go away without treatment.

Symptoms Bleeding is the most common symptom of ITP. Bleeding under the skin may cause bruises to appear on your skin. You may have nosebleeds or you may bleed from your gums. You will probably feel fine.

Diagnosis Blood tests can determine if your platelet count is low and rule out other causes of your symptoms.

Treatment If you are diagnosed with ITP, your doctor will prescribe high doses of the steroid drug prednisone, which can usually reduce the binding of the antibodies to the platelets. Bleeding usually diminishes within 1 day of treatment. Long-term use of prednisone may reduce your spleen's production of the platelet-destroying antibodies. For a person with recurring ITP, surgical removal of the spleen may be recommended.

DEEP-VEIN THROMBOSIS

Deep-vein thrombosis is the formation of blood clots in veins deep inside the legs. The condition is usually caused by sluggish blood flow when a person lies or sits still for long periods of time, such as during prolonged bed rest after surgery or in cases of paralysis. Prevention of thrombosis is one of the reasons you are told to get up and walk around as soon as possible after having an operation.

Deep-vein thrombosis is more common among women over 35 who smoke and take birth-control pills, or women who are or recently have been pregnant. Deep-vein thrombosis is not always a serious condition but, if a piece of a blood clot breaks off and travels to your lungs, it can block an artery, which can be life threatening. A blood clot in a lung is called a pulmonary embolism (see page 511).

Symptoms A clot in a vein in your leg can cause a variety of symptoms, including pain, tenderness, swelling, redness, and a feeling of warmth on the skin over the clot.

Diagnosis Deep-vein thrombosis can be diagnosed by radionuclide scanning (see page 512) or an ultrasound (see page 405). These imaging tests can provide information about the condition of the veins in your legs and the flow of blood through them.

Treatment If the blood clots are small and confined to your calf, you may not need any treatment. The clots may break up and dissolve by themselves, especially if you walk around frequently. If you have a serious case of thrombosis, your doctor may prescribe drugs that thin your blood and prevent clotting, especially if there is a risk of a pulmonary embolism. Clots that are located in the deep veins in the thigh or behind the knee are more likely to break off and travel to the lungs. Surgery to remove a clot is sometimes necessary.

VARICOSE VEINS

Varicose veins, which are extremely common, are veins just under the skin that become enlarged and twisted, and may look unsightly. Varicose veins result from a weakening of the valves in the veins that usually keep blood flowing in one direction. Gravity tends to put pressure on the valves, sometimes making them become weak or defective, which can cause the blood to collect, or pool, in the veins. This pooling of blood makes the veins swollen and distorted.

Varicose veins are most visible on the legs, but they can occur in the rectal area as hemorrhoids (see page 522) and in the esophagus. A number of factors—including obesity, the hormonal changes that accompany pregnancy or menopause, or standing for long periods of time—can contribute to the development of varicose veins. Varicose veins tend to run in families and are more common in women than men.

Reducing your risk of varicose veins

Here are some things you can do to help prevent varicose veins or relieve discomfort if you have them:

- Keep your weight under control. Extra weight, especially in your abdominal area, presses on veins in the upper thigh or groin area, causing them to collapse and slowing down the circulation of blood.
- Exercise regularly. Walking, bicycling, or jogging several days a week strengthens your leg muscles and helps push blood through your veins.
- Elevate your legs when you sit or lie down to help move the blood from your legs back to your heart.
- Wear support stockings. Try the support stockings available in stores or ask your doctor to recommend a special kind for varicose veins. Do not wear knee-high stockings, which can constrict the area just below the knee.

Symptoms Varicose veins are blue, prominent, swollen, kinked veins that usually appear on the back of the calf or anywhere on the inside of the leg. You may not feel any discomfort from a varicose vein, but the affected area may ache, your feet and ankles may swell, and your skin may itch and become dry. The symptoms often become progressively worse during the day but can be relieved by elevating your legs.

Diagnosis A doctor can diagnose varicose veins by their appearance alone.

Treatment In most cases, the only treatment necessary for varicose veins is wearing elastic support stockings, walking

VARICOSE VEINS
A healthy vein (right) in the leg has a series of valves that keep blood flowing up toward the heart. In a varicose vein (far right), the valves are weakened, allowing blood to pool in the vein, causing it to become swollen and distorted.

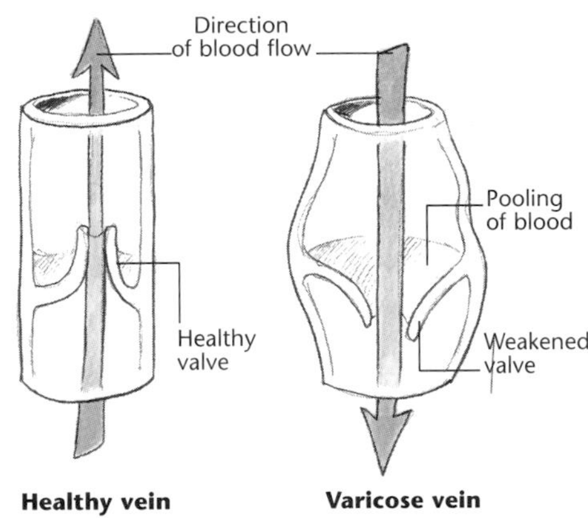

regularly, and avoiding standing for long periods of time. When you sit, prop your feet up to allow blood to drain out of your legs. Varicose veins that are very painful may be treated by removing them surgically. This procedure, called stripping, usually takes about half an hour for each leg and is done using local anesthesia (see page 260).

Your doctor may recommend a nonsurgical procedure called sclerotherapy. In sclerotherapy, an irritating solution is injected into the varicose vein, which causes the walls of the vein to stick together, closing off the flow of blood. The vein then becomes less visible under the skin. Other veins nearby take over the work of the treated vein. After either stripping or sclerotherapy, you may still develop varicose veins elsewhere.

ONE WOMAN'S STORY
VARICOSE VEINS

I have always liked the way my legs looked, so I was horrified last year to notice one of the veins in my thigh begin to bulge and turn purple. It kept getting worse and growing more unsightly. It didn't hurt and I didn't pay much attention to it during the winter months but, when summer came, this vein had gotten even bigger. I was embarrassed to wear shorts because this vein made me look so much older than my age.

At first, I didn't want to go to the doctor. I had heard that you have to have surgery to correct varicose veins and I didn't want surgery. But I was worried that the vein might burst or something, so I finally went.

I was relieved to find out that varicose veins are not a serious condition. The veins in our legs have little valves that keep blood flowing in one direction—up to the heart. When these valves grow weak—from pregnancy, aging, or lack of activity—the blood pools in the veins causing the swollen blood vessels that you can see through the skin.

"My varicose vein was corrected without surgery right in my doctor's office."

My varicose vein was corrected without surgery right in my doctor's office. My doctor performed a simple procedure called sclerotherapy. He injected a chemical solution into my varicose vein, which closed it off. The blood that formerly flowed through that vein simply rerouted itself through another vein.

I'm quite happy with the way my legs look now and I'm relieved to know that, if this happens again, there is a simple solution. I also know that keeping your leg muscles in good shape helps prevent varicose veins, so now I'm walking at least three mornings every week.

CHAPTER 18

Your lungs

Contents

Your lungs and respiratory system have a vital job—they take in oxygen from the air you inhale and allow it to pass into your bloodstream. The red blood cells in your bloodstream transport the oxygen to all parts of your body. A waste product of this process—carbon dioxide—builds up in your bloodstream; your lungs eliminate carbon dioxide when you exhale.

As each breath brings air into your lungs, it also brings in dust, bacteria, and pollutants that can cause infection or disease. To sweep out these impurities, your lungs and air passages are lined with microscopic hairs called cilia. Glands in your air passages constantly secrete mucus. Dirt and germs adhere to the layer of mucus, and the mucus is moved out of your lungs by the cilia. Inside your lungs, scavenger cells digest any remaining dirt or germs.

Your respiratory defense system is extremely efficient but it cannot protect you from every infection or from the effects of long-term exposure to cancer-causing substances such as those found in tobacco smoke.

Protecting your lungs

Each lung is made of spongy tissue that expands with air with each breath. When you inhale, air travels into lung tissue through a system of airways. From a single tube—the trachea (windpipe)—the airways branch into two main bronchial tubes. The bronchial tubes branch into smaller and smaller passageways that eventually end in tiny, fragile air sacs called alveoli. From the alveoli, oxygen passes into tiny adjacent blood vessels called capillaries and is taken up by red blood cells, which deliver the oxygen to cells in all of your tissues. At the same time, the waste product carbon dioxide passes from the red blood cells into the alveoli. Carbon dioxide is eliminated from your body when you exhale.

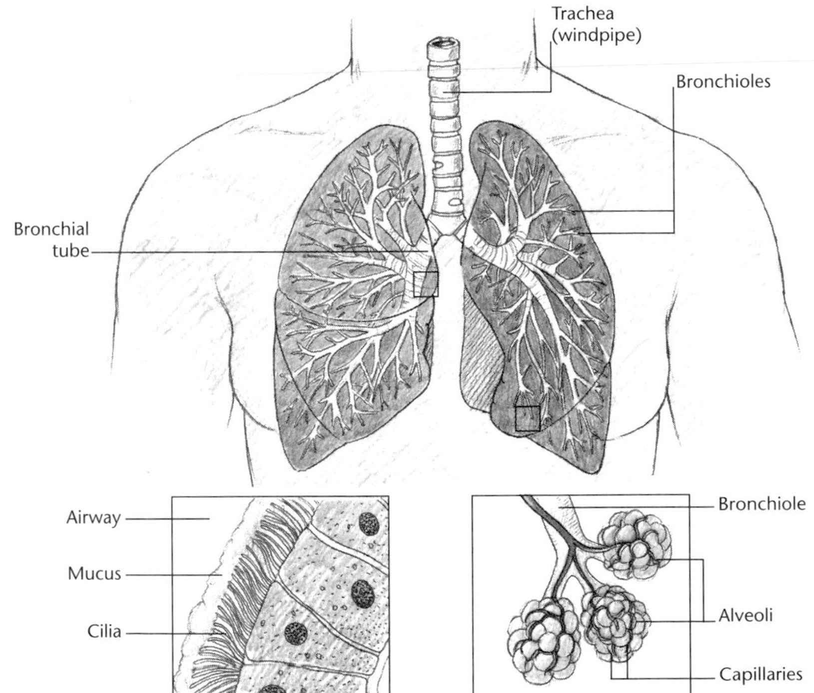

YOUR AIRWAYS

The air that you breathe passes through your trachea (windpipe), which divides into two smaller tubes called bronchial tubes, each of which leads to one of your lungs. The bronchial tubes branch into smaller and smaller tubes called bronchioles. At the ends of the bronchioles are tiny clusters of air sacs called alveoli (below right), where oxygen is absorbed into your bloodstream and carbon dioxide is eliminated from your bloodstream. Glands in your airways constantly secrete mucus, to which dirt, germs, and other impurities adhere. Tiny microscopic hairs called cilia (below left) keep your airways clean by sweeping out the impurities.

HARMFUL SUBSTANCES

Unlike the rest of your body, which is protected by your skin, the thin, fragile tissues that line your lungs are sometimes directly exposed to substances that you breathe in from the air around you. That is, these substances can bypass the mucous barrier in your nose and bronchial tubes and the hairlike cilia that are supposed to sweep them out. A number of these substances (described below) can cause lung disease.

Cigarette smoke Cigarette smoke is the major cause of lung cancer, chronic bronchitis, and emphysema. Smoking makes your lungs susceptible to infections, including colds. An excessive amount of mucus may accumulate in your air passages, which impairs the cleansing action of the cilia. Smoking also constricts air passages, making breathing more difficult. If smoking has severely damaged your lungs, they will not be able to pass as much oxygen into your blood.

Exposure to secondhand smoke from someone else's cigarette can also be harmful. This kind of smoke can cause irritation to the eyes and upper airways. Secondhand smoke contains toxic substances including carbon monoxide, cancer-causing agents, and materials that can cause allergic reactions and lung disease. Children of people who smoke have more respiratory infections than other children. A person whose spouse smokes has an increased risk of lung cancer and heart disease.

Occupational hazards You may be breathing in substances at work that can cause lung problems. In severe cases, these substances cause hypersensitivity pneumonitis, a condition that has symptoms similar to those of allergies and asthma (see page 635). You may feel shortness of breath, wheezing, and fatigue that occurs during the workweek but subsides on weekends or vacations. Some common substances that cause occupational lung disease include organic solvents (such as those used in dry cleaning and other industries), cotton dust (in textile manufacturing), or feathers (in

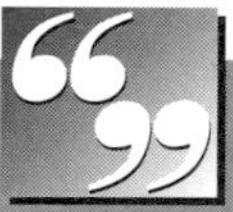

ONE WOMAN'S STORY
SMOKING AND LUNG CANCER

I started smoking when I was 16 and smoked a pack of cigarettes a day for 29 years. I tried to quit many times but each time, as soon as I started to gain weight or whenever something stressful happened, I went back to smoking. When I was 45, I developed a smoker's cough, so I cut back to half a pack a day. I wasn't too worried about lung cancer because my mother smoked all of her life and she never got cancer. In spite of all that I knew about the dangers of smoking, I felt that somehow it wasn't going to affect me. I was wrong.

A year later, my cough got a lot worse. My doctor recommended a chest X-ray, which showed a tumor in my right lung. Then I had to have a CT scan and a biopsy of the tumor. The biopsy showed that the tumor was cancerous. My doctor told me I was lucky that the cancer was in only one lung and did not appear to have spread to the nearby lymph nodes. I had surgery to remove part of that lung and, thank heaven, the lymph nodes weren't cancerous. It took a long time to recover. My chest hurt a lot, I had trouble breathing, and I had to do lots of exercises and physical therapy to get back on my feet.

"In spite of all that I knew about the dangers of smoking, I felt that somehow it wasn't going to affect me. I was wrong."

I'm now back at work. My doctor tells me the cancer is in remission, but I know it can come back at any time or that a new tumor might develop. I finally quit smoking and regret that I didn't do it years ago. But my biggest regret is the pain I have caused my family.

Warning signs
Lung disease

The symptoms of several different kinds of lung disease are similar. If you notice any of the following warning signs, call your doctor immediately:

- **Persistent cough** Any cough that lasts more than a month is an important early sign that something may be wrong with your respiratory system.
- **Shortness of breath** It is normal to be short of breath during strenuous exercise. However, you should not be short of breath for longer than a few minutes after you stop exercising or when doing something that other people your age can do with ease; nor should you experience shortness of breath when you are not exerting yourself.
- **Persistent production of phlegm** Phlegm, a thick mucus, is produced in your air passages to fight infection. Normally, the production of phlegm subsides as soon as the infection clears up. If you cough up phlegm or mucus for more than a month, you may have a condition that requires medical attention.
- **Wheezing** If you hear wheezing or another noise when you breathe, something may be obstructing your airways.
- **Coughing up blood** If you are coughing up blood, it may be coming from your lungs. This can be a sign of a serious respiratory disease such as lung cancer.
- **Frequent chest colds** If you have more than two colds a year with chest congestion that lasts longer than usual, or if you have a cold that lasts more than 2 weeks, you could have a condition that requires medical attention.
- **Chest pain** Chest pain that increases when you breathe or cough may be a sign of lung inflammation or pleurisy (inflammation of the membrane that surrounds the lung).

poultry handling). If you are exposed to any of these substances on the job or elsewhere and you have a chronic cough or symptoms similar to those of asthma, see your doctor immediately.

Other environmental hazards Outdoors, industrial pollutants, automobile exhaust fumes, and pollen from plants and trees can aggravate a person's asthma or bronchitis. Even in your own home, your lungs may be exposed to substances that can irritate them or, over the long term, contribute to lung disease. For example, a poorly ventilated furnace or stove can produce poisonous, odorless, carbon monoxide fumes, which can be lethal. Radon gas seeping out of the ground into your basement may slightly increase your risk of lung cancer.

Controlling indoor air pollution Here are some relatively simple things you can do to keep the air in your home clean:

- Get an annual inspection of your furnace, hot water heater, and gas appliances. Poorly ventilated equipment can result in a buildup of poisonous carbon monoxide gas.
- Purchase a carbon monoxide detector for your home that will warn you if this gas is present.
- Make sure wood or coal stoves are ventilated to the outside and that the exhaust system does not leak. Never cook with charcoal inside your home.
- To reduce your exposure to allergens, clean your air conditioners, humidifiers, and dehumidifiers regularly. Wash bedding materials in hot water to reduce dust mites.
- Carefully read the warning labels on household products, hobby materials, and pesticides. Use them only in well-ventilated areas. Use pump sprays instead of aerosols whenever possible.
- Reduce the concentration of formaldehyde gas that may come from carpets, paneling, and drapes by keeping rooms well ventilated to improve the mix of fresh air with recirculated air.
- You can purchase a radon detector to check the level of radon gas in your home. If the radon level is elevated, sealing up cracks in your basement and ventilating the basement can markedly reduce it.

Germs You breathe into your lungs many different kinds of organisms—bacteria, viruses, and fungi—that have the potential to cause disease. Most of the time, they are expelled or neutralized by your body's immune system. But, if your body's defenses are impaired, many of these organisms can cause colds, influenza, pneumonia, or bronchitis.

There are some steps you can take to help prevent lung diseases. Most importantly, do not smoke. If you smoke, quitting is the most important thing you can do for your health. (For information about how to quit, see page 157.) Avoid exposure to secondhand smoke at home and at work. You should be immunized against influenza and pneumonia (see page 138) if you are over 65 or have asthma or another lung disease, or if you have a chronic disease such as diabetes (see page 617).

Disorders that obstruct airflow

Millions of Americans—nearly all of them over 40—are affected by chronic bronchitis or emphysema. These conditions, which are almost always caused by years of cigarette smoking, result in a restriction of airflow out of the lungs. Asthma is another common lung condition that also obstructs airflow. Asthma attacks are often triggered by an allergic reaction that causes spasm of the muscles of the bronchial tubes and inflammation of the lining of the smaller airways (bronchioles). For more about asthma, see page 635.

CHRONIC BRONCHITIS

Bronchitis is inflammation of the lining of the bronchial tubes. This inflammation often results in severe coughing with heavy mucus. Bronchitis is considered to be chronic when it occurs for at least 3 months a year for 2 years. Chronic bronchitis is usually caused by smoking; other causes include infection, air pollution, and industrial dusts.

People often fail to seek treatment for chronic bronchitis because they consider it more of a nuisance than an ailment, and they do not think the disease is serious. In addition, if they are smokers, they may be reluctant to acknowledge that they have to quit smoking in order to cure their bronchitis. In fact, bronchitis can lead to life-threatening respiratory diseases and heart failure. Over a period of months and years, bronchitis damages the protective, hairlike structures (cilia) that move mucus out of your lungs. As a result, mucus collects in your lungs and creates an environment favorable to infection and inflammation, which can result in permanent damage to your lungs.

Symptoms Chronic bronchitis often starts as a cold. But long after the other symptoms are gone, a cough that produces mucus lingers. The condition may go away but then may return and last even longer with each new cold. Gradually, the cough and mucus become constant, occurring without other cold or flu symptoms. Smokers often dismiss bronchitis as a "smoker's cough." The cough may be worse in the morning and in damp, cold weather.

Diagnosis Bronchitis is usually diagnosed from a pattern of symptoms, particularly a persistent cough with mucus.

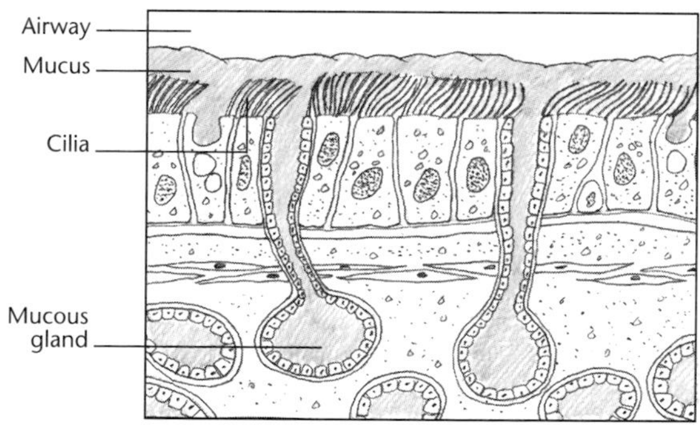

Wall of healthy bronchial tube

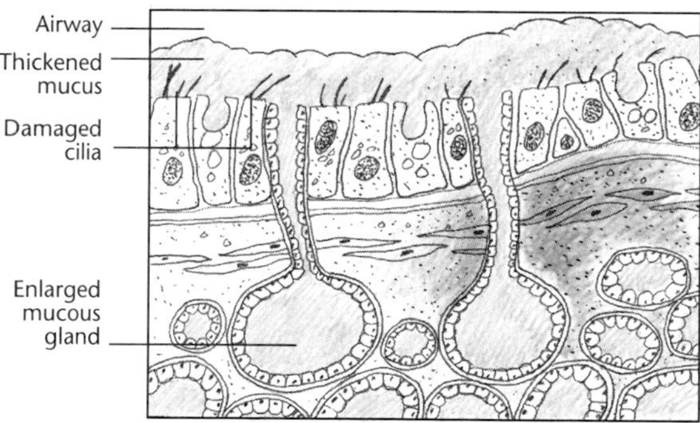

Wall of tube affected by chronic bronchitis

EFFECTS OF CHRONIC BRONCHITIS
The bronchial tubes of a normal lung (left) are lined with tiny hairlike structures called cilia that sweep mucus up and out of the lung in a constant flow. In a lung with bronchitis (right), mucous glands grow larger and produce more mucus. The cilia become damaged by irritants such as tobacco smoke and are no longer able to sweep away the thickening mucus. The lining of the bronchial tubes becomes inflamed. Bacteria that lodge in the relatively immobilized mucus can cause infection and congestion.

Treatment Chronic bronchitis is treated by reducing the inflammation of the bronchial tubes. If you smoke, your doctor will tell you that you need to quit. (For information about how to quit smoking, see page 157). You may also need to avoid secondhand smoke (see page 155) and dusty and polluted environmental conditions that are irritating your airways.

If you develop an infection in your lungs, your doctor may prescribe medications, including antibiotics. Drugs called bronchodilators (see page 637) can help open your air passages. Your doctor may also recommend that you have vaccinations against influenza and pneumococcal pneumonia (see page 138) because both of these lung infections can make bronchitis worse.

EMPHYSEMA

Emphysema is a disease in which the structure of the alveoli (tiny air sacs in the lungs where the exchange of oxygen and carbon dioxide takes place) is permanently changed. When these changes are extensive, the critical transfer of oxygen and carbon dioxide between the air and the blood inside the lungs is inadequate. Even before this process breaks down, the normal elasticity of lung tissue may be reduced so that an expanded, inflated lung is less able to spring back, or to expel air rapidly. One consequence of this decreased elasticity is diminished airflow out of the lungs. The inability to move air into and out of the lungs rapidly and the greatly increased effort required to breathe causes shortness of breath and a sensation of labored breathing at levels of activity that healthy people can handle with ease.

Emphysema is usually caused by long-term exposure to tobacco smoke and other irritants. A rare, inherited form of emphysema can develop in people who are missing an enzyme that normally helps the fibers in the walls of the alveoli retain their elasticity.

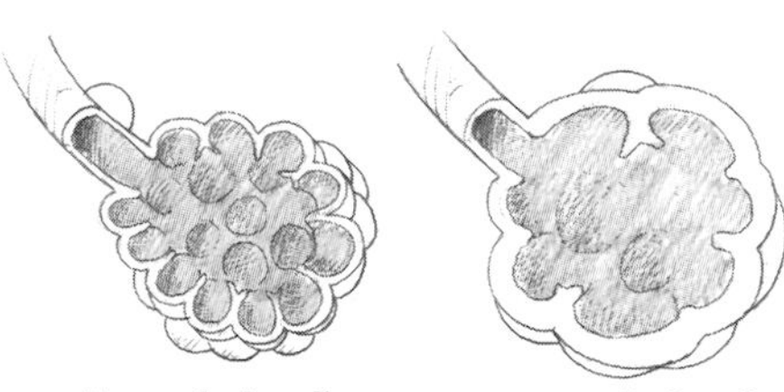

EFFECTS OF EMPHYSEMA
Normal alveoli (left) look like a tiny bunch of grapes. When tobacco smoke damages and breaks down the walls of the alveoli (right), they merge to form fewer, larger sacs with thicker walls. This process reduces the surface area that is available for essential oxygen to be absorbed into the body and for carbon dioxide to be removed.

Symptoms The most common symptom of emphysema, shortness of breath, may first occur only during exercise or exertion. However, gradually you may begin having shortness of breath even during moderate activity. Many people with emphysema also have chronic bronchitis and continually cough up mucus. However, in late, advanced stages of emphysema, coughing is less common.

Diagnosis To diagnose emphysema, your doctor may use several tests. A chest X-ray (see page 504) can show whether your lungs are overinflated. However, you can have emphysema even if your lungs are not overinflated and your chest X-ray looks perfectly normal. Tests called pulmonary function tests can determine how much air your lungs can hold and how quickly you can exhale.

Treatment Emphysema cannot be cured, but treatment can improve the length and quality of your life. Quitting smoking (see page 156) is the first and most important thing you must do. Your doctor may prescribe bronchodilators, medications that you can take in tablets or by inhaler (see page 638). Bronchodilators relax the muscles of your bronchial tubes and reduce inflammation, making it easier for you to breathe. In some cases, corticosteroid drugs (synthetic hormones that reduce inflammation) can help reduce shortness of breath. If you develop a bacterial infection such as pneumococcal pneumonia (see page 509), your doctor will prescribe an antibiotic. Some people with severe emphysema eventually develop congestive heart failure (see page 492) because of the increased work the heart must do to pump blood through the damaged lungs.

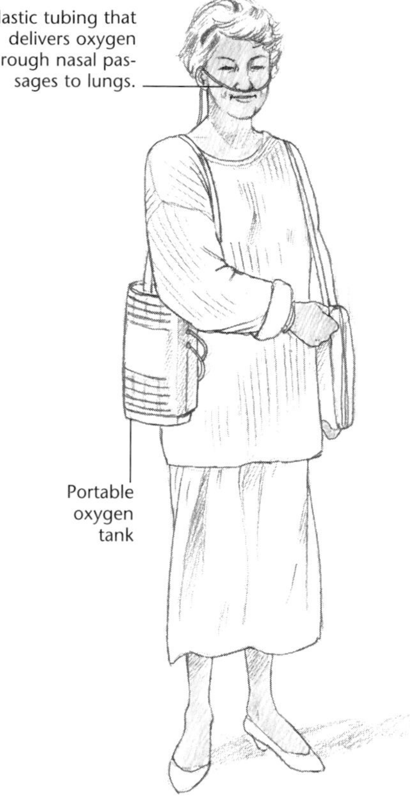

Physical therapy and breathing exercises may help. Your doctor may recommend that you join a pulmonary rehabilitation program to help improve your general physical conditioning. Improved conditioning can reduce your breathing needs during ordinary activities.

If you have severe emphysema or chronic bronchitis, your doctor may prescribe supplemental oxygen. You can have oxygen tanks delivered to your home or use an oxygen concentrator, which extracts oxygen from the air. You breathe the oxygen through plastic tubes attached to your nose. The treatment does not interfere with your ability to talk, eat, or drink. You should use the oxygen at least 15 hours a day and have a portable oxygen supply available when you go out.

USING A PORTABLE OXYGEN TANK
People whose lungs have lost the ability to absorb a sufficient amount of oxygen may need to use supplemental oxygen from either a portable oxygen supply that they can take with them wherever they go, or from a supply in a larger, stationary tank kept at home. Although cumbersome, portable oxygen provides mobility to a person who would otherwise be confined to his or her home.

Other lung disorders

Lung cancer, pneumonia (infection in the lungs), and pulmonary embolism (a blood clot in an artery that leads to the lungs) are common lung disorders that can be fatal. Pneumonia and pulmonary embolism are especially dangerous for people whose health has already been weakened by age or heart disease or other chronic illnesses. Cystic fibrosis (see page 512) is the most common inherited genetic disorder among whites (mostly those of European descent); sarcoidosis (see page 513) is a chronic disease that is most common among black women.

LUNG CANCER

Lung cancer is the leading cause of cancer deaths in American women. Seven out of eight cases of lung cancer are caused by years or decades of cigarette smoking. In rare cases, when lung cancer develops in a nonsmoker, the cause may be long-term exposure to secondhand smoke or to other cancer-causing substances in the air. An increase in the number of people who have diseases that weaken the immune system—such as AIDS or chronic diseases (such as diabetes)—may also be a factor in the rising incidence of lung cancer.

Symptoms Lung cancer can grow very slowly for many years with no symptoms. It is sometimes discovered by a routine chest X-ray, but more often it is detected only after symptoms begin. The symptoms of lung cancer are similar to those of other lung diseases. A cough is often the first sign. You may begin to cough when the cancerous growth (tumor) irritates the lining of your airways or blocks the passage of air. You may have a "smoker's cough" that becomes progressively worse. As the tumor grows and blocks your air passages, you may experience shortness

Warning signs
Lung cancer

The symptoms of lung cancer are similar to those of other lung diseases. Call your doctor if you experience any of the following:

- Persistent cough
- Coughing up blood
- Constant chest pain
- Shortness of breath and wheezing
- Repeated bouts of pneumonia or bronchitis
- Weight loss
- Swollen neck and face
- Pain and weakness in your shoulder, arm, or hand

of breath, wheezing, or repeated bouts of pneumonia or bronchitis. You may begin coughing up blood or your voice may become hoarse.

Once a lung cancer grows or spreads, the symptoms vary depending on the site to which it has spread. If a tumor presses on a large vein near your lung, it may block the flow of blood returning to your heart, causing your neck or face to swell. A tumor that presses on nerves inside your chest can cause pain in your chest or back and weakness in your shoulder, arm, or hand. Like other cancers, lung cancer can cause fatigue, loss of appetite, and weight loss. Cancer that has spread to more remote parts of your body can cause headache, pain, mental confusion, bone fractures, and other symptoms that appear to be unrelated to the cancer. These symptoms result when particular substances made by the cancerous cells enter your bloodstream.

Diagnosis If your doctor suspects that you might have lung cancer, he or she will ask you about your symptoms and your personal and family health histories. Your doctor will want to know if you smoke or if you work in a place where you are exposed to substances that are potentially cancer causing. Your doctor will perform a physical examination that includes listening to your lungs with a stethoscope.

In many cases, a chest X-ray (see below) or computed tomography (CT) scan (see page 572) can determine if there is a tumor in the lung. If a tumor is detected, a sample of tissue (biopsy) from the tumor must be taken to determine if the tumor is benign (noncancerous) or malignant (cancerous). The tissue sample is usually removed in an outpatient procedure called bronchoscopy.

Chest X-ray

A chest X-ray is a simple, painless procedure that provides an image of your lungs, usually on film. A chest X-ray is often the first test to be done when a person has symptoms of lung disease. If you have a chest X-ray, you will be asked to remove your clothes and jewelry from the waist up and you will be given a hospital gown to wear. While you are standing in front of the X-ray machine, the technician will ask you to take a deep breath, hold it in, and remain still.

Two views are usually taken in a chest X-ray—one from the front and one from the side. Other views may be taken as well. The image produced on a chest X-ray shows the bones (such as the ribs), air-filled structures (such as the lungs and bronchial tubes), and the heart. A tumor may appear as a round, white lump or a white area with radiating spikes.

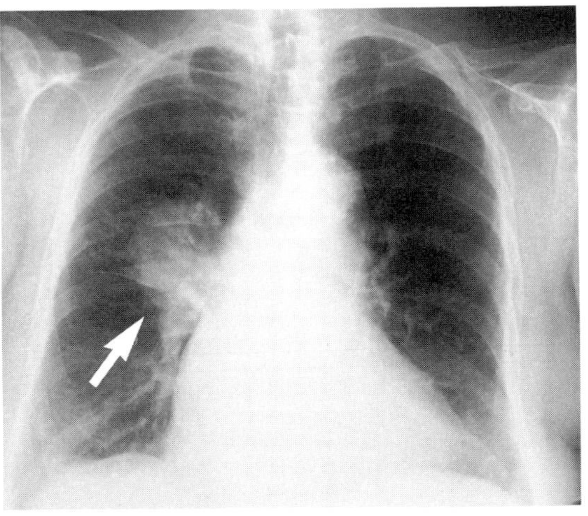

CANCEROUS TUMOR
The light area (arrow) shown on the X-ray indicates a cancerous tumor in the lung.

WHERE LUNG CANCER CAN SPREAD

At an early stage, lung cancer is confined to the lung. But lung cancer may metastasize (spread) to other areas of the body—including the bones, liver, lymph nodes, adrenal glands, or brain. The symptoms then vary widely, depending on the sites to which the cancer has spread. For example, a bone weakened by a tumor may fracture, or cancer that spreads to the brain may cause partial paralysis.

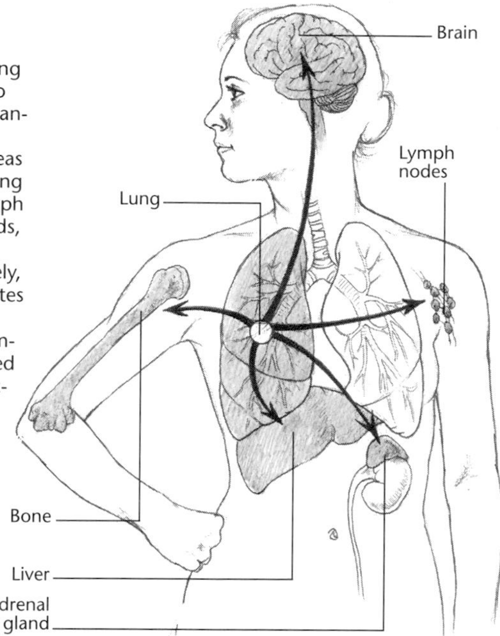

Bronchoscopy Doctors use bronchoscopy to help them diagnose an abnormal shadow or spot found on a chest X-ray, or the cause of symptoms such as coughing, wheezing, or coughing up blood. The procedure is also used to investigate a tumor in the lung or to take a tissue sample from it for laboratory examination to determine if it is cancerous.

For bronchoscopy, a long, thin (about 1/4 inch in diameter), flexible tube with a light at its tip (bronchoscope) is inserted through your mouth or nose into your lung. Before the procedure, you will be given a sedative to relax you or a local anesthetic that is sprayed into your throat to numb it. When the doctor inserts the bronchoscope through your nose or mouth, you may feel a slight pulling. The scope is guided through your larynx (voice box) into your windpipe, which may cause you to cough. As the instrument is passed into the bronchial tubes, your doctor examines all of these structures for signs of tumors, inflammation, narrowing, or other abnormalities.

Coping with the side effects of treatment for lung cancer

The side effects of different treatments for lung cancer can vary. Following are descriptions of the side effects you can expect and the ways in which they are managed:

Surgery After you have surgery for lung cancer, your doctor will prescribe medication to help relieve the pain. If the medication your doctor prescribes does not reduce your discomfort or pain, tell your doctor immediately; the dosage or the medication itself may need to be changed. During the first 4 or 5 days after surgery, fluid that collects in the area of your chest from which your lung was removed will be drained through flexible tubes put in place during the surgery. As you recover from the surgery, a nurse will help you to turn in bed to allow you to cough and breathe deeply; this helps to expand your remaining lung tissue and eliminate excess air and fluid that accumulate in the space in your chest created by the removal of lung tissue.

Once you are stronger, after about 1 or 2 weeks, you will be taught a set of exercises that expand your lungs and prevent the buildup of fluids in your chest. If the surgery has weakened the muscles in your chest and arm, a physical therapist will help you to strengthen them with special exercises. You must continue to do these exercises at home. Because you now have less lung tissue with which to breathe, you may experience some shortness of breath. Limit your activities until you gradually recover your strength.

Radiation therapy Radiation therapy often causes extreme fatigue. Rest frequently but try to stay as active as you can. Your skin near the site of radiation may become red, dry, tender, and itchy. You will be given instructions about how to care for your skin; do not use any lotion without your doctor's permission or expose your skin to the sun. The effects of the radiation may make it difficult for you to swallow. Eat soft foods and drink plenty of fluids until the problem goes away. For more about coping with the effects of radiation therapy, see page 255.

Chemotherapy The side effects of chemotherapy depend on which anticancer medications you are taking. You may have less energy, bruise or bleed easily, or get more frequent infections. You may lose some or all of your hair or experience digestive problems such as nausea and vomiting. These side effects usually go away gradually after treatment stops. For more about coping with the effects of chemotherapy, see page 255.

UNDERSTANDING CANCER

IF YOU HAVE BEEN DIAGNOSED with cancer (or if someone close to you has cancer), you probably have many questions. You want to know what is happening inside your body and why. How should your cancer be treated and what does your future hold? You may find it difficult to understand explanations from your doctors, articles you have read, or conversations with other people. Cancer is a complex disease and much is still unknown about it. But having a good understanding of what cancer is will enable you to take a more active role in your treatment.

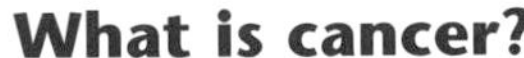

What is cancer?

Cancer is caused by changes, or mutations, in genes that control healthy cell division. When these genes are altered or damaged, cells divide out of control and become cancerous tumors. Basically, two types of genes are involved—oncogenes and tumor suppressor genes. Oncogenes promote normal cell division—in the same way the accelerator of your car makes it move. When an oncogene is damaged, it acts like an accelerator that gets stuck to the floor, and the cells continue dividing out of control.

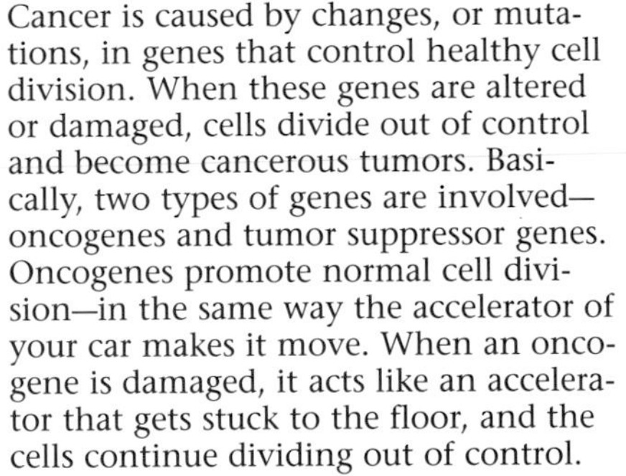

Mutations in tumor suppressor genes can also lead to cancer. When they are healthy, tumor suppressor genes tell cells when to stop dividing. When a tumor suppressor gene becomes disabled, it acts like a faulty brake on a car and can no longer control runaway cell division.

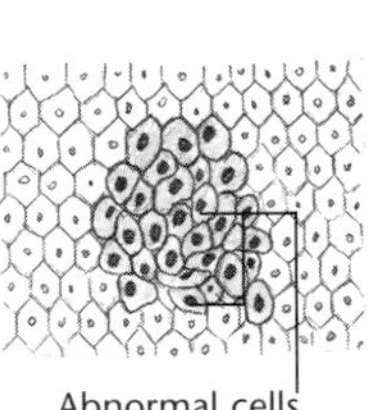

These two types of genes can become damaged by substances in the environment called carcinogens, which include cigarette smoke, chemicals, radiation, and some viruses. Other factors that can cause the genetic changes that lead to cancer include hormones, the aging process, diet, an inefficient immune system, and a hereditary susceptibility.

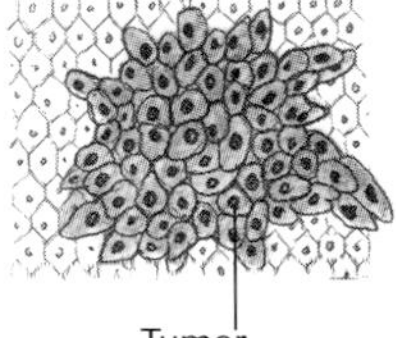

Cancer terms

Here are some common terms you may read or hear in discussions about cancer:

Benign tumor An abnormal growth that is not cancerous and does not spread to other parts of the body

Biological therapy Treatment using substances produced by your own body to help your immune system fight disease; also called immunotherapy

Biopsy Removal of a sample of tissue for examination under a microscope for the presence of cancer cells

Carcinogen Any substance that can cause a genetic change (mutation) that leads to cancer

Chemotherapy Treatment using powerful drugs to kill cancer cells throughout the body

Hormone therapy Treatment of cancer by either providing specific hormones that can affect the growth of cancer cells or blocking the production of these hormones by the body

Malignant tumor A group of rapidly dividing cancer cells, which can invade nearby tissues or travel to other parts of the body

Metastasis The spread of cancer cells from one part of the body to another

Oncogenes Genes that promote normal cell division

Radiation therapy Treatment using high-energy X-rays to kill cancer cells

Remission Temporary or permanent disappearance of the signs and symptoms of cancer

Tumor suppressor genes Genes that normally tell cells when to stop dividing

How cancer can spread

The site in which a cancer begins is called a primary tumor. When a cancerous tumor extends to a small blood vessel, it can grow through the wall of the vessel and enter the bloodstream. Cancer cells may then travel through the body to other sites and form what are called secondary tumors. Cancer cells can also enter the lymph nodes and travel to other parts of the body through the lymphatic vessels. This process of spreading is called metastasis. Because a cancer sometimes spreads to other areas of the body, surgery to remove the primary tumor may fail to prevent a recurrence of the cancer at the same site or elsewhere. Chemotherapy, biological therapy, and hormone therapy are possible treatments for cancer that has spread beyond the site of the original tumor.

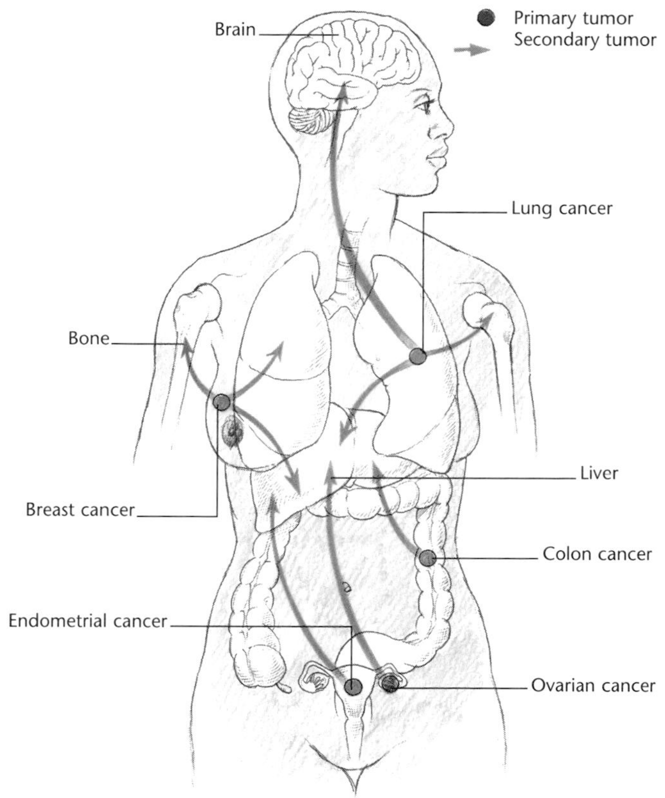

COMMON SECONDARY TUMORS
Cancers that begin in one area of the body (primary tumors) can spread to other sites (secondary tumors). Tumors that develop in the brain, bone, lung, and liver have often spread there from another part of the body.

How cancer can affect the body

Cancer can have widespread effects. It depletes the body's resources, including the ability of the immune system to fight off disease. Healthy cells weaken, causing damage to organs and preventing them from performing their usual job. Impaired organ function can cause symptoms such as loss of appetite, weight loss, anemia, fever, and fatigue.

In recent years, the increase in tests to diagnose many forms of cancer at an early, more treatable stage and the development of more effective treatments have dramatically improved the outlook for many people with cancer. Talk to your doctor and take advantage of all the recommended screening tests—such as Pap smears and mammograms—so that any cancer you have can be detected in time for a possible cure.

If you have cancer

If you have been diagnosed with cancer, you and your doctor will need to discuss the various treatment options. Include your family in these discussions. It may take some time before you and your family come to accept the idea that you have cancer, particularly if it is not causing pain or other symptoms. You may need several sessions with your doctor to go over the information, ask questions, and decide the best treatment for you. Seek out other sources of information as well. The more you know about your condition, the better you will be able to take an active role in the many decisions that lie ahead.

It is a good idea to join a support group of other people who also have cancer. Learning about their experiences with cancer and treatments can help you make decisions about your own treatment and can give you a more positive outlook. Having a positive attitude can significantly increase your chances for a cure.

BRONCHOSCOPY

Your doctor can look directly inside your lungs using a bronchoscope, a flexible tube with a light at its tip. The tube is gently inserted through your mouth (or nose) down into your bronchial tubes. Through a bronchoscope, a doctor can view the inside of the bronchial tubes and observe changes caused by inflammation or congestion, take a tissue sample from an abnormal growth, or retrieve an inhaled object.

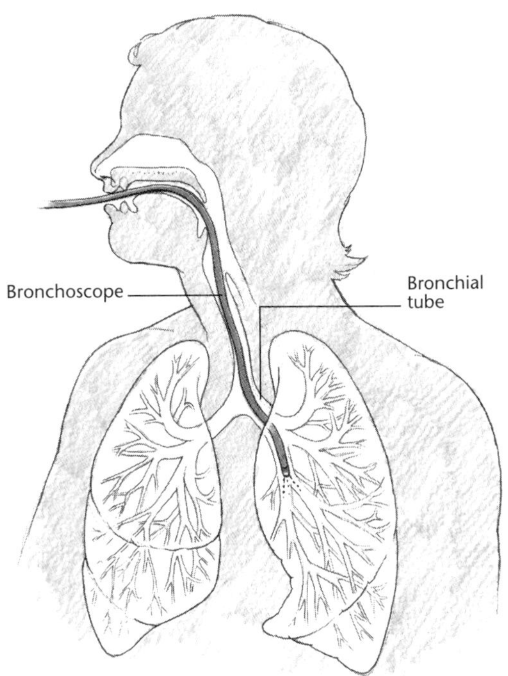

If a biopsy is necessary, the doctor takes a very small tissue sample with an instrument that he or she inserts through the bronchoscope; you will not feel any pain. The doctor then gently pulls the bronchoscope out. The entire procedure takes 20 to 30 minutes. You may feel a little groggy from the sedative but you should feel no pain or discomfort after the procedure. Because of the effects of the sedative, you should not drive home from the hospital; arrange for someone to pick you up.

Complications from bronchoscopy are rare but may include reactions to the anesthesia, bleeding from the nose or the site from which the tissue sample was taken (you might cough up blood), or temporary shortness of breath. In extremely rare cases, fever, pneumonia, injury to the larynx, abnormal heart rhythms, or a collapsed lung may result.

If a tissue sample cannot be removed through a bronchoscope, a sample can be taken through a needle inserted into your chest. You will be given a local anesthetic to numb the area in which the needle is inserted.

If the tumor is found to be malignant, your doctor will evaluate the stage of the cancer—how far it has advanced—in order to determine treatment options. Your doctor will want to determine if your cancer has spread to the lymph nodes in your chest or to other sites in your body. The lymph nodes must be removed and examined under a microscope to determine if they contain cancer cells.

Treatment If you are diagnosed with lung cancer, your treatment will depend on the size, location, and stage of the tumor, as well as your age and general health. Treatment may involve surgery, radiation therapy, chemotherapy, or a combination of any of these. For information about these cancer treatments and their side effects, see page 505.

To help you make informed decisions about the cancer treatments that your doctor recommends, ask him or her for educational materials about your type of cancer. Contact the local branch of organizations such as the American Cancer Society and the American Lung Association. Join a support group of people with cancer; most hospitals can direct you to such groups. Members of your family will also need information and support.

If the cancer is limited to one lung or to one lung and nearby lymph nodes, surgery to remove the cancer is the most common treatment. People who cannot undergo surgery because the tumor is very large or they have other health problems, such as heart disease, are often given radiation therapy. Radiation therapy is also the usual treatment for people whose cancer has spread inside the chest to many lymph nodes.

In some cases, surgery and radiation therapy are combined. If your cancer has spread to more distant parts of your body or to other organs, your doctor may recommend a combination of radiation and chemotherapy. Once a cancer has spread, it is much harder to control. In this case, the goal of treatment may be to shrink the tumor to relieve pain and other symptoms.

PNEUMONIA

Pneumonia is an infection in the lungs caused by bacteria, viruses, or other organisms. Before the development of antibiotics in the 1940s, pneumonia was the leading cause of death in the US. Although pneumonia is no longer a major cause of death, new strains of bacteria are emerging that are resistant to the standard antibiotics used to treat the infection. As a result, pneumonia is still a potentially fatal disease that can be difficult to treat.

Anyone can get pneumonia but people with a weakened immune system are at increased risk. You should be vaccinated against pneumonia if you are over 65, have a chronic illness such as diabetes that reduces your immunity, or work in a hospital or other health care environment that exposes you to people with lung infections. Having a flu shot every year can also help reduce your risk of pneumonia because pneumonia may develop as a complication of the flu or other viral infections.

Bacterial pneumonia A type of bacteria called pneumococcal bacteria is the most common cause of pneumonia. These bacteria exist in the throats of many healthy people. However, when your immune defenses are weakened or you develop other, usually mild, infections, the bacteria can multiply in your lungs. Your lung tissue becomes infected and inflamed. The bacteria can multiply rapidly and cause congestion in your lungs and a buildup of fluid in your chest. In a severe infection, the bacteria may enter the bloodstream, which can be life threatening.

The symptoms of bacterial pneumonia may appear gradually or suddenly. Common symptoms include shaking chills, fever, severe chest pain, and a cough that produces a yellow, green, or rust-colored mucus. Your temperature may go higher than 102°F and you may sweat heavily. Your breathing and pulse rates increase rapidly. Your lips and the skin under your nails may appear blue from the lack of oxygen in your blood.

If the doctor suspects or determines that bacteria are the cause of your pneumonia, you will be treated with antibiotics. Unless your condition is severe, you may not require hospitalization. However, if tests show your blood is not receiving enough oxygen or if you require intravenous antibiotics, you will have to be hospitalized in order to receive appropriate treatment. It can take several weeks or months to recover completely from a severe case of pneumonia.

Legionnaires' disease Legionnaires' disease is a form of bacterial pneumonia that is caused by bacteria that have been found in water supplies; large, water-cooled, air-conditioning systems; and plumbing systems. Legionnaires' disease sometimes affects groups of people who are clustered together at a single site. The pneumonia was named for a group of American Legion members who acquired the infection at a convention in a hotel in Philadelphia in the 1970s. Symptoms of legionnaires' disease include a high fever, chills, and muscle aches, followed by a cough that produces only a small amount of clear mucus. The infection is usually treated in the hospital with antibiotics given intravenously and is rarely fatal.

Aspiration pneumonia Aspiration pneumonia can occur when food or vomit is inhaled (aspirated) directly into the lungs. People who are unconscious as a result of intoxication, anesthesia, or drug use, or who have an illness such as a stroke can experience this because the gag reflex that normally prevents food or secretions from entering their windpipe is not working. Bacteria from the mouth or from food, or acidic stomach contents can cause infection and irritation in the lungs.

WARNING SIGNS
PNEUMONIA

Call your doctor immediately if you experience any of the following symptoms:

- Fever, chills, or heavy sweating
- Cough
- More rapid breathing and pulse
- Severe chest pain

This type of pneumonia is usually treated with antibiotics given intravenously and with supplemental oxygen (see page 503). If your lungs cannot provide sufficient oxygen or if the condition has reduced your ability to breathe, a mechanical ventilator may be required to take over your breathing while you are undergoing treatment. If your doctor suspects that pieces of food or other foreign objects may be lodged in the air passages of your lungs, bronchoscopy (see page 508) may be performed to remove them.

Viral pneumonia Many viruses have been identified as a cause of pneumonia. A virus can invade the lungs and multiply there. Viral pneumonia, like other infections, is most common in people whose immune system is weakened from age, heart disease, or a chronic, debilitating disease.

The symptoms of viral pneumonia are similar to those of the flu, including a dry cough, headache, muscle pain, and weakness. You may experience increasing shortness of breath and your cough may become severe and produce bloody mucus. You may also have a high fever. Your lips and the skin under your nails may appear blue because of a lack of oxygen in your blood.

There is no effective treatment for viral pneumonia because no drugs have yet been developed that can kill the common types of viruses that cause pneumonia. However, antibiotics may be used to treat viral pneumonia because it is sometimes not possible to rule out bacteria as the cause in a person with symptoms of pneumonia. In addition, people with viral pneumonia are often at risk of being infected with bacteria as well. In most cases, even without treatment, the person's immune system can eliminate the infection in days or weeks. In severe cases, intravenous fluids and supplemental oxygen may be necessary to help maintain the person's body functions during the recovery period.

Mycoplasmal pneumonia Pneumonia can be caused by a tiny disease organism called a mycoplasma. This form of pneumonia is most common in children and young adults and often spreads among young people who are living together in close quarters, such as dormitories or military barracks.

The most common symptom of mycoplasmal pneumonia is a violent cough. If your infection is mild, you may feel only slightly ill and may continue your usual daily activities. For this reason, the infection used to be called walking pneumonia. You may also feel short of breath and develop a rash, headache, stiff neck, and inflamed joints. Although mycoplasmal pneumonia is resistant to penicillin, it can be effectively treated with other antibiotics taken by mouth. Depending on the severity of the infection, recovery may take a week or longer.

TUBERCULOSIS

Tuberculosis (TB) is a highly contagious disease caused by a type of bacterium that primarily infects the lungs. The incidence of TB, which had been declining steadily for more than 20 years, began to increase in the 1980s. TB has always been more common among people who have a diminished capacity to fight disease, such as the very young, the very old, and people who have chronic, debilitating illnesses such as cancer. An increasing number of people who are infected with the AIDS virus, which weakens the immune system and its ability to fight infections of all kinds, are also becoming infected with TB.

TB is transmitted in minute particles of respiratory secretions that become suspended in the air when an infected person coughs or sneezes. You are unlikely to become infected through casual contact with an infected person, but more intimate and repeated contact, such as among members of a household, increases your risk of contracting the disease. Whenever a person is diagnosed with TB, all of his or her family members and other close associates should be tested (see page 133) to determine if they are also infected.

Symptoms Some people who acquire a TB infection do not become sick or develop any symptoms. When your body's defenses work normally, they suppress the TB organisms and render them harmless. The symptoms of an active infection are common to many other diseases. In the early stage of a TB infection, you may experience gradual weight loss, a cough, and a fever (especially at night). If the infection is more advanced, you may have symptoms such as chills, coughing up blood, and chest pains.

Diagnosis A diagnosis of TB is made from a combination of tests, including a positive (abnormal) tuberculin skin test (see page 133), laboratory testing of a sample of sputum, and a chest X-ray. In severe cases, the bacteria may be found in other parts of the body, including spinal fluid and urine.

Treatment Many of the medications available to treat TB are very effective if they are taken properly. People with TB must take the medication for at least 6 months (sometimes longer), depending on the severity of their infection. Taking the medication improperly, starting and stopping it, or discontinuing it before you complete the prescribed treatment can result in the development of a strain of the disease-causing bacterium that is resistant to that class of antibiotic. This is especially dangerous because drugs that would otherwise work become ineffective, and your infection progresses. People to whom you transmit this now drug-resistant infection will not be able to receive effective treatment with standard antibiotics. Because TB is so contagious, people with active infections are isolated in hospitals, and health care workers are required to wear face masks in all situations in which they may be exposed to infection.

PULMONARY EMBOLISM

A pulmonary (lung) embolism is an obstruction of one of the arteries that supply blood to the lungs. The blockage, usually a blood clot, originates in a remote area of the body and is carried in the bloodstream to the lungs. In the lungs, a clot can lodge in an artery and block the delivery of blood and oxygen to part of one of the lungs. The most common site of blood clot formation is in a vein in the legs. In a small percentage of people, a pulmonary embolism causes death within a few minutes, but people who survive the initial attack are likely to recover fully with treatment.

Symptoms If you have a pulmonary embolism, the severity of your symptoms will depend on the size of the blood clot and the general health of your cardiovascular system. When a clot lodges in one of your lungs, you may have sudden chest pain or simply shortness of breath and a feeling of anxiety. Other symptoms of a pulmonary embolism include a rapid heartbeat and a cough that produces some blood-streaked mucus. A large embolism, or one that occurs in a person who has a heart condition, can cause a sudden loss of consciousness or death.

Diagnosis Diagnosing a pulmonary embolism is not always easy because the symptoms may be confused with that of a heart attack, particularly in a person known to have heart disease. Your doctor may recommend a chest X-ray (see page 504), a blood test to measure the amount of oxygen in your blood, an imaging procedure called radionuclide scanning (see page 512), an electrocardiogram (ECG; see page 132), or a pulmonary angiogram.

A pulmonary angiogram, which provides the most definitive diagnosis, is the

Who is at risk of blood clots?

The most common cause of blood clots is sluggish blood flow through the veins of the legs and pelvis that results from inactivity. People who are confined to bed by illness often develop blood clots. Other factors that can increase your risk of developing a blood clot are being pregnant, being obese (more than 20 percent over your ideal weight; see page 99), or using birth-control pills if you are over 35 and a smoker (see page 156). You are also at increased risk of blood clots if you have cancer or heart failure or are over 70. Blood clots are more common after surgery or a serious injury (especially in the legs) because, in these circumstances, people are more likely to be confined to bed and the physical stresses of surgery or injury increase the production of clotting proteins in the blood.

WARNING SIGNS
PULMONARY EMBOLISM

A pulmonary embolism can be confused with other conditions, including a heart attack. Call an ambulance or have someone call for you if you experience any of these symptoms, especially if you already have a lung or heart condition:

- Sudden chest pain
- Sudden shortness of breath and rapid breathing
- Sudden, persistent, severe feelings of anxiety
- Cough that produces blood-streaked mucus

most complicated of the diagnostic tests. A liquid dye that is visible on X-rays is injected into a vein in your arm or leg. X-ray images are taken at rapid intervals as the dye passes through your heart and into your lungs. If a blood clot is obstructing any of the major blood vessels in your lungs, it will show on the X-ray.

Treatment If your doctor suspects you have a pulmonary embolism, he or she will start you on medication even before the diagnosis is definite. You are likely to be given an injection or intravenous drip of a drug that will prevent your blood from clotting. You may also be given drugs that may help dissolve the existing clot. Your doctor will prescribe a medication in pill form that you take for the next 3 to 6 months to prevent new clots from forming.

If your clot is large, it may have to be removed surgically. If you cannot take anticlotting medication or if you have recurring clots in spite of taking anticlotting medication, a small filter may be placed in a vein in your groin to strain out any clots that may form there before they can move to your lungs or heart.

Radionuclide scanning

Radionuclide scanning is a painless imaging procedure that is very effective in diagnosing pulmonary embolism. In this procedure, two scans are done: a blood-flow scan shows the distribution of blood throughout your lungs and a ventilation scan shows the distribution of air throughout the bronchial tubes. Together, the two scans take less than an hour.

For the blood-flow scan, a radioactive substance is injected into your bloodstream; the substance circulates through your bloodstream and into the blood vessels in your lungs. A special camera is used to take a picture of the distribution of blood in your lungs. For the ventilation scan, you inhale a radioactive gas or spray that spreads to all the functioning areas of your lungs. The camera is used to immediately take a picture that shows how uniformly your lungs fill with (and then empty) the radioactive gas.

In healthy lungs, the two scans match—the air and the blood go into the same places in the lungs. If the scans show that some areas fill with air but not with blood, there is a strong possibility that you have a pulmonary embolism. The radioactive substance breaks down into harmless materials that are eliminated from your body. A diagnosis of pulmonary embolism from radionuclide scanning can be confirmed with a pulmonary angiogram.

CYSTIC FIBROSIS

Cystic fibrosis is a genetic disorder that prevents the mucus-secreting glands in the lungs from functioning normally. When healthy, these glands secrete thin, slippery mucus. In people with cystic fibrosis, the glands produce thick, sticky secretions that can block passageways in the lungs and interfere with breathing. These sticky secretions can interfere with vital body functions, including breathing and digestion. Thick mucus accumulates in the lungs, which can cause frequent lung infections. Recurring lung infections are the most common, life-threatening effect of cystic fibrosis.

Although the life expectancy of people with cystic fibrosis is shortened, it is much longer today than it once was and it continues to improve with advances in medical technology. More than half of all people born with cystic fibrosis now live into their late 20s and some live into their 40s and 50s.

The gene for cystic fibrosis is a recessive gene (see page 373); to have the disorder you must inherit a copy of the defective gene from both parents. If you inherit the gene from only one parent, you are a carrier of the gene but do not have the disease. However, you can transmit the disease to your children if your partner is also a carrier. Cystic fibrosis does not result from anything the parents did before or during pregnancy. Some people have the mistaken impression that cystic fibrosis is contagious because coughing is one of the most common symptoms.

Cystic fibrosis is the most common genetic disorder among whites. If anyone in your family (including aunts, uncles, and cousins) has cystic fibrosis and you are planning to become pregnant, you and your partner should have a blood test to determine if you are carriers of the defective gene. When you do become pregnant, a prenatal diagnostic test—amniocentesis (see page 406) or chorionic villus sampling (see page 407)—can determine if the fetus has the disease.

Symptoms A person born with cystic fibrosis may not develop symptoms for several years. At birth, about 15 percent of babies with the disease have an intestinal blockage called meconium ileus. Meconium is a baby's first bowel movement; ileus is a condition in which normal bowel movements do not occur because of an absence of normal intestinal contractions. The obstructed stool causes a blockage in the intestine, which can rupture if it is not treated with medicated enemas. Replacement fluids, enzymes, and vitamins are also necessary for babies with this condition.

Cystic fibrosis causes excessive secretion of salt from the sweat glands. During exercise or in hot weather, the depletion of salt in the body can cause fatigue, weakness, fever, muscle cramps, abdominal pain, and vomiting. The thick, sticky secretions in the lungs can cause labored breathing and wheezing and frequent lung infections. The person may have a persistent cough, which may or may not produce mucus.

The lung secretions also prevent adequate amounts of digestive juices secreted by the pancreas from reaching the intestines. Food is not digested completely, and nutrients and calories from the food are not absorbed in sufficient amounts. As a result, a child with cystic fibrosis does not gain weight at a normal rate, in spite of a healthy appetite. He or she may experience diarrhea, abdominal pain caused by bowel obstruction, and excess gas.

Diagnosis A test of the concentration of salt in a child's sweat can be used to diagnose cystic fibrosis at any time after a child is a few months old. The child may also have a test to determine if he or she has the gene for cystic fibrosis.

Treatment Because there is no cure for cystic fibrosis, the goal of treatment is to control the symptoms. Supplements of the missing pancreatic enzymes can improve digestion. In some cases, thick mucus may obstruct the intestines; medications, digestive enzymes, and enemas may be required to help break up the mucus and stool and allow them to pass through the digestive tract.

The most common and serious complication of cystic fibrosis is chronic lung infections that result from the abnormally thick mucus in the lungs, which promotes the growth of disease-causing organisms. Medications taken through an inhaler can thin the mucus, open the bronchial tubes, and help clear the airways, thereby reducing the risk of infection. Physical therapy is also important; thumping on the person's chest and back can help dislodge mucus from the blocked air passages and allow his or her lungs to drain. If a severe lung infection occurs, hospitalization is necessary to give the person intravenous antibiotics. Antibiotics taken by mouth may not be absorbed in the stomach in sufficient quantities to reach the infected lung tissue.

SARCOIDOSIS

Sarcoidosis is a disorder characterized by inflammation in lymph nodes (infection-fighting glands) and other organs—usually the lungs, liver, skin, or eyes. The cause of the disease is unknown, but it may have a genetic component. Sarcoidosis occurs primarily between ages 20 and 40 and is most common among blacks. The disease can appear suddenly, possibly triggered by an immune reaction. Most people recover fully from sarcoidosis, with or without treatment, within 2 years. However, in some people, the disease remains active and progresses; in about 10 percent of people it is fatal.

Symptoms Almost half of people who have sarcoidosis do not have any symptoms. When symptoms occur, the first one may be a red eye, a skin rash, arthritis, or a vague feeling of being ill. Most cases involve the lungs and lymph nodes. When the lungs are affected, the disease is more likely to become chronic. As the patches of inflammation (called granulomas) grow, the lung tissue becomes hard and inelastic, making it difficult to breathe. You may feel short of breath during exertion.

Diagnosis In some cases, sarcoidosis can be diagnosed only by a chest X-ray (see page 504) that shows enlarged lymph nodes. But a biopsy of lung tissue, taken via bronchoscopy (see page 505), may be necessary to make a definitive diagnosis. Examination of affected tissues, such as lung tissue, lymph nodes, or skin, under a microscope shows the characteristic granulomas. A blood test can determine if the level of an enzyme called angiotensin-converting enzyme is elevated; an elevated level of this enzyme is a possible sign of sarcoidosis.

Treatment Most cases of sarcoidosis gradually clear up on their own and cause little or no permanent damage. Before beginning treatment, your doctor may recommend waiting to see if the disease progresses or begins to subside. If your symptoms persist or are severe, your doctor may prescribe corticosteroid medications to reduce inflammation and help relieve the symptoms, primarily breathing difficulty. In severe cases in which there is extensive scarring of lung tissue, supplemental oxygen (see page 503) may be necessary. In some people, especially young people, who have an extreme, life-threatening form of the disease, lung transplants have been successful.

CHAPTER 19

Your digestive system

Contents

The major function of your digestive system is to break down the food that you eat into molecules that your body can absorb and use for energy and growth. Food passes from your mouth down a tube called the esophagus to your stomach, where the digestive process converts it into a thick liquid. The liquefied food then passes through the small and large intestines; most of the nutrients from the digested food are absorbed from your small intestine into your bloodstream through tiny blood vessels called capillaries. Your large intestine absorbs water from the remaining material, and this undigested waste leaves your body through the rectum.

Your body is remarkably good at extracting the calories it needs for energy from the food you eat. Although the digestive system works efficiently most of the time, a variety of disorders or conditions can arise that may cause discomfort or pain. Some disorders of the digestive system organs can be life threatening. For this reason, it is important to tell your doctor if you experience any pain or symptoms.

Disorders of the esophagus and stomach

Your esophagus and stomach form the upper gastrointestinal tract. The esophagus is a tube that connects your mouth to your stomach. Your stomach stores and partially digests food. Muscles in your stomach wall grind the food and turn it into a pulp, while powerful enzymes and acid digest it further. The muscle between your esophagus and stomach normally prevents digested food and stomach acid from backing up into your esophagus from the stomach. If this muscle (called the lower esophageal sphincter) is not functioning properly, you may experience the burning sensation in your chest called heartburn. Stomach acids, which are essential for digesting food, may erode the lining of the stomach and duodenum (the part of the small intestine that leads out of the stomach). This erosion of the linings can cause sores called ulcers.

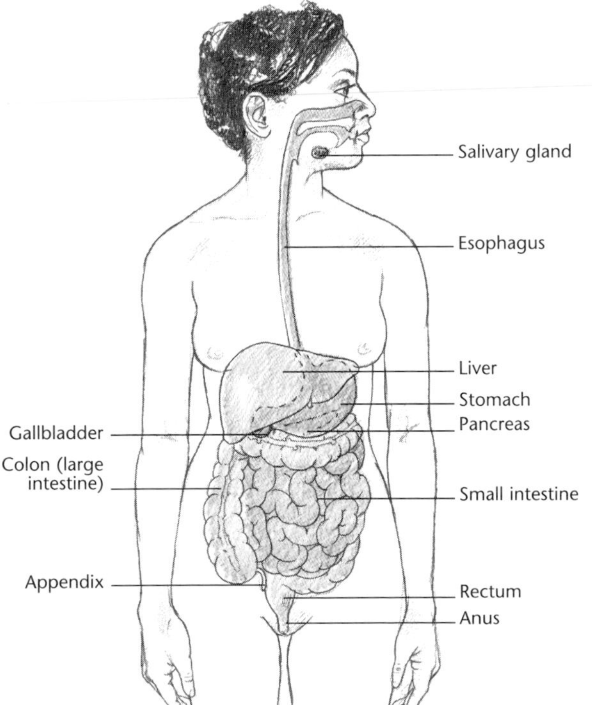

YOUR DIGESTIVE SYSTEM
Saliva secreted inside your mouth begins the digestive process of breaking down the food you eat. The food is moved through your digestive tract by waves of muscular contractions—through your esophagus, stomach, small intestine, colon (large intestine), and rectum—to your anus, from which it is eliminated from your body. Along the way, other organs of your digestive system—the liver, gallbladder, and pancreas—secrete juices that promote digestion. The appendix, attached to the large intestine, has no known function.

ESOPHAGEAL REFLUX

A muscle called the lower esophageal sphincter keeps the opening between the esophagus and stomach closed. This muscle opens momentarily after you swallow to allow food into your stomach, but quickly closes again to ensure that the food stays in your stomach. In a condition called esophageal reflux, the esophageal sphincter muscle is too relaxed and allows the contents of the stomach, including digestive acids, to enter the esophagus. The main symptom of esophageal reflux is heartburn, a burning sensation in your chest.

Reflux can be worsened by smoking, drinking caffeinated beverages or alcohol, or by eating acidic foods such as citrus fruits or tomatoes. Chocolate, fat, and peppermints can also cause the lower esophageal sphincter muscle to relax. Reflux is common during the later months of pregnancy because increased levels of the female hormone progesterone in a pregnant woman can cause the esophageal sphincter muscle to relax. In addition, the expanding uterus increases pressure inside the woman's abdomen during the late stages of pregnancy and may also contribute to reflux.

Long-term esophageal reflux can sometimes have serious consequences. Continual irritation of the lining of the esophagus by acidic stomach juices may cause pain and bleeding; in rare cases, this bleeding can lead to anemia (see page 493). Persistent irritation may also lead to scarring and narrowing of the lower esophagus, which can cause food to stick in your esophagus after you swallow. A moderate degree of narrowing causes solid food to stick momentarily; more severe narrowing may result in obstruction of the esophagus by larger pieces of food.

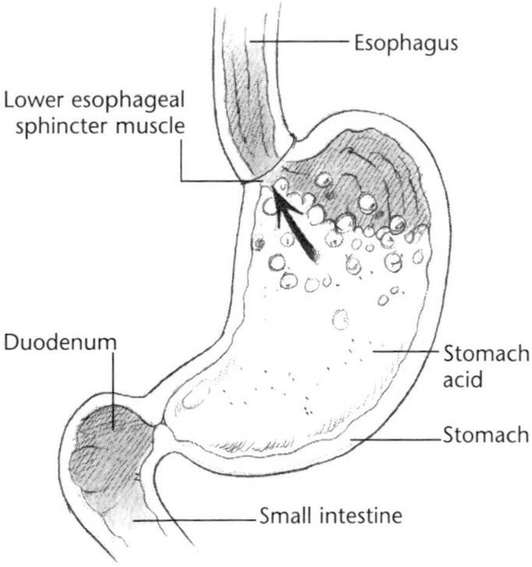

ESOPHAGEAL REFLUX

Esophageal reflux occurs when the muscle that normally prevents stomach acid from entering the esophagus, called the lower esophageal sphincter, does not function properly and allows stomach acid to escape into the esophagus. The acid can irritate the lining of your lower esophagus, causing a burning sensation in your chest (heartburn).

Symptoms The symptoms of esophageal reflux include a burning sensation in your upper abdomen or chest (heartburn) caused by irritation of the lining of your esophagus by stomach acid. The burning sensation may start in your upper abdomen and move up. You may experience backing up of acid and food into your throat and mouth, or a feeling of pressure or pain in your chest. You may regurgitate sour-tasting, partially digested food from your stomach into your throat or mouth. You may notice stomach irritation or pain when you eat citrus fruits or tomatoes, or drink caffeinated or alcoholic beverages.

Diagnosis A doctor can usually diagnose esophageal reflux by the symptoms. If your condition is severe or does not respond to treatment, your doctor may examine your esophagus and stomach using an endoscope, a tube that he or she inserts through your mouth and esophagus to directly view the lining of the esophagus. In some cases, an endoscopic examination detects a hiatal hernia, which occurs when part of the stomach bulges upward through the diaphragm into the chest cavity. Many people have minor hiatal hernias that cause no symptoms and do not require treatment. However, a large hiatal hernia may make you more susceptible to developing esophageal reflux or heartburn.

Treatment If you are diagnosed with esophageal reflux, your doctor will recommend quitting smoking (if you are a smoker) and reducing your consumption of certain foods and beverages, such as citrus fruits and coffee, that may worsen the condition. It also helps to divide your daily food intake into more frequent meals with smaller portions to prevent your stomach from getting too full. Avoid eating anything for 3 hours before bedtime. If you are overweight, losing weight will reduce the pressure on your stomach and lessen reflux. Elevate the head of your bed at least 6 inches by placing books, blocks, or bricks under

HIATAL HERNIA
Normally, the stomach is positioned below the diaphragm (right). A hiatal hernia (far right) occurs when a portion of the stomach bulges up into the chest cavity through an abnormally enlarged opening in the diaphragm. This condition often causes heartburn.

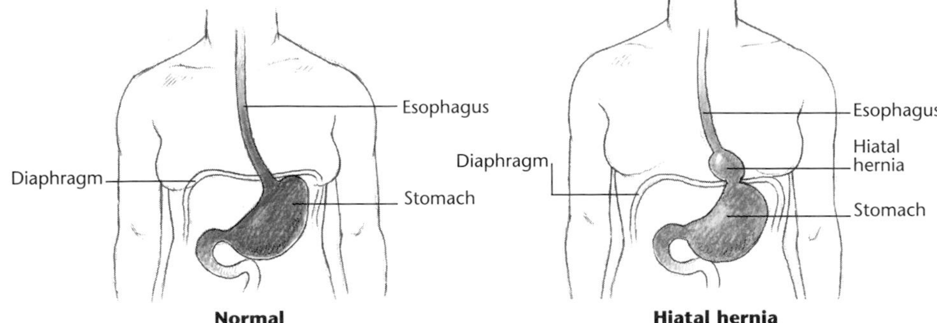

the front legs; this elevation can help prevent stomach acid from entering your esophagus while you sleep. If you cannot elevate your bed, you can purchase an antireflux pillow at a medical supply store; the pillow keeps your upper body raised slightly.

If you have heartburn only occasionally, an over-the-counter liquid antacid can be helpful, especially if you take it after meals or at bedtime. If you have heartburn often, your doctor may prescribe medication that reduces the amount of acid your stomach produces or that increases the strength of your esophageal sphincter muscle. In rare cases, surgery may be necessary to strengthen the sphincter muscle or to repair a severe hiatal hernia.

PEPTIC ULCERS

A peptic ulcer is a hole or break in the lining of your stomach or duodenum (the part of the small intestine that leads out of the stomach). Peptic ulcers that occur in the stomach are called gastric ulcers; peptic ulcers in the duodenum are called duodenal ulcers. Peptic ulcers are very common, affecting 1 in 10 Americans at some time in their life. Your risk is slightly increased if you have a family history of peptic ulcers.

Normally, a layer of mucus protects the lining of your stomach and duodenum from acid and other digestive secretions. Peptic ulcers occur when this protective barrier breaks down and digestive juices and acids come into contact with cells of the stomach lining, injuring them.

Although the exact cause of peptic ulcers is unclear, a number of factors contribute to their development. Infection with bacteria called *Helicobacter pylori* increases your risk of peptic ulcers. However, many people have these bacteria in their digestive tract and do not have peptic ulcers. It is not known how people acquire this bacteria. Smoking increases your risk of peptic ulcers and can worsen an existing ulcer and slow its healing.

In some cases, over-the-counter nonsteroidal anti-inflammatory drugs—including aspirin, ibuprofen, and naproxen—can irritate the stomach lining if they are taken in large doses for long periods of time. Drinking alcohol does not contribute to the development of peptic ulcers; nor do any specific foods (including spicy ones) have a harmful effect on the lining of the stomach. Although it is widely believed that emotional stress causes ulcers, the role of stress in the development of ulcers is not clear.

WARNING SIGNS
PEPTIC ULCERS

Seek emergency treatment if you vomit bright red blood. If an ulcer is bleeding excessively, your skin will feel clammy or you may feel faint.

Symptoms Symptoms of peptic ulcers include burning or a gnawing sensation in your upper abdomen or lower chest; uncomfortable hunger pains (which may ease during meals, worsen 1 to 3 hours after meals, and intensify during the night as levels of irritating stomach acid rise or fall); discomfort that is relieved by consuming milk, food, or antacids; nausea and (especially bloody) vomiting; and black, tarry, foul-smelling stools—a sign of bleeding in the stomach.

Diagnosis Peptic ulcers can be diagnosed by an X-ray or by gastroscopy (see page 519).

Treatment The goal of treatment is to reduce the amount of irritating acid in the stomach to allow the ulcer to heal. Most ulcers can be treated with medication. Over-the-counter liquid antacids help neutralize stomach acids. Your

Gastroscopy

Gastroscopy is a diagnostic procedure that enables your doctor to directly view the upper part of your digestive tract through a viewing tube called a gastroscope. The gastroscope is inserted through your mouth down into your esophagus, stomach, and duodenum (the part of the small intestine that leads out of the stomach). A variety of instruments can be attached to the end of the gastroscope to allow your doctor to take a sample of tissue or fluid for laboratory examination, or to perform other procedures. You will be told not to eat anything for several hours before you have gastroscopy. Ask your doctor if you should make arrangements ahead of time for someone to drive you home after the procedure.

A local anesthetic may be sprayed into your mouth just before the procedure to numb the back of your throat and suppress the reflex that makes you gag when something touches the back of your throat. Your doctor will also give you an injection of a mild sedative to relax you during the procedure. You may feel some mild discomfort or fullness as the tube is inserted. The gastroscope is passed all the way into the duodenum. A small amount of air is delivered through the tube to expand your stomach, which allows the doctor to view internal structures. As the gastroscope moves through your digestive tract, the doctor examines an image of the interior of your digestive organs on a video monitor.

After the procedure, your throat may feel sore for a few hours. Your doctor will give you guidance about what to eat after the procedure. Gastroscopy is very safe. Complications are extremely rare but may include mild bleeding (if a large tissue sample is taken or a polyp is removed). If there is bleeding, you may notice that your stool is black. This bleeding usually clears up on its own without treatment. Call your doctor if you have any concerns after the procedure.

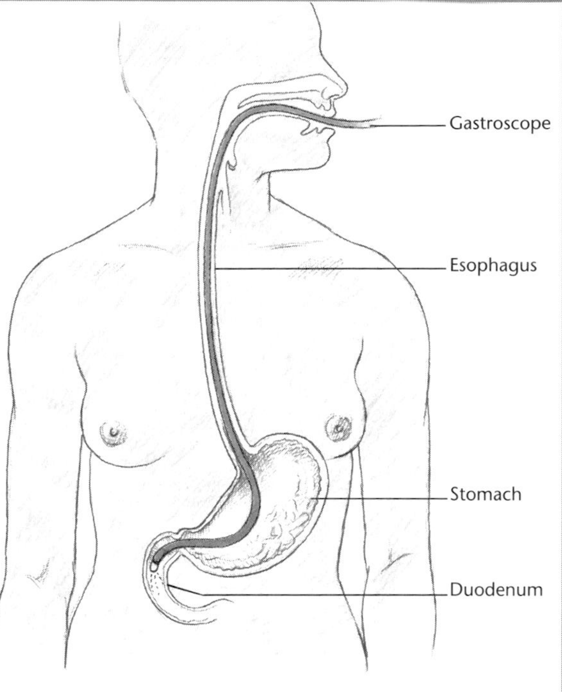

GASTROSCOPY
To diagnose a disorder in the upper digestive tract, your doctor uses a gastroscope, a long, flexible, lighted viewing tube. He or she inserts the tube through your mouth down into your esophagus, stomach, and duodenum (the part of your small intestine that leads out of your stomach). Through the gastroscope, the doctor can see the lining of your upper gastrointestinal tract.

doctor may prescribe a medication that reduces the secretion of acid in your stomach or one that coats the ulcer itself to protect it from stomach acid. If your doctor detects the presence of *H pylori* bacteria in a sample of tissue from your stomach or from a blood test, he or she will prescribe antibiotics. This treatment allows the ulcer to heal and usually prevents a recurrence. Without treatment with antibiotics, almost all ulcers associated with *H pylori* bacteria recur within 1 to 2 years after they heal.

For severe cases of peptic ulcers that are bleeding, have perforated (ruptured through the wall of the stomach or duodenum), or have not responded to treatment with medication, surgery may be necessary. The particular surgical procedure a doctor performs depends on the size of the ulcer, its location, and whether or not you have any associated complications, such as a rupture. Severe bleeding of a duodenal ulcer may be stopped by closing the hole in the duodenum with stitches.

Disorders of the small and large intestines

Most of the food you eat is absorbed in the 12 to 22 feet of tubing that makes up your small intestine. Your small intestine is divided into three parts—the duodenum, which leads out of the stomach; the jejunum, the middle and largest potion in which most nutrients are absorbed; and the ileum, which also absorbs some nutrients. By the time food passes into your large intestine (colon), nearly all its nutrients have been absorbed. The function of your colon is to absorb excess fluid from the liquid product of the digestive process and convert that product into a solid form. This solidified waste, or stool, collects in your lower colon until it is expelled through the anus. Disorders that can affect the intestines range from the discomfort of occasional diarrhea or constipation to serious diseases such as colon cancer.

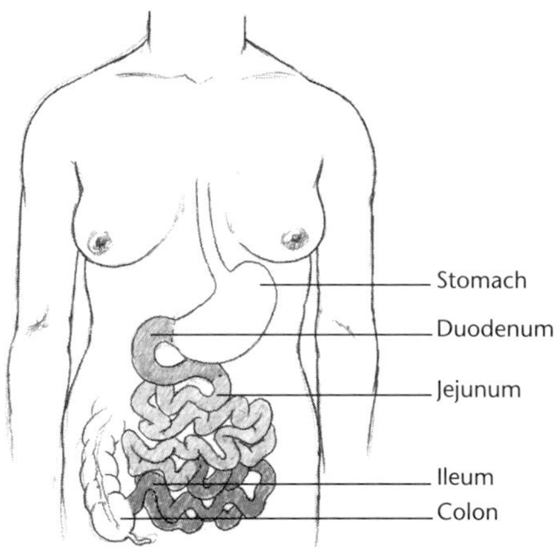

PARTS OF THE SMALL INTESTINE
Your small intestine is divided into three parts—the duodenum, jejunum, and ileum.

CONSTIPATION

Constipation is defined as fewer than three bowel movements a week. Constipation is often extremely uncomfortable. When a bowel movement occurs, the stool is usually hard and difficult to pass. Constipation is a symptom, not a disease. Some common causes of constipation include lack of adequate liquid or fiber in the diet or overuse of laxatives. You can become constipated if you put off defecating when you have the urge. A number of disorders, such as irritable bowel syndrome (see page 526), or medications, such as iron supplements, can

Preventing constipation without laxatives

You should not take laxatives regularly unless your doctor recommends them. Regular use of some laxatives over a long period of time may make you dependent on them to have a normal bowel movement. When taken in excess, laxatives can cause diarrhea and even dehydration. Instead of taking laxatives, try the following self-help measures to prevent constipation or relieve it:

- Drink at least 8 to 12 (8-ounce) glasses of water or other fluid every day.
- Get plenty of fiber in the form of whole-grain cereals and breads. You should take in 25 to 30 grams of fiber every day (see page 50). Fruits and vegetables are also rich in fiber and they contain a large amount of water as well.
- Take a psyllium-based fiber supplement daily with a large (8-ounce) glass of water if altering your diet is not possible or has not been helpful. Psyllium is not a laxative but, when combined with sufficient fluid, it increases the water content of your stool, making it softer and easier to pass.
- Respond promptly to the urge to have a bowel movement.
- Take a brisk walk every day; try to walk for at least 45 minutes, but even a 15-minute walk is beneficial.
- Do not use enemas or laxatives unless your doctor recommends them.
- If your constipation does not improve with these measures, see your doctor.

also cause constipation. Older people are much more likely to have constipation because they often do not drink enough fluids or get enough fiber in their diet, and many get little exercise. Older people are also more likely to use medications that cause constipation.

If you experience occasional constipation, prevention is the best approach (see page 520). If your constipation is caused by a disease or by a particular medication you are taking, your doctor will recommend a treatment to correct those problems. For example, he or she may want to determine if you have an obstruction in your colon or if you have hypothyroidism (see page 624), a thyroid disorder that can cause constipation. If a medication you are taking regularly is causing your constipation, your doctor will adjust the dosage or prescribe a different drug.

DIARRHEA

Diarrhea is the frequent passing of loose, watery stools. Usually, your intestines absorb most of the liquid from stool before it leaves your body. When illness or infection interferes with this absorption process, you can have frequent, liquid stools. Most cases of diarrhea clear up quickly without treatment. However, if diarrhea is prolonged or severe, it can lead to dehydration.

The most common kind of diarrhea is called nonspecific diarrhea. This type of diarrhea begins and ends so quickly that the particular bacterium or virus that caused it is never identified. Traveler's diarrhea is a more serious condition caused by a type of bacteria called *Escherichia coli*, which secretes a toxin into the intestine, or by other disease-causing bacteria present in contaminated food or water. As its name implies, traveler's diarrhea often occurs when people travel to countries in which the bacteria are present in water or food.

Diarrhea can result from the use of some drugs, including some over-the-counter antacids and laxatives. Using large amounts of artificial sweeteners such as sorbitol, which is found in some sugar-free gums and candies, can also cause diarrhea. Discontinue use of these products if you suspect they may be causing your diarrhea.

For nonspecific diarrhea, try taking an over-the-counter medication for treating diarrhea. In order to avoid becoming dehydrated, it is important to drink plenty of liquids (water, juice, or broth) until the problem clears up. Avoid caffeine, alcohol, and dairy products because they can make the diarrhea worse. If you have diarrhea for more than 48 hours or if it is accompanied by a fever, see your doctor. Recurring diarrhea may be a symptom of a more serious intestinal disorder or of an infection that must be treated.

Lactose intolerance Lactose intolerance is caused by the absence of the enzyme that digests lactose, a sugar found in milk and other dairy products. People who are missing this digestive enzyme have gas, bloating, or diarrhea when they eat dairy products. Nearly 30 million Americans—mostly people of African, Asian, Jewish, or Native American descent—have lactose intolerance. Most affected people have a mild case that rarely causes symptoms. Lactose intolerance is more common in older people and tends to worsen with age.

If you have lactose intolerance, decrease the amount of dairy products you eat. To get sufficient calcium, eat low-fat yogurt and cheese, which contain less lactose than milk. You will probably also need to take a calcium supplement to bring your intake up to the recommended daily amount (see page 58). You can buy lactose-reduced milk and other products in many grocery stores. Lactose pills are available to aid the digestion of dairy products. Ask your doctor whether or not you need to take lactose pills or calcium supplements.

Food poisoning Food poisoning is a very common condition—characterized by nausea, vomiting, diarrhea, and fever—that results from eating food that is contaminated with bacteria. The bacterium *Staphylococcus aureus* is a common cause of food poisoning. Other bacteria that cause food poisoning include campylobacter and salmonella organisms and *Escherichia coli*. Bacteria are usually spread to food from the hands of the person who prepares it; the bacteria then multiply in the food. Undercooked poultry, meats, fish, and raw eggs are the foods most likely to cause food poisoning. Chicken that has been left out of the refrigerator to thaw, that has not been properly washed,

Flatulence

All people produce gas, or flatus, in their intestines during digestion. Most intestinal gas is a combination of oxygen, nitrogen, hydrogen, carbon dioxide, and methane. The unpleasant odor is usually caused by small amounts of the gases methane, hydrogen sulfide, and ammonia. Gas is usually expelled during a bowel movement and most people expel some at other times during the day. In some cases, an excessive amount of gas can result from a disorder of the digestive tract, such as irritable bowel syndrome (see page 526), lactose intolerance (see page 521), or some forms of diarrhea. You can also develop gas from eating certain foods, such as dried beans, wheat, oats, bran, brussels sprouts, cabbage, and corn. You may experience an increase in intestinal gas if you increase the fiber in your diet. Gradually increasing the amount of fiber you eat can give your intestines time to adjust, limiting the amount of gas you have.

If your problem with gas results from a disorder of your digestive tract, treating the disorder often reduces or eliminates the problem. While excess gas may be annoying or embarrassing, it is not a serious condition that should cause you to be concerned about your health

or that has been undercooked is a common source of food poisoning.

The symptoms of food poisoning usually subside after several hours. After you stop vomiting and can hold down some liquid, drink clear fluids such as diluted fruit juice or broth for about 12 hours. For the next 24 hours, eat increasing amounts of starchy foods, such as bread, rice, or crackers. Avoid dairy products and fat because they can worsen your symptoms.

To prevent food poisoning, keep food refrigerated at all times. Thaw frozen foods in the refrigerator overnight or in the microwave. When cooking stuffed poultry, allow extra time for the stuffing to cook completely inside the bird. Do not eat raw eggs or anything containing raw eggs, such as homemade eggnog; use egg substitutes when you prepare these foods. When picnicking, pack foods in insulated coolers with ice packs. Thoroughly wash all poultry before you cook it and use soap and water to wash all surfaces (including your hands) and utensils that come into contact with raw poultry.

HEMORRHOIDS

A hemorrhoid is a swollen (varicose) vein that protrudes from the lining of the anus. A hemorrhoid may occur inside the anus or rectum or on the outer rim of the anus. Hemorrhoids are not dangerous to your health, but they can be annoying or, in some cases, painful. Some people are more susceptible to hemorrhoids than others. Hemorrhoids are common during pregnancy and occur more often in obese people than in people of normal weight. Both pregnancy and obesity increase pressure inside the abdomen, which causes the veins of the lower pelvis to become swollen. In many cases, the cause of hemorrhoids is unclear.

Symptoms Hemorrhoids can cause pain, particularly during a bowel movement, or persistent discomfort or itching in your anal area. Hemorrhoids also can cause bleeding. If you see blood in your stool or on toilet paper, report it to your doctor immediately. Bleeding can also be a sign of colon cancer (see page 529). A prolapsed hemorrhoid (a hemorrhoid that is elongated and protruding from the anus) may itch or discharge mucus.

Diagnosis Doctors diagnose hemorrhoids by examining the anus and rectum with a finger. The diagnosis is usually confirmed by a direct visual examination of the inside of your rectum and anus using a flexible viewing instrument called an endoscope. To rule out cancer, the doctor may want to examine your colon farther up using a longer viewing instrument in a procedure called sigmoidoscopy (see page 130). In some cases, colonoscopy (see page 530) is used to examine more of the colon.

Treatment To ease the discomfort of hemorrhoids and to help prevent them, eat lots of high-fiber foods and drink plenty of fluids. Avoid alcohol or caffeinated beverages, which can aggravate hemorrhoids. Fiber and fluids help make the stool bulky and soft and easier to pass through your rectum and anus. Bathe once or twice a day in warm water and cleanse the area once a day with mild soap. Taking a warm bath or applying an ice compress or an over-the-counter pain-relieving cream may help reduce irritation. Some people find sitting on a doughnut-shaped pillow more comfortable. If the pain persists for more than 12 hours, see your doctor.

Severe pain from a hemorrhoid can be a sign that a blood clot has formed inside it. In this case, your doctor may recommend surgery. He or she may use a local anesthetic to numb the area and make a small incision in the hemorrhoid to remove the clot. Because a blood clot in a hemorrhoid usually goes away without treatment, surgery is performed only in severe cases to relieve pain.

If you have a persistent prolapsed hemorrhoid that is protruding outside your anus, your doctor may need to manipulate it back inside with his or her fingers. However, this is not always effective with large hemorrhoids, which tend to protrude again. Hemorrhoids that cause persistent symptoms can be treated in a variety of ways. A procedure called infrared coagulation uses heat to seal a hemorrhoid and prevent it from bleeding. In another procedure, rubber bands are placed around the base of the hemorrhoid to cut off its blood supply, causing it to shrink and fall off. If a hemorrhoid is very large, surgery may be necessary to remove it.

APPENDICITIS

Appendicitis is inflammation of the appendix, a small, worm-shaped organ that projects out from the beginning of the colon (see page 516). The appendix has no known function. For reasons that are not understood, the appendix can become inflamed, causing severe pain that may start in the middle of your abdomen and move to the lower right part of your abdomen. Appendicitis can also cause loss of appetite, fever, nausea, vomiting, or diarrhea.

Diagnosis Appendicitis can be difficult to diagnose. The infection is usually suspected on the basis of your symptoms, particularly the site of pain in your abdomen, and an examination of your abdomen. The doctor presses gently on your abdomen to locate the site of inflammation and listens through a stethoscope placed on your abdomen for the sounds of normal digestive activity. (There are no sounds if you have a severe infection.)

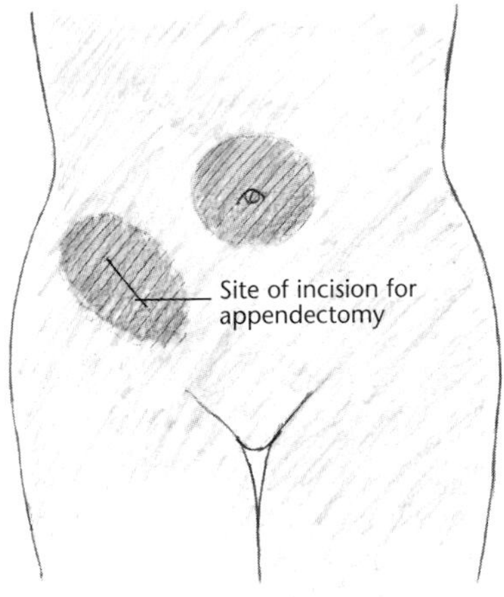

APPENDICITIS
The shaded areas show where you are likely to feel pain if you have appendicitis (inflammation of the appendix). You may first feel pain around your navel. As the appendicitis progresses, the pain moves to the lower right part of your abdomen. If your doctor makes the diagnosis of appendicitis, your appendix will be removed in a surgical procedure called an appendectomy. The diagonal line shows the usual site of the incision that is made to remove the appendix.

Treatment If your doctor thinks that you may have appendicitis based on your symptoms and an examination of your abdomen, he or she will admit you into the hospital for careful observation or for surgery to remove your appendix. If surgery is not done soon enough, your appendix can rupture, spilling its infected contents into your abdominal cavity. This spread of infection, called peritonitis, causes severe pain throughout your abdomen and can be life threatening.

Before removing your appendix, the doctor may need to confirm the diagnosis in a procedure called laparoscopy (see page 263), which is done through a small incision in your abdomen. In some cases, an appendix that has not ruptured can be removed through the laparoscope (a viewing tube that is inserted through the incision in your abdomen). Alternatively, the diagnosis of appendicitis and the removal of the appendix sometimes has to be done through a larger incision in

SYMPTOM CHART

Recurring abdominal pain

Abdominal pain that occurs on several days for a week or longer.

START

Is the pain in the upper part of your abdomen?

YES → Is it a burning pain that gets worse when you bend over?

YES → *Call your doctor.* You may have esophageal reflux or a hiatal hernia, both of which can cause heartburn. See Esophageal reflux, page 517. See also Hiatal hernia, page 518.

NO → Is the pain relieved when you take an antacid?

YES → *Call your doctor.* You may have an ulcer in your stomach or small intestine. See Peptic ulcers, page 518.

NO → Does the pain come in waves mainly in the upper right side of your abdomen or around your ribs?

YES → ***Call your doctor NOW.*** Your gallbladder may be inflamed and you may have gallstones (see page 532).

NO → If you are unable to make a diagnosis from this chart, talk to your doctor.

NO (upper part of abdomen) →

continued on next page

continued from previous page

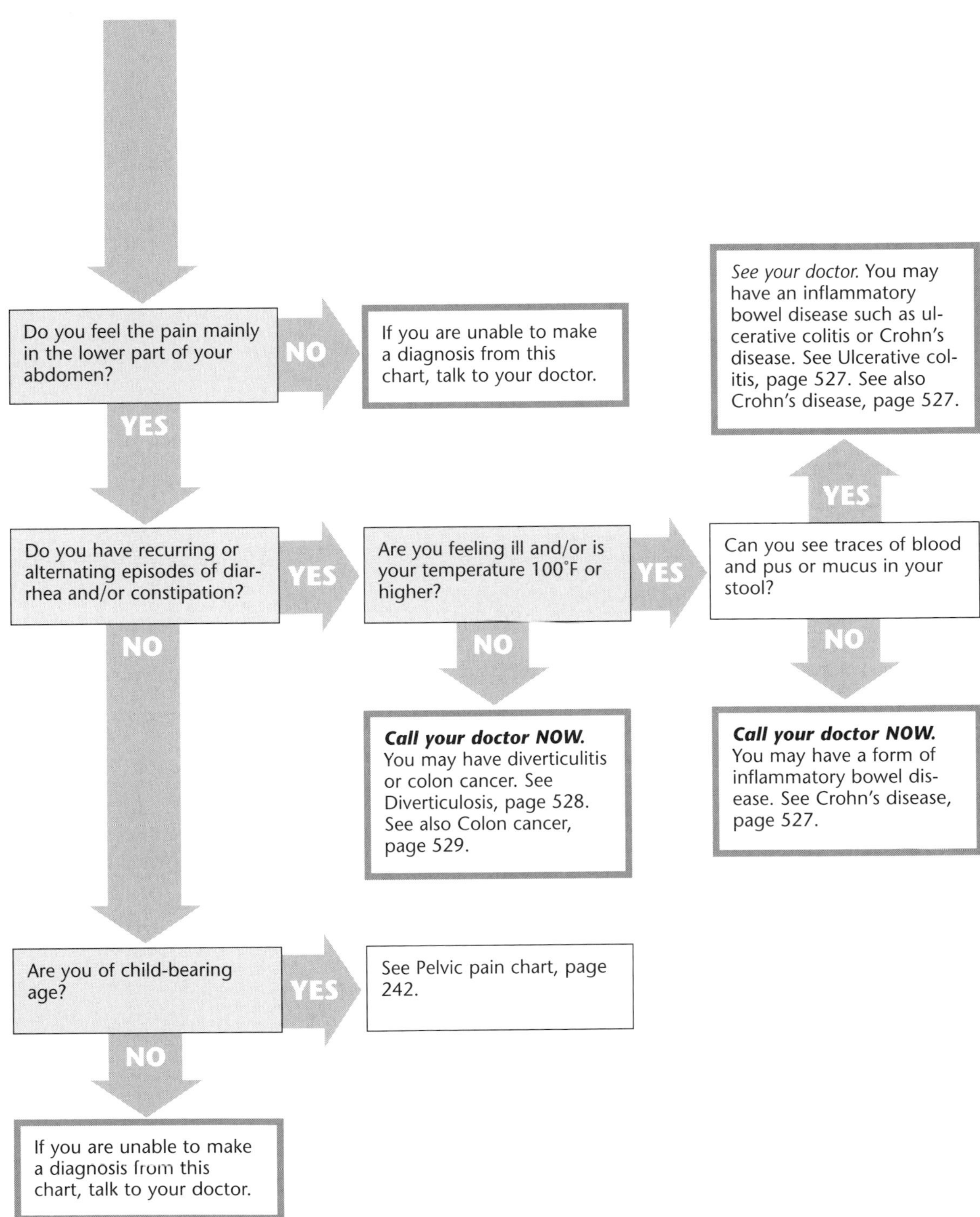

the abdomen in a procedure called laparotomy (see page 264).

Surgery of any kind to remove an appendix is performed in the hospital using general anesthesia (see page 261). Depending on the severity of your condition, you will be in the hospital for 1 to 3 days and will probably be able to resume eating and drinking within 24 hours after the operation.

IRRITABLE BOWEL SYNDROME

Irritable bowel syndrome is a collection of symptoms that include periodic abdominal discomfort or pain, constipation, or alternating periods of constipation and diarrhea. Irritable bowel syndrome has no obvious cause, but stress is known to play a role in triggering symptoms. Consuming caffeine, alcohol, or dairy products may also bring on symptoms. Irritable bowel syndrome is also referred to as irritable colon, spastic colon, spastic bowel, mucous colitis, or functional bowel disease.

Symptoms Irritable bowel syndrome often causes abdominal pain, bloating, gas, constipation, diarrhea, and alternating periods of constipation and diarrhea. In rare cases, a person has severe but painless diarrhea. High-fat foods (especially fried foods, meats such as bacon and sausage, and dairy products) and caffeine can trigger episodes. Stress can also bring on symptoms, probably because the functioning of the colon and the digestive process are controlled by the nervous system.

Diagnosis Irritable bowel syndrome is usually diagnosed by ruling out other possible causes of your symptoms. If you have irritable bowel syndrome, an examination of your colon—either directly through a viewing tube (endoscope) inserted through your rectum or on an X-ray—will rule out inflammation or other signs of disease. Blood tests and other laboratory tests will also be normal.

Gastrointestinal series

Diagnostic examinations called gastrointestinal (GI) series are X-ray procedures that are used to help doctors detect or monitor disorders of the digestive tract (esophagus, stomach, and intestines). These tests use the mineral barium, which shows up on a video screen or X-ray, to highlight the area of the digestive tract that is being examined. These barium X-ray procedures are painless and do not require an overnight stay in the hospital.

- **An upper GI series**—which examines the esophagus, stomach, and duodenum (the part of the small intestine that leads out of the stomach)—is used to detect disorders such as ulcers, tumors, and polyps. When you have an upper GI series, you drink a liquid containing barium and the doctor observes on a video screen the movement of the barium through your esophagus, stomach, and duodenum.
- **A small bowel series** is a set of X-rays taken of the small intestine. For a small bowel series, barium is introduced through a flexible tube that has been inserted into your mouth and down through your esophagus and stomach into your small intestine. A small bowel series can take up to 2 hours because it may take that long for the barium to go through your small intestine to the colon.
- **A lower GI series** is used to examine your colon (the large intestine) and rectum. When you have a lower GI, you are given a barium enema: a diluted barium liquid is introduced into your colon through a catheter (a flexible tube) that has been inserted into your rectum. Air is then introduced through the catheter into your colon. This enables the doctor to see the walls of the colon better and find any abnormal growths, such as polyps or tumors, that may be present. Most of the barium solution is expelled from your body immediately after the procedure; the rest is later eliminated in feces.

Treatment Irritable bowel syndrome does not cause serious long-term health problems and can usually be managed with a combination of a healthy diet, stress management techniques (see page 186), or, in some cases, medication. Restrict your consumption of foods that may be causing your symptoms, especially those that are high in fat. Eat lots of fruits, vegetables, and whole-grain breads and cereals; a diet rich in fiber can help keep stool bulky and soft so it moves more easily through your system.

Try to reduce the level of emotional stress in your life. Regular exercise is a very effective way to help reduce stress. If diet, exercise, and other stress management techniques do not work, your doctor may prescribe antispasmodic drugs to relieve the spasms in the bowel that are thought to cause the cramping and abdominal pain.

INFLAMMATORY BOWEL DISEASE

Inflammatory bowel disease includes two conditions—Crohn's disease and ulcerative colitis—that cause inflammation of the intestines. The cause of these disorders is unknown; in some cases, they are triggered by a bacterial infection or by taking antibiotics to treat a bacterial infection. Crohn's disease can affect any part of the digestive tract but most often affects the area where the small intestine and colon (the large intestine) meet. Ulcerative colitis always involves the rectum (the lowest part of your colon) and may extend to any part of the colon.

Symptoms The symptoms of inflammatory bowel disease include diarrhea, fever, and abdominal pain. The stool may contain blood, mucus, or pus. In Crohn's disease, abnormal connecting channels called fistulas can develop between your intestines or from your intestine to the skin in your genital area. If you have a fistula that connects to your skin, the liquid contents of your intestine may leak out of your body. If the fistula prevents digested food from being absorbed by the small intestine, you will experience diarrhea and weight loss.

For reasons that are not clear, inflammatory bowel disease may cause symptoms in areas of your body other than your intestines. For example, the irises of your eyes may become red and inflamed, or your joints may become inflamed or swollen. These symptoms may be the result of an abnormal immune response that occurs when your immune system mistakenly identifies normal body tissues as foreign and attacks them.

Diagnosis Your doctor may suspect that you have inflammatory bowel disease based on your symptoms and a physical examination. To confirm the diagnosis, the doctor may need to directly examine the inside of your colon using a flexible viewing instrument called an endoscope, which is inserted through your rectum. You may also have X-rays done of your intestines (gastrointestinal series, see page 526).

Treatment There is no cure for inflammatory bowel disease, but several medications are available that can help control the symptoms. Drugs such as cortisone and sulfasalazine can reduce inflammation of the intestine. In some cases, drugs are used to suppress the body's abnormal immune reaction and to treat complications, such as fistulas. Surgery is sometimes necessary to repair a fistula or a part of the colon that has become narrowed from scarring caused by inflammation. Surgery to remove the affected part of the colon may also be required for people who have severe ulcerative colitis that is not responding to medication or if the doctor finds that the cells in the colon show early changes that could turn into cancer.

Some people with inflammatory bowel disease find that their symptoms worsen when they drink milk or alcohol or eat spicy or high-fiber foods. Look for patterns in your diet and avoid foods that seem to trigger symptoms. Your doctor may recommend a high-calorie nutritional supplement if you are losing weight because your body is not absorbing a sufficient amount of nutrients from your intestines. If you have severe weight loss, diarrhea, or bleeding, your doctor may recommend temporary intravenous feeding in the hospital to provide you with the nutrients your body needs.

In severe cases of chronic ulcerative colitis that do not respond to medication, or when colon cancer is found, it is necessary to remove the entire colon. When your colon is removed, the end of the small intestine is brought through a small opening in your abdomen (a procedure called an ileostomy). A bag for collecting feces is attached to your skin around the opening. In an alternative surgical procedure, called ileoanal anastomosis, the small intestine is attached to the anus. A pouch is created surgically from a portion of the small intestine to take over the colon's job of holding stool before it is passed from the body. The person can then pass stool in a nearly normal way.

DIVERTICULOSIS

Diverticulosis is the formation of small pouches that bulge out of the lining of the intestine, particularly the lower colon. Diverticulosis is very common; it is estimated that half of all people over age 60 may have the disorder. In most people, diverticulosis causes no symptoms and does not require treatment. The cause of diverticulosis is not clear, but doctors believe that it may result from eating a diet low in fiber, which may increase pressure in the colon.

Symptoms Most people with diverticulosis have no symptoms. In some cases, a person feels tenderness in the affected area or some pain in the lower left side of the abdomen. If a diverticulum becomes inflamed and ruptures, you will have a fever and feel intense pain in the lower left side of your abdomen.

Diagnosis Because diverticulosis usually causes no symptoms, it is often not diagnosed until it is detected by chance during a procedure such as a gastrointestinal series (see page 526) or a colonoscopy (see page 530) performed for another reason. These tests are also used to diagnose diverticulosis if you do have symptoms. However, if you have pain and fever caused by diverticulitis (inflammation of a diverticulum), you will not be given these tests until your symptoms subside or have been treated because the tests may worsen your symptoms.

Treatment If you have diverticulosis and you are not experiencing any symptoms, you do not need treatment. Eating a nutritious diet that is high in fiber and low in fat can help keep your colon healthy.

Sometimes a diverticulum becomes infected or ruptures. In either case, you may be hospitalized and given intravenous fluids and antibiotics. If the infection forms an abscess (a pus-filled sac), your doctor may have to drain the pus in a procedure called laparotomy (see page 264). If an infected diverticulum ruptures, surgery may be necessary to remove the affected section of your colon. Depending on the severity of the rupture, the two remaining ends of the colon may be rejoined. In cases in which the rupture is extensive, a colostomy (see page 530) is required.

DIVERTICULA
Small bulges or pouches called diverticula often develop in the colon (right). If these pouches cause no pain or other symptoms, the condition is called diverticulosis. When they become blocked with particles of undigested food and inflamed, they can cause pain and fever, and they may rupture (far right). When a diverticulum becomes inflamed, the condition is called diverticulitis. Diverticulitis may be treated with antibiotics or, in severe cases, with surgery.

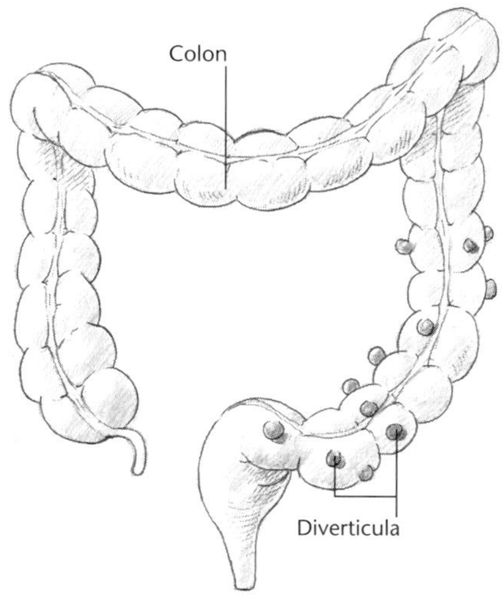

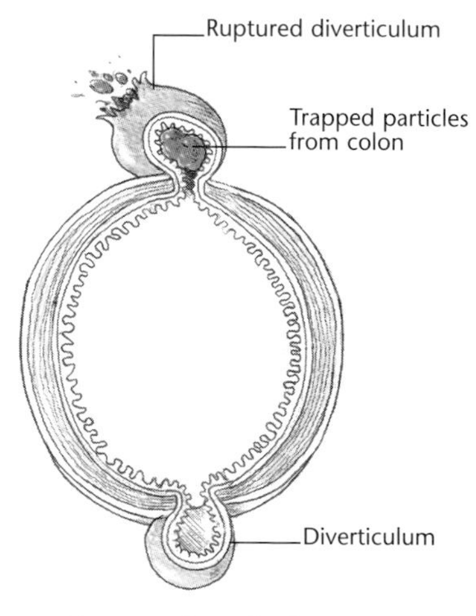

Cross section of colon

COLON CANCER AND POLYPS

Cancers of the colon and rectum—often referred to jointly as colorectal cancer or simply colon cancer—are two of the most common forms of cancer. Colon cancer is the third most common cause of cancer deaths in women—after cancers of the lung and breast. The cause of colon cancer is not fully understood, but a diet that is high in animal fat, particularly red meat, and low in fiber is linked to an increased incidence of the cancer. Eating a fiber-rich diet with lots of fresh fruits, vegetables, and whole grains may help protect you from colon cancer. (For a list of foods that are high in fiber, see page 50.)

A family history of colon cancer or a personal history of extensive ulcerative colitis (see page 527) increases your risk of developing colon cancer. In either case, you will need to have more frequent checkups. Small, benign (noncancerous) growths called polyps that are common in the colon pose no risk to health. However, a type of polyp in the intestine called an adenomatous polyp, or adenoma, can become cancerous. If your doctor detects these polyps during an examination, he or she will recommend that they be removed before they have a chance to develop into cancer.

Symptoms The symptoms of colon cancer include blood in the stool; constipation; stool that is narrower than usual; general stomach or abdominal discomfort such as bloating, fullness, or cramps; frequent gas pains; a feeling that your bowel does not empty completely; unexplained weight loss; or constant fatigue. Always report any of these symptoms to your doctor. These symptoms can indicate disorders of the colon and rectum other than cancer.

Diagnosis If your doctor suspects you have colon cancer or adenomatous polyps, he or she may recommend a diagnostic procedure called colonoscopy (see page 530). For a colonoscopy, the doctor inserts a flexible, lighted viewing tube through your rectum into your colon to directly view the lining of your colon and look for abnormal growths. Sigmoidoscopy (see page 130) is similar to colonoscopy but it allows the doctor to see only into the lower part of the colon (the sigmoid colon).

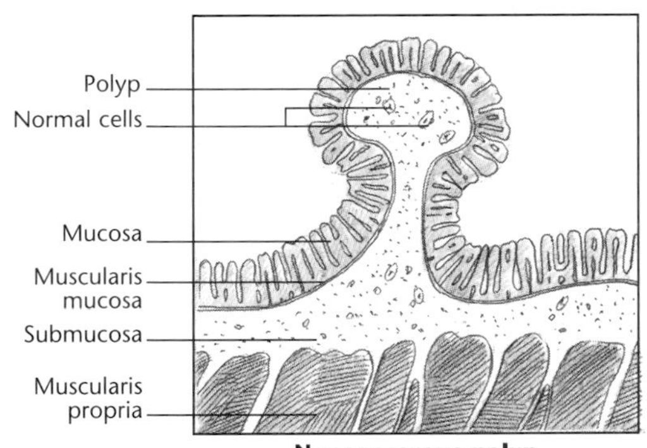

Noncancerous polyp

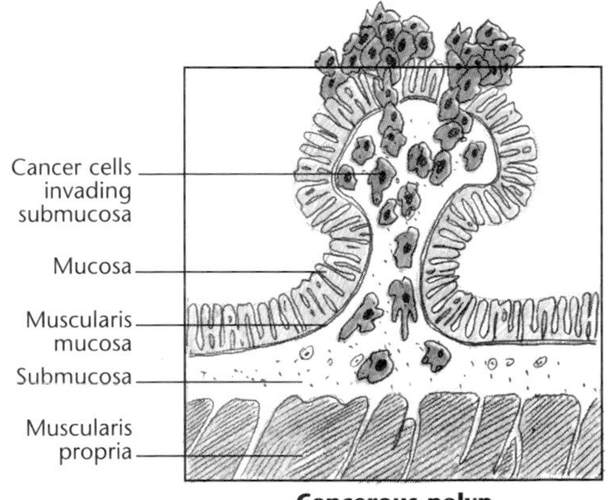

Cancerous polyp

WHEN POLYPS BECOME CANCEROUS

Polyps are growths of tissue in the inner lining of the wall of the colon, called the mucosa (right). The most common type of polyp, called an adenomatous polyp, is noncancerous (above left), but it can grow and become cancerous. When a polyp in the colon becomes cancerous, its cells multiply in a disorganized, unchecked way, and the abnormal cells break through the muscularis mucosa and grow into the next layer of the colon wall, the submucosa (above right). If the cancer cells continue to grow unchecked, they may grow through the outer layer of the colon wall. Cancer cells that escape through the outer wall of the colon may invade blood vessels and travel to the liver and lymph nodes, spreading the cancer further.

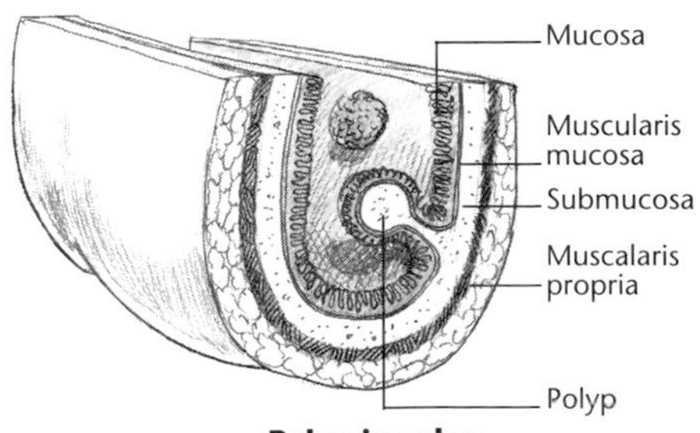

Polyp in colon

Warning signs
Colon cancer

If you notice any of the following symptoms, see your doctor immediately:

- Bleeding from your rectum
- Blood in or on your stool
- Recent change in bowel movements—including constipation, diarrhea, narrower-than-usual stool, or a feeling that your bowel does not empty completely
- Abdominal cramps or pain
- Unexplained weight loss

If you are 40 or older, you should regularly have a screening test called a fecal occult-blood test (see page 130). This test can detect microscopic amounts of blood in the stool, which helps doctors diagnose colon cancer at an early, curable stage, even before symptoms develop. Colon cancer may also be suspected if a routine blood test shows anemia (see page 493), which can result from bleeding in the colon.

Colonoscopy

In a diagnostic procedure called colonoscopy, your doctor can examine the full length of your colon. A flexible, lighted, viewing tube called a colonoscope is passed through your rectum to the beginning of your colon. While slowly withdrawing the tube, the doctor examines the inside of your colon directly through the colonoscope or on a video monitor. Colonoscopy can be used to diagnose polyps or cancer in the colon or to look for inflammation in the lining of the colon. Instruments can be passed through the colonoscope to take a tissue sample or to remove polyps.

If you are going to have a colonoscopy, you will be told not to eat anything except clear liquids (such as water or broth) for 24 hours before the procedure. You will be instructed to drink a gallon of liquid the night before the procedure to flush all the stool out of your colon. Before the colonoscopy, the doctor will give you a sedative to relax you and pain medication to make you more comfortable. Ask your doctor if you should make arrangements ahead of time for someone to drive you home after the procedure. You will feel sore for a few hours afterward but you can eat as soon as you like.

Complications from colonoscopy are rare but can include perforation of the wall of the colon or bleeding. Colonoscopy is not done if you are having an attack of colitis (see page 527) or if you have diverticulitis (see page 528).

Treatment If you have been diagnosed with cancer of the colon or rectum, your doctor will first determine how far the cancer has advanced. This process is called staging. A variety of tests and X-rays—usually a computed tomography (CT) scan (see page 572)—can be used to determine if the cancer has spread to other parts of your body. Depending on the stage, colon cancer is treated with surgery, radiation therapy, chemotherapy, or a combination of these methods.

Surgery Surgery is the most common treatment for colon cancer. The type of surgery depends on how quickly the cancer cells are multiplying and how far the cancer has spread. In a surgical procedure called a bowel resection with reanastomosis, the doctor cuts out (resects) the segment of colon that contains the cancer and rejoins the remaining healthy sections (reanastomosis). Lymph nodes (infection-fighting glands that can carry cancer cells throughout the body) near the cancer site are also removed to determine if the cancer has spread to them.

If the cancer is blocking your colon, your doctor may have to do an operation called a colostomy. A colostomy creates an opening in your abdominal wall to allow feces to be eliminated without passing through your lower colon and rectum. The cancerous part of your colon is removed and the remainder is attached to the opening in your abdomen, called a stoma. You attach a special bag to the stoma to collect feces. The bag adheres to your skin in a watertight fit without causing irritation to your skin.

In some cases, a colostomy is temporary. After the lower colon and rectum heal, the doctor can do a second operation to rejoin the healthy parts of the colon and restore normal bowel function. Before you have a colostomy, you may be given radiation therapy to help shrink the tumor. Radiation therapy alone is not adequate for treating colon cancer. (For more about radiation therapy, see page 253.)

Chemotherapy Chemotherapy, the use of powerful drugs to kill cancer cells, may be used to treat colon cancer that has spread to other parts of the body. Your doctor may recommend chemotherapy after surgery or radiation therapy if he or she suspects that some cancer remains in your

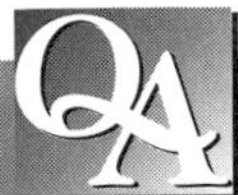

QUESTIONS WOMEN ASK
COLON CANCER

Q I was recently diagnosed with inflammatory polyps. Does this increase my risk of developing colon cancer?

A No, having inflammatory polyps does not increase your risk of colon cancer. These common polyps in the colon are associated with inflammatory bowel disease (see page 527).

Q My mother has colon cancer. She told me several of her aunts and uncles died of it. It sounds like this runs in our family. Is there anything I can do to avoid getting the cancer myself?

A Yes, and preventive measures are important for you because having a close relative with colon cancer does increase your risk of developing the same type of cancer. Eat a low-fat, high-fiber diet, including foods such as fruits, vegetables, and whole grains to help reduce your risk. Limit your consumption of animal fat, particularly red meats and high-fat dairy products. Make sure your doctor knows of your family history of colon cancer so that he or she can examine you regularly for polyps or cancer. Like all cancers, the earlier colon cancer is detected, the more effective treatment is likely to be.

Q My doctor says I need to have a colostomy to surgically remove the cancer in my colon. I'm worried about what it will be like to live with a colostomy.

A Many people dislike the idea of having a colostomy bag. But after using one for about 2 months, most people become comfortable with it, pausing only once or twice a day at regular intervals to empty and clean it. In fact, many people find that a colostomy is preferable to the pain and discomfort they experienced from their cancer or other disorder. While you are still in the hospital after the operation, nurses can help you learn how to take care of your colostomy.

body. Chemotherapy drugs may be administered by mouth or by injection into a vein. While undergoing chemotherapy, you may have to stay in the hospital for a few days and continue taking the medication after you return home. Most people have several cycles of treatment; for example, you may take the medication for a few weeks, stop for a few weeks, and then begin the cycle again.

Cancer treatments have a variety of side effects. Coping with these side effects (see page 255) can be difficult. Joining a support group of other people who are undergoing a similar experience or seeking counseling can be helpful.

Diseases of the gallbladder, pancreas, and liver

The gallbladder, pancreas, and liver play vital roles in the digestion of food and your body's absorption of nutrients. An essential digestive juice called bile is produced by the liver and stored in the gallbladder. When you eat, fat is broken down by enzymes secreted from the pancreas. The pancreas produces a variety of enzymes that digest carbohydrates and proteins as well as fat. Bile flows out of the gallbladder into the intestine, where it mixes with and dissolves the fat in your food. The liver breaks down and filters out any potentially harmful substances that you consume, including alcohol and other drugs.

GALLSTONES

Gallstones are lumps of solid material that form inside the gallbladder. Most gallstones consist of cholesterol, but some are made up of other substances such as calcium salts or bile pigments. Gallstones often cause no symptoms but they may eventually block the opening of the gallbladder and cause severe pain and inflammation.

The cause of gallstones is not fully understood. Women are more likely than men to develop them, as are people of Native American ancestry. Other factors that increase your risk include being overweight, having several pregnancies, or losing a large amount of weight in a short period of time.

Symptoms Gallstones often cause no symptoms, but the longer you have them, the more likely they are to cause complications. The primary symptom of gallstones is persistent pain that may fluctuate and increase in intensity in the upper or upper right side of your abdomen. The pain may spread to your chest, shoulders, or back. You may also experience indigestion, nausea, or vomiting. If a gallstone blocks the drainage of bile from the liver to the intestine, you will develop jaundice (yellowing of your skin and the whites of your eyes), chills, and fever. If a gallstone blocks the cystic duct (the duct that leads out of the gallbladder), pressure builds up in the gallbladder and causes infection and severe pain.

GALLSTONES
Gallstones are solid lumps, consisting mostly of cholesterol, that form in the gallbladder. Gallstones often do not cause any symptoms. In some cases, a small gallstone passes on its own out of the gallbladder through the bile duct and out of the body in stool, causing no pain. But if a large stone blocks the cystic duct, which causes intense pain, both the duct and the gallbladder are removed surgically.

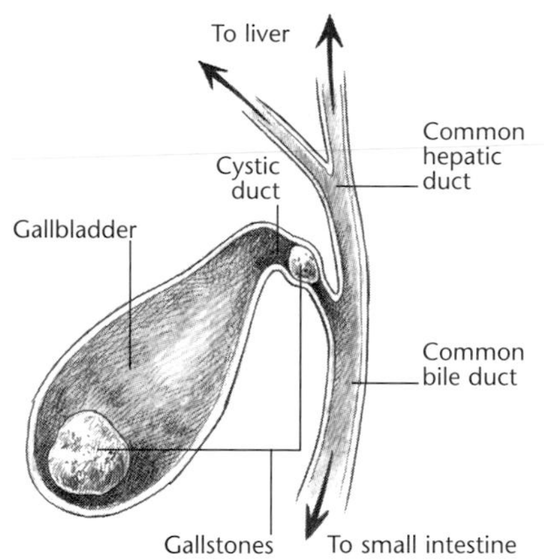

Diagnosis Your doctor can tell whether you have gallstones by your symptoms and by an ultrasound (see page 405) of the gallbladder. Gallstones that have traveled into the common bile duct (which empties into the small intestine) can be detected with an X-ray procedure called endoscopic retrograde cholangiography. In this procedure, dye is injected into the duct through a viewing tube (endoscope) inserted through your mouth, esophagus, and stomach to the area of the small intestine.

Treatment Gallstones can be treated by surgically removing your gallbladder in a procedure called cholecystectomy. Cholecystectomy is one of the most frequently performed surgical procedures in the world. The gallbladder can often be removed through several small incisions in your abdomen (see page 533). Once your gallbladder has been removed, bile flows directly from your liver to the small intestine. This rerouting of bile usually has little, if any, effect on the digestive process.

In some cases, if the gallstones are small and composed entirely of cholesterol, a medication that dissolves them may be effective. This medication, called ursodiol, is a naturally occurring bile acid that slowly dissolves gallstones over a period of 6 months to 2 years. You take the drug by mouth each day. However, this medication is not always successful and gallstones frequently recur after treatment.

PANCREATITIS

Pancreatitis is a disease that results when, for unknown reasons, digestive enzymes begin attacking the pancreas, causing inflammation. There are two forms of pancreatitis—acute and chronic. Acute pancreatitis occurs suddenly and can be life threatening. Most cases of acute pancreatitis are caused by alcohol abuse, gallstones, injury to the abdomen, high levels of harmful fats in the blood called triglycerides, or use of some medications. Chronic pancreatitis usually follows many years of alcohol abuse.

Symptoms The symptoms of acute pancreatitis include severe, constant pain in the upper abdomen that spreads to the back. The pain usually comes on rapidly

Laparoscopic cholecystectomy

Laparoscopic cholecystectomy is a common surgical procedure to remove the gallbladder. The operation is performed while you are under general anesthesia.

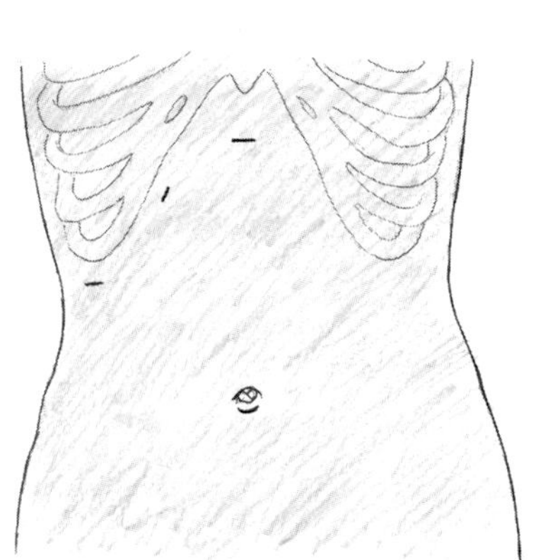

INSERTING THE INSTRUMENTS

Rather than making a large incision, the surgeon makes four small incisions (left) for inserting a lighted viewing tube called a laparoscope and surgical instruments (right) for performing the procedure. The laparoscope allows the surgeon to view the inside of the body on a monitor during the procedure.

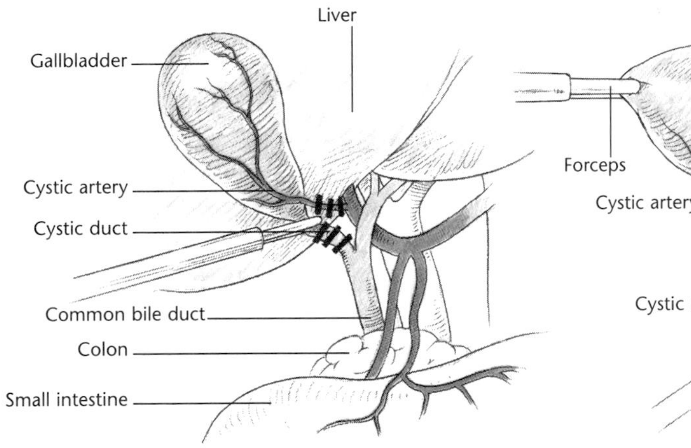

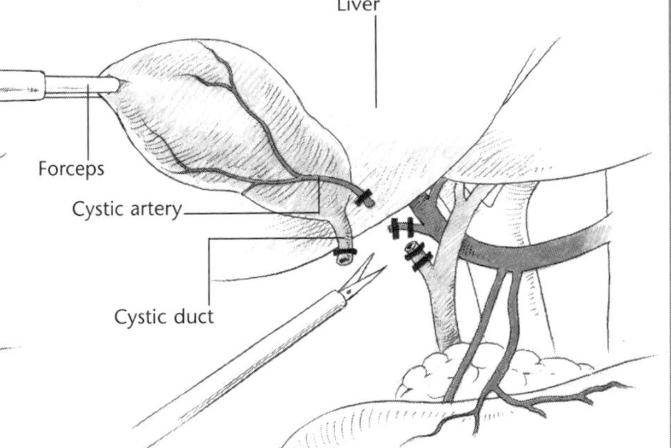

FREEING THE CYSTIC ARTERY AND CYSTIC DUCT

The surgeon uses forceps to push the gallbladder up away from the small intestine and colon. Using tiny scissors, he or she frees the cystic artery that feeds the gallbladder with blood and the cystic duct that connects the gallbladder with the liver. An X-ray is taken to confirm that the common bile duct does not contain any hidden gallstones. The surgeon then puts clips on the artery and the cystic duct.

REMOVING THE GALLBLADDER

The surgeon uses tiny scissors to cut the cystic artery and cystic duct and to separate the gallbladder from the liver. He or she then seals off the blood vessels to the gallbladder, draws the gallbladder out through the incision beneath the navel, and stitches the incisions close.

and may last several days. You may also have a mild fever, nausea, vomiting, and bloating. In a severe attack, which can be life threatening, you may have a rapid pulse and low blood pressure.

Diagnosis Pancreatitis is usually diagnosed from the symptoms and a physical examination. If you have pancreatitis, a blood test will show elevated levels of amylase or lipase, two digestive enzymes that are normally produced by and stored in the pancreas. When the pancreas is inflamed, these enzymes are released into your bloodstream.

Treatment Treatment of either form of pancreatitis depends on the severity of the condition. An attack of acute pancreatitis often subsides on its own without treatment. You may be hospitalized and given intravenous fluids to prevent dehydration. Surgery may be necessary if a complication occurs, such as the development of pseudocysts (collections of fluid) in the pancreas. Attacks of pancreatitis may be triggered by the passage of a gallstone down the common bile duct (which leads to the small intestine). In this case, surgery may be required to remove the gallbladder and to remove the gallstone from the common bile duct. You should not drink alcohol during an attack of pancreatitis, and you should never drink alcohol again if the pancreatitis was caused by alcohol.

Treatment of chronic pancreatitis involves controlling pain and correcting nutritional deficiencies that result from the condition. Your doctor may tell you to cut down on fat in your diet; your pancreas may not be producing enough enzymes to digest fat. He or she may prescribe digestive enzymes to reduce pain and improve the digestion or breakdown of fats, proteins, and carbohydrates. If you have chronic pancreatitis, you should not drink alcohol.

VIRAL HEPATITIS

Hepatitis is a contagious infection of the liver caused by one of the hepatitis viruses—hepatitis A, B, C, or D. These viruses cause inflammation of the liver. Each of the hepatitis viruses is spread in a different way and causes a different pattern of symptoms. Most people recover from a hepatitis infection, but some have mild flare-ups that may recur for months or years. Some people die of the initial infection; the hepatitis B and D viruses are the most deadly.

An infection with the hepatitis A virus is most common in adolescents and young adults. The virus is present in the feces of an infected person. You can contract the virus by consuming contaminated water or food. Hepatitis A causes only a mild illness in children, which may go unnoticed. In adults, the infection can vary from mild to severe.

Treatment of hepatitis A consists mostly of controlling the symptoms—primarily fever and dehydration—with over-the-counter painkillers, such as aspirin, and fluids. Once you recover from a hepatitis A infection, you are immune to the virus for life.

Infection with the hepatitis B virus is the most serious form of hepatitis. The virus is present in the blood of infected people. Many people infected with hepatitis B have no symptoms but are carriers of the virus—they can spread it to others. The virus can be transmitted through sexual intercourse, through sharing of needles during intravenous drug use, or through a transfusion of contaminated blood. All blood banks screen donors and donated blood for all the hepatitis viruses, but there is still a very small risk of infection from a transfusion. A pregnant woman can transmit hepatitis B to her child at birth.

The hepatitis C virus is a common cause of hepatitis. Many people carry the hepatitis C virus and have no symptoms. Hepatitis C is spread through transfusions of contaminated blood or through sharing of contaminated needles during intravenous drug use. Although the flu-like symptoms of hepatitis C are less severe than those of hepatitis B, hepatitis C is more likely to become chronic (long term).

About 1 out of 10 people with hepatitis B and nearly half of people with hepatitis C develop chronic infections that can lead to cirrhosis of the liver (a disease caused by widespread destruction of liver cells) and increase the risk of liver cancer. If you have chronic hepatitis B or C, your doctor may recommend testing at regular intervals to rule out liver cancer. Such testing may include an ultrasound (see page 405) of the liver or a liver biopsy (taking a sample of tissue from the liver for examination under a microscope).

Hepatitis D (delta hepatitis) is spread primarily through blood transfusions or needle sharing during intravenous drug use. Hepatitis D causes illness only when it occurs simultaneously with a hepatitis B infection or in people who already have hepatitis B. However, when it does occur, hepatitis D is usually very severe.

Symptoms Many people, especially younger people, have no symptoms when they acquire a hepatitis infection. When symptoms do occur, they are similar to those of the flu. For this reason, many cases of hepatitis are undetected. Possible symptoms of an infection with any of the viruses include fatigue, fever, nausea, vomiting, loss of appetite, weight loss, mild abdominal pain, muscle or joint aches, and diarrhea.

During an early stage of the initial hepatitis infection, you may develop jaundice—your skin and the whites of your eyes become yellow and your urine may be dark and your stools pale. Jaundice also occurs in people who have a chronic hepatitis infection from which they have developed cirrhosis of the liver.

Diagnosis To diagnose a hepatitis infection, your doctor will first ask about your medical history and will want to know any risk factors you may have that exposed you to the virus. He or she will examine you for physical signs of a hepatitis infection, such as jaundice and liver enlargement. A simple blood test can determine whether you have hepatitis or carry one of the hepatitis viruses. If you have hepatitis A, inform members of your family and other people with whom you have close contact; they should have an injection of a protein substance called gamma globulin to protect them from contracting the virus. If you have hepatitis B, your sexual partner should be vaccinated.

Treatment Treatment of a hepatitis infection depends on the particular disease-causing virus. Most people recover from a hepatitis infection without treatment in a few weeks to 6 months. Medications are available for people who develop a chronic infection from hepatitis B or C, but these drugs are only partially effective. Your doctor will ask you about any medications you are taking and determine whether or not you

Avoiding hepatitis

If you understand how a particular hepatitis virus is transmitted, you can take measures to help protect yourself against infection. The hepatitis A virus is present in the feces of infected people. To avoid infection, always practice good personal hygiene by washing your hands frequently with soap and water, and washing dishes, utensils, and clothing thoroughly with hot water and detergent. If you are traveling to a country with a poor sanitation system, talk to your doctor several months beforehand. He or she may recommend an injection of gamma globulin (which protects against hepatitis A for about 3 months) or a vaccination (which provides protection for at least 20 years). The vaccination is given in two doses 6 to 12 months apart.

The hepatitis B, C, and D viruses are transmitted through contact with infected blood. Hepatitis B can also be transmitted sexually through semen and vaginal secretions (see page 346). You cannot acquire these viruses from casual contact such as using a drinking fountain or toilet that an infected person has used. However, you should avoid contact with that person's blood. Do not have unprotected sexual intercourse with a person who is infected with hepatitis B. Do not share personal items—such as toothbrushes, razors, needles, nail files, nail scissors, washcloths, or towels—that may expose you to infected blood.

Effective vaccines are available to protect you against hepatitis B. All children are now vaccinated against hepatitis B. People who are exposed to blood or blood products on the job, such as health care workers, should be vaccinated. Ask your doctor if you should be vaccinated. There is no vaccine for hepatitis C.

should continue taking them. Some medications, such as acetaminophen, may worsen the injury to your liver. Your doctor will tell you to take it easy, but that does not mean you have to stay in bed. Eating a nutritious diet is important when you have hepatitis. You should avoid alcohol and other drugs that can put a strain on your liver's already limited functioning.

CHAPTER 20

Your urinary tract and kidneys

Contents

The urinary tract consists of the bladder, the urethra (a short tube that empties urine from the bladder), and two kidneys, which are each connected to the bladder by a tube called a ureter. Your urinary tract filters waste from your bloodstream and expels it from your body in the form of urine. Your urinary tract also regulates your body's balance of important chemicals such as sodium and potassium. Urinary tract problems, such as infections and incontinence (involuntary leaking of urine), are common in women and can occur at any age. Although these conditions can adversely affect the quality of your life, most are not life threatening and can be treated effectively.

Your urinary tract and kidneys

The function of your urinary tract is to filter waste products and excess fluid from your bloodstream and expel them from your body in the form of urine. Oval organs called kidneys, each about the size of a fist, have an intricate system of filters that remove excess water, salts, and waste products from your blood. The remaining substances are reabsorbed into your blood in precisely the amounts your body needs. The waste product urine is then propelled from the kidneys down two delicate tubes called ureters into your bladder, a muscular organ that stores the urine until you feel the urge to urinate. Urine leaves your body through a narrow tube called the urethra.

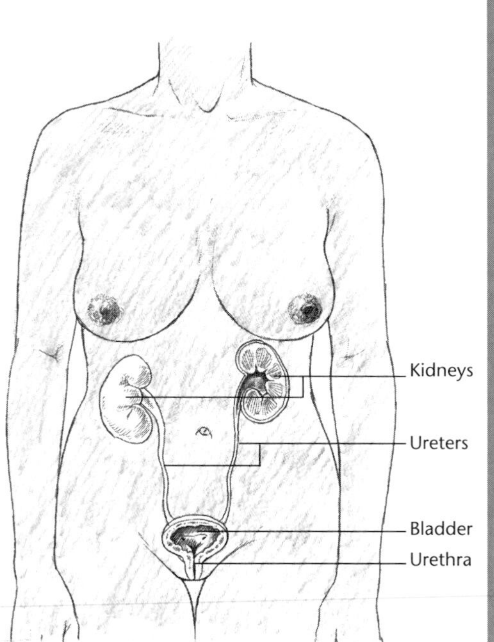

Urinary incontinence

Urinary incontinence is the involuntary loss of urine from your bladder. It is characterized by the leaking of urine when you sneeze or cough; sudden, uncontrollable urges to urinate; or trickling of urine throughout the day. Millions of women, including one out of three women 60 and older, experience some degree of urinary incontinence during their lifetime. They may feel a growing sense of isolation as they gradually restrict their social activities for fear of having an embarrassing accident. But most cases of urinary incontinence can be treated. If you experience incontinence, talk to your doctor. Surgery, medication, or a program of bladder training to increase the capacity of your bladder can help you regain control of the functioning of your urinary system.

DIAGNOSING URINE LOSS

There are several different forms of urinary incontinence that have different causes and require different treatments. The first step in getting treatment for incontinence is to get an accurate diagnosis. Describe your problem as precisely as you can to your doctor. Talking to your gynecologist is a good place to start. Tell him or her under what circumstances you have incontinence. Your doctor may ask if you feel a sense of urgency or frequency about urinating. Urgency is not just the sensation that you need to urinate, but that you must do so immediately. Frequency is feeling the need to urinate more often than usual—even when your bladder is not full or not holding much urine.

Before you see your doctor, it is a good idea to keep a diary of your urinary habits for 2 days. Write down when you urinate and when you experience leaking, and note the activities that may have triggered the leaking, such as sneezing, coughing, or exercising. When you see your doctor, be prepared to answer the following questions:

- How often do you leak urine?
- Does any activity, such as coughing or sneezing, make you lose urine?
- How much urine leaks each time—a few drops or a gush?
- Is the condition severe enough for you to have to wear an absorbent pad?
- When you urinate, do you have the feeling that you are not emptying your bladder completely?
- Do you have any warning or urge before the leaking?
- Do you have to get up in the middle of the night to urinate? How many times?
- When did you first experience incontinence (even if it was many years ago)?
- How much fluid do you drink during a regular day?
- Do you drink fluids shortly before going to bed?
- Do you notice that urine loss occurs after you have had a particular medication, food, or drink (such as coffee, tea, or caffeine-containing soft drinks)?
- Have you ever been treated for incontinence? If so, what kind of treatment did you have?
- Do you have frequent urinary tract infections?

Your doctor may perform some relatively simple tests to evaluate your problem further. He or she will examine your vagina and urethra to determine if the muscles have relaxed. Relaxing of the muscles occurs in some women after a vaginal delivery. You will be asked to provide a sample of urine for laboratory

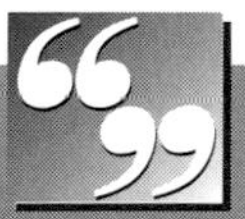

One woman's story
Urine loss

I first noticed I had a problem with leaking urine while I was taking an exercise class after my third child was born. Over the next few weeks, I found that I frequently leaked urine when I coughed or jumped. I used to enjoy playing tennis, but I stopped because I was too nervous about having an accident on the court. I had to wear a large pad whenever I went out, to avoid leaking through my clothes. I found myself avoiding all kinds of social situations and activities for fear of embarrassment.

I went to my doctor and she asked me a lot of questions about when and how often I leaked urine. She examined me and determined that I have a condition called stress incontinence. She said it usually gets worse with each vaginal delivery a woman has. My doctor first recommended that I do pelvic-floor exercises called Kegels to strengthen the muscles in my pelvis. She told me that these exercises can be effective for mild cases of stress incontinence, but that more severe cases require surgery.

"I found myself avoiding all kinds of social situations for fear of embarrassment."

I was very diligent about doing the exercises—I wanted my problem to go away. At first I couldn't contract the muscles for the recommended 10 seconds each time, but I gradually improved. Throughout the day I did my Kegels whenever I could—before I got out of bed, standing in the shower, sitting at my desk at work, and even sitting in my car at stoplights.

After several months of hard work, I noticed some improvement in my incontinence. I still leak some urine occasionally, so I always wear a panty liner. If my problem gets worse, my doctor has reassured me that, if I decide to have surgery to correct my type of incontinence, it should be highly effective.

analysis to rule out a urinary tract infection, which can also cause loss of urine, frequent urination, or urgency.

Cystoscopy You may have an examination called cystoscopy, in which a thin, flexible, viewing tube called a cystoscope is gently inserted into your urethra (the tube that empties urine from your bladder). The doctor looks through the cystoscope to examine your bladder and urethra for abnormalities such as malformations, inflammation, or muscle weakness. You may have some discomfort during a cystoscopy, but usually not enough to require an anesthetic or sedative. For a day or two after the procedure, you may experience some mild discomfort when you urinate.

Cystometry Your doctor may also recommend a diagnostic procedure called cystometry. In this procedure, a catheter (a hollow, flexible tube) with a pressure-sensitive device is inserted through your urethra into your bladder and your bladder is filled with water. A series of pressure measurements is made to determine how much urine your bladder can hold before the pressure in your bladder becomes higher than that in your urethra; at this pressure point, urine will leak out of the bladder. This evaluation can help the doctor determine how effective any planned surgical procedure to treat your incontinence is likely to be. For a day or two after this test, you may experience some mild discomfort when you urinate.

STRESS INCONTINENCE

Stress incontinence is the involuntary leaking of urine during activities that increase pressure inside your abdomen, causing organs in the abdomen to press against your bladder. Common triggers of stress incontinence include coughing, sneezing, and high-impact exercises such as jogging. Stress incontinence occurs when the muscles that support the urethra relax, allowing the urethra to sag from its normal position in the pelvis. The supporting muscles can be weakened by pregnancy and childbirth, a persistent cough, or frequent constipation—all of which increase pressure inside the abdomen. Lack of the female hormone estrogen after menopause can also cause a weakening of pelvic muscles that can contribute to incontinence.

Treatment Most cases of stress incontinence can be treated with surgery. If your incontinence is caused by prolapse of the uterus (see page 234), in which your uterus has dropped from its normal position because of weakened supporting tissues, your doctor may recommend surgery to lift the bladder back up to its normal position. This surgery is often performed in addition to a hysterectomy

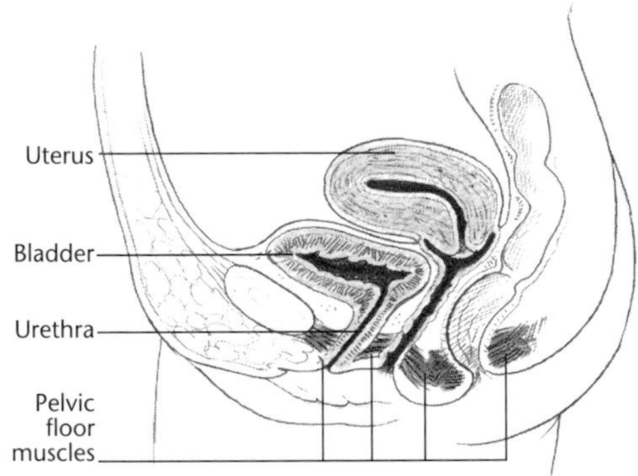

Normal position of pelvic organs

Sagging uterus puts pressure on bladder

Bladder

Urethra

Leaking urine

Weakened pelvic floor muscles

Position of pelvic organs in stress incontinence

WHAT CAUSES STRESS INCONTINENCE?

Pelvic floor muscles support the organs in your lower abdomen (left). Stress incontinence occurs when these supporting muscles are weakened (right). Under pressure from displaced organs, the muscle that circles the urethra cannot adequately stop the flow of urine, which may leak when you cough, sneeze, or jump.

(surgical removal of the uterus; see page 256). The results of this type of surgery for stress incontinence are excellent, as long as the other forms of incontinence, such as urge incontinence (see below) or overflow incontinence (see page 542), have been ruled out. Surgery cannot treat urge incontinence or overflow incontinence.

If you are past menopause and your doctor finds, during a pelvic examination, that the walls of your urethra have become thin or dry because your body is no longer producing the female hormone estrogen, he or she may prescribe estrogen cream (see page 363). You apply estrogen cream to the inside of your vagina and to your urethral opening three or more times a week to help restore elasticity to the tissues of your vagina and urethra and to improve muscle tone. Estrogen taken in pills (hormone replacement therapy, see page 359) also improves muscle tone in your vaginal area, but it may take longer than the cream to have an effect.

Mild stress incontinence may be treated with exercises to strengthen the supporting muscles in your pelvis (see page 238). These exercises (sometimes referred to as Kegels or pelvic-floor exercises) are done by tightening your urinary sphincter muscles as if you were stopping the flow of urine. To treat or prevent mild stress incontinence, you may need to work up to 150 Kegel exercises a day, holding the muscles tense for 10 seconds each time.

Your doctor may also recommend using weighted vaginal cones to strengthen these muscles. You insert a small cone (about the size of a tampon) into your vagina, tighten your pelvic muscles to hold the cone in place, and walk around for about 15 minutes (with the cone still in place). As your muscles gradually get stronger and tighter, you use increasingly larger and heavier cones. Alternatively, your doctor may recommend using an electrical device (see page 238) that can be inserted into your vagina to stimulate the muscles to contract, which strengthens them.

URGE INCONTINENCE

Urge incontinence is the involuntary leaking of urine after a sudden, uncontrollable urge to urinate. The leaking is caused by an involuntary contraction of the bladder muscle. In most cases, the cause of these spontaneous contractions of the bladder muscle is unknown. However, they can be triggered by activities such as running, laughing, or changing position; by an infection; or by a medication you are taking. For reasons that are unclear, in some women, urge incontinence may result from a reduced ability of their bladder to hold urine. In rare cases, people with neurological conditions such as stroke (see page 569) or multiple sclerosis (see page 586) can experience urge incontinence.

Your doctor may recommend a medication that helps suppress the contractions of the bladder muscle that trigger the incontinence. Bladder training (see below) can help increase the capacity of your bladder and reduce accidents. In some cases, medication and bladder training together are more effective than either one alone.

Bladder training

Bladder training can be an effective treatment of mild urge incontinence and overflow incontinence that are not caused by major anatomical problems, such as weakening of the pelvic muscles. The purpose of bladder training is to improve the ability of the bladder to hold urine by establishing a predictable pattern of urination. For example, if you record how often you urinate and find that you can usually go 90 minutes without an accident, urinate every 90 minutes for the next few days whether or not you feel the urge.

Use an egg timer or a wristwatch with a beeper to know when to urinate. After several days without an accident, increase the timing of urination to every 2 hours. Add half an hour every week until you reach a goal set by you and your doctor, and continue on this schedule. Eventually, you may find that you can go through the night without having to urinate.

OVERFLOW INCONTINENCE

Overflow incontinence is the periodic leaking of urine when your bladder is full to a point at which it cannot hold any more. Overflow incontinence can result from one of two causes—either the signal that your bladder is full is failing to reach your brain, or the muscles that allow your bladder to empty are unable to work properly to allow urine to flow out completely.

Overflow incontinence may occur in people who have disorders—such as diabetes (see page 617) or multiple sclerosis (see page 586)—that can damage the nerves that supply the bladder. Damage to these nerves can prevent them from relaying the signal to your brain that your bladder is full, or prevent the muscles in your bladder from functioning properly.

Overflow incontinence is difficult to treat with medication or surgery alone. A complete medical evaluation is necessary to determine the underlying cause of the incontinence (such as diabetes). Treating the underlying cause may be helpful in reducing the incontinence. Some women with overflow incontinence have to learn to urinate by straining or bearing down to help the bladder muscles expel urine. Other women with this form of incontinence may have to periodically insert a catheter (a hollow tube) into their urethra to allow urine to empty.

Urinary tract infections

Infections of the urinary tract are extremely common in women. Some women have them repeatedly. Urinary tract infections can be annoying, painful, and persistent, but they rarely cause a serious threat to your health. Infections most often affect the bladder, but they can also spread up the ureters (the tubes connecting the bladder and kidneys) to the kidneys. Most urinary tract infections occur when bacteria from the skin around the anus enter the urethra (the tube that empties urine from the bladder), usually during sexual intercourse, or from wiping incorrectly after using the toilet (always wipe from front to back).

Because urinary tract infections are caused by bacteria, they can be treated effectively with antibiotics. Treating an infection promptly is important because, if it is not treated, it can spread to the kidneys, where the infection is more

WARNING SIGNS
URINARY TRACT INFECTIONS

Urinary tract infections must be treated with antibiotics prescribed by your doctor. See your doctor if you experience any of the following symptoms:

- Pain or burning sensation during urination
- A sudden, strong urge to urinate
- Frequent need to urinate
- Fever or chills
- Soreness in your lower abdomen, back, or sides

Preventing urinary tract infections

You can take several relatively simple steps to reduce your risk of getting a urinary tract infection:

- After using the toilet, always wipe from front to back to avoid spreading bacteria from your anus to your urethral opening.
- Practice good hygiene by washing your genital and anal areas daily with soap and water, always wiping from front to back. Wash these areas before and after you have sexual intercourse.
- Drink plenty of fluids to flush bacteria out of your urinary system.
- Urinate frequently to help eliminate bacteria before they have a chance to multiply; urinating after you have sexual intercourse may help eliminate any bacteria that have entered your urethra.
- Follow the guidelines for safer sex (see page 337) to avoid contracting sexually transmitted diseases that can also cause urinary tract infections.

serious. Prompt treatment for a urinary tract infection is especially important if you have diabetes (see page 617), an obstructed kidney, or a suppressed immune system from a condition such as AIDS (see page 344). In people with these conditions, a severe infection in the kidneys is more likely to result in kidney damage, which can lead to kidney failure (see page 548).

CYSTITIS

Cystitis, an infection of the bladder caused by bacteria, is more common in women than men because a woman's shorter urethra enables bacteria to travel up to the bladder more quickly and easily. A woman's urethra is only 1 to 2 inches long (a man's urethra is about 4 to 6 inches long, running the length of his penis). In addition, the opening to a woman's urethra is very close to the openings to her vagina and anus, so that bacteria normally present in this area can easily enter the urethra during sexual intercourse.

Symptoms The symptoms of cystitis include an urge to urinate more frequently than usual, even when your bladder is not full; a painful, burning sensation during urination; a strong urge to urinate that occurs suddenly and without warning; or blood in your urine.

Diagnosis If your doctor suspects that you have cystitis, he or she will want to confirm the diagnosis by examining a sample of your urine under a microscope for the presence of bacteria and infection-fighting white blood cells.

Treatment Most urinary tract infections are cured quickly with antibiotics. If you have recurring bladder infections, your doctor may prescribe an antibiotic that you take after each time you have sexual intercourse. Your doctor may recommend that you drink plenty of fluids to help flush the bacteria out of your bladder and reduce burning when you urinate. Drinking large amounts of cranberry juice may help reduce the growth of bacteria, but it cannot totally eliminate bacteria when you have a urinary tract infection—only antibiotics can do that.

URETHRITIS

Urethritis is an infection of the urethra, the tube that carries urine from your bladder out of your body. In women, it is often difficult for doctors to differentiate urethritis from cystitis (infection of the bladder) because a woman's urethra is short, allowing bacteria easy access to the bladder. If urination is painful and frequent but a urinalysis finds no bacteria present in your urine, the infection may be in your urethra.

If you have recurring infections, your doctor may want to examine your urethra for small abnormal pockets of tissue called urethral diverticula. One of these pockets can trap urine, creating an environment favorable for the growth of bacteria. The presence of bacteria can lead to inflammation, which can cause tenderness in the area around your urethral opening.

Urethral diverticula may also contribute to urinary incontinence (see page 538) because urine can leak out of the pocket and out of your body at any time, such as when you change position or have intercourse. Your doctor can confirm the presence of a diverticulum by feeling the wall of your urethra with his or her hand for an abnormal bulge or by placing a thin viewing tube called a urethroscope into your urethra to examine it directly. If detected, a diverticulum is usually removed by cutting out the abnormal tissue through a small incision at the opening of the vagina.

Urinalysis

A urinalysis is a diagnostic evaluation of a sample of urine. Urinalysis helps doctors diagnose kidney disorders and urinary tract infections. The test is also used to measure substances in the urine that may indicate the presence of other disorders, such as diabetes (see page 617). If you are having a urinalysis, you will be asked to urinate directly into a small sterile container provided by your doctor. To avoid contaminating the urine sample with bacteria from your vagina, you must clean your vaginal area first with a moist cloth (wiping from front to back). Expel a small amount of urine into the toilet and then urinate into the container, making sure not to touch the container to your vaginal area.

If the urinalysis shows a high level of bacteria in your urine, a drop of urine will be cultured (the bacteria in the sample are grown in the laboratory and examined under a microscope). The culture is treated with various antibiotics to find the one that is most effective in destroying the bacteria.

Questions women ask
Urinary tract infections

Q Are my urinary tract infections in any way related to my sexual activity?

A They could be. The thrusting motion of intercourse can massage bacteria from the skin around your vagina and anus into the opening of your urethra. Urinating immediately after you have intercourse may help flush out the bacteria and help you avoid this type of sex-related urinary tract infection, which is sometimes referred to as honeymoon cystitis. Washing your genital and anal areas before and after you have intercourse (wiping from front to back) can also help. In any case, talk to your doctor about your infections.

Q Why does my urinary tract infection keep returning?

A If you have taken preventive measures, such as always wiping from front to back after using the toilet and urinating immediately after having intercourse, and you still get these infections, you may have an abnormality in your urinary tract that is interfering with the flow of urine. An inadequate flow of urine or a urethral diverticulum (a small pouch bulging out of the lining of the urethra) can encourage bacteria to become established and multiply. Your infection may be recurring because you did not take all of the antibiotic your doctor prescribed to treat the infection and, as a result, the bacteria have not been completely eliminated from your system.

Q I am planning to become pregnant. I have had several bladder infections. If I have one while I'm pregnant, could it cause miscarriage or infect my fetus?

A No. However, it is possible for an undetected urinary tract infection to cause a pregnant woman to go into labor early (preterm labor, see page 427). You are more susceptible to urinary tract infections during pregnancy (see page 420) because of hormonal changes that may cause the muscles in your urinary tract to relax, allowing more bacteria to reach your bladder. During your pregnancy, tell your doctor immediately if you have any symptoms of a urinary tract infection.

Q I went through menopause about 2 years ago and since then I have had several painful urinary tract infections. What can I do to avoid them?

A If you are not taking estrogen in hormone replacement therapy (see page 359), you should consider it. The lack of estrogen can cause the tissues of your urethra and vagina to become dry and thinned out, which makes them more prone to injury or infection. Estrogen improves circulation in all the tissues of your genital tract and makes them more resilient and less susceptible to infection. Talk to your doctor about your choices.

PYELONEPHRITIS

Pyelonephritis is a kidney infection, and it is more serious than an infection in your lower urinary tract. In rare cases, a kidney infection can damage the kidneys and lead to kidney failure (see page 548). Prompt treatment of a bladder infection is essential to prevent it from spreading to your kidneys.

Symptoms The symptoms of a kidney infection are similar to those of other urinary tract infections—including frequent urination; pain during urination; and sudden, strong urges to urinate. However, a kidney infection usually also causes fever, chills, and pain in your back or sides.

Diagnosis Your doctor can diagnose a kidney infection by a physical examination in which he or she taps gently on your back to see if you feel any tenderness in the area around your kidneys and by a urinalysis (see page 543). Your doctor may also want to determine if you have

SYMPTOM CHART

Painful urination

Discomfort when urinating, sometimes accompanied by pain in the lower abdomen.

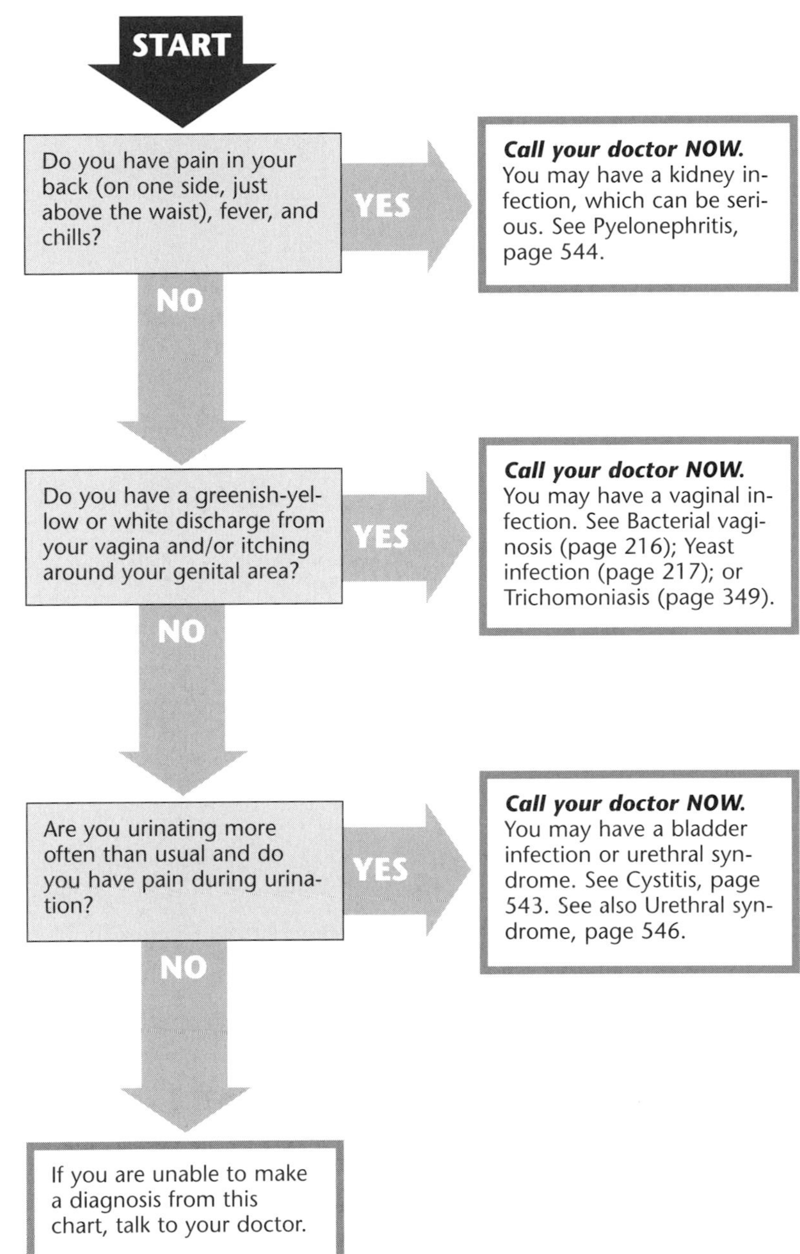

Preventing urinary tract infections

Here are some tips for avoiding urinary tract infections:

- Always wipe from front to back after using the toilet
- Wash your genital area daily
- Urinate frequently
- Urinate after sexual intercourse
- Drink plenty of fluids, including cranberry juice
- Don't use deodorant tampons or pantyliners
- Practice safer sex (see page 337)

an underlying problem that is contributing to the infection. For example, you may be more likely to have urinary tract infections if you have reflux, a condition in which urine occasionally flows backward from your bladder through the ureters and up toward your kidneys instead of exiting your body through the urethra. Inside your bladder, some of the bacteria in the urine, which are usually eliminated when you urinate, may multiply enough to cause an infection in your kidneys. Kidney stones (see below) can also make you more susceptible to infections in your urinary tract.

Treatment If you have a kidney infection, you are likely to be hospitalized for at least 24 hours and given intravenous antibiotics. Antibiotics taken by mouth may not reach the kidneys in sufficient amounts to cure the infection.

URETHRAL SYNDROME

Urethral syndrome is a condition in which you experience the symptoms of a urinary tract infection repeatedly, but standard testing (urinalysis, see page 543) does not detect a bacterial infection. You may experience burning, tingling, or irritation during urination; a persistent feeling of urgency to urinate; and unusually frequent urination. In many cases, the symptoms occur after sexual intercourse.

A number of factors can cause urethral syndrome, including an undiagnosed urinary tract infection or a sexually transmitted disease caused by an organism called chlamydia (see page 339). Urethral syndrome can also result from injury to the urethra (usually during sexual intercourse) or a deficiency of the female hormone estrogen, which makes the tissues of the urethra thinner and more fragile.

It is often difficult to find the cause of urethral syndrome or a treatment that works. If a urinalysis does not show that you have a urinary tract infection but the symptoms continue, your doctor may recommend treatment with antibiotics in case you have a mild infection that has not shown up on tests. Your doctor may also prescribe anti-inflammatory drugs to reduce inflammation and irritation of your urethra. In some cases, a cream containing estrogen that you apply directly to the area around the urethra may be helpful.

Kidney disorders

The kidneys remove waste and excess fluid from your body in the form of urine. The kidneys also regulate your body's balance of important chemicals, including sodium and potassium, and produce hormones and vitamins that affect the function of many other organs in your body. An imbalance of these vital chemicals can cause you to either retain water or lose water abnormally. Kidney stones and kidney failure are common kidney disorders.

KIDNEY STONES

A kidney stone is a mass of crystallized substances in urine that form a clump in the kidney. A kidney stone can be as small as a speck of dust or as large as a golf ball. Kidney stones are most common among young and middle-aged adults; they are more common in men than in women. The cause of kidney stones is not known but factors that can increase your risk of developing them include not drinking enough fluids, a family history of kidney stones, recurring urinary tract infections, limited physical activity for several weeks, or pregnancy. Kidney stones often occur in the area where a ureter joins a kidney or in one of the ureters. Many people have repeated occurrences.

Symptoms Some people with kidney stones have no symptoms. But most people experience at least some symptoms, many of which are similar to the symptoms of a kidney infection (pyelonephritis, see page 544). These include severe, sudden pain in your back or lower side; fever, chills, and weakness; burning during urination; a frequent need to urinate in small amounts; cloudy or foul-smelling urine; blood in your urine; nausea and vomiting; and an inability to urinate when you have the sensation that

Intravenous pyelography

Intravenous pyelography (IVP) is an X-ray examination that is used to diagnose structural defects or abnormalities of the kidneys and urinary tract, and some forms of kidney disease. An IVP can also show obstructions, such as kidney stones, in the urinary tract.

If you are scheduled to have an IVP, your doctor will ask you not to drink fluids for 8 to 12 hours before the test. You will also be given a laxative to take the day before the test to empty your bowels, which allows the doctor to get a better image of your urinary tract, including your kidneys. During the IVP, you lie on an examining table while a series of X-rays is taken of your abdomen. A special dye (called a radiocontrast agent) is then injected into a vein in your arm; the dye travels to your kidneys and urinary tract. Another set of X-rays is taken 5, 10, and 20 minutes later to follow the path of the dye out of your kidneys. When the dye has filled your bladder, you will be asked to urinate, and another set of X-rays will then be taken to determine if your bladder has emptied completely.

your bladder is full. If you notice any of these symptoms, call your doctor immediately.

Diagnosis A specialized X-ray called an intravenous pyelogram (see above), an ultrasound (see page 405), or a simple X-ray of the kidney and lower abdomen can often detect a stone.

Treatment Even without treatment, most small kidney stones are carried out of your kidney in urine and passed from your body within 3 weeks of their formation. Depending on the size of the stone, it can be extremely painful when you pass one. To help this process along, drink plenty of fluids—at least eight 8-ounce glasses of water a day. In some cases, medication may help dissolve stones that do not pass.

Lithotripsy Most kidney stones that do not pass can be removed in a procedure called extracorporeal (outside the body) shock wave lithotripsy. The procedure usually does not require an overnight stay in the hospital, but it can be painful. You will be given intravenous sedatives, an epidural (see page 260), or, less often, general anesthesia (see page 261). In lithotripsy, high-energy shock waves are directed at your kidneys from different angles to break up a stone into small pieces that can be passed out of your body in urine. X-rays are used to precisely locate the stone and guide the procedure.

Lithotripsy usually uses water to conduct the shock waves through the surface of the skin to the kidney stone. During the procedure, you will be positioned in a water bath or on top of a cushion filled with water. When the shock waves coming in from different angles meet at the kidney stone, they produce a burst of energy that shatters the stone.

After the procedure, you will be asked to drink lots of fluids and walk around to encourage the pieces of the stone to be passed in your urine. You may experience some temporary discomfort as the stones are passed; most will be passed within 8 to 10 hours in the hospital.

Removing a stone If you have an infection, obstruction, or kidney damage, kidney stones can be removed surgically. Your doctor can remove a kidney stone using a thin, flexible viewing tube (cystoscope, see page 540) inserted through your urethra and bladder to reach a stone in your ureter. In an alternative procedure, the doctor may insert a tube through an incision in your back and guide it through your kidney to remove a stone in your ureter.

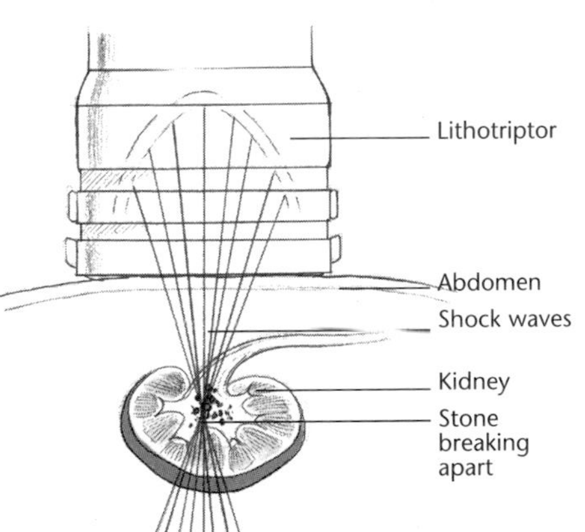

LITHOTRIPSY
Lithotripsy is a procedure used to destroy kidney stones. A machine called a lithotriptor, which is placed on the abdomen, emits shock waves and focuses them on the kidney stone to break it into fragments.

ACUTE KIDNEY FAILURE

In acute kidney failure (or renal failure), the kidneys suddenly lose their ability to filter waste from the blood. Acute kidney failure is life threatening. However, immediate treatment is often effective. The most common causes of acute kidney failure include severe bleeding, dehydration, or shock, which can reduce circulation to such an extent that the blood supply to the kidneys is interrupted. This interruption in blood flow can cause some of the tissue to die.

Acute kidney failure can also result from severe infection with streptococcal bacteria, from a variety of diseases that affect the whole body (such as lupus, see page 641), or from severe, uncontrolled high blood pressure. Your kidneys can fail if you ingest toxic substances such as solvents or heavy metals (such as lead), or if your kidneys have a reaction to a particular medication such as an antibiotic or antiseizure medication.

WARNING SIGNS
ACUTE KIDNEY FAILURE

Acute kidney failure is an emergency that requires immediate hospital treatment. Call your doctor or an ambulance immediately if you have any of the following symptoms:

- Fluid retention; you are urinating much less than usual
- Blood in the urine or urine that is dark or black
- Drowsiness or confusion
- Seizures
- Loss of appetite and nausea or vomiting with any of the above symptoms

Treatment If you have acute kidney failure, you need immediate treatment in the hospital. With prompt treatment, acute kidney failure can usually be reversed. Many people recover within 6 weeks, although their kidneys may not regain their total function for as long as a year. Your doctor will regulate your intake of fluids and measure your urine output to ensure that your body is not retaining fluids. If you are retaining fluids, your intake of liquids will be restricted.

You will be put on a diet that is high in carbohydrates and low in protein, potassium, and salt; this diet relieves the kidneys from the extra effort required to process protein. In the early stages of acute kidney failure, you may need to have dialysis, a treatment that takes over the function of your kidneys while they recover. Dialysis can remove excess fluid and acid from your body and establish normal levels of chemicals such as salt and potassium. Dialysis can also prevent such complications of kidney failure as water retention and congestive heart failure.

CHRONIC KIDNEY FAILURE

Chronic kidney failure is the loss of kidney function over a period of time. In some cases, chronic kidney failure has no symptoms in the early stage and may go undiagnosed and untreated for years. But over time chronic kidney failure can have an effect on most systems of your body. Eventually, your kidneys stop functioning altogether. Chronic kidney failure is usually the result of another chronic disease a person has, particularly diabetes (see page 617). If you have diabetes, it is extremely important to regulate the level of sugar in your blood because high sugar levels can lead to kidney damage. People who have lupus (see page 641) or sickle-cell anemia (see page 493) may also develop chronic kidney failure. Kidney stones, high blood pressure (see page 480), glomerulonephritis (inflammation of the kidneys), or other conditions that directly affect the kidneys can also lead to chronic kidney failure.

Symptoms The symptoms of chronic kidney failure can occur gradually over a period of several years. You may not have any warning that the functioning of your kidneys is decreasing. Chronic kidney failure causes uremia, a buildup in your blood of urea and other waste products that are normally excreted in urine. You may develop anemia (see page 493) or stomach ulcers (see page 518). Abnormal levels of potassium, calcium, and other chemicals may affect your memory or ability to concentrate or may cause muscle twitching in your arms and legs.

Your bones may fracture easily because the condition causes calcium to be lost from your bones, making them weak. Some people with chronic kidney failure also have a bad taste in their mouth and itching all over their body. Fluid retention is a common symptom of chronic kidney failure that can lead to congestive heart failure (see page 492).

Diagnosis If you have chronic kidney failure, both of your kidneys may appear smaller than normal on an ultrasound (see page 405). Blood tests will show elevated levels of two waste products—urea and creatinine—that your kidneys usually excrete in urine. Your doctor will compare the levels of urea and creatinine in your blood to the levels of these waste products in your urine to evaluate how well your kidneys are filtering your blood.

Treatment There is no cure for chronic kidney failure, but measures can be taken to slow its progress and reduce complications. The underlying cause of chronic kidney failure—such as high blood pressure, urinary tract infections, or diabetes—must be treated. Severe anemia may require a blood transfusion or an injection of a hormone called erythropoietin. Erythropoietin is made by the kidneys and signals the bone marrow to make more blood. In people with chronic kidney failure, the level of erythropoietin may be low or their kidneys may not make enough of the hormone to maintain the blood at a normal level.

Nutrition is an important part of treatment for chronic kidney failure. You will be placed on a diet that restricts fluids, proteins, potassium, salt, and phosphorus but provides the calories and nutrients your body needs. A restriction of protein in your diet can help prevent nausea, vomiting, and a decreased appetite. Limiting your consumption of salt may help lower your blood pressure if you have high blood pressure. If necessary, your doctor will give you guidelines about how to regulate your intake of water.

If your kidneys have completely or almost completely stopped functioning, you will require regular dialysis, a treatment in which an artificial kidney takes over the functioning of your kidneys, or you may need a kidney transplant (see page 550). Although dialysis is sometimes a temporary measure for treating acute kidney failure, it is usually used on a regular basis by people who have chronic kidney failure.

Dialysis In a person whose kidneys are not functioning adequately, a machine called a dialyzer functions as an artificial kidney. It takes over the kidneys' job of removing waste and excess water and acid from the blood and restoring the body's chemical balance. Most people with kidney failure need to have dialysis three times a week; the procedure usually takes about 3 to 4 hours. In addition to filtering wastes and excess water from your blood, a dialyzer adjusts the balance of calcium, potassium, and acid in your blood.

Peritoneal dialysis Another kind of dialysis, called peritoneal dialysis, is a procedure that you can perform at home. In peritoneal dialysis, your blood is filtered inside your abdomen, without the use of

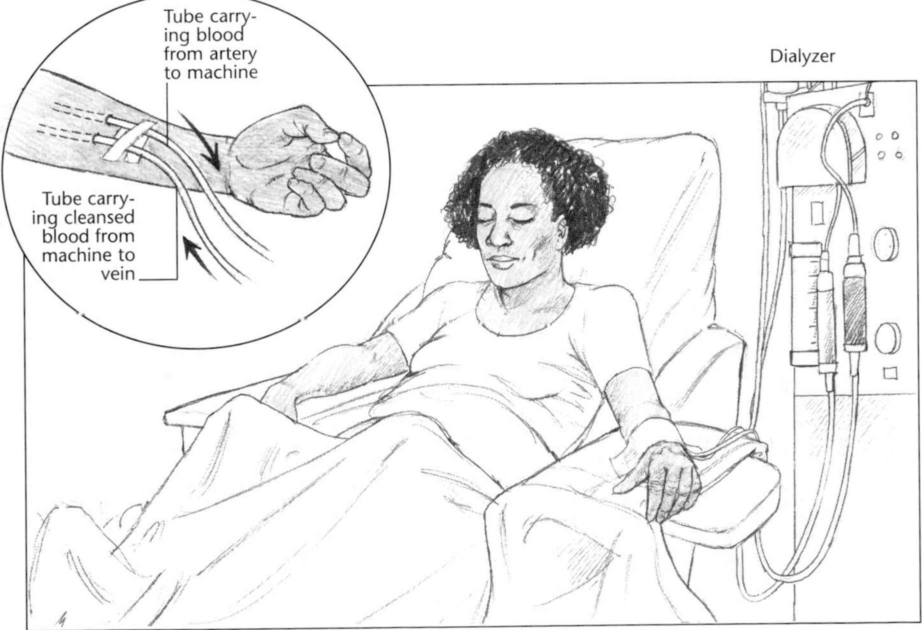

HOW KIDNEY DIALYSIS IS DONE
In kidney dialysis, blood from an artery in your arm or leg (inset) flows through a thin plastic tube to a machine called a dialyzer. In the dialyzer, the blood passes through a porous membrane filter that serves as the artificial kidney. The cleansed blood then flows out of the machine through another tube that has been inserted into a nearby vein in the same arm or leg.

a complicated machine. Before you begin regular treatments with peritoneal dialysis, a plastic tube called a catheter is permanently implanted in your abdomen. When you give yourself a treatment, you attach a special bag containing a cleansing fluid to the catheter.

During peritoneal dialysis, the cleansing fluid flows through the catheter into your abdominal cavity and is left in place for several hours. The cleansing fluid draws waste products and excess water and salt, potassium, and other chemicals out of the blood vessels lining your abdomen. When you release a clamp on the tube that leads to the bag, the mixture of the cleansing fluid, excess water, waste products, and chemicals drains from your abdomen through the catheter and out into the bag.

You will need to perform this procedure, called continuous ambulatory peritoneal dialysis, four or five times a day. In another type of peritoneal dialysis, called continuous cycling peritoneal dialysis, a machine introduces the fluid into your abdomen and drains the fluid and other materials automatically several times during the night while you sleep.

Kidney transplant Kidney transplants are successful in most cases. A person who receives a new kidney in a transplant can function well. If you have a serious medical condition, such as heart disease (see page 461), you may not be able to undergo the major surgery required for a transplant.

It can be difficult to find a compatible donor—that is, a person whose blood type and tissue type match yours. Finding as close a match as possible reduces the likelihood that your body will reject the new kidney. A brother, sister, or parent is the most likely to be a compatible donor. Because a person needs only one kidney to function, a donor who gives up one kidney can live in good health with his or her remaining kidney. (For information about how to become an organ donor, see page 711.)

If a relative cannot donate a kidney, you may be able to find a compatible kidney from a center that receives kidneys from people who died in accidents or of other causes. However, you might have to wait a long time (an average of 2 years) before a compatible kidney can be found.

After you have a kidney transplant, you must take medication every day to prevent your immune system from rejecting the new kidney. This medication also suppresses the ability of your immune system to fight off invading disease-causing organisms, so you will be more susceptible to infections. You may experience anxiety about the continuing possibility that your body will reject the new kidney. However, most people who are eligible for a kidney transplant choose it over long-term dialysis because a transplant significantly improves the quality of their life.

KIDNEY TRANSPLANT

A kidney transplant can be an effective treatment for people who have kidney failure. Your body can function well with only one kidney. In most cases, the transplanted kidney is implanted in the right lower corner of the abdomen and connected to the iliac artery and iliac vein, which provide its circulation. The ureter (the tube that carries urine from the kidney to the bladder) of the transplanted kidney is connected to your bladder. In most cases, the damaged kidneys are left in place because they are small, shrunken, scarred, and harmless and removing them requires a difficult surgical procedure. They are removed before a transplant only if they cause recurring infections or bleeding.

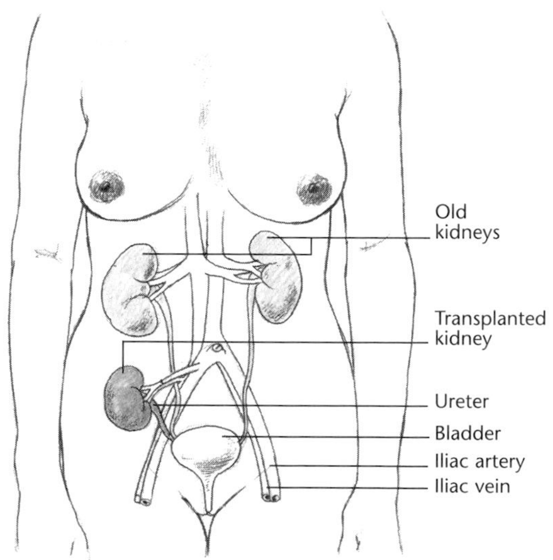

CHAPTER 21

Your bones and joints

Contents

Osteoporosis, a disorder that causes bones to become thin and weak, and osteoarthritis, a disorder that causes joints to deteriorate, are two potentially debilitating conditions that are very common among women.

Half of all women over 50 eventually develop a fracture as a result of osteoporosis. These fractures are not only painful, they can severely limit a woman's activity and threaten her independence. Although osteoporosis most noticeably affects older women, the disease develops over a lifetime. Taking steps to prevent this debilitating disorder is extremely important, no matter what your age.

Osteoarthritis is a degenerative disorder of the joints. Although the exact cause is unknown, osteoarthritis may result from wear and tear on the joints that occurs over time, causing the smooth lining of the joint (called cartilage) to gradually deteriorate. Although little can be done to reverse the effects of osteoarthritis, you can take measures to reduce symptoms such as pain and inflammation.

Osteoporosis

Osteoporosis is a disease that causes bones to become thin, porous, and weak and, therefore, prone to fracture. Almost all women who are 75 and older, and many women who are approaching menopause, have bones that show signs of osteoporosis. A broken hip and curved upper spine are often thought to be a consequence of old age but they are, in fact, effects of osteoporosis.

One in three women who lives to be 90 will fracture a hip, usually as the result of osteoporosis. One out of five women who breaks a hip dies of complications from it, such as pneumonia or a blood clot that travels to her lungs. Many women who survive a hip fracture are unable to walk without help or to return to their former level of physical activity and independence.

Although you are unlikely to experience the effects of osteoporosis until you are past menopause, the eating and exercise habits you acquired during your childhood, adolescence, and young adulthood make an important difference in whether or not you will develop the disorder. Getting enough calcium in your diet and exercising regularly are essential for building and maintaining the strength of your bones throughout your life. The stronger your bones are before you reach menopause, the less they will be weakened by the loss of bone strength and density that normally occurs after menopause.

Bone is living tissue that undergoes constant change. Throughout your life, your bones—into which calcium is deposited—continually break down and rebuild themselves. Until you are about 30, the rate of bone formation is greater than the rate of breakdown; this process gradually builds up your bones to their peak density. In women, the hormone estrogen plays a key role in keeping bones strong. Estrogen causes bones to absorb calcium from the blood and slows the loss of calcium from bone. After age 30, both men and women begin gradually to lose more bone than their body makes. In women, menopause causes a decline in estrogen that rapidly accelerates the loss of bone tissue. The highest rate of bone loss occurs in the first 5 to 7 years after menopause.

As osteoporosis progresses, your bones gradually become more porous, like a sponge with tiny holes that grow larger and larger. The percentage of calcium stored in your bones decreases, resulting in brittle bones that break easily. When your estrogen level falls at menopause, your bones weaken quickly and continue to lose density for the rest of your life unless you take estrogen in hormone replacement therapy (see page 359) to replace the estrogen your body no longer produces. Estrogen slows bone loss significantly and may even increase bone density.

Most women have no symptoms of osteoporosis until they fracture a bone. Although osteoporosis can affect any bone in your body, fractures are most common in the vertebrae (the small bones of the spinal column), the hip, or the wrist. Most fractures in the hip or wrist are the result of a fall, but vertebrae can deteriorate gradually and fracture simply from the physical stress of everyday activities, such as bending over.

Living, changing bone

The 206 bones in your body may seem like permanent structures but they are, in fact, living tissue that is constantly changing. Inside the hollow center of bones is the marrow, which produces all the blood cells in your body. The marrow is surrounded by spongy bone called the medullary canal, which in turn is surrounded by a layer of dense bone called cortical bone. Cortical bone, which is made of the protein collagen, contains cells that maintain bone tissues. Dense deposits of calcium give bone its strength. Your bones are covered by a thin, hard membrane called the periosteum, which contains nerves and blood vessels; the periosteum is essential for the growth and formation of new bone.

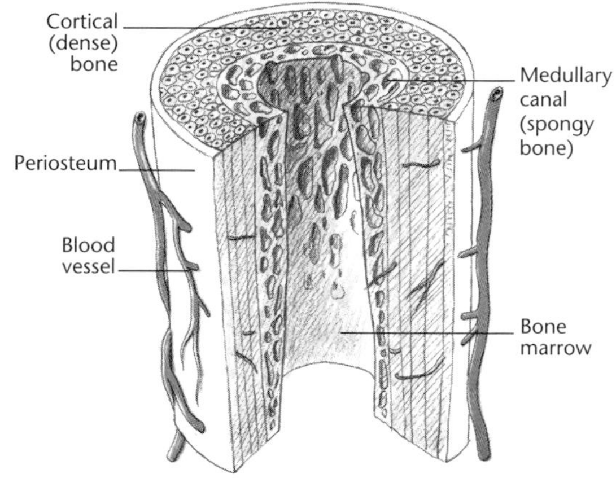

BONE—A LIVING TISSUE

Bone is covered by a hard outer membrane called the periosteum, which is interwoven with a system of blood vessels and nerves that provides for the formation of new bone. Beneath the periosteum is dense cortical bone, which is filled with circular structures that contain blood vessels and nerves. Inside cortical bone is a layer of spongy bone called the medullary canal that surrounds a center filled with bone marrow. Bone marrow produces all of your blood cells.

OSTEOPOROSIS

In osteoporosis, bone gradually becomes more porous, like a sponge with tiny holes that grow larger and larger. Age and the loss of estrogen at menopause decrease your body's ability to absorb calcium and deposit it in your bones. If the percentage of calcium stored in your bones decreases, the area of spongy bone grows larger while the area of dense bone becomes smaller, making the bone hollow and weak and more susceptible to fracture. The top illustration shows healthy, dense bone tissue. The bottom illustration shows bone that has become porous and weakened by osteoporosis.

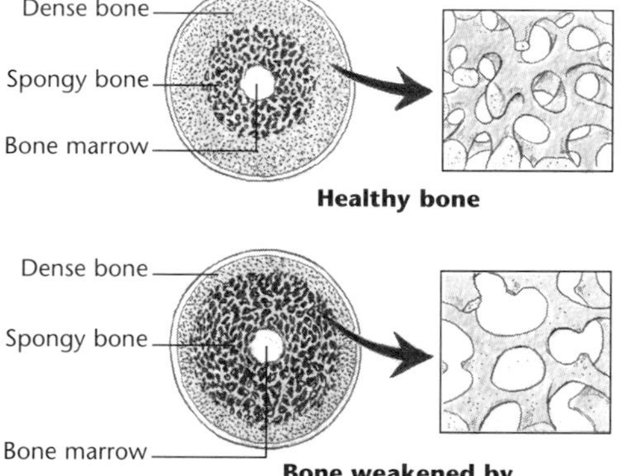

Healthy bone

Bone weakened by osteoporosis

PREVENTING OSTEOPOROSIS

Every woman needs to be concerned about preventing osteoporosis. Effective treatments of the disease are available for many women. But if the disease has already significantly thinned your bones and made them fragile, it is not always possible to restore enough strength to them to prevent fractures. Therefore, it is important to maximize the density of your bones throughout your life so that the effects of bone loss as you age are less severe. Adequate intake of calcium and vitamin D (which helps your body absorb calcium) and regular weight-bearing exercise (such as walking) and strengthening exercises (such as lifting weights) are the most important preventive measures you can take.

If you are past menopause, taking estrogen in hormone replacement therapy (HRT; see page 359) to replace the estrogen your body no longer produces is the most effective way to help prevent osteoporosis. Even if you already have osteoporosis, these measures may help stop further bone loss and restore some of your bone.

Calcium Getting sufficient amounts of calcium throughout your life can help keep your bones strong. About 99 percent of the calcium your body needs is stored in your bones. Calcium is necessary not only to maintain bone structure but also for other body functions such as contractions of the heart and other muscles. When you do not get enough calcium from your diet, your body withdraws calcium from your bones to meet its needs. This bone-robbing process accelerates after menopause.

Most women get less than 500 milligrams of calcium a day, far below the recommended requirement of 1,000 to 1,500 milligrams. An 8-ounce glass of skim milk provides about 300 milligrams of calcium; other good sources of calcium (see page 58) include calcium-fortified orange juice; nonfat yogurt; and dark green, leafy vegetables such as turnip greens.

For women who do not get an adequate amount of calcium from their diet, doctors may recommend calcium supplements to bring their daily calcium intake up to the suggested level. Calcium supplements are available in tablets, chewable tablets, and liquid preparations. Make sure you read the label on the supplement to determine how much elemental calcium each dose contains; elemental calcium is the actual amount of calcium your body absorbs.

Your daily calcium needs throughout life

You can get 1,200 milligrams (mg) of calcium by drinking four 8-ounce glasses of skim milk. Other good sources include nonfat yogurt; low-fat cheese; tofu; sardines; and dark green, leafy vegetables, such as turnip greens.

Ages 11 to 24

1,200-1,500 mg

Over 24

1,000 mg

1,200-1,500 mg if you are pregnant or breast-feeding

Ages 50 to 65 (past menopause)

1,000 mg if you are taking hormone replacement therapy

1,500 mg if you are not taking hormone replacement therapy

Over 65

1,500 mg

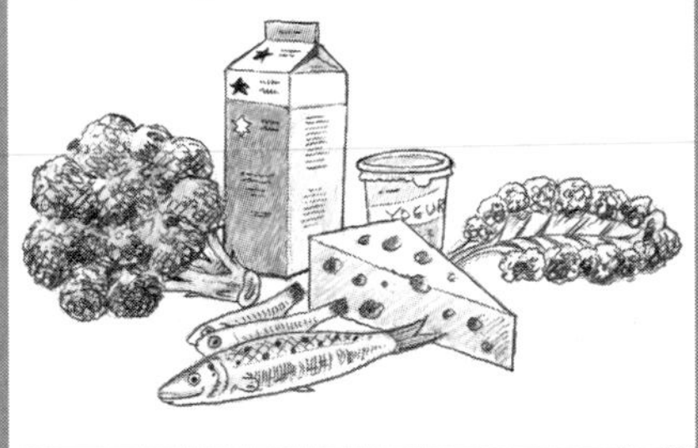

Vitamin D Vitamin D plays an important role in preventing bone loss—it helps your body absorb calcium from the intestinal tract into your bloodstream. It is relatively easy to get sufficient amounts of vitamin D from foods such as fortified dairy products, eggs, and oily fish such as salmon. Skim milk fortified with vitamin D is an especially good source and it does not have the fat and calories of low-fat and whole milk. The dietary requirement for vitamin D is 400 international units a day; an 8-ounce glass of milk contains 100 international units. Although your body manufactures vitamin D when your skin is exposed to the sun, you are unlikely to get enough of the vitamin without consuming some in your diet. If you are on a very strict low-fat diet, your doctor may recommend that you get your allowance of vitamin D from a multivitamin or calcium supplement.

Weight-bearing exercise To build strong bones, you must do activities in which you are putting weight on your bones—called weight-bearing exercise. Walking, jogging, stair climbing, weight lifting, and push-ups are excellent weight-bearing exercises. Bones respond to weight-bearing exercise by adding new calcium and becoming denser and stronger. Activities in

Who is at risk of osteoporosis?

Women are far more likely to get osteoporosis than men. A number of factors other than being female can increase your risk. You are more likely to develop osteoporosis if you:

- Are past menopause (either naturally or as a result of the surgical removal of your ovaries) and are not taking estrogen in hormone replacement therapy
- Have a family history of osteoporosis
- Are white or Asian
- Have a small body frame
- Have a thin or lean body or are underweight
- Lead a sedentary lifestyle
- Get an insufficient amount of calcium in your diet
- Have a history of smoking
- Have undergone long-term therapy with corticosteroids (synthetic hormones) for such conditions as rheumatoid arthritis or inflammatory bowel disease
- Consume an excessive amount of alcohol or caffeine
- Have a gastrointestinal disorder, such as peptic ulcers or lactose intolerance, that interferes with the body's ability to absorb calcium

which your weight is supported, such as swimming, are less likely to help maintain or increase your bone density.

Active people of all ages have a higher bone density than people who are sedentary. Weight-bearing exercise can help girls and young women increase their bone density during the critical years (ages 2 to 20) when 95 percent of their bone is being built. The more bone you have built up during childhood, the more protection you will have against osteoporosis and debilitating fractures later in life.

It is never too late to start exercising. Even after you reach menopause, walking 45 minutes a day several days a week may help slow bone loss. Doing moderate weight-lifting exercises can also help you maintain strength in your bones and muscles and your ability to do everyday tasks. To be most effective in maintaining strength in your bones, exercise must be combined with a calcium-rich diet and, after menopause, with hormone replacement therapy (see page 359).

If you are diagnosed with osteoporosis, your risk of bone fractures is extremely high. Your doctor may recommend that you do only low-impact exercises, such as walking, and avoid activities—such as golf, bowling, tennis, or racquetball—that involve twisting or unbalanced movement.

TREATING OSTEOPOROSIS

Although prevention is best when it comes to osteoporosis, medical science is working to find new treatments for the disease. As the population ages, increasing numbers of women will develop osteoporosis. Many promising new treatments are being developed that are likely to substantially reduce the incidence of fractures and disability that result from the disease.

Hormone replacement therapy Because estrogen is so important in maintaining bone density in women, doctors usually prescribe hormone replacement therapy (HRT; see page 359) at menopause for women who are at risk of developing osteoporosis. If you begin taking estrogen as menopause begins, it can prevent the dramatic bone loss that occurs during the first few years after menopause. Estrogen can also help restore bone in older women who have already experienced bone loss.

However, estrogen works only as long as you are taking it. If you stop, bone loss will begin—at the same rate as if you had never taken it. Estrogen also significantly reduces your risk of heart disease (see page 461) and prevents many unpleasant symptoms of menopause (see page 353), such as hot flashes.

Calcitonin If a bone density test (see page 558) shows signs of osteoporosis and you are unable to take HRT, your doctor may recommend calcitonin, a naturally occurring hormone produced by the thyroid gland. You take a synthetic form of the hormone (calcitonin salmon) in a nasal spray (once a day) or in an injection (every day or every other day). Calcitonin slows bone loss and can increase bone density in some women with osteoporosis. The drug may also relieve disabling back pain in women with osteoporosis.

Calcitonin is not a substitute for estrogen and it is not intended for long-term use. The drug is not as effective as estrogen in preventing fractures; nor does it have the beneficial effects against heart disease and Alzheimer's disease that

Is your medication causing bone loss?

A number of common medications contribute to bone loss by reducing your body's ability to absorb calcium from your intestines. This limits the amount of calcium that is available for your bones. If you are taking any medication on a regular basis, ask your doctor if it could be affecting your bone density. You may be able to reduce this problem by taking the medication through an inhaler or in an injection. When taken in either of these forms, the drug bypasses your intestines.

To maintain your bone density, your doctor may recommend that you increase your intake of calcium and have hormone replacement therapy (see page 359). Do not discontinue your medication or decrease the dosage without talking to your doctor. You may also want to ask your doctor if you should have a bone density test (see page 558) to evaluate your risk of osteoporosis. You may be at risk of bone loss if you are taking any of the following medications:

- **Glucocorticoids** Glucocorticoids are corticosteroid drugs (synthetic hormones that reduce inflammation) that are prescribed for rheumatoid arthritis (see page 645), severe asthma, allergies, inflammatory bowel disease (see page 527), liver disease, lupus (see page 641), and cancer, and to prevent rejection in organ transplants. These drugs can weaken bones by reducing the ability of your digestive tract to absorb calcium from the food you eat, thereby depriving your body of the calcium it needs to maintain strong bones. Glucocorticoids also stimulate cells that destroy bone and inhibit cells that build bone. Because of these side effects, glucocorticoids are prescribed only in severe cases for which other medications are not likely to be as effective.
- **Thyroid hormone** High doses of thyroid hormone, which is often prescribed for people who have hypothyroidism (see page 624), cause accelerated bone loss. If you are being treated with thyroid hormone, your doctor will periodically monitor the level of the hormone in your blood to make sure it is not excessive.
- **Antiseizure medications** Phenytoin and phenobarbital—medications that are used to control seizures in people who have epilepsy (see page 578)—may contribute to the development of osteoporosis if they are taken in high doses over a long period of time. Antiseizure medications can interfere with your body's use of vitamin D, which promotes calcium absorption.
- **Antacids that contain aluminum** Some antacids contain aluminum. If they are taken in large quantities, the aluminum replaces some of the calcium in your bones, potentially weakening them. Some antacid tablets actually contain calcium. Check the label on any antacid that you are taking and try to avoid those than contain aluminum.
- **Gonadotropin-releasing hormones** Gonadotropin-releasing hormones, which are used to treat endometriosis (see page 230), contribute to bone loss if they are used for a long time by women who already have low bone density. These medications reduce bone density by lowering the level of estrogen in women who take them. For this reason, they are usually not prescribed for periods of more than 6 to 9 months.
- **Cholestyramine** Cholestyramine is a medication that is frequently used to lower cholesterol level. However, the drug also reduces the body's ability to absorb vitamin D, which helps the body absorb calcium from foods.

estrogen does. Treatment with calcitonin sometimes causes side effects such as bloating and gastrointestinal discomfort, which usually subside over time.

Alendronate sodium A newer, nonhormonal treatment for osteoporosis is a medication called alendronate sodium, which can build healthy bone and restore some bone that has already been lost. Alendronate sodium can reduce the incidence and severity of fractures in women who have osteoporosis. Like calcitonin, alendronate sodium is recommended primarily for women who are not good candidates for hormone replacement therapy because it does not provide the additional health benefits that estrogen does, such as protection against heart disease. For example, a doctor might recommend alendronate sodium to a woman who has been recently diagnosed with breast cancer.

You take alendronate sodium in a pill each morning along with a 6- to 8-ounce glass of water at least 30 minutes before you eat or drink anything else or take another medication.

The most common side effects of this treatment, which are usually mild, are abdominal discomfort and muscle pain. Less common side effects include digestive problems such as nausea and heartburn.

BONE FRACTURES

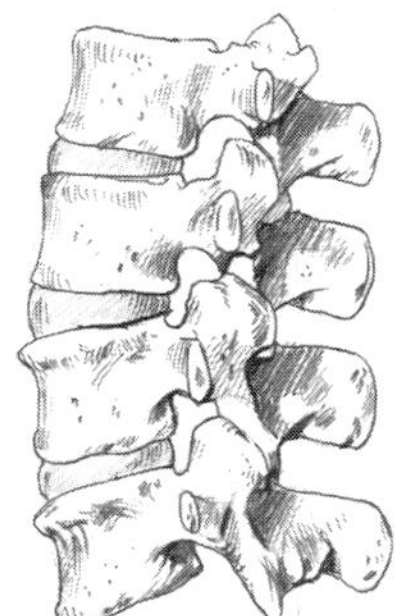

Normal vertebrae

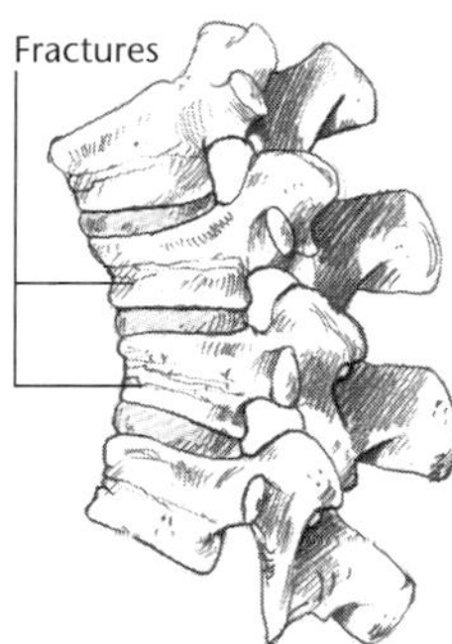

Vertebrae collapsed from osteoporosis

SPINAL FRACTURES
Tiny fractures in the vertebrae of a spine that is weakened by osteoporosis can cause the vertebrae to collapse. This collapse, called a compression fracture, is painful and can cause curving of the upper spine, a weakening of the spine, and a reduction in height.

Osteoporosis usually causes no symptoms until a bone weakened by the disorder fractures. Fractures occur most often in the wrist, vertebrae (the small bones of the spinal column), and hip. Some women who have osteoporosis first notice a decrease in their height, or they experience persistent pain along their spine or muscle spasms in their back.

Fractures in the spine When your bones are weakened by osteoporosis, even an ordinary movement such as bending over or sneezing can cause a tiny, hairline crack in one or more vertebrae. Over time, tiny hairline fractures can accumulate in vertebrae, eventually causing the weakened bone to collapse from the weight of your body. This injury is called a compression fracture. Several compression fractures can severely weaken your spine. Your posture may begin to shift gradually and subtly and you may notice a reduction in your height and curving of your upper spine. A compression fracture may press on a spinal nerve, causing immediate, severe pain or a persistent, dull pain.

A fractured vertebra cannot be repaired with surgery or set in a cast. Because the bone has collapsed, not broken, it must heal on its own, but it will never regain its original height and density. A compression fracture forces the nearby muscles, ligaments, and nerves to realign themselves. In some cases, this shifting can cause nagging pain.

If you are diagnosed with a compression fracture, your doctor will recommend bed rest for the first 2 or 3 days, during which the pain should lessen. After that, you can speed your recovery by resuming as much activity as you can. The bone may take 6 to 8 weeks to mend and up to 12 weeks to heal completely. To help reduce the pain while your fracture is healing, your doctor may recommend an over-the-counter nonsteroidal anti-inflammatory medication (such as aspirin, ibuprofen, or naproxen) or a prescription pain reliever. You may find that applying a heating pad or ice to the affected area also helps relieve the pain.

Exercises to improve flexibility and strength in your back and torso may help reduce the curvature of your upper spine that can result from fractured vertebrae. Your doctor may recommend the temporary use of a back brace to help prevent you from bending strenuously and to help reduce the pain in your back and the curvature of your spine. A cane or walker may help you get around more confidently while your fracture is healing. A very firm mattress is the best choice for sleeping because it provides more support for your back.

Learn to move without putting stress on your back. When you pick up an object, bend at the knees rather than at your waist. Avoid activities, such as golf or tennis, that require excessive twisting from the waist. Never lift anything heavier than 15 pounds.

Wrist fracture In women younger than 75, the wrist is the most common site of bone fracture. Wrist fractures usually occur when a woman puts out her hand in an attempt to break a fall. A wrist fracture is a warning sign of low bone density but it is sometimes mistaken for a sprain. If you have persistent pain after a fall, swelling of your wrist, or less movement in your fingers, see your doctor immediately. An X-ray can determine if your wrist is broken. Your doctor will probably

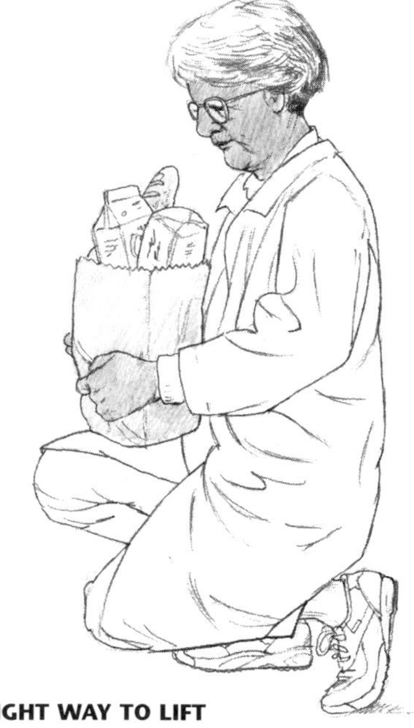

THE RIGHT WAY TO LIFT
It is always important to protect your back when lifting objects, but proper lifting becomes even more important when you have osteoporosis. To pick something up, bend at your knees rather than at your waist. If you have osteoporosis, never lift anything heavier than 15 pounds.

Bone density tests

Because the early stages of osteoporosis seldom cause symptoms, the only way to know you are at risk or have the disease is through an evaluation of the density of your bones. This evaluation can be done using one of several imaging methods, which are painless procedures similar to having a standard X-ray. A bone density study helps your doctor and you understand your risk of developing osteoporosis so that you can make decisions about how best to maintain strength in your bones. If you are in your 40s and have no signs of osteoporosis but are weighing the decision of whether or not to take estrogen in hormone replacement therapy (HRT; see page 359) when you reach menopause, knowing the current density of your bones could help you make that decision.

If you have already had a bone fracture, a bone density test may show that an underlying decrease in your bone density is the cause. Your doctor may recommend repeating the test 1 year later to determine the rate at which you are losing bone in order to make decisions about treatment or, if you are already undergoing treatment for osteoporosis, to monitor the success of that treatment.

- **Dual energy X-ray absorptiometry** Dual energy X-ray absorptiometry (DEXA) is the most effective imaging technique for determining bone density. DEXA produces a measurement of your bone density using a very low dose of radiation and can detect bone loss of as little as 1 percent. The test takes only about 3 to 7 minutes to perform.
- **Dual photon absorptiometry** Dual photon absorptiometry (DPA) is an imaging technique that measures bone density in the spine, neck, and hips using a very low dose of radiation. The technique evaluates bone density in these areas of your body by passing a beam of photons (particles of light) across them. DPA is used to determine the need for HRT in women who are past menopause and have experienced a bone fracture. The procedure takes about 20 to 40 minutes.
- **Single photon absorptiometry** Single photon absorptiometry (SPA) is an imaging technique that can detect signs of bone loss in the wrist or heel, but not in the hip or spine. In this imaging method, which takes about 15 minutes, a single beam of photons is passed across the limb.
- **Quantitative computed tomography** Quantitative computed tomography is an imaging procedure that uses X-rays to detect evidence of low bone density in the spine. This procedure takes 10 to 15 minutes and is performed on women who have osteoporosis to monitor their rate of bone loss and evaluate the effectiveness of any treatment they are receiving.

recommend a bone density test (see above) to determine if osteoporosis caused the fracture. You may also have other tests, such as vision and hearing tests, to see if another health problem may have been the cause of your fall.

Treatment of a wrist fracture depends on the location and severity of the break in the bone. In a simple fracture, the edges of the broken bone can be manipulated back together. A cast that extends beyond your elbow will immobilize your wrist and elbow joint and allow the broken bone to mend. If you have more than one fracture, or if your wrist joint is damaged, you may need to have surgery to reset the bones before your arm is set in a cast. A physical or occupational therapist will give you instructions about exercises you can do while your cast is on to help prevent your fingers from becoming stiff. While your wrist is healing, you may need help with your daily routine, particularly if the fracture is in the arm you use most often.

You will have periodic X-rays to determine if the bone is healing properly. Surgery may be necessary if the bone is not healing correctly. The cast is removed after 6 to 8 weeks, and you can then begin a program of exercises to strengthen your hand, wrist, and forearm.

Hip fracture A hip fracture can cause an older woman who is active and independent to become dependent on others for much of her care or to have to move into a nursing home. Hip fractures can also have life-threatening complications. A broken hip is almost always caused by a fall. The break is usually in the upper, narrow part of the thighbone closest to the pelvic bone. The most common treatment for a hip fracture is surgery in which

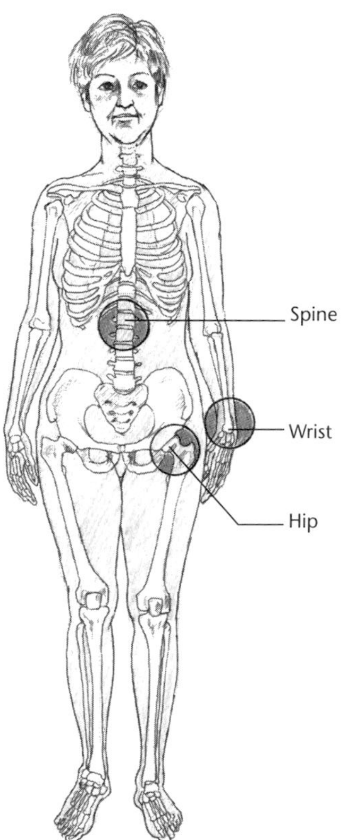

screws or pins are inserted to hold the bone together. Artificial implants can be used to replace areas of bone that have worn away, thereby restoring strength and function to the hip.

Recovery may be slow and, in some cases, the implants or screws do not hold, or they loosen with long-term use or further injury. When this occurs, a total hip replacement (see page 566) is required to place an artificial joint in the area of the unstable bone.

COMMON SITES OF FRACTURES FROM OSTEOPOROSIS
The bones weakened by osteoporosis that are most likely to break are those in the spine, wrist, or hip. If you break your wrist or hip, your doctor will identify the break with a physical examination and confirm it with an X-ray. Fractures in the wrist can be set; those in the hip usually require surgery to repair or replace the joint. A fractured vertebra is less obvious and can be diagnosed only by an X-ray. Compression fractures in vertebrae cannot be set because the bone has collapsed completely and must heal on its own.

Joint disorders

Most of your joints, where two or more bones meet, allow movement. Freely moving joints are lubricated by fluid and cushioned by a set of small liquid-filled sacs called bursae. The ends of the bones that meet at a joint are covered by a tough, smooth tissue called cartilage. Because you use your joints thousands of times each day, some may eventually wear down, resulting in a type of arthritis called osteoarthritis ("osteo" means bone, "arthritis" means inflammation of the joint). Because of its name, osteoarthritis is sometimes confused with osteoporosis or rheumatoid arthritis but is very different from both of these.

OSTEOARTHRITIS

Osteoarthritis results from thinning or destruction of cartilage in the joints. A major cause of osteoarthritis, sometimes called wear-and-tear arthritis, is damage to joints that occurs over time from injury or overuse. Osteoarthritis is extremely common, affecting almost everyone over age 60 to some degree. In many people, osteoarthritis causes no symptoms and goes unnoticed unless it is detected by chance on an X-ray performed for another reason. But in some people the disorder causes irritation and pain in the joints and adjacent bone.

Athletes who have injured a joint and physical laborers who do heavy work are at increased risk of developing osteoarthritis. However, there is no evidence that repetitive physical exercise such as running, bicycling, or walking causes arthritis in uninjured joints. If you have a family history of osteoarthritis, you are at increased risk. You are also at greater risk if you are obese. Being overweight tends to put more stress on all the joints.

The areas of the body most often affected by osteoarthritis are the hip, knees, fingers, feet, and spine. The

SYMPTOM CHART

Back pain

Pain and/or stiffness in your back that may be constant or intermittent.

START

Did the pain start suddenly?

YES → Did the pain start after a fall or other injury to your back?

YES → Since then have you noticed any of the following symptoms?
- Loss of bladder or bowel control
- Difficulty moving an arm or leg
- Numbness or tingling in an arm or leg

YES → ***EMERGENCY Get medical help immediately.*** You may have damaged your spinal cord.

NO → Your back pain is probably the result of bruising or a muscle spasm. Talk to your doctor if the pain is severe or if it continues for more than 3 days.

(Did the pain start after a fall or other injury to your back?) NO → Have you been lifting heavy weights and/or exercising more strenuously than usual?

YES → Does the pain shoot down the back of your leg?

YES → Call your doctor if the pain lasts more than 3 days or is not relieved with anti-inflammatory medication such as aspirin or ibuprofen. You may have a condition called sciatica, which is caused by pressure on a major nerve.

NO → continued on next page, second column

(Have you been lifting heavy weights and/or exercising more strenuously than usual?) NO → continued on next page, second column

(Did the pain start suddenly?) NO → continued on next page, first column

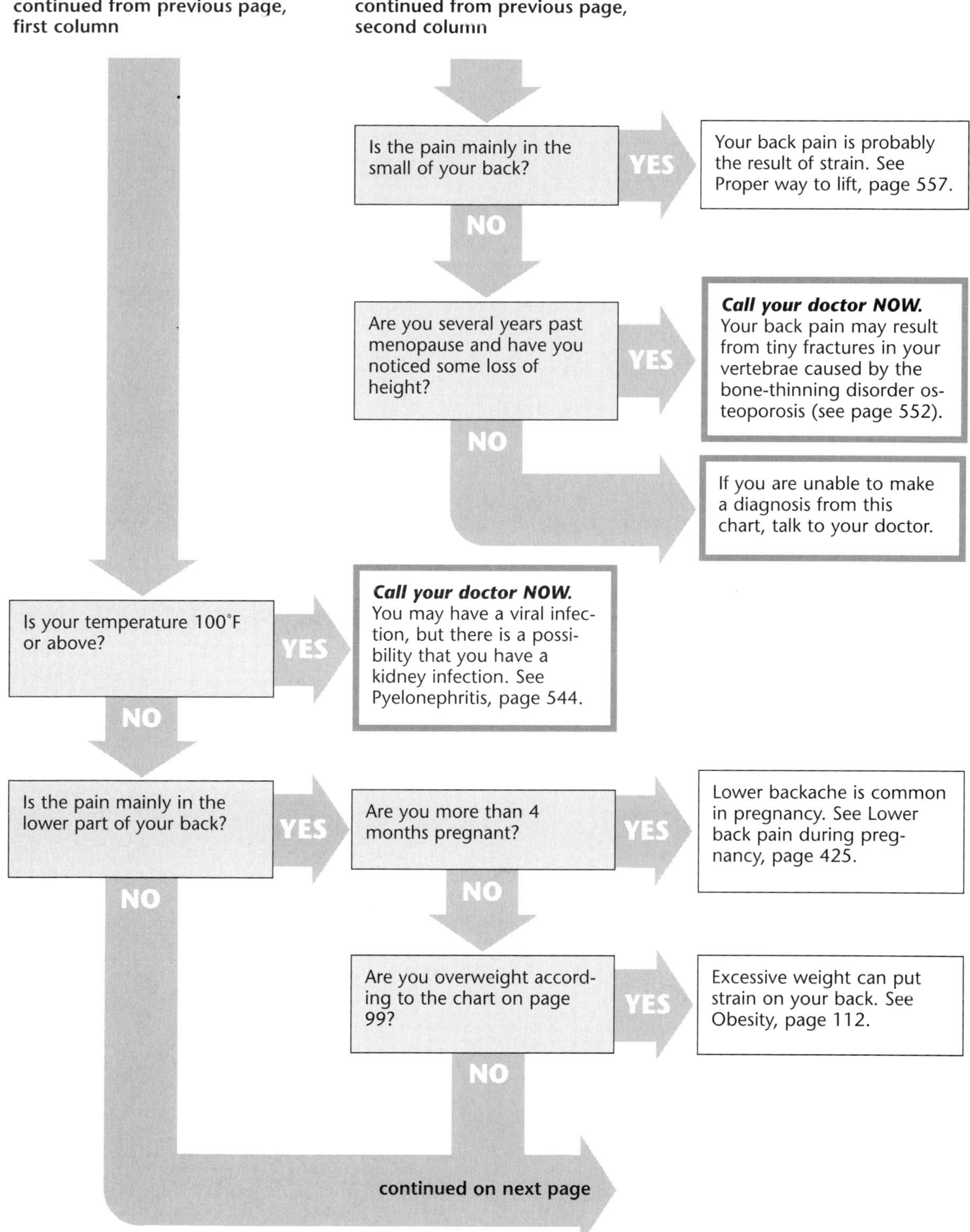
continued from previous page, first column
continued from previous page, second column
Is the pain mainly in the small of your back?
YES
Your back pain is probably the result of strain. See Proper way to lift, page 557.
NO
Are you several years past menopause and have you noticed some loss of height?
YES
Call your doctor NOW. Your back pain may result from tiny fractures in your vertebrae caused by the bone-thinning disorder osteoporosis (see page 552).
NO
If you are unable to make a diagnosis from this chart, talk to your doctor.
Is your temperature 100°F or above?
YES
Call your doctor NOW. You may have a viral infection, but there is a possibility that you have a kidney infection. See Pyelonephritis, page 544.
NO
Is the pain mainly in the lower part of your back?
YES
Are you more than 4 months pregnant?
YES
Lower backache is common in pregnancy. See Lower back pain during pregnancy, page 425.
NO
Are you overweight according to the chart on page 99?
YES
Excessive weight can put strain on your back. See Obesity, page 112.
NO
NO
continued on next page

continued from previous page

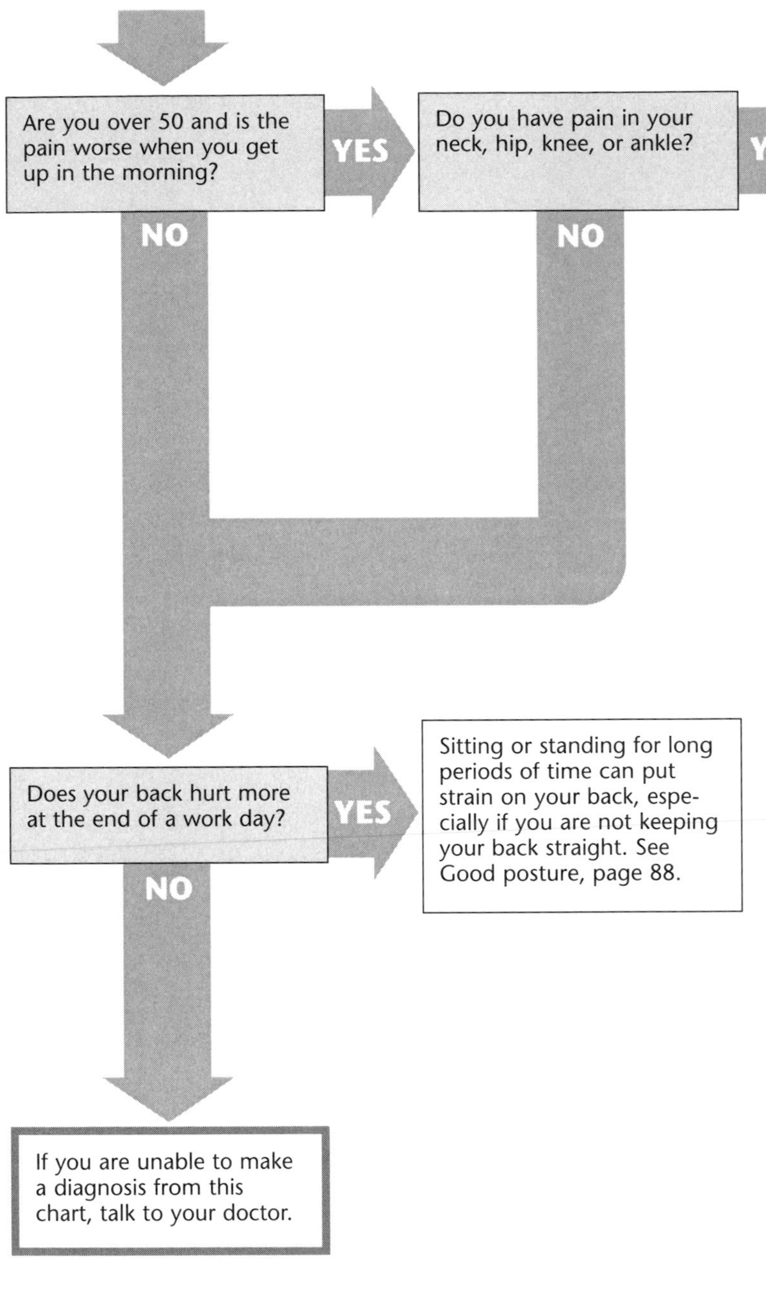

Your mattress may not be firm enough to give your back sufficient support, or you may have osteoarthritis. See Osteoarthritis, page 559.

Sitting or standing for long periods of time can put strain on your back, especially if you are not keeping your back straight. See Good posture, page 88.

Tips for avoiding back pain

- Exercise regularly.
- Get adequate calcium (see page 58).
- Wear well-cushioned shoes when you exercise.
- Don't jog on pavement.
- Don't bend from the waist when lifting objects (see page 557).
- Maintain good posture.
- Wear low-heeled shoes.

See your doctor if you have persistent back pain.

disorder affects each joint differently but symptoms can include stiffness, pain, weakness, or numbness. You may experience pain in only one joint or in several joints. Having osteoarthritis in one joint does not mean you will get it in other joints, but the affected joint may gradually deteriorate. Although there is no way to stop or reverse the effects of osteoarthritis, there are several things you can do, including exercise, to control the symptoms.

Symptoms You may experience the following symptoms in your joints:

- **Hips** Pain or aching in your thigh, groin, hip, or buttocks
- **Fingers** Red, swollen, tender, aching joints in your fingers; numbness or tingling in your fingertips
- **Knees** Feeling of tenderness when you bend; a grating or rubbing feeling inside your knee; pain when you walk up or down stairs
- **Spine** Pain at the base of your neck or in your arms or legs; stiffness in your lower back; weakness or numbness in your arms or legs

Diagnosis If your doctor suspects you have osteoarthritis based on your medical history and a physical examination, he or she will recommend an X-ray of the affected joints to confirm the diagnosis. If an abnormal amount of fluid accumulates in a joint, your doctor may want to rule out other possible causes of your symptoms by withdrawing some of the fluid through a needle and sending it to a laboratory for examination. Blood tests can also help rule out diseases with similar symptoms, such as rheumatoid arthritis (see page 645) or lupus (see page 641).

Treatment There is no cure for osteoarthritis, but there are things you can do to control the symptoms and, in some cases, slow the progression of the disease.

Protect your joints It is especially important to protect your joints from injury by reducing any activity or motion that causes pain or pressure. Your doctor can help you determine how best to do this. He or she may recommend the temporary use of splints to help take pressure off some joints, such as those in your fingers; using a cane or walker may help relieve stress on your hips and knees. Losing weight can also reduce stress on your joints. Ask for help if you need to lift or move something heavy.

Get regular exercise Although you may hesitate to move a joint when it hurts, inactivity can cause a joint to become stiff and even more painful. You and your doctor can work out a regular exercise program to keep your joints flexible without putting extra stress on them. Moving your joints will also maintain

DAMAGED HIP
In a healthy hip (right), smooth cartilage cushions the thighbone and pelvis so the ball can glide easily inside the socket. When the cartilage becomes damaged, the bones rub together and become rough and irregular (far right). Movement becomes stiff and painful.

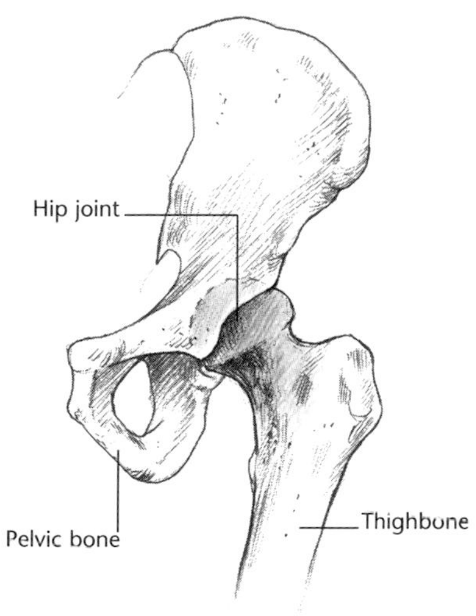

Healthy hip

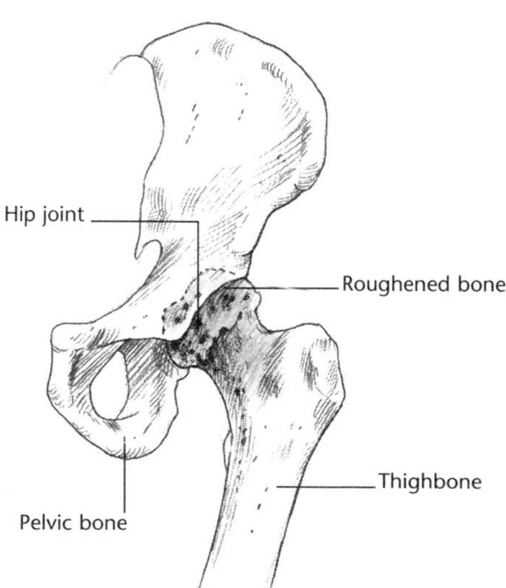

Hip damaged by osteoarthritis

SYMPTOM CHART

Painful or swollen joints

Pain, stiffness, or swelling in or around a joint, or limitation of movement of a joint.

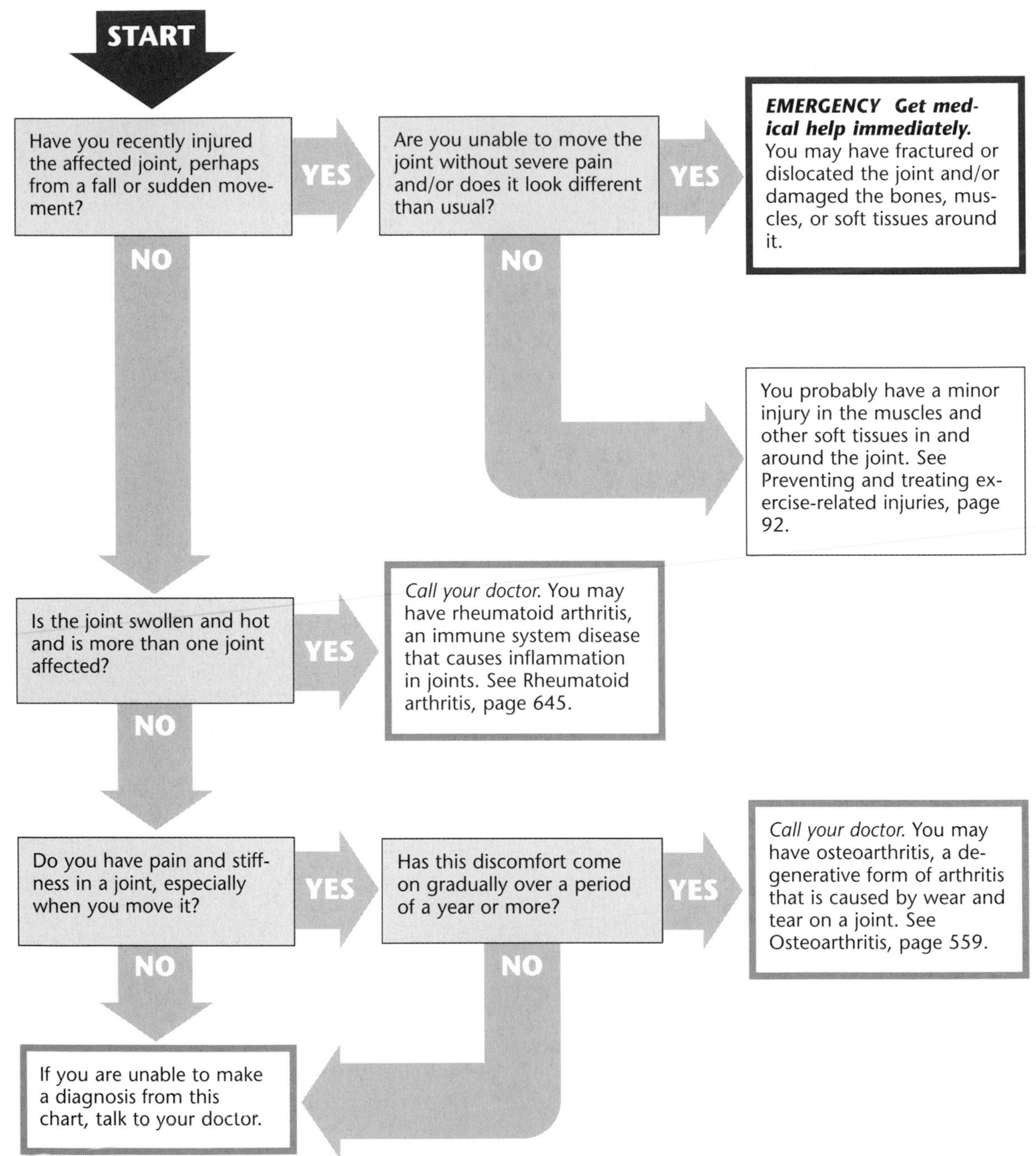

strength in the muscles that support them, which helps protect them from further damage and pain. Your doctor may recommend low-impact activities such as walking, swimming, or biking.

Pain medications To relieve pain and tenderness in joints affected by osteoarthritis, your doctor may first recommend an over-the-counter anti-inflammatory pain medication such as aspirin, ibuprofen, or naproxen. Aspirin is very effective for relieving the pain of osteoarthritis. If aspirin irritates your stomach, you may want to try coated aspirin tablets, which cause less irritation. If you cannot take aspirin, ask your doctor to recommend a different medication. Any anti-inflammatory medication should be taken with food to reduce irritation to your stomach lining.

Over-the-counter pain medications can usually control pain as effectively as more expensive prescription medications. However, some people have periodic painful flare-ups that require stronger prescription pain medication. Talk to your doctor if your pain medication is not effective.

Weight control If you are overweight, losing weight will help slow the progression of osteoarthritis by taking excess physical stress off your already painful joints. The best way to lose weight is to reduce your consumption of calories and fat and increase the amount of regular exercise you do. For more about losing weight, see page 106.

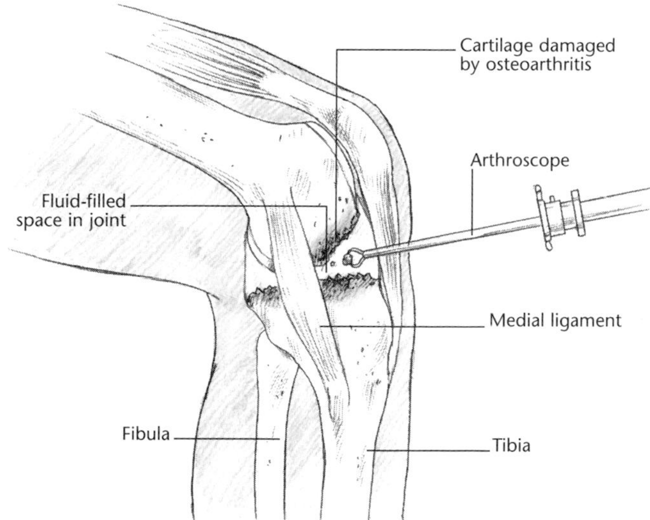

ARTHROSCOPIC KNEE SURGERY
Damaged joints can be diagnosed and repaired using an arthroscope, a long viewing tube with a light and a tiny video camera at its tip. The arthroscope can be inserted into the fluid-filled space in the knee joint. In this illustration, the arthroscope is being used to look at the jagged cartilage of a knee affected by osteoarthritis.

Heat treatments Applying heat can temporarily relieve pain in a joint. Heat relaxes muscles around the affected joint that can become tense and painful when they strain to protect the joint. A hot shower in the morning can relax your muscles and reduce the tightness that accompanies tender joints. A heating pad, hot water bottle, or heat lamp can also help reduce pain. You may want to look for a health center in your area that offers exercise sessions in a warm pool.

Surgery In some cases, surgery may be necessary to correct a deformity, to improve the movement in a joint, or to replace a joint with an artificial device. These operations are performed by an orthopedic surgeon. Artificial joints have been developed for most of the body's major joints. Hip replacements (see page 566) and knee replacements are common.

Although rare, complications from hip surgery can include infection in the hip socket or dislocation of the new hip. Because of the slight risk of developing blood clots in your legs after the surgery, your doctor will prescribe anti-clotting medication or a special compression stocking to help keep your blood flowing. You will be in the hospital for about 4 to 7 days after hip-replacement surgery. You are likely to experience some soreness in the replaced joint, which will gradually subside as you exercise the joint. Your doctor will prescribe painkillers to help relieve the discomfort.

You will be able to stand and begin to walk—at first with the support of a walker—a few days after the surgery. During this time, you will begin physical therapy and learn exercises that you will continue to do at home. Physical therapy can help strengthen the muscles and ligaments that support your hip.

Make arrangements with family and friends to be available once you return home; you will need to rely on them as you gradually regain your mobility. Setting up your bedroom on the same floor as the kitchen may make it easier for you to maintain some independence.

It is also important to make changes in your home that minimize your risk of falling (see page 179). You will probably be able to resume all your usual activities within 3 to 4 months of the surgery. Depending on the severity of your problem before you had hip replacement surgery, you should regain nearly full motion in your new joint.

In some cases, instead of replacing the joint, a surgeon can improve functioning of the joint by removing damaged tissue. This type of surgery (called arthroscopy) can be performed through a small incision and does not require an overnight stay in the hospital. Recovery from arthroscopic surgery on the knee or another joint is rapid. Most people can resume all of their usual activities within a few days.

Hip replacement

A hip replacement is an artificial ball-and-socket joint made of metal and plastic that is a common solution for the pain and immobility caused by osteoarthritis, osteoporosis (see page 552), fractures, or inherited hip disorders.

Surgery to replace a hip is most frequently performed in people over age 60 who have chronic, debilitating pain and severe difficulty walking. Although hip replacements are performed in younger people when necessary, they tend to wear out more quickly because younger people are usually more active than older people. For people under 50, "cementless" joints are used that have a rough, porous surface that allows bone to grow directly into and around the new joint, holding it in place. Most artificial hip joints last at least 20 years.

An artificial hip imitates the natural ball-and-socket hip joint. One part of the implant is a metal shaft that is anchored into the thighbone. The other end of the shaft resembles the ball of the natural joint and fits into an artificial socket that has been implanted into the pelvic bone. You will be given general anesthesia (see page 261) for this surgery.

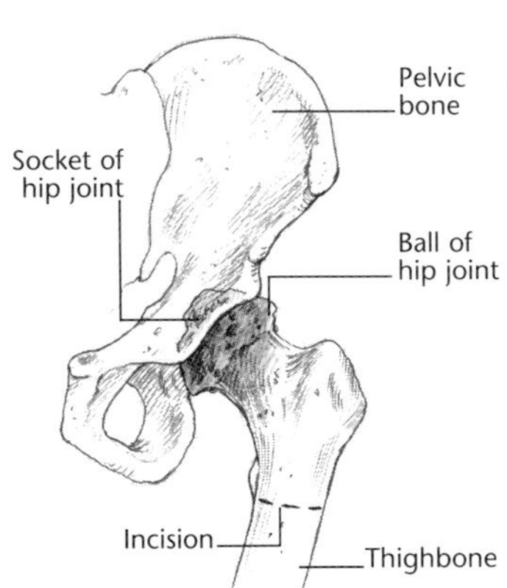

1. The surgeon cuts the thighbone and removes the top portion, which forms the ball of the joint.

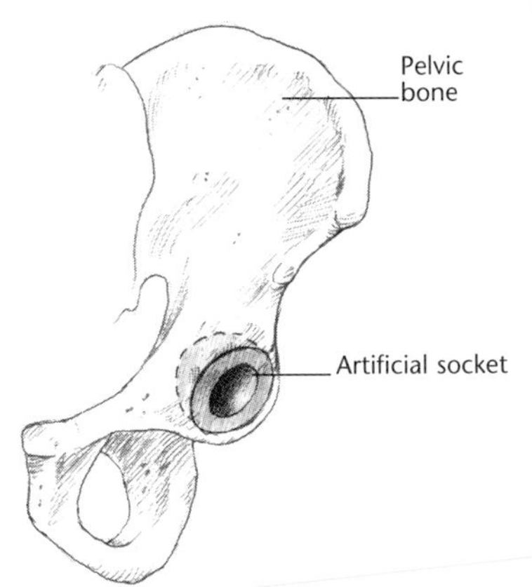

2. An artificial socket is implanted into a cavity in the pelvic bone that has been formed by the surgeon.

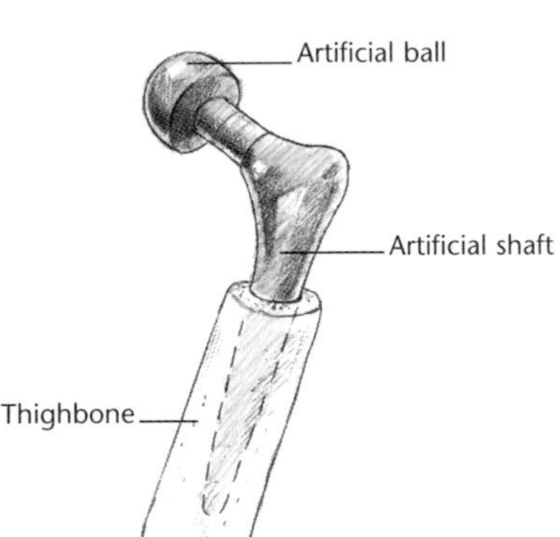

3. A metal shaft with a ball-shaped head is inserted into a hollow canal that the surgeon has made in the thighbone.

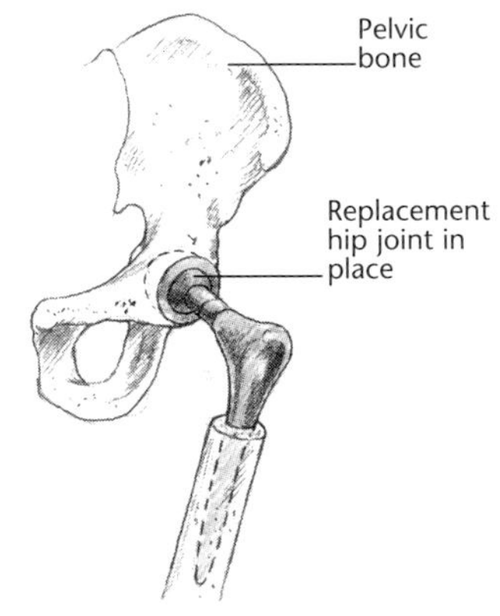

4. The ball at the top of the artificial shaft is fitted into the artificial socket to form the new hip joint.

CHAPTER 22

Your brain and nervous system

Contents

Your brain and nervous system

Your nervous system has two major parts—the central nervous system and the peripheral nervous system. Your brain and spinal cord make up your central nervous system, which coordinates all your body's interactions with your environment. Your brain, the most complex organ of your body, regulates most of your body's functions. Each area of the brain is responsible for different functions, such as language, vision, movement, or emotions. Your peripheral nervous system consists of nerves that radiate out from your brain and spinal cord to all parts of your body. These peripheral nerves convey information from different parts of your body to your brain and send messages back to those parts from the brain. Your brain is always working, even when you are asleep.

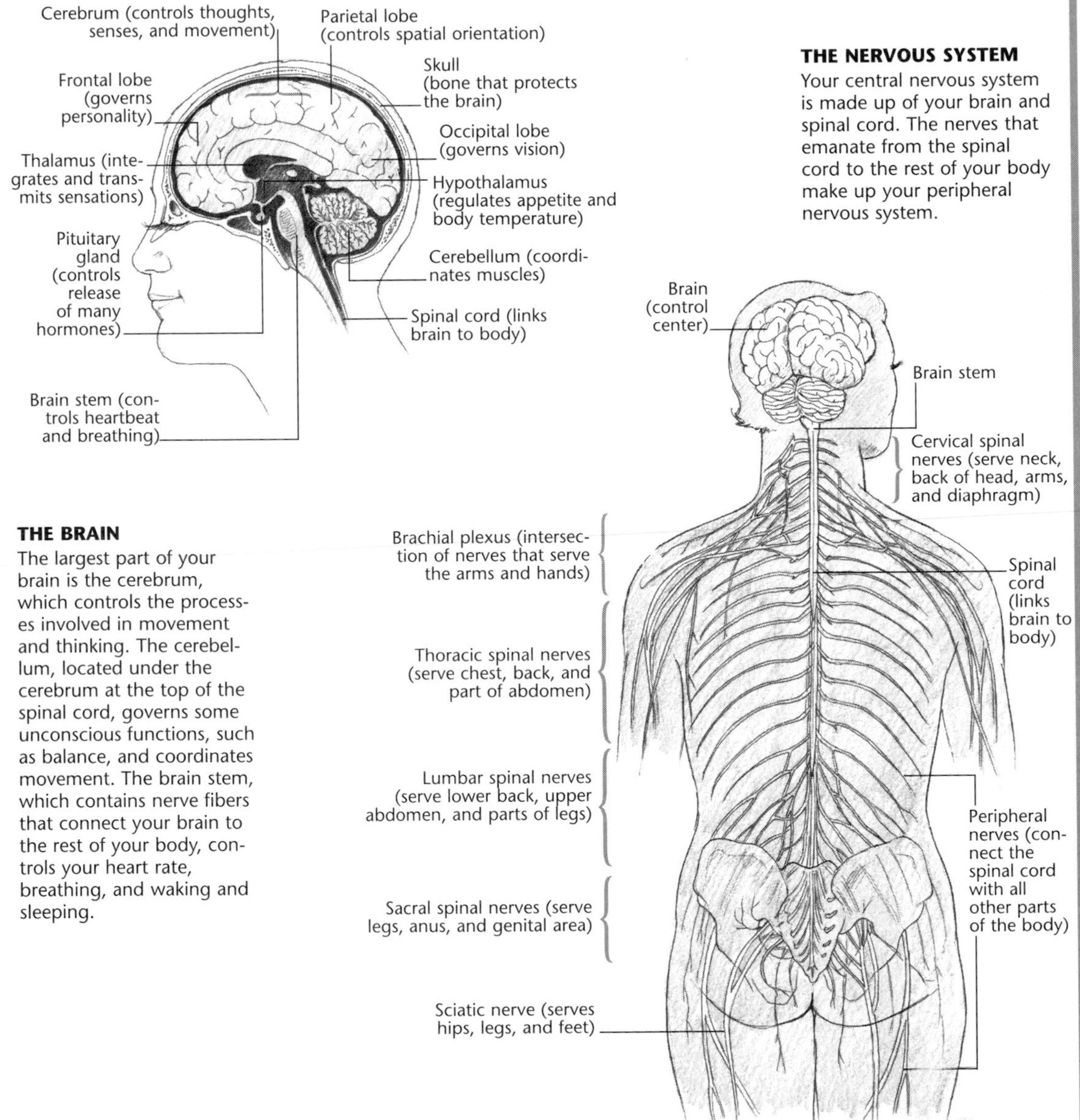

THE NERVOUS SYSTEM

Your central nervous system is made up of your brain and spinal cord. The nerves that emanate from the spinal cord to the rest of your body make up your peripheral nervous system.

THE BRAIN

The largest part of your brain is the cerebrum, which controls the processes involved in movement and thinking. The cerebellum, located under the cerebrum at the top of the spinal cord, governs some unconscious functions, such as balance, and coordinates movement. The brain stem, which contains nerve fibers that connect your brain to the rest of your body, controls your heart rate, breathing, and waking and sleeping.

Your brain and nervous system are the most important and complex parts of your body. Together, they regulate and coordinate all the functions of your body and your responses to your environment. A disorder that affects your nervous system (called a neurological disorder) can be especially difficult to deal with because it can impair both your physical and mental abilities. The most common disorder of the nervous system—stroke—is the leading cause of serious disability in the US. Each year, about 500,000 Americans have strokes.

Stroke

A stroke occurs when part of the brain is deprived of blood. This usually happens when an artery is blocked by a buildup of fatty deposits (a process called atherosclerosis) or by a blood clot. A stroke that results from a blockage in a blood vessel is called an ischemic stroke (see page 573). A stroke can also result from rupture of an artery in the brain. This type of stroke is called a hemorrhagic stroke. If an artery in the brain ruptures, blood flow to the brain from the artery is interrupted. Bleeding from the rupture can irritate other blood vessels in the brain, causing them to go into spasm and damage surrounding areas of the brain.

In just a few seconds, a stroke can cause vision or speech difficulties, paralysis in part of the body, or loss of consciousness. A stroke that continues for a few minutes may destroy brain cells, which can result in permanent impairment or death. Although stroke is more common in men, women are more likely to die of a stroke, probably because they tend to be older at the time it occurs.

The right side of your brain controls the left side of your body and the left side of your brain controls the right side of your body. A stroke that damages an area on the left side of your brain usually affects the right side of your body; conversely, a stroke that damages the right side of your brain affects the left side of your body.

The effects of a stroke can take many forms and can be different for each person, depending on the area of the brain that is damaged and the extent of the damage. For example, one woman may find that the right side of her body is paralyzed and that she has difficulty understanding what people are saying to her. Another woman may have no paralysis but find that, although she can understand what people are saying to her, she has a hard time coming up with the right words with which to respond. Another woman may lose sensation on one side of her body. She may not even recognize that part of her body as hers and may forget to move it, dress it, or wash it. Depression may accompany any of these conditions.

Depending on the severity of a stroke and the areas of the brain that it damages, different parts of the body can be affected in various ways. In addition to paralysis and loss of speech, results of a stroke can include poor circulation and fluid retention (edema) and reduced bladder control. A person who has had a stroke may develop other problems as well—including pneumonia, urinary tract infections, and bed sores (sores that result from prolonged pressure on one area of the skin)—as a result of the general weakness and loss of mobility that can follow a stroke. All of these conditions can be treated, but they can make recovery longer and more difficult.

Although a stroke can be devastating, new treatments have made it possible for doctors to help limit the damage to the brain and speed recovery. Most importantly, doctors now know how to help people reduce their risk of a stroke. Some people are able to recover completely

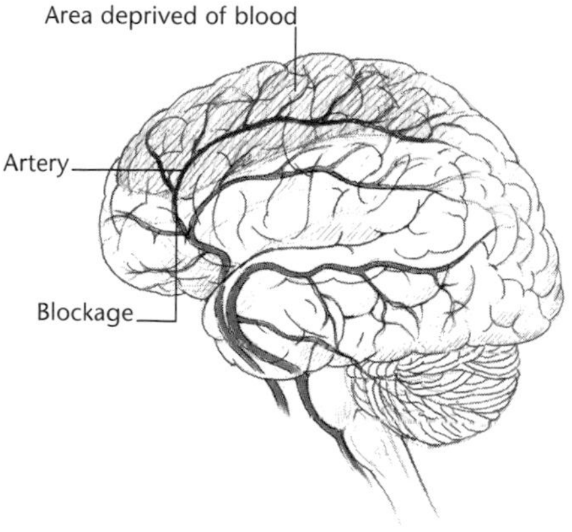

HOW STROKE CAN DAMAGE THE BRAIN
When an artery becomes completely blocked by the buildup of fatty deposits or a blood clot, the blood that artery normally supplies to a portion of the brain does not reach it. The result can be damage in the entire area of the brain supplied by the artery.

from a stroke; other people can gradually regain much of the functioning they have lost. The key to successful treatment is to get to the hospital as quickly as possible if you are having a stroke. The longer the delay in getting treatment, the greater the risk of permanent brain damage.

ARTERIES OF THE BRAIN

The vertebral and carotid arteries run up the neck to bring blood to the brain. Inside the brain, they branch into the anterior cerebral, middle cerebral, and posterior cerebral arteries, which run to all parts of the brain.

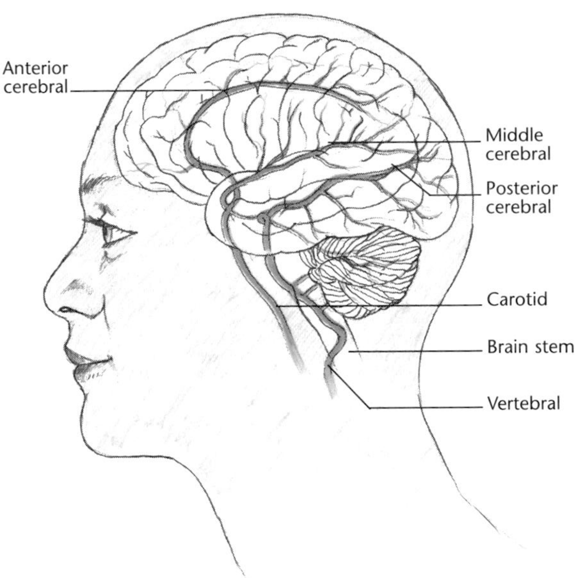

REDUCING YOUR RISK

You cannot control some risk factors for a stroke, including your age, race, or family history. The older you are, the greater your risk of having a stroke. Women tend to have strokes later in life than men, usually after menopause. Blacks are at increased risk of stroke because they have a higher incidence of high blood pressure, which is a major cause of stroke. Your risk is also increased if you have diabetes (see page 617). These conditions weaken blood vessel walls and make the vessels more susceptible to rupture or blockage. If you have already had one stroke or if you have had a transient ischemic attack (TIA; see page 571), your chance of having a stroke is many times higher than a person who has not had a stroke or a TIA. A TIA results from a temporary lack of blood flow to the brain. However, you can influence many risk factors for stroke by taking the following steps:

- **Lower your blood pressure.** High blood pressure increases your risk of having a stroke more than any other factor. The higher your blood pressure, the more likely you are to have a stroke. People with moderately high blood pressure—between 140/85 and 170/95 millimeters of mercury (mm Hg)—may be able to lower it by losing weight (see page 106), eating a diet low in salt and fat (see page 107), and exercising regularly (see page 78). More severe high blood pressure (see page 481) must be treated with medication.
- **If you smoke, quit.** Smoking cigarettes can increase your blood pressure, reduce the oxygen supply to all of your organs and tissues, and increase the tendency of your blood to clot. If you smoke, quitting is the most beneficial thing you can do for your health. For information about how to quit smoking, see page 157.
- **Call your doctor if you think you have had a TIA.** Days, weeks, or months before you have an actual stroke, you are likely to experience one or more small strokes (TIAs). Because a TIA is a warning sign that you are at risk of having a stroke, informing your doctor as quickly as possible can be lifesaving. Your doctor may recommend treatment—such as medication or surgery or a combination of the two—to reduce your risk.

■ **Take anticlotting medication if your doctor prescribes it.** If blood tests show the number of platelets or clotting proteins in your blood is abnormally high, your blood is more likely to clot and block an artery. Your doctor may prescribe medications called anticoagulants to prevent your blood from clotting.

TRANSIENT ISCHEMIC ATTACKS

A transient ischemic attack (TIA) is a small stroke that results from a temporary (transient) disruption in blood flow (ischemia) to the brain when a blood vessel that supplies the brain is blocked or narrowed. This disruption in blood flow is often caused by a small blood clot that travels through the bloodstream and lodges in an artery in the brain. The clot may dissolve quickly, allowing blood to flow through again and avoiding permanent damage to the brain. A TIA is a warning that a stroke may occur in days, weeks, or months. TIAs occur most often before ischemic strokes.

A TIA can last from seconds to several hours; most last from 2 to 15 minutes. You may have one isolated TIA or many over a period of a few days or weeks. Although you may not feel anything at all, TIAs usually cause symptoms such as temporary blindness in one or both eyes, numbness or weakness in an arm or leg, or difficulty speaking or using words correctly. Because the symptoms of a TIA are likely to go away soon after they appear, many people ignore them. But taking these symptoms seriously and getting prompt medical attention can mean the difference between having a severely disabling stroke, having a mild stroke, or preventing a stroke altogether.

If you think you may have had a TIA, call your doctor immediately. If your doctor determines that you have had a TIA, he or she will prescribe treatment that is designed to prevent you from having a major stroke. Your doctor may recommend that you change your lifestyle—quit smoking, eat a diet low in fat, lose weight, and exercise.

The cause of your TIA may be investigated with an imaging procedure such as a computed tomography (CT) scan (see page 572) or magnetic resonance imaging (MRI; see page 572). Another imaging procedure, called a carotid ultrasound (see page 573), may be used to evaluate the carotid arteries in your neck (which supply blood to your brain). A carotid ultrasound can measure blood flow in these arteries to determine if they have been narrowed by a buildup of plaque. If a carotid ultrasound shows significant narrowing of the artery, you are likely to undergo an imaging procedure called cerebral angiography (see page 573), which can provide more detailed information about the blockage.

If the blockage is significant, your doctor may recommend a surgical procedure called carotid endarterectomy (see page 574) to remove the plaque from the artery. Alternatively, he or she may prescribe anticlotting medications called anticoagulants to prevent potentially dangerous blood clots from forming in your blood.

WARNING SIGNS
STROKE

The sooner you get treatment for a stroke, the more likely you are to recover without serious disability. If circulation to the damaged area of your brain is restored quickly, you are likely to regain partial or even complete functioning. If you are at high risk of stroke, make sure your family and friends are also aware of the following symptoms so that they can recognize them and help you get immediate medical attention. Call your doctor or an ambulance immediately if you experience any of the following symptoms:

- Sudden numbness or weakness in your face, in an arm or a leg, or on one side of your body
- Sudden dimness or loss of vision, particularly in one eye
- Loss of speech, or difficulty talking or understanding speech
- Sudden, severe headache with no apparent cause
- Dizziness, unsteadiness, or a sudden fall, especially in combination with any of the above symptoms

DIAGNOSTIC TESTS

If you have had a stroke or TIA, your doctor will ask about your symptoms and medical history. A series of tests can reveal any damage to the brain. You will have vision tests, hearing tests, and tests of your sense of touch and your balance, strength, coordination, and reflexes. You are likely to have one or more of the imaging scans described in the following pages.

Computed tomography scan A computed tomography (CT) scan is a painless procedure that produces cross-sectional images of organs in your body. A computer converts these "slices" into a detailed picture of the area of the body that is being examined. A CT scan is the best way to determine if a stroke was caused by a ruptured artery and bleeding into the brain. A CT scan can also show the location and size of a damaged area of the brain.

For a CT scan, you will lie on a narrow table that slides through a large doughnut-shaped ring, which rotates around you as you go through it. Narrow X-ray beams pass through a cross section of your body and are picked up by detectors in the ring to produce an image of that cross section. A series of several images is taken.

The whole procedure takes about 30 minutes. A CT scan exposes you to little radiation. However, if there is any chance you may be pregnant, you should tell your doctor and the radiology technician. If you are pregnant and your doctor considers the scan absolutely necessary, you will be given a lead apron to shield your abdomen, pelvis, and fetus from radiation.

Magnetic resonance imaging Like a CT scan, magnetic resonance imaging (MRI) produces images from cross-sectional "slices" of the part of your body that is being investigated. Instead of X-rays, MRI uses a powerful magnetic field to create a signal that a computer processes into an image. MRI is useful in diagnosing strokes caused by either rupture of an artery or a blockage. An MRI scan provides a sharp image of any injury to the brain and can detect smaller injuries than a CT scan can. However, an MRI may not detect bleeding that is present.

To have an MRI, you lie on a table that slides through a cylindrical magnetic tube. The procedure is painless, but you must lie completely still for 30 minutes to an hour in order to ensure a clear image. This restriction and the confinement in the tube make some people

CT scanner

Rotating X-ray source

Detectors

X-ray beam

HAVING A CT SCAN
To have a CT scan, you lie on a table that slides through a large, doughnut-shaped scanning machine that takes a series of cross-sectional images of some areas of your body. The amount of X-rays absorbed by different tissues is recorded by detectors in the scanner and transformed by a computer into an image that is interpreted by a radiologist. The procedure takes about 30 minutes.

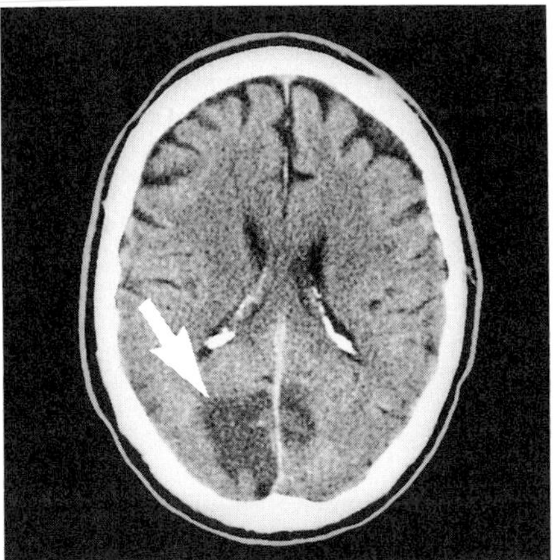

CT SCAN OF THE BRAIN
The darkened area (arrow) on this CT image of the brain indicates damage from a stroke caused by a blockage in an artery that supplies blood to the back of the brain. Because this area of the brain is important for vision, this stroke would have impaired the person's ability to see to one side of his or her body.

uncomfortable. If you are concerned about feeling confined during an MRI, discuss it with your doctor. He or she can give you a sedative to help relax you during the procedure.

Carotid ultrasound A carotid ultrasound is a painless procedure that uses sound waves to determine the location and extent of blockages in the carotid arteries in your neck. These arteries supply blood to your brain, so a blockage in one of them can cause a stroke. The procedure does not require anesthesia or a hospital stay. The ultrasound technician places a device that emits sound waves (called a transducer) on various parts of your neck. A computer receives the signals after they echo back out from the blood vessel and interprets them into an image on a video monitor. When an artery is narrowed, the blood flows faster through that part of it. An ultrasound can detect these changes in the rate of blood flow through a carotid artery and can also evaluate the severity of the blockage. The test takes about 20 to 30 minutes.

Cerebral angiography If an ultrasound has found a blockage in a carotid artery in your neck, your doctor is likely to recommend cerebral angiography to evaluate it further. Cerebral angiography is a procedure that produces an image of the arteries in your brain and the carotid arteries in your neck. This image can show the location and severity of blockages of any of these arteries. An angiogram provides a better image than carotid ultrasound (above) and allows doctors to see arteries located farther inside the brain.

Cerebral angiography helps doctors diagnose blood vessel abnormalities such as an aneurysm (a bulging out of a thinned area of an artery wall), arteriovenous malformation (a group of fragile blood vessels that may rupture), or dislocation of blood vessels caused by a tumor in the brain. A cerebral angiogram is also performed before a surgical procedure such as a carotid endarterectomy (see page 574), which removes a blockage in an artery. The cerebral angiogram pinpoints the site of the blockage for the surgeon.

For a cerebral angiogram, your doctor inserts a hollow needle into an artery in your groin. A thin, hollow tube called a catheter is then threaded through the needle up into the carotid arteries in your neck. A special dye, called a contrast agent, is injected through the catheter into your arteries. The dye shows up on an X-ray of the arteries in your brain, allowing the doctor to see any blockages or narrowing. You are given local anesthesia (see page 260) to numb the area in your groin into which the needle is inserted, and a mild sedative to relax you. The procedure itself takes about 1 hour but you will remain in the hospital for several hours afterward or, in some cases, overnight. During this time, you will be closely monitored to make sure you do not have any complications from the angiogram, such as bleeding from the site the needle was inserted into your groin.

ISCHEMIC STROKES

An ischemic stroke occurs when an artery that brings blood and oxygen to part of your brain is completely blocked. (The term "ischemic" refers to a decreased blood supply to a body organ or tissue.) Ischemic strokes are the most common type. Brain tissues that are normally nourished by that artery die. Parts of one side of your body become weak or numb for days or weeks or permanently. You may experience some improvement a few weeks after your stroke as your damaged brain tissue begins to recover.

Most ischemic strokes result from atherosclerosis (see page 468), a process in which fatty deposits (called plaque) build up inside artery walls. This accumulation of fatty material causes damage to and narrowing of the artery walls. A blood clot may then form in the damaged, narrowed area and block the artery. Some strokes occur when a clot that has formed elsewhere in the body travels to the brain and lodges in a cerebral artery already narrowed by atherosclerosis.

The carotid arteries in the neck are common sites of blockage from atherosclerosis. If the buildup of plaque caused by atherosclerosis reduces blood flow to part of the brain, you may have a transient ischemic attack (TIA; see page 571) or a stroke. Pieces of plaque can also break off and travel to the brain, lodging in an artery there and causing a TIA or stroke.

Treatment Treatment of a stroke often begins while the stroke is under way. The goal of treatment is to increase blood flow

Carotid endarterectomy

A carotid endarterectomy is a surgical procedure in which a buildup of fatty material called plaque in a carotid artery is peeled off the wall of the artery to restore the flow of blood to the brain. The carotid arteries are two major blood vessels that run up the front of your neck and deliver oxygen-rich blood to your brain. The carotid arteries are common sites for the buildup of plaque, which can narrow and block the arteries, causing a stroke.

Carotid endarterectomy is most often recommended for people who have had either a mild ischemic stroke (see page 573) or a transient ischemic attack (TIA; see page 571). The procedure is usually recommended only when an artery is at least 70 percent (but not completely) blocked. If your artery is less than 70 percent blocked, the benefit of the surgery may not be worth the risk. If your artery is completely blocked, it is not possible to reopen it using this procedure. If you have other health problems such as heart disease, uncontrolled diabetes, or high blood pressure, you may not be able to undergo a carotid endarterectomy. These conditions increase your risk of complications from the surgery.

Before you have a carotid endarterectomy, you will have a cerebral angiogram (see page 573) to locate the exact site of the blockage. The endarterectomy procedure requires general anesthesia (see page 261). For an endarterectomy, the surgeon makes a vertical incision down the side of your neck to expose the main artery and temporarily shuts off the blood flow around the blockage. He or she then makes an incision along the artery at the blockage, peels the plaque from the wall of the artery, and stitches close the incisions in the artery and in the skin.

Your doctor will probably recommend that you make arrangements ahead of time to have someone drive you home after the surgery. You should not drive for several hours after you have had general anesthesia. The procedure takes about 30 to 45 minutes. After you wake up from the anesthesia, you may have a headache or feel light-headed. You may also notice a slight, temporary loss of feeling in the area around the site of the incision in your neck. These effects of the procedure are nothing to worry about and usually pass quickly. You will remain in the hospital for 1 or 2 hours after the procedure so your condition can be monitored.

Although a carotid endarterectomy can be highly effective for reopening a narrowed artery, the process that caused the narrowing—atherosclerosis—must be treated to prevent your arteries from narrowing again. To achieve this, your doctor will recommend changes in your diet (such as reducing your intake of fat) and lifestyle (such as getting regular exercise).

to the brain. Getting to the hospital immediately is crucial. Call an ambulance or, if you think you can get there more quickly by car, have someone drive you. Once you get to the hospital, you may have a computed tomography (CT) scan (see page 572) so doctors can diagnose the type of stroke you are having and determine the appropriate treatment. You may be given drugs to dissolve a possible blood clot. If you are dehydrated, you may be given intravenous fluids to make sure that a sufficient amount of blood reaches your brain.

After a major stroke, your brain may swell. This swelling, called edema, occurs when fluid leaks from damaged blood vessels and accumulates in surrounding tissues. Edema can cause further injury to your brain, worsen your symptoms, and may cause nausea or vomiting. In some cases, medications are effective in reducing brain swelling caused by a stroke.

Once your condition stabilizes, doctors will determine the best way to improve blood flow to your brain over the long term. Anticoagulant medications (sometimes called blood thinners) may be able to prevent future clots from forming in the arteries of your brain or in other arteries in your body. A drawback to taking anticoagulants is that they may slightly increase your risk of hemorrhage (bleeding) after an injury.

Your doctor may recommend that you take aspirin daily to help prevent clots from forming. Many people can safely take aspirin on a regular basis, but some people develop stomach discomfort or ulcers from it. Enteric-coated aspirin (aspirin that has a special coating) dissolves more slowly than regular aspirin and causes less stomach discomfort. If aspirin does not work for you, your doctor may prescribe a medication called ticlopidine, which causes fewer problems in the digestive system. However, because ticlopidine may reduce your level of infection-fighting white blood cells, your doctor will recommend periodic blood tests to monitor the level.

HEMORRHAGIC STROKES

A hemorrhagic stroke occurs when a blood vessel in your brain ruptures, preventing the blood vessel from supplying oxygen to a part of your brain and causing tissues in that area of the brain to die. In addition, blood that leaks from the rupture can damage surrounding tissues. Although hemorrhagic strokes are less common than ischemic strokes, they are usually more severe.

Some hemorrhagic strokes occur when a weakened area of the blood vessel wall (called an aneurysm) suddenly gives way. In many cases, aneurysms are present from birth and gradually enlarge. High blood pressure can make an aneurysm more threatening by putting increased pressure on the already weak artery wall. One type of hemorrhagic stroke is caused by leakage of blood into the space between the brain and the surrounding skull (the subarachnoid space); this is called a subarachnoid hemorrhage. Another type of hemorrhagic stroke is caused by bleeding deep inside the brain (intracerebral hemorrhage). High blood pressure is usually a contributing factor in hemorrhagic strokes.

Symptoms A hemorrhagic stroke is characterized by a sudden, unusually severe headache. You may also experience weakness, dizziness, confusion, extreme sensitivity to light, or a stiff neck. A major hemorrhage can cause paralysis or even unconsciousness.

Diagnosis A hemorrhagic stroke is diagnosed from the symptoms, from a computed tomography (CT) scan (see page 572) that detects blood in the brain, and from a test called a lumbar puncture that shows blood in the fluid that surrounds the brain and spinal cord (cerebrospinal fluid).

Treatment The goal of treatment of a hemorrhagic stroke is to limit the amount of damage to the brain. The person is kept calm, his or her blood pressure is controlled, and medication may be given to reduce swelling in the brain. If necessary, blood is drained from the brain to prevent further damage.

In many cases, a subarachnoid hemorrhage is treated with immediate surgery to repair the aneurysm that caused it. In this case, you will first have a cerebral angiogram (see page 573) to locate the site of the rupture. The damaged area of the artery is then surgically repaired to stop the bleeding and to prevent the artery from rupturing again.

Because high blood pressure is the cause of many hemorrhagic strokes, the most effective treatment is to reduce blood pressure gradually and then maintain it at a safe level. If your blood pressure drops too quickly, there may not be enough circulation to supply blood to the outer, smaller blood vessels (capillaries) in your brain.

A hemorrhagic stroke may cause hematomas (blood clots) to form in the brain. A hematoma in the brain often is surrounded by an area of swollen, bruised brain tissue that has been damaged by blood that has leaked from a ruptured blood vessel. The swelling and pressure of an expanding hematoma on the brain can cause even more damage. If the hematoma is in an area of the brain in which tissue damage can be life threatening, and if the hematoma is accessible, it may be drained. In some cases, a hematoma clears up on its own and the body gradually reabsorbs the blood. A hematoma that is very large or that affects an entire hemisphere of the brain can often be fatal.

RECOVERING FROM A STROKE

In the first few hours, days, or months after a stroke, many people recover most of the functions they lost from the stroke and are able to live independently and return to work. About 20 percent of people who have strokes continue to need help with some of the tasks of daily life, such as bathing; about 15 percent become permanently dependent on others. If your recovery is not complete, you have to learn to adapt to your disabilities and try to regain as much of your independence as possible.

It is well worth the time and effort to work with trained therapists who can help you recover some of the functioning you may have lost. Physical therapy can keep the joints of your paralyzed limbs flexible. A series of range-of-motion exercises can help prevent contracture, a painful condition in which a joint becomes permanently stiffened from lack of use. If your ability to walk has been impaired, a major goal of physical therapy is for you to be able to walk again. You will learn to rely on the strength of your healthy leg and arm and use a cane or a walker. An occupational therapist can teach you how to perform daily tasks such as dressing, bathing, preparing food, and writing. With time and practice, you will be able to transfer many of the tasks you previously performed with one hand to the other hand. If you have difficulty speaking or understanding language, you will have speech therapy that may help

Adapting your home after a stroke

Most people are able to go home from the hospital after a stroke and resume many of their usual activities. If you will be using a wheelchair, or if you have limited use of your hands, following are some things you can do to adapt your home to your needs. If these measures are not feasible, depending on your circumstances, you may want to consider moving to a home that is designed for a person with a wheelchair.

Access to your house If you are in a wheelchair, you will need to have a ramp constructed over a set of outside stairs. The ramp and your driveway should slope no more than 4 to 5 degrees to make it easier for you to control your wheelchair. All pathways and walks should be smooth and wide. Make sure there are handrails next to all the ramps.

Inside your home It is a good idea to have your bedroom, kitchen, and living areas on one floor. If you cannot get through the doorways with your wheelchair, have the doors removed from their hinges to give you more space. Remove throw rugs from floors. Wall-to-wall carpeting should be short and dense. Remove unnecessary or unstable furniture.

Bathroom Accessibility to the bathroom is a top priority. Install grab bars on the walls by the toilet and tub to give you support when getting out of your wheelchair. Install vertical and horizontal bars in the tub or shower. Make sure the lighting is bright. Use a rubber mat or nonskid surface on the floor of the tub or shower. Put a sturdy stool or chair in the shower to sit on while showering.

Kitchen To have some independence in your kitchen, place frequently used items where they are easy to reach. Make sure the room is well lighted and light switches are within reach. If you have trouble with your hands, install handles on the faucets that you can turn off with your wrists or arms. If you are in a wheelchair, a table or counter with leg room under it makes it easier for you to eat your meals.

you recover at least some of your ability to talk. A speech therapist can also help you and your family learn new ways to communicate.

Stroke and depression Up to one half of people who have a stroke become depressed at some time afterward. For unknown reasons, depression is sometimes a direct result of a stroke that has damaged tissue in the left hemisphere of the brain. Signs of depression include withdrawal, sleeplessness, and indifference to therapists and family members who are trying to help. Many people who have had a stroke may feel isolated from friends and relatives and avoid formerly pleasurable activities. They may be overly concerned about financial matters. If you have had a stroke, you may be disappointed in the progress of your rehabilitation therapy. People who have language problems are particularly susceptible to depression because their difficulty communicating adds to their feeling of isolation. At times, it may seem that the person has given up or is unwilling to try to get better.

In most cases, this depression is temporary. Participating in a support group with other people who have had strokes (and their families) may be helpful for you and your family. Joining a support group is a good way to gather information, share common experiences, and learn positive ways of coping with your situation. You may also want to see a psychiatrist or other mental health professional, who can help you overcome your depression. If your depression is prolonged, your doctor may prescribe medication to treat it (see page 595).

People who have had a stroke may also experience uncharacteristic moods. They may feel uncontrollably sad or angry, irritable or tearful, withdrawn or indifferent. Because emotions are controlled by the brain, unpredictable and inconsistent emotional changes are often one of the aftereffects of stroke. For example, a person may laugh or cry easily without feeling any true happiness or sadness. Friends and family need to learn to adjust to these inconsistent moods and understand that the person cannot control them.

Disorders of brain function

Some common disorders of the nervous system appear to be caused by a problem in the way in which the brain and the blood vessels that nourish it work. The physical causes of tension headaches and migraines are not fully understood, even though they have been studied extensively and are very common. Similarly, in many cases of epilepsy, a condition characterized by excessive electrical activity in the brain, the cause is unknown; however, medication can usually control it.

HEADACHE

Headache is one of the most common types of pain. Headaches can be temporarily disabling or recurring, but they are rarely a sign of serious underlying illness. Millions of people have headaches on a regular basis. Most headaches are your body's response to a physical stress such as tension, hunger, an allergy, or a cold. Almost all headaches are temporary and can be treated with over-the-counter pain relievers—including aspirin, ibuprofen, or acetaminophen. If you have frequent headaches that do not respond adequately to over-the-counter medications, talk with your doctor. He or she can usually determine the kind of headache you have from a description of your symptoms and your medical history.

More than 90 percent of headaches are tension headaches, which are also called muscle contraction headaches, because they are caused by a tensing of muscles in the scalp and neck. This type of headache is usually triggered by anxiety and stress. Muscle strain resulting from poor posture can also cause tension headaches; people who are in jobs that require them to bend or lean forward, such as assembly line workers and hairdressers, frequently get tension headaches.

A tension headache can cause your whole head to hurt, from your forehead to the back of your neck. The pain may feel like a dull ache, a throb, or tight squeezing. This type of headache can last for as little as an hour or for several days. A tension headache can usually be treated with over-the-counter pain relievers, such as aspirin or ibuprofen. Some people find that gently massaging their scalp and neck helps relieve the pain.

Frequent tension headaches can cause a change in your personality or even depression. Talk with your doctor if you are feeling depressed. Treating the pain from the headaches is the first step, but your doctor may also recommend medication to treat your depression.

Some tension headaches are caused by other medical conditions, such as strain or dysfunction in the joints and muscles of the jaw, a blow to the head, arthritis, whiplash, or a metabolic disorder such as hyperthyroidism (see page 625). In these cases, once the condition is treated, the headaches usually clear up.

WARNING SIGNS
SERIOUS HEADACHE

Most headaches are not a sign of a serious medical problem such as a stroke, but some can be. If your headache is more severe or lasts longer than any headache you have ever had, or if it is accompanied by any of the following conditions, call your doctor immediately:

- Pain in your eye or ear
- Fever or nausea
- Stiff neck
- Confusion, dizziness, weakness, or paralysis
- Convulsions

Keeping a headache diary

A diary of your headaches may help you and your doctor find the triggers that cause them. Answer the following questions whenever you feel a headache coming on; write your answers down, along with the date; and note any patterns you find. Bring your notes with you to the doctor.

- What were you doing when your headache began? Some headaches are triggered by strenuous exercise or by sexual activity.
- Where were you? Indoors or outdoors? In an air-conditioned room or car?
- Were you around any potential allergens, including tobacco smoke, dust, pets, pollen, disinfectants, industrial pollutants, or solvents?
- What were you drinking or eating before your headache began?
- Do your headaches occur more often right before, or after, your period?
- Were you feeling tense or emotionally upset?

MIGRAINE

A migraine headache can cause pounding, throbbing pain. This intense pain can be located in your forehead, temple, ear, jaw, or around your eyes. Most migraines occur on one side of the head, or they start on one side and spread to the other. You may have diarrhea, nausea, or vomiting at the same time. Some people who have migraines get them several times a week; other people have them once every few years. Twice as many women as men have severe, disabling migraines. A susceptibility to migraines appears to be inherited.

Although the cause of migraines is not clear, they may result from narrowing of the blood vessels in the scalp, which reduces the oxygen supply to the brain. When the blood vessels respond to the need for more oxygen by widening, they release chemicals that cause pain, inflammation, and swelling. Many doctors believe that migraine headaches result from changes in blood flow in the brain. A brain chemical called serotonin may also play a role in migraines by causing a reduction in blood flow to some areas of the brain. A migraine can be triggered by stress, fatigue, glaring lights, noise, a change in the weather, some foods (such as cheese or chocolate), red wine, or foods or beverages that contain caffeine.

Symptoms Some people who have migraines experience recognizable symptoms that precede the onset of the headache. These symptoms, called auras, may include seeing dots, flashing lights, or jagged lines in front of the eyes or a "pins and needles" sensation on one side of the face or body. You may also experience nausea or vomiting. The migraine itself usually starts as an intense, gripping pain on one side of your head; in some cases, it affects both sides of the head.

Diagnosis Doctors can usually diagnose migraine headaches by the symptoms they cause. In some cases, it is necessary to perform diagnostic tests such as a computed tomography (CT) scan (see page 572) to rule out other, more serious causes of the headache, such as a tumor.

Treatment Migraine headaches can be treated or prevented with a number of medications. When a migraine starts, you may be able to relieve the pain with over-the-counter anti-inflammatory medications such as aspirin, acetaminophen, ibuprofen, or naproxen. If these medications are not effective, your doctor may prescribe stronger drugs such as ergotamine, which you take in a pill that is dissolved under your tongue. Ergotamine prevents blood vessels from widening and causing the throbbing pain that often accompanies a migraine. Your doctor may prescribe a drug called sumatriptan, which is taken in a pill or in an injection that you give yourself as soon as a migraine begins; your doctor will show you how to administer the shot.

If you have several headaches a month, your doctor may prescribe medication to prevent them. Calcium channel blockers and beta blockers, prescription drugs that are also used to treat high blood pressure and heart disease, are effective for preventing migraines in some people. Both beta blockers and calcium channel blockers prevent migraines by maintaining adequate blood flow to the brain. Some antidepressant medications are also effective in preventing migraines.

EPILEPSY

In a person with epilepsy, electrical activity in the brain sometimes occurs in bursts in a large number of nerve cells instead of in small, regular pulses. This abnormal electrical activity disturbs the normal functioning of the brain. When this electrical activity is excessive, it can cause seizures (temporary lapses in

How to help someone during a seizure

A grand mal seizure usually involves a loss of consciousness and involuntary shaking movements of the arms and legs. The person may fall to the ground. If you witness a person having a seizure, here are some things you can do to help:

- The most important step is to make sure the person is not in any physical danger during the seizure. Clear away any furniture or sharp objects that might cause injury.
- Do not try to restrain the person and do not place anything in his or her mouth.
- If the seizure lasts longer than about 5 minutes, or if another seizure begins within a few minutes of the first, get medical help immediately.
- Once the shaking movements have stopped, place the person on his or her side and make sure nothing is blocking his or her airway.
- The person may pass urine during a seizure. Although this may be embarrassing, it is not dangerous.
- When the person regains consciousness, help him or her to a comfortable place to lie down. He or she will feel exhausted, dazed, and temporarily disoriented.

SYMPTOM CHART

Headache

Pain in your head that can range from mild to so severe that it affects your ability to function.

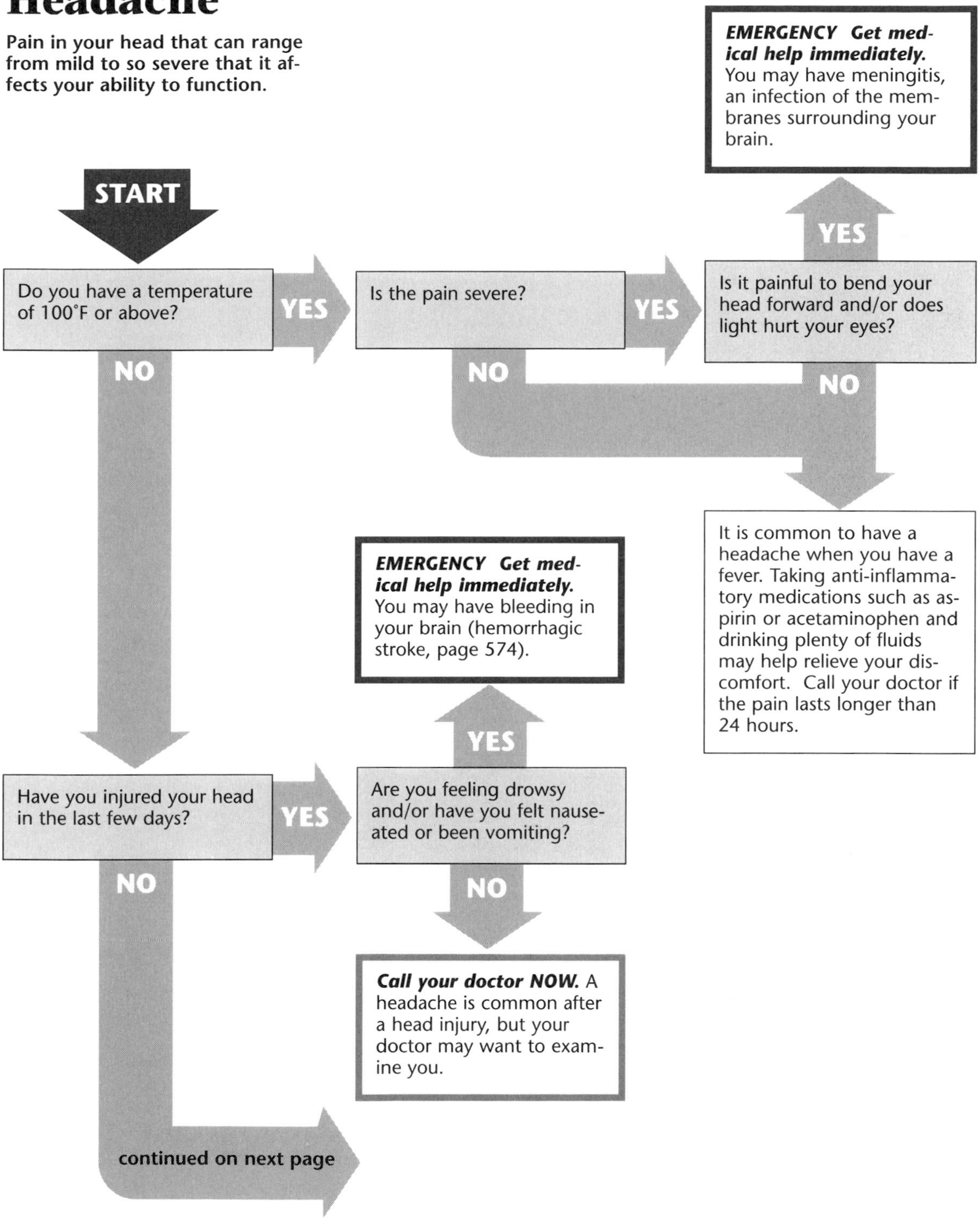

START

Do you have a temperature of 100°F or above?

YES → Is the pain severe?

YES → Is it painful to bend your head forward and/or does light hurt your eyes?

YES → ***EMERGENCY Get medical help immediately.*** You may have meningitis, an infection of the membranes surrounding your brain.

NO (from "Is the pain severe?" or "Is it painful to bend your head forward...") → It is common to have a headache when you have a fever. Taking anti-inflammatory medications such as aspirin or acetaminophen and drinking plenty of fluids may help relieve your discomfort. Call your doctor if the pain lasts longer than 24 hours.

NO (from temperature question) → Have you injured your head in the last few days?

YES → Are you feeling drowsy and/or have you felt nauseated or been vomiting?

YES → ***EMERGENCY Get medical help immediately.*** You may have bleeding in your brain (hemorrhagic stroke, page 574).

NO → ***Call your doctor NOW.*** A headache is common after a head injury, but your doctor may want to examine you.

NO → continued on next page

continued from previous page

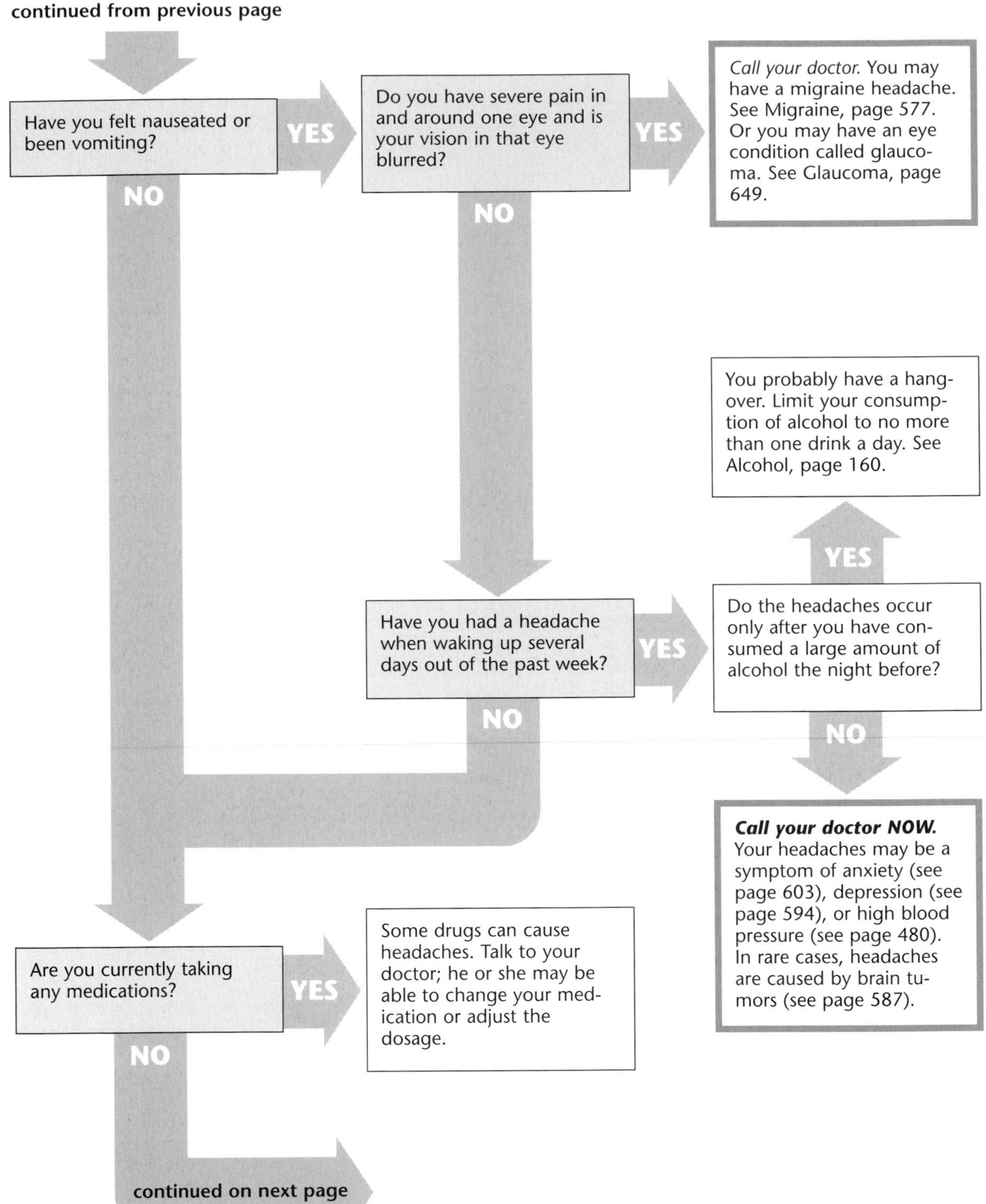

continued on next page

continued from previous page

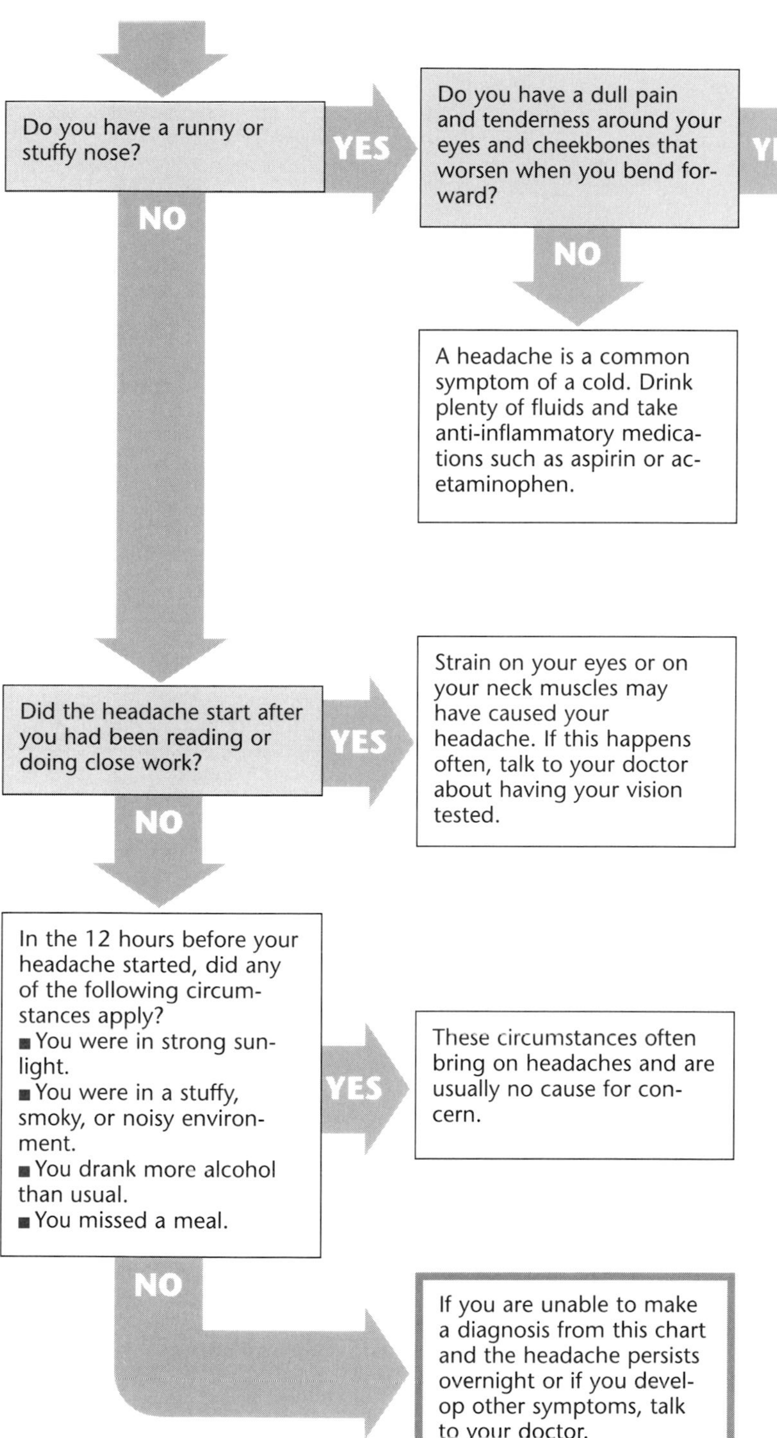

Stroke

Get immediate medical attention if you experience any of the following symptoms of a stroke:

- Sudden, excruciating headache
- Sudden numbness or weakness in your face, an arm or leg, or on one side of your body
- Sudden loss of vision in one eye
- Loss of speech or difficulty speaking
- Dizziness or unsteadiness

consciousness or memory, or uncontrolled movements).

After stroke, epilepsy is the most common neurological disorder in the US, affecting more than 2 million Americans. The condition often appears first during childhood or adolescence, but it can begin at any age. In many cases, the cause of epilepsy is unknown. Although epilepsy is not an inherited disorder, having a family history increases your risk. If you or a family member has a seizure for the first time, see a doctor as quickly as possible to get a diagnosis. It is important to rule out potentially life-threatening causes of seizures, such as an infection or bleeding in the brain. If the diagnosis is epilepsy, the condition can usually be treated effectively with medication that prevents seizures.

Symptoms Epilepsy can cause different kinds of seizures. A grand mal seizure is characterized by loss of consciousness, uncontrollable limb movements, and loss of coordination and balance. In some cases, a grand mal seizure can cause loss of bladder or bowel control. In this type of seizure, the loss of consciousness can last several minutes. Afterward, the person feels exhausted and dazed. Some people who have grand mal seizures have a recognizable warning sign that precedes the seizure itself. Such a warning sign, called an aura, is often a distinct sensory perception, such as a characteristic sound, smell, or visual image.

An absence seizure, also called a petit mal seizure, is a temporary lapse in consciousness that can last for only a second or can occur in several bursts. A person may also experience brief confusion, muscle twitches, or rapid eye movements during an absence seizure. In some cases, these symptoms are so subtle that they are unnoticeable, but they can occur so often—hundreds of times a day—that it is difficult for the person to concentrate or complete ordinary activities. Absence seizures are more common in children.

Psychomotor epilepsy is the least common form of epilepsy. The affected person laughs, talks strangely, walks around in circles, or makes other automatic responses such as lip smacking or chewing that he or she is not aware of. These episodes are brief; afterward, the person feels confused and cannot remember what happened.

Diagnosis The first step in diagnosing epilepsy is to evaluate the pattern and type of seizures you are having. Your doctor will need to know in great detail your symptoms, when they occur, and how long they last. Because you most likely will not remember what happened during a seizure, you may need to get some of this information from people who were present. You are likely to have an electroencephalogram (EEG), which

Coping with epilepsy

Because epilepsy can take many forms, it can affect people in many different ways. If you have frequent seizures, your daily life can be difficult. In some cases, frequent seizures occur when people with epilepsy stop taking their medication because it makes them feel drowsy or causes them to gain weight. If this is the case, talk to your doctor; it may be possible to change your medication or dosage. Because antiseizure medications can reduce your coordination and make you drowsy, you should not use alcohol, which can increase these effects.

Most doctors recommend that people who have epilepsy not drive a car unless their medication has prevented seizures for at least 1 year. You should also refrain from driving for a year after the dose of your medication has been changed to make sure your seizures are under control. Different states have different requirements for drivers who have epilepsy. Check with your state licensing bureau regarding the regulations in your state.

If you cannot drive a car (because your seizures are not under control) or if you occasionally experience seizures in public or at work, you may begin to feel isolated or "different." This can lead to anger, frustration, or depression, which in turn can lead to more frequent seizures. It is important to take care of your psychological and emotional needs. Call a local hospital or ask your doctor if there are any support groups in your area for people with epilepsy and their families. You may also find it helpful to talk to a therapist about your difficulties and frustrations. Ask your doctor to recommend a qualified therapist.

evaluates the electrical activity of your brain. You will probably have a computed tomography (CT) scan (see page 572) or magnetic resonance imaging (MRI; see page 572) to rule out the presence of a tumor, cyst, or excess fluid in your brain. If you have any of these conditions, treating them may stop the seizures.

Treatment Epilepsy can usually be treated successfully with medication that prevents most or all of the seizures. Finding the right medication in the right dosage may take some time. You may need to try more than one drug before you and your doctor find the one that works best for you.

In some cases, if medication fails to eliminate seizures, epilepsy can be treated with surgery to remove the part of the brain in which the seizures occur. This procedure frees the rest of the brain from the constant disruption caused by the seizures. Surgery is seldom done in areas of the brain that involve speech, language, hearing, and other major functions.

Electroencephalogram

An electroencephalogram (EEG) is a painless test that detects and records patterns of electrical impulses in the brain. An EEG is used to help diagnose brain disorders—including epilepsy, tumors, an injury such as a concussion, internal bleeding, inflammation, the effects of various drugs, and some psychiatric disorders.

For an EEG, several electrodes are attached to your scalp to record the electrical activity that naturally occurs inside your brain. The electrical brain waves are then translated into a reading on a printout.

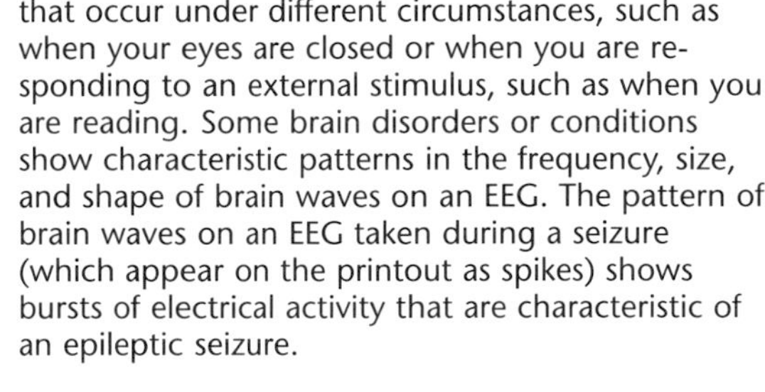

An EEG picks up different types of brain waves that occur under different circumstances, such as when your eyes are closed or when you are responding to an external stimulus, such as when you are reading. Some brain disorders or conditions show characteristic patterns in the frequency, size, and shape of brain waves on an EEG. The pattern of brain waves on an EEG taken during a seizure (which appear on the printout as spikes) shows bursts of electrical activity that are characteristic of an epileptic seizure.

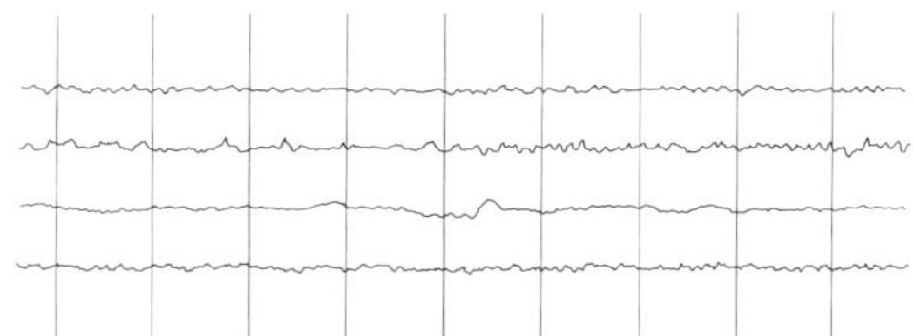

Normal electrical patterns in the brain

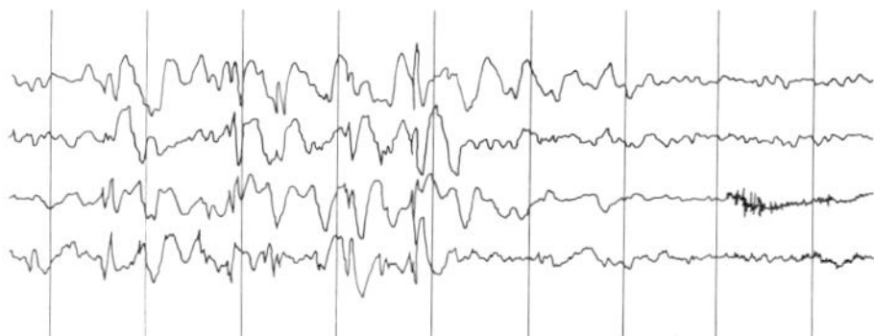

Patterns during a grand mal seizure

ELECTRICAL ACTIVITY IN THE BRAIN DURING A SEIZURE
An electroencephalogram (EEG) is a recording of the electrical activity in the brain. Using EEGs, doctors can compare brain wave patterns that occur during seizures (right) with normal patterns (left). An EEG is used to help diagnose epilepsy and some other brain disorders.

Other disorders

Some neurological diseases—such as Alzheimer's disease and multiple sclerosis—cause changes in the nervous system that worsen over time. Brain tumors can be cancerous or benign but are always serious because they can grow into and destroy brain tissue. Bell's palsy and carpal tunnel syndrome result from injury to nerves that transmit impulses between the brain and other areas of the body. Bell's palsy is caused by injury to the facial nerve. Carpal tunnel syndrome results from injury to the nerve that transmits impulses to the hand.

ALZHEIMER'S DISEASE

Alzheimer's disease is a progressive, degenerative disease that destroys brain cells, eventually causing death. The disease is the most common cause of dementia, the deterioration of a person's mental faculties. Alzheimer's disease gradually causes the loss of intellectual abilities such as memory, thinking, reasoning, judgment, orientation, and concentration, and it can cause drastic changes in personality, mood, and behavior. Alzheimer's is a disease, not a normal part of aging. Although memory loss is a hallmark of Alzheimer's disease, ordinary forgetfulness is not a sign that you have the disorder. It is very common to forget where you put your keys; you have cause to be concerned if you forget what the keys are for.

Although men and women are thought to be at equal risk of Alzheimer's disease, it affects more women. This is at least partly because women live longer than men and Alzheimer's occurs at older ages. As life expectancy increases, more people will develop Alzheimer's disease. The disease has no known cause but genes are linked to a rare form of the disease that begins at a younger age—during a person's 40s or 50s. However, most people who develop Alzheimer's have no family history of the disease. No substance in the environment or anything you eat, drink, or breathe has been found to cause Alzheimer's disease.

Although the cause of Alzheimer's disease is still not known, doctors are learning about ways to delay its effects. People who have many years of education and who stay mentally active throughout their life may be able to postpone the onset of symptoms of Alzheimer's disease or to reduce the severity of early symptoms. Intellectually stimulating activities increase the number of connections between your brain cells. These additional connections may provide a buffer against the destructive effects of Alzheimer's disease. Women who are undergoing hormone replacement therapy (HRT; see page 359) after menopause may have a reduced risk of Alzheimer's because the female hormone estrogen nourishes many types of brain cells.

Alzheimer's disease has a great impact on women not only because more women than men are affected but also because women are most likely to be caregivers for a person with Alzheimer's. Most people with Alzheimer's disease are cared for at home during the early to middle phases of the disease. During the later stages, people with Alzheimer's disease may become extremely confused, disoriented, unaware of their surroundings, irritable, suspicious, fearful, or even violent. They may become unable to perform daily functions, such as dressing, eating, or using the toilet. During the later stages, the caregiver for a person with Alzheimer's disease often can no longer provide the necessary care. He or she is then faced with the difficult decision of turning over the care of their loved one to others.

Symptoms In its early stages, Alzheimer's disease has symptoms similar to those of depression—including withdrawal, apathy, loss of concentration and interest, memory failure, intellectual impairment, anxiety, agitation, and delusions. But whereas depression usually comes on suddenly and rapidly gets worse, the symptoms of Alzheimer's disease appear gradually and worsen over a period of years.

Diagnosis Alzheimer's disease is difficult to diagnose and is often misdiagnosed. Doctors recognize the disease mainly from the symptoms reported by the affected person and family members and by a series of tests. These tests evaluate the person's mental functioning, such as the ability to remember things in the recent past (short-term memory). No brain scan or blood test can diagnose Alzheimer's disease with certainty, although tests such as a computed tomography (CT) scan (see page 572) or magnetic resonance imaging (MRI; see page 572) may show the degeneration of brain tissues that is characteristic of the disorder. A CT scan or MRI can also help rule out other possible causes of dementia, such as a brain tumor (see page 587).

An important step in diagnosing Alzheimer's disease is to rule out other possible causes of the symptoms, including depression (see page 594), adverse effects from some medications, excessive consumption of alcohol, thyroid disorders (see page 624), liver failure, kidney failure (see page 548), a vitamin deficiency, bleeding inside the skull, and infections that can affect the brain. Parkinson's disease can also cause degrees of mental impairment.

Treatment There is no cure for Alzheimer's disease. Treatment of a person with Alzheimer's primarily involves caring for him or her and dealing with the worsening symptoms. Good nutrition is important because deficiencies of vitamins and other nutrients can intensify the symptoms of Alzheimer's disease.

The only medication available for treating Alzheimer's disease, called tacrine, is not effective in all people. Tacrine can reduce symptoms slightly in some people. The drug replaces acetylcholine, a brain chemical that is missing in people who have the disorder. Acetylcholine transmits messages between brain cells and is important for memory.

But tacrine can cause side effects such as nausea and vomiting and liver damage in some people. Because of these poten-

If you are a caregiver

Most people in the early stages of Alzheimer's disease live at home and are cared for by members of their family. Caring for an adult who has become completely dependent can be intensely stressful. It is important to prepare yourself emotionally and physically and to be realistic in your expectations of how much you can do. In addition, you need to prepare yourself for the future. Here are some things to consider:

- **Get a diagnosis early.** Do not ignore the first warning signs, such as confusion, forgetfulness, or withdrawal. These may be symptoms of another disorder, such as a nutritional deficiency, that can be reversed if treated early.
- **Take care of legal and financial planning.** Make sure that a will and advance directives (see page 708) such as a living will are in place, and that someone the person loves and trusts has durable power of attorney to act on his or her behalf. Determine how much home care is covered by health insurance or Medicare. Consider the costs of a nursing home or hospice.
- **Get as much information as you can.** Call the local chapter of the Alzheimer's Association. This national organization provides a broad range of services and programs, including educational materials and support groups for families affected by the disorder. Trained staff at the local chapter can help you learn how to deal with your loved one's symptoms.
- **Learn how to protect your loved one.** People with Alzheimer's disease may lack the judgment to protect themselves from potential dangers such as a hot stove or electrical shock, or wandering out of the house and getting lost. You will need to take precautions such as locking away medicines and dangerous substances in your home. The Alzheimer's Association has a national program—called Safe Return—that registers people with Alzheimer's disease and provides them with an identifying bracelet or necklace, clothing labels, and wallet cards. If the person wanders away from home and gets lost, he or she can be identified through a 24-hour toll-free number and returned home safely. Ask your doctor for information about how to register your loved one in the Safe Return program.
- **Get help.** Look for adult day-care programs, some of which provide transportation to and from a facility where people with Alzheimer's disease can spend several hours a day in a supervised setting. Other resources that may be available in your community include in-home assistance, visiting nurses who can temporarily relieve you and give you some time for yourself, and delivery of meals to your home. Do not try to do it all alone. Share the responsibilities with family members and friends by accepting help and asking for it when you need it. When asking for help, be specific about what you need.
- **Don't neglect your own needs.** Make sure to take time to do the things you have to do or want to do, including work, hobbies, or social activities. Eat a nutritious diet, exercise regularly, and get enough rest.
- **Face reality.** The progression of Alzheimer's disease is certain. Grieve for the loss of the companion you once had and your future together. A support group can help you overcome the difficulty of grieving for a person who is still alive.
- **Know when to let go.** One of the most difficult decisions you will eventually have to make is when to turn the care of your loved one over to others. There are no standard guidelines for knowing when to seek help because each family has a unique situation. As soon as your loved one is diagnosed with Alzheimer's disease, begin educating yourself about nursing homes in your community and their requirements for admission. The more information you have, the easier it will be for you to make informed decisions about appropriate long-term care for your loved one. For more about how to find a nursing home, see page 148.

tial side effects, a person who is taking tacrine is closely monitored by his or her doctor. In some cases, medications can be used to lessen symptoms such as sleeplessness.

Families and caregivers often experience a high degree of stress and anxiety as they watch a loved one succumb to the debilitating effects of the disease, including a complete lack of recognition of family members. All people with Alzheimer's disease eventually reach a point at which they cannot be left alone. In some cases, this forces a spouse or adult child to quit a job or give up regular activities to stay home to care for the person. In other cases, the painful, difficult decision must be made to place the person into a setting where he or she can be cared for by trained professionals.

A person who becomes a full-time caregiver may experience increasing isolation and stress, which often leads to depression. If you are a caregiver, getting support from other family members and friends as well as help from counselors and organized support groups is an essential part of coping (see page 189).

MULTIPLE SCLEROSIS

Multiple sclerosis (MS) is a progressive, disabling disease of the central nervous system. In most cases, MS first appears between ages 20 and 40. Two out of three people with the disorder are women. The cause of MS is not clear, but it may result from a genetic susceptibility that is triggered by infection with a virus contracted early in life. A family history of the disease increases your risk.

MS causes a breakdown of communication in your nervous system. The disease destroys the protective, fatty coating (myelin) on nerve cells in your brain or spinal cord, reducing the ability of your brain to transmit messages to the rest of your body. MS may be a type of autoimmune disease in which the body mistakenly reacts against and destroys its own tissues—in this case, the myelin sheaths that surround nerve cells.

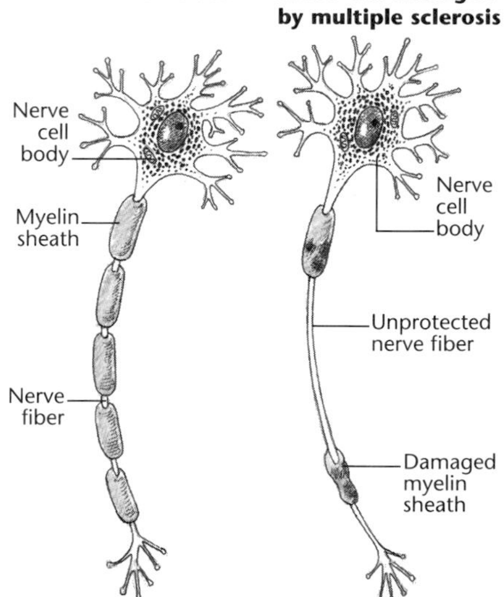

NERVE DAMAGED BY MULTIPLE SCLEROSIS
Multiple sclerosis is a progressive disease in which the protective coatings (myelin sheaths) that normally surround nerve fibers are damaged and worn away. The nerves are then exposed and cannot properly transmit messages to and from the brain.

Most women who have MS live a normal lifespan. In a small percentage of cases, the disease progresses very rapidly and leads to premature death from complications such as pneumonia or other infections. In some people, MS is so mild that they do not know they have it; evidence of damage to their central nervous system is only discovered in an autopsy after they die.

Symptoms The first symptoms of MS usually include severe fatigue; weakness or paralysis in one or more limbs; blurred vision, pain when you move one eye, or rapid, involuntary eye movements; a sudden change in bladder control, such as urinating more frequently or feeling stronger urges to urinate; lack of coordination, dizziness, unsteady walk, or trembling in a hand or limb; and decreased sensation during sex. The symptoms may worsen when your body heats up from exercise or a hot bath.

MS is characterized by recurring attacks in which the symptoms become severe for weeks or months. The attacks are followed by periods of remission during which the symptoms lessen. It is not fully understood what triggers these attacks, but in some cases they result from exposure to a virus.

MS affects each person differently. In some people, the symptoms of MS remain mild and never become serious. In other people, the symptoms become progressively and steadily worse. Gradually, recovery from each attack is less complete and you may eventually become permanently disabled. A person in whom the effects of the disease are limited mostly to nerve cells that control the arms and legs may experience weakness or even paralysis in those limbs. Another person may have permanent blindness caused by damage to the optic nerve in the eye.

Diagnosis To diagnose MS, your doctor must eliminate causes of similar symptoms such as a stroke (see page 569) or brain tumor (see below). One difference between these other disorders and MS is that, while only one part of the brain is affected by a stroke or tumor, MS affects major portions of the entire nervous system. Although no laboratory test can confirm that a person has MS, magnetic resonance imaging (MRI; see page 572) can detect damaged areas of the brain that are often present in people with the disease.

A second test, called a lumbar puncture (or spinal tap), is often used to help diagnose MS. For a lumbar puncture, cerebrospinal fluid (the fluid that surrounds your brain and spinal cord) is drawn out of your spinal column through a hollow needle that is inserted between vertebrae in your lower spine. The procedure is done using local anesthesia and takes about 20 minutes. The presence of particular antibodies in the cerebrospinal fluid indicates a very strong likelihood that you have MS. Antibodies are proteins that the body normally produces to fight foreign invaders such as bacteria and viruses, but, in MS, they are produced for no known reason.

You may also have an evoked response test. In this test, electrodes are placed on your head to record the electrical responses of your brain while you are exposed to a variety of stimuli, such as flashing lights.

Treatment There is no cure for MS. However, treatment can help prevent attacks or lengthen the time between them. Many drugs for treating MS are currently under study. For now, the only medication that helps prevent attacks is a synthetic version of interferon beta, a naturally occurring protein that the body uses to enhance the immune response.

Some medications can be taken during an attack to reduce symptoms; these drugs include corticosteroids (synthetic hormones) such as prednisone or dexamethasone, or adrenocorticotropic hormone, which acts on the adrenal gland to stimulate the body's production of steroids. Steroids are hormones that reduce inflammation and swelling. During an attack, corticosteroids may be administered intravenously or taken by mouth in high doses that are gradually reduced over a period of 3 to 4 weeks.

Your doctor may prescribe an antiviral medication called amantadine or stimulants such as epinephrine and methylphenidate to help reduce fatigue. Staying cool with air-conditioning can also help decrease fatigue. To relieve other symptoms, such as muscle spasms, your doctor may prescribe medications such as muscle relaxants. If you are experiencing urinary incontinence (see page 538), your doctor may prescribe an antispasmodic medication that relaxes the bladder muscle and prevents the contractions that may be causing urine to leak. Physical therapists can help you build strength in your muscles and improve your coordination, balance, and stamina. An occupational therapist can teach you ways to make daily tasks easier to perform.

BRAIN TUMORS

A brain tumor is a mass of abnormal tissue in the brain that may be cancerous (malignant) or noncancerous (benign). Because any tumor that grows in the brain can be dangerous, the distinction between cancerous and benign may not be as important with a brain tumor as it is with tumors in other parts of the body.

So-called primary brain tumors originate in the brain or spinal cord and, in some people, are present from birth. A cancerous tumor that originates in the brain seldom spreads to other parts of the body. A secondary brain tumor is a cancer that has spread (metastasized) from another area of the body. In women, secondary tumors have usually spread from a cancer in the breast or lung. Secondary brain tumors are the more common type.

A brain tumor can occur at any age. Although brain tumors are relatively rare, they present a difficult problem because they are next to or in tissues that control all your body's functions, including your intellect, memory, and emotions. However, in some cases, a tumor can be treated successfully, leaving the brain with no permanent damage.

Symptoms A brain tumor may grow slowly for years without causing any symptoms. Once a tumor becomes large enough to affect brain function, problems can develop rapidly. An expanding tumor increases pressure inside the skull, causing compression of brain tissue, nerves, and blood vessels. When the pressure becomes strong enough, you may experience symptoms—including headaches, vision problems, numbness in your arms and legs, and seizures (abnormal electrical activity in your brain that can cause a temporary loss of consciousness).

Diagnosis A variety of tests can help diagnose a brain tumor. A computed tomography (CT) scan (see page 572) or magnetic resonance imaging (MRI; see page 572) is usually the first step. A CT scan or MRI can produce a computerized image of the brain and each is nearly 95-percent accurate in detecting a tumor. If a tumor is found on a CT scan or MRI, you may have a cerebral angiogram (see page 573) to further evaluate the nature of the tumor. For example, an angiogram can determine if the tumor is pushing on normal blood vessels or if there are numerous blood vessels in the tumor. The number of blood vessels in a brain tumor helps doctors determine the type of tumor it is and how large it is. In some cases, an electroencephalogram (EEG; see page 583) is done to see if the tumor is altering the functioning of the brain or causing seizures.

Treatment Surgery is often the first treatment for a brain tumor. Procedures vary widely depending on the location and accessibility of the tumor. During surgery, a doctor may be able to remove the tumor and determine whether it is benign or malignant. If the tumor is malignant and cannot be removed completely, you are likely to have radiation therapy (see page 253) or chemotherapy (see page 254). In some cases, high-frequency sound waves (ultrasound), lasers (powerful, highly focused beams of light), or focused radiation can be used to destroy brain tumors.

WARNING SIGNS
BRAIN TUMOR

See your doctor if you have any of the following symptoms:

- Prolonged, continuous headaches that are often worse in the morning
- Blurred or double vision
- Weakness or numbness in your arms or legs
- Loss of sensation below a certain level of your body
- Seizures

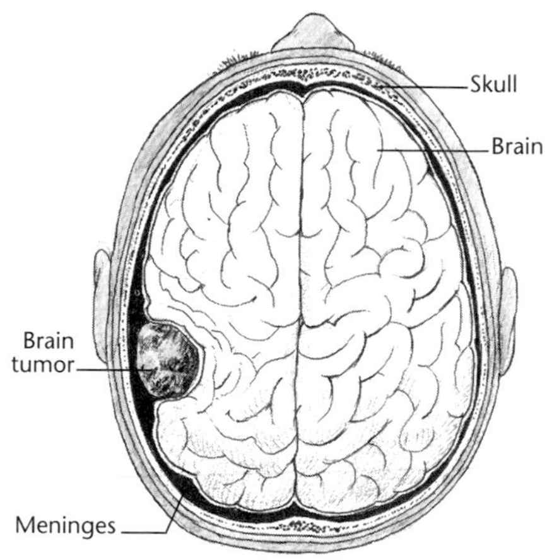

MENINGIOMA: A NONCANCEROUS BRAIN TUMOR

A meningioma is a noncancerous brain tumor that is located in the outer layer of tissue (the meninges) that encloses and protects the brain. The pressure created by a tumor in this area causes loss of some brain functions such as the ability to speak and understand language. Doctors usually try to remove a meningioma surgically, depending on its size and location.

BELL'S PALSY

Bell's palsy is temporary paralysis of the muscles in the face caused by inflammation of the facial nerve. In most cases, only one of the two facial nerves is affected and the paralysis affects only one side of the face. Bell's palsy is sometimes confused with stroke because strokes often affect only one side of the body. But, unlike a stroke, Bell's palsy does not result from damage to the brain; it is caused by damage to the facial nerve, which is outside the brain. Although the symptoms can be alarming, in many cases they are only temporary and last no longer than several months. The cause of Bell's palsy is not clear, but it may result from infection with a virus that makes the nerve swell at the point where it leaves the brain through a small opening in the skull. Because the nerve has no room to expand inside this bony canal, pressure builds up and damages the nerve.

Symptoms Bell's palsy may cause complete paralysis on one side of your face, making it impossible for you to change expression on that side. The muscle on one side of your face may sag. You may be able to only partially close the eye on that side and your eye may water excessively. The corner of your mouth may turn down and saliva may drain out of it. The paralysis in your face may be preceded a day or two by a feeling of pain behind your ear on that side. You may have a decreased sensation of taste on that side of your tongue or some difficulty eating or speaking. These symptoms often occur suddenly or over a period of 1 to 2 days.

Diagnosis Because a number of conditions, including stroke, can affect function on one side of the body, your doctor must evaluate your symptoms carefully. If your symptoms begin suddenly and you do not have any other neurologic problems (such as weakness in muscles other than those in your face), you are likely to have Bell's palsy. Your doctor may recommend electromyography (EMG), a test that can evaluate the functioning of your facial nerve. EMG may help predict how fast and complete your recovery will be.

Treatment Although, in most cases, Bell's palsy clears up on its own, many doctors prescribe an anti-inflammatory drug such as the corticosteroid (synthetic hormone) prednisone to help reduce inflammation and swelling and speed recovery. In rare cases, a person must have surgery to relieve pressure in the canal through which the nerve exits the skull. If you cannot close your eye, you will need to take measures to prevent it from drying out to avoid permanent damage. Your doctor may recommend eyedrops to use during the day and a patch or ointment to protect your eye while you are sleeping.

CARPAL TUNNEL SYNDROME

Carpal tunnel syndrome is a condition in which pressure on a nerve that leads from your spinal cord to your hands causes numbness, pain, or tingling in your hand or fingers. The carpal tunnel is a narrow passage formed by ligaments in your wrist through which nerves and tendons pass. When the muscles and ligaments of the carpal tunnel become swollen or inflamed, they compress the median nerve, which leads to your thumb and first two fingers. This pressure causes pain or numbness. In some cases, both wrists are affected.

Carpal tunnel syndrome is more common in women than men. The disorder usually occurs in people who do work that causes repetitive stress on one or both wrists—such as word processing operators, computer operators, chefs, factory workers, librarians, and violinists. The condition can occur in pregnant women and in women who have recently given birth, because the buildup of fluid in their body during pregnancy puts extra pressure on nerves. In some cases, carpal tunnel syndrome is caused by a disease—such as diabetes (see page 617), rheumatoid arthritis (see page 645), or hypothyroidism (see page 624)—that affects the blood vessels of the median nerve or the connective tissue (the carpal tunnel or ligaments) in the wrist.

CARPAL TUNNEL SYNDROME

Carpal tunnel syndrome is pain or numbness in your thumb and first two fingers that results from excessive, prolonged pressure on the median nerve as it passes through a narrow channel (called the carpal tunnel) in the wrist. This pressure on the median nerve is usually caused by repetitive manual activities, such as typing on a computer keyboard, that put excessive stress on surrounding tendons and other tissues in the wrist.

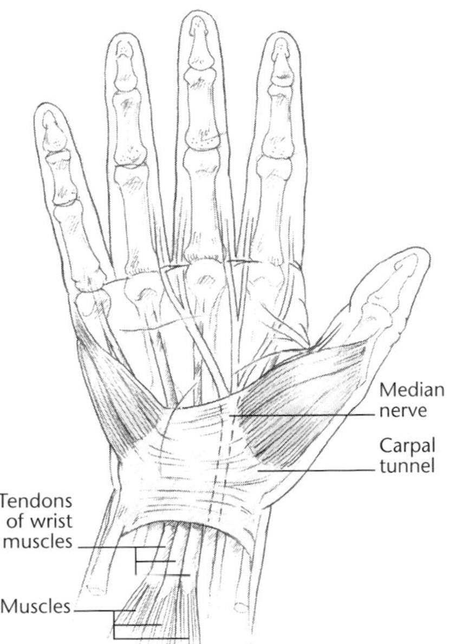

Palm of right hand

Sleeping with your wrist bent sharply inward can worsen the condition.

Symptoms The symptoms of carpal tunnel syndrome may come and go, and include the following: numbness in your hand or fingers (especially the thumb and first two fingers); pain that starts in your wrist and shoots down into the palm of your hand or the surface of your fingers, or up into your forearm; pain or numbness that increases at night, particularly after a day during which you have used your hands more than usual in a repetitive activity; and pain or numbness in your hand during pregnancy or shortly after.

The symptoms are often progressive. At first, you may be bothered only at night, partly because fluids are more likely to accumulate in your arms and legs while you sleep. The symptoms may begin to occur at other times. Gradually, even simple tasks become painful. In some cases, the disorder goes away on its own. In other cases, if the condition is not treated, it can progress until you cannot use the affected hand.

Diagnosis Carpal tunnel syndrome is usually identified by pain and numbness that occur only in your thumb and first two fingers and nowhere else in your hand. Your doctor may tap lightly on the front of your wrist. If pain shoots into your hand or forearm, it is a strong indication that you have carpal tunnel syndrome. Your doctor may recommend nerve conduction tests, such as electromyography (EMG), to determine if you have any nerve damage. EMG can also show if nerve impulses are impaired as they pass through your wrist.

Treatment If you are diagnosed with carpal tunnel syndrome, your doctor may first recommend slowing down the

Preventing carpal tunnel syndrome

Making periodic, minor adjustments in the position of your hands or wrists while you perform a repetitive activity can make a difference and help you avoid carpal tunnel syndrome. If you work at a keyboard, type with your wrists straight, bent neither up nor down. To make this adjustment, you may have to raise or lower your seat. Stop your work periodically to rest your hands by doing the following:

1. Make a loose fist and open and gently stretch your hand. Repeat several times.
2. Stand up and place your hands palms down on a table. Press firmly with both of your hands against the table. Hold for 5 seconds and release. Repeat four times.
3. Lay your forearm on a table with your hand dangling off the edge. Bend your wrist back as far as it goes. Gently pull your fingers back using your other hand. Hold for 5 seconds. Repeat four times with each hand.

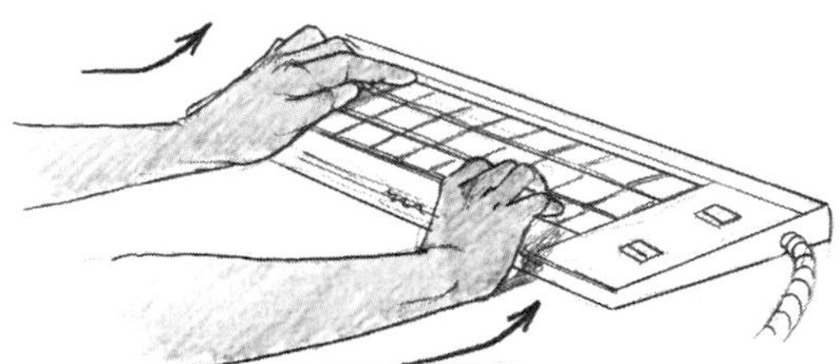

Improper angle of wrists

POSITION YOUR WRISTS PROPERLY AT YOUR KEYBOARD

Many keyboard typists and computer users are affected by carpal tunnel syndrome. Position your keyboard at a height where your wrists do not bend up or down while you type. Your elbows should be at a 90-degree angle, with your forearms parallel to the floor. To achieve the correct position, try lowering your keyboard or raising your chair.

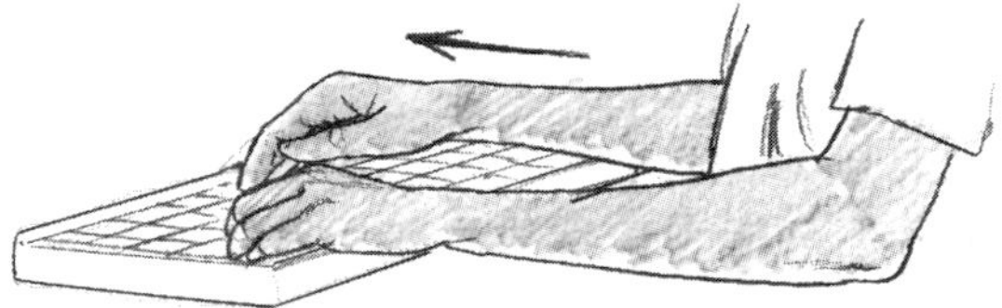

Proper angle of wrists

pace at which you work, or resting the joint by avoiding the repetitive activity with your wrists that caused the problem. You will be given advice about how to modify your work area to put less strain on your wrists. Your doctor may recommend taking time off from work altogether to allow the inflammation to subside.

Using a splint at night to keep your wrist straight can help relieve pain and other symptoms and allow you to get a good night's sleep. Your doctor may recommend that you also wear the splint during the day to immobilize your wrist while still allowing your hand to function. If pain is a problem, ask your doctor about over-the-counter anti-inflammatory medications (such as aspirin or ibuprofen or, if you are pregnant, acetaminophen). If you are pregnant, your symptoms will probably subside gradually after the pregnancy.

If your pain persists, your doctor may prescribe injections of a corticosteroid (synthetic hormone) such as cortisone into your wrist to reduce pain and inflammation. If the problem does not clear up after two injections of corticosteroids, you may want to consider surgery.

The surgery for treating carpal tunnel syndrome, called carpal tunnel release, is a relatively fast and simple procedure that is performed to relieve the pressure on the median nerve. The surgery is done using local anesthesia (see page 260) and usually does not require an overnight stay in the hospital. In this procedure, the surgeon cuts the ligaments that form the carpal tunnel, freeing the compressed median nerve. After 2 or 3 weeks, you can begin to use your hand again. You may not gain complete function for about 3 months because the nerves must regrow past the wrist into the muscles of the hand and fingers.

CHRONIC FATIGUE SYNDROME

Chronic fatigue syndrome (CFS) is a disorder characterized by unexplained, persistent, debilitating fatigue. Other symptoms can include difficulties with memory and concentration, sleep disturbances, and pain in muscles and joints. CFS appears to involve the central nervous system (the brain and spinal cord) and the immune system. The average length of time for a person to have CFS is 2 years, but many people have it much longer than that. CFS occurs in people of all ages and both sexes, but it is most common among women under 45. The cause is unknown.

Symptoms The most prominent symptom of CFS is excessive fatigue that can result from even moderate exertion. This incapacitating fatigue lasts for 6 months or more and substantially reduces your ability to function in your job and personal life. Some people with CFS improve with time, but most have a reduced ability to function for several years. Other symptoms include poor concentration, impaired short-term memory (not remembering something you did a few minutes or hours ago), unrefreshing sleep, or fatigue that lasts more than 24 hours after exertion. You also may experience symptoms similar to those of an infection, such as a sore throat, tender lymph nodes in your neck and under your arms, unusual headaches, or pain in your muscles or joints.

Diagnosis CFS is difficult to diagnose because many of the symptoms are similar to those of various other disorders. There are no specific laboratory tests or imaging procedures that can diagnose CFS. Your doctor will ask about your health history and give you a physical examination. He or she will evaluate your mental state to rule out disorders such as depression. You may also have a blood test or other laboratory tests to rule out disorders such as hypothyroidism (see page 624), chronic hepatitis B or C (see page 534), multiple sclerosis (see page 586), lupus (see page 641), or AIDS (see page 344). If you are in your middle to late 40s, your doctor may want to rule out menopause (see page 352) as a cause of your symptoms. Some symptoms of CFS—including difficulty sleeping, impaired memory and concentration, and reduced energy level—are similar to those of menopause.

After ruling out other possibilities, your doctor is likely to diagnose CFS if you have debilitating fatigue that has lasted longer than 6 months and four or more of the other symptoms listed above.

Treatment No specific treatment or medication can cure CFS, but medications can control some of the symptoms. For example, if you have headaches, sore throat, tender lymph nodes, or pain in your muscles or joints, your doctor may prescribe a pain reliever or a nonsteroidal anti-inflammatory medication, such as aspirin. In addition, your doctor may recommend a medication that you take at bedtime to improve your sleep.

You will need to learn your limits and how to function within them. Determine your priorities and try to spend your available energy on those, letting go of less important responsibilities. Have your spouse or another family member or friend go with you to the doctor to learn about your condition.

Your symptoms may be worsened by anxiety and emotional stress and may be improved with rest. Practice techniques for reducing stress (see page 186). Do not blame yourself for not meeting your expectations or those of other people. Joining a support group for people with CFS is a good way to share information and learn coping strategies.

CHAPTER 23

Your mental health

Contents

Mental disorders used to be something that you did not discuss, even with your own family. But the stigma of mental illness has decreased significantly with major advances in understanding of the causes of these disorders. New knowledge has led to the development of more effective treatments for many mental illnesses, which can affect people of all ages and socioeconomic groups.

Like most illnesses, the earlier mental disorders are diagnosed, the more effectively they can be treated. If you recognize the symptoms of one of the disorders described in this chapter—in yourself or in someone you love—see a doctor as soon as possible. Depending on the disorder, your doctor may treat you or he or she will refer you to a psychiatrist or another qualified mental health professional.

Mood disorders

Mood disorders, also called affective disorders, are extreme, persistent disruptions of your usual emotional state. It is normal to feel down or blue for a period of time after you experience a traumatic event, such as the death of a loved one or loss of a job. Even a major positive change in your life, such as the birth of a baby or a new job, can be stressful. (For information about postpartum depression, see page 449.) But a prolonged depression that interferes with your ability to work, sleep, eat, or socialize usually requires evaluation and treatment by a doctor. Most mood disorders can be relieved relatively quickly with medication or psychotherapy or a combination of these two treatments.

DEPRESSION

Depression is a common but serious illness that affects both your mind and your body. Depression can disable you emotionally, physically, socially, and professionally. Depression occurs in twice as many women as men, usually between ages 18 and 44. The illness is not a sign of personal weakness. If you are depressed, you cannot just "pull yourself together" or will yourself to get better. Effective treatment is available; the important first step is getting the help you need, as you would for any other medical problem.

Depression usually results from a combination of genetic, biological, psychological, and environmental factors. In some cases, depression results from an imbalance of brain chemicals (called neurotransmitters) that carry messages between the cells in the brain that affect behavior, emotions, and thought. Severe stress, grief, or other difficult changes in a person's life may contribute to this chemical imbalance. Some people inherit a susceptibility that makes them more likely than other people to become depressed when they are exposed to a stressful event, such as the death of a loved one.

Family history is also a factor. If you have a parent or sibling or other close relative who has had depression, you are more likely than other people to develop it at some time in your life. However, depression also occurs in people who have no family history of the illness. A person's psychological makeup may make him or her more vulnerable or less vulnerable to depression than others. People who have low self-esteem, who are pessimistic about themselves and the world, are overly dependent on others, or are readily overwhelmed by stress are more prone to depression.

In older people, depression can result from a serious illness—such as a stroke, diabetes, or some types of cancer—or from some medications, such as those used to treat high blood pressure or arthritis. It is important for your doctor to know about all medications you are taking and their dosages; always have this information with you when you go to a doctor.

Doctors classify depression into several categories. Clinical, or major, depression is considered severe and usually requires treatment. Unlike milder feelings of sadness or the blues, major depression seldom goes away with time or an improvement in circumstances. Without treatment, the symptoms of depression can last for months or years.

Less severe forms of depression

People who have less severe, but long-term, recurring symptoms of depression have a form of depression called dysthymia. Dysthymia can prevent you from functioning at your normal level or from feeling good. In some cases, people who have dysthymia also experience periods of major depression.

Another type of depression—called an adjustment disorder with a depressed mood—is an unusually strong reaction to a single event, such as a death, divorce, or loss of a job. It is normal to feel angry, confused, or sad when you are going through a stressful time. If you have an adjustment disorder, you may have symptoms such as extreme sadness, difficulty sleeping, inability to concentrate at work, or inability to show interest in your family. These symptoms usually subside gradually over a period of weeks or months as you adapt to your new situation. If the symptoms last longer than 6 months, you may have a more serious mood disorder, such as major depression, that requires treatment.

Symptoms The symptoms of major depression and their severity vary substantially from person to person. Some people have only a few symptoms, while others experience many. You may feel persistently low, sad, anxious, or irritable; hopeless or pessimistic; or guilty, worthless, or helpless. You may have no interest in activities that you used to enjoy. You may experience a significant change in your appetite or weight or have sleep problems (inability to sleep, sleeping too much, or waking up in the middle of the night or early in the morning and being unable to go back to sleep). You may feel a loss of energy or fatigue or be unable to concentrate or make a decision. You may even think about death or suicide. Some people with depression have persistent aches and pains—such as headaches, digestive problems, or abdominal or pelvic pain—that do not respond to treatment.

Diagnosis A thorough medical and psychiatric evaluation is necessary to diagnose depression. Your doctor will give you a physical examination that includes a neurological examination. A neurological examination tests the functioning of your brain and nervous system by evaluating your coordination, reflexes, and balance. You may also have laboratory tests to rule out other illnesses—such as a thyroid disorder (see page 624) or anemia (see page 493)—that can cause or worsen the symptoms of depression.

The doctor will ask about your symptoms, whether or not you have been treated for them previously, and if any members of your family have had depression. He or she will ask about your use of alcohol and other drugs and if you have had thoughts of suicide or ever tried to commit suicide. Be honest in answering these questions; your doctor needs information to help you.

Treatment If you are diagnosed with depression, your doctor will need to evaluate the severity of your depression in order to plan the most appropriate treatment or to determine whether to refer you to a mental health professional, such as a psychiatrist, for treatment. Nearly all people who undergo treatment for depression experience at least some relief from their symptoms. Treatment of depression usually involves medication or psychotherapy or both of these together. The combination of medication and psychotherapy is usually the most effective treatment. If you do not start to feel better after several weeks of treatment, your doctor may recommend a change in your treatment plan.

Antidepressant medications In many cases, depression is treated with medications called antidepressants. The drugs that are used most often to treat depression are tricyclic antidepressants, serotonin reuptake inhibitors (SRIs), monoamine oxidase inhibitors (MAOIs), and bupropion. These medications affect people in different ways and some people need to take more than one at the same time to improve their condition. You may have to try several different medications before you and your doctor find the particular drug or combination of drugs that works best for you.

Antidepressant medications are not addictive, and they are not stimulants that artificially elevate mood. Antidepressants relieve depression by altering the balance of neurotransmitters—chemical messengers in your brain that influence mood, concentration, sleep, energy levels, and appetite. You may not notice any improvement until you have been taking the medication for several weeks.

It is important to see your doctor regularly while you are taking antidepressants

SYMPTOM CHART

Depression

A feeling of sadness, hopelessness, inadequacy, despair, or guilt that may make you unable to cope with normal life.

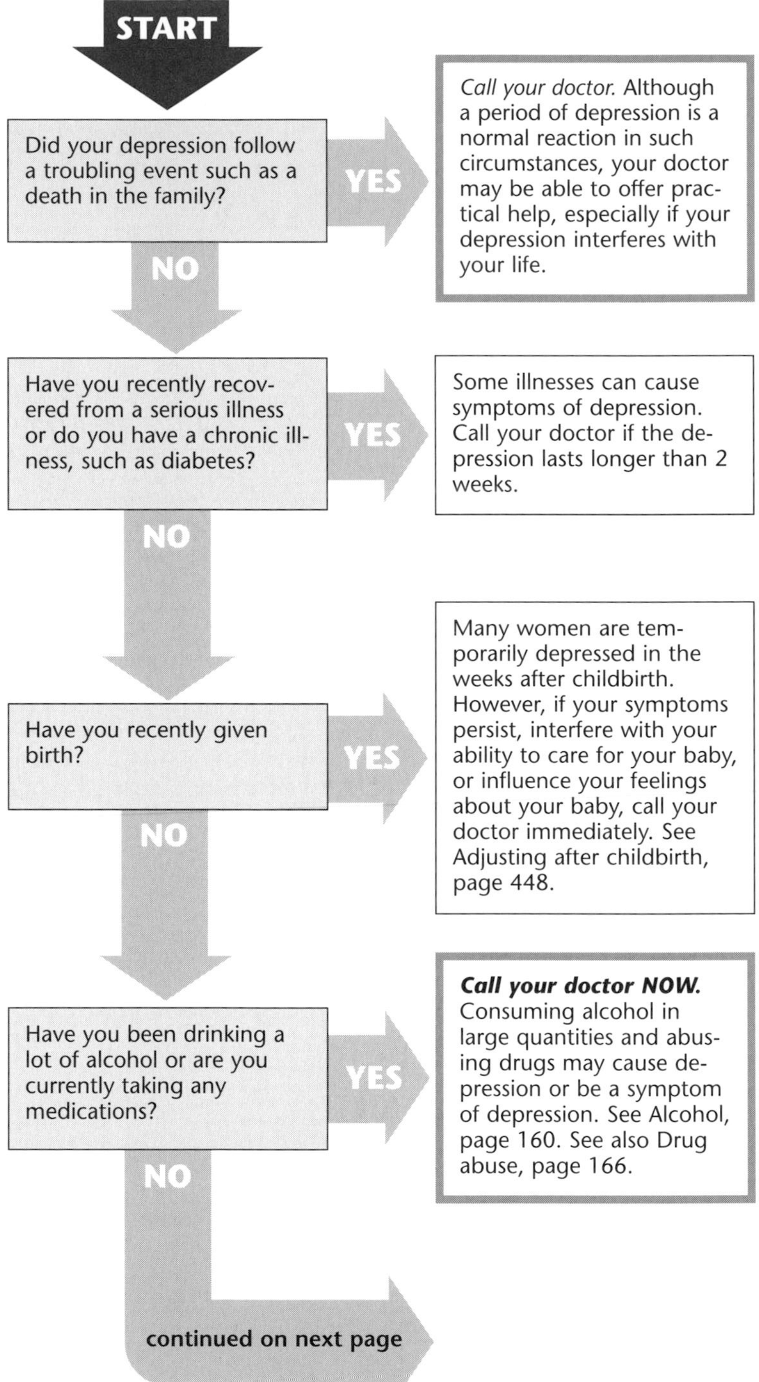

Depression

See your doctor immediately if you experience any of the following symptoms of major depression that last for more than 2 weeks:

- Sad or anxious mood
- Loss of interest in formerly pleasurable activities
- Feelings of hopelessness or pessimism
- Sleeping problems
- Change in appetite; weight loss or gain
- Decreased energy; fatigue
- Difficulty concentrating
- Physical symptoms, such as digestive problems, that do not respond to treatment

continued from previous page

Do you consider life no longer worthwhile or have you considered committing suicide?

YES → ***EMERGENCY Get medical help immediately.*** See Suicide, page 599. See also Depression, page 594.

NO ↓

Do you have two or more of the following symptoms?
- Difficulty sleeping or getting out of bed in the morning
- Loss of appetite
- Loss of energy
- Difficulty concentrating or making decisions

YES → ***Call your doctor NOW.*** You may have major depression, which can be treated. See Depression, page 594.

NO ↓

If you are unable to make a diagnosis from this chart, talk to your doctor.

Offering your help

If you have a friend or family member who is depressed, the most important thing you can do is to help the person get a diagnosis and appropriate treatment. Depression can almost always be treated successfully. Encourage the person to continue treatment once it has begun. Offer the person emotional support as well—understanding, patience, and affection—and encourage him or her to engage in conversation and activities he or she always found enjoyable. Assure the person that he or she will feel better with time.

so that he or she can monitor their effects. If you experience any side effects from the medication, tell your doctor. Side effects—which can include dry mouth, drowsiness, constipation, headaches, nausea, nervousness, or insomnia—usually subside after a few weeks as your body adjusts to the medication. If side effects persist, your doctor may be able to adjust the dose or prescribe a different medication.

Although the side effects of antidepressants are often temporary, the beneficial effects of the medication can be long lasting, continuing even after you stop treatment. It is important to continue taking the medication until you and your doctor decide it is time for you to stop. Antidepressants are usually taken for 6 to 18 months, under the careful guidance of a doctor.

Because anxiety (an exaggerated feeling of apprehension or fear) and insomnia often accompany depression, your doctor may also prescribe an antianxiety medication or a mild sedative. Lithium (a mood stabilizer), thyroid hormone (see page 625), and stimulants are sometimes used in addition to antidepressants to enhance the effectiveness of the antidepressant. Other drugs that may be prescribed in addition to antidepressants include antipsychotic medications (see page 613); these medications are used to treat extreme agitation or psychotic symptoms (such as hearing voices, seeing visions, or feeling persecuted), which can accompany some forms of severe depression.

Psychotherapy Psychotherapy, also called talk therapy, involves meeting regularly with a trained, qualified therapist to discuss all aspects of your emotional and behavioral problems and learn how to make positive changes in your life. Like antidepressant medications, psychotherapy can relieve depression by altering the balance

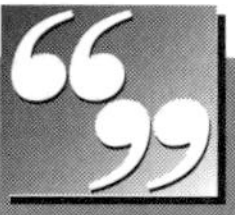

ONE WOMAN'S STORY
DEPRESSION

It took me awhile to realize what was happening to me. I was living alone. My children had grown and moved out of state and my husband had died a couple of years before. I was working full-time as a librarian. I found myself becoming more and more isolated. I didn't feel like calling friends or doing anything social. I started turning down invitations because I just didn't feel like going out.

I found it difficult to drag myself out of bed in the morning, let alone get to work each day. I became less and less interested in my job. I was just showing up for work and putting in my time. I let chores slide at home. I ate only canned soup and crackers. I would sit staring at the TV for hours, feeling hopeless, like my life was over.

Then, several months ago, my good friend Ellen came for a visit. She noticed something was wrong and urged me to see a psychiatrist who had helped a member of her family. In fact, Ellen made an appointment and took me to see the psychiatrist the next week. I started seeing the psychiatrist regularly and she helped me recognize the negative thought patterns I had developed that had led to my depression. She prescribed an antidepressant medication, which I took every day.

I had psychotherapy sessions once a week for a few months. The therapy helped me understand how to make adjustments in my life that would help me deal with situations in more positive and constructive ways. The medication improved my mood. With the medication and psychotherapy I began to get my life back on track. I gradually regained my energy and I can enjoy my friends again. I'm still struggling to understand how things got so bad, but at least now I can work at doing things differently.

"I found it difficult to drag myself out of bed in the morning, let alone get to work each day."

The hardest part about being depressed was getting up the energy and motivation to do something about it. I was lucky I had a good friend who saw how ill I had become and helped me get the treatment I needed. It made all the difference. I can now look forward to the rest of my life.

of neurotransmitters—chemical messengers in your brain that influence mood, concentration, sleep, energy levels, and appetite. You can undergo psychotherapy with a psychiatrist, a psychologist, or a social worker. For information about how to choose a qualified mental health professional, see page 194.

For psychotherapy, the therapist applies techniques based on established principles to gain insight into your difficulties and to help you understand them. Depending on your particular problem, your therapist may use one or more different techniques. Interpersonal psychotherapy may be used if you have difficulties in relationships. Problems in social and personal relationships may cause or precede depression, which in turn can cause more difficulties in these relationships. In interpersonal therapy, you and your therapist discuss your behavior patterns and your interactions with your spouse and other family members and other important people in your life. The goal of this form of therapy is to help you deal more effectively with others. Many people with depression find that improving their relationships gives them an important source of support and often helps reduce their symptoms.

Cognitive-behavioral therapy for depression is a form of psychotherapy based on the belief that thought patterns can lead to depression. A therapist can help you learn to recognize your negative thought patterns and behaviors and replace them with positive ones. This form of therapy is usually short term, highly focused, and goal-oriented.

Psychodynamic therapy is based on the idea that your behavior and emotions are influenced by an internal psychological conflict, such as wanting to be both independent and cared for, or feeling angry when you believe you should always be kind and loving. The goal of psychodynamic therapy is to understand these unconscious conflicts, which may be rooted in your early childhood, and resolve them.

Hospitalization Hospitalization is sometimes required for people who have severe periods of depression that involve serious weight loss, extreme agitation, psychosis (loss of touch with reality), or thoughts of suicide. While the person is in the hospital, doctors can perform comprehensive evaluations of the person's condition and begin treatment with medication and psychotherapy. At the same time, the person is protected and prevented from harming himself or herself by receiving 24-hour care.

When you are ready to leave the hospital, your doctor may recommend a day-hospital program to help you make a gradual transition back to home life. A day-hospital program provides you with intensive treatment during the day but you return home to spend the night.

Electroconvulsive therapy In some severe cases of depression in which a person is suicidal, psychotic (out of touch with reality), or malnourished, cannot take antidepressant medication, or has not responded to any other treatments, electroconvulsive therapy can be helpful and even lifesaving. Current therapy is more effective and has fewer side effects than earlier forms of this treatment.

Suicide

About twice as many women as men attempt suicide. However, women are less likely than men to actually kill themselves. In many cases, a failed suicide attempt is a cry for help from a person who desperately wants to overcome his or her problems. No suicide attempt should be ignored or dismissed simply as an attempt to get attention. Instead, it should be seen as a clear signal that the person needs professional help immediately. It is important to remember that the vast majority of people with depression can be treated successfully.

A common misconception is that a person who talks about committing suicide will not actually do it. In reality, any conversation about suicide should be taken very seriously. If you think about suicide or a person you know talks about suicide, get help. Call your doctor or your local hospital emergency room, where a suicide crisis worker should be available 24 hours a day to evaluate the situation and intervene. If you feel someone is in immediate danger, call 911.

Helping yourself if you are depressed

Treatment for depression often takes some time to be effective. Depression can make you feel tired, worthless, helpless, and hopeless—and you may feel discouraged about your treatment. But these negative views of yourself and your life do not accurately reflect your situation; they are caused by your depression. As your treatment progresses, these symptoms will subside. Don't give up. Here are some things you can do to help make your treatment more effective:

- Do not expect too much of yourself too soon; this can increase your feelings of failure.
- Set realistic goals for yourself and do not take on additional responsibility at this time.
- Break large tasks into small ones; set priorities.
- Try to be with other people, especially friends, as much as you can.
- Engage in activities that may make you feel better; for example, exercise, go to a movie, or participate in religious or social activities.
- Whenever possible, postpone important decisions (such as changing your job or getting married or divorced) until your depression has subsided.

Electroconvulsive therapy is performed by a psychiatrist and anesthesiologist (a doctor who administers anesthesia), usually in a hospital. Anesthesia is used so that the person is relaxed and asleep during the treatment, which takes seconds or minutes. Electrodes are placed on one or both sides of the scalp; an electrical pulse is delivered from a small machine to the electrode to induce a seizure (abnormal electrical activity in the brain). Doctors believe that electroconvulsive therapy works by altering the balance of chemicals in the brain.

After a brief recovery period (30 minutes to 2 hours), the person returns to normal functioning and has no memory of the procedure. The number of treatments varies from person to person but at least six treatments are usually necessary. After the initial series of treatments, periodic sessions of electroconvulsive therapy may be necessary to prevent recurring depression.

MANIC-DEPRESSIVE ILLNESS

Manic-depressive illness, also called bipolar disorder, is a chemical imbalance in the brain that causes wide mood swings—from times of extreme elation and irritability (mania) to times of depression. The length of these episodes varies widely from person to person; some people have a brief period of normal mood in between. The disorder usually begins in early adulthood and continues with periods of mania and depression, which may occur closer together over time. In some people, one phase (usually depression) may predominate for months at a time.

Manic-depressive illness is relatively common; at least 1 percent of Americans have it. Your risk is increased if you have a close relative with manic-depressive illness. Doctors believe the illness results from faulty regulation of chemical messengers in the brain (called neurotransmitters) that help nerve cells communicate with each other. Stressful events in a person's life may trigger changes in neurotransmitters that affect their ability to regulate mood.

Manic-depressive illness is often not recognized as an illness until it has caused substantial damage to a person's life—including marital breakup, loss of a job, abuse of alcohol and other drugs, or suicide. Many people have the disorder for years before they finally seek treatment. In the early stage, people with manic-depressive illness may enjoy the way they feel during the manic phase of the disease—energetic, self-confident, productive—and they usually deny that anything is wrong.

But if manic-depressive illness is not treated, it can be severely disruptive and disabling. Treatment with medication often makes it possible for a person who has the disorder to live a normal, productive life. If a family member or friend has this disorder it is important to encourage him or her to get treatment as soon as possible. Like most physical and mental disorders, manic-depressive illness is easier to treat in its early stages. Talking to your family doctor about how to get help for your loved one is an important first step.

Symptoms The manic phase of manic-depressive illness is a period of elation, euphoria, or irritability. Many people with the disorder require little sleep or food, become easily distracted, or experience sudden rage or paranoia (excessive or irrational suspiciousness). Some people with manic-depressive illness engage in a whirlwind of activity that is very different from their usual behavior. For example, they may spend their family into bankruptcy, engage in multiple sexual relationships, pick fights with their boss, begin grandiose projects that have no chance of success, or drink too much alcohol or use other drugs. Their self-confidence may become so extreme that they think nothing can stop them from accomplishing anything they want. They may even think they can step off the top of a building or out of a moving car without getting hurt.

In the depressive phase of the disorder, people may feel hopeless, worthless, or totally indifferent about life in general. They may lose their appetite, have difficulty sleeping, or have unexplained aches and pains. Prolonged sadness, unexplained crying spells, irritability, and jumpiness are also common during the depressive phase of the illness. Affected people may be unable to concentrate or remember details and may think about death or suicide.

Diagnosis A comprehensive medical and psychiatric evaluation is often necessary to diagnose manic-depressive illness. Your doctor will give you a physical examination that includes a neurological examination to test your coordination, reflexes, and balance. You may also have laboratory tests to rule out other illnesses—such as a thyroid disorder or anemia—that can cause or worsen the symptoms of depression.

The doctor will ask about your symptoms and whether or not you have been treated for them previously and if any members of your family have had manic-depressive illness. He or she will ask about your use of alcohol and other drugs and if you have ever thought about suicide or tried to commit suicide. Be honest in answering these questions; the doctor needs information to help you.

Recognizing the symptoms of manic-depressive illness

Although many conditions cause symptoms similar to those of manic-depressive illness, see your doctor if you experience any of the following symptoms to an extent that interferes with your ability to function:

During the manic phase:

- Extreme irritability and distractibility
- Excessive euphoria or elation
- Increased energy, activity, or restlessness
- Racing thoughts and ideas and rapid speech
- Unrealistic belief in your abilities and powers
- A prolonged period of behavior that is different than usual
- Uncharacteristically poor judgment
- Increased sexual drive
- Abuse of drugs
- Intrusive, obnoxious, or provocative behavior
- Denial that anything is wrong
- Paranoia (excessive or irrational suspiciousness)

During the depressive phase:

- Feeling sad or anxious
- Feeling hopeless, empty, or pessimistic
- Feeling guilty, worthless, or helpless
- Loss of interest or pleasure in activities you used to enjoy, including sex
- Sleep disturbances—including insomnia (see page 609), early-morning waking, or sleeping too much
- Change in appetite and a resulting weight loss or gain
- Decreased energy or fatigue, or feeling slowed down
- Thoughts of death or suicide; a suicide attempt
- Restlessness or irritability
- Difficulty concentrating, remembering, or making decisions
- Persistent physical problems—such as headaches, digestive problems, or aches and pains—that do not respond to treatment

After ruling out other illnesses, your doctor is likely to refer you to a psychiatrist, who is trained in treating manic-depressive illness. A psychiatrist can evaluate your mental state by asking you about changes in your moods, speech, thought patterns, memory, and social or work-related activities.

Treatment In about 70 percent of people with manic-depressive illness, a medication called lithium is effective in reducing the frequency and intensity of episodes of mania or depression. Lithium prevents mood swings by balancing the chemicals (neurotransmitters) that carry messages between brain cells. In some people, lithium eliminates symptoms completely. Most people who have manic-depressive illness must take lithium throughout their life to prevent recurring episodes.

Tell your doctor about any side effects you experience while taking lithium, including weight gain, loss of coordination, digestive problems, hand tremors, and muscle weakness. If lithium does not improve your symptoms, your doctor may recommend a different medication to enhance or replace lithium.

Because manic-depressive illness can cause a great deal of stress and disruption in your life and in the lives of people close to you, psychotherapy (see page 194) with a qualified therapist will be an important part of treatment for you and your family. Joining a support group of people who have similar problems is a good way to share information and experiences and learn coping strategies.

SEASONAL AFFECTIVE DISORDER

Seasonal affective disorder (SAD) is depression that affects a person each year during the fall and winter months, when the days are shorter and provide less sunlight. The deficiency of light during the winter months is thought to decrease the level of a brain chemical called serotonin, which affects emotions, behavior, and thought. Women are four times as likely as men to have SAD, which usually appears between ages 20 and 50. Because SAD seldom occurs before puberty and is uncommon in women after menopause, the female hormone estrogen may also play a role. SAD is much more common in northern latitudes, which have fewer hours of daylight than tropical, southern areas. Cold winter weather adds to the problem by encouraging people to spend more time indoors, out of the sun.

Symptoms The symptoms of SAD usually begin in October or November and subside in March or April. SAD causes symptoms similar to those of depression (see page 595), including sadness or anxiety, decreased energy or fatigue, difficulty concentrating and accomplishing tasks, and withdrawal from friends and family. People with SAD may experience other symptoms as well, including increased drowsiness, increased appetite, food cravings, and weight gain. The symptoms of depression that occur during the fall and winter months alternate with less depressed moods, normal moods, or sometimes even elevated moods during the spring and summer.

Diagnosis SAD is diagnosed primarily by a pattern of depression that recurs each year during the winter months. Your doctor will ask about your symptoms and if you have a family history of mood disorders, including SAD. He or she will give you a physical examination that includes a neurological examination to test the function of your brain and nervous system. You may also have laboratory tests to rule out other medical conditions—such as a thyroid disorder or anemia—that can cause or worsen the symptoms of depression. After ruling out other illnesses, your doctor is likely to refer you to a psychiatrist who is trained in treating the various forms of depression, including SAD.

Treatment If you are diagnosed with SAD, your psychiatrist is likely to prescribe daily light treatments using a special box that emits high-intensity fluorescent light (which is 5 to 20 times brighter than ordinary indoor lighting). Your doctor will tell you how to obtain a light box and how to use it. (Some insurance plans cover the cost of the box.)

Do not attempt light therapy on your own without the guidance of a psychiatrist. You should not use light therapy if you have eye problems that are affected by light or if you are taking medications that increase the sensitivity of your skin to light. For this reason, your doctor will recommend a thorough eye examination with an ophthalmologist (a doctor who specializes in eye care) and ask about your medical history before he or she prescribes light therapy. Possible side effects of light therapy include headaches, eyestrain, irritability, and insomnia. If you have any of these reactions, tell your doctor. He or she may recommend reducing the amount of time you are exposed to the light or sitting a little farther away from the light source.

Your doctor may prescribe medication in addition to light therapy. Antidepressant medications called serotonin reuptake inhibitors (see page 595), especially a drug called fluoxetine, are often prescribed for treating SAD. Tricyclic antidepressants are not used as frequently to treat SAD because these drugs can cause side effects, such as drowsiness and weight gain, that can already be problems for people who have the disorder. In addition to light therapy or medication, your doctor is likely to recommend stress management techniques (see page 186), exercise, and psychotherapy (see page 598) to help you deal with your depression.

Anxiety disorders

Anxiety is a normal emotion that helps you rise to life's challenges. If you have an anxiety disorder, this normally helpful emotion actually prevents you from coping and, in fact, interferes with your ability to function. Anxiety disorders are characterized by unrealistic or excessive worry about a particular situation or for an unidentifiable reason. You may feel anxious most of the time for no apparent reason. You may begin to avoid activities that you think may bring on these uncomfortable feelings. Or you may have occasional periods of anxiety that are so intense that they terrify and immobilize you. Several common anxiety disorders are described here. Effective treatments are available for most of them.

GENERALIZED ANXIETY DISORDER

Generalized anxiety disorder—the most common anxiety disorder—is characterized by persistent, exaggerated worry and tension. You may be constantly anticipating disaster, often worrying excessively about your health, finances, family, or job. You may not be able to identify the source of your worry; just getting through the day makes you feel anxious. People with generalized anxiety disorder seem unable to eliminate their worries, even though they may realize their anxiety is exaggerated.

Unlike more serious anxiety disorders, generalized anxiety disorder usually causes only mild impairment that does not cause people to avoid situations or prevent them from participating in social activities or functioning on their job. However, in severe cases, the disorder can be debilitating, impairing a person's ability to perform ordinary daily tasks.

Generalized anxiety disorder occurs gradually, usually during childhood or adolescence, but it can also begin in adulthood. Generalized anxiety disorder is more common in women than men and it has a genetic component—you are more likely to have generalized anxiety disorder if other members of your family have had it. For most people, the symptoms of the disorder diminish with age.

Symptoms Generalized anxiety disorder can make you excessively anxious or worried most of the time, often for no known reason. You may be unable to relax or have trouble falling asleep or staying asleep. You may have physical symptoms as well, including trembling, muscle tension, headaches, sweating, or hot flashes. You may feel light-headed or out of breath, startle easily, or have difficulty concentrating. Some people with generalized anxiety disorder also experience depression (see page 594).

Diagnosis Generalized anxiety disorder is usually diagnosed when a person has been excessively worried about a number of everyday problems for most days during a period of at least 6 months. Your doctor will ask about other symptoms (such as depression or substance use), your medical history, and your family medical history, and give you a physical examination. You may also have laboratory tests to rule out other causes of your symptoms, such as hyperthyroidism (see page xxx) or a medication you are taking.

Treatment Although the symptoms of generalized anxiety disorder usually diminish with time, they can be successfully treated with medications called benzodiazepines or an antianxiety medication called buspirone. Generalized anxiety disorder can also be treated with psychotherapy, including psychodynamic therapy or cognitive-behavioral therapy (see page 599). Relaxation techniques (see page 190) can be helpful in relieving muscle tension, which often accompanies the disorder.

OBSESSIVE-COMPULSIVE DISORDER

Obsessive-compulsive disorder is an anxiety disorder in which you are trapped in a pattern of disturbing, anxious thoughts and repetitive behaviors, which are senseless and distressing but extremely difficult to overcome. The disturbing thoughts or images are called obsessions; the repetitive behaviors, or rituals, are called compulsions. For example, you may be obsessed with germs, so you wash your hands over and over throughout the day. In severe cases, people may wash their hands so much that they become raw and bleed.

You may constantly fear that harm will come to you or a loved one, so you continuously check to make sure the stove is off, the doors are locked, or the emergency brake on your car works. You may have an unreasonable fear that you have a serious medical disorder and continuously examine your body for signs of illness. You may be preoccupied by order or symmetry and spend long periods of time touching things or counting or arranging them.

Obsessive-compulsive disorder is not ordinary fussy, neat, clean, methodical, or meticulous behavior. Many people have these traits and do not have the illness. In obsessive-compulsive disorder, these rituals can take up hours of the day, interfering with a person's ability to live a normal life. Most people with obsessive-compulsive disorder recognize that their behavior is senseless, but they cannot stop it.

The disorder is more common than you might expect, affecting as many as 1 out of every 50 people—men and women equally. Obsessive-compulsive disorder is thought to result from an interaction of brain chemistry and personality. The illness can begin in childhood but usually first appears during adolescence or early adulthood.

Recognizing the symptoms of obsessive-compulsive disorder

Obsessive-compulsive disorder affects people differently. In some people, the symptoms come and go; in others, symptoms subside over time or grow progressively worse. Although obsessive-compulsive disorder can persist throughout your life, it can be treated effectively with a combination of medication and behavioral therapy. Many people who have obsessive-compulsive disorder are secretive about their symptoms and wait many years before seeking help or do not ever seek help. If you recognize your behavior in any of the following descriptions, talk to your doctor:

- **Cleaning** Spending hours each day cleaning, scrubbing walls, washing your hands, or showering to avoid germs.
- **Repeating** Performing routine actions—such as getting in and out of a chair or going through a doorway—or saying certain phrases over and over to relieve anxiety.
- **Completing** Performing a series of actions in a specified order until the ritual is complete as a means of relieving fears and anxiety. For example, you may feel you must walk or drive to a particular destination along the same route every time.
- **Checking** Repeatedly checking to see if doors are locked or the stove is turned off even though you remember you just checked.
- **Being overly meticulous** Arranging and rearranging your desk, closets, or dresser drawers countless times.

Diagnosis Obsessive-compulsive disorder is diagnosed by the symptoms after a medical and psychiatric history, laboratory tests, and physical examination have ruled out other causes, such as another illness or a medication you may be taking. If you are diagnosed with obsessive-compulsive disorder, your doctor is likely to refer you to a psychiatrist for treatment.

Treatment The primary treatment for obsessive-compulsive disorder is a combination of medication and a type of behavioral therapy called exposure and response prevention. Your doctor may prescribe an antidepressant called a serotonin reuptake inhibitor (see page 595), such as clomipramine or fluoxetine. These medications affect the level in the brain of a chemical called serotonin, which affects thought, emotions, and behavior.

Using exposure and response prevention therapy, you and your therapist will work together to determine the specific anxieties or obsessions that trigger your compulsive, ritualistic behavior. The goal of exposure and response prevention therapy is to lower your anxiety to a tolerable level. You will be exposed to the feared object or idea, either directly or using your imagination, and then discouraged or prevented from carrying out the usual ritual associated with it. For example, if you fear germs, you may be asked to pick up dirt from the floor or touch a doorknob and then be denied the opportunity to wash your hands.

The therapy usually requires regular sessions over a period of weeks to months. For most people, exposure and response prevention therapy provides long-lasting improvement in their symptoms. They gradually experience less anxiety from their obsessive thoughts and become able to prevent the compulsive actions.

You and family members may benefit from joining a support group of other families who are dealing with obsessive-compulsive disorder. It is a good way to exchange information and learn effective ways to cope with the disorder.

PANIC DISORDER

Panic disorder is characterized by brief periods of intense fear accompanied by physical symptoms such as a pounding heart, chest pains, or dizziness. These periods, called panic attacks, occur for no obvious reason. They are thought to result when the brain's normal mechanism for responding to fear (called the "fight-or-flight" response) becomes inexplicably aroused. Most people who have panic disorder develop irrational fears, or phobias (see page 606), of the specific situations they think will bring on an attack and begin to avoid those situations. This fear and the resulting avoidance can have a serious impact on a person's daily life.

Twice as many women as men have panic disorder. Heredity plays an important role; if you have family members with panic disorder, you are at significantly increased risk of developing it.

The first time you have a panic attack, it may occur suddenly while you are engaged in a routine activity such as driving your car or going for a walk. Suddenly, a barrage of frightening and uncontrollable symptoms—including a sense of terror or unreality or a fear of losing control—comes over you. The symptoms may last for a few seconds or several minutes. A first attack often occurs when a person is under unusual stress, such as an extremely heavy workload or the death of a loved one. Excessive use of caffeine or stimulant drugs (including some appetite suppressants) may trigger an attack. Use of cocaine (see page 167) has also been linked to panic attacks.

Panic disorder sometimes occurs in people who have agoraphobia—fear of being in public places or in situations from which escape might be difficult or help unavailable. People with agoraphobia often restrict themselves to a self-imposed zone of safety that is usually limited to their home and immediate neighborhood. In severe cases, the person may never leave home or will go out only with a trusted companion.

Symptoms If panic disorder is affecting your ability to function, it is important to get professional help. If you experience several of the following symptoms more than once in a 2-week period for no obvious reason and they are accompanied by feelings of intense fear or discomfort, talk to your doctor:

- Racing or pounding heartbeat
- Difficulty breathing or a choking sensation
- Sweating, shaking, or flushing
- Chest pains
- Dizziness, light-headedness, or nausea
- Fear of losing control and doing something embarrassing
- Tingling or numbness in the hands
- Sense of unreality
- Sense of impending doom or a fear of dying

Diagnosis To diagnose panic disorder, your doctor will ask about your symptoms of panic and anxiety or depression and your health history. He or she may ask if you have a family history of panic disorder. You are likely to have a physical examination and laboratory tests to rule out other possible causes of your symptoms, such as hyperthyroidism (see page 625), some forms of epilepsy (see page 578), or heartbeat abnormalities.

Treatment Treatment of panic disorder, which usually involves psychotherapy and medication, can be effective in preventing panic attacks or substantially reducing their severity and frequency. Treating the condition at an early stage can prevent it from becoming incapacitating. A form of psychotherapy called cognitive-behavioral therapy (see page 599) is usually part of the treatment. The cognitive part of cognitive-behavioral therapy helps you identify thoughts that might trigger a panic attack and learn to change them. For example, you might learn to replace an alarmist thought such as "I'm going to die!" with a more appropriate one, such as "It's only uneasiness I feel. It will pass." Behavioral therapy helps you change your behavior. It may include relaxation techniques (see page 190), such as breathing exercises, to help reduce your anxiety. Hypnosis is also sometimes used to help treat panic disorder.

Your doctor may prescribe an antidepressant medication (see page 595)—such as a tricyclic antidepressant, a serotonin reuptake inhibitor, or a monoamine oxidase inhibitor—or an antianxiety medication. You and your doctor will work together to find the medication and dose that works best for you and that causes the fewest side effects. These medications are taken for several months to treat the symptoms of panic disorder and for longer periods to prevent recurring panic attacks.

Panic disorder often recurs, sometimes for no obvious reason. Many people who have previously been treated for the condition are able to use the skills they learned in therapy to help them overcome or deal with an occasional panic attack. Their ability to cope with the disorder prevents it from curtailing their activities and reducing the quality of their life again.

Self-help for panic attacks

Together with your therapist, you will work on ways to recognize and overcome the triggers of your panic attacks. Here are some techniques that are effective for many people:

- Stay in the present; focus on what is happening now rather than what might happen.
- Remember that, although your feelings and symptoms are frightening, they are not dangerous or harmful and will pass.
- Notice that when you do not add frightening thoughts to your fear it begins to fade.
- If you feel fear, don't fight it; expect it and accept it. Try to stay calm and give it time to pass.
- Give yourself credit for how well you have progressed in accepting and dealing with your fears, and think about how good you will feel when you succeed this time.

PHOBIAS

A phobia is an intense, irrational fear of an object or situation that may cause anxiety that is so extreme that it can interfere with your ability to work or socialize. Phobias occur in different forms. A simple or specific phobia is fear of a particular object or situation—such as spiders, heights, elevators, tunnels, water, flying, or driving. Social phobia is fear of being humiliated or embarrassed in social situations. The most common social phobia is fear of public speaking. Agoraphobia is a fear of being in public spaces from which escape might be difficult or help unavailable. Claustrophobia is fear of being in cramped spaces.

Specific phobias are common; more than 1 in 10 people has a specific phobia. Phobias tend to run in families and are more common in women. If the object of the fear is easy to avoid, a person may not feel the need to seek treatment. However, if a phobia interferes with your life in any way—such as influencing important career or personal decisions—treatment can be helpful.

Symptoms The symptoms of phobias include sudden, uncontrollable, and irrational fear when you are exposed to a particular situation or object. You may recognize that your fear is excessive. You

Common phobias

Phobias occur in different forms. Following are some of the most common types of phobias:

- Insects or animals (spiders, snakes, mice, or dogs)
- Natural environment (storms, heights, or water)
- Situations (elevators, flying, enclosed spaces, or crowds)
- Social contact or performance (such as public speaking)
- Blood or injury

may experience rapid heartbeat, shortness of breath, trembling, and an overwhelming desire to flee a particular situation or place. Or you may avoid situations that trigger your fear, which can interfere with your ability to function normally.

Diagnosis The symptoms of a phobia are often obvious to the person with the phobia and his or her doctor. The medical evaluation will include a medical and psychiatric history, physical examination, and a psychiatric evaluation to rule out underlying or coexisting depression (see page 594). The doctor will also ask about the person's memories of exposure to the frightening object or situation and his or her response.

Treatment Phobias can usually be treated effectively with cognitive-behavioral therapy (see page 599), medication, or a combination of the two. Many people who are able to overcome a phobia through treatment find that they are cured of it for life. In a type of cognitive-behavioral therapy called exposure therapy, you will be exposed to the feared object or situation in a controlled setting until your fear of it subsides. This therapy can be done either gradually in several sessions or all at once for as long as it takes for you to overcome your anxiety.

In some cases, antianxiety medications are used to treat phobias, but a careful balance must be struck. For some people with phobias, taking medicine when needed may be helpful. But taking medication that completely masks your symptoms may backfire because some discomfort caused by the symptoms can be helpful in stimulating you to work at overcoming them. If depression is part of your problem, your doctor may also prescribe antidepressants (see page 595).

POSTTRAUMATIC STRESS DISORDER

Posttraumatic stress disorder is a debilitating condition that can follow a terrifying event—such as a rape—that involves intense fear, helplessness, and horror. The illness is characterized by recurring memories of the traumatic event, withdrawal from friends and family, and emotional numbness. Once referred to as shell shock and considered a disorder that affected only war veterans, posttraumatic stress disorder is now known to affect many more women than men. In addition to rape, common causes of posttraumatic stress disorder in women include being a victim of childhood sexual abuse (see page 727) or domestic violence (see page 721). As many as 10 percent of all Americans are thought to have posttraumatic stress disorder and many more people may have some symptoms of it.

Posttraumatic stress disorder can occur at any age, including childhood. In severe cases, a person may have difficulty functioning at work or in social situations. Many people who have posttraumatic stress disorder abuse alcohol or other drugs. They may be trying to medicate themselves with excessive amounts of these drugs to avoid painful memories and emotional responses. Some people with the disorder are at high risk of suicide. For this reason, it is essential to seek treatment promptly.

Symptoms The symptoms of posttraumatic stress disorder usually begin within 3 months of the traumatic event and can vary from mild to severe. You may have recurring dreams or vivid memories of the event (called flashbacks) that are triggered by ordinary situations. A flashback can make you feel like you are reliving the experience. You may avoid places or situations that remind you of the traumatic event. You may feel emotionally numb and withdraw from people you were once close to. Some people with the disorder act as if they are constantly being threatened by the trauma they experienced and may become irritable or easily startled. The disorder may also cause sleep problems, depression, or difficulties with concentration or memory. If you have any of these symptoms, it is important to talk to your doctor as soon as possible and get help.

Attention-deficit/hyperactivity disorder

Attention-deficit/hyperactivity disorder is a behavior disorder that begins during childhood (usually before age 7) and sometimes continues into adolescence and adulthood. The disorder is characterized by an abnormal, persistent pattern of inattention, hyperactivity, and impulsiveness. This pattern of behavior interferes with the person's ability to function at home, at school or work, or in social situations. The disorder is common, affecting about 6 percent of all school-age children, mostly boys. Attention-deficit/hyperactivity disorder has a genetic component; it is more common in people who have a close relative with the disorder. In most people, the symptoms decrease in severity during late adolescence and adulthood.

People with the disorder may not be able to concentrate on a task for any length of time or may make careless mistakes. Their work is often messy, performed carelessly, and they may shift from one uncompleted task to another. They are easily distracted and forgetful. In social situations, they may frequently change the subject in conversation or not listen to others.

In children with attention-deficit/hyperactivity disorder, signs of hyperactivity can include fidgeting, squirming in their seat or getting up from their seat in the classroom and walking around, running or climbing in inappropriate situations, or talking excessively. In adolescents and adults, hyperactivity takes the form of feelings of restlessness and difficulty engaging in quiet, sedentary activities. Signs of impulsiveness include blurting out answers before questions have been completed, difficulty waiting their turn, or interrupting or intruding on others.

If you notice these symptoms in your child, or in yourself or an adult family member, talk to your doctor. Attention-deficit/hyperactivity disorder can be treated with a combination of changes in the person's environment (such as establishing structure and routine), education, medication, or individual and family psychotherapy (see page 194). For both children and adults with the disorder, learning how to organize and schedule tasks and activities and to think before they respond can help increase their sense of accomplishment and self-esteem.

Diagnosis To diagnose posttraumatic stress disorder, a doctor will ask about the history of the traumatic event and the symptoms or feelings that are bothering you.

Treatment Individual psychotherapy may help you resolve conflicts you may have about the event and enable you to regain your self-esteem and take control of your life. Family therapy can help members of your family understand your disorder and cope with your condition and its impact on all of you. Support from family and friends often speeds a person's recovery.

Group therapy is an important part of treatment of posttraumatic stress disorder. Many people who have the disorder feel alone in their experience and are usually relieved to know that other people have experienced similar horrors and share their symptoms and their pain. Group therapy with other people who have been through similar experiences can provide an opportunity to express your feelings and to begin to heal.

Medication may help control some of the symptoms of posttraumatic stress disorder. Antidepressants (see page 595) or antianxiety medications may be prescribed for relieving the symptoms of depression, anxiety, or panic that can accompany the disorder. However, medication alone is usually not effective in treating posttraumatic stress disorder.

Sleep disorders

Sleep disorders affect millions of Americans. Some people may not get enough sleep or sleep fitfully, while others may sleep too much. If you occasionally are sleepy during the day or have trouble falling or staying asleep, see page 191 for ways to help you get a good night's rest. If your sleep problems continue after trying those self-help tips, you will find useful information in this section about how your doctor may treat more serious sleep disorders. Do not try any over-the-counter sleep medications without talking to your doctor first.

INSOMNIA

Insomnia—difficulty falling asleep or staying asleep long enough to feel rested and alert the next day—affects one out of three adults in the US. Lack of sleep can cause not only fatigue and lack of energy, but irritability, difficulty concentrating, memory loss, and low productivity. Several weeks of insomnia can follow a stressful event, such as the loss of a loved one, but normal patterns of sleep usually return with time. Insomnia is considered chronic if it occurs every night, or regularly for several months.

Sleep can be disturbed by a variety of medical conditions—including incontinence (see page 538), arthritis (see page 645), and heart disease (see page 461)—or by taking some medications. Mood disorders (see page 594) are often linked to insomnia. Together, mood disorders and insomnia tend to reinforce each other and create a vicious cycle.

Older people often have trouble getting a restful night of sleep because they sleep lightly and wake up many times throughout the night. During menopause, many women are awakened by hot flashes or drenching night sweats. Pregnant women may find their sleep disrupted by the need to urinate frequently or by leg cramps. Mothers wakened by young children during the night often find it difficult to fall back asleep.

If you are repeatedly unable to get enough sleep at night, see your doctor. He or she may first recommend some things you can do on your own to improve your sleep. Do not attempt to solve your sleep problem with over-the-counter sleeping pills or alcohol. They do not provide any real or sustained relief and can contribute to other problems. Your doctor may refer you to a doctor or clinic that specializes in sleep disorders.

Symptoms You may have insomnia if you have any of the following symptoms for at least 1 month:

- Inability to fall asleep at night within 30 minutes of going to bed
- Frequent waking during the night
- Inability to fall back to sleep after you have awakened in the middle of the night or early in the morning
- Inability to sleep for more than 5 hours a night

Diagnosis The symptoms of insomnia are often obvious. Your doctor will ask when you began having problems sleeping and about any significant events or factors in your life that could be the cause. For example, a change in your daily routine (such as a new job) or a recent stressful event may cause a change in your sleep pattern.

Treatment Part of the treatment of your insomnia will be determining how many hours of sleep you actually need each night. Eight hours is the average, but you may need fewer or more than that. Your doctor may ask you to keep a diary for several weeks of how much sleep you get each night and how you feel the next day. If you find that you need only 6 hours of sleep each night and you go to bed at 10 PM and plan to get up at 7 AM, you can expect to spend 3 hours tossing and turning. After you know the number of hours you need to sleep, set specific times for going to bed and getting up, and stick to these times to set your body's internal clock.

If you and your doctor find that you are not getting enough sleep, the next step is to determine the cause. Stress is the most common cause of insomnia in adults. Your doctor may recommend relaxation exercises (see page 190) or self-help tips such as those on page 191 to help you sleep better. These methods have longer-lasting effects than sleep medications. If the cause of your insomnia is a medical problem—such as depression (see page 594), incontinence, pain from arthritis, or diabetes (see page 617)—your doctor will prescribe appropriate treatment for that particular condition. In most cases, once the underlying medical problem is cleared up, normal sleep patterns resume.

Sleeping pills Your doctor may prescribe sleep-promoting medications, but only after other treatments have failed, and only as part of a long-term sleep program. All sleep medications are hypnotics—they induce sleep by depressing the central nervous system. Medications called benzodiazepines are prescribed most often for treating insomnia. Your doctor is likely to first prescribe a so-called short-acting benzodiazepine, which is effective for no more than about 6 hours. Medications that last longer than that are also available, but these can make you feel groggy the next day. You and your doctor can choose the medication that is best for you.

Some sleep medications are addictive or habit-forming or may require increasingly larger doses to have the same effect. For this reason, sleep medications are considered only a temporary solution for insomnia. You should use them only under your doctor's guidance—for the shortest possible time and in the smallest dose that is effective for you. Make sure your doctor knows if you are pregnant or planning to become pregnant, because some sleep medications may be harmful to the fetus. If you are taking any other medications, make sure your doctor knows; combining sleeping pills with other drugs can be dangerous. It is also dangerous to combine sleep medications with alcohol or illicit drugs.

You should stop taking sleeping pills as soon as you have reestablished an acceptable sleep pattern. But do not stop taking the medication until you talk to your doctor. He or she will help you gradually reduce the dose of the medication and discontinue it. Stopping the medication suddenly can cause insomnia that may be worse than you had before you began taking the medication.

NARCOLEPSY

Narcolepsy is a sleep disorder that causes excessive sleepiness during normal waking hours. Periods of intense, deep sleep (called sleep attacks) may occur several times a day even though you have had adequate sleep the night before. During an attack, you may find it impossible to stay awake and fall asleep for periods ranging from a few seconds to half an hour. You may fall asleep during inappropriate or even dangerous moments such as while engaging in conversation, eating, walking, or driving a car.

Narcolepsy may be linked to depression or to a disorder called sleep apnea, which causes breathing difficulties during sleep. Although as many as 1 in 100 people may have narcolepsy, the majority do not seek treatment for many years. Narcolepsy usually begins during adolescence with mild symptoms that increase in severity over several years.

Symptoms The major symptom of narcolepsy is excessive daytime sleepiness that makes you fall asleep at unusual times, such as in the middle of a conversation. Many people with narcolepsy experience vivid dreams or hallucinations (illusions) and short episodes of muscle weakness that may cause them to drop things or even fall to the floor.

Diagnosis Your doctor will diagnose narcolepsy by your symptoms. If you have experienced sudden attacks of extreme sleepiness, muscle weakness, and intense dreams or hallucinations several times a day for at least 3 months while getting adequate sleep at night, you may have narcolepsy.

Treatment If you are diagnosed with narcolepsy, your doctor is likely to prescribe a medication that will increase your alertness throughout the day. If you have depression or muscle weakness, your doctor may also prescribe another medication, such as an antidepressant (see page 595).

Eating disorders

An eating disorder is a complex psychological illness characterized by a distorted body image, an intense fear of gaining weight, and an obsession with food. The two major eating disorders—anorexia nervosa and bulimia—are widespread, together affecting up to 4 percent of all adolescent and young adult women. Women in these age groups are vulnerable to eating disorders because many go on strict diets to achieve the unrealistically thin figure of a fashion model.

BULIMIA AND ANOREXIA NERVOSA

Bulimia is the most common eating disorder. A woman who has bulimia eats huge quantities of food in one sitting (called binge eating) and then forcibly rids her body of the excess calories (called purging). She may purge by vomiting, taking large doses of laxatives to stimulate bowel movements or diuretics to increase urination, or giving herself enemas. She may exercise excessively. A woman with bulimia may be extremely concerned about controlling her weight, but food is so psychologically important in her life that she has difficulty limiting her consumption.

A woman who has anorexia may starve herself, which can damage vital organs such as the heart and brain, shut down important body functions such as menstruation, and eventually cause death. The underlying cause of anorexia is not always obvious. The illness may be a response to stress inside or outside the family that causes a young woman to feel a desperate need to control at least one part of her life—in this case, her weight. For more about the causes of eating disorders, see page 113.

Like many other illnesses, eating disorders are treated most effectively when they are diagnosed at an early stage. The longer your abnormal eating behavior continues, the more difficult it will be to overcome the psychological hold the disorder has on you and its damaging effects on your body. It is sometimes hard to convince a woman who has an eating disorder that she needs help because many who are affected deny that they have a problem. For this reason, many young women with anorexia do not receive treatment until they have become dangerously malnourished and thin. Many people who have bulimia are of normal weight and are therefore able to hide their illness for years.

Symptoms Recognizing the following symptoms in yourself (or a loved one) and getting immediate treatment can be lifesaving. Some people have both anorexia and bulimia and have symptoms of both disorders. Call your doctor immediately if any of the following symptoms apply to you:

Bulimia

- Binge eating—consuming large quantities of food in a short period of time and feeling you have no control over it
- Vomiting or using drugs to induce vomiting (emetics), bowel movements (laxatives), or urination (diuretics)
- Disappearing into the bathroom for long periods of time (usually to induce vomiting after a meal)
- Failure to gain weight even though you regularly binge (eat huge quantities of food at one time)
- Abnormal interest in food; practicing strange eating rituals, such as making elaborate plans for an eating binge
- Eating in secret
- Absence of at least three menstrual periods in a row
- Exercising obsessively
- Feeling seriously depressed
- Abusing alcohol or drugs

Anorexia nervosa

- Losing 15 percent or more of your normal body weight in a relatively short period of time
- Continuing to diet even though you are extremely thin
- Believing you are fat, even though you are severely underweight
- Abnormal interest in food; practicing strange eating rituals, such as eating tiny morsels of food one at a time and very slowly
- Eating in secret
- Absence of at least three menstrual periods in a row
- Exercising obsessively
- Feeling seriously depressed

Diagnosis Eating disorders are diagnosed by their symptoms and by a complete medical and psychiatric evaluation, including a physical examination and laboratory testing, to rule out other illnesses. The doctor will also evaluate any

Learning to eat again

Once you are in treatment with a doctor and a trained mental health professional, try using some or all of these tips to help you reestablish normal eating patterns:

- See your recovery as an ongoing, lifelong process. Being free of binges for several months means that you are successfully recovering—not that you are "cured."
- Make changes in your eating patterns gradually. Recovery is not going to happen overnight.
- Keep a journal of how much you are eating and how often you vomit or use laxatives or other agents for purging.
- Gradually incorporate healthy foods into your diet that you previously omitted.
- Try to eat at regular mealtimes and eat moderate portions of a variety of nutritious foods.
- Rejoin social eating situations. Eating at a table with others will gradually become a pleasure again.

physiologic abnormalities that may have resulted from the disorder, including dehydration, malnutrition, or chemical imbalances.

Treatment If you are diagnosed with an eating disorder, your doctor will first determine if your health is in immediate danger. In some cases, hospitalization is necessary to prevent a person who has anorexia from starving or committing suicide. Treatment of eating disorders is complex—usually involving a medical doctor, a nutritionist, and a psychotherapist (for both the individual and the family). The major goals of your treatment are to help you reach a normal weight if you have become dangerously underweight, to learn to control your abnormal eating behaviors, and to increase your ability to express your emotions. A nutritionist will work with you to help you establish healthy eating habits so that you can regain your health.

Psychotherapy is crucial for a lasting cure. The focus is on resolving the underlying psychological issues that triggered your eating disorder so that you will be able to continue a healthy eating and exercise routine after you stop treatment. Psychotherapy may help you recognize the feelings of anxiety or depression that trigger your abnormal eating behaviors and learn how to respond to those feelings differently. Psychotherapy also helps improve your self-esteem and self-confidence, which enables you to broaden your interests and social activities and take control of your life.

Family therapy will be another important part of your treatment. Your family and friends may feel confused, frustrated, or scared about your illness. They can learn how to help you gain a sense of individuality that is crucial to your developing a positive self-image. If you have bulimia, group therapy with other women who have the disorder can be helpful. In group therapy, you share experiences and information, which can help you learn to express your feelings and realize you are not alone. If you are depressed, your doctor may prescribe an antidepressant medication, which can help improve the way you feel about yourself and reduce compulsive behaviors, such as binge eating and purging.

In some cases of anorexia, even with psychotherapy and support from family, hospitalization is required, usually when weight loss continues beyond a critical point. You may not be consuming enough calories for your body to function and you may experience life-threatening irregular heart rhythms and heart failure. Hospitalization is not an admission of failure. It simply means that you need medical help to control the progression of your illness. Most young women respond well to treatment in the hospital and return to their home and school or work within a few weeks. It is essential to continue your treatment outside of the hospital to avoid a relapse, which often occurs in women who have anorexia.

Psychotic disorders

A psychosis is a severe mental disorder in which a person loses touch with reality and is unable to distinguish real experiences from unreal ones. Schizophrenia—the most common psychotic disorder—is the most chronic (continuous or recurring) and disabling of the major mental illnesses.

SCHIZOPHRENIA

Schizophrenia is a complex, poorly understood condition that is usually characterized by disordered thinking, abnormal perception of reality, hallucinations (illusions) or delusions (false beliefs that are not subject to reason), inappropriate emotional responses, or abnormal behavior. Schizophrenia is the most common major mental disorder, affecting 1 percent of the population—men and women equally. In women, the first symptoms of schizophrenia usually appear in their 20s or early 30s. In men, it occurs earlier—during their teens or 20s.

The cause of schizophrenia is not fully understood but is thought to be linked to an imbalance of interrelated chemicals in the brain. Schizophrenia may be one disorder or many disorders, with different causes. People who have a family history of schizophrenia are at increased risk of the illness. Doctors believe that people inherit genes that make them susceptible to developing schizophrenia, but they are not sure which environmental factors during a person's life cause those genes to "switch on" the disorder.

Schizophrenia affects people in different ways and to varying degrees. Some people have only one period of psychosis; other people have many episodes of psychosis during their lifetime, but in the periods in between they lead a relatively normal life. Less obvious symptoms—such as social isolation or withdrawal, or unusual speech, thought processes, or behavior—may precede or follow the periods of psychosis.

Symptoms The symptoms of schizophrenia can be devastating to the individual who is affected as well as to family and friends. A person with the disorder may show different kinds of behavior at different times. People who have schizophrenia may sense things that do not actually exist. For example, they may hear voices that tell them to do unusual things, see people or objects that are not really there, or feel invisible fingers touching their body.

They may have delusions, such as believing that their thoughts are controlled by another person or that people on television are sending special messages directly to them. Their thinking may become disorganized and fragmented, which makes it difficult for other people to follow their conversation. Their emotional responses may be blunted or inappropriate. Some people with schizophrenia appear distant or detached and may sit for hours without moving or saying a word. They may also become agitated or violent toward themselves or others.

Diagnosis Because symptoms similar to those of schizophrenia can be caused by other conditions—including abuse of alcohol or other drugs, a physical blow to the head, a brain tumor, a mood disorder (see page 594), or severe emotional trauma (such as the death of a parent, abandonment, or abuse)—a doctor will want to rule them out. After ruling out other illnesses, your doctor will refer you to a psychiatrist. Some people with a particular symptom that might occur in schizophrenia—such as talking out loud to a family member who has died—may be merely eccentric. The context of such a symptom is essential to understanding its significance in diagnosing schizophrenia. For example, if it is the only symptom the person has or if it has occurred only one time, he or she probably does not have schizophrenia.

Treatment Treatment of schizophrenia is focused on relieving the symptoms and reducing the likelihood that the symptoms will recur. A variety of treatments or combinations of treatments can be used. People with schizophrenia vary considerably in their need for treatment, but most people require some form of continuing therapy. Some people who have the disorder require constant care and attention, while other people can learn to function more independently.

Antipsychotic medications Antipsychotic medications can partially correct the chemical imbalances in the brain of a person with schizophrenia, significantly reducing hallucinations and delusions and helping the person think more clearly. Although the medications do not cure schizophrenia, they may make it possible for the person to live at home with his or her family and participate in many normal daily activities, including holding down a job. The doctor will prescribe antipsychotic medication in the lowest dose that is effective in preventing psychosis in that person. With continued treatment, the medication can reduce the frequency of future episodes of psychosis. The doctor will monitor the person's condition closely while he or she is taking the medication. The person must not stop taking the medication unless the doctor recommends it and then only under the doctor's supervision.

Antipsychotic medications have side effects, particularly during the first few weeks. These side effects can include dry mouth, blurred vision, drowsiness, lowered blood pressure, muscle spasms or cramps in the head and neck, restlessness, or stiff muscles. Most of these side effects can be relieved by lowering the dose, or trying another medication or combination of medications.

Some antipsychotic medications can cause a more serious long-term problem—called tardive dyskinesia—in about 10 percent of people who take them, especially when they have been taking high doses of the drugs for many years. Tardive dyskinesia is a condition characterized by abnormal muscle movements—including tongue, mouth, and lip movements; facial tics; and abnormal jaw movements. These symptoms may reach a plateau and not get any worse or be so mild that the person is unaware of the unusual movements.

Striking the proper balance between medications that relieve symptoms in psychotic disorders and their side effects is complicated and is based on an individual's distinct needs. Many people with schizophrenia are willing to risk the side effects of antipsychotic medication because the medication relieves them of their debilitating symptoms.

Other forms of treatment Once antipsychotic medications have controlled the most severe symptoms of schizophrenia in a person, his or her doctor will recommend other forms of therapy. With the combination of medication and psychotherapy, many people who have schizophrenia can live at home, work, and continue to participate in many daily activities. Rehabilitation programs can help a person with schizophrenia learn to establish and maintain relationships and develop work skills and other abilities that enable him or her to function independently—including problem solving, money management, or using public transportation.

Individual and group psychotherapy can help the person deal with current or past problems, experiences, thoughts, feelings, or relationships. During treatment, people with schizophrenia may gradually come to understand more about themselves and their problems. The therapist can also help them distinguish between the real and the unreal or the distorted.

Family therapy provides an opportunity for the individual and his or her family members to learn more about the disorder and understand the effects of the illness on each of them. The therapist can give them emotional support, and encourage them to help plan and participate in the treatment of their loved one.

DELUSIONAL DISORDER

Delusional disorder is a mental disorder in which people have delusions (false beliefs that are not subject to reason) that something is happening to them that is not actually happening. For example, they may believe that they are being deceived by their spouse or harmed. Paranoia (excessive or irrational suspiciousness) is common in people who have delusional disorder. They exaggerate small slights, and a perceived injustice may become the focus of the delusion.

Symptoms Other than having delusions, a person with delusional disorder may behave normally. But, in some cases, a delusion may be severe enough to impair a person's ability to function at work or in social situations. A delusion can make a person angry, violent, or disruptive, particularly if it involves paranoia or jealousy. Some people become irritable or depressed. Other people with the disorder undergo numerous unnecessary medical tests based on a belief that they have a condition that requires treatment.

Diagnosis To diagnose delusional disorder, a psychiatrist will talk with the person and try to evaluate his or her delusions. The psychiatrist will also usually talk with people who are close to the person to distinguish the truth from the delusion. If the person's delusions involve physical ailments, the psychiatrist will consult with the person's internist. Because delusions can also occur in people who have other mental disorders, the psychiatrist will rule these out before making a diagnosis of delusional disorder.

Treatment Treatment of delusional disorder usually combines medication and psychotherapy. Although many people with delusional disorder resist treatment, antipsychotic medications can be helpful. It is important for family members, friends, and doctors to give the person support and understanding, rather than confront him or her about his or her false beliefs. Psychotherapy can help the person feel supported and safe, and may uncover the cause of his or her delusions and help him or her learn to tell the difference between a false belief and reality.

CHAPTER 24

Your endocrine system

Contents

Your endocrine system is made up of glands that secrete hormones. These powerful hormones control numerous essential body functions, including the chemical activity of cells, growth, the balance of salt and fluid, sexual development, and the response to illness or stress. The major endocrine glands are the hypothalamus, pituitary gland, thyroid gland, adrenal glands, ovaries, and, in pregnant women, the placenta. Some cells in the pancreas—called islet cells—are also an important part of the endocrine system.

Disorders of the endocrine glands can have wide-ranging effects throughout your body. A malfunctioning gland influences all of the parts of the body that are stimulated or controlled by the hormones that the gland secretes. This chapter discusses disorders of the endocrine system, focusing on those that are most common in women—diabetes and thyroid disorders. For information about the ovaries and the hormones that regulate the reproductive system, see the chapters on the female reproductive system, planning a pregnancy, and menopause.

The endocrine system

Each endocrine gland secretes hormones directly into the bloodstream. The hormones influence the function of specific organs and tissues throughout the body:

- The **hypothalamus** in the brain secretes a number of hormones that regulate the production and release of hormones by the pituitary gland.
- The **pituitary gland** in the brain secretes hormones that stimulate other glands to produce hormones. The pituitary is often called the master gland because it regulates and controls other endocrine glands and many body processes, including growth and reproduction.
- The **parathyroid glands** secrete parathyroid hormone, which maintains the level of calcium in your blood.
- The **thyroid gland** secretes thyroxine and triiodothyronine (which regulate metabolism and body temperature) and calcitonin (which helps bones absorb calcium).
- The **adrenal glands** secrete corticosteroid hormones (which are important for many cell activities and are secreted in response to stress), epinephrine (which is also called adrenaline and helps your body react immediately to stressful or frightening situations), and aldosterone (which controls the level of salts in your body).
- The **pancreas** secretes insulin and glucagon, which control your body's use of sugar (glucose), fats, and proteins.
- The **ovaries** secrete estrogen and progesterone, which regulate your reproductive system.

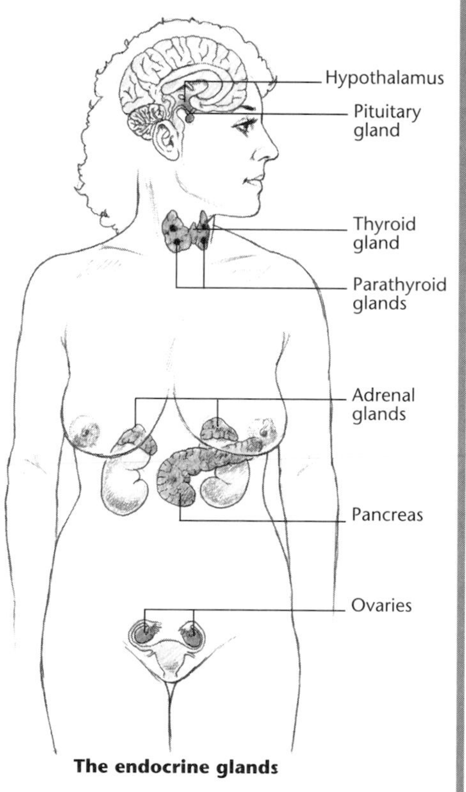

The endocrine glands

Disorders of the pancreas

The pancreas, a long, flat organ about the size of your hand, is located behind your stomach. Your pancreas produces chemicals called enzymes that help break down the food you eat as it passes through your digestive system. Inside the pancreas are small islands of cells called islet cells that secrete the hormone insulin. Insulin regulates your body's use of sugar in the form of glucose, which is a major source of energy for the chemical processes that take place inside your body. Insulin has another very important role—it regulates your body's use of fat and amino acids, which are essential for storing energy and building proteins. When insulin is not available or is not able to do its job, the result is one of two forms of diabetes—a very common, debilitating disease.

TYPE I DIABETES

Type I diabetes—also called insulin-dependent diabetes or juvenile diabetes—occurs when the pancreas stops producing sufficient amounts of the hormone insulin. Insulin is essential; it enables your body to convert food into energy that it can use right away or store as fat for future needs. Your body gets energy from glucose, the major form of sugar in the foods you eat. Insulin acts as a key that unlocks doors on cells to allow glucose to enter and be used properly. If your body is not producing enough insulin, glucose cannot enter the cells and builds up in the blood. The excess glucose enters the urine and passes out of your body unused. The accumulation of glucose in your bloodstream causes symptoms such as frequent urination, excessive thirst, increased hunger, or unexplained weight loss.

Between 500,000 and 750,000 Americans have type I diabetes. A person usually develops type I diabetes during childhood or adolescence, but the disease can occur at any age. Type I diabetes is an autoimmune disease, a term that describes a disorder in which a person's immune system reacts against the cells in his or her own body. In type I diabetes, the immune system mistakes the insulin-producing cells (islets) in the pancreas for foreign cells and attacks and destroys them. The reason for this reaction is not yet known. Doctors believe that it results from an interaction of genes and environmental factors.

Some people are born with genes that make them susceptible to developing diabetes. However, most people with these genes do not develop the disease. In susceptible people, exposure to one or more factors in the environment (such as a virus) may trigger their immune system to attack the insulin-producing cells of their pancreas.

Tests are now available to screen family members, especially children or siblings, of people who have type I diabetes to evaluate their risk of developing the disease. A blood test is used to detect the presence of specific antibodies that are associated with the autoimmune destruction of the insulin-producing cells of the pancreas. Doctors are currently testing techniques that may be effective in preventing type I diabetes in susceptible people.

Type I diabetes can have life-threatening complications. If you have type I diabetes, you cannot survive unless you take injections of insulin every day to control the level of glucose in your blood. Over time, excessive amounts of glucose in your blood can cause a variety of problems that can lead to blindness, kidney failure, nerve damage, heart

WHAT IS DIABETES?
In a healthy person (top), the hormone insulin "opens doors" on cell surfaces to allow cells to take in glucose from the bloodstream to use for energy. A person with type I diabetes (center) does not produce enough insulin; the cells cannot take in glucose, and glucose builds up in the bloodstream. In a person with type II diabetes (bottom), cells are resistant to the effects of insulin; the pancreas produces more and more insulin but eventually cannot produce enough to overcome the cells' resistance, and glucose builds up in the bloodstream.

Insulin allows glucose to enter cell

Cell of healthy person

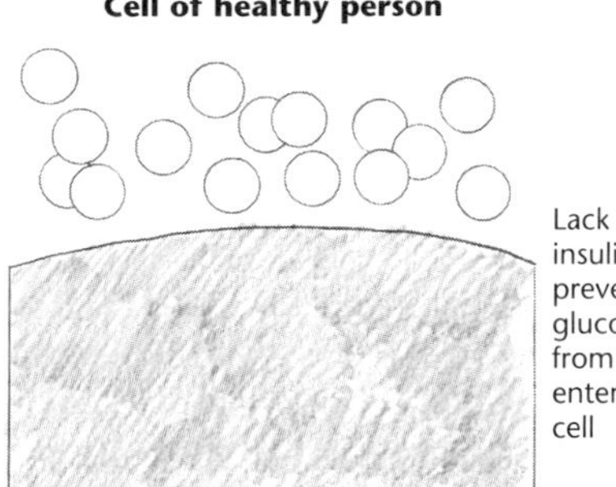

Cell of person with type I diabetes

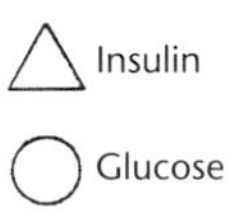

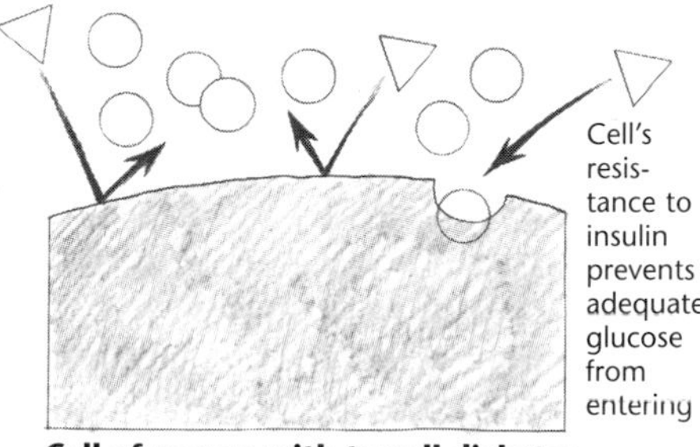

Cell of person with type II diabetes

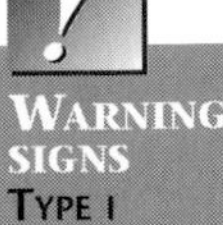

WARNING SIGNS
TYPE I DIABETES

The symptoms of type I diabetes usually appear suddenly in people under age 20. Without immediate treatment, this form of diabetes can be fatal. If you have any of the following symptoms, see your doctor immediately:

- Frequent urination
- Excessive thirst
- Extreme hunger
- Weight loss despite increased appetite
- Blurred vision

ALWAYS CARRY YOUR ID

If you have diabetes, always wear an identifying bracelet or necklace, or carry a card in your wallet to alert doctors or other emergency health-care personnel of your diabetes in case you become unconscious.

disease, high blood pressure, cholesterol abnormalities, and early death. However, with careful control of your glucose level, you can prevent or delay these serious complications and lead an active, healthy life.

Symptoms The symptoms of type I diabetes usually occur suddenly, after significant numbers of insulin-producing cells in the pancreas have been destroyed and the pancreas has stopped producing sufficient amounts of insulin. In most cases, early symptoms of type I diabetes include frequent urination accompanied by unusual thirst, extreme hunger, unexplained weight loss, or blurred vision. If you notice any of these symptoms, see your doctor immediately.

In some cases, the first indication of type I diabetes is a life-threatening condition called ketoacidosis (see page 619), the buildup in the blood of acids called ketones, which can poison the body. Ketones can build up in your blood and appear in urine when your body does not have enough insulin. Without insulin, your body burns fat instead of glucose for energy. Ketones are the waste products of this breakdown of fats.

Diagnosis To diagnose type I diabetes, your doctor will ask about your symptoms, health history, and your family health history and will give you a physical examination. If you have the disorder, blood tests will show persistently high levels of glucose in your blood. You may have a urine test to detect acids called ketones, which can accumulate in your urine if your body does not have enough insulin.

Treatment If you are diagnosed with type I diabetes, you will need to give yourself injections of insulin every day for the rest of your life. Your doctor will teach you how to give yourself insulin. Insulin is not a cure for diabetes, but it controls the level of glucose in your blood, prevents complications from the disease, and allows you to live a normal, active life.

Your doctor will tell you how often you should test your glucose and take your insulin injections. Using a home glucose meter, you can accurately measure your blood glucose level from a small drop of blood taken from a finger prick. Most people find this test easy to do and relatively painless and they like the control that frequent testing of their blood glucose level gives them over their treatment.

The amount of insulin you need to control your glucose level can change dramatically at puberty and during adolescence. Many women find that their insulin requirements change during their menstrual cycle. Stress or an illness can also affect the amount of insulin you need. As people get older, their insulin requirements may change as their eating habits and level of activity change.

Diet Diet is an important part of the treatment of diabetes. A dietitian will work with you to design a meal plan that is right for you—one that includes foods you enjoy and that fits into your schedule and eating habits. The meal plan tells you how much you can eat and when, and what kinds of foods to choose for meals and snacks. Your diet should include mostly complex carbohydrates (such as starchy vegetables, whole grains, and fruits) and high-fiber foods (such as vegetables, dried beans and peas, and whole grains).

It is important to eat about the same amount of carbohydrates, protein, and fat at each meal from day to day. This consistency in your intake of food will help ensure a proper balance between insulin and glucose in your blood. Your doctor will give you guidelines about balancing these important nutrients and limiting fat in your diet. The goal is to keep your glucose level as close to normal as possible.

Exercise Regular exercise—even as little as a 20-minute walk four times a week—is extremely beneficial if you have diabetes. Exercise helps lower glucose levels in the blood by improving your body's ability to efficiently convert the food you eat into energy. Exercise also improves the health of your heart and blood vessels, which uncontrolled diabetes can damage over time. Consult your doctor before you begin any exercise program. He or she will help you decide which type of exercise—and how much—is best for you. Your activity must be planned around your meal schedule and your insulin injections to maintain the balance of your insulin requirements and your blood glucose level.

Long-term complications of diabetes
Both type I and type II diabetes can have serious long-term complications. Generally, these complications are more severe in people with type I diabetes and they occur at an earlier stage of the disease. Maintaining rigorous control of the level of glucose in your blood is the best way to prevent or delay these complications. Over time, uncontrolled diabetes can cause significant damage to your blood vessels, kidneys, and nerves. Diabetes is the leading cause of blindness and kidney failure and is the most common reason for amputation of limbs.

It is important to recognize the early signs of these complications and to seek prompt treatment. If you have diabetes, you should see your doctor regularly, even when you are feeling fine. Have your eyes tested every year by an ophthalmologist (a doctor who specializes in eye care); make sure he or she knows that you have diabetes. If you carefully follow the treatment program recommended by your doctor, you should be able to live a healthy, active life.

Heart disease Diabetes is a major risk factor for heart disease (see page 461), as are high blood pressure (see page 480), high cholesterol level (see page 131), and cigarette smoking. If you have diabetes, it is essential to maintain your blood pressure and cholesterol levels in a healthy range and to not smoke. Many people with diabetes have cholesterol abnormalities—such as a low level of helpful high-density lipoprotein (HDL) cholesterol and a high level of harmful low-density lipoprotein (LDL) cholesterol—that can lead to narrowing and blocking of arteries that supply blood to the heart, causing a heart attack. They are also twice as likely to have high blood pressure. In people with diabetes, smoking even less than half a pack of cigarettes a day significantly increases the risk of dying of heart disease.

Short-term complications of diabetes

Diabetes that is not carefully controlled can cause acute problems that require immediate medical attention. Ketoacidosis, which is life threatening, can occur if the level of insulin in the blood becomes dangerously low. An insulin reaction can occur when the level of glucose in the blood is abnormally low.

Ketoacidosis Ketoacidosis is a condition in which excessive levels of acids called ketones build up in your blood. The buildup occurs because, without insulin to help cells take in glucose to use for energy, the body breaks down stored fats to use for energy instead. As fats are broken down, they are converted into ketones. Ketoacidosis can poison your body and lead to coma and death. The lack of insulin also causes glucose to build up in the blood (hyperglycemia). Ketones accumulate to a high level in urine. Symptoms of ketoacidosis include constant fatigue; dry or flushed skin; nausea, vomiting, or abdominal pain; fast breathing; breath that smells fruity; or confusion.

Insulin reaction An insulin reaction, also called hypoglycemia, occurs when the level of glucose in the blood is abnormally low. You can develop an insulin reaction if you take too much insulin, do not eat enough, do not eat on schedule with your insulin injections, or exercise too much. You may feel shaky, sweaty, dizzy, hungry, irritable, light-headed, or confused. This reaction can take place while you are exercising or up to 12 hours later. Make sure you know these signs so you can recognize them if they occur. As soon as you feel a reaction coming on, stop your activity immediately and test your glucose level. If it is low, treat it immediately by eating or drinking some form of sugar.

Peripheral vascular disease People with diabetes are at increased risk of peripheral vascular disease, which is a narrowing of blood vessels that deliver blood to tissues in the feet and legs. The main symptom of peripheral vascular disease is pain in your thigh, calf, or buttocks that occurs during exercise and is relieved by rest. Peripheral vascular disease can lead to infections that heal poorly because of the lack of nourishing oxygen-rich blood provided to the tissues. If these infections are not treated, they can result in amputation of a foot or leg. You can avoid serious problems by carefully monitoring your feet for sores and having your doctor examine your feet regularly. Any infection in your foot should be examined promptly by your doctor.

Taking care of your feet

Over time, diabetes can damage nerves and blood vessels in your feet. Small cuts can become infected and, if blood flow is severely limited, can lead to gangrene (tissue death). In some cases it is necessary to amputate the toes in order to save the rest of the foot and leg. The following guidelines can help you prevent this serious complication of diabetes:

- Inspect your feet every day for scratches, cuts, blisters, ingrown toenails, warts on the soles of your feet (plantar warts), or puncture wounds. See your doctor if you notice any of these problems.
- Immediately report to your doctor any signs of infection, burning, tingling, or numbness in your feet.
- Do not cut or treat corns or calluses yourself. Have a doctor remove them.
- Make sure your doctor examines your feet at each visit.
- Wash your feet every day and dry them well, especially between the toes.
- Check inside your shoes for pebbles, gravel, or other objects that could cause a cut or blister.
- Wear comfortable, well-cushioned shoes that do not pinch at the toes or scrape at the heel. Try wearing shoes that are a half-size larger than you normally wear. Do not wear high heels.
- Change your socks every day. Cotton socks, which absorb moisture, are best. Smooth your socks or panty hose over your feet carefully, leaving no bumps or lumps that could cause chafing or blisters.
- Do not walk barefoot.

HOW TO CUT YOUR TOENAILS

To prevent ingrown toenails and infections, be extra careful when you trim your toenails. Cut your nails straight across the top. If you have numbness in your feet, you should not trim your own nails.

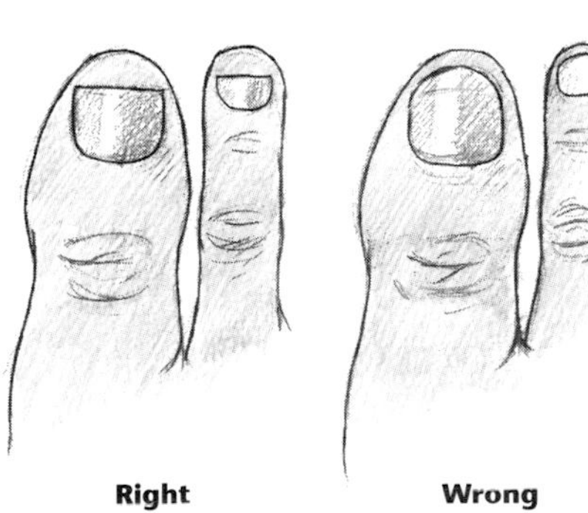

Stroke Diabetes increases your risk of stroke (see page 569) because it makes you more likely to have high blood pressure—the major cause of stroke. Diabetes can also cause abnormalities of cholesterol and other fats in your blood, which can lead to narrowing and blocking of arteries that supply blood to your brain. This process, called atherosclerosis (see page 468), makes the arteries weak and susceptible to rupture.

Nerve damage Neuropathy—damage to nerves—is one of the most common long-term complications of diabetes. At least half of people with diabetes eventually have nerve damage, particularly in their feet and legs. Neuropathy can affect any area of your body, including your bladder, digestive tract, or reproductive organs. Depending on the nerves that are affected, you may experience loss of feeling, pain, muscle weakness, or decrease in a function, such as digestion or the ability to achieve orgasm. The loss of feeling can have serious consequences. When you lose feeling in your feet and toes, you can injure your foot and not realize it because you do not feel the pain. Such injuries increase the likelihood of foot infections that can lead to gangrene (tissue death) and amputation. Your risk of neuropathy is even higher if you smoke cigarettes or if you have uncontrolled high glucose levels.

Eye disorders Diabetes is a major cause of blindness in people between 25 and 74. The disease causes abnormalities of the small blood vessels that supply the retina in the back of the eye. These blood vessel abnormalities in the eyes are called diabetic retinopathy (see page 654). High blood pressure and cigarette smoking increase your risk of diabetic retinopathy. Diabetes also increases your risk of cataracts (see page 652), which is clouding of the lenses of your eyes, and the eye disorder glaucoma (see page 649), which is caused by increased pressure inside the eye.

Notify your doctor immediately of any changes in your vision. Have your eyes examined every year; make sure your ophthalmologist (a doctor who specializes in eye care) knows you have diabetes. Early detection and treatment can often prevent retinopathy from progressing to an advanced stage and causing blindness.

Kidney disease Kidney disease is a major cause of illness and death in people with diabetes. Diabetes causes kidney disease by gradually damaging and obstructing small blood vessels in the kidneys. Over time, uncontrolled high blood pressure and high levels of glucose in the blood can lead to kidney failure.

The presence of protein in your urine is often the first sign of kidney damage from diabetes. To detect this at an early stage, your doctor may ask you to collect your urine over a 24-hour period. If the level of protein is elevated, your doctor will prescribe medications to control your blood pressure and your glucose level. These measures can help prevent further damage to your kidneys.

TYPE II DIABETES

In type II diabetes—which is also called non–insulin-dependent or adult-onset diabetes—your body is resistant to the actions of the hormone insulin. Insulin enables your body to convert food into energy that it can use right away or store as fat for future needs. Your body gets energy from glucose, a form of sugar that it makes from the foods you eat. Insulin acts as a key that unlocks doors on cells (primarily in your muscles), enabling the cells to take in glucose.

The resistance to insulin that is characteristic of type II diabetes is caused primarily by obesity, which makes it harder for insulin to push glucose into cells because they are already filled with fat. Initially, the cells in your pancreas can overcome this resistance to insulin by producing more insulin. But eventually, your pancreas cannot produce enough insulin to overcome the resistance.

In type II diabetes, even higher-than-normal levels of insulin cannot open the cell doors and, as a result, glucose builds up in the blood. This accumulation is usually gradual, but it eventually causes symptoms such as frequent urination, excessive thirst, increased hunger, unexplained weight loss, frequent vaginal infections, or slow healing of wounds.

The vast majority of people with diabetes have type II diabetes. Because this disorder can progress for years without causing any noticeable symptoms, half of the people who have it have not yet been diagnosed.

Most people who develop type II diabetes are over age 40 and overweight. The disease has a genetic component—the more relatives you have with the disease, the higher your risk of developing it. In spite of the strong genetic influence, type II diabetes can often be prevented or delayed by maintaining a healthy weight and exercising regularly. Excess body fat increases your risk of type II diabetes because it causes resistance to insulin. If insulin cannot get glucose into your cells, glucose builds up in your blood. In many cases, losing weight is all it takes to bring your glucose level down to normal. Exercise helps reduce your risk of type II diabetes by increasing your body's sensitivity to insulin.

Symptoms Type II diabetes may cause no symptoms and go undiagnosed for 5 to 7 years. When symptoms do occur, some are the same as those of type I diabetes—frequent urination, excessive thirst, increased appetite, unexplained weight loss, and fatigue. In addition to these symptoms, you may also experience blurred vision; numbness, tingling, or pain in your legs, feet, or fingers; or frequent infections of your vagina, bladder, or skin.

Diagnosis Type II diabetes can be diagnosed in one of three ways. You are considered to have type II diabetes if you have any of the following:

- Two or more fasting glucose tests (see page 623) that show the level of glucose in your blood is higher than 140 milligrams per deciliter (mg/dL).
- One blood test that shows your level of glucose is higher than 200 mg/dL and you have symptoms of diabetes.
- An oral glucose tolerance test (see page 623) that shows your glucose level is higher than 200 mg/dL 2 hours after you ingest a special glucose drink and a blood

Gestational diabetes

Some women who do not have diabetes develop high sugar levels in their blood while they are pregnant. This form of diabetes is called gestational diabetes (see page 418).

test (at a different time) that shows a glucose level higher than 200 mg/dL.

Treatment If you have type II diabetes, careful control of the level of glucose in your blood is important. Type II diabetes, like type I, can have serious complications (see page 619), including heart disease, stroke, and blindness. The initial treatment for type II diabetes usually involves a diet plan, weight reduction, and regular exercise. In many cases, these measures are enough to maintain normal glucose levels. If they are not effective, your doctor may prescribe hypoglycemic medication (drugs that lower your blood glucose level) that you take by mouth every day. Some people with type II diabetes have to take insulin injections to control the level of glucose in their blood.

Even if you do not have to take insulin or hypoglycemic medication, your doctor may recommend testing your glucose level regularly with a home test that measures your glucose level from a drop of blood taken from a needle prick of your finger. People get used to this relatively painless procedure and find it helps them evaluate the effectiveness of their diet, exercise, and medication therapy.

Diet Because obesity is the major cause of type II diabetes, the first line of treatment is usually weight loss. Being overweight also increases your risk of complications from diabetes, such as high blood pressure and heart disease. Work closely with your doctor and nutritionist to develop a diet plan that fits into your life and includes the foods you enjoy. As with type I diabetes, your diet should include mostly complex carbohydrates (such as starchy vegetables, whole grains, and fruits) and high-fiber foods (such as vegetables, dried beans and peas, and whole grains). Limit your daily intake of fat to no more than 25 percent of your total calories (see page 107).

Immediately after you eat, your blood glucose level rises. Regulating your food intake by eating about the same amount of food at the same time every day may help you keep your glucose levels consistent and normal. Even if you are not overweight and you have type II diabetes, you need to closely follow a meal plan that provides good nutrition and sufficient calories to maintain your ideal weight.

Exercise Exercise is extremely important for people with type II diabetes. Exercise

WARNING SIGNS
TYPE II DIABETES

The onset of type II diabetes is usually gradual and the symptoms often go unnoticed for years. If you experience any of the following symptoms, see your doctor immediately:

- Frequent urination
- Unusual thirst
- Extreme hunger
- Unexplained weight loss in spite of increased appetite
- Fatigue
- Blurred vision or any change in your eyesight
- Numbness, tingling, or pain in your legs, feet, or fingers
- Frequent infections of the vagina, bladder, or skin

Risk factors for type II diabetes

When diabetes is detected and treated at an early stage, it is possible to prevent or delay many of the debilitating complications, such as heart disease and high blood pressure, that can result from the disease. Talk to your doctor about being tested for diabetes if you have any of the following risk factors:

- A family history of type II diabetes (parent or sibling with the disease)
- Obesity—you are more than 20 percent over your ideal weight (see page 99)
- Race; you are at increased risk if you are Native American, Hispanic, or black
- A condition called impaired glucose tolerance (see page 623), indicated by a test showing a higher-than-normal level of glucose in your blood
- A history of diabetes during a pregnancy, called gestational diabetes (see page 418), or having delivered a large baby (9 pounds or heavier)

Tests for type II diabetes

A number of tests are used to screen for, diagnose, and monitor the effectiveness of treatment for type II diabetes.

- **Screening test** If you do not have any symptoms of diabetes, but you are at risk of type II diabetes (see page 622), your doctor will recommend a blood test to measure the level of glucose in your blood. If this test shows the level of glucose is high or low, your doctor may recommend further testing.
- **Fasting glucose test** If a screening blood test shows that your glucose level is too high or too low, you will have a fasting plasma glucose test. This blood test measures your glucose level after you have not eaten for 10 to 16 hours (overnight). For this test, a sample of blood is taken from a vein in your arm. In general, glucose levels of less than 115 milligrams per deciliter (mg/dL) are considered normal. Levels of more than 140 mg/dL on two or more fasting glucose tests indicate a diagnosis of diabetes. Your blood glucose level can be influenced by your general health and some medications you may be taking, such as diuretics.
- **Oral glucose tolerance test** If your fasting blood glucose level is between 115 and 140 milligrams per deciliter (mg/dL) or if your fasting blood glucose level is normal but you have symptoms of diabetes, your doctor will recommend further testing. You will probably have a blood test called an oral glucose tolerance test. Before this test, your doctor will tell you to eat a diet rich in carbohydrates for 2 or 3 days and then to fast overnight—for at least 10 hours, but not more than 16 hours. You will first have a fasting glucose test. After that, you will be given a sweet-tasting glucose drink and blood will be taken every 30 minutes for 2 hours. During this time, you will be asked to lie or sit quietly because any amount of exercise can lower your glucose level and alter the results of the test.

  If your glucose level is more than 200 mg/dL between the first and last test and is still over 200 mg/dL on the last test, you have diabetes. If your glucose level is 200 mg/dL at any point during the test but less than 200 mg/dL at the end of the test, you have a condition called impaired glucose tolerance. This condition puts you at high risk of developing diabetes. Your doctor will recommend losing weight if you are overweight and exercising regularly to help prevent or postpone symptoms of the disease. He or she will also recommend regular testing of your blood glucose level.

can lower the level of glucose in your blood and reduce your risk of heart disease and stroke, which are common in people with type II diabetes. Exercise also reduces your risk of heart disease by helping you lose weight and lowering the level in your blood of harmful low-density lipoprotein (LDL) cholesterol. Before starting your exercise program, talk with your doctor about how often and for how long you should exercise.

Medication Many people who have type II diabetes do not need to take medication if they carefully follow their diet, weight loss, and exercise program. However, if these measures do not keep your level of glucose in the normal range, your doctor may prescribe hypoglycemic medication (in pills), which lowers your blood glucose level by stimulating your pancreas to make more insulin. The insulin enables your cells to take in more glucose. Make sure your doctor knows of any other medications you are taking.

Side effects of hypoglycemic medications include hypoglycemia (low blood sugar), which can result if you take too much of the drug, or loss of appetite, skin rashes, or itching. Tell your doctor right away if you have any kind of reaction to the medication. Some people with type II diabetes eventually have to take insulin injections every day to control their glucose level.

Disorders of the thyroid gland

Your thyroid gland lies in the lower part of your neck just in front of your windpipe (trachea). The thyroid gland secretes the hormones thyroxine (also called thyroid hormone), triiodothyronine, and calcitonin. Thyroid hormone controls the rate of your metabolism. The more thyroid hormone you have in your blood, the greater the speed of your metabolism. If your thyroid gland produces too little of the hormone, you have a condition called hypothyroidism; if the gland produces too much of the hormone, you have hyperthyroidism. Women are eight times more likely than men to develop a thyroid disorder.

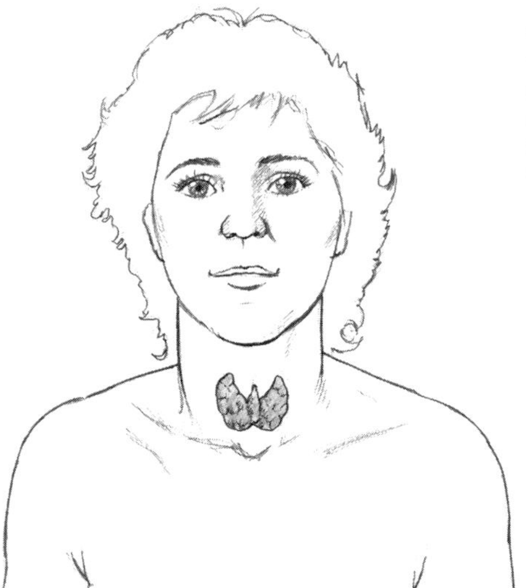

THE THYROID GLAND

The thyroid gland is a butterfly-shaped gland at the base of your neck. The thyroid gland secretes the hormones thyroxine and triiodothyronine, which regulate metabolism, and calcitonin, which helps bones absorb calcium.

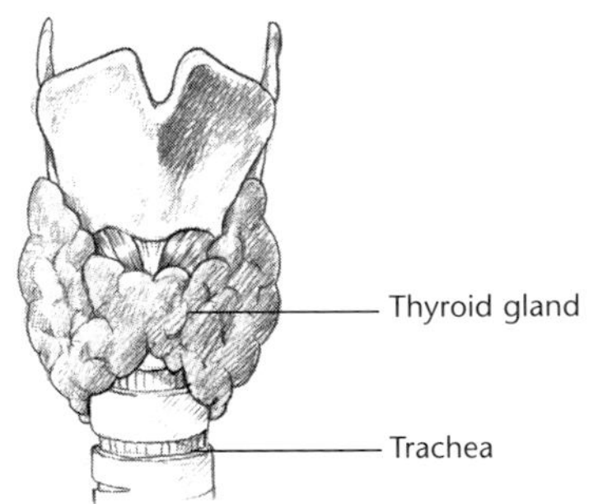

HYPOTHYROIDISM

Hypothyroidism is a condition that results when the thyroid gland is underactive and secretes too little of the hormone thyroxine. Thyroxine, or thyroid hormone, regulates the rate of your body's metabolism. Hypothyroidism—which is more common in women than men—is often caused by a disorder called Hashimoto's disease. Hashimoto's disease is an autoimmune disease in which the immune system mistakes cells in the thyroid gland for potentially harmful invaders and sends out white blood cells to destroy them. The white blood cells gradually replace normal thyroid tissue, which reduces the amount of thyroid hormone the gland can produce.

The pituitary gland responds by secreting more of another hormone, called thyroid-stimulating hormone, to encourage the thyroid gland to try to produce more thyroid hormone. The increased demand on the thyroid gland can cause it to enlarge; this condition is called a goiter (see page 626).

Because hypothyroidism caused by Hashimoto's disease is an inherited condition, other family members may be at risk. Let them know you have the disorder so that they can inform their doctor, who can examine them regularly for it. Hypothyroidism can also result from treatments for an overactive thyroid (hyperthyroidism, see page 625), including surgery or radioactive iodine treatments.

Symptoms Thyroid hormone affects almost every organ of your body, so a reduction in the amount of the hormone in your bloodstream can cause a wide variety of symptoms. These symptoms can include:

- Goiter (an enlarged thyroid gland that looks like a swelling in the neck)

- Weight gain even though you have lost your appetite
- Unusually heavy or light periods
- Sensitivity to cold
- Slowed heart rate
- Fatigue
- Constipation
- Dry skin and brittle fingernails
- Anemia
- Swollen ankles
- High cholesterol level
- Stiff or weak muscles or muscle cramps
- Depression

These symptoms can be so subtle in the beginning and increase so gradually that many people mistake them for the normal signs of overwork, stress, or aging. But the fatigue, aches, and pains of hypothyroidism can have serious effects on your ability to function and on the quality of your life.

Diagnosis Hypothyroidism is diagnosed by its symptoms, a physical examination, and blood tests that measure the level of thyroid-stimulating hormone and thyroid hormone. If your doctor suspects you have hypothyroidism, he or she will recommend a blood test to measure the level of thyroid-stimulating hormone. If the level of thyroid-stimulating hormone is increased, your doctor may recommend a blood test to measure the level of thyroid hormone. If your level of thyroid hormone is abnormally low, you have hypothyroidism.

Treatment Hypothyroidism is usually treated with pills that contain a synthetic form of thyroid hormone. The dose of the hormone is gradually increased until it reaches a normal level in your blood. If you are older or if you have a heart condition, your doctor will start you on a low dose of the hormone until your body gets used to more normal levels of the hormone in your blood; this will prevent a rapid rise in your heart rate.

Obesity and thyroid disorders

Many people believe that because hypothyroidism lowers your metabolism, it can cause obesity. In fact, hypothyroidism usually causes only a moderate weight gain of 5 to 10 pounds, most of it in excess fluid. After starting treatment with thyroid hormone, people often lose this extra weight.

If you are severely overweight when you develop hypothyroidism, you will lose only a few pounds after you begin treatment. Treatment for an underactive thyroid gland is not a cure for obesity. It is dangerous to try to lose weight by taking high doses of thyroid hormone because excessive doses can damage your heart, weaken your bones, and cause mood swings and indigestion.

If you develop hypothyroidism, it is likely to be a permanent condition. For this reason, you will probably have to take thyroid hormone every day for the rest of your life. The dose may need to be adjusted periodically. In some cases, excessive doses of thyroid hormone taken for a long period of time may cause bone loss that can lead to osteoporosis (see page 552). Taking too much thyroid hormone may also cause symptoms of hyperthyroidism (see below). To make sure the level of the hormone in your blood is not too high, your doctor will monitor it with regular blood tests.

If any of the symptoms of hypothyroidism return or continue to bother you while you are taking thyroid hormone, tell your doctor. He or she will increase the dose of medication until blood tests show that your hormone levels are normal.

HYPERTHYROIDISM

Hyperthyroidism occurs when the thyroid gland produces too much thyroid hormone. The most common cause of hyperthyroidism is Graves' disease, also called diffuse toxic goiter. Normally, the activity of the thyroid gland is regulated by thyroid-stimulating hormone, which is produced in your pituitary gland. The thyroid gland itself produces thyroid hormone, which controls your body's rate of metabolism.

In Graves' disease, your body produces antibodies that attach to cells of the thyroid gland. These antibodies mimic thyroid-stimulating hormone, so, when they attach to cells in the thyroid gland, the gland responds by growing and secreting more thyroid hormone. This

Goiter

A goiter is an enlarged thyroid gland that looks like a swelling in your neck. A goiter can be a symptom of hypothyroidism (see page 624) or hyperthyroidism (see page 625). A goiter can also result from taking antithyroid drugs for hyperthyroidism. If a goiter is large, it can press on your esophagus or trachea, making it uncomfortable or painful to swallow or breathe.

The thyroid gland may grow slightly larger but still function normally under some circumstances, such as during puberty or pregnancy. When these conditions are no longer present, the gland usually shrinks to its normal size.

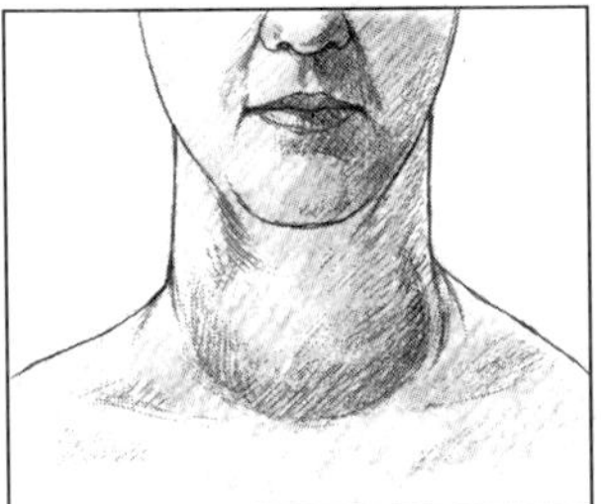

GOITER
A goiter, an enlarged thyroid gland that looks like a swelling in the neck, can range in size from a barely noticeable lump to a swelling the size of a grapefruit.

condition runs in families and is most common in women of childbearing age.

Symptoms The symptoms of hyperthyroidism develop gradually and often include mood swings, anxiety, and irritability. The excessive level of thyroid hormone in your blood boosts your metabolic rate and increases your heart rate. Your body may burn calories more quickly, causing you to lose weight even though you are eating the same amount of food as usual. The increased rate of your metabolism can make you feel warmer than usual in temperatures that you used to find comfortable.

Other symptoms of hyperthyroidism may include light or irregular menstrual periods, increased sweating, indigestion, diarrhea, swelling of your ankles, faster-than-usual nail growth and cracking nails, hair loss, goiter (enlarged thyroid gland that looks like a swelling in your neck), and protruding eyes. Over the long term, hyperthyroidism can cause heart damage, abnormal heart rhythms, and loss of calcium from the bones.

Diagnosis Hyperthyroidism is diagnosed by its symptoms, a physical examination, and blood tests that measure the level of thyroid hormone and thyroid-stimulating hormone. You have hyperthyroidism if the level of thyroid hormone in your blood is increased and the level of thyroid-stimulating hormone is abnormally low.

Treatment Treatment of hyperthyroidism depends on the cause and severity of the condition, and your age and general health. Medications called beta blockers (see page 475) are often prescribed to reduce symptoms such as a rapid heartbeat. However, these drugs do not reduce the excessive level of thyroid hormone in the blood.

Other medications, called antithyroid agents, reduce the amount of thyroid hormone the thyroid gland makes by preventing the gland from using the iodine it needs to make the hormone. These medications are usually taken for about 3 months to a year. At first, you may take both antithyroid agents and beta blockers. As the antithyroid agents decrease the amount of thyroid hormone your thyroid gland is producing, you can stop taking the beta blockers.

If treatment with these medications does not clear up the condition, your doctor may recommend treatment with radioactive iodine to reduce the amount of hormone the thyroid gland produces. For this treatment, you take a single dose of radioactive iodine in a liquid or pills. Within 24 hours, most of the iodine accumulates in your thyroid gland, where the radiation destroys tissue and reduces

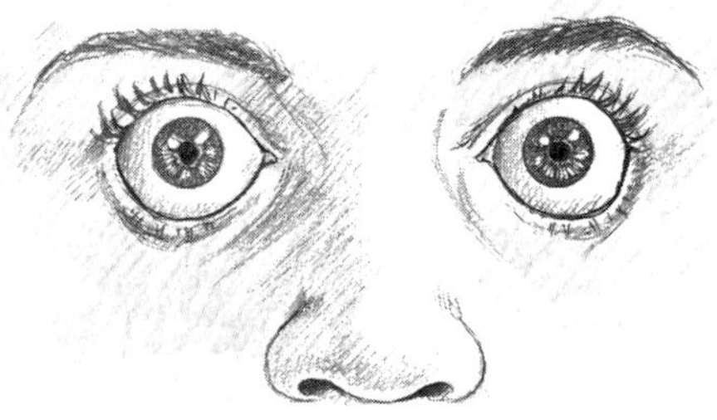

GRAVES' DISEASE
Graves' disease causes your body to produce excessive amounts of thyroid hormone, a condition called hyperthyroidism. A wide-eyed stare, which results from a pulling back of the upper eyelids, is very common in people who have hyperthyroidism. In some people, Graves' disease can cause swelling of the muscles that control eye movement, which can cause the eyes to protrude.

the gland's ability to produce thyroid hormone. Your doctor will carefully calculate the proper dose because too high a dose can cause hypothyroidism (an underactive thyroid gland). You will probably have to take antithyroid agents for up to 6 months after you have a radioactive iodine treatment because it can take that long for the medication to have the full effect. Some people need to have a second or third treatment with radioactive iodine.

If only part of your thyroid gland is enlarged, your doctor may recommend surgery to remove that part of the gland. He or she will refer you to a surgeon who specializes in this kind of surgery. The procedure will be performed in the operating room under general anesthesia (see page 261).

THYROID NODULES

Sometimes small lumps, or nodules, grow in the thyroid gland. You may have one nodule or many. Most thyroid nodules are noncancerous and contain a harmless gelatinous substance or functioning thyroid tissue. However, a small percentage of nodules are cancerous. People are more likely to develop thyroid nodules as they age and, as with most disorders of the thyroid gland, the nodules are much more common in women than men.

If you have been exposed to radiation—such as X-ray therapy for acne or enlarged adenoids or tonsils (which was common medical practice in the 1950s and 1960s) or radiation therapy to your neck for other reasons—you are at increased risk of developing nodules in your thyroid gland. If you have had any of these treatments, tell your doctor.

Symptoms Nodules that are composed of functioning thyroid tissue can produce thyroid hormone, which may reach an excessive level in the blood, causing hyperthyroidism (see page 625). The symptoms of hyperthyroidism can include increased metabolism and heart rate, mood swings, anxiety, and irritability.

Diagnosis Although some people discover a nodule in their neck while they are buttoning their collar, most of the time thyroid nodules are detected by a doctor during a physical examination. Your doctor may perform a test called a thyroid scan. For this test, you drink a small amount of radioactive iodine. You then lie under a special camera that detects areas of the thyroid gland that take in the radioactive iodine. Nodules that are composed of functioning thyroid tissue will absorb the iodine and be detected by the camera.

Nodules that contain a gelatinous substance or cancer cells do not absorb radioactive iodine and, therefore, are not detected on the thyroid scan. Nodules that do not show up on the film are further evaluated using a procedure called fine needle aspiration. In this procedure, the doctor inserts a small needle into the nodule and uses a syringe to withdraw a small amount of tissue and fluid. The tissue sample is then examined under a microscope for cancer cells. In some cases, fine needle aspiration is performed as the first step in evaluating a thyroid nodule.

Treatment If no cancer is detected in a fine needle aspiration, your doctor may prescribe thyroid hormone to decrease the size of the nodule. This treatment is effective in about half of the people who receive it. If the nodule is very small and does not bother you, you and your doctor may decide to do nothing except monitor the nodule for changes in size every 6 months to a year. If the nodule enlarges, your doctor may recommend another fine needle aspiration to make sure that the nodule has not become cancerous.

Nodules that produce too much thyroid hormone can be destroyed with radioactive iodine treatment (see page 626) similar to that used for treating hyperthyroidism. In some cases, thyroid nodules are removed surgically. Surgery is usually performed in the hospital using general anesthesia. The surgeon makes a small incision over the thyroid nodule and removes it. The tissue is sent to a laboratory for examination under a microscope to determine if it is cancerous. If cancer cells are found, the surgeon will probably remove all of the thyroid gland on the side of the nodule and take a tissue sample from the other side of the gland. If the cancer has spread to the other side of the gland, you will be treated with high doses of radioactive iodine to kill the remaining cancer cells.

Disorders of the pituitary gland

The pituitary gland is a pea-sized gland at the base of your brain. It regulates and controls the activities of many other endocrine glands and produces several hormones that control growth, metabolism, and reproduction. Two of these hormones—prolactin and oxytocin—are involved in the production of breast milk. Along with the female hormone estrogen, prolactin stimulates the breasts to produce milk; oxytocin triggers the release of milk during breast-feeding. Oxytocin also stimulates contractions of the uterus during labor and childbirth.

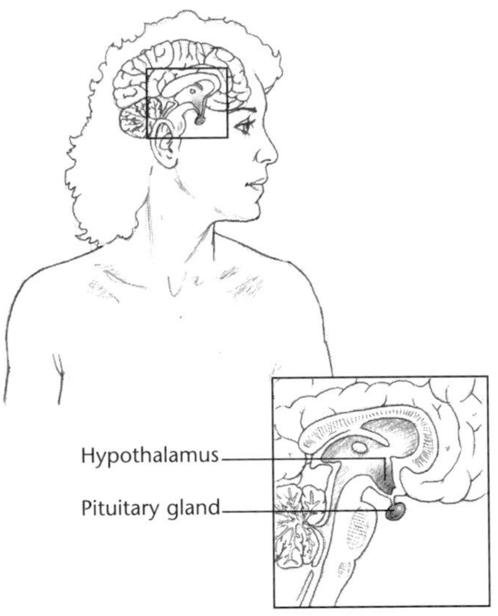

THE PITUITARY GLAND

The pituitary gland is a tiny gland that is suspended from the base of the brain (inset). It secretes growth hormone (which promotes the growth of muscles and bones), antidiuretic hormone (which helps control your body's water balance), follicle-stimulating hormone and luteinizing hormone (which regulate the ovaries' production of estrogen and progesterone), thyroid-stimulating hormone (which regulates the production of thyroid hormone by the thyroid gland), oxytocin (which stimulates contractions of the uterus during labor and release of milk during breast-feeding), and prolactin (which stimulates milk production). The secretion of hormones by the pituitary gland is regulated by hormones secreted by a part of the brain called the hypothalamus, which is located just above the pituitary gland.

PROLACTINOMAS

A prolactinoma is a noncancerous tumor of the pituitary gland that causes the gland to make an excessive amount of the hormone prolactin. Prolactin stimulates a pregnant woman's milk ducts to begin producing breast milk a few days before delivery and to continue producing milk for as long as the woman nurses a child. But a prolactinoma can stimulate milk production in a man as well as in a woman who is not pregnant or breast-feeding.

Any type of fluid leaking from your nipple should be evaluated by your doctor. In addition to giving you a breast examination, your doctor will take a sample of the fluid from the nipple for laboratory testing to rule out the presence of cancer cells.

In most cases, abnormal milk production is not a serious threat to health but it can be annoying and unpleasant. If there are no abnormal cells in the nipple discharge and the level of prolactin in your blood is normal, there is no cause for concern. Milk production can also result from repeated stimulation of the nipples by rubbing against clothing or during lovemaking.

Symptoms In some cases, a prolactinoma causes no symptoms other than abnormal milk production and does not require treatment. However, if the level of prolactin in your blood is increased, it may stop your ovaries from producing estrogen, which can be serious. The lack of estrogen can cause irregular or absent menstrual periods, infertility, and bone loss. The pressure of the pituitary tumor on the brain can cause headaches. If a prolactinoma enlarges, it can crush the other cells of the pituitary gland and prevent them from secreting their hormones. A large tumor can put pressure on the optic nerves (which carry images from the eyes to the brain) and cause peripheral (side vision) blindness.

Diagnosis A prolactinoma is diagnosed by a blood test that shows an elevated level of prolactin. If the level is high or if you have symptoms such as headaches or changes in your peripheral vision, your doctor will recommend a computed tomography (CT) scan (see page 572) or magnetic resonance imaging (MRI; see page 572) to rule out a tumor.

Treatment In many people who have a prolactinoma, hormone levels gradually return to normal without treatment. If the level of prolactin in your blood remains high and a CT scan or MRI shows a small tumor, your doctor will prescribe a medication called bromocriptine, which you take in pills every day. Bromocriptine blocks the production of prolactin by the pituitary gland and can decrease the size of the tumor and lower the level of prolactin in your blood. This stops the production of breast milk and restores normal function to your ovaries.

Side effects from bromocriptine can include dizziness or light-headedness (especially when you get up rapidly from a lying or sitting position), nausea, constipation, or loss of appetite. Tell your doctor of any problems you may be experiencing.

You may have to take bromocriptine indefinitely because stopping may result in an increase in prolactin production and a return of your symptoms. However, in some people, the level of prolactin in the blood stays normal after they stop taking bromocriptine. For this reason, your doctor will ask you to stop taking the medication once every 2 years to determine if the level of prolactin in your blood remains normal without the drug.

Rarely, a prolactinoma does not respond to treatment with bromocriptine. In this case, it may have to be removed surgically or treated with radiation therapy (see page 253) to shrink it.

Disorders of the adrenal glands

The adrenal glands are two triangular glands that sit on top of each kidney. The glands produce a variety of hormones that affect nearly every system of your body. Adrenal hormones help control metabolism, regulate salt and water levels in your body, and help you respond to stress. The stress hormone epinephrine (adrenaline) increases your heart rate, blood pressure, and other body functions to help you deal with stressful situations.

CUSHING'S SYNDROME

Cushing's syndrome results from an excessive level in the blood of corticosteroids, hormones produced by the adrenal glands. Cushing's syndrome can be caused by long-term treatment with synthetic corticosteroids, drugs used to reduce inflammation in disorders such as rheumatoid arthritis (see page 645) or asthma (see page 635) or to prevent a person's body from rejecting a transplanted organ.

Cushing's syndrome may also result from a tumor in one of the adrenal glands that causes it to secrete excessive amounts of corticosteroids, or from a tumor in the pituitary gland. The pituitary gland controls the activity of the adrenal glands by producing a hormone that stimulates the adrenal glands to grow. A tumor in the pituitary gland can cause it to produce too much of this hormone, which stimulates the adrenal glands to produce excessive amounts of corticosteroids.

Cushing's syndrome can occur at any age, but is most common in middle age. If not treated, the disorder may lead to high blood pressure (see page 480), diabetes (see page 617), weight gain, easy bruising, or osteoporosis (see page 552).

Symptoms The symptoms of Cushing's syndrome usually occur gradually over a period of several months. Your face may look more round and redder than usual and you may gain weight. In some people with the disorder, a pad of fat develops between the shoulder blades, making the shoulders look rounded. You may lose muscle from your arms and legs and feel weak and tired. You may develop high blood pressure. Cushing's syndrome causes some people to bruise easily. Excessive levels of corticosteroids may cause irregular or absent menstrual periods or an increase in body hair.

Diagnosis If your doctor thinks you may have Cushing's syndrome, he or she will probably refer you to an endocrinologist (a doctor who specializes in disorders of the endocrine system). If you are not taking prescription corticosteroids, Cushing's syndrome is diagnosed by your symptoms, a physical examination, and tests to measure the levels of corticosteroids in your blood or urine. You may also have a computed tomography (CT) scan (see page 572) or magnetic resonance imaging (MRI; see page 572) of your adrenal glands and pituitary gland to look for any abnormalities, such as tumors.

Treatment If the disorder resulted from taking corticosteroid drugs for another condition, your doctor may decrease the dose of medication, if possible. Do not discontinue taking corticosteroids unless your doctor recommends it. Suddenly stopping this medication after using it for an extended time can lead to shock, which is life threatening. Because the adrenal glands are not working while you are taking corticosteroids, it will require a period of time, as the dose of medication is slowly decreased, for the glands to regain their normal function.

If you have a tumor in an adrenal gland, that gland will be removed surgically. This treatment is usually successful in clearing up the disorder because the remaining gland can produce sufficient amounts of hormones for you to function normally. If both adrenal glands have to be removed, your doctor may prescribe synthetic hormones to replace the essential hormones no longer provided by your adrenal glands. You will need to take these replacement hormones every day for the rest of your life.

CHAPTER 25

Your immune system

Contents

Your immune system is a complex network of cells and organs that protects your body from foreign invaders, such as bacteria and viruses, and diseases of many kinds. If your immune system malfunctions, a wide variety of problems can result. For example, if your immune system is weakened by a condition such as severe stress, you are more vulnerable to infection. If your immune system inappropriately responds to a normally harmless substance (such as ragweed pollen), you develop an allergic reaction to that substance. If your immune system mistakenly identifies your own cells as potentially harmful invaders and launches an attack against them, you develop an autoimmune disease, such as rheumatoid arthritis (see page 645) or lupus (see page 641).

The immune system

The major organs of the immune system are called lymph nodes. Lymph nodes—clustered in your neck, armpits, abdomen, and groin—contain small white blood cells called lymphocytes that mount the immune response against potentially harmful invading organisms, such as viruses or bacteria. Like all blood cells, white blood cells are made in the soft marrow inside bones. White blood cells leave the bone marrow and are carried in the blood to the lymph nodes.

A system of fluid-filled ducts, called lymphatic vessels, channels white blood cells from the lymph nodes back into the bloodstream. White blood cells patrol the entire body—circulating between the blood, lymph nodes, and lymphatic vessels—to watch for germs and to remove damaged cells.

Another important organ of the immune system is the thymus, which lies behind the breastbone. The thymus is the site in which one group of lymphocytes, called T cells (see page 633), grows into maturity. The spleen, a fist-sized organ in the upper left corner of your abdomen, contains enormous numbers of white blood cells, including many lymphocytes. The tonsils and nearby adenoids (not shown) and the appendix are clumps of lymphoid tissue that provide lines of defense at sites in the body where potentially harmful organisms are likely to enter or multiply.

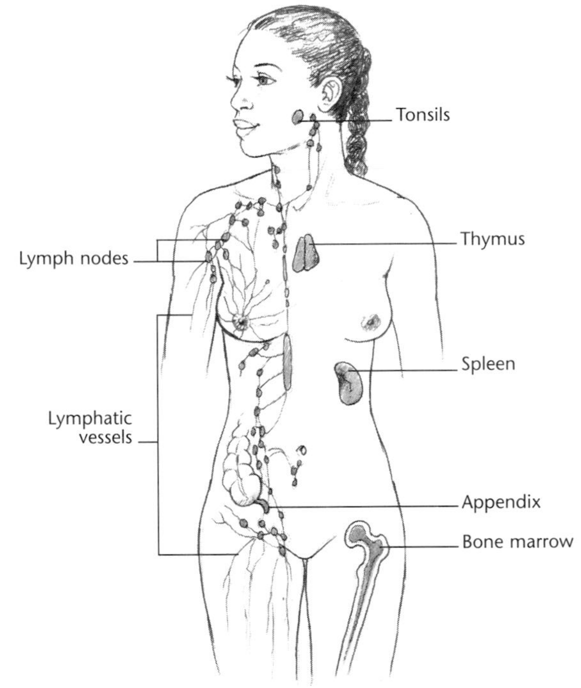

The organs of the immune system

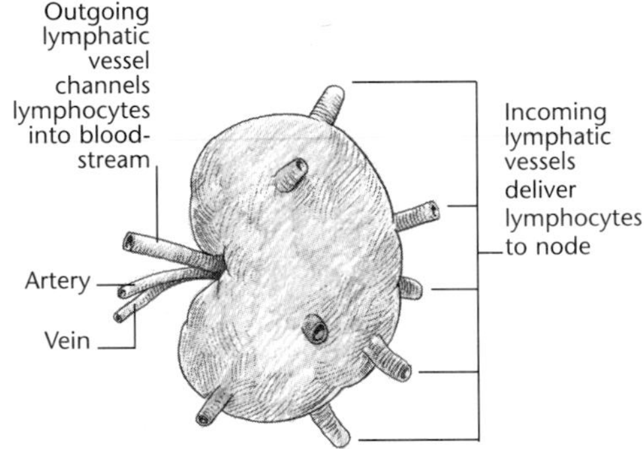

LYMPH NODES

Lymph nodes are glands that are clustered in your neck, armpits, abdomen, and groin. Infection-fighting white blood cells called lymphocytes circulate throughout your body—between the bloodstream, lymph nodes, and lymphatic vessels—and are on guard against disease-causing organisms. The lymphocytes enter and return from the bloodstream through the lymph nodes. Inside lymph nodes, lymphocytes can trap and destroy disease-causing organisms. The node's blood circulation is supplied by an artery and a vein.

The immune response

The main function of your immune system is to distinguish between your body's own normal cells and potentially harmful foreign substances. When a substance such as a bacterium, virus, or fungus enters your body, the cells of your immune system—which are called lymphocytes—recognize it as potentially harmful and try to eliminate it. During this process, some of the lymphocytes develop a memory of a unique protein, called an antigen, on the surface of the invading organism. These memory cells enable your immune system to recognize the same organism if it enters your body again and to be better able to fight it.

This type of protective immune system memory is called immunity. The ability of your immune system to produce memory cells is why you get some infections, such as chickenpox, only once and why vaccines are effective in protecting you against specific infections. A vaccine exposes you to a small amount of a specific disease-causing organism (such as polio), which stimulates your body to produce lymphocytes with memory that will be able to recognize the organism in the future. Your immune system is then prepared to respond quickly and effectively should the actual disease-causing organism enter your body.

HOW YOUR IMMUNE SYSTEM WORKS

Your immune system functions in two fundamental ways to fight disease—using proteins called antibodies and lymphocytes called T cells. Your immune system can produce antibodies, or immunoglobulins, which circulate in the blood to fight off disease-causing organisms. When a potentially harmful organism, such as a virus or bacterium, enters your body, one group of lymphocytes (called B cells) manufactures antibodies to neutralize or destroy it. Each antibody recognizes a uniquely shaped protein (called an antigen) on the surface of the invading organism. When antibodies bind to specific antigens, they trigger a process that destroys the organism.

The second basic mechanism of the immune system involves lymphocytes called T cells. Helper T cells recognize antigens of a potentially harmful organism and call in killer T cells. The killer T cells rapidly converge on the organism and destroy it. After the organism is de-

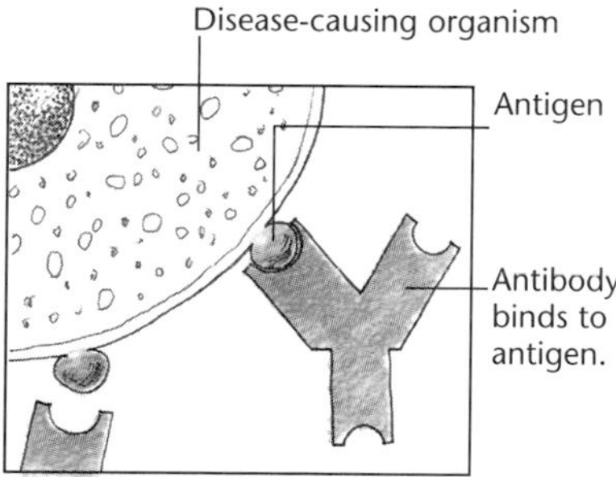

ANTIBODY BINDS TO ANTIGEN: A PERFECT FIT

An antibody in the blood has a unique shape that fits, or binds to, a specific protein (called an antigen) on the surface of an invading disease-causing organism, such as a virus or bacterium. When the antibody binds to an antigen on a specific organism, it initiates the destruction of that organism.

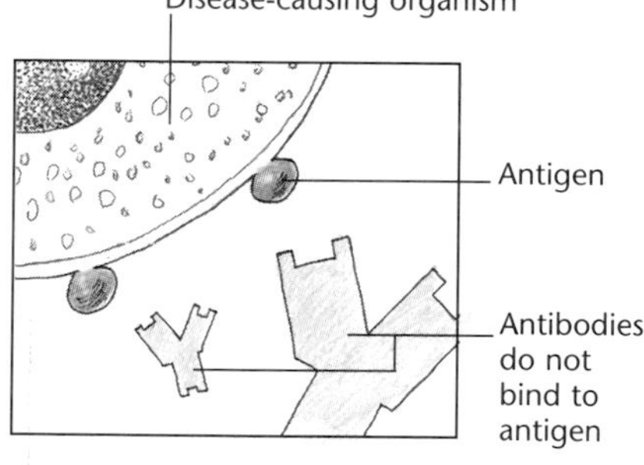

ANTIBODY DOES NOT BIND TO ANTIGEN: A BAD FIT

These antibodies do not have the same shape as the antigens on the surface of this particular disease-causing organism, and do not bind to them. Therefore, these antibodies will not cause the destruction of this organism. They will continue to watch for other disease-causing organisms that have antigens to which they can bind. When they find these antigens, they will alert the immune system to produce more antibodies like themselves to fight the organism.

stroyed, a small number of the T cells become memory cells. If the same organism enters your body again, your immune system will be better prepared to destroy the organism because the immune cells remember the organisms from the first encounter.

The effectiveness of your immune system is influenced by your genes. In some people, the immune system may have a strong response to a particular disease-causing organism, while in others the immune system responds weakly to that same organism. Babies are born with a weak immune system, but receive a boost in their immunity from their mother through breast-feeding (see page 452). The antibodies contained in breast milk help protect infants from early infections. In all babies, the immune system steadily grows stronger as they develop.

Doctors do not yet know how to improve the effectiveness of an individual's immune system. However, there is some evidence that exercising regularly, eating a nutritious diet, reducing stress, and avoiding risky behaviors, such as smoking, might help keep your immune system functioning at peak performance.

IMMUNODEFICIENCY

A variety of health conditions can suppress your immune system, making you vulnerable to disease and infection. Your body's ability to mount an effective immune response can be temporarily impaired by factors such as common viral infections (including influenza, infectious mononucleosis, and measles); malnutrition (including excessive dieting); or stress. Having a blood transfusion or undergoing major surgery or treatment for cancer can also temporarily reduce the functioning of your immune system.

Some people are born with immune system defects that involve abnormalities in the number or functioning of infection-fighting B cells, T cells, or both. These disorders are often genetic in origin, but in some cases are acquired during fetal development. The disorder usually becomes apparent during infancy or childhood, when the child develops an unusual number of infections. In less severe cases, the disorder may not be detected until the person becomes an adult.

Treatment of these disorders depends on the particular immune system defect. In some cases, a person may take antibiotics regularly to prevent recurring infections. Some people may be given specific antibodies intravenously to replace those that their immune system does not produce. In severe cases, a transplant may be necessary to replace the thymus (the gland in which infection-fighting T cells mature) or bone marrow (which produces all the blood cells of the body, including the immune system's white blood cells).

Allergic reactions

An allergy occurs when the immune system attacks a substance that is normally harmless—such as ragweed pollen, a medication, or a food—as if it were a disease-causing organism. Your immune system remembers this encounter and, when that substance enters your body again, you develop an allergic reaction.

HAY FEVER

Hay fever, or allergic rhinitis, is an allergic reaction to the airborne pollen of one or more specific seasonal plants. Despite its name, hay fever is seldom caused by hay and does not cause a fever. Most people experience symptoms in the spring or fall when pollen is abundant. If your symptoms continue at other times, you may be allergic to airborne substances that you encounter indoors, such as mold spores, animal dander, feathers, or dust mites.

A person can develop hay fever at any age. You are at increased risk if you have a personal or family history of asthma (see page 635), atopic eczema (see page 673), or other allergies.

Symptoms Hay fever causes frequent sneezing, a stuffy or runny nose, itchy eyes, dry throat, and coughing. It is sometimes mistaken for a cold or influenza. The symptoms may become intense for periods of 15 to 20 minutes.

Diagnosis To diagnose hay fever, your doctor will ask about your symptoms. He or she may perform a skin test to find the specific plant substance that is causing your reaction. For a skin test, the doctor places small drops of various substances on your arm; you are allergic to a substance that turns your skin red.

Treatment During the time you have symptoms of hay fever, stay inside as much as you can. Keep the windows and doors closed and use an air conditioner with a filter if possible.

Your doctor may recommend over-the-counter medications called antihistamines to help relieve your symptoms. Many antihistamines cause drowsiness; if this is a problem for you, ask your doctor about medications that do not have this side effect.

Your doctor may prescribe a stronger medication containing corticosteroids (synthetic hormones that reduce inflammation) that is delivered in a nasal spray. This medication is designed to reduce symptoms during a severe attack and is not to be used for a long period of time.

If a skin test has determined the specific allergen that is causing your problem, your doctor may recommend that you have allergy shots to suppress your allergic reaction over the long term. For this treatment, you receive a series of injections of the allergy-causing substance for 3 to 5 years. Treating allergies with shots is effective in about three out of four cases.

An allergic reaction

Most people have no reaction when they encounter a harmless substance such as ragweed pollen. However, in some people, the immune system responds to a harmless substance as though it is a harmful organism that needs to be destroyed. The immune system produces proteins called antibodies that attach to cells of the immune system called mast cells (top), which are present in skin and in the linings of the stomach and of the airways in the lungs (bronchial tubes) and the upper respiratory tract.

The next time that particular substance (allergen) enters the person's body, it binds to these antibodies and stimulates the mast cells to release powerful chemicals (bottom). The release of these chemicals, such as histamine, causes the characteristic symptoms of an allergic reaction—hives (a red, patchy, raised rash); watery, itchy eyes; a runny nose; sneezing; or wheezing.

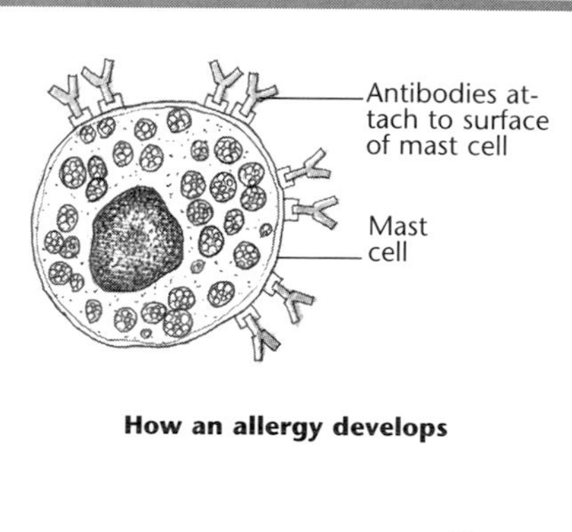

How an allergy develops

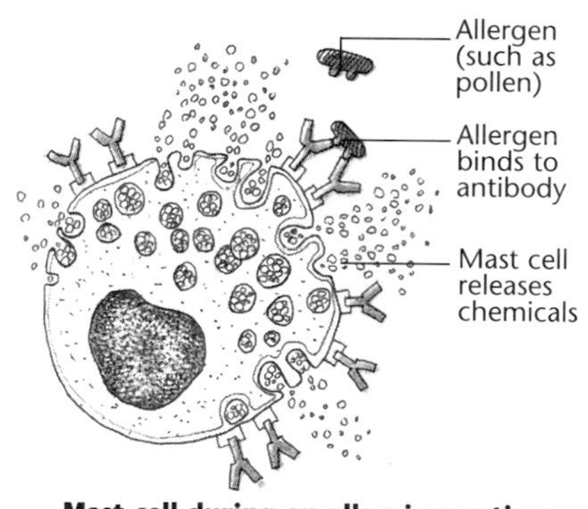

Mast cell during an allergic reaction

ASTHMA

Asthma is a common chronic condition in which the bronchial tubes of the lungs periodically narrow, making breathing difficult. Millions of people in the US have asthma and the numbers are increasing. One reason for the increase may be the worsening quality of the air we breathe indoors and out. A family history of asthma increases your risk of developing the disorder. Although most cases occur before age 25, asthma can develop at any age.

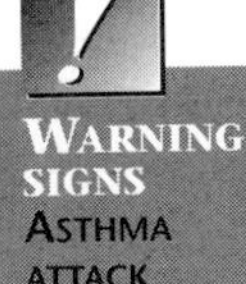

WARNING SIGNS
ASTHMA ATTACK

Do not wait until you are in the middle of an asthma attack to use your inhaler (see page 638) or call for help. Watch for these early warning signs:

- Difficulty breathing
- Tightness in your chest
- Wheezing when you breathe
- Coughing or congestion
- Awakening at night short of breath and wheezing

An asthma attack is often an exaggerated response of the airways to an airborne substance that a person inhales. Asthma attacks can be triggered by irritants such as tobacco smoke; an allergy to pets, plants, or chemicals; cold air; overexertion; or stress. During an attack, you have trouble breathing air in and even more difficulty breathing out. The cells lining your air passages begin secreting a thick, sticky mucus that can further plug up your air passages. An attack can last minutes, hours, or days.

Symptoms The primary symptom of asthma is difficulty breathing. You may experience tightness in your chest, wheezing, coughing, restlessness, or difficulty sleeping. Most asthma attacks are mild, but a severe attack can be life threatening and requires immediate medical attention. A severe attack causes extreme shortness of breath—to the point that even talking is difficult. Your neck muscles become tight and your lips and the skin under your nails may appear pale, gray, or blue because they are not receiving enough oxygen.

Although the symptoms of a severe asthma attack may subside with treatment, the inflammation of tissues in your lungs may persist and can lead to a recurring attack that may last a day or longer unless it is also treated. These recurring episodes of asthma are responsible for most hospitalizations for asthma. An attack can also increase your sensitivity to the allergens that trigger your attacks; this increased sensitivity may last for days or weeks.

Diagnosis To diagnose asthma, your doctor will give you a physical examination and ask you about your symptoms and your personal and family health histories. You may have a chest X-ray (see page 504) and pulmonary function tests that measure how much air your lungs can expel in one breath and how fast the air flows out of your lungs.

Treatment If the tests suggest that you have asthma, your doctor may refer you to a doctor who specializes in lung diseases or allergies for continuing management of your condition. If your doctor does not refer you to a specialist, you may want to ask him or her to recommend one. The goal of treatment for asthma is to control the symptoms so that you can lead a normal life, sleep through the night, and be able to exercise. Your doctor will explain how you can reduce the number of attacks you have, and how to control them when they occur.

You may have to make changes in your lifestyle to help prevent attacks. Do not smoke, and try to avoid occupations or activities that might expose you to fumes, dust, or other potential allergens. Avoid the allergens—such as animals with fur or feathers, or foods or food additives such as some dyes—that trigger your attacks. Some medications—including beta blockers, aspirin, and ibuprofen—can also trigger attacks. To reduce irritating dust in your home, use a double-filter vacuum cleaner to trap more of the microscopic dust particles. (There is no medical evidence that a negative ion generator, which manufacturers claim draws dust out of the air, reduces a person's risk of having an asthma attack.)

You may find that the onset of your menstrual period is accompanied by an asthma attack. If this is the case, your doctor may prescribe a medication you can take a few days before your period begins to prevent an attack.

WHAT HAPPENS DURING AN ASTHMA ATTACK?

In healthy bronchial tubes (top), muscles in the wall keep the airways open. Mucus secretions help keep the airways clean. Asthma causes inflammation of the lining of the bronchial tubes and tightening of the outer layer of smooth muscle that surrounds the airways (bottom). The inflammation and muscle contractions narrow the air passages and increase their secretion of mucus. Blood vessels in the walls of the airways widen in response to substances that are released by cells in the airways when inflammation occurs. All of these changes obstruct airflow, making it harder for you to breathe.

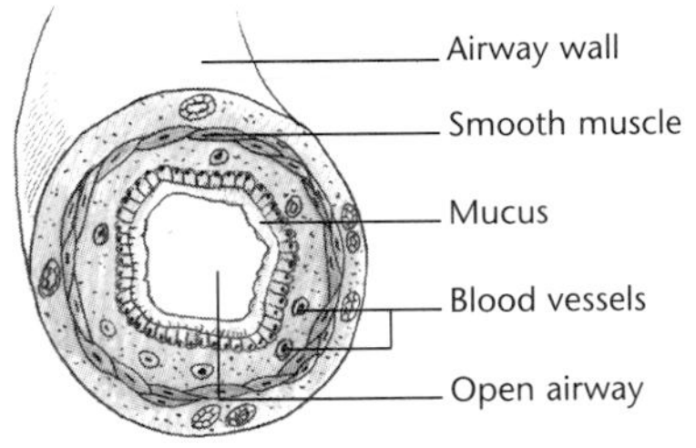

Healthy bronchial tube

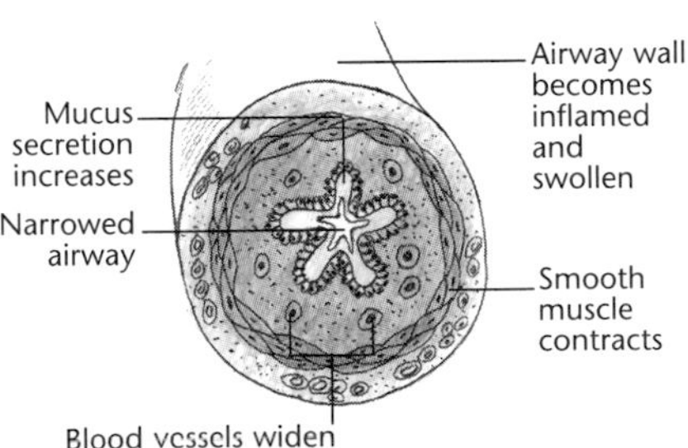

Bronchial tube in an asthma attack

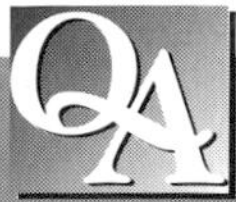

Questions women ask
ASTHMA

Q I have asthma. I don't smoke, but my husband does. Is his smoking making my asthma worse?

A It could be. Both smoking and breathing secondhand smoke are known to trigger asthma attacks. People with asthma should not be exposed to smoke. Talk with your husband about quitting. If he cannot or will not quit smoking, ask him to step outside when he smokes or confine his smoking to a closed room in the house. You might also suggest that he talk with your doctor about how his smoking is affecting your health as well as his. The doctor may tell him about medication that can help him quit (see page 158). Look for a support group in your area for people with asthma and their families. A support group may also be able to help your husband quit smoking.

Q My whole family is very attached to our golden retriever, but I have asthma. Do we have to get rid of our dog?

A The dander from an animal's skin is an allergen that triggers asthma attacks in some people. If exposure to animal dander contributes to your attacks, there are steps you can take to reduce your exposure. Have someone else in your family wash your pet once a week. Restrict your dog to one or two rooms of your home, and do not allow it in your bedroom at all. You should not have wall-to-wall carpeting because it traps dander and other allergens. Whenever possible, have someone else vacuum and dust, and make sure that it is done frequently.

Q Often my inhaler doesn't seem to work and I have ended up in the hospital several times as a result. What's wrong?

A You may not be using your inhaler correctly. In order to get the medication you need, you have to use your inhaler properly. Ask your doctor or pharmacist to show you how to use your inhaler and carefully read the instructions that come with it. Use your inhaler at the first sign of any symptoms of an asthma attack; do not wait until an attack is underway. You may need to take other medication, in addition to the medication that you take in your inhaler, to control your asthma. Talk to your doctor.

In some people, exercise triggers asthma attacks. The amount of air that moves into and out of your lungs is increased when you exercise. This additional breathing cools your airways just as perspiration cools your skin. If you have asthma, this cooling of the airways may cause an attack. But exercise is as important for you as it is for everyone else. Here are steps you can take to help avoid attacks while you are exercising:

- Take your medication shortly before you exercise.
- Engage in exercise that does not tend to trigger asthma attacks. For reasons that are not entirely clear, swimming is less likely than running or bicycling to trigger an attack.
- During cold weather, try to exercise indoors.
- Always warm up before you exercise (see page 87).

Asthma medications To keep your asthma under control, you and your doctor will work together to determine the right combination of medications for you. Many drugs used to treat asthma are taken through an inhaler (see page 638).

Bronchodilators Bronchodilators are drugs that quickly relax and open bronchial tubes that have become constricted, or narrowed. Bronchodilator drugs can be delivered with an inhaler or in pills.

Using an inhaler

An inhaler is a device that people with asthma use to deliver a specific dose of medication into their lungs to open their airways. Many people use their inhaler on a regular schedule, two to four times a day. You can also use your inhaler as soon as you develop any symptoms or believe an attack is beginning. Do not wait until your symptoms are severe. Always have your inhaler with you; you might want to keep a spare one at work.

Inhalers are available in a variety of shapes and sizes and can be used in different ways. Make sure your doctor or pharmacist shows you how to use your inhaler correctly. In addition, you should carefully read the instructions and check the illustrations that come with your inhaler. Your inhaler is effective only if you use it correctly.

Devices called spacers can be used with most inhalers. A spacer is a small tube or chamber that attaches to your inhaler and serves as a reservoir for the medication before it enters your mouth. Many people find that a spacer makes it easier for them to use their inhaler correctly because it eliminates the need to carefully coordinate the timing between squeezing the inhaler and taking a deep breath. Ask your doctor about using a spacer with your inhaler.

Some people who are unable to use an inhaler effectively, such as young children or people who cannot use their hands, use a device called a nebulizer. A nebulizer is an electric pump that disperses the medication in a fine mist that is delivered through a mask applied to the person's face.

Mast cell stabilizers Mast cell stabilizers help prevent narrowing of the bronchial tubes caused by substances called histamines. Histamines are released by specialized cells in the body called mast cells in response to an allergic trigger. When mast cell stabilizers are taken by inhaler, they block the release of histamine and related substances that cause inflammation and narrowing of the airways. Your doctor may recommend that you take a dose of medication 1 hour before you exercise or before you go anywhere you expect to be exposed to an allergen, such as the home of a person who has pets.

Corticosteroids Corticosteroids are synthetic hormones used to limit inflammation of the airways. When taken through an inhaler, corticosteroids have almost no side effects because little or no medication is absorbed into the blood. When they are taken in pill form, they can cause unpleasant side effects in some people, including fluid retention, acne, facial redness, muscle weakness, peptic ulcers (see page 518), weight gain, and an increased risk of the bone-thinning disorder osteoporosis. However, if you have moderate to severe asthma, taking corticosteroids in pill form at the beginning of an attack can prevent it from progressing to a serious episode that requires prolonged use of the drugs, a visit to a hospital emergency room, or even longer hospitalization.

ALLERGIES TO MEDICATIONS

Many people have unpleasant reactions to medications. In fact, almost any medication can cause a reaction in some people. Women experience adverse reactions to drugs more often than men. However, most reactions to medications are not true allergic reactions—that is, they do not involve the immune system. They are most often side effects from medications that affect some people more than others.

Some people do have true allergic reactions to particular medications. Penicillin and similar antibiotics are the most common causes of medication allergies, producing symptoms that can range from a mild rash to shock. Medications are most likely to provoke a reaction when they are delivered by injection through a muscle or intravenously because they enter the bloodstream directly. Medications are less likely to cause an allergic reaction when they are taken by mouth because the digestive process breaks down some of the potentially allergy-causing substances.

Symptoms The symptoms of an allergic reaction to medication include a skin rash or hives (a patchy, raised rash), wheezing or difficulty breathing, itching, or, in extreme cases, shock.

Diagnosis To evaluate a possible allergy to a medication, your doctor will ask you

WARNING SIGNS
ALLERGY TO MEDICATION

When taking a medication, report any unpleasant side effects to your doctor. If you have severe symptoms—including vomiting; mental confusion; slurred speech; unconsciousness; swelling of your mouth, tongue, or throat; wheezing or difficulty breathing—you need immediate medical help. In extreme cases, an allergic reaction can lead to shock. If you have any of the following milder symptoms, call your doctor:

- Itching
- Hives (a red, patchy, raised rash)
- Skin rash
- Swelling of your lips

detailed questions about your symptoms. He or she may refer you to an allergist (a doctor who specializes in the treatment of allergies), who can help with the evaluation. The allergist may give you skin tests in which small amounts of specific medications are applied to the surface of your skin to see if they cause a reaction, including swelling or redness. Your doctor may send a sample of your blood to the laboratory to detect the presence of antibodies that your body may have produced against the suspected allergy-causing medication.

Treatment Allergies to medications cannot be cured. The symptoms (such as hives) are treated with medications called antihistamines or, in some cases, corticosteroids (synthetic hormones that reduce inflammation). Make sure that you tell all your doctors about your allergy so that they will not prescribe that medication. If you must have treatment using a specific drug that causes you to have an allergic reaction, your doctor will refer you to a certified allergy specialist. The allergist may be able to help you prevent or control the reaction. Always wear a medical alert bracelet or necklace that informs people of your allergy in case of an emergency.

Anaphylactic shock

Anaphylactic shock is an extreme allergic reaction that is most often triggered by an injected drug, such as penicillin, or by an insect bite, such as a bee sting. Less often, it occurs after taking a particular medication by mouth or eating a particular food. An anaphylactic reaction is an emergency that requires immediate medical treatment.

In an anaphylactic reaction, your body releases an extremely large amount of histamine and related chemicals. These chemicals make your blood vessels widen, which causes a sudden drop in blood pressure. You may develop itchy hives (a patchy, raised rash) over several areas of your body, and your tongue, lips, throat, or breathing passages may swell, making breathing difficult.

This condition requires immediate injection of a medication called epinephrine, which quickly counteracts the dangerous reaction. If you have not had such a reaction before, call the local emergency number (usually 911). If you know you have a severe allergy and you carry a self-injecting device containing epinephrine, use it as soon as your symptoms begin. If you are with a person who goes into anaphylactic shock, call 911 immediately. If the person becomes unconscious, lay him or her down with legs raised to improve circulation to the heart and brain.

FOOD ALLERGIES

An allergic reaction to a particular food you have eaten can occur while you are eating the food, immediately after you eat it, or 1 to 2 hours later. The symptoms of a food allergy can range from mild to severe. Contrary to popular belief, food allergies are rare.

A food allergy is a potentially serious condition that can, in some cases, be fatal. Foods that most often cause allergies include nuts (especially peanuts, walnuts, and Brazil nuts), legumes (such as soybeans), fish and shellfish (especially whitefish and shrimp), egg whites, milk, and wheat. In many cases, a person has to eat a large amount of the food before it triggers an allergic response. However, in people whose allergy is highly developed, even one bite of the food can cause a severe, potentially fatal allergic reaction.

Symptoms Common symptoms of food allergies can include abdominal pain, diarrhea, nausea, or vomiting; hives or other skin rashes; swelling of the lips, tongue, and throat; nasal congestion; and wheezing or difficulty breathing.

Diagnosis To evaluate a possible food allergy, your doctor will ask about your symptoms, including when they occur, which foods seem to cause problems, and the amount of food needed to trigger symptoms. Your doctor may refer you to an allergist. The allergist may give you skin tests to help find the problem food. For this type of testing, extracts of foods that have the potential to cause an allergic reaction are applied to the surface of your skin (which has been pricked or scratched), usually on the inside of your arm. You are allergic to a food if it causes a reaction, including redness or swelling.

Tests in which extracts of suspected allergy-causing foods are injected into or under your skin or placed under your tongue can be misleading and dangerous, especially if you have a severe allergy. You should not have such tests. The safest allergy testing is on the surface of your skin, which is the kind used by highly experienced allergy specialists.

Alternatively, the allergist or your primary care doctor may send a sample of your blood to a laboratory to test for the presence of antibodies that your body may have produced against the suspected food.

Treatment If your doctor determines that you have a true food allergy that provokes a severe reaction, you must avoid that food. At home, read all food labels carefully. When you eat out, ask about all the ingredients used to prepare a dish you are considering. Allergy-causing foods are often hidden in unexpected places. For example, peanuts are used frequently in Asian cooking as seasoning and as a base for sauces, but their flavor can be masked by accompanying spices. Peanuts are also used in some commercially prepared pasta sauces and to thicken chili. Soybeans are used in a variety of substances including soy sauce, tofu, meat substitutes, and a Japanese flavoring called miso.

If you are extremely allergic to a food, make sure that you always carry with you a self-injecting device that contains

WARNING SIGNS
FOOD ALLERGY

If you experience any of the following symptoms, call your doctor. If the symptoms are severe, call 911 or go immediately to a hospital emergency room:

- Abdominal pain, diarrhea, nausea, or vomiting
- Hives (a patchy, raised rash) or swelling beneath your skin
- Swelling of your lips, eyes, face, tongue, mouth, or throat
- Difficulty swallowing
- Wheezing or difficulty breathing

Food intolerance and other nonallergic reactions

Food allergy is often confused with food intolerance, which is much more common. A food intolerance is an adverse reaction to a food, but it does not involve the immune system. Most cases of food intolerance, such as lactose intolerance (see page 521), result from digestive system abnormalities that make it difficult for the person's body to break down a particular food or substance in food (such as the milk sugar lactose). Symptoms of food intolerance include gas, bloating, abdominal pain, or diarrhea.

Some people have an abnormal reaction to eating particular foods, beverages, or food additives—including alcohol, aged cheese, chocolate, cured meats (such as salami), organ meats (such as liver), nitrates used as preservatives, and sulfites found in some red wines. Reactions to these substances cause chemical disturbances in the body but do not involve the immune system. Therefore, they are not allergic reactions. A headache is the most common symptom of this type of reaction. In some people, eating food that contains the additive monosodium glutamate (MSG) may cause tingling around their mouth, a rash on their face, or a burning sensation in their upper body.

epinephrine, a medication that quickly counteracts a dangerous reaction called anaphylactic shock (see page 639) if you inadvertently eat the food. Your doctor, or the nurse who works with your doctor, will show you how to use the device. As soon as the symptoms of a severe food allergy attack develop, give yourself an injection of epinephrine and go to the nearest emergency room.

Autoimmune diseases

Autoimmune diseases result when the immune system mistakenly identifies the body's own cells and tissues as foreign and attacks them. Although the exact cause of autoimmune diseases is not clear, they are thought to result from a combination of genetic and environmental factors. You may be born with genes that make you susceptible to developing a particular autoimmune disease. However, you will not develop the disease unless you are exposed to a specific trigger, such as a common virus or a medication, at some time in your life. For reasons that are not yet understood, many autoimmune diseases are far more common in women (especially after menopause) than in men. A family history of an autoimmune disease increases the risk for both women and men.

In the future, doctors may discover ways to prevent and cure these diseases. For now, medications are available that can reduce the symptoms and complications and enable you to lead a normal life. Early detection is the key to successful treatment. Increasingly sensitive diagnostic tests have made it possible for doctors to more accurately diagnose autoimmune diseases at an earlier stage.

This chapter describes the autoimmune diseases lupus, scleroderma, Sjögren's syndrome, and rheumatoid arthritis. Other diseases that involve an autoimmune response include type I diabetes (see page 617), Crohn's disease (see page 527), multiple sclerosis (see page 586), Graves' disease (see page 625), psoriasis (see page 680), and idiopathic thrombocytopenic purpura (see page 494).

LUPUS

Lupus (systemic lupus erythematosus) is an autoimmune disease in which the immune system can attack the connective tissues and numerous organs. The disorder can cause inflammation in any part of the body, including the joints, skin, kidneys, lungs, heart, nervous system, and blood. Most people with lupus experience symptoms in only a few organs. Lupus affects ten times as many women as men, usually between ages 13 and 45. Women of Asian, African, and Hispanic origin are more likely to get the disease than women of European descent.

The cause of lupus is unknown and the disease affects people in different ways. In some people, lupus may begin with a skin rash triggered by exposure to the sun. In other people, the disease is activated by an infection, such as a cold, or by a medication they are taking. Symptoms may first appear during pregnancy or soon after delivery. Some people with lupus have mild symptoms that flare up only occasionally. (Flare-ups can be triggered by factors such as exposure to sunlight, infection, surgery, injury, stress, or exhaustion.) Other people with lupus have life-threatening complications, such as internal bleeding or kidney failure.

Symptoms The symptoms of lupus can be vague and come and go over a long period of time. The disease can be difficult to diagnose because no two cases are alike. When asked about their symptoms, people sometimes respond that they "feel achy all over." Even though this is an accurate description of how many people with lupus feel, it is too vague to help the doctor make a definitive diagnosis. In addition, the symptoms of lupus are similar to those of other illnesses. See your doctor if you experience some of the following symptoms:

- Butterfly-shaped rash over your nose and cheeks.
- Round, scaly, raised patches of skin on your face, arms, upper back, scalp, and ears. If the rash appears on your scalp, it may result in permanent hair loss.
- Sensitivity to sunlight that triggers a rash and possibly fever, fatigue, joint

pain, and other symptoms of lupus when you are exposed to the sun.

- Painless ulcers (open sores) on the roof of your mouth that resemble cold sores.
- Arthritis that causes pain and swelling of your joints (particularly your hands and toes) but no permanent damage.
- Pain in your chest when you breathe deeply, caused by inflammation of the lining of the lungs.
- Neurologic abnormalities including seizures, confusion, or memory loss.

Diagnosis To diagnose lupus, your doctor will examine you and ask about your symptoms and your personal health history as well as your family health history. You may have a variety of tests, including blood tests, a urinalysis, or a chest X-ray. However, the results of the tests and your symptoms may suggest only that you have an autoimmune disease, not which one you have. Depending on your symptoms and test results, your doctor may diagnose lupus or recommend more tests. If you have several of the symptoms mentioned previously or if the following test results apply to you, your doctor is likely to tell you that you have lupus.

- Blood abnormalities, including low counts of platelets (blood cells that promote clotting), red blood cells, or infection-fighting white blood cells.
- Antibody abnormalities, including high levels of infection-fighting antibodies or high levels of antinuclear antibodies (which attack a person's own cells rather than invading organisms).
- Urine abnormalities, including the presence of protein and/or red blood cells in the urine.

Treatment Even without a definitive diagnosis of lupus, your doctor can prescribe treatment to reduce inflammation and relieve other symptoms. Because of the variety of side effects and long-term health effects from many of the medications used for treating lupus, you and your doctor may have to try different drugs and doses or combinations of drugs to find the treatment that is best for you. The medications most often prescribed for lupus include the following:

Nonsteroidal anti-inflammatory drugs Nonsteroidal anti-inflammatory drugs are the most common treatment for lupus, especially for mild cases. These medications—including aspirin, ibuprofen, and naproxen—can help reduce pain and inflammation in your joints and elsewhere in the body. Because aspirin can cause stomach upset in some people, your doctor may recommend taking it with meals, with a glass of milk, or with antacids.

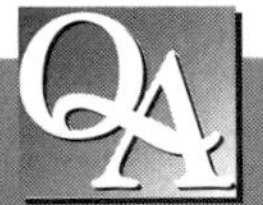

QUESTIONS WOMEN ASK

LUPUS

Q Because of my lupus, do I need to take any extra precautions during sexual intercourse?

A Yes. Having lupus makes you more susceptible to infection, so your partner (even in a mutually monogamous relationship) should always use a condom during sexual intercourse, unless you are trying to conceive. Painless ulcers (open sores) in the vagina that are sometimes a symptom of lupus may provide an opening for viruses or bacteria that cause sexually transmitted diseases, including AIDS, herpes, gonorrhea, and syphilis.

Q I have lupus. How long is it safe for me to be outdoors in the sunlight?

A Although excessive exposure to sunlight can cause a flare-up of lupus, you can spend time outdoors. However, you should try to avoid or limit your outdoor activity between the hours of 10 AM and 3 PM, when the sun is strongest. When you go out, always wear sunscreen with a sun protection factor (SPF) of at least 15, protective clothing, and a hat or visor that shields your face.

Corticosteriods Corticosteroids are synthetic hormones that reduce inflammation and suppress the activity of the immune system. Corticosteroid cream applied to the skin may help relieve rashes. An injection of the medication into an affected joint may help relieve pain in that area. Taken by mouth, corticosteroids may reduce extreme fatigue, severe arthritis, uncontrolled fever, or kidney disease. Corticosteroids can cause serious side effects, such as bone thinning, high blood pressure, and increased risk of infection and stomach ulcers. For this reason, your doctor will carefully monitor the dose to maximize the beneficial effects of the medication and minimize the potentially harmful side effects.

Antimalarial drugs Antimalarial drugs, which were designed to treat malaria, can help control rashes, mouth ulcers (open sores), and joint symptoms in some people with lupus. Side effects from these medications are rare, but may include occasional diarrhea, rashes, or vision problems.

Immunosuppressive drugs Immunosuppressive drugs are medications that reduce inflammation and tend to suppress the immune system. Because these drugs can cause side effects such as anemia (see page 493) and a reduction in the level of infection-fighting white blood cells, they are used only for severe cases. Immunosuppressive drugs are used when major organs, such as the kidneys or brain, are being damaged, when a person's muscles are severely inflamed, or when a person's arthritis has not responded to other treatment.

Lupus and pregnancy If you have lupus and are planning a pregnancy, talk to your doctor. If possible, you should time your pregnancy to coincide with periods of good health—when you have had no symptoms for at least 1 year before becoming pregnant and your blood pressure is normal. Many women who have lupus give birth to healthy babies without having a flare-up of the disease.

Self-help for lupus

If you have lupus, you can reduce your risk of a flare-up by following these guidelines:

- Maintain good health by eating a balanced, nutritious diet and exercising regularly.
- Limit your exposure to sunlight, halogen lamps, and fluorescent light.
- Practice good dental hygiene (see page 142)—brush your teeth twice a day, floss every day, and visit your dentist once every 6 months to be checked for mouth ulcers (open sores), abscesses (collections of pus), or gum infections.
- Wash your hands frequently.
- Limit your contact with people who have infections.

However, it is especially important for you to receive excellent prenatal care throughout your pregnancy. Your doctor will closely monitor your blood pressure, kidney function, and the growth of the fetus. A flare-up of lupus while you are pregnant can cause miscarriage, stillbirth, or premature birth. If the disease affects your kidney function, it can slow the growth of the fetus.

The presence in the blood of a particular type of antibody that is produced by some people who have lupus can also cause miscarriage or premature birth. If you are planning a pregnancy, your doctor will give you a blood test to detect this antibody. Your doctor will also check for another type of antibody produced by some people who have lupus. This particular antibody can affect the fetus's heart during pregnancy. Because women with lupus are susceptible to a flare-up of the disease during delivery and the first few weeks after delivery, your doctor is likely to recommend preventive treatment with medication during this time.

SCLERODERMA

Scleroderma (which means "hard skin") is an autoimmune disease that is characterized by thickening and hardening of the skin. This thickening and hardening results from the accumulation of excessive amounts of the protein collagen in connective tissues. The extent and severity of the disease can vary widely. In many people, scleroderma may affect only isolated patches of skin and cause no serious problems. But in some people, it is a life-threatening condition that restricts movement and can damage the kidneys, lungs, heart, or digestive tract. Depending on the tissues that are involved, scleroderma can cause major complications, including kidney failure (see page 548), heart failure (see page 492), or disabling joint impairment.

Scleroderma affects four times as many women as men. The disease has no known cause or cure, but some of the symptoms respond to treatment. The first symptoms of scleroderma usually appear between ages 20 and 40, although the disease occasionally occurs in children and older people.

Symptoms Scleroderma often begins with a condition called Raynaud's phenomenon, which causes the fingers and toes to become cold and pale when exposed to cold air or cold water. Raynaud's phenomenon occurs when changes in blood vessels prevent blood from flowing adequately to the hands and feet. Other, more severe symptoms include thickening and tightening of your skin (especially on your arms, face, or hands), loss of flexibility of your hands or face (which results from thickening and tightening of your skin), pain and stiffness in your joints, or heartburn and other digestive problems (which result from thickening and hardening of tissues of the digestive tract).

WARNING SIGNS
SCLERODERMA

As with other autoimmune diseases, the earlier scleroderma is diagnosed, the better the chances for relief of your symptoms. See your doctor if you experience any of the following:

- Cold hands and feet (which first turn white, then blue, then pink) after exposure to cold air or cold water
- Thickening and tightening of your skin, especially on your arms, face, or hands
- Loss of flexibility of your hands or face from thickening and tightening of the skin
- Puffy hands or feet, especially in the morning
- Pain and stiffness in your joints
- Heartburn and other digestive problems

Diagnosis To diagnose scleroderma, your doctor will examine you and ask about your symptoms, your health history, and your family health history. If your skin is thickened or hardened, your doctor may take a small tissue sample for laboratory examination under a microscope. An accumulation of excess collagen in the tissue sample confirms the diagnosis.

Treatment Treatment for scleroderma consists of controlling the symptoms. If you have symptoms of Raynaud's phenomenon (your fingers and toes become unusually cold when exposed to cold air or water), your doctor may prescribe a medication to widen your blood vessels and help improve the circulation of blood to your hands and feet. In addition, you will need to wear gloves whenever your hands will be subjected to cold. Nonsteroidal anti-inflammatory drugs—such as aspirin, ibuprofen, or naproxen—can help reduce pain in your joints. Your doctor will recommend exercises to help keep your skin and joints flexible and improve your circulation. To avoid the heartburn that is sometimes associated with scleroderma, do not eat less than 3 to 4 hours before bedtime and take other measures to prevent stomach juices from entering your esophagus (see page 517). If you smoke, quit. Smoking can cause further damage to small blood vessels and decrease blood flow to affected areas of your body, which can worsen your symptoms.

SJÖGREN'S SYNDROME

Sjögren's syndrome is an autoimmune disease in which the immune system attacks the salivary glands (glands inside the mouth that secrete saliva) and the lacrimal glands (glands that secrete tears into the eyes). The resulting decrease in the secretion of saliva causes your mouth to be dry; the decrease in the secretion of tears causes dryness, itching, burning, and redness of your eyes. You may have the sensation that you have something in your eye that you cannot remove.

Sjögren's syndrome can affect other parts of the body as well. If glands of your respiratory system are affected, your nose and throat may be dry and irritated.

If glands in your vagina are affected, you may experience vaginal dryness and painful intercourse. If the disorder affects your skin, your skin will become excessively dry.

Sjögren's syndrome often accompanies other autoimmune diseases, including rheumatoid arthritis, lupus, and scleroderma. Women, usually after age 45, are nine times more likely than men to develop Sjögren's syndrome. The disease affects about 2 million Americans.

Symptoms Most of the symptoms of Sjögren's syndrome result from the decrease in secretions from the mouth and eyes. You may have Sjögren's syndrome if you experience any of the following symptoms:

- Swollen salivary glands (glands on the sides of the mouth that secrete saliva)
- Difficulty swallowing
- Dryness of your mouth or eyes
- Frequent constipation
- Dryness of your nose and throat
- Hoarseness
- Persistent or recurring cough
- Dry, scaly skin
- Vaginal dryness and itching; painful intercourse

Diagnosis To diagnose Sjögren's syndrome, your doctor will examine you and ask about your symptoms and your health history. Your doctor may recommend a blood test to detect particular antibodies that are present in most (but not all) people who have the syndrome.

Treatment Treatment for Sjögren's syndrome involves controlling the symptoms and preventing permanent damage. To prevent permanent damage to your eyes, you must keep them lubricated. Your doctor will recommend drops that you put in your eyes to help relieve the irritating, scratchy feeling. You can stimulate the production of saliva by sucking on hard candy or by chewing gum. Your doctor may also recommend saliva substitutes and other mouth lubricants, such as mineral oil or glycerin water. In the winter months, a humidifier in your home can help reduce dryness in your mouth, eyes, and breathing passages. If you have vaginal dryness, using water-based lubricants during intercourse can help relieve the discomfort. If you are past menopause, estrogen cream (see page 360), which you apply directly into your vagina, can help restore the lubricating ability of your vaginal tissues. For severe cases of Sjögren's syndrome, corticosteroids (synthetic hormones that reduce inflammation) or other medications may be prescribed.

RHEUMATOID ARTHRITIS

Rheumatoid arthritis is an autoimmune disease in which the immune system attacks the smooth lining of joints (the synovium). The joints become inflamed, which causes pain and swelling. The disease can be disabling—it often leads to deformity and decreased mobility of the joints. Rheumatoid arthritis can also affect the heart, lungs, and eyes. The disease is more common among women than men and usually first appears between ages 20 and 40. Although rheumatoid arthritis is usually chronic (long term) and incurable, it has cycles in which symptoms worsen and then subside.

Rheumatoid arthritis is very different from the more common form of arthritis, osteoarthritis (see page 559), which results from wear and tear on joints over time. The cause of rheumatoid arthritis is unknown, but there is a genetic component. People who have a close relative with the disease are more likely to develop it themselves. The severity of rheumatoid arthritis varies from one person to the next, and it is difficult to predict who will be affected most seriously. If you have nearly continuous symptoms for 4 to 5 years, you are more likely to have a lifelong serious problem with rheumatoid arthritis.

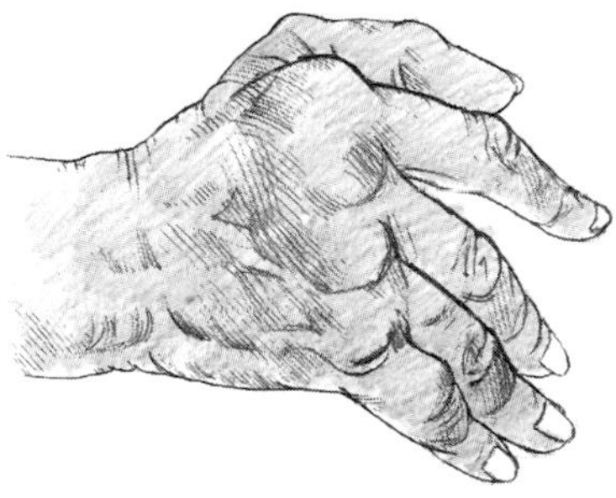

ADVANCED RHEUMATOID ARTHRITIS
In advanced rheumatoid arthritis, joints become deformed. This deformity results from both inflammation of the joints and weakening of the muscles, tendons, and ligaments that support them.

Symptoms Rheumatoid arthritis usually affects more than one joint at a time, causing achiness throughout the body.

RHEUMATOID ARTHRITIS
A healthy joint (right) is composed of supporting structures—ligaments, tendons, muscles, and cartilage—that allow it to function normally. A thin membrane called the synovial lining produces a liquid that lubricates and helps nourish the joint. Rheumatoid arthritis causes inflammation of the synovial lining (far right). The synovial lining gradually thickens, the cartilage deteriorates, the bone erodes, and the supporting ligaments, tendons, and muscles weaken.

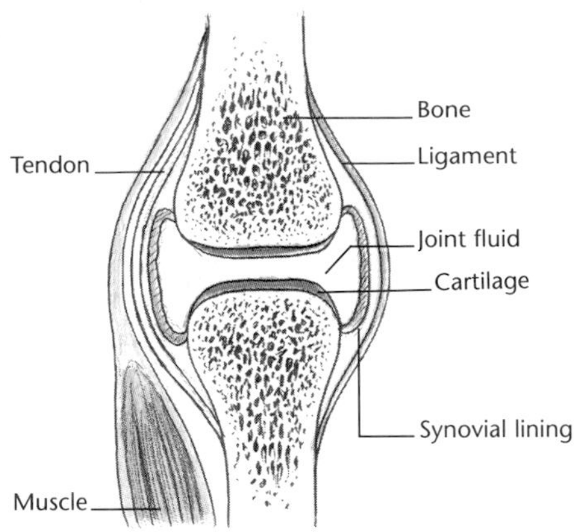

A healthy joint

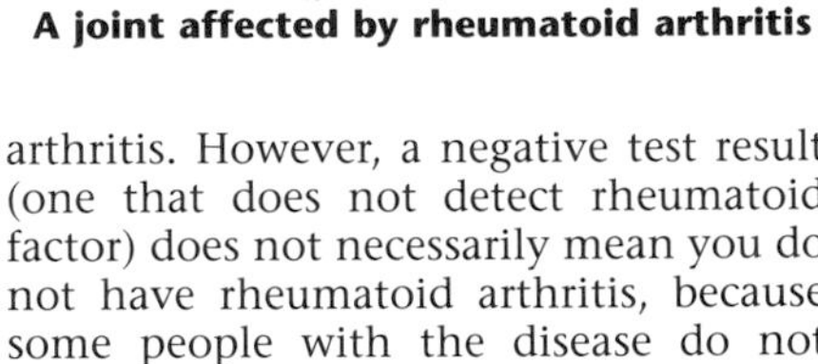

A joint affected by rheumatoid arthritis

When it affects the joints of one arm or leg, the matching joints of the other arm or leg are usually affected as well. Small lumps called rheumatoid nodules may form under the skin around your knees, elbows, ears, or nose, on the back of your scalp, or under your toes. These lumps are not painful and do not cause serious problems. When the disease is active, it can cause fever and subsequent sweating, and a loss of muscle strength.

Diagnosis Rheumatoid arthritis is tentatively diagnosed by your symptoms and a physical examination of your joints. X-rays can identify characteristic changes, such as the erosion of bones in your joints. Your doctor may recommend a blood test to detect an antibody called rheumatoid factor, which is present in most people who have rheumatoid arthritis. However, a negative test result (one that does not detect rheumatoid factor) does not necessarily mean you do not have rheumatoid arthritis, because some people with the disease do not have the antibody in their blood.

Treatment Treatment of rheumatoid arthritis can help many people with the disease live a nearly normal, active life. Aspirin and other anti-inflammatory medications have traditionally been the first line of medical treatment for rheumatoid arthritis. But more powerful medications, such as methotrexate and corticosteroids, are now being used more frequently in the early stages of the disease to slow or stop its progress. The use of these medications has proven to be the most effective way to prevent long-term disability from rheumatoid arthritis. However, because these medications can have significant side effects, your doctor will monitor your condition closely while you are taking them. In addition, these drugs work so well that you may be tempted to overuse your joints. Such overuse can damage your joints even more.

In some cases, surgery may be necessary to repair or replace a severely damaged joint (see page 566). Regular exercise can help maintain and restore flexibility and strength to your joints. Your doctor will give you guidelines about the best kinds of exercise for you. During flare-ups of the disease, you should rest your joints; your doctor may recommend using splints to help keep them immobile.

WARNING SIGNS
RHEUMATOID ARTHRITIS

Rheumatoid arthritis primarily affects your joints, but you may have other symptoms as well. If you have any of the following symptoms, see your doctor:

- Pain, swelling, and warmth in your joints, especially the smaller joints of your feet
- A general feeling of aching or stiffness throughout your body, particularly after you wake up or after you have been motionless for a while
- Excessive fatigue, especially right after you wake up in the morning

CHAPTER 26

Your eyes, ears, and teeth

Contents

Your eyes and ears are highly complex organs that enable you to take in and respond to information from your environment. Your teeth are essential to your ability to eat and to speak clearly, and they give shape to your face. Disorders that affect any of these parts of your body can dramatically reduce the quality of your life. Many of these problems can develop as a person ages. But taking preventive measures, such as having regular medical and dental examinations, can help you preserve your sight and hearing as well as the health of your teeth. For information about routine medical examinations and screening tests and when you should have them, see chapter 4.

Eye disorders

Your eyes are extremely intricate sensory organs. They capture and focus a continuous stream of images that are instantly transmitted to your brain for interpretation. When you look at an object, its image enters each eye through a dark opening in the center called the pupil, which widens or narrows according to the brightness of the light. The cornea (the transparent, dome-shaped outer coating of your eye) and lens (located behind the colored part of your eye, the iris) focus the image. Inside the back of each eye, the retina contains millions of nerve cells that receive the focused image and transmit it via the optic nerve to your brain for interpretation. The eyelids protect your eyes and tears keep the eyes lubricated and clean.

For many people, vision worsens with age. The lens may become cloudy, forming a cataract, or the pressure of fluid inside the eyeball may increase, causing a disorder called glaucoma. Diabetic retinopathy is a major cause of blindness in people who have diabetes (see page 654).

If you are under 40 and you do not have any eye diseases or need corrective lenses, you should have your eyes examined by an ophthalmologist (a doctor who specializes in eye care) once every 2 or 3 years. If you wear corrective eyeglasses or contact lenses, have an examination every year. You should also have an annual eye examination if you are over 40, because your risk of glaucoma increases after that age. Your ophthalmologist may recommend more frequent or less frequent testing, depending on your risk of glaucoma or other eye diseases. For more about eye examinations, see page 140.

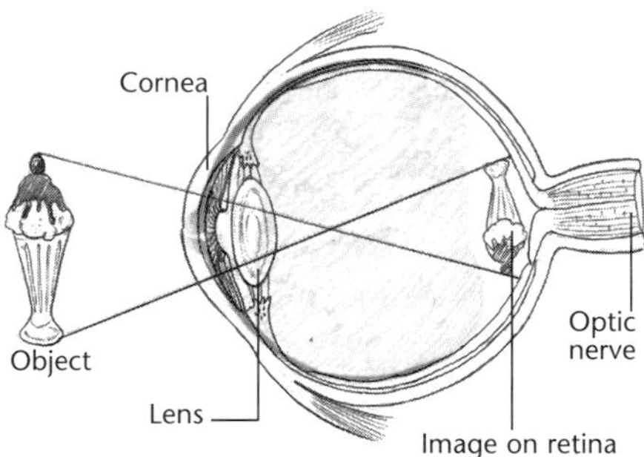

VISION

When you look at an object, light rays from the object pass through the cornea and lens of your eye and are focused upside down on the retina in the back of your eye. The retina transmits information about the object via the optic nerve to your brain, which interprets the image right side up.

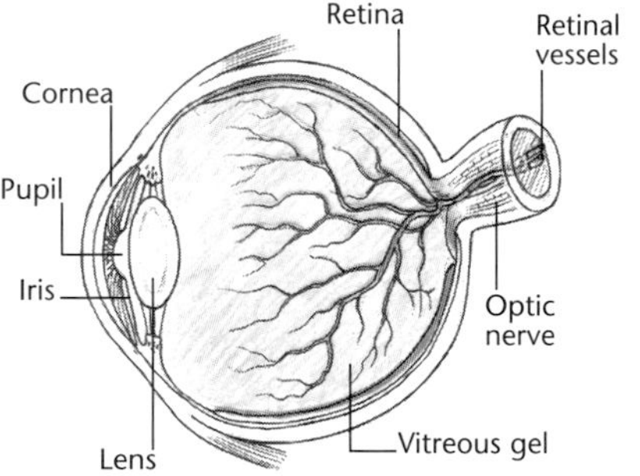

STRUCTURE OF THE EYE

The pupil, the opening at the center of your eye, controls the amount of light that enters your eye. The cornea and lens focus light rays through a clear, liquid gel (the vitreous gel) to the retina. The retina converts the image into nerve impulses that are sent to the optic nerve, which transmits them to the brain. A thin network of branching blood vessels (called retinal vessels) provides a constant supply of blood to the retina.

Aging and vision problems

After age 40, you should have an eye examination every year by an ophthalmologist (a doctor who specializes in eye care). Many people need corrective lenses as they get older, and screening for more serious eye problems, including glaucoma and cataracts, becomes more important. You should also see your ophthalmologist if you experience any of the following vision problems:

- Difficulty reading or seeing objects up close while your ability to see at a distance remains the same.
- Gradual vision loss even though you already wear glasses. You may need a new prescription to correct any changes in your eyes and your ophthalmologist can rule out a serious condition that may be affecting your vision.
- Gradual blurring of vision that is not helped by moving closer or farther away from the object you are looking at. You may have cataracts (clouding of the lens of the eye).
- Change in your vision while you are taking a medication. Call your doctor to find out if the medication could be affecting your vision.
- Sudden blindness in one eye, even if it is only temporary. Call your doctor immediately or go to the emergency room. You may have had a stroke (see page 569), or you may have a condition called temporal arteritis (inflammation and thickening of some of the arteries that supply blood to the eye).

GLAUCOMA

Glaucoma is a condition that results in damage to the optic nerve, which carries images from the eye to the brain. This damage can reduce your vision and even cause blindness. Glaucoma can occur in one of two main forms—acute or chronic. Chronic glaucoma, called chronic open-angle glaucoma, is the most common form of the disease. Chronic glaucoma develops gradually over a period of several years from the pressure of excess fluid inside the eyeball. Acute glaucoma, called acute closed-angle glaucoma, develops rapidly, usually with no warning.

Normally, a clear fluid called the aqueous humor circulates in and out of the front of your eyeball, delivering nutrients and washing away wastes. If the area of the eye through which the fluid normally drains becomes blocked, the fluid builds up inside the eye. This buildup of fluid increases pressure inside the eye, potentially causing irreversible damage to the optic nerve. If the optic nerve is damaged, its ability to transmit images to the brain is reduced, potentially leading to blindness.

Glaucoma is the third most common cause of blindness in the US. Chronic glaucoma develops gradually as you age. Unless you have a regular eye examination that includes a test for glaucoma, you may not realize you have a problem until the disease has caused considerable injury and your sight is affected. Damage caused by glaucoma is irreversible, but, if the condition is detected early and treated, the harmful buildup of pressure inside the eye can be prevented. For this reason, you should be tested for glaucoma every year after age 40. You are more likely to develop chronic glaucoma if you are over 40, black, have a family history of glaucoma, are nearsighted, or have diabetes (see page 617).

Symptoms Chronic glaucoma develops very slowly. Most people have no symptoms until the disorder has damaged the optic nerve and impaired their vision. Chronic glaucoma is usually detected during a regular eye examination by an ophthalmologist.

By contrast, acute glaucoma occurs suddenly and requires immediate medical attention to reduce the buildup of pressure inside the eye. Acute glaucoma may cause symptoms such as blurred vision, severe eye pain, a headache, rainbow halos around lights, nausea, or vomiting.

Diagnosis Your ophthalmologist can examine your eyes and perform tests to determine if you have glaucoma or are at

ACUTE GLAUCOMA

In a healthy eye (right), a clear liquid called the aqueous humor flows out of the eye through a channel called the drainage angle, located at the front of the eye.

The acute form of glaucoma, called acute closed-angle glaucoma (far right), develops suddenly when the drainage angle becomes completely blocked and causes pressure to build up rapidly inside the eye. Acute glaucoma is a medical emergency that requires immediate treatment to reduce the pressure inside the eye and save the person's vision.

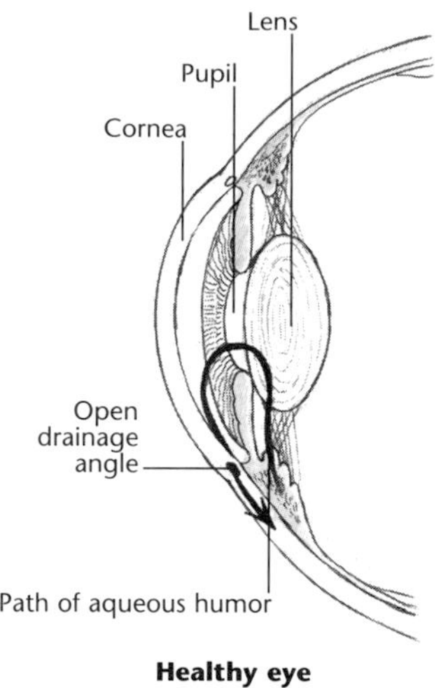

Healthy eye

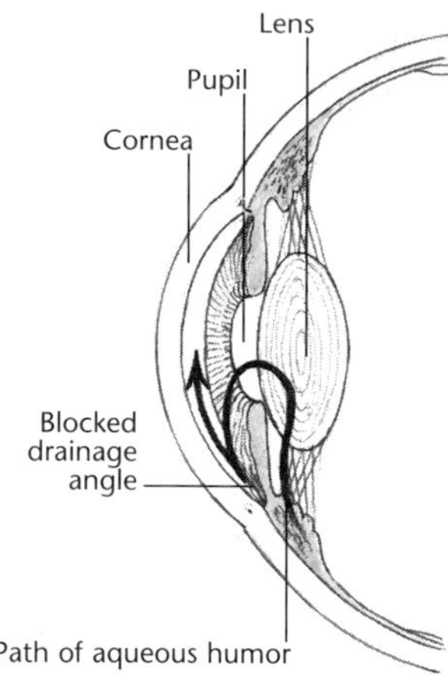

Eye with acute closed-angle glaucoma

WARNING SIGNS
ACUTE GLAUCOMA

Unlike chronic glaucoma, which usually causes no symptoms until your vision is impaired, acute glaucoma occurs suddenly. Acute glaucoma requires emergency medical treatment to save your vision. If any of the following symptoms occur suddenly, call your doctor or go to the nearest emergency room:

- Blurred vision
- Severe eye pain
- Rainbow halos around lights
- Severe headache
- Nausea and vomiting

risk of developing it. He or she will measure the pressure inside your eye, examine the drainage angle (the channel through which fluid leaves the eyeball) for signs of blockage, and examine the optic nerves for signs of damage. Your doctor may also evaluate the completeness of your vision in each eye to see if the disease has affected your sight.

The test for measuring the pressure inside your eyes, called tonometry, is quick, safe, and painless. Your ophthalmologist will put a drop of a local anesthetic on each cornea to numb it before putting a drop of an orange liquid called fluorescein in each eye. Then he or she will place an instrument called a tonometer against your cornea (the transparent, dome-shaped covering of the front of your eye) to flatten it. The amount of force needed to flatten the cornea indicates the pressure inside your eyeball. During this test, which takes a few seconds for each eye, you will see a small circle of bright blue light coming closer to your eye.

Your ophthalmologist will also look into your eye through the cornea to evaluate the depth of the front of your eyeball. A shallow or narrow drainage angle suggests that the drainage of fluid from the eye may eventually become obstructed—a condition that can lead to acute closed-angle glaucoma.

To evaluate the health of the optic nerve, the doctor may use a hand-held viewing instrument called an ophthalmoscope, which has a very bright light to look through your pupil (the dark opening in the center of your eye). The optic nerve, located in the back of your eye, transmits images from the eye to your brain. Glaucoma can cause irreversible damage to this nerve, which can lead to blindness.

Your doctor may want to test the visual field (peripheral, or side, vision) of each eye to determine if your sight has been affected by glaucoma. To do this, he or she will move an object, such as a pencil, into your view from the side, while you look straight ahead. If you cannot see the object until it is almost directly in front of you, your peripheral vision may have been impaired by glaucoma.

If your doctor suspects you have glaucoma, he or she is likely to recommend additional tests, including gonioscopy. Your ophthalmologist examines the drainage angle of your eye with a special contact lens called a gonioscope, which he or she places on your eye. This lens has mirrors and facets that enable the doctor to view the drainage angle and look for any changes or signs of blockage. Your eye will first be numbed with anesthetic drops to reduce any discomfort during the procedure.

Your doctor may also use a special camera to take photographs (called disc photos) of each optic nerve. These pictures are used to document and monitor any changes in or damage to the nerves.

Treatment Damage caused by glaucoma cannot be reversed, but treatment with medication or surgery can prevent or slow further damage.

Medication If you have glaucoma, your doctor will first prescribe medication in the form of eyedrops. This medication decreases pressure inside the eye either by slowing the amount of fluid produced in the eye or by improving the flow of fluid out of the eye. You must take the eyedrops regularly, usually several times a day, for the rest of your life to prevent damage from glaucoma and to preserve your vision. Do not stop taking the drops because the medication is effective in preventing glaucoma only for as long as you use it. Tell your doctor if you experience any side effects from the eyedrops, which may include a stinging sensation in your eyes, redness in your eyes, blurred vision, headaches, or changes in your pulse or heartbeat. In some cases, the dose of medication can be adjusted to reduce these side effects.

Medication taken in pills can also reduce pressure inside the eye. However, because this medication may have more serious side effects than the eyedrops, it is used only if eyedrops have not been effective. Side effects of the pills may include tingling of your fingers and toes, drowsiness, loss of appetite, constipation, kidney stones, or reduced ability of your blood to clot. If you experience any of these side effects, call your ophthalmologist immediately. He or she may be able to adjust the dose or prescribe a different medication.

Surgery If you have acute closed-angle glaucoma, or you are at risk of developing it, treatment is likely to include a surgical procedure called an iridotomy. Iridotomy, which is usually performed using laser beams (high-energy beams of light), creates a tiny drainage hole in the iris. The procedure is painless, takes only

Using eyedrops for glaucoma

Because the surface of your eye can hold only a limited amount of fluid, when you use eyedrops any excess liquid will run out of your eye. This extra fluid also pools in the corner of your eye and a small amount may even drain into your nose, where it can enter your bloodstream and possibly cause side effects. In addition, these medications can be expensive so you do not want to waste any. Here are some tips for taking your eyedrops correctly:

- Ask your doctor for drops that come in a metered dose dispenser, which carefully controls the amount of medication in each drop.
- Take your drops while lying down or tilting your head back.
- Look up and pull your lower lid away from your eye to form a small pouch to catch the drop.
- After putting the drop in, close your eye and gently press your finger against the inner corner of the eyelid to prevent the medication from draining out to the nasal passage.
- Wait 5 minutes between drops if your doctor has prescribed more than one drop for each eye.

a few minutes, and is done in the doctor's office or an outpatient facility.

If you have chronic open-angle glaucoma that cannot be controlled with eyedrops or pills, your doctor may recommend laser surgery to create a better flow of fluid through the drainage angle. This relieves the dangerous pressure inside the eye. The procedure, which is painless, takes a few minutes and is done in the doctor's office or in an outpatient facility.

In some cases, traditional surgery in a hospital operating room may be necessary to create an opening in the front of the eye to allow excess fluid to drain out. The procedure, which is done using general or local anesthesia, takes about 1 to 1½ hours. Complications may include pressure inside the eye that is too high or too low, or bleeding. In some cases, the procedure is not effective and must be repeated.

CATARACTS

A cataract is clouding of the normally clear and transparent lens of the eye. A cataract occurs when the structure and alignment of the protein fibers that make up the lens change, gradually causing the lens to become cloudy or opaque. This clouding often causes blurred vision. A cataract often appears first in one eye and then, eventually, the other eye. Cataracts are the leading cause of blindness, but they can almost always be effectively treated with surgery (see page 653).

Cataracts are usually the result of aging. They can also result from exposure to the rubella virus (see page 138) before birth or from a serious injury to the eye. You may also be at increased risk of cataracts if you have diabetes (see page 617) or a family history of cataracts, if you have taken corticosteroid medications to treat inflammatory diseases such as rheumatoid arthritis (see page 645), or if you have had surgery on the inside of your eye. Exposing your eyes to sunlight or the high-intensity light inside tanning booths for extended periods of time without wearing protective sunglasses may also increase your risk of cataracts. You should never stare at the sun, even for short periods, because doing so can cause permanent changes in your retina, which can reduce your vision.

You cannot get cataracts from overusing or straining your eyes. They do not spread from one eye to the other, or from person to person. Cataracts are neither a form of cancer nor a cause of irreversible blindness. Most people experience some gradual clouding of their lenses as they age. In some cases, a person may have a mild cataract that does not interfere with his or her vision, never gets worse, and does not require treatment. If the clouding does not cover the center of the lens, the person may not even be aware of it. However, if a cataract begins to interfere with your normal activities, treatment may be necessary.

Symptoms A cataract can develop so gradually that you do not notice it. Cataracts are often detected in a regular eye examination or after a person fails to pass a vision test for a driver's license. See your ophthalmologist if you experience any of the following symptoms:

- Painless blurring of vision
- Glare in bright sunlight or from oncoming headlights
- Frequent changes in prescription for corrective lenses
- Double vision in one eye
- Need for brighter light to read
- Poor night vision
- Changes in your perception of colors; colors may appear faded or yellow

Diagnosis Cataracts are diagnosed with a comprehensive eye examination by an ophthalmologist. He or she examines your eye with a variety of instruments to determine the type, size, and location of the cataract, and to rule out any other problems that can affect vision.

The doctor will dilate (widen) your pupils with eyedrops to examine the interior of your eyes with a biomicroscope (also called a slit lamp), which magnifies the structures inside your eye. The doctor shines a beam of light into each eye and looks for signs of clouding of the lens.

Treatment Currently, there are no eyedrops or other medications that can reverse or slow the progression of cataracts. If your impaired vision cannot be improved with new eyeglasses, the only treatment for vision loss caused by a cataract is surgery to remove the clouded lens. You will then need an artificial replacement lens. In most cases, a permanent replacement lens is implanted inside the eye during the cataract surgery. Most people who have a lens implant also need to wear bifocals. If you do not have a permanent lens implanted in your eye during cataract surgery, you will have to wear special thick eyeglasses or a contact lens.

If your vision is only slightly impaired by a mild cataract, wearing prescription eyeglasses may be enough to improve it. Cataract surgery is sometimes necessary to prevent inflammation or glaucoma (see page 649), or to enable the doctor to examine the inside of the eye. Your ophthalmologist will help you make a decision about having cataract surgery, based in part on whether the problem is interfering with your daily activities, such as driving a car or reading. Do not delay surgery to the point that your cloudy lens affects the quality of your life. Cataract surgery has a very high success rate.

If the cataracts are not significantly impairing your vision, discuss with your doctor the benefits and risks of delaying surgery. In rare cases, people who have cataract surgery develop swelling or detachment of the retina in the back of the eye, glaucoma, an infection in the eye, or displacement of the lens implant. If the new lens is displaced, additional surgery may be necessary.

Cataract surgery In cataract surgery, which is the most common surgical procedure performed on people over 65, the cloudy lens of the eye (the cataract) is removed and usually replaced with a permanent plastic lens implant. The procedure is relatively short and painless and is usually performed using local anesthesia (see page 260) in an operating room.

Before the procedure, you may receive a mild sedative in a pill or by injection to relax you. A local anesthetic may be administered to the area around your eye. The anesthetic prevents your eye from moving and prevents you from feeling anything that touches it. You may not be able to see well from the eye during the surgery and, if you had a sedative, you may doze off during the procedure or be only vaguely aware of your surroundings.

Because of the delicacy of the eye and the intricacies of cataract surgery, the procedure is performed under a special operating microscope using tiny instruments. The ophthalmologist makes a small incision on the front of the eye, and removes the cataract. The back membrane of the lens, called the posterior capsule, is usually left in place if a plastic lens implant is going to be used. The replacement lens implant is then inserted into the eye and permanently held in place with soft, flexible springs.

Your vision will probably be blurry immediately after the surgery, but will gradually clear. Most people are able to go home the same day as the surgery.

CATARACT SURGERY
A cataract is usually removed through a small incision in the front of the eye. The ophthalmologist uses tiny instruments to remove small pieces of the cataract (right). In most cases, an artificial replacement lens is then implanted into the eye (center). The lens implant is held in place with soft, flexible springs. Months or years later, if the membrane in back of the lens (the posterior capsule) becomes cloudy and causes blurring of your vision, your doctor may correct it using a laser. The laser beam passes harmlessly through the surface of the eye to form an opening in the posterior capsule (far right).

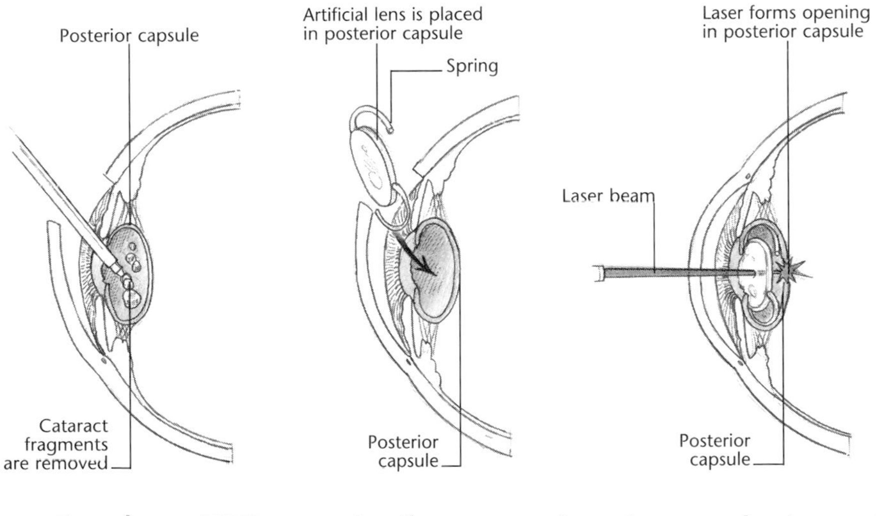

Removing a cataract

Inserting a permanent artificial lens

Laser procedure to correct blurring of lens

However, if you have a serious medical condition (such as heart disease) or if your surgery is more complicated than usual, your doctor may recommend staying overnight in the hospital. He or she will monitor your eye for potential problems, such as inflammation, infection, bleeding, or glaucoma.

Your doctor may recommend using eyedrops or wearing a protective shield for a short time after the surgery. You can resume your usual activities soon after the surgery, but it may take a few weeks or months to regain your optimal vision. Call your doctor immediately during this time if you have pain, loss of vision, nausea, vomiting, excessive coughing, or injury to your eye. Most people who have had cataract surgery still need to wear corrective lenses even if they have a lens implant. If you need corrective lenses for both distance vision and near vision, bifocals may be a good choice because they take care of both vision problems at the same time.

Several months or years after cataract surgery, the posterior capsule (the membrane of the back of the lens) may turn cloudy, blurring your vision. If this occurs, your ophthalmologist can eliminate the blurring by making an opening in the membrane using a laser (a high-energy beam of light). This is a painless procedure (eyedrops that contain an anesthetic will be applied to your eye beforehand) that can be done in a short time in the doctor's office or in an outpatient facility.

DIABETIC RETINOPATHY

Diabetic retinopathy is a complication of diabetes (see page 620). Diabetes is a chronic disease that can damage and weaken blood vessels, including those in the retina (a thin membrane that lines the inside of the eye). In the back of your eye, the retina records images of objects and sends information about the images to your brain for interpretation. In diabetic retinopathy, the weakened blood vessels may begin to leak blood or fluid and develop tiny, fragile branches and scar tissue that can blur your vision or distort the information that the retina sends to your brain.

Retinopathy usually affects both eyes (although unequally) at the same time. If it is not treated, retinopathy can lead to blindness. The longer you have diabetes, the more likely you are to eventually develop retinopathy. Many people who have had diabetes for more than 15 years have some degree of retinopathy.

Early detection and treatment of retinopathy can often prevent serious vision problems. If you have diabetes, the best way to prevent retinopathy may be to carefully control the level of glucose in your blood. Test your blood glucose level regularly, take medication if necessary, rigorously follow your diet plan, and exercise regularly. You should also make sure your blood pressure is under control. People who have both diabetes and high blood pressure have more problems with their eyes. (For more about controlling diabetes, see page 622.)

The only way to detect retinopathy is through an examination by an ophthalmologist. Make sure your ophthalmologist knows you have diabetes. He or she will regularly monitor your eyes for

DIABETIC RETINOPATHY

In a healthy eye (right), the blood vessels of the retina branch out in a regular pattern to supply blood to the eye. In people who have had diabetes for many years, the disease can cause the blood vessels in the retina at the back of the eye to leak fluid or to grow fragile, brushlike branches and form scar tissue (far right). This process can blur and distort vision and may lead to blindness.

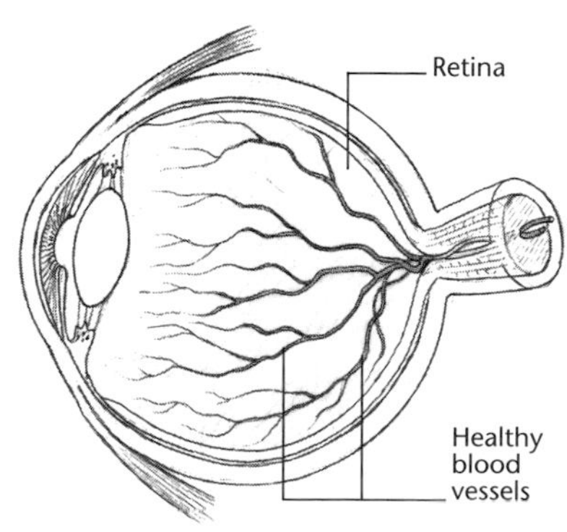

Healthy eye

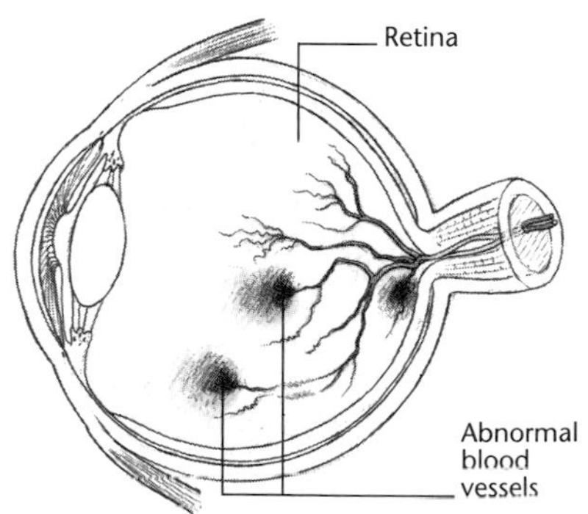

Eye with diabetic retinopathy

LASER SURGERY FOR DIABETIC RETINOPATHY
A painless laser procedure is sometimes used to treat damage to blood vessels caused by diabetic retinopathy. In this procedure, the ophthalmologist directs high-energy beams of light (called lasers) at the abnormal blood vessels of the retina to seal the vessels.

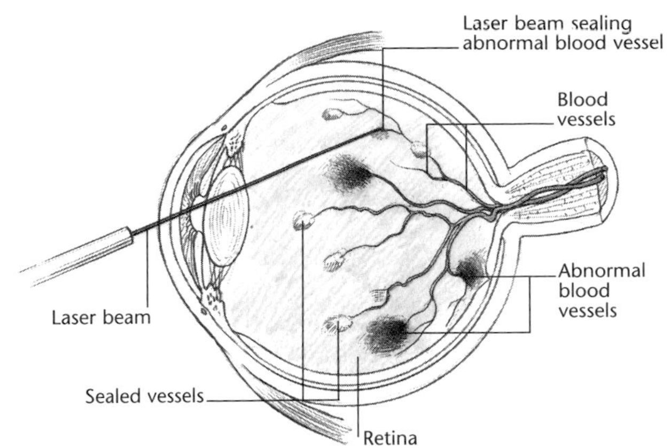

changes that are characteristic of retinopathy. If you have diabetes, have an eye examination every year (or more often if your doctor recommends it) to ensure that any problem can be treated early, before your vision is impaired.

Symptoms Diabetic retinopathy may not cause obvious symptoms in the early stages, or you may notice a gradual blurring of your vision. As the disease progresses, the abnormal blood vessels can begin to bleed or leak fluid. This leaking can cause your sight to become hazy, you may see spots in front of your eyes, or you may suddenly lose your vision completely. See your ophthalmologist immediately if you experience any of the following symptoms:

- Blurred vision
- Seeing spots in front of your eyes
- Fluctuating vision—your vision alternates between being clear and diminished
- Sudden loss of vision
- Pain in your eyes

Diagnosis To determine if you have retinopathy, your doctor will examine your retina with an ophthalmoscope (an instrument that shines a light into the back of your eye) to look for any abnormal blood vessels or bleeding. To find if any blood vessels are leaking, your doctor may take photographs of the retina and the blood vessels of the retina. Before taking the photographs, the doctor injects a special dye into a vein in your arm. The dye travels through your bloodstream to your eyes, where it highlights the blood vessels and can reveal if any are leaking.

Treatment If you are diagnosed with diabetic retinopathy, you will need to have regular eye examinations at least once a year to monitor the health of your eyes. Maintaining strict control of the level of glucose in your blood may help slow the progress of the disease (see page 622). In some cases, surgery is recommended. Ask your doctor what you can expect from such surgery, including the recovery time, level of pain, or effects on your vision.

Laser surgery An ophthalmologist can seal leaking blood vessels in the retina using small bursts of high-energy light (laser beams). If the retinopathy is caused by abnormal growth of blood vessels, the laser bursts are scattered across the surface of the retina to seal off the abnormal blood vessels and prevent damage to the eye. This procedure, which is painless, may be done in the doctor's office, in an outpatient facility, or in a hospital.

Cryotherapy If the clear, jellylike substance that fills the eye (called the vitreous gel) is clouded by blood from leaking vessels, laser surgery cannot be used to treat the retinopathy. Instead, cryotherapy (freezing) may be used to freeze the retina and shrink the abnormal blood vessels. This procedure is performed using local anesthesia (see page 260) and may be done in the doctor's office, in an outpatient facility, or in the hospital. You may experience some discomfort or mild pain.

Vitrectomy For diabetic retinopathy that is at an advanced stage, microsurgery (delicate surgery that is done under a microscope) can remove the blood-filled vitreous gel and replace it with a clear solution. This procedure, called vitrectomy, can reverse the loss of vision caused by the accumulation of blood in the vitreous gel. Vitrectomy is performed in an operating room using local or general anesthesia (see page 260). The procedure may take several hours and can cause discomfort. The recovery time is extremely variable and depends on how severe the problem was before the surgery.

Reattaching the retina If scar tissue pulls on the retina and detaches it from the back of the eye, blindness can result. Your ophthalmologist may recommend surgery to reattach the retina. This procedure is performed in an operating room using local or general anesthesia. The procedure may take several hours and can cause discomfort. This surgery may be combined with vitrectomy or laser surgery.

Ear disorders

Your ears have two functions—hearing and balance. The structures of the outer and middle ear collect sound and transmit it to the brain. The inner ear has tiny fluid-filled structures that are sensitive to position and movement and help you keep your balance. The ear is susceptible to a variety of disorders. Some ear disorders can lead to deafness; others can cause dizziness or loss of balance

HEARING LOSS

There are two types of hearing loss: conductive and sensorineural. If sound waves are not properly transmitted, or conducted, to your inner ear, the resulting hearing loss is called conductive hearing loss. It can result from a buildup of earwax, a perforated eardrum, injury, or an infection in your middle ear (otitis media). Conductive hearing loss can also result from problems with the three small bones of your middle ear (the malleus, incus, and stapes). Abnormalities of these small bones can be present at birth or acquired later from a disease or an injury.

Sensorineural hearing loss occurs when sound waves are not picked up in the inner ear and transmitted to the brain. This type of hearing loss can result from injury, tumors, previous infections, aging, or exposure to some antibiotics or excessively loud noise. (For information about the long-term effects of loud noise on hearing, see page 180.) Some people are born with a susceptibility to developing sensorineural hearing loss.

Hearing loss can be a frightening and isolating experience at any age. Many people whose hearing is failing simply do not realize they have a problem; others deny it. Because people with hearing loss have difficulty following conversations they cannot hear, they may appear to be withdrawn or confused. Family members and friends may not know why they are behaving differently. In many cases, family and friends feel they need to protect the person from embarrassment so they pretend the problem does not exist. But, for many hearing problems, treatment can significantly improve a person's hearing and quality of life. If you are having problems with your hearing, do not hesitate to talk to your doctor about it and ask about treatment options.

Symptoms If you have conductive hearing loss, you may experience the following symptoms:
- People seem to be speaking too softly.
- You hear voices better in noisy surroundings than in quiet ones.
- You can tolerate loud noises that bother most people.

If you have sensorineural hearing loss, you may experience the following symptoms:
- People seem to be speaking more softly than usual.
- You have difficulty hearing speech in noisy places.
- You hear the pitch of a sound differently in each ear.

Diagnosis If you notice any loss of hearing, see your doctor. He or she will take your medical history and give you a physical examination and may order laboratory tests to rule out a serious illness that could be causing your hearing loss.

If other causes have been ruled out, your doctor will set up a hearing test for you. Hearing tests are usually conducted by audiologists, specialists who are trained in the science of hearing. An audiologist can use a variety of tests to evaluate hearing impairment and help determine treatment. For more about hearing tests, see page 141.

Treatment Treatment for hearing loss depends on the cause. For example, if a plug of wax in your ear is causing your hearing problem, your doctor can remove it. Do not put anything, including a cotton swab, in your ear to try to remove earwax yourself because you can force the wax farther in and possibly damage your eardrum. Your doctor may

Structure of the ear

The cuplike part of your ear outside your body (called the pinna) collects sound waves from your environment and channels them into the ear canal. The sound waves vibrate the tympanic membrane (eardrum), a thin, fibrous membrane covered with skin. These vibrations are passed to three tiny interconnecting bones in the middle ear—the malleus (hammer), incus (anvil), and stapes (stirrup). The sound vibrations then enter the cochlea, a snail-shaped passage filled with fluid. Inside the cochlea, the vibrations in the fluid move microscopic hairs that stimulate nerve cells to send sound information via the vestibulocochlear nerve to the brain.

Your inner ear controls your sense of balance. The inner ear consists of a maze of passages called the labyrinth (shaded area). The labyrinth is made up of the semicircular canals, the cochlea, and the vestibule, all of which are fluid-filled chambers. The semicircular canals and the vestibule contain cells that interpret the position and movement of the fluid to gather information about gravity, balance, posture, movement, and position. These cells transmit this information in sensory impulses to your brain via the vestibulocochlear nerve.

The eustachian tube connects your middle ear to your throat. The eustachian tube is usually closed, but contractions of the small muscles of the head and neck open it whenever you yawn or swallow.

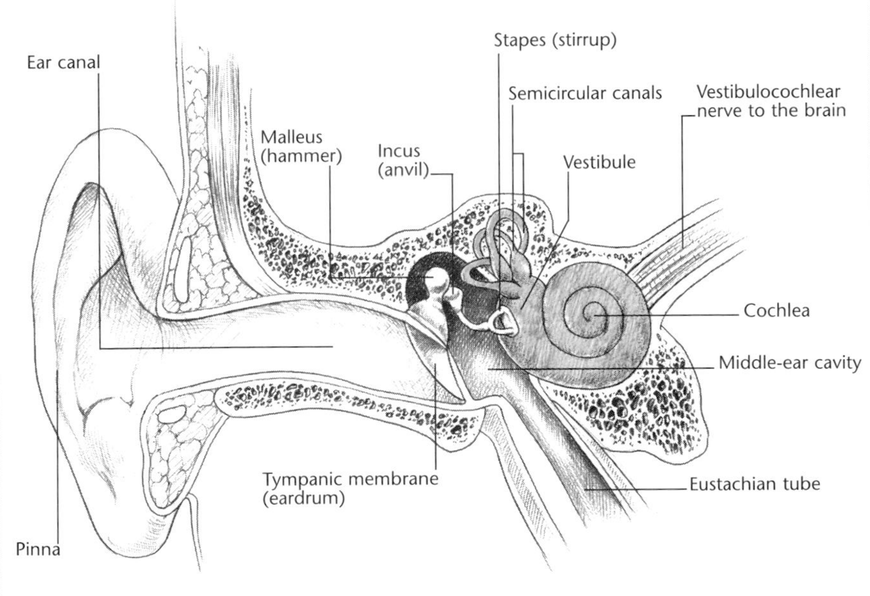

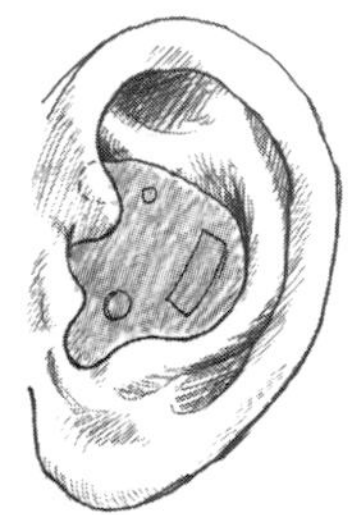

In-the-ear hearing aid

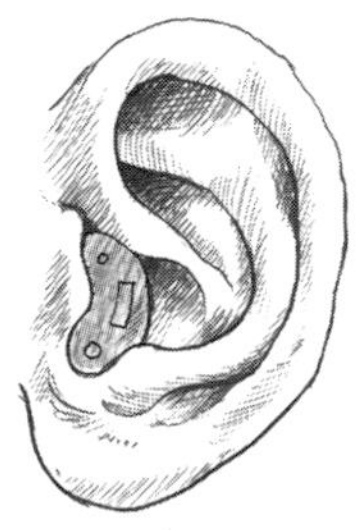

In-the-canal hearing aid

HEARING AIDS THAT FIT IN THE EAR
An in-the-ear hearing aid fits snugly in your outer ear (top); an in-the-canal hearing aid fits into your ear canal (bottom).

recommend over-the-counter eardrops to help relieve the problem. Eardrops soften the wax and loosen it.

Hearing aids Some types of hearing loss can be corrected with a hearing aid. A hearing aid is a small, battery-powered device that picks up sounds and amplifies them for your ear. Many hearing aids today are so small that they are hardly noticeable. If your doctor thinks you need a hearing aid, he or she will probably refer you to an audiologist. The audiologist will do a comprehensive hearing test to evaluate your hearing and your need for a hearing aid. He or she will perform tests to determine which kind of hearing aid is best for you. Because of the variety of devices available, the audiologist is likely to ask about your lifestyle, your financial situation, and any concerns you may have about using a hearing aid.

If you need a hearing aid, a wax impression will be made of your ear and sent to a laboratory that will make a hearing aid that conforms to the shape of your ear. During the first few weeks, you will learn how to use it correctly. After that, your hearing aid should be adjusted and tested regularly by the audiologist to make sure it is working correctly.

The recommended schedule for adjustments and checkups depends on the type of hearing aid you have. Most states authorize a 30-day trial period during which you can return your hearing aid if you are not satisfied for any reason. Be sure to ask your doctor or audiologist about any such trial period. Even after the trial period, make sure your doctor knows about any difficulties you have with your hearing aid.

There are several different kinds of hearing aids. The most common are those that fit snugly into the ear. In-the-ear devices are remarkably small and have an outer covering that makes them barely visible. In-the-ear hearing aids can be worn comfortably during strenuous physical activity and do not interfere with your eyeglasses.

In-the-canal hearing aids are the least visible type because they fit inside the ear canal. They are effective in people who have mild-to-moderate hearing loss. Some people cannot use this type of hearing aid because their ear canals are too small to accommodate them comfortably. In-the-canal hearing aids are comfortable during strenuous physical activity. They are the most expensive

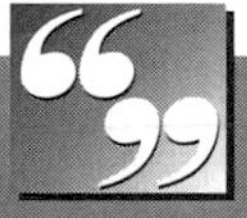

ONE WOMAN'S STORY
HEARING AIDS

Last spring, when my daughter was visiting me from out of town, she kept turning down the volume on the TV. At first I thought she just didn't like it that I kept the television on in the kitchen while I made supper. But then she said it was so loud she couldn't stand it.

I knew my hearing wasn't as good as it used to be. I found myself getting annoyed with other people when they didn't speak up. I often couldn't understand the point of conversations because I had missed important details. I hated always asking people to repeat themselves. I dropped out of some of my social groups and began staying home more, reading, gardening, and doing housework. I guess I was unwilling to face the fact that, at age 67, my hearing was failing.

"Now that I can hear again, I realize how much I was missing."

My daughter convinced me to talk to my doctor. He sent me to an audiologist to have my hearing tested. It turned out that I have the kind of hearing loss that can be corrected with a hearing aid. I worked with the audiologist to pick out the type of hearing aid I wanted. I chose an in-the-ear aid, which fits perfectly in my ear. It took a little while for me to get used to the hearing aid. Now that I can hear again, I realize how much I was missing. I feel alive again; my life is so much more interesting now. I even started going back to my bridge club. I was self-conscious about wearing the hearing aid at first but people don't seem to notice. Even if they did, it wouldn't bother me. My hearing aid is my lifeline—I depend on it.

Hearing loss and aging

Most people experience some degree of hearing loss after age 50. Hearing loss is such a gradual process that you will probably be unaware of it. Your family members are likely to be the first to notice and bring it to your attention or to the attention of your doctor. If you or your family thinks you may be losing your hearing, see your doctor for an evaluation and, if necessary, get a hearing aid—that is usually all it takes to improve your hearing immediately.

If you experience hearing loss:

- Have your doctor test your hearing to determine if a hearing aid would help.
- Have your doctor check your ears for a buildup of wax, which can interfere with hearing. Your doctor may recommend that you have your ears cleaned at regular intervals to prevent buildup.
- During conversation, try to eliminate or reduce background noise or sounds from a television or radio, or from machinery.
- In noisy places, seat yourself near surfaces that absorb sound—such as curtains, books, or upholstered furniture. Stay away from expanses of glass, plaster, or tile, which can cause echoing.

type and, because they are very small, they are easy to drop, lose, or break. They also require more frequent adjustments by the audiologist.

If you have severe hearing loss, a behind-the-ear hearing aid may be the best choice. Behind-the-ear hearing aids are often more sophisticated, powerful, and comfortable than other hearing aids. The microphone and amplifier hang behind the ear and are connected by a tube to an ear mold that sits inside your ear canal. You can adjust the sound level yourself. Most people find that this type of hearing aid does not interfere with their eyeglasses. You may need to hold the telephone receiver differently if it is uncomfortable. If you are very physically active, you may find this type of hearing aid cumbersome. Discuss your concerns with your doctor or audiologist.

Surgery In some cases, surgery is required to improve hearing. Your doctor may recommend one of the following surgical procedures:

- **Tympanoplasty and stapedectomy** Tympanoplasty and stapedectomy are two surgical procedures that may be performed to repair an eardrum or to replace bones of the middle ear that have been damaged. This damage can result from infection or from an inherited ear disorder, such as otosclerosis (overgrowth of bone in the middle ear). The affected bones may be replaced with an artificial implant that takes over the job of transmitting sound waves to the inner ear.

  Tympanoplasty and stapedectomy are performed using local or general anesthesia (see page 260) and, in many cases, the surgery does not require an overnight stay in the hospital. After having this type of surgery, your doctor will ask you to relax at home for about 7 to 10 days. You may have mild pain for a few days after the surgery. It usually takes about 8 weeks for the ear to heal completely. Your hearing may be much better in 2 weeks, or it may improve gradually over several months.
- **Myringoplasty** Myringoplasty is a surgical procedure to repair a perforated eardrum with tissue taken from another part of the ear or an area near the ear. An eardrum can become perforated by a severe infection or an injury to the ear. The surgery is usually done using local anesthesia and may require an overnight stay in the hospital. You will experience very little pain after this procedure. Your doctor will recommend that you rest at home for 1 week after the surgery. Your hearing will be completely restored within about 6 weeks.
- **Mastoid surgery** Surgery that involves the mastoid process, the bone that you can feel just behind your ear, may be necessary in some circumstances. In rare cases, a person may develop a destructive ingrowth of skin (called a cholesteatoma) in the middle ear and mastoid process.

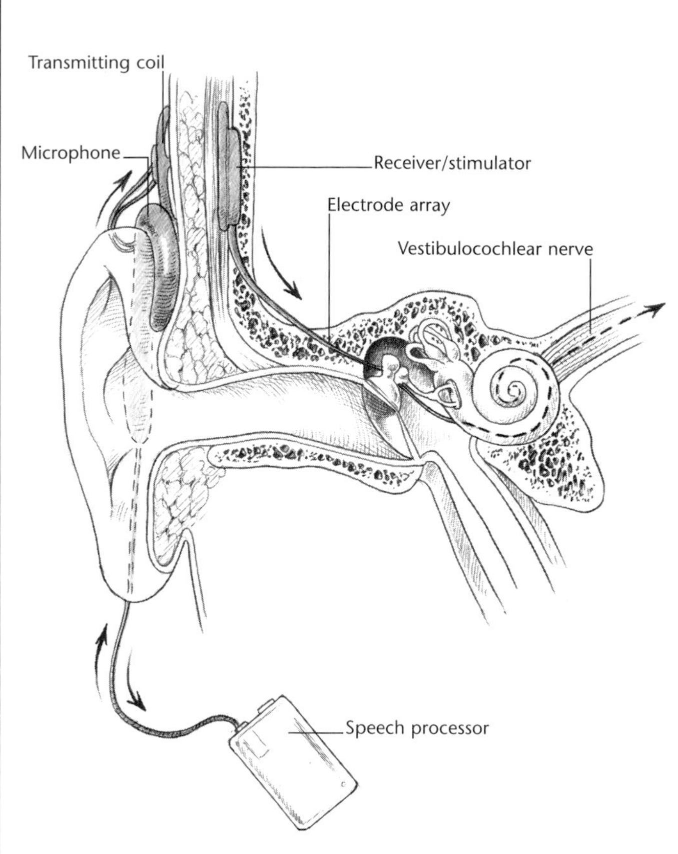

HOW A COCHLEAR IMPLANT WORKS
A cochlear implant is an electronic device that enables adults and children who have severe deafness in both ears to distinguish among sounds and to understand speech. The implant has both external and internal components. The microphone, which is worn like a behind-the-ear hearing aid, receives incoming sound and transmits it via a thin cord to the speech processor. The speech processor, which can fit into a pocket or be worn on a belt or in a harness underneath or over clothing, converts the sounds into electrical signals that it sends to the transmitting coil in the headset. The transmitting coil, which is held in place against the skin by magnetic attraction to the implanted receiver/stimulator, sends the electrical signals through the skin to the receiver/stimulator. The receiver/stimulator activates individual electrodes in the electrode array, which then directly stimulate specific nerve fibers in the ear. The vestibulocochlear nerve transmits the signals to the brain, which interprets them as sound.

An infection in your middle ear can become so severe that it spreads to the mastoid bone from your middle ear. Either of these conditions can impair your hearing and, in some cases, can damage the eardrum and ear canal and cause life-threatening infections.

A cholesteatoma can be corrected with surgery to remove the ingrown skin. To prevent an infection from spreading into your inner ear or brain, the doctor may need to surgically drain pus from your middle ear.

Because an important goal of mastoid surgery is to restore hearing, it is sometimes necessary for a person to also have a tympanoplasty (see page 659). Mastoid surgery usually requires an overnight stay in the hospital. After the surgery, your doctor may recommend 1 or 2 weeks of rest at home. You will experience little pain during the healing process; complete healing and restoration of hearing may take up to 4 months.

Cochlear implants For people who have sensorineural hearing loss that is severe enough to cause total deafness (for which hearing aids provide no help), a cochlear implant may be used. A cochlear implant transforms sound into electrical impulses that can be transmitted to the brain. Cochlear implants are showing promise in enabling children who were born completely deaf to learn to speak. However, the implants are most effective in people who lack useful hearing in both ears but who were once able to hear well enough to learn to speak and understand language. Cochlear implants cannot produce completely normal sounds, but they can enable you to understand speech or, at least, to distinguish among different kinds of sound. For this reason, the implants can enhance a person's ability to read lips.

A cochlear implant consists of internal and external components (see illustration at left). The internal component—a unit called a receiver/stimulator and a flexible coil of electrodes, called an electrode array—is surgically implanted into one of your ears while you are under general anesthesia. This procedure takes about 2 to 4 hours and usually requires a hospital stay of 1 to 2 days.

After your ear has healed completely (usually in about 4 to 6 weeks), your doctor fits you with the external components—a headset (which contains a microphone, connecting cords, and a transmitting coil) and a speech processor. An audiologist will carefully adjust the settings on your implant to allow the best level of hearing. You will work with the audiologist for several weeks or months after you receive your implant to learn how to use it most effectively.

TINNITUS

A person who has tinnitus hears ringing, buzzing, or hissing in one or both ears even when there is no external source of sound. Although many people experience ringing in their ears occasionally, a person with tinnitus may experience ringing that becomes louder and more persistent as he or she ages. Although tinnitus can be annoying and stressful, it is not a threat to your health. However, in some cases, tinnitus is a symptom of a more serious ear disorder or an illness such as anemia or heart disease. Tinnitus is often associated with loss of hearing.

Symptoms The symptoms of tinnitus include ringing, buzzing, hissing, or whistling in the ears. A person may also experience some degree of hearing loss.

Diagnosis To diagnose tinnitus, your doctor will first rule out more serious disorders. He or she will examine your ears for signs of infection, a blockage, or Meniere's disease. You are likely to have a hearing test and you may have a computed tomography (CT) scan (see page 572) to look for any abnormalities that could be affecting your hearing.

Treatment Treatment of tinnitus depends on the cause, which can vary widely and cannot always be determined. Surgery may be required if the cause is a perforated eardrum or otosclerosis (an overgrowth of bone in the middle ear). If you have a buildup of wax or dirt in your ear, your doctor will remove it. If you have an infection of the middle ear, your doctor is likely to prescribe antibiotics.

If the condition cannot be treated effectively, your doctor may recommend things you can do to make the condition easier to live with. For example, playing background music can help drown out the annoying sounds in your head. If you have hearing loss, the low-level sounds picked up by a hearing aid can help diminish the sounds of tinnitus. Your doctor may recommend a device called a tinnitus masker, which you wear like a hearing aid; a tinnitus masker emits a steady, monotonous noise that masks the internal ringing of tinnitus. If your tinnitus sometimes interferes with your sleep, your doctor may prescribe a medication that you can take occasionally to help you sleep better.

MENIERE'S DISEASE

Meniere's disease is characterized by fluctuating or sporadic hearing loss and periods of dizziness that result when excess fluid builds up in the labyrinth, the structure of the inner ear that controls hearing and balance. The effects of Meniere's disease can range from mild to incapacitating. The disease can occur at any age but is rare in children. The cause is unknown but many doctors believe that a virus that infects the ear may cause damage that appears years later in the form of Meniere's disease. No specific virus has been identified.

There is no cure for Meniere's disease, but treatment can usually relieve the symptoms. In most cases, the spells of dizziness go away within 5 to 10 years, but a severe hearing loss will usually be permanent.

Symptoms The three characteristic symptoms of Meniere's disease include attacks of dizziness, hearing loss (usually in one ear), and ringing, buzzing, or roaring sounds in an ear (tinnitus). An attack may begin with the sensation of pressure inside your ear and tingling or ringing in the ear. Within a few minutes, you may become very dizzy and you may lose some of your ability to hear in that ear. An attack may last for hours and make you vomit or feel nauseous. Attacks may recur frequently for months and then not occur again for several years.

Diagnosis Meniere's disease is usually diagnosed from the symptoms. If the diagnosis is in question, your doctor may recommend tests to help confirm it. You may also have an auditory brain-stem response test or magnetic resonance imaging (MRI; see page 572) to rule out other possible causes of your symptoms, such as a brain tumor. An auditory brain-stem response test provides a computerized measure of how long it takes the vestibulocochlear nerve to carry a sound impulse from your ear to your brain stem. An unusually slow reaction time may indicate pressure on the nerve, such as from a tumor.

Treatment Treatment for Meniere's disease depends on the severity and nature of your symptoms. Lying still during an attack can help reduce the dizziness and other symptoms. Because Meniere's disease is caused by fluid buildup inside the ear, your doctor may recommend limiting your intake of salt and taking diuretics (medications that help the body eliminate excess fluid). These measures can usually decrease the severity and frequency of attacks. Many people with Meniere's disease also find that eliminating caffeine provides some relief. If your attacks cause nausea and vomiting, your doctor can prescribe medication to reduce these symptoms.

If your symptoms are severe and recurring, and if you have already lost hearing in the affected ear, your doctor may recommend surgery to relieve the dizziness. This type of surgery involves cutting the nerves that are responsible for the dizziness, while sparing the nerve that is necessary for hearing.

Disorders of the teeth and mouth

Problems with your teeth can disrupt your daily life more than you might think. Your teeth and mouth are necessary for good nutrition—they start the digestive process when you eat food. Your mouth also enables you to communicate with speech or with expressions, such as a smile or frown, that show your emotions. You can keep your teeth healthy for life by brushing and flossing them every day; eating a nutritious, balanced diet; and having regular checkups and cleanings by your dentist. For more about keeping your teeth and gums healthy, see page 142.

Gum disease occurs when plaque, a sticky substance that contains bacteria, builds up in and around the gums and teeth, often causing swollen or bleeding gums. Gum disease is usually painless, unless it forms an abscess (a pus-filled pocket). For this reason, many people may not be aware that they have a problem until the disease reaches an advanced stage and threatens loss of teeth. Gum disease is the leading cause of tooth loss after age 35.

Gum disease is common in all adults, but it occurs more frequently in women than men because of fluctuating hormone levels during puberty, pregnancy, breast-feeding, and menopause. Gum disease can take the form of gingivitis, which, if left untreated, can lead to the most serious form called periodontitis.

GINGIVITIS

Gingivitis is inflammation and bleeding of the gums, usually resulting from an infection. Most people experience gingivitis at some time in their life. The most common cause of gingivitis is a buildup of plaque and a hard, crustlike deposit called tartar, or calculus. Plaque is a soft, sticky deposit of bacteria (which is naturally present in your mouth) mixed with proteins from your saliva. Plaque can build up above or below the gums. Brushing and flossing your teeth can remove the plaque, but it rapidly reforms within 24 hours. The buildup of plaque and tartar results from failure to brush your teeth and floss regularly.

In many cases, the symptoms of gingivitis are temporary and clear up with careful brushing and flossing. Using an over-the-counter antibacterial mouthwash after you brush your teeth can also help reduce the buildup of plaque and prevent gingivitis. If you have inflammation or bleeding of your gums that does not clear up with brushing and flossing, see your dentist.

Medications that thin the blood, including aspirin, can contribute to bleeding gums. Diseases that reduce the blood's ability to clot, including liver diseases such as hepatitis (see page 534), can also cause gingivitis. Some medications that are used to treat epilepsy, depression, or heart disease may cause swollen gums. Tell your dentist about any medications you are taking and see him or her if your gums are bleeding.

Symptoms See your dentist if you notice any of the following signs of gingivitis:

- Your gums bleed easily.
- Your gums bleed when you eat.
- Your toothbrush or dental floss turns pink or red when you use it.
- You have bad breath.

Diagnosis To diagnose gingivitis, a dentist places an instrument called a periodontal probe between the gums and teeth to measure the space between them and to check for bleeding or swelling.

Treatment An early case of gingivitis can be cured by brushing your teeth at least twice daily with a soft bristle toothbrush and flossing every day to remove food debris and soft plaque deposits from between your teeth. Devices called oral irrigators—which use a thin, forceful stream of water to clean between teeth—are not as effective as dental floss; they remove large pieces of food between the teeth but do not remove plaque. Your dentist may prescribe a mouth rinse that contains the antibacterial ingredient chlorhexidine to help reduce the buildup of plaque. If the plaque and tartar are firmly established on your teeth, the only way to remove them is to have your teeth cleaned at your dentist's office.

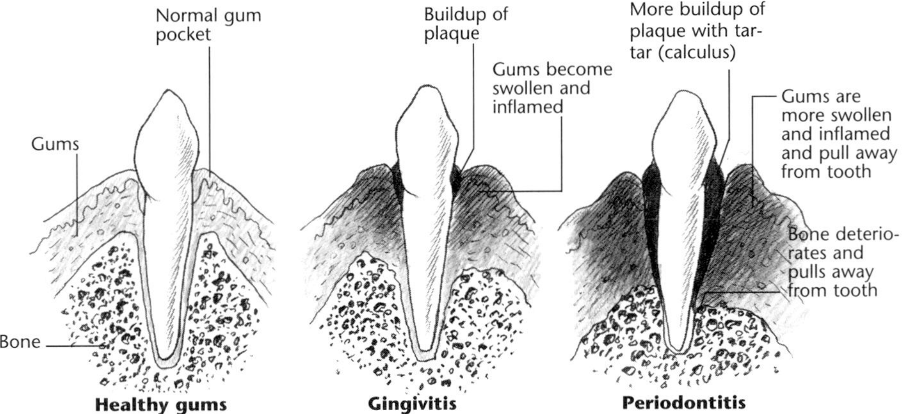

HOW GUM DISEASE PROGRESSES

Healthy gums (left) adhere firmly to your teeth. They are firm and pale pink and do not bleed when you brush them. When a bacteria-containing substance called plaque builds up between your teeth and gums (center), the gums become irritated and inflamed and may bleed easily. If the plaque is not regularly cleaned away, it can become hardened, forming a substance called tartar, or calculus, and lead to a more serious form of gum disease called periodontitis. In periodontitis (right), the supporting gum tissues and jawbone pull away from the tooth, eventually causing the tooth to loosen or fall out.

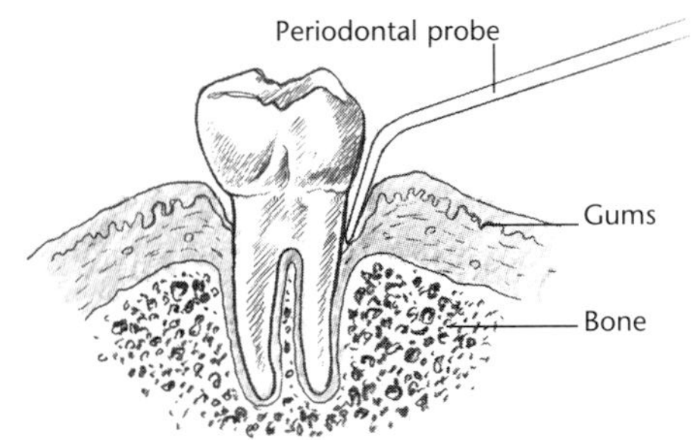

EVALUATING GUM DISEASE

At your regular visits to the dentist, he or she examines your mouth for signs of gum disease and evaluates the extent of disease by measuring the space between your teeth and gums with an instrument called a periodontal probe. X-rays are also used to monitor the health of your teeth and gums.

PERIODONTITIS

When gingivitis is not treated, it can advance to a more serious stage of gum disease called periodontitis, in which the tissue surrounding the tooth becomes infected. Plaque-filled pockets form between the tooth and gum and the gums become inflamed; this inflammation causes the pockets to enlarge further and collect even more plaque, which can gradually detach the gums from the teeth. Bacteria can invade the pockets, causing more infections, and pus may ooze from around your teeth. Over time, the bony sockets that hold the teeth in place can erode and cause the teeth to loosen and fall out.

Symptoms See your dentist immediately if you notice any of the following symptoms of periodontitis:

- Swollen or recessed gums
- Pain in a tooth when you eat hot, cold, or sweet foods
- A loose tooth or change in your bite
- Bad breath or unpleasant taste in your mouth

Diagnosis A dentist diagnoses periodontitis by placing an instrument called a periodontal probe between the gums and teeth and checking for bleeding, swelling, or pus. The probe can measure the space between the teeth and gums and help the dentist evaluate the extent of disease. Periodontitis can also be diagnosed from an X-ray that shows deterioration of the bone that surrounds and supports the tooth.

Treatment The first step in treating periodontitis is a thorough cleaning of your teeth by a dental hygienist. Your dentist will instruct you in a strict daily program of dental hygiene to improve your condition. Your gums may bleed when you brush and floss, but this usually stops within 2 weeks if the disease was diagnosed at an early stage. If your gums become less red and swollen and more firm after several weeks of diligent daily care, you may be able to avoid having surgery to treat the disease.

In more advanced cases, surgery is usually necessary. In one surgical treatment for periodontitis, the dentist opens a flap of gum to remove deposits from around your teeth below the gum line or to remove infected tissue. The flap of tissue is then stitched in place. In another procedure, called a gingivectomy or gingivoplasty, your dentist trims away part of your gum to decrease the size of the pocket in which tartar and bacteria are collecting. After the procedure, the surface of the gum is coated with a protective putty to allow it to heal. This coating should not interfere with your ability to eat or drink; if it causes any problems, call your dentist. After about a week, your dentist will remove the putty and examine your gums to evaluate how well they are healing.

In addition to either of these surgical procedures, and depending on the site of your periodontal disease, your dentist may place a thin fiber that is coated with an antibiotic medication into the affected gum pocket to eliminate the bacteria. The antibiotic fiber is removed after 10 days and your gums are allowed to heal normally.

If gum disease has caused the loss of gum tissue and supporting jawbone, transplants of gum and bone taken from a healthy part of your mouth may be necessary to replace the damaged tissue.

TEMPOROMANDIBULAR DISORDER

Temporomandibular disorder (TMD) is a disorder of the temporomandibular joint, which is located between the temporal bone (part of the skull above the ear) and the mandible (lower jawbone). TMD causes pain or clicking sounds when you open and close your jaw. Although the condition is not dangerous to your health, it can be uncomfortable.

For unknown reasons, women are much more likely than men to have TMD. The cause of TMD is unclear. Many people who clench or grind their teeth (usually at night while sleeping and often in response to emotional stress) have TMD. Teeth that do not fit together properly can cause the jaw to become misaligned, which in turn can cause TMD. TMD can also result from injury to the jaw, osteoarthritis (see page 559), poor posture (particularly thrusting the head and jaw forward), chewing gum, or eating too many chewy foods.

Symptoms TMD causes pain or clicking or grating sounds when you open and close your jaw. The disorder can also cause headaches, toothaches, earaches, or neck pain. You may have difficulty opening and closing your mouth or your jaws may lock in an open or closed position. Other symptoms of TMD can include dizziness or ringing in your ears.

Diagnosis TMD can be difficult to diagnose. Diagnosis is usually based on your symptoms. Your dentist will ask if you have any habits, such as grinding your teeth or chewing gum, that can cause TMD. Although some dentists may take X-rays or do a magnetic resonance imaging (MRI) scan (see page 572), these tests

Cosmetic dentistry

Crooked, cracked, or discolored teeth can affect the way you feel about yourself. Cosmetic dental procedures are not medically necessary but are done to make teeth look better. Most people who have cosmetic dentistry are happy with the results and find it boosts their self-confidence. However, many of these procedures can be expensive and are often not covered by dental insurance. Like any medical procedure, cosmetic dental procedures have risks. If you are considering having a cosmetic dental procedure, such as the following, make sure you ask your dentist to explain the risks and potential benefits:

Bleaching Bleaching is a cosmetic dental procedure that is done to lighten the color of teeth that are severely stained from decay or damage. The most common bleaching method involves using a custom-fitted mouth guard that you fill with a bleaching gel and wear in your mouth overnight, usually for about 2 weeks. While you are undergoing this process, your dentist will monitor your mouth regularly for any changes in the health of your teeth and gums. He or she will evaluate the degree of whitening by comparing the shades of your teeth before and after the bleaching procedure.

Another bleaching procedure, which provides results more rapidly, is done in one visit to your dentist's office. In this procedure, the dentist applies a bleaching solution to your teeth after placing a covering over your gums to protect them. The solution remains on your teeth for about 30 minutes to an hour. The results are noticeable immediately. Bleaching can cause irritation to your gums or other tissues that line your mouth, including your cheeks, tongue, or throat, but the irritation usually goes away in a short time.

Composite bonding Composite bonding is used to cover stains or to build up a chipped tooth using the same tooth-colored material that is used to fill a cavity in a highly visible tooth. Before applying the composite, the dentist roughens the tooth surface and applies adhesive to it. The composite, which the dentist matches as closely as possible to the natural color of your teeth, is then applied in layers to the tooth and sculpted to create the correct shape. Composite bonding can last 3 to 5 years before it needs to be touched up to correct any discoloration or damage from excessive wear.

Veneers Teeth that are severely damaged or discolored can be restored by covering the entire visible surface of the tooth with a thin layer of composite material or porcelain. Porcelain veneers resist abrasion and discoloration and are more durable and long-lasting than veneers made of composite material.

Aesthetic contouring Teeth that are too large, misaligned, or overlapping can sometimes be made smaller and shaped to look more even and matched. The enamel of healthy teeth is usually thick enough to be reshaped to make the teeth look more attractive. Reshaping is also used for other purposes, such as improving your bite so your teeth mesh properly.

often show a normal joint even in people who have obvious symptoms of TMD. However, these images can help evaluate the anatomy of the jaw and rule out tumors or other abnormal growths.

Treatment If you are diagnosed with TMD, your dentist will recommend eating soft foods for a specified period of time. Avoid hard, crunchy, or chewy foods, gum, or foods (such as corn on the cob or a large sandwich) that require opening your mouth wide. To relieve pain and muscle spasms, take an over-the-counter pain reliever, such as aspirin, ibuprofen, or acetaminophen. If these over-the-counter medications are not effective in relieving your discomfort, your dentist may prescribe muscle relaxants. Placing cold or hot compresses on your jaw may also help; experiment to see which works best for you. Rest your jaw

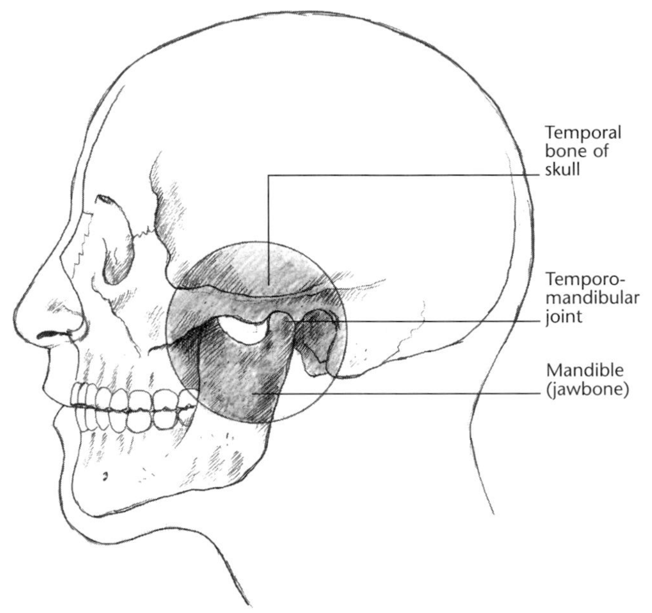

THE TEMPOROMANDIBULAR JOINT
The temporomandibular joint is a hinged joint located on each side of your head where your lower jawbone (mandible) connects with your skull (the temporal bone). Temporomandibular disorder, which causes pain or clicking noises when you open and close your jaw, occurs when the joint or supporting ligaments and muscles become inflamed, injured, or dislocated.

Corrective dentistry

Teeth that are decayed (have cavities) can cause infections, pain, and tooth loss. Tooth decay can also make it difficult, or even impossible, to eat or speak or embarrassing to smile. Corrective, or restorative, dental procedures can repair the areas of decay and restore the teeth to complete functioning. Following are some corrective dental procedures that your dentist may perform:

Fillings Fillings are usually used to repair small to moderate-sized cavities. The dentist drills away the area of decay and fills it with a strong material such as silver, gold, or tooth-colored materials called composites.

Crowns Crowns, also called caps, are used to replace the natural enamel of teeth that are damaged too extensively to be restored with fillings. Crowns are stronger and last longer than bonding or veneers and can also improve the appearance of teeth. Porcelain crowns are used for the more visible front teeth; for back teeth, many people choose gold crowns, which last longer than porcelain crowns but look less natural.

Replacing missing teeth Replacement of missing teeth, in front or back, is important for maintaining the health of your mouth. When teeth are missing, the adjacent remaining teeth can shift and crowd together, which increases the risk of tooth decay and gum disease and interferes with normal chewing. In addition, if back teeth are missing, your cheeks can sink in, altering your appearance. Tooth loss is a common cause of wrinkles in the lower part of the face.

Two or more crowns can be fitted together to replace missing teeth. This structure is called a bridge. Implants are permanent artificial tooth supports that are surgically positioned in the jaw to anchor single-tooth crowns, multiple-tooth bridges, or dentures (artificial teeth). Dentures that are anchored with implants are significantly more stable and secure than traditional dentures, which are held in place by suction that forms between them and the upper or lower gums. Dentures that are held in place with implants also make chewing, eating, talking, and smiling much easier.

as much as you can by avoiding excessive chewing and maintaining your jaw in the teeth-apart, lips-closed position. This position is the jaw's physiological rest position. Try to reduce neck strain by maintaining good posture (see page 88); do not carry heavy shoulder bags or use the side of your head to hold a telephone on your shoulder.

Your dentist may prescribe gentle exercises to relax your jaw and neck muscles, or he or she may refer you to a physical therapist. To prevent you from grinding your teeth at night, your dentist may recommend a device, such as a bite guard or splint, that fits over the biting surfaces of your teeth and stabilizes your bite (the way in which your upper and lower teeth fit together). It is sometimes necessary to adjust or stabilize your bite with braces, porcelain or gold crowns, or by grinding down parts of any teeth that may be interfering with the normal closing of your jaw.

ORAL CANCER

Cancer may develop in any part of the mouth, but is most common on the lips, the lining of the cheeks, the gums, and the floor of the mouth. Oral cancer usually occurs after age 45 and is most common in people who use tobacco (including chewing tobacco) or who drink excessive amounts of alcohol. If you smoke cigarettes and drink alcohol, you are at even greater risk of oral cancer. Long-term, persistent irritation of tissues inside the mouth from jagged teeth or dentures may also cause oral cancer.

Like most cancers, oral cancer is treated most successfully when it is detected at an early stage. But more than half of all oral cancers are at an advanced stage when they are detected and many have spread to the nearby lymph nodes in the neck, making treatment more difficult and less likely to succeed. One of the most important benefits of regular visits to your dentist is an examination of the inside of your mouth for signs of oral cancer.

You should also do a regular self-examination of your mouth every month. This monthly examination is extremely important if you smoke or use other forms of tobacco, or if you drink alcohol. Examine the tissues that line your mouth, particularly along the sides or the bottom of your tongue and on the floor of your mouth underneath your tongue, where most oral cancers occur. Look for any changes, lumps, or patches of red or white tissue and report anything unusual to your dentist or doctor immediately. He or she will do a more thorough examination.

Symptoms The symptoms of oral cancer can include a number of changes in the tissues that line your mouth, especially on the sides or bottom of your tongue and on the floor of your mouth, under your tongue. See your doctor immediately if you notice any of the following symptoms of oral cancer:

- A small, pale lump or thickening of tissue inside your mouth, particularly along the sides or bottom of your tongue or on the floor of your mouth
- Bleeding from a sore, small lump, or patch in your mouth
- Unusual growth or change in the color of the tissue anywhere in your mouth
- Any sore in or around your mouth that does not heal within 2 weeks
- A lump or thickening in your cheek that you can feel with your tongue
- Soreness or a feeling that something is caught in your throat
- Difficulty chewing or swallowing
- Difficulty moving your jaw or tongue
- Numbness of your tongue or other areas of your mouth

Diagnosis If your dentist suspects that you have oral cancer, he or she will perform a biopsy to confirm the diagnosis. For a biopsy, a small amount of tissue is removed from the suspicious area of your mouth and sent to a laboratory for examination under a microscope to look for cancer cells.

Treatment Treatment for oral cancer is usually done by an oral surgeon (who is a dentist) or by an oncologist (a doctor who specializes in cancer). If your cancer is diagnosed at an early stage and has not spread to surrounding tissues or the lymph nodes in your neck, surgery can usually remove all the cancerous tissue. The type of surgery you have will depend on the location and size of the tumor and may involve removing parts of your tongue, gums, jaw, or teeth. After the surgery, you may need to have therapy to help restore your ability to speak and chew normally.

When a tumor is too large to remove surgically, radiation therapy is often used to shrink the tumor. (For more about radiation therapy and its effects, see page 253.) If the cancer has spread to the lymph nodes in your neck or to other parts of your body, your dentist or doctor will recommend chemotherapy—treatment with powerful drugs that kill cancer cells throughout your body. (For more about chemotherapy and its effects, see page 254.)

CHAPTER 27

Your skin

Contents

Your skin is the largest organ of your body. It is a barrier against dirt, germs, irritants, heat, and cold. It seals in moisture and controls your body's temperature by cooling it with perspiration and evaporation. Nerves in your skin respond to touch, pain, pressure, and temperature.

The structure of your skin

Your skin has three layers—the epidermis (the outer layer), dermis (middle layer), and the subcutaneous layer (the inner layer). Cells in the lower layer of the epidermis (the basal layer) produce the pigment melanin, which gives skin its color. The more melanin you have, the darker your skin. Your skin contains hair follicles from which hairs grow, sebaceous glands that produce oil, and sweat glands that help cool your body with perspiration. The thickness of your skin varies in different parts of your body, ranging from the thinness of your eyelids to the thickness of the soles of your feet. The average thickness of the top two layers of your skin is less than 1/5 of an inch.

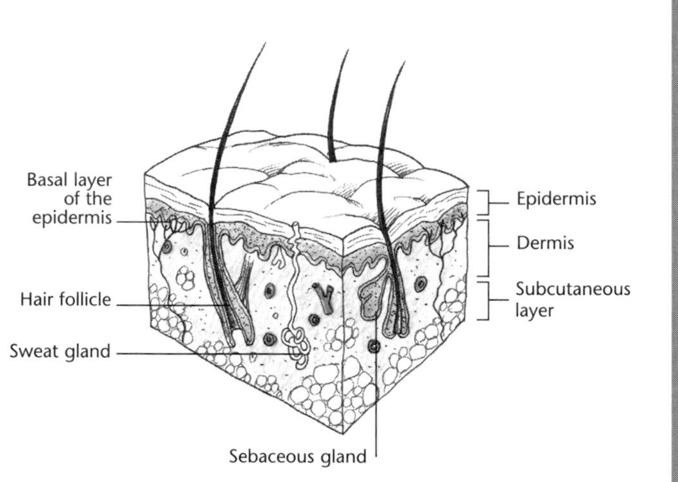

Caring for your skin

The most important thing you can do for the health of your skin is to protect it from the sun. You can also keep your skin healthy by eating a balanced diet, cleansing your skin when it is dirty, and moisturizing your skin when it is dry. Do not smoke cigarettes—smoking causes premature wrinkles. Avoid substances that irritate your skin or cause allergic reactions and try to protect your skin from cuts, abrasions, and burns, which can lead to infection or scarring.

CLEANSING AND MOISTURIZING

Cleansing your skin every day lowers your risk of skin infections by reducing the amount of oil, debris, and bacteria that accumulate. If the skin on your face is especially oily, you can wash it two times a day. Always cleanse your skin with gentle soaps or cleansers to avoid excessive drying and irritation. Be extra gentle when washing around your eyes to avoid damaging the delicate skin. If your skin tends to be sensitive or to react to cosmetics, use cosmetics that do not contain a fragrance. Fragrances are common ingredients in many cosmetics and they often cause irritation.

Dry skin results when the layers of your skin lose too much water through evaporation. The top layer becomes brittle and flakes. Many people have dry skin in the winter, caused both by heated, dry indoor air and by cold, dry outside air. Skin also tends to become drier with age. Practicing these guidelines can help keep your skin healthy and prevent it from becoming dry:

- Use warm (not hot) water for washing and bathing.
- Use mild soaps such as a fatted soap.
- Do not bathe for longer than is necessary to get your skin clean.
- Use a moisturizer every day.
- Apply moisturizer immediately after bathing to seal water in your skin.
- In winter, cover your hands and face by wearing gloves and a scarf to keep in moisture and protect against cold.

Moisturizers can temporarily restore moisture and smoothness to the outside

Itching

A number of factors can cause your skin to itch. Itching caused by dryness can usually be relieved by following the steps described on page 670. A fungal infection (such as athlete's foot) or dermatitis (see page 676), both of which may appear as red patches or spots on your skin, can also cause itching. Over-the-counter antifungal creams or the anti-inflammatory cream hydrocortisone may help relieve these conditions. Itching that is caused by insect bites or poison ivy or poison oak can be relieved with calamine lotion, cold compresses, or hydrocortisone cream. Some over-the-counter preparations that are promoted for relieving itching are not effective. Check with your doctor before using these products.

Try not to scratch itchy skin; doing so can break the surface of the skin, allowing bacteria to enter and cause infection. Scratching can also make the itching worse. If the itching does not go away with any of the above measures, see your doctor.

layer of your skin. The best choice is a moisturizer that has a sun protection factor (SPF) of 15. Many inexpensive moisturizers are as effective as—and sometimes more effective than—more expensive products. Petrolatum, an ingredient used in many lotions and creams, is an excellent moisturizer because it helps seal in the skin's natural moisture. Because moisturizers contain different ingredients, no particular product is best for everyone. You may have to try several before you find the one that is most effective for you. Moisturizers work best when you apply them every day.

Many moisturizing creams contain alpha-hydroxy acids (substances that are present in milk, fruit, and sugar), which may help diminish fine wrinkles. However, the solution of acid may not be strong enough in over-the-counter preparations to have a significant effect; the solution of alpha-hydroxy acid in these preparations is only 2 to 8 percent. The chemical peels (see page 672) used by dermatologists to diminish fine wrinkles and even out irregular skin pigmentation contain alpha-hydroxy acid in solutions of 20 percent or greater. Ask your doctor for more information about the benefits of using these products.

If you are concerned about your wrinkles, your dermatologist may prescribe a moisturizer that contains tretinoin, a substance that is chemically related to vitamin A. Tretinoin, which is also used for treating acne, can somewhat diminish fine wrinkles that result from years of exposure to the sun. You can usually see results from tretinoin after applying it daily for several months (usually before going to bed at night). Do not use tretinoin if you are pregnant because its effect on the fetus is not known.

PROTECTING YOUR SKIN FROM THE SUN

Ultraviolet (UV) rays from the sun can cause changes in your skin that may lead to cancer (see page 683). Sun exposure is especially dangerous if your skin is fair; light skin is more susceptible to cancer than darker skin.

To protect your skin, avoid excessive exposure to the sun between the hours of 10:00 AM and 3:00 PM, when radiation from the sun is most intense. When you are in the sun, wear protective clothing, such as hats and long sleeves, and use sunscreen. Most dermatologists recommend using a sunscreen on exposed areas of your skin every day, especially if you have fair skin. Even in moderation, any exposure to the sun is damaging to your skin. The use of tanning beds is an increasing source of skin damage and aging. Doctors recommend that you never use them.

When choosing a sunscreen, select one that protects you from both kinds of ultraviolet radiation—UVA and UVB. (This information is indicated on the label.) Both kinds of radiation cause your skin to age and wrinkle prematurely and increase your risk of skin cancer. Most sunscreens contain chemicals that protect your skin by absorbing UV rays.

Use a sunscreen that has a sun protection factor (SPF) of 15 or greater. (The SPF is indicated on the label.) An SPF of 15 means that you can stay in the sun 15 times longer than you normally could before your skin begins to burn. If you are planning to be in the sun for a long period of time, reapply sunscreen frequently (especially if it gets washed off from swimming or sweating) to achieve the maximum protection. Note, however, that reapplying sunscreen does not lengthen the total amount of time you are protected.

Apply sunscreen liberally; many people apply only a thin layer that does not provide sufficient protection. Whenever possible, apply the sunscreen half an hour before you go out in the sun so that the sunscreen is well absorbed into your skin.

If you become sensitive to a particular sunscreen, try another one that has different active ingredients listed on the label. You may have to try several before you find one that does not cause any skin reactions. Some sunscreens contain titanium dioxide, a substance that blocks UV rays by providing a physical barrier (like wearing a T-shirt). Titanium dioxide used to be available only in a very visible thick, white cream. It now comes in a preparation that is transparent on your skin. But remember, the best protection against skin cancer is to avoid the sun.

PREVENTING OR DIMINISHING WRINKLES

Long-term exposure to the sun is the major cause of wrinkles. The sun's ultraviolet (UV) rays weaken the elastic collagen fibers in skin, which make your skin resilient and give it support. When your skin loses its resiliency, it is more likely to sag and form wrinkles. Fair skin is more susceptible to damage from the sun because it has less of the pigment melanin, which gives skin a darker color and protects it against the harmful effects of UV rays.

Smoking cigarettes can also contribute to premature aging and wrinkling of your skin by damaging the collagen fibers. Over time, smoking causes deep creases and wrinkles in your skin, primarily around your mouth and eyes. No specific foods or vitamins are known to either cause or prevent wrinkles.

Although wrinkles are not a medical problem and do not require treatment, some people choose to have them reduced or eliminated for cosmetic reasons. Following are some procedures that a dermatologist might recommend for diminishing wrinkles. To reduce your risk of complications, make sure the doctor who performs the procedure is a qualified, trained dermatologist or plastic surgeon.

Chemical peel In a procedure called a chemical peel (see page 695), your dermatologist applies a mild form of acid directly to your skin to diminish roughness and wrinkles and lighten minor discoloration resulting from sun damage. After the procedure, you will feel pain and burning for several hours in those areas of your skin to which the acid was applied. Scabs may form. The effects of a chemical peel can last for several years. Although complications from chemical peels are uncommon, they may include slight skin discoloration or scarring. Discoloration is more common in people who have dark skin. If your skin is dark, your dermatologist is not likely to recommend a chemical peel.

Collagen injections Collagen is the structural protein that gives skin its resiliency and support. Injections of a purified form of bovine (cow) collagen into major creases or wrinkles on your face can help smooth out these areas. In some cases, collagen injections are effective in diminishing scars from acne. After the injections, the area will be red and swollen for a few days. The effects usually last from 4 months to a year because your body eventually absorbs the collagen. In some cases, allergic reactions can occur that cause long-term redness and swelling. For this reason, your dermatologist will test a small area of skin before performing the procedure.

Cosmetic surgery A variety of surgical techniques can be used to eliminate areas of sagging, wrinkled skin on the face and other parts of the body. For example, in a facelift (see page 690), excess facial skin is removed and the remaining skin is tightened to reduce wrinkles. In a procedure called blepharoplasty (see page 692), excess skin on the eyelids is removed. For more about cosmetic surgical procedures, see chapter 28.

If you have dark skin

Black or dark brown skin resists the effects of sun exposure better than lighter skin because it has more of the pigment melanin, which protects it against damage from the sun. People with dark skin have a lower rate of skin cancer than people with light skin, and they tend to wrinkle less with age. But having dark skin does not make you immune to skin cancer. You should wear a sunscreen with a sun protection factor (SPF) of at least 15 whenever you spend time in the sun. Most skin diseases that occur in whites also occur in blacks. However, the following skin problems are more common among people with dark skin or may affect them differently:

Dry skin If your skin is dark, dryness may make it look gray. You can reduce dryness by applying a moisturizer (see page 670) liberally every day. However, if you have acne, try to limit the use of lotions that contain oil on your face; it is best to use water-based products.

Skin discoloration A cut, abrasion, or acne can cause some areas of your skin to be darker or lighter. This problem usually goes away on its own. Do not scrub or pick at the discolored area.

Dermatosis papulosa nigra Dermatosis papulosa nigra, a condition that occurs almost exclusively in blacks, is characterized by brown or black areas of skin that look like moles or flat warts. These abnormalities, which usually occur on the face and neck, are not painful and do not become cancerous. However, many people have them removed for cosmetic reasons.

Keloids A keloid is an abnormal scar that is raised, firm, and irregularly shaped. Keloids are the result of an abnormal healing process in which excessive amounts of the structural protein collagen collect at the site of healing. Although keloids also develop in whites, they are much more common in blacks. Keloids can form anywhere the skin has been cut or broken, but they are most common on the chest and shoulders. They may also form over a vaccination or surgical incision or on pierced ears.

Various treatments are available to decrease the size of a keloid if you find it unattractive. Talk to your doctor. Treatment may include injections of corticosteroids (synthetic hormones) into the keloid to soften it and make it smaller. Surgery is not always successful because the new scar that forms is also likely to be a keloid. In an alternative treatment, small sheets of silicone gel are placed over the keloid and held in place with an adhesive. The sheets look like large, clear bandages. Although doctors are not sure exactly how the silicone works, this treatment is effective in decreasing the size of keloids in some people. At first, you wear the silicone sheet, which you cut to fit the size of your scar, for 4 hours a day, and then gradually increase the time to 24 hours a day. People usually use this treatment for about 3 to 6 months. Radiation therapy (see page 253) is also sometimes used to help shrink a keloid.

Dermatitis

Dermatitis is a term that means inflammation of the skin. The condition can take different forms and have different causes. Although most forms of dermatitis are not a threat to health, in some cases the disorder can be an indication of a serious, long-term illness or a future health problem.

ATOPIC ECZEMA

Atopic eczema, also called atopic dermatitis, is a common form of dermatitis that causes itching, redness, flaking, thickening, or, sometimes, blistering of the skin. The condition can occur in localized patches, on the arms or legs, or, in severe cases, over wide areas of the body. Atopic eczema can range from mild and short-lived to severe and recurring. The condition has a genetic component; most people with atopic eczema have a family history of the disorder or other allergies, including asthma (see page 635) or hay fever (see page 634).

Symptoms Atopic eczema is characterized by intense itching and scaly, thickened skin, most often on the elbows, backs of the knees, face, neck, upper chest, hands, or feet. The symptoms can be worsened by excessive sweating; rapid temperature changes; bathing in hot

SYMPTOM CHART

Common skin problems

Any change in the skin, including pimples, rashes, and bumps.

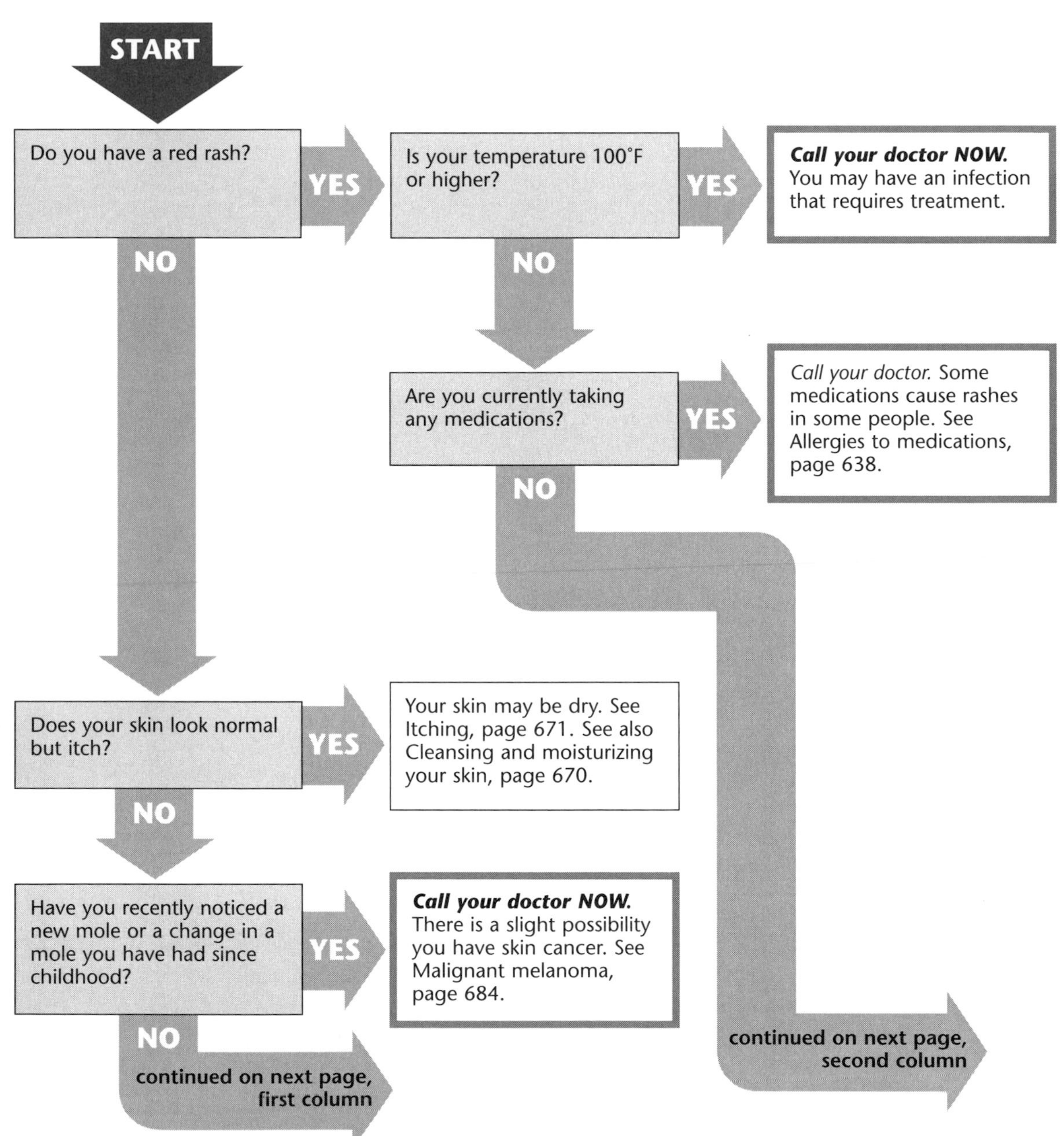

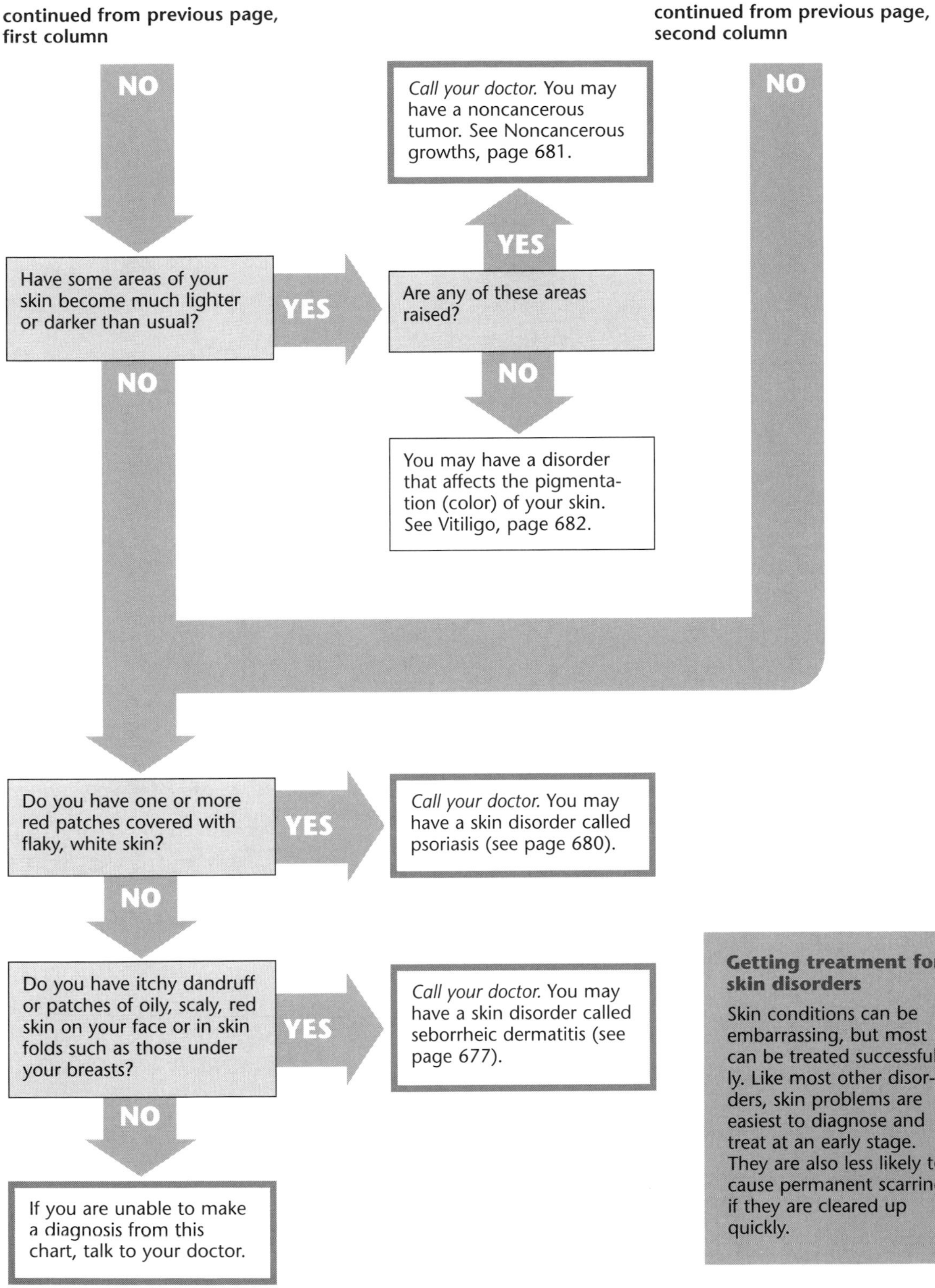

continued from previous page, first column

NO

Have some areas of your skin become much lighter or darker than usual?

YES → Are any of these areas raised?

YES → *Call your doctor.* You may have a noncancerous tumor. See Noncancerous growths, page 681.

NO → You may have a disorder that affects the pigmentation (color) of your skin. See Vitiligo, page 682.

NO

continued from previous page, second column

NO

Do you have one or more red patches covered with flaky, white skin?

YES → *Call your doctor.* You may have a skin disorder called psoriasis (see page 680).

NO

Do you have itchy dandruff or patches of oily, scaly, red skin on your face or in skin folds such as those under your breasts?

YES → *Call your doctor.* You may have a skin disorder called seborrheic dermatitis (see page 677).

NO

If you are unable to make a diagnosis from this chart, talk to your doctor.

Getting treatment for skin disorders

Skin conditions can be embarrassing, but most can be treated successfully. Like most other disorders, skin problems are easiest to diagnose and treat at an early stage. They are also less likely to cause permanent scarring if they are cleared up quickly.

water; exposure to rough, scratchy, tight clothing (especially woolens); use of harsh soaps; or emotional stress or nervousness.

Diagnosis Atopic eczema can often be diagnosed by the symptoms. In some cases, it is necessary for the dermatologist to rule out other disorders—such as contact dermatitis (see below), a fungal disease (such as athlete's foot), or a bacterial infection—that may cause similar symptoms.

Treatment If you are diagnosed with atopic eczema, your doctor will recommend preventing exposure of your skin to irritants, such as harsh soaps and wool clothing. He or she may also recommend that you avoid frequent or long showers or baths and bathe only in lukewarm (not hot) water. You should use a good moisturizer and apply it generously and frequently, including immediately after bathing. An over-the-counter hydrocortisone cream may help reduce the inflammation and itching. Topical preparations that contain coal tar are also sometimes used for treating eczema. In severe, chronic cases, a doctor may prescribe synthetic hormones called corticosteroids (either in a topical solution or in pills), which reduce inflammation, or ultraviolet light therapy.

CONTACT DERMATITIS

Contact dermatitis, sometimes called allergic dermatitis, is a reaction of the skin to exposure to a particular substance (allergen). Contact dermatitis is triggered by a substance that does not cause a reaction in most people.

The following substances are common causes of contact dermatitis:

- Poison ivy or poison oak
- Nickel or copper, which are metals often used in jewelry (especially earrings), zippers, and belt buckles
- Rubber, often used in shoes, belts, and stretchy garments
- Hair dyes
- Chromates, which are chemicals found in paints, glues, disinfectants, and bleaches

If you have a persistent rash, see a dermatologist. You and your doctor can work together to determine the cause of your allergic reaction so that you can avoid contact with it in the future.

Symptoms Contact dermatitis usually begins with redness and swelling of the skin in the affected area; small, raised areas; or fluid-filled blisters. The blisters may break and crust over. If the irritation persists, your skin may become leathery, dark, and cracked.

Diagnosis It is sometimes difficult to distinguish contact dermatitis from other forms of dermatitis or rashes. A thorough medical history and a physical examination can often uncover the source of the problem. Your doctor will ask about your possible exposure to common allergy-causing substances.

If the diagnosis is uncertain, your doctor may perform a biopsy of the affected area of skin. For a biopsy, a small sample of skin is sent to a laboratory for evaluation. If it looks like you have contact dermatitis, your doctor may recommend a skin test to determine the specific allergen that is causing your problem. In this test, your skin is exposed to a small amount of a particular substance and examined to see if it reacts.

Treatment The main treatment of contact dermatitis is to avoid exposure to the substance that is causing your skin reaction. If necessary, wear gloves or other protective clothing to reduce your exposure. For many people, switching to different detergents, cosmetics, or other products eliminates the problem.

Do not scratch the affected area, because you may open the blisters and

Rashes

A rash is an area of red, inflamed skin or a group of spots on the skin. A rash can be a symptom of many different problems or disorders—such as contact with a substance to which you are allergic (contact dermatitis), eczema (see page 673), or an infectious disease, such as measles. In some cases, the cause of a rash is not determined. If you have an unfamiliar rash and the cause is not obvious to you, see your doctor immediately.

allow bacteria to enter them and cause infection. Applying an over-the-counter cream or ointment that contains hydrocortisone to the affected area may help relieve the itching. In severe cases, a doctor may prescribe pills that contain corticosteroids (synthetic hormones that help reduce inflammation).

SEBORRHEIC DERMATITIS

Seborrheic dermatitis is characterized by inflammation in areas of the skin that have the most sebaceous glands, which secrete oil into the skin. The cause of seborrheic dermatitis is unknown, but it is often triggered by stress. Moisture from perspiration that remains trapped between folds of skin (such as those under the breasts or arms or in the genital area) may encourage the growth of a yeast or other fungus, which can worsen the symptoms.

Symptoms The condition causes persistent, itchy dandruff on the scalp or patches of oily, scaly, red skin, usually on the sides of the nose, behind the ears, along the eyebrows or eyelids, or in the middle of the chest.

Diagnosis Seborrheic dermatitis is diagnosed by an examination of the affected areas of skin. Your doctor will rule out other causes of your symptoms, such as a yeast infection.

Treatment Seborrheic dermatitis may subside without treatment, but usually recurs. If you have seborrheic dermatitis, your doctor may recommend an over-the-counter hydrocortisone cream or ointment to help reduce the redness and itching. If you have dandruff, your doctor may recommend an over-the-counter antidandruff shampoo. Use the shampoo every day, making sure to rinse it out thoroughly. Avoid scratching or picking the affected areas, which can worsen the problem.

Other common skin disorders

Acne and noncancerous growths, such as moles and warts, are some of the most common skin problems. Acne can now be treated effectively with medication, but it is extremely important to see a doctor as soon as signs of acne appear. The earlier acne is treated and cleared up, the less likely it is to cause permanent scarring.

ACNE

Acne is a common disorder that causes blemishes on the skin, usually on the face, chest, and back. An acne blemish, which appears on your skin as a whitehead or blackhead, occurs when a plug of an oily substance called sebum becomes blocked inside a hair follicle. Your skin contains millions of hair follicles—tiny tubelike structures through which hairs grow. Each hair follicle has a sebaceous gland that secretes sebum, which lubricates the hair and the surrounding skin.

Most women have acne at some time in their life. People with oily skin are more likely to have acne than other people. You are also more likely to have acne if your parents or siblings had it. Acne is especially common during adolescence, when hormonal changes stimulate the sebaceous glands to produce more sebum. For both teens and adult women, the hormonal fluctuations of the menstrual cycle can cause a flare-up of acne around the time of their period. In many people, acne can be triggered by stress.

For some people, acne is a persistent problem from adolescence through early adulthood that causes permanent scarring and a loss of self-esteem and confidence that deeply affects their life. Some people continue to experience severe acne long after adolescence or develop acne for the first time in their 20s or 30s.

Some medications can affect acne. Most birth-control pills decrease outbreaks of acne, particularly if the pills contain a higher dose of the female hormone estrogen and a smaller dose or milder form of the hormone progestin. Pills with more estrogen decrease the production of oil, which can reduce acne. Pills with a larger amount or stronger form of progestin can trigger new outbreaks of acne or worsen the condition. Other medications that can make acne worse include corticosteroids,

HOW A BLEMISH FORMS

In healthy skin (top), the sebaceous gland in a hair follicle secretes an oily substance called sebum to lubricate the hair and the surrounding skin. A pimple or blemish forms when sebum secreted from the sebaceous gland mixes with dead skin cells and forms a blockage in a hair follicle. A blockage that occurs near the skin's surface becomes a blackhead (center); a blockage deeper in the skin becomes a whitehead (bottom).

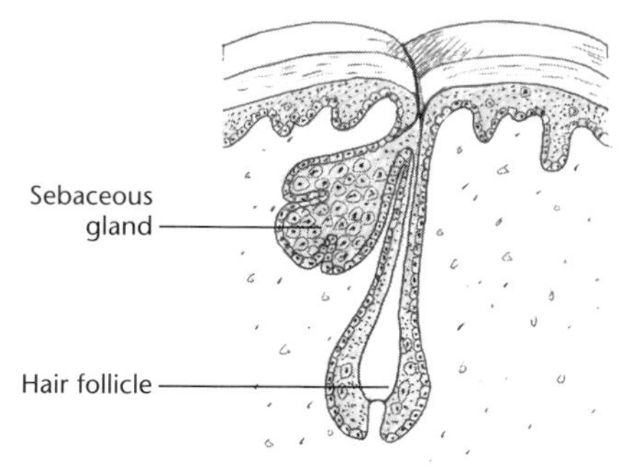

Healthy skin

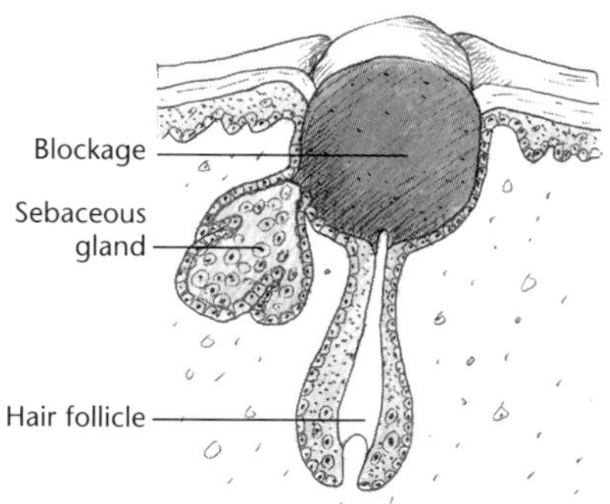

Blackhead

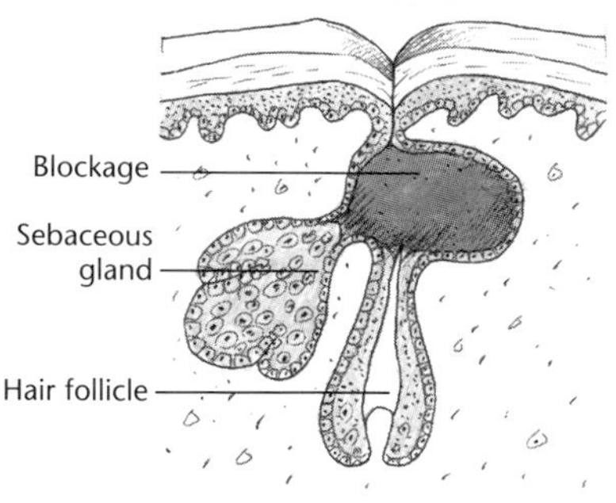

Whitehead

synthetic hormones used for treating inflammatory illnesses; lithium, used for treating some mental disorders (see page 602; and phenytoin, used for treating epilepsy (see page 578).

Many people with acne, especially teens, do not seek treatment from a doctor. But getting treatment as early as possible increases your chances of clearing up the condition and preventing permanent scarring. Many effective medications are available for treating acne.

Symptoms Acne can cause several kinds of blemishes. A blackhead results when dead skin cells and sebum block a hair follicle near the surface of the skin. The mixture of pigment (the protein that gives skin its color) from the dead skin cells and sebum makes a blackhead dark; it is not dirt that can be washed away. A whitehead occurs when a plug of sebum blocks a hair follicle deeper in the skin. Whiteheads and blackheads sometimes develop into pus-filled blemishes called pustules. Pustules that are near the surface of the skin usually break and disappear quickly. Deeper, larger pustules require treatment by a dermatologist.

Diagnosis Acne is diagnosed by its characteristic appearance.

Treatment If your acne is severe, see a dermatologist. He or she can answer your questions and recommend appropriate treatment. If you are prone to acne, your doctor is likely to recommend keeping your skin clean and free of oil. You may need to wash it two or three times a day with mild soap. Soap and water remove sebum, bacteria, and dead skin cells that can contribute to the problem. Wash your skin gently. Keeping your skin clean does not prevent acne but dirty, oily skin can aggravate acne if you already have it. Scrubbing or using harsh soaps or abrasive cleansers can irritate your skin and make acne worse. Do not use oil-based moisturizers on blemished areas.

Although some people who have acne find that moderate exposure to the sun improves their skin's condition, do not consider this a treatment. Any exposure to the sun increases your risk of developing skin cancer later in life. For the same reason, sun lamps or tanning beds are not recommended for treating acne.

Some over-the-counter preparations that you apply to blemishes can be effective for treating acne. Medications that contain a chemical called benzoyl peroxide kill bacteria inside hair follicles, reduce inflammation, and help dry up oil on the surface of the skin. Your doctor may recommend starting with a 2.5 percent solution of benzoyl peroxide and then increase it to a 5- or 10-percent

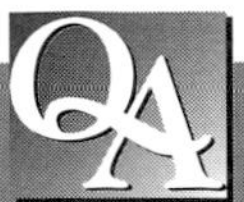

Questions Women Ask
Acne

Q My friend says that eating chocolate gives her pimples, and another friend won't eat french fries for the same reason. Do these foods cause acne?

A No. You cannot get acne from eating chocolate or fatty foods. Diet has little or no influence on outbreaks of acne. Your production of sebum, the oil in your skin that contributes to acne blemishes, is influenced by your hormones rather than by any fat in your diet. For help in treating acne, see a dermatologist, a doctor who specializes in skin disorders.

Q Whenever final exams come around, my skin breaks out. Does stress cause acne?

A Yes, emotional stress can cause acne to flare up. In addition, many people pick at their blemishes when they are under stress, which can cause more damage and scarring. Wash your hands frequently and try to keep them away from your face.

Q When I became pregnant, my acne cleared up. Why?

A The increased level in your body of the female hormone estrogen during pregnancy improved the condition of your skin. An increase in estrogen can cause the sebaceous glands in the skin to produce less oil. However, in some women, pregnancy makes acne worse. You must not take acne medications, such as isotretinoin, during pregnancy because of the risk of birth defects in the fetus. Make sure you ask your doctor about any acne medications you are taking if you plan to become pregnant.

solution if necessary. Benzoyl peroxide can cause your skin to become dry and peel. If so, talk to your doctor about the concentration of the solution you are using and how often you should apply it. Your doctor may recommend a gentle, nonoily moisturizer to help reduce the dryness and peeling.

Your doctor may prescribe a medicated cream, gel, or liquid that contains tretinoin, a substance that is chemically related to vitamin A. Tretinoin speeds up the process by which old skin cells are sloughed off and replaced by new cells. The medication—which you apply to the affected skin—is safe and effective for preventing blackheads and whiteheads. However, if you are using tretinoin, you must protect the treated areas of skin from exposure to the sun because the treated skin is more susceptible to sun damage. Always use a sunscreen with a sun protection factor (SPF) of 15 or more, and wear a hat and protective clothing. Do not use tretinoin during pregnancy because its effects on the fetus are not known.

Your doctor may prescribe an antibiotic in a liquid that you apply to the affected skin. The antibiotic penetrates the hair follicles and decreases inflammation by eliminating the bacteria that can contribute to the development of acne blemishes. If the antibiotic liquid does not adequately control your acne, your doctor may prescribe antibiotics in pill form to help reduce the inflammation.

Blackheads and whiteheads should be treated only by a doctor to avoid infection or scarring. He or she can carefully

When you get a pimple

As tempting as it may be, do not squeeze a whitehead or blackhead. Doing so can damage your skin or spread bacteria. Using a needle or other device to open a blemish can cause infection or permanent scarring. If the blemish does not go away on its own, see a dermatologist, who can treat it easily.

squeeze out the plug of sebum and dead skin cells from the blocked hair follicle using instruments that will not harm your skin. For some blemishes, minor surgery using local anesthesia may be necessary. Pus-filled blemishes (pustules) may be treated by injecting corticosteroids into them to reduce inflammation. After your acne is under control, your doctor may recommend a procedure, such as a chemical peel (see page 695) or dermabrasion (see page 697), to diminish scarring.

A powerful medication called isotretinoin is used to treat severe cases of acne that can be disfiguring. Isotretinoin is prescribed only after other acne medications have been tried and have not been effective in clearing up the condition. Your doctor will caution you that you must not use isotretinoin if there is any possibility that you may become pregnant while you are taking the medication or for 1 month after you stop taking it because the drug can cause birth defects in a fetus. Before prescribing isotretinoin, your doctor will carefully discuss these serious risks. You will probably be asked to have a pregnancy test 2 weeks before you begin taking the medication and at regular intervals while you are taking it.

ROSACEA

Rosacea is a skin disorder that makes the nose and cheeks red and blotchy. It usually occurs in people who have a tendency to flush. The disorder may begin with occasional flare-ups that are triggered by a number of factors—including hot or cold air, a strong wind, hot beverages, alcoholic beverages, vigorous exercise, exposure to sunlight, hot flashes during menopause, spicy foods, or emotional stress. Flare-ups may gradually become more frequent; in some cases, the condition becomes persistent.

Rosacea, which is most common among women who have fair skin, usually appears after 35. The cause is not fully understood, but it may be an allergic reaction to the tiny insects (mites) that live in the hair follicles of the skin.

Symptoms Occasional flushing around the nose and cheeks gradually becomes more frequent and progresses to blotches and bumps. In the advanced stage of rosacea, small blood vessels called capillaries appear on the skin and the nose may swell.

Diagnosis Rosacea is usually diagnosed by the symptoms and the appearance of the skin.

Treatment Rosacea is most easily treated in the early stages. In later stages, the symptoms and damage to the skin can be difficult or even impossible to treat. Your doctor is likely to recommend limiting or avoiding exposure to those things that trigger your flare-ups, such as alcohol, hot beverages, or spicy foods. In addition, your doctor may prescribe an antibiotic in pill form that you take every day or an antibiotic ointment that you apply every day to the affected area of your skin. You may have to use the antibiotic for several months or indefinitely. It is also important to protect your skin by applying sunscreen with a sun protection factor (SPF) of at least 15 and a moisturizer every day.

PSORIASIS

Psoriasis is a skin disease that causes thick, scaly, itchy, dry skin, usually on the scalp, elbows, or knees. In psoriasis, new cells in the epidermis (the outermost layer of cells) are made faster than old cells are shed in affected areas of the skin, causing dead skin cells to accumulate in those areas. This accumulation of cells causes the skin to thicken. The condition can range from mild and hardly noticeable to severe and covering the entire body. Psoriasis is not contagious. The condition has a genetic component; it tends to run in families.

In many people, psoriasis has periods (called flare-ups) in which it is active and periods in which it causes no symptoms (called remissions). Flare-ups can be triggered by stress, excessive consumption of alcohol, or an infection.

Symptoms Psoriasis often begins with red patches on the skin. These patches gradually grow and silvery-white scales appear on them. The surfaces begin to flake off and the patches grow and may merge together to cover a large area of skin on your elbows, scalp, knees, genitals, arms, or legs. Psoriasis usually appears in the same place on both sides of the body. Your fingernails and toenails may also be affected. Psoriasis can cause pitting, thickening, or crumbling of the nails, or separation of the nail from the skin. Psoriasis sometimes appears in folds of skin, such as those under the breasts, between the buttocks, or in the genital area.

Diagnosis Psoriasis is usually diagnosed by its characteristic appearance. In rare cases in which the symptoms are not obvious, a sample of tissue (biopsy) may be sent to a laboratory for examination under a microscope.

Treatment If you have psoriasis, avoid picking or scratching at the affected areas of your skin and do not use hot water or strong soaps. Use moisturizing creams or lotions to reduce dryness and itching. Over-the-counter shampoos, soaps, lotions, creams, and ointments that contain salicylic acid or coal tar may help reduce itching and redness. The shampoos work best if you leave the lather on your head for at least 5 minutes before rinsing.

Although moderate exposure to sunlight may improve some areas of psoriasis, a sunburn can make the condition worse. If psoriasis affects more than a third of your body, your doctor may prescribe treatments with ultraviolet light (phototherapy). Prescription creams or ointments that contain corticosteroids may help relieve inflammation and other symptoms. However, long-term use of corticosteroids may cause thinning of the skin or changes in skin color. When you stop taking the medication, the psoriasis may return.

In severe, disabling cases, psoriasis may be treated with a powerful medication called methotrexate or a form of vitamin A called etretinate. You can take these medications in pills for as long as your symptoms persist or your doctor thinks is necessary. Your doctor will monitor your condition closely while you are taking either of these drugs because they can cause serious side effects such as liver damage. You cannot take them if you are pregnant, if you are planning to become pregnant, or if you are not using reliable birth control because both drugs are linked to birth defects. If you are ever planning to become pregnant in the future, talk to your doctor about these serious but potential risks before you make a decision about using either of these medications for your psoriasis.

NONCANCEROUS GROWTHS

Abnormal growths on the skin—such as moles, age spots (also called liver spots), and warts—are common. Most of these growths are noncancerous (benign) and harmless and do not require treatment.

Actinic keratosis Actinic keratosis is a skin disorder characterized by patches of reddish brown, raised, scaly skin that result from long-term overexposure to the sun. Actinic keratosis is most common in people with fair skin. The patches appear most often on the face and hands. Although the condition is not serious, you should have your doctor examine any abnormalities on your skin. These skin patches are a sign of early skin changes that could lead to skin cancer. In a small percentage of cases, actinic keratosis develops into squamous cell skin cancer (see page 684).

To prevent these areas of actinic keratosis from becoming cancerous, your doctor is likely to recommend removing them by applying medication to them, or freezing, burning, or cutting them out surgically. If your doctor feels it necessary, he or she may perform a biopsy and send a small tissue sample to the laboratory to rule out the presence of cancer cells.

Cherry angiomas Cherry angiomas are small, harmless, red bumps that may appear on the skin, usually on the trunk, arms, or legs. Cherry angiomas, which usually begin to appear after age 30, are composed of tightly packed clusters of very small blood vessels, which give them their red color. You should avoid scratching a cherry angioma because it can bleed heavily. Angiomas do not need to be treated or removed for medical reasons. But some people have them removed because they find them unattractive. Cherry angiomas are usually removed by electrical burning or laser surgery (which uses high-energy beams of light to destroy tissue).

Skin tags Skin tags are small, protruding flaps of skin that usually appear on the neck, armpits, upper trunk, or in folds of skin, such as those under the breasts. Skin tags are soft and may be the same color as your skin or dark like a mole. Skin tags are common and usually appear after age 20. They are harmless but may be irritated by friction. If your skin tag is in a location where it is constantly being irritated or if it bleeds, you may want to have it removed. Your doctor can remove it by cutting it out or burning it. People rarely have a scar after either treatment.

Age spots Age spots, also known as liver spots, are flat, brown or black spots on the hands or face. These harmless spots are areas of increased pigmentation (coloring) that can be as small as a freckle or several inches across. Age spots, which result from long-term exposure to the sun, do not need to be treated. However, some people find them unattractive and choose to have them lightened by bleaching or removed by freezing (cryotherapy) or laser therapy (treatment using high-energy beams of light). Use sunscreen with a sun protection factor (SPF) of 15 or higher to prevent age spots from reappearing. Have your doctor examine any age spots because, in rare cases, they may be early changes that could lead to the most serious form of skin cancer, malignant melanoma (see page 684).

Moles Most moles are harmless clusters of cells that produce the pigment melanin, which gives them their dark color. Some moles contain dark hairs. Many moles appear during childhood and do not need to be removed unless they begin to change in appearance, which may indicate they are cancerous. Moles that are present at birth, especially larger ones, are more likely than other moles to develop into cancer. If you have a mole that has been present since birth, ask your dermatologist if you should have it removed. Moles are removed by cutting them out.

It is important to monitor all of your moles for changes in their color, size, or shape, which can be a sign of malignant melanoma (see page 684), the most deadly form of skin cancer. During pregnancy, your moles may darken or enlarge; these changes are usually nothing to worry about. However, it is a good idea to ask your obstetrician or dermatologist to evaluate any moles that change during your pregnancy. The moles may or may not return to their usual color or size after pregnancy.

Seborrheic keratosis Seborrheic keratosis is a common skin disorder that is characterized by yellow, brown, or black growths that usually appear on the face, hands, shoulders, and chest. The cause is unknown. Seborrheic keratosis occurs most often in adults who have fair skin. The growths are waxy, oval, and slightly elevated and often look like warts. They may appear in clusters. The growths are painless and seldom require treatment unless a person finds them unattractive, itchy, or irritating. They can be removed by freezing, scraping, or cutting.

Warts Warts are small, firm, flesh-colored lumps that can appear anywhere on the skin, but occur most often on the hands and feet. Warts are caused by a virus that infects skin cells, making them grow rapidly. Because warts are contagious, you should avoid touching warts on someone else's skin. If you have warts, keep them from coming into contact with other people's skin. Warts that occur on the soles of the feet, called plantar warts, tend to grow inward, causing pain. Warts may go away on their own within about 2 years, or you may be able to dissolve the wart with an over-the-counter medication. If this treatment fails, your doctor can prescribe a stronger medication for you to use at home. Your doctor can remove a wart by cutting, freezing, or burning it, or by laser surgery (treatment using high-energy beams of light to destroy tissue).

VITILIGO

Vitiligo is a common disorder of skin pigmentation in which areas of skin lose their color. The disorder is thought to be an autoimmune disease (a disease in which the immune system attacks the body's own cells); the immune system mistakenly identifies the pigment-producing cells (melanocytes) as foreign cells and attacks them. The resulting lack of melanocytes causes areas of the skin—most often in symmetrical areas on the face, hands, armpits, and groin—to look lighter or white. These areas are most noticeable on people with dark skin. Although vitiligo can occur at any age, it usually develops in early adulthood.

In mild cases, vitiligo requires no treatment. You may want to use makeup to hide the affected skin. Because these areas of skin do not have the pigment melanin, which provides protection against damage from the sun, you should avoid exposing them to the sun. Wear protective clothing and always wear sunscreen with a sun protection factor (SPF) of at least 15.

Creams that contain corticosteroids (synthetic hormones) may help restore some of the natural pigment to the skin. Your doctor may recommend treatment using ultraviolet light (phototherapy), which is effective in many cases. For phototherapy to be successful, you must have several treatments.

Skin cancer

Skin cancer, which usually results from prolonged exposure to the sun, is the most common type of cancer. Most skin cancers are treatable and curable, but one form, malignant melanoma, can be fatal. Malignant melanoma is increasing at a faster rate than any other cancer because of the popularity of outdoor recreation and suntans. Skin cancer occurs most often on those areas of the body that are repeatedly exposed to the sun—the face, chest, back, shoulders, and legs.

Skin cancer is easy to avoid. You can prevent skin cancer by protecting your skin from the sun (see page 671). If you do develop skin cancer, the earlier it is detected the easier and more effective treatment is likely to be. Because women tend to discover skin cancer at an earlier stage than men, the overall cure rate of skin cancer in women is higher than that in men. Whenever you have a checkup, ask your doctor to examine your skin for signs of cancer.

BASAL CELL CANCER

Basal cell cancer, the most common form of skin cancer, occurs in cells in the top layer of the skin. Long-term exposure to the sun is the major cause of basal cell cancer. You are at increased risk of developing this form of skin cancer if you have a family history of the cancer or if you have fair skin. Because basal cell cancer rarely spreads from the original site to other parts of the body, it is seldom life threatening. However, if it is not detected at an early stage and treated, it can advance and spread to nearby tissues, including nerves, bones, or the brain.

Symptoms You may notice a firm, pearly, or waxy-looking lump, or a flat, skin-colored or brown spot that resembles a scar. A basal cell cancer sometimes looks like a sore that never heals.

Diagnosis Your doctor may suspect basal cell cancer by its appearance. To diagnose the cancer, he or she will do a

Examine your skin regularly

Examine all the skin on your body every month for signs of new growths or changes in existing ones. Pay closest attention to those areas of your body that are most frequently and directly exposed to the sun and are, therefore, the most susceptible to cancer—including your scalp, face, ears, shoulders, chest, back, arms, legs, the backs of your hands, and the tops of your feet. Follow these steps each time you do a self-examination:

- Examine your body, front and back, in a mirror. Look at your shoulders, and raise your arms and look at your right and left sides.
- Still standing in front of a mirror, use a hand mirror to look at the back of your neck and the top and back of each ear. Lift parts of your hair all over your head to examine your scalp. Examine your back and buttocks.
- Bend your elbows and look carefully at your forearms, the backs of your upper arms, and the backs of your hands.
- Examine the tops and bottoms of your feet and the spaces between your toes.

biopsy. For a biopsy, the doctor removes all or part of the suspicious lump or spot and sends it to a laboratory to be examined under a microscope for cancer cells.

Treatment Treatment of basal cell cancer depends on the size, depth, and location of the cancer. In most cases, a tumor is cut out surgically in a simple procedure using local anesthesia. You will probably have a flat, white scar afterward.

In an alternative procedure, the tumor is shaved off one layer at a time. As each layer is removed, it is examined under a microscope for cancer cells until all the cancerous layers have been removed. Other treatments for basal cell cancer include freezing (cryosurgery) or electrosurgery, which uses an electrical device to destroy cancer cells.

If the tumor is large, you may need to have a skin graft using skin from another part of your body to replace the missing tissue. Radiation therapy (see page 253) can also be an effective treatment for basal cell cancer. In most cases, basal cell cancer is completely cured. However, you should continue to see your doctor for regular checkups to monitor your skin for abnormal growths.

SQUAMOUS CELL CANCER

Squamous cell cancer, which occurs in cells in the top layer of skin, begins as a small, firm, painless lump or patch on the skin that slowly enlarges. Squamous cell cancer is much less common than basal cell cancer. Like basal cell cancer, it is caused by exposure to the sun and occurs in areas of the skin that are most often exposed to the sun, especially the face, lips, ears, or backs of the hands. Squamous cell cancer is more aggressive than basal cell cancer—it spreads more rapidly and can be fatal. However, when the cancer is detected and treated at an early stage, it is almost always curable. Your risk of squamous cell cancer is increased if you have fair skin.

Symptoms A squamous cell tumor is a firm, skin-colored or red lump or a scaly or crusted patch on the skin that is usually painless. It may look like a sore that never heals. It may become painful if it forms an ulcer (open sore) or bleeds. A squamous cell tumor usually begins in normal skin, but it can also develop in a burn, a scar, or a precancerous skin tumor that can occur in a condition such as actinic keratosis (see page 681).

Diagnosis Your doctor may suspect squamous cell cancer by its appearance. To diagnose the cancer, he or she will perform a biopsy. For a biopsy, a small sample of tissue is removed from the tumor and sent to the laboratory for examination under a microscope for the presence of cancer cells.

Treatment Most squamous cell tumors are removed by cutting them out or burning (electrocautery). The cure rate for squamous cell cancer is very high if it is detected at an early stage.

MALIGNANT MELANOMA

Malignant melanoma is the most serious form of skin cancer; it affects the pigment-producing cells of the skin (called melanocytes). When not detected early, malignant melanoma often spreads to the lymph nodes (infection-fighting glands) and other parts of the body. Unlike squamous cell and basal cell cancers, melanoma often develops in a mole that has been present since childhood. Moles that are present at birth, especially larger ones, are more likely than other moles to eventually become cancerous. If you have a mole that has been present since birth, ask your dermatologist if you should have it removed. However, melanoma can also develop in a newer mole or in normal skin.

The incidence of malignant melanoma is increasing dramatically—faster than any other kind of cancer—because more people are spending their leisure time outdoors in the sun. Long-term exposure to the sun or a family history of melanoma increases your risk of developing malignant melanoma. Melanoma is most common in people with fair skin and usually occurs on the trunk, arms, or lower legs. But blacks and other people with dark skin are not immune to malignant melanoma; in people with darker skin, the cancer usually develops on the palms of the hands or soles of the feet.

Melanoma has the potential to spread rapidly and be fatal. Do not delay seeing your doctor if you notice any of the symptoms of malignant melanoma described here.

Symptoms The most common sign of malignant melanoma is a change in the size, shape, or color of a mole. The mole may begin to grow or to have an irregular shape or to become lighter or darker in color. It may develop a darker border that spreads into the surrounding skin. It may bleed without being scratched, or become itchy. In time, the mole may become thicker and lumpy. Be especially vigilant about watching for changes in a mole that you have had since birth, which is more likely to develop into malignant melanoma than other moles.

Diagnosis If your doctor thinks a spot on your skin may be melanoma, he or she will recommend removing all or part of it for examination.

WARNING SIGNS
MALIGNANT MELANOMA

See your doctor immediately if you notice a change in a mole or any of the following signs of melanoma. These are the "ABCDs" of skin cancer detection:

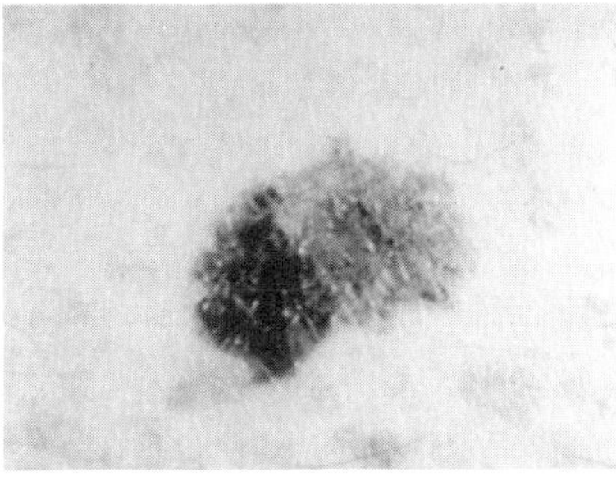

ASYMMETRY
A mole is asymmetrical if you draw an imaginary line down the middle of it and each side is a different size and shape.

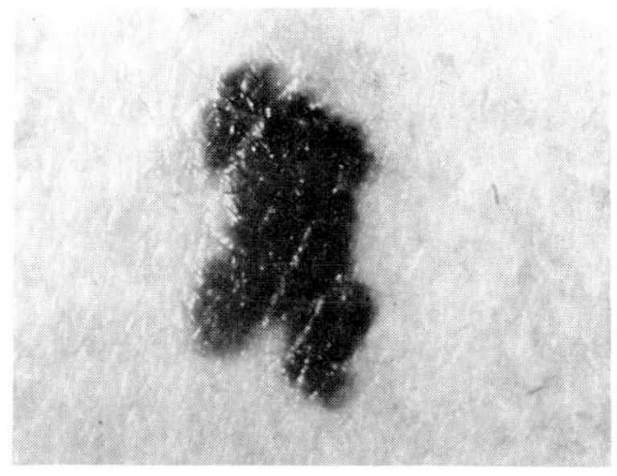

BORDER
The border of the mole is irregular or blurred, not smooth and distinct.

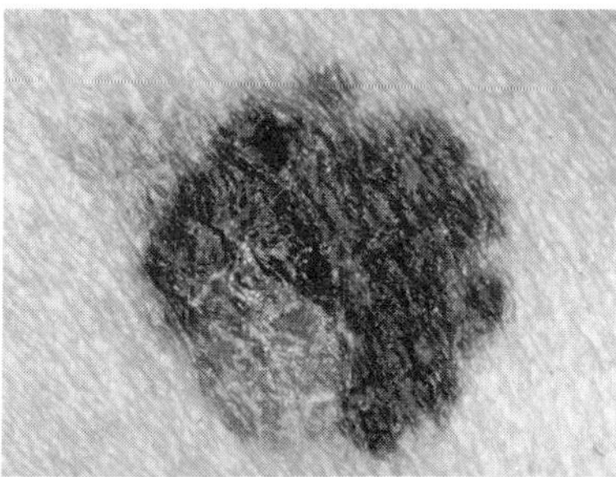

COLOR
While most moles are a solid color, a melanoma has more than one shade or color, including black, blue, brown, red, and white.

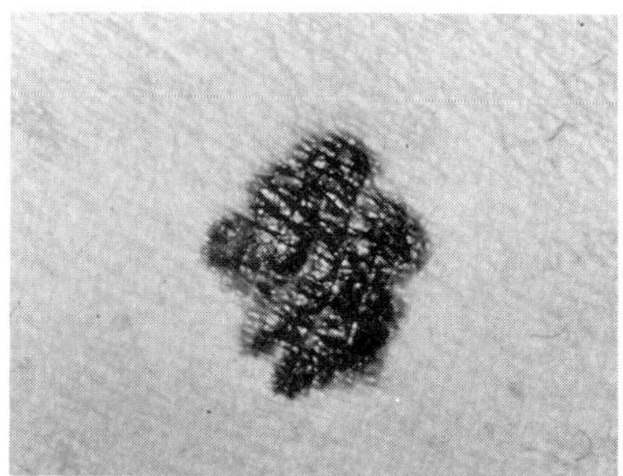

DIAMETER
Consider suspicious any mole that is larger around than a pencil eraser, especially if it is growing.

Treatment If laboratory examination of the suspicious area of your skin detects melanoma, your doctor will need to evaluate the stage of the cancer. The stage of the cancer is determined by its thickness and depth, and whether or not it has spread to lymph nodes or other parts of your body. In most cases, treatment of melanoma involves cutting out the cancerous tissue and some of the tissue surrounding it. If a large area of your skin is removed, you may need to have a skin graft using skin from another part of your body. With or without a skin graft, you are likely to have some scarring after the surgery.

If the melanoma is deep or has spread to other parts of your body, it is likely to recur after treatment. In this case, your doctor may recommend chemotherapy, treatment with powerful drugs that can kill cancer cells throughout your body. For more about chemotherapy and its side effects, see page 254. For information about coping with cancer treatments, see page 255.

CHAPTER 28

Elective cosmetic surgery

Contents

Cosmetic surgery is plastic surgery that is usually performed to improve a person's appearance. This includes procedures to tighten aging or sagging skin, improve the appearance of scars, reshape the nose, change the size or shape of breasts, or remove body fat. Cosmetic surgery is not essential for maintaining good health. This chapter does not discuss plastic surgery that is considered medically necessary, such as a skin graft to replace skin after a severe burn or reconstructive surgery after an accident. For information about breast reconstruction after mastectomy, see page 286.

Considering cosmetic surgery

If you are thinking about having a cosmetic surgical procedure, consider your expectations and choose your surgeon carefully. As with any elective (nonessential) surgical procedure, it is important to recognize and fully understand both the benefits and the risks of any cosmetic procedure you are considering.

YOUR EXPECTATIONS

If you have realistic expectations about what cosmetic surgery can do for you, you are much more likely to be pleased with the results. Before you have any cosmetic surgical procedure, talk to your plastic surgeon about your reasons for wanting to have the surgery and about your expectations. A procedure that might be right for one person may not suit another. Ask your doctor to describe the procedure in detail, including the use of anesthesia and the recovery period. Before you make your decision, consider the following:

- **Your reasons** The decision to have cosmetic surgery is a personal one. You are more likely to be comfortable with the results of a cosmetic surgical procedure if you are having it to satisfy yourself, rather than to please another person or in response to peer pressure. If you feel that a cosmetic surgical procedure will improve a feature you are unhappy with, cosmetic surgery may be an appropriate choice. However, you will be disappointed if you expect a procedure to help you find the perfect mate or earn you a job promotion. (For information about improving your self-esteem and emotional well-being, see page 183.)
- **The results you expect** It is possible for a person who has had cosmetic surgery to be disappointed with the results, even though the surgeon considers the procedure highly successful. For example, eyelid surgery (blepharoplasty, see page 692) can reduce the amount of sagging skin above and below your eyes, but it will not make you look 30 if you are 50. Gathering as much information as you can and knowing what to expect before the surgery can help prevent such disappointment.
- **Recovery** Some people assume that because cosmetic procedures are elective, recovery from them will be quicker or easier than from other forms of surgery. This is not true. As with any type of surgery, after cosmetic surgery you may feel tired or even exhausted as your body heals. Although you will not feel pain during the procedure itself, you may feel discomfort or pain afterward. At first, you may not be able to do some of your usual activities. You may choose to limit your social activities for a period of time after the procedure because bruising and swelling can affect your appearance.

Planning ahead

Here are some steps to take before cosmetic surgery so you know what to expect afterward:

- Ask your doctor how extensive the surgery will be and how long it will take for you to feel perfectly normal again.
- Let your family know in advance about any bruising, swelling, or scarring you may have on your face or body after surgery. Make sure that family members understand that you will need a period of time to recover fully.
- Find out what kinds of activities you will need to avoid and for how long.
- Prepare yourself for postoperative letdown; the immediate results of your surgery may not be apparent until all the swelling or bruising is gone. Ask your doctor how long it will take before you will see the full effects of the surgery.

Smoking and cosmetic surgery

If you are going to have cosmetic surgery, your doctor will ask you to stop smoking for at least 1 to 2 weeks before and after the surgery. Smoking slows the healing process. If you are having surgery on your face, quitting can improve the long-term results of the surgery. Smoking can cause the skin on your face to wrinkle and sag prematurely (see page 672). Your surgery may be the motivation you need to give up cigarettes permanently. For information about how to quit smoking, see page 157.

■ **Cost** Elective cosmetic procedures are expensive and are seldom covered by health insurance. Make sure you ask your doctor about all the costs of a cosmetic procedure you are considering. Find out what portion, if any, is covered by your health insurance.

After you have carefully weighed the benefits and risks of having cosmetic surgery, you may decide it is the right choice for you. The next step is to carefully select a skilled plastic surgeon who is experienced in performing the procedure.

CHOOSING A PLASTIC SURGEON

To find a skilled doctor to perform cosmetic surgery, begin by asking your primary care doctor or gynecologist for a recommendation. Some doctors who use the title "cosmetic surgeon" may not have undergone specialized training in the field. Look for a plastic surgeon who is trained in reconstructive surgery and is certified by the American Board of Plastic Surgery. Ask doctors what type of board certification they have.

Another qualification to look for is an office or clinic that has been inspected and certified by the American Association for Accreditation of Ambulatory Plastic Surgery Facilities. Ask if the doctor is affiliated with a hospital, even if your procedure will be done in his or her office; hospitals require surgeons to meet a variety of criteria before granting them operating room privileges.

After training and board certification, experience is the most important qualification to look for in a skilled plastic surgeon. Choose a doctor who has performed your particular procedure many times. In your initial consultation with the surgeon, ask specific questions about the procedure you are considering and its risks. Be wary if the doctor plays down the risks. He or she should ask why you want the procedure. An experienced doctor will try to make sure your expectations are realistic and, if they are

New techniques for cosmetic surgery

Newer medical techniques, such as laser surgery, are frequently described as technological breakthroughs that reduce scarring, bruising, and recovery time after cosmetic surgery. It is important to carefully weigh the risks and potential benefits when you are considering a procedure performed with laser surgery or any other new technique. New is not necessarily better. Traditional surgical methods have the advantage of time and experience and proven value.

■ **Laser surgery** A laser is a powerful, highly focused beam of light that can cut and remove tissue, and control bleeding. For many cosmetic procedures, the benefits of using laser surgery have not yet been well established.

Laser techniques may be used in some types of cosmetic procedures on the face (such as the removal of a large birthmark) because lasers can reduce the amount of bleeding and swelling. The results of laser surgery and the recovery time are often the same as those of traditional surgery. In some cases, laser surgery can cost more and cause more complications, such as burns or tissue damage.

■ **Endoscopy** Endoscopy—a technique that has been widely used to diagnose and treat gynecologic and digestive disorders—enables a surgeon to view the surgical site using a lighted instrument (endoscope) with a tiny camera at its tip. The endoscope can be inserted through a very small incision, thereby avoiding the large scars that sometimes result from traditional methods. Endoscopy is now being used in some cosmetic procedures, such as brow lifts (see page 693). However, the technique has not yet been perfected for most cosmetic procedures and, like any surgical procedure, carries risks. Before having a cosmetic surgical procedure that uses endoscopy, make sure your plastic surgeon has extensive experience with this technique.

not, may recommend against having the procedure.

The cost of cosmetic procedures varies widely but can run into thousands of dollars. Shop around, but do not make price your primary concern. Having the procedure done properly by a skilled surgeon is more important than the cost.

Facial surgery

The best approach to a more youthful appearance is to prevent wrinkling and other signs of aging by avoiding exposure to the sun and not smoking. Still, as you grow older, you will begin to notice signs of aging on your face, and facial surgery is one way to counteract them. If you are considering cosmetic facial surgery to diminish the effects of aging, keep in mind that wrinkles and sagging will gradually reappear, especially if you continue to subject your skin to damage from the sun or smoke cigarettes. For more about how to prevent wrinkles, see page 672. For more about reducing your exposure to the sun, see page 671.

Do facial exercises work?

Facial exercises and massage are sometimes recommended as "natural facelifts" to help you look younger. However, the benefits of facial exercises and massage are unproven and these measures should be viewed with skepticism. Excessive movement of the muscles of your face and the application of pressure to your skin may actually cause wrinkles by damaging the protein collagen, which gives skin its support.

FACELIFT

A facelift (rhytidectomy) is a surgical procedure that tightens loose skin and sagging muscles on your face, jaw, and neck. Excess fat in these areas is often removed at the same time. A facelift cannot stop or reverse the aging process, but it can create a more youthful appearance. A facelift does not eliminate wrinkles or smile lines, but it may diminish them slightly.

Ask your surgeon about the best time for you to have this surgery. The results of a facelift are not permanent; your face will continue to age. Many people who have a facelift eventually have another one, usually within 5 to 15 years, depending in part on their age. Women over 65 sometimes return within a year or two for a less extensive follow-up procedure because their skin is less resilient and may stretch out more quickly. The results of the follow-up procedure are more long lasting. In women under 50, a facelift may help prevent some of the sagging of skin and muscles that normally occurs with aging. A facelift is often, but not always, combined with eyelid surgery (blepharoplasty, see page 692).

The procedure A facelift may be performed in a surgery clinic or in a hospital operating room. You will probably not stay overnight unless you have a medical condition, such as high blood pressure, that needs to be monitored after surgery. Depending on how extensive your facelift will be, you may be given local anesthesia (see page 260) to numb your face and sedatives to make you drowsy, or general anesthesia (see page 261). The procedure can take from 2 to 4 hours. A facelift is a highly individualized procedure, focusing on the features that can benefit the most from surgery.

After surgery You will experience little pain after a facelift. If you do feel significant pain, tell your doctor immediately; it could be a sign of a possible complication. Your bandages will be removed after 1 to 5 days and you will notice some swelling and bruising, which will gradually fade over the next 1 to 2 weeks. Your cheeks or ears may feel numb for a few weeks or months. After the bandages and draining tubes have been removed, you can take a shower and wash your hair with a mild shampoo. In the meantime, your doctor will recommend being extra careful while you are bathing to avoid getting your bandages wet.

The stitches around your ears and under your chin will be removed after about 5 days. If you are concerned about the bruising, tell your doctor. He or she

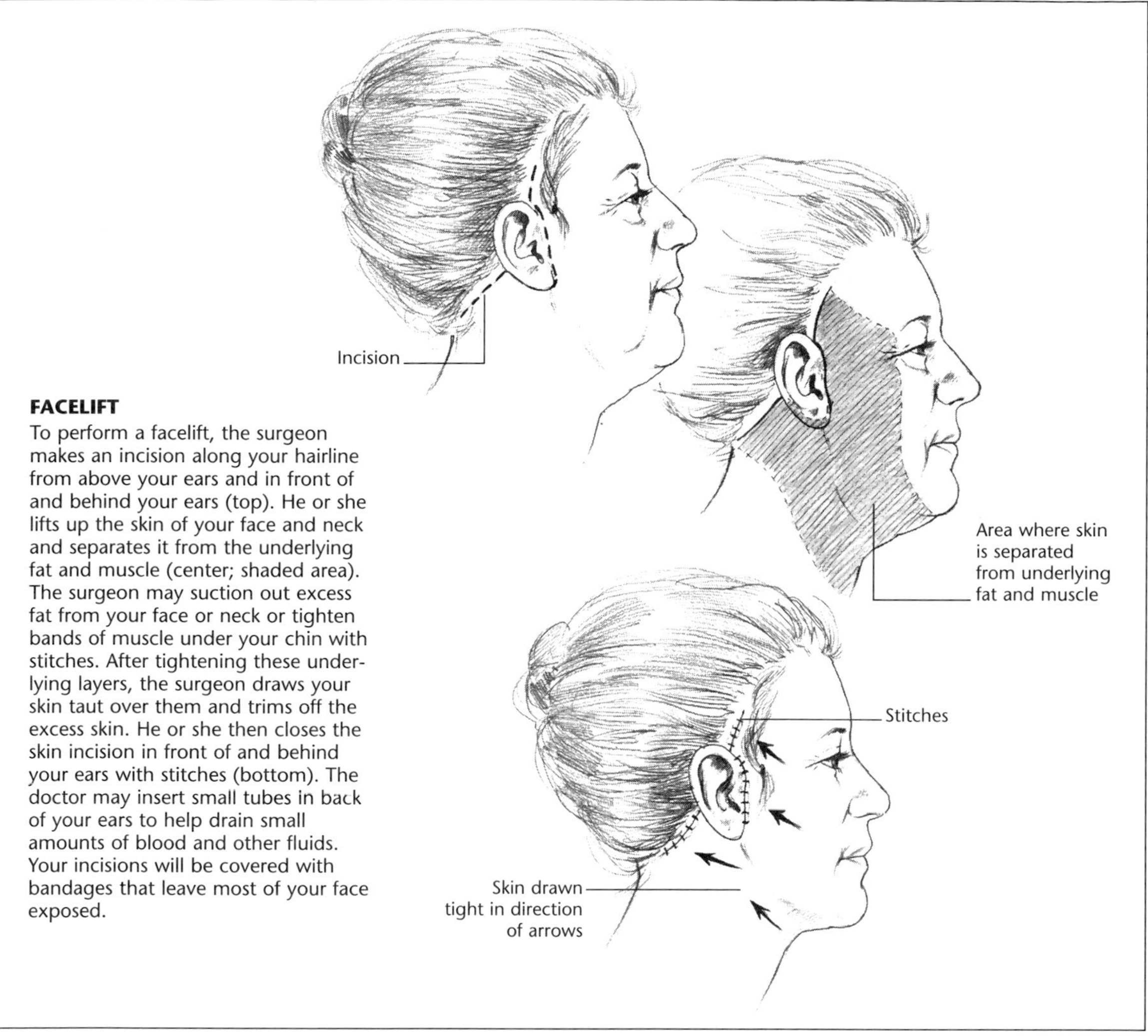

FACELIFT
To perform a facelift, the surgeon makes an incision along your hairline from above your ears and in front of and behind your ears (top). He or she lifts up the skin of your face and neck and separates it from the underlying fat and muscle (center; shaded area). The surgeon may suction out excess fat from your face or neck or tighten bands of muscle under your chin with stitches. After tightening these underlying layers, the surgeon draws your skin taut over them and trims off the excess skin. He or she then closes the skin incision in front of and behind your ears with stitches (bottom). The doctor may insert small tubes in back of your ears to help drain small amounts of blood and other fluids. Your incisions will be covered with bandages that leave most of your face exposed.

can recommend makeup to hide it. For 1 to 2 weeks, you should avoid strenuous physical activity or exercise, including housework and sexual activity. Do not use a steam bath, whirlpool bath, or sauna, or drink alcohol. All of these activities can increase blood flow to your face, which increases the risk of oozing from small blood vessels. Your facial movements may feel stiff at first, usually because of the swelling. The swelling and stiffness will gradually subside.

Most women who have a facelift can return to work and resume their other activities in about 2 weeks. Any remaining scars, particularly behind the ears, will gradually heal over a period of several months.

Complications Complications from a facelift are rare. If excessive bleeding occurs beneath your skin and causes a small blood clot (called a hematoma) to form, your doctor may remove the blood through a tiny needle inserted through the skin. In rare cases, swelling after the operation causes paralysis of facial nerves that can affect the lower lip or, after an extensive facelift procedure, larger muscles of the face. This paralysis is rarely permanent and gradually goes away over a period of weeks or months. In most people, healing is quick and complete. In rare cases, a poorly or slowly healing patch of skin may require minor corrective surgery at a later time.

EYELID SURGERY

Eyelid surgery, called blepharoplasty, reduces sagging of the upper or lower eyelids by removing excess skin and fat. Some older people may have this procedure if aging has caused their eyelids to sag and interfere with their vision. Some teenagers have blepharoplasty to correct an unusually heavy upper eyelid that interferes with their vision, a condition that runs in some families. The results of blepharoplasty last 5 years or more.

Talk to your doctor about whether both your upper and lower lids need to be done, and whether you should consider having a facelift (see page 690) or brow lift (see page 693) at the same time. Your doctor will evaluate your health to rule out medical conditions—such as diabetes, high blood pressure, heart disease, or thyroid disorders (which can cause changes in the tissues around your eyes)—that can increase your risk of complications from surgery.

Before surgery Your plastic surgeon may recommend that you have a comprehensive eye examination by an ophthalmologist (a doctor who specializes in disorders of the eye) before you have eyelid surgery. The ophthalmologist can make sure you do not have any problems, such as inadequate flow of tears, that might interfere with the results of the surgery.

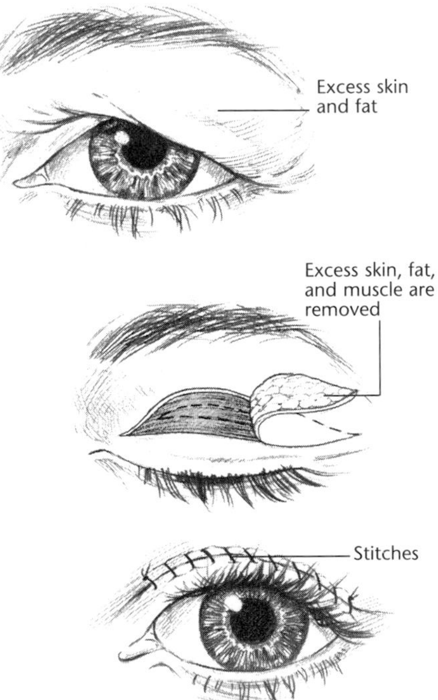

UPPER EYELID SURGERY
In upper eyelid surgery, excess skin and underlying fat are removed to make the eyes look younger or to improve vision that may have been impaired by drooping lids (top). The surgeon makes an incision in the fold of the upper eyelid and removes excess skin and some underlying fat and muscle (center). The incision is closed with stitches (bottom).

The procedure Eyelid surgery can be done in a surgeon's office, a surgery clinic, or a hospital outpatient surgery unit; it does not require an overnight stay. Local anesthesia (see page 260) is often given to numb the area around your eyes and sedatives are given to relax you. You will not feel pain during the procedure, but you may feel some pulling or occasional discomfort while the surgeon removes fat from under your eyelids. The procedure takes from 1 to 2 hours.

For the upper lid, the surgeon makes a 1-inch incision in the fold of your lid. The excess skin and some of the underlying muscle are cut away. Excess fat is removed. The surgeon closes the incision with fine stitches, which are usually concealed in the fold of the eyelid. The scar is rarely visible.

For the lower lid, the surgeon makes an incision just below your bottom lashes, separates underlying fat from muscle, removes excess fat, and trims away the excess skin. He or she then closes the incision with stitches, which are usually concealed underneath the eyelashes. The scar is barely noticeable. After the procedure, the surgeon lubricates your eyes with antibiotic ointment to keep your eyes moist and to prevent infection. Cold compresses may be applied to the area for several hours to reduce swelling.

After surgery After eyelid surgery, your lids may throb as the anesthesia wears off. If the pain is severe, tell your doctor immediately. You will probably be allowed to go home after spending about an hour or so in the recovery room. For the first 24 hours, rest as much as you can and use cold packs to reduce swelling and bruising; the skin on your eyelids is thin and bruises easily. For several days after surgery, avoid excessive activity and keep your head elevated above the level of your heart, especially while you are sleeping (put extra pillows under your head and shoulders) to help reduce swelling.

After about 2 or 3 days, you should be able to watch television or read, but your eyes will feel irritated at first. You cannot wear contact lenses for about 1 to 2 weeks; even then, they may feel slightly uncomfortable. Your stitches will be removed in

LOWER EYELID SURGERY

Lower eyelid surgery is done to remove excess skin and fat from under the eyes. The surgeon makes an incision beneath the lower lashes (top), separates the fat from the muscle, and removes excess fat and skin (center). The skin is pulled together and the incision is closed with stitches (bottom).

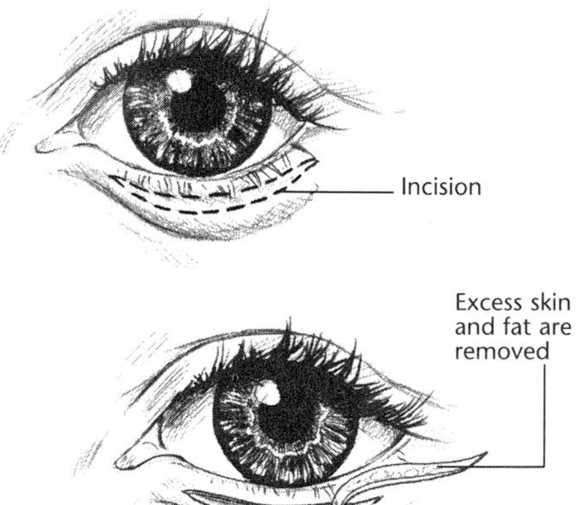

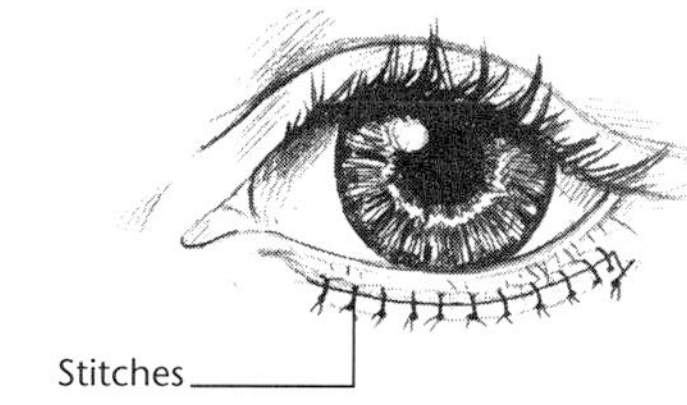

2 to 6 days, but your eyelids may be swollen for several days longer. Most people can return to work after a week but some choose to stay at home until the bruising is less visible or until they can cover it with makeup—usually in 1 to 2 weeks. Do not exercise or engage in sexual activity for 2 weeks. Do not wear makeup for 7 to 10 days. If you have a small amount of discharge from your incision, rinse it off gently with water. Otherwise, avoid touching your incisions.

You may have a small scar that extends to the outer corner of your eye and looks like one of the fine lines in your eyelids. The scars may remain pink for about 6 months and then gradually fade and become almost invisible.

Complications Serious complications are extremely rare with cosmetic eyelid surgery. As with any surgery, there is a slight risk of infection. If you develop an infection, your doctor will prescribe antibiotics that you take by mouth. To help prevent infection after the surgery, wash your hands frequently, especially before you touch your eyes. Try to avoid touching your eyes.

One eye may heal faster than the other and you may notice that one eye looks different from the other. As the eyes heal, this difference will diminish. You may have some difficulty shutting your eyes when you sleep. In some cases, this condition may persist for months; in rare cases, it is permanent. Occasionally, the lower eyelid can pull down too far as it heals, making the white of the eye below the iris visible. This condition is usually temporary. In rare cases, additional minor surgery may be necessary to correct the problem.

BROW LIFT

A brow lift, sometimes called a forehead lift, raises drooping eyebrows and slightly smooths out fine wrinkles on the forehead. In some people, this type of surgery may also raise the upper lids, producing effects similar to those of eyelid surgery (see page 692). Most people have a brow lift to diminish some of the effects of aging. Some people who are born with a heavy, drooping brow may have the surgery earlier in life to help "open up" their eyes. The effects of brow surgery are subtle. To get an idea of what a brow lift might do for you, place your fingers at the outer edge of your eyes above your eyebrows and gently draw the skin upward, raising the whole brow area. A brow lift is often done in conjunction with a facelift.

Because the incision for a brow lift is made in the forehead just above the hairline, it may make a particularly high forehead look even larger. The incision can be made below your hairline, but it leaves a scar.

The procedure Brow-lift surgery can be done in a surgery clinic, a doctor's office, or a hospital outpatient surgery unit and seldom requires an overnight stay. The procedure is usually done using local anesthesia (see page 260) that is injected into the area above your eyebrows. The procedure takes about 1½ hours.

Your surgeon will make an incision that starts at one ear and runs across the top of your forehead (behind the hairline) and down to the other ear. The scalp area has many blood vessels and may bleed heavily. Your surgeon will stop the bleeding by sealing the blood vessels with heat or delicate stitches that will eventually be absorbed by your body. The surgeon then gently lifts up the skin of your forehead and removes portions of the underlying muscle, depending on which areas are being treated. He or she removes any excess tissue and closes the incision with stitches or metal clips. The incision is covered with gauze padding and your head is wrapped in bandages. A tiny tube may be inserted under your scalp to drain any excess blood that may gradually accumulate after the procedure.

After surgery After you have brow-lift surgery, you will feel some pain around the incision and you may have headaches. Tell your doctor before the surgery if you are prone to headaches because he or she can give you an additional anesthetic during the procedure that may help prevent them. For the first 2 to 3 days after the surgery, keep your head elevated, especially while you sleep, to prevent swelling. The bandages will be removed a day or two after surgery. You can shower and wash your hair with a mild shampoo after the bandages are removed. You are likely to have some swelling and bruising around your eyes and on your cheeks. This will fade after about 2 weeks. The stitches or clips will be removed in about 2 weeks.

You can probably return to work after about a week, hiding any visible signs of the surgery with makeup. Growth of hair in the area of the incision may be slower than usual for about 6 months. Avoid vigorous physical activity, including sex, for about 10 days after the surgery. Stay out of the sun for at least 6 weeks because your healing skin is delicate and more susceptible to damage.

Complications Excessive bleeding is a rare but possible complication of brow-lift surgery. A small blood clot (hematoma) may form under your skin. Your doctor can withdraw the blood through a tiny needle inserted into your skin, which is a painless procedure. Because some nerves in your forehead are cut during the procedure, the area may be temporarily numb. In extremely rare cases, the nerve that controls eyebrow movement may be permanently injured.

Most of the scars can be hidden by your hair, unless your hair is very fine. The scars sometimes widen; hair will not regrow in the scar itself. A follow-up procedure can be performed to narrow the width of a scar. When a brow lift is performed using endoscopy (see page 689), scarring is significantly reduced. The use of endoscopy techniques allows doctors to make a series of short vertical incisions along the hairline instead of one long, horizontal incision. Recovery is much easier and quicker after a brow lift using endoscopy.

NOSE RESHAPING

Surgical reshaping of the nose (called rhinoplasty) is done to create a smaller or narrower nose or to correct visible features such as a hump. Nose reshaping is a common cosmetic surgical procedure.

Many people who have surgery to reshape their nose are teenagers. The surgery can be done safely after age 13 or 14, when the nose is almost completely developed. Doctors will sometimes recommend delaying the surgery until the nose is fully formed, at about age 16. However, many surgeons believe that corrective surgery such as nose reshaping is best performed in early adolescence, before the person's self-esteem has been affected negatively.

Some people make a decision later in life to have their nose reshaped. A plastic surgeon usually makes more subtle changes in adults than in teens because adults often have a harder time adjusting to their new appearance.

Nose reshaping can be done in a variety of ways. A hump can be removed; the base of the nose can be made narrower. Other cosmetic possibilities include shortening the length of the nose, reducing the overall size of the nose, reshaping a large tip, or increasing the angle between the nose and the upper lip.

Before surgery If you are considering having your nose reshaped, the first thing you should do is ask your plastic surgeon about whether or not your nose can be changed the way you want. If you are a teenager, your surgeon can evaluate whether your nose is sufficiently developed for you to have the surgery. A young teenage girl who is considering this surgery should discuss her reasons and expectations with her doctor and a parent or other adult who can help her make the final decision. If you have seasonal allergies, such as hay fever (see page 634), your doctor is likely to recommend scheduling your surgery for a time of the year when you are less likely to have symptoms, such as a runny nose or sneezing.

The procedure Nose reshaping is usually done in the doctor's office or in an outpatient surgery unit in a hospital and does not require an overnight stay. However, if you have a complicated nasal problem, such as an obstructed passageway, you may need to stay in the hospital overnight so your condition can be carefully monitored. You will be given local anesthesia (see page 260) to numb the area around your nose and a sedative to relax you during the procedure.

A plastic surgeon can use a number of different techniques to change the appearance of a nose. The incision is usually made inside the nostril, and the skin and soft tissue are separated from the underlying cartilage or bone and mucous membrane. To create the desired effect, the surgeon shaves down the bone and cartilage or builds it up (usually using bone or cartilage from another part of your body). To narrow a nose, the nasal bones are surgically separated from their base near the cheeks and brought closer together. The tip of the nose is reshaped from within. If the nostrils are being made smaller, small wedges of skin are removed from their base, leaving small scars at the base of each nostril. These scars will gradually fade.

After all the incisions have been closed with stitches, a splint of tape and plaster is applied to your nose to stabilize it during healing. Your surgeon may also cover the area beneath each eye with a pressure bandage the first day to help reduce swelling.

After surgery The day after surgery, your nose and face may be puffy and your nose and head may ache. You will probably have to breathe through your mouth. Your doctor will ask you to keep your head elevated for the first day or two to reduce swelling. You will also be told to eat only a liquid or soft-food diet to reduce facial movement from chewing. Your teeth may be sensitive at first and may hurt when you chew. Periodically place cold packs on and below your eyes for the first 2 days to reduce swelling and bruising. You can get up and walk around after 2 days, but ask your surgeon when you can resume your usual activities.

Discharge from your eyes may dry and build up; gently rinse it away with water or a commercial eye moisture solution. Your stitches will be removed in 4 to 6 days.

Complications Complications from nose reshaping are rare. You may have a small amount of bleeding (or a larger amount if the surgery was extensive) from your nostrils for the first 24 hours. This bleeding usually stops by itself. But if it persists longer than a day or does not stop after you apply firm pressure to the site of bleeding for 5 minutes, call your surgeon.

Occasionally, a small blood clot develops under the skin, causing swelling and bruising. Your surgeon may allow the clot to be absorbed naturally by your body or he or she may drain it through a small needle. Small broken blood vessels may appear on your skin but these usually fade with time. In some cases, a minor follow-up operation or revision is necessary to smooth out flaws, such as a small bump on the nose or a slight unevenness in the tip of the nose. Follow-up procedures are usually not done for at least 6 months after the original nose reshaping surgery to allow enough time for the swelling to subside and complete healing to take place.

CHEMICAL PEEL

A chemical face peel (chemabrasion) smooths fine lines on the face by removing the outer layer of skin. A chemical peel does not tighten the skin or remove deeper lines, wrinkles, or scars (such as those resulting from acne). A chemical peel can be performed on the entire face or on one area, such as the forehead or around the mouth. The procedure is most often done on people in their 40s and 50s. The procedure can help diminish fine lines in older people, but their skin heals more slowly.

Because a chemical peel lightens skin color and may cause skin discoloration, people with fair skin have the best results because the color change is less noticeable. If you have dark skin, it may not be wise to have a chemical peel. Some newer peeling techniques lighten the skin less but may have fewer long-term benefits. Make sure the doctor you choose has extensive experience performing chemical peels and has been recommended by another doctor or by a former patient who is satisfied with the results of his or her own procedure.

Before the procedure If you smoke, you should stop for at least 2 weeks before and after you have a chemical peel to improve the healing process. (This is an excellent opportunity to quit smoking for good. For information about how to quit, see page 157.) Many people have the procedure in the spring or fall, when it is easier to avoid extremely hot or cold air, which can irritate healing skin. Because of the risk of skin damage from the sun, most doctors recommend against having a chemical peel in the summer. Do not plan an outdoor vacation during your recovery because you will have to stay out of the sun for a few months after the procedure.

You and your doctor should evaluate whether or not this procedure will give you the effect you are looking for. You may want only a partial face peel that concentrates on the lines on your forehead or around your mouth, or you may want a full-face treatment. You may choose to have a strong solution containing a chemical called phenol or a milder treatment using trichloroacetic acid.

The recovery time is longer after a peel using phenol and the chemical may cause more bleaching of the skin, but the results are usually more dramatic in terms of diminishing wrinkles. Peels using trichloroacetic acid in combination with other chemicals have fewer undesirable side effects, such as bleaching of the skin, than peels using phenol.

Some peeling techniques use fruit acids (alpha-hydroxy acids), which produce an effect similar to that of a sunburn. Peels using alpha-hydroxy acids may be beneficial for a short period, but there is controversy over whether or not they produce long-term benefits even when they are done repeatedly.

The procedure A partial chemical peel is usually done in the doctor's office; a full-face peel is usually done in a surgery facility or hospital and does not require an overnight stay. You will be given a sedative to relax you during the procedure, but probably not an anesthetic. Your face will first be washed with antiseptic solutions that cleanse and remove oils from your skin.

The doctor then applies the chemical slowly and carefully to specific areas of your face. The peel usually goes only to the edge of the jaw. At first, you will feel a slight burning but then the chemical acts as an anesthetic, blocking the sensation of pain. Your doctor may end the procedure by covering your face with petroleum jelly or another ointment to allow the solution to penetrate deeply into your skin.

After the procedure Shortly after the procedure, you may feel tingling or throbbing, which can be relieved with over-the-counter painkillers, such as aspirin or ibuprofen. If the pain is severe, your doctor can prescribe stronger pain-relieving medication. Plan to spend the first 2 days in bed after you have had a chemical peel. If you have had a full-face peel, your eyes may be swollen shut. You will be asked to avoid touching your face with your hands so that your skin can heal evenly and cleanly. Your doctor may ask you to wash the treated area repeatedly and apply ointment. Ointment prevents crusts from forming, which can be stiff and limit facial movement.

The outer surface of your skin will gradually dry to a brown crust that will flake off within 1 to 3 weeks. Your doctor may prescribe an antibiotic cream to help keep your skin moist and free of infection. The swelling will gradually subside over a period of 2 to 3 weeks and the redness will fade to pink. After about a week, you can resume moderate exercise or other activities. After 2 weeks you can wear light makeup; ask your doctor to recommend one.

Your doctor will ask you to stay out of the sun for at least 6 months while your skin is healing. If you cannot avoid the sun, protect your skin completely by wearing a hat and sunscreen that has a sun protection factor (SPF) of at least 15. Exposing your skin to the sun in the months after you have a chemical peel may cause your skin to become blotchy.

Complications When performed by an experienced, skilled doctor, face peels rarely have complications. If whiteheads appear on your skin, you can sometimes remove them with thorough washing. If they persist, your doctor may have to remove them. When performed by an inexperienced doctor, a chemical peel may be allowed to go too deep in the skin and cause permanent scarring. If the chemical is applied too superficially, it may be ineffective.

DERMABRASION

Dermabrasion is a procedure that uses an instrument with a rough burr or brush at the tip to scrape away the outer layer of skin to reduce fine lines on the skin and scars from acne (see page 677). Although the results are usually permanent, the procedure does not slow the aging process or the development of new wrinkles. On a person with dark skin, dermabrasion can make the skin blotchy.

Before the procedure Before you decide to have dermabrasion, talk with your doctor about which areas of your skin are most likely to benefit from the procedure. Many people have the procedure in the spring or fall, when it is easier to avoid extremely hot or cold air, which can irritate healing skin. Because of the risk of skin damage from the sun, most doctors recommend against having the procedure in the summer. Do not plan an outdoor vacation during your recovery because you will have to stay out of the sun for a few months after the procedure. Your doctor will ask you to shampoo your hair and wash your face with an antibacterial soap the morning of the surgery.

DERMABRASION
Dermabrasion is a procedure to reduce fine lines, wrinkles, and acne scars on the face. The doctor uses an electrical instrument that rotates a fine wire brush or diamond tip to scrape away the surface layer of the skin until the wrinkles or scars become less visible.

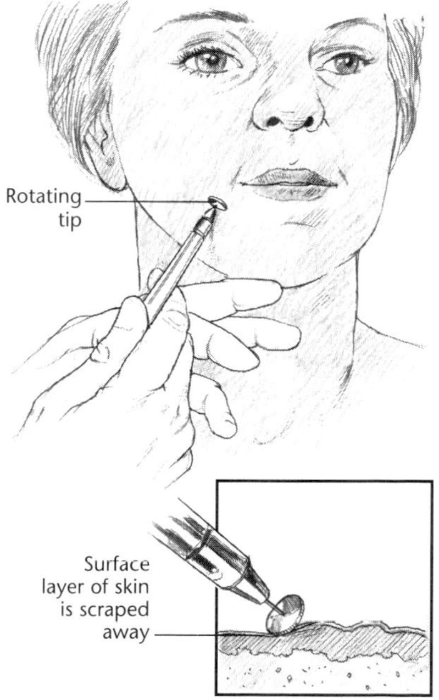

The procedure Dermabrasion is usually performed in the doctor's office but, if the area to be treated is extensive, the procedure may be done in an outpatient surgery unit at a hospital. You may have the entire procedure in one session or several. You will be given local anesthesia (see page 260) to numb the area and a sedative to relax you during the procedure. In some cases, a super-cold gas is used instead of a local anesthetic to numb the face.

Using an electrical instrument with either a fine wire brush or a delicate diamond tip, the surgeon gradually scrapes away at the affected skin to a depth that will make the wrinkles or scars less visible without harming the skin. Warm air may be blown over your face during the procedure to prevent bleeding and help form a protective crust.

After the procedure You may experience some discomfort or pain after dermabrasion. If the pain is severe, your doctor can prescribe pain-relieving medication. Doctors use various methods to promote healing after dermabrasion. Your doctor may cover your face with a wet bandage or waxy gauze, or leave your skin open to the air and ask you to apply ointment frequently. A crust will form on the treated skin and flake off as new skin begins to grow in from beneath. Your skin may itch slightly as new skin grows in.

The new skin will look bright pink and may be swollen at first. The pinkness will gradually fade until its color matches that of the surrounding skin; the swelling will gradually subside over about a week. Most people can return to work within 2 weeks but it may take up to 3 months for the pinkness to fade. For the first 2 weeks, avoid any kind of activity that might cause you to bump your face.

Complications After dermabrasion, exposure to the sun can cause the new, delicate skin to discolor. Protect your skin with sunscreen that has a sun protection factor (SPF) of at least 15 and wear a wide-brimmed hat.

Tiny whiteheads may appear on your skin, which you can usually remove with thorough washing. If they persist, your doctor may have to remove them. Although rare, an infection can delay healing from dermabrasion and cause scarring. Ask your doctor what you can do to reduce your risk of infection. Scars can form if too much skin has been removed. The best way to avoid complications is to choose a doctor who has extensive experience and is skilled in performing dermabrasion.

Breast surgery

The size of your breasts is determined by the genes you inherited from your parents. No exercises, creams, or machines can change the size of your breasts. Breast surgery can enlarge small breasts using implants, reduce the size of large breasts, or lift sagging breasts. For information about breast reconstruction after mastectomy for breast cancer, see page 286.

Any surgical procedure done on your breasts will leave scars. Surgeons can hide many scars by making the incisions under the fold of the breast or around the edge of the nipple. Before you make a decision about having breast surgery, ask your doctor to show you some photographs so you can see what the scars will look like.

Some forms of breast surgery, especially breast reduction, can make it impossible to breast-feed. If you are concerned about not being able to breast-feed, talk to your surgeon before you have any type of breast surgery.

Many women have one breast that is slightly larger than the other. Some women's breasts differ so much in size that their bras and other clothing do not fit properly and they feel self-conscious. A surgeon can perform surgery on one or both breasts to make them look more alike. Your surgeon will help you decide whether you would feel more comfortable making the smaller breast larger (using a breast implant) or making the larger breast smaller.

BREAST ENLARGEMENT

Breast enlargement is a surgical procedure in which a synthetic implant is inserted into the breast to make it larger. Breast implants usually feel like a natural breast. The major disadvantage of implants is that they sometimes become surrounded by scar tissue that makes the breast feel hard, or areas around the nipples or the incisions feel numb.

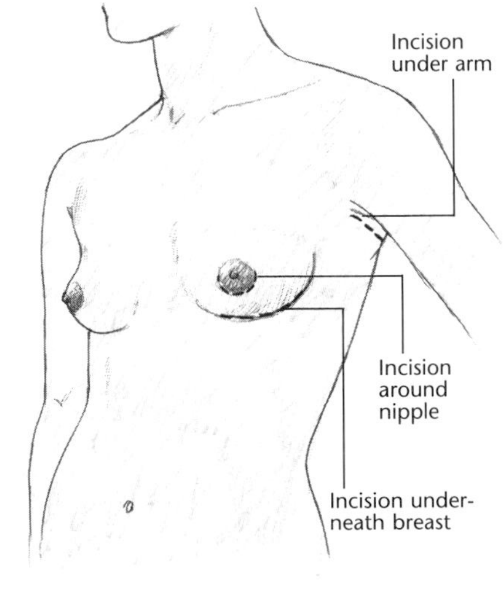

As you age, the breast implant may stay in place while the rest of your breast droops. A surgical procedure called a breast lift (see page 700) can correct this problem, but most women who have implants remain satisfied with the appearance of their breasts over time.

POSSIBLE SITES FOR BREAST ENLARGEMENT INCISIONS

Before breast enlargement surgery, discuss with your surgeon the location of the incisions you will have. Incisions can be made in the crease underneath the breast, around the nipple, or in the armpit.

Before surgery Talk with your surgeon about the results that you desire—it may help to bring in a picture of a woman whose breast size you like. Ask what types of implants are available and discuss the advantages and disadvantages of each.

Ask your doctor where he or she will make the incisions to best hide the scars. The most common incision site is in the fold under the breast. Another possible location is around the outer edge of the areola (the dark area around your nipple). When the procedure is performed properly, it should not affect the sensation in your nipples or any other part of your breasts. Although loss of nipple sensation is rare, it is possible, especially when a very large implant is used. No breast implants or breast enlargement procedures have been linked to breastfeeding problems.

Breast enlargement is sometimes done through an incision in the armpit, which reduces the risk of loss of sensation in the nipples and does not leave a scar on or under the breast. However, this procedure is more difficult because the implant must be inserted over a longer distance to its final position in the breast. In rare cases, the implant may end up slightly too high. Endoscopy (see page 689) has made it easier for doctors to perform this type of breast-enlargement procedure.

The location of the implants—under the chest muscle or over it—is a personal decision that you must make with your surgeon. Implants placed under the chest muscle interfere less with detection of tumors on a mammogram and are less likely to cause tissues around the implant to become hard or change in shape. In some cases, a surgeon may feel that a more natural shape is possible when the implant is placed over the muscle. You and your doctor together can determine the best option for you.

The procedure Breast enlargement surgery is performed in an outpatient surgery facility or in a hospital operating room and usually does not require an overnight stay in the hospital. You are likely to be given local anesthesia (see page 260) to numb your chest and a sedative to relax you during the procedure. General anesthesia (see page 261) to put you asleep during the surgery is an option. The procedure takes about $1\frac{1}{2}$ to 2 hours.

For breast enlargement, the surgeon makes an incision at the predetermined site (in your breast or armpit) and separates the tissues to create a pocket for the implant. The newly formed pocket may be rinsed with an antibiotic solution to reduce the risk of infection. During the procedure, your surgeon may tilt the position of the operating table to observe the effect of gravity on the position of the breast when your body is upright. The surgeon then inserts the implant and closes the incision with stitches. Tape and a gauze bandage may be applied after the incision is closed and you may be dressed in a special bra that provides good support and light pressure to reduce swelling.

After surgery After breast enlargement surgery, you may feel substantial discomfort or pain, especially if the implant is placed under your chest muscle. If your pain is severe, your doctor can prescribe pain-relieving medication. You can bathe normally soon after the surgery. The stitches will be removed after about a week, but the area will still be swollen and bruised. Each breast may heal at a different rate. Most of the swelling is likely to subside within 6 weeks. The scars will be pink for about 6 weeks and

DIFFERENT POSITIONS FOR BREAST IMPLANTS

Breast implants may be positioned either under the chest muscle (right) or over the chest muscle (far right). Placing implants under the chest muscle may make it easier to detect tumors on a mammogram and reduce the risk that the tissues around the implant will become hard or change in shape.

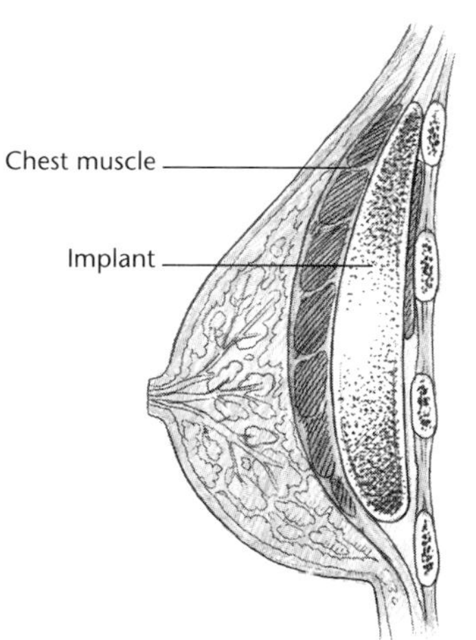

Implant positioned under chest muscle

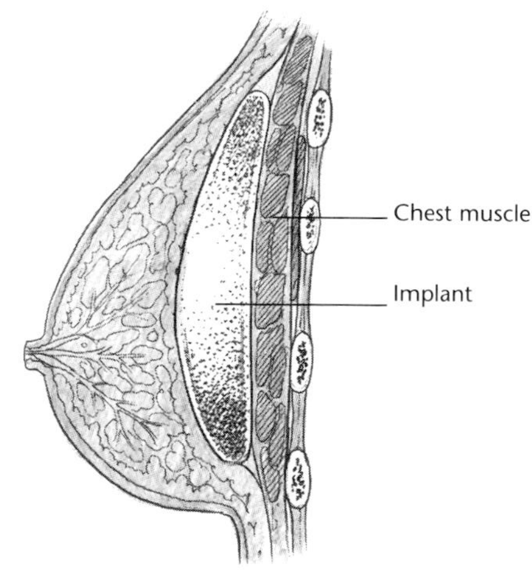

Implant positioned over chest muscle

Safety of breast implants

Safety issues have been raised about breast implants, especially those filled with silicone gel. Occasionally an implant leaks. If you have implants filled with saline (salt solution), one breast may look slightly flatter than the other as the implant leaks and deflates. Saline that leaks from an implant is safely absorbed by your body. If you have a silicone gel implant, you may not realize it is leaking.

The consequences of silicone leaking from breast implants are not yet clear. Research has not shown that silicone from breast implants causes illness of any kind. However, because of concerns about leakage, silicone implants, which were once widely available and preferred, are currently used only for scientific studies. Implants that are filled with saline are now the only kind available in the US for most breast enlargement procedures.

Having breast implants does not increase your risk of breast cancer. Implants do not affect your ability to feel a lump during a breast self-examination (see page 276) because all of your own breast tissue is in front of the implant. However, an implant placed over the chest muscle may make it more difficult to detect a tumor on a mammogram (see page 127). Make sure the technician who performs the mammogram and the radiologist who interprets it know that you have breast implants and that they have experience working with women who have implants.

will begin to fade in about 6 months. Avoid sexual arousal for a week after the procedure because it can increase blood circulation to the breasts and cause swelling. After that, sexual activity without breast contact is fine until your breasts no longer feel sore—about another 2 to 4 weeks.

Complications Although breast enlargement is a simpler form of surgery than other cosmetic breast procedures, complications can occur. Many women who have breast implants have them replaced in another procedure at some time in their life, usually because of capsular contraction. Capsular contraction occurs when the tissue surrounding a breast implant becomes tight, forming a capsule around the implant and causing the breast to feel unusually hard. Some women are not bothered by this hardness; others find it extremely uncomfortable and unattractive. You may feel a firmness in your chest when you hug someone or when you lie on your stomach.

To correct this problem, the surgeon may need to perform a procedure called an open capsulotomy in which he or she reopens the incision and makes a cut in the tissue capsule to relieve the pressure. If this procedure does not provide sufficient relief, the implant and the surrounding scar tissue will be removed. The scar tissue may adhere to the breast tissue, making removal difficult. Implants that contain saline (salt) solution have a lower rate of capsular contraction than silicone implants.

Various other problems can occur with breast implants. Your nipples may feel overly sensitive or less sensitive than before; both conditions are likely to improve over time. Implants can sometimes leak. Saline that leaks from an implant is safely absorbed by your body. Although research has not found a link between silicone from breast implants and illness, in most cases in which a silicone implant ruptures or leaks, a surgeon will recommend replacing it with a saline-filled implant. If you have silicone implants that are not painful, hard, leaking, or causing you any other problems, you do not need to have them removed.

Infection is an extremely rare complication of breast-enlargement surgery. If an infection develops, the implant must be removed and the surgically created pocket must be cleansed thoroughly. A new implant can be inserted after about 3 to 6 months.

BREAST LIFT

A breast lift, or mastopexy, is a surgical procedure to reposition breasts that have sagged. Sagging of the breasts is common and normal in women of all ages, and tends to increase with pregnancy, breastfeeding, and age. A breast lift is a complicated procedure that leaves noticeable scars. In many cases after a breast lift, the breasts will sag again over time. In women who receive breast implants (to increase the size of their breasts) at the same time they have a breast lift, the lift may last longer because the implants hold their breasts in place.

Before surgery At the initial consultation with your surgeon, discuss the results you would like. The scars from a breast lift are noticeable. It is a good idea to ask your surgeon to show you pictures before you have the surgery so that you know what to expect. Your doctor will measure your

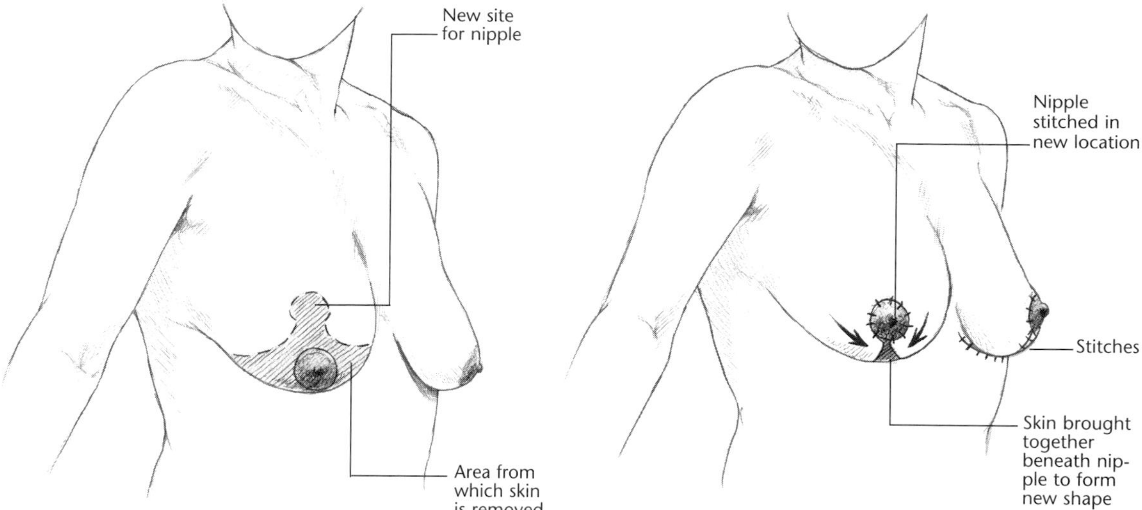

BREAST LIFT
The surgeon makes a keyhole-shaped incision (broken line; left) above your nipple (which will be the new location of the nipple) and extends the incision to each side of your breast and along the crease under your breast. The incision outlines the area of skin (shaded area) that will be removed. The nipple and areola are relocated to the higher position (right). The surgeon then repositions the underlying breast tissue to a higher level, removes excess skin from the lower portion of the breast, and draws the remaining skin together under the nipple to form the shape of the new breast. The skin is stitched together in a vertical line below the nipple and along the crease underneath your breast.

breasts while you are sitting or standing up. If you have small breasts or your breasts have lost volume and you are considering having implants at the same time, talk to your doctor.

The procedure A breast lift removes only skin—not underlying tissue—because breast sagging usually results from stretching of the skin. A breast lift is usually performed in a hospital, outpatient surgery facility, or the surgeon's office and does not require an overnight stay. In most cases, local anesthesia (see page 260) is given to numb the area around your breasts and a sedative is given to relax you during the procedure. In some cases, general anesthesia (see page 261) may be used. The procedure takes about 2 to 3 hours.

After surgery After having a breast lift, you will have considerable bruising and swelling as well as some discomfort or pain. If the pain is severe, your doctor can prescribe pain-relieving medication. To minimize swelling and discomfort, you will wear a surgical support bra all the time (including while you sleep) for a few days. The skin of your breasts may be unusually dry; your doctor will recommend a moisturizing lotion to help relieve this problem and will instruct you to avoid putting the lotion on the healing incisions. Avoid scented or harsh, potentially irritating soaps.

You will have numbness in your breasts. This numbness usually fades gradually, but may be permanent in some areas. Do not stretch your arms too wide or lift anything over your head for a few weeks (or until your surgeon says you can) to avoid opening your incisions. Your stitches will be removed after 1 or 2 weeks.

Plan to be out of work for at least a week after your surgery. Avoid sports or any strenuous activity for 2 to 3 weeks. Avoid sexual activity for at least a week because sexual arousal can increase blood circulation to your breasts and cause swelling. After that, you can resume gentle sexual activity during which you continue to wear your bra. Do not allow direct breast contact until your breasts are no longer overly sensitive.

Complications Like any surgical procedure, a breast lift can have complications. In some cases, bleeding under the skin and infection may occur, which can cause the scars to widen slightly. The scars usually fade to thin, less visible, lines over time. Your breasts or nipples may not be perfectly symmetrical.

BREAST REDUCTION

Women who have unusually large breasts sometimes choose to have their size reduced surgically. If you are overweight, you may be able to reduce the size of your breasts somewhat by significantly decreasing your overall body fat with diet and exercise. But for many women with very large breasts, no amount of weight loss can sufficiently reduce the size of their breasts.

Large, heavy breasts can cause severe discomfort when you run or perform other physical activities and sports. Many women with unusually large breasts develop orthopedic problems such as back pain and poor posture, or rashes underneath the breasts, where skin touches skin. Over time, the weight of excessively heavy breasts can cause ridges from bra straps to develop on the shoulders. If you and your doctor can demonstrate that your breasts are causing physical problems, your health insurance plan may cover the cost of the surgery.

The goal of breast reduction surgery is to reduce the overall bulk and size of your breasts by moving the nipple to a higher location and removing excess skin and underlying tissue. You will have some scars, but your surgeon will try to hide them as much as possible. Most women who have breast reduction surgery will not be able to breast-feed because a substantial amount of breast tissue is removed and the milk ducts often have to be cut to reposition the nipples.

Many women, especially teenagers, with very large breasts may feel self-conscious. Some girls with very large breasts are teased by their classmates and may become withdrawn and even more self-conscious. Women who undergo breast reduction surgery are usually very satisfied with the results because of the positive physical and emotional impact it has on their life.

Before surgery If you are overweight, your doctor will recommend losing some weight before you have breast reduction surgery so that he or she can judge more accurately how much reduction is

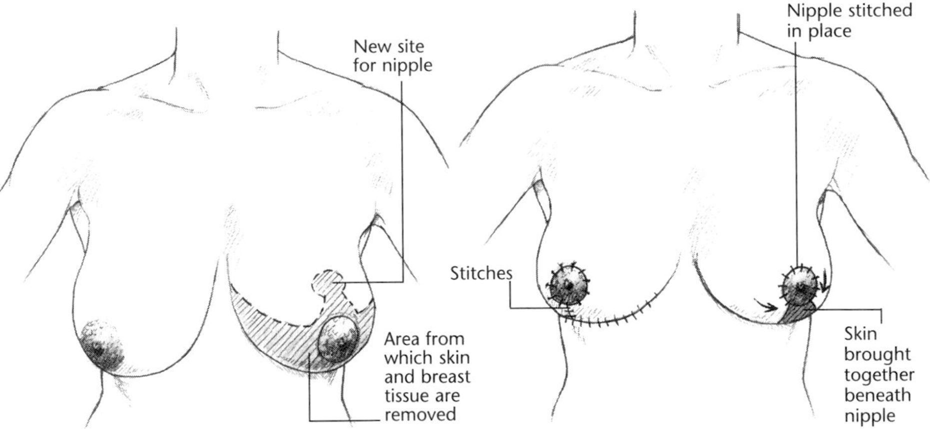

BREAST REDUCTION
The surgeon makes a keyhole-shaped incision (broken line; left) above the nipple (where the new location of the nipple will be) and extends the incision to each side of the breast and along the crease under the breast. The incision outlines the area of skin, breast tissue, and fat (shaded area) that will be removed. After separating the skin from the underlying breast tissue, the surgeon removes excess breast tissue and skin, wraps the skin around the reformed breast mound, and repositions the nipple to the higher area (right). (The nipple always remains attached to breast tissue.) The nipple and breast skin are stitched in place in a vertical line that descends from the nipple and along the crease underneath the breast.

needed. You will lose some breast fat if you follow an overall weight-loss program. However, most women need to lose 20 pounds or more before the size of their breasts or their bra size decreases.

Discuss your expectations and desires with your doctor before you have breast reduction surgery to make sure that you both agree about the final result. Ask your doctor to show you pictures of what the scars will look like after the procedure. Your doctor will measure and diagram your breasts while you sit or stand.

The procedure Breast reduction surgery is usually performed in a hospital operating room using general anesthesia (see page 261) and may require an overnight stay in the hospital. In some cases, liposuction (see page 704) is used to help remove fat from the breasts and from the armpit area. The procedure takes about 2½ to 4 hours.

After surgery When the procedure is complete, your incisions will be covered with bandages and you will be dressed in a surgical bra. You will probably feel a substantial amount of pain in the area of the incisions for the first 2 days. It may hurt to sit up or move around. Your doctor can prescribe medication to help relieve the pain. The pain should subside completely within about 10 days.

You may shower normally after about a week. You are likely to experience some numbness and random shooting pains in your breasts for several months. Wait about 4 to 6 weeks after surgery before you buy new bras to be sure all the swelling has subsided. Avoid stretching your arms wide or lifting anything over your head for 3 to 4 weeks to avoid opening the incisions. You can resume normal work and social activities in 1 to 2 weeks. But you should avoid all sexual activity for about 3 weeks because sexual arousal can increase blood circulation in your breasts and cause swelling. During the fourth to sixth weeks after surgery, you can engage in gentle sex that does not involve direct breast contact. You can then resume your usual sex life.

Adjusting to your smaller breasts

Most women who have their breasts reduced feel relieved because they no longer have bothersome symptoms (such as backaches) and they feel better about their appearance. If you are concerned about other people noticing the sudden change in your shape, tell them you have lost weight, which is true. Give yourself time to get used to your new figure.

Complications Like any surgical procedure, breast reduction surgery can have complications. Some women may lose some sensation in their nipples and breasts. This problem is often temporary, but your sensitivity may return very slowly.

You may find that the area beneath your nipples heals more slowly than the rest of your breast. The skin of your breasts may be unusually dry after surgery. Your doctor will recommend a moisturizing lotion to help relieve this problem and will instruct you to avoid putting the lotion on the healing incisions. Avoid scented or harsh, potentially irritating soaps.

The scars left by breast reduction surgery are usually visible and sometimes prominent for months. After 6 to 18 months, the scars may fade to pale pink, brown, or white. On the other hand, some women who had noticeable stretch marks on their breasts before the surgery see a significant improvement.

Body contouring

A weight-loss program (see page 106) that combines diet and regular exercise is the best way to alter the natural contours of your body. You cannot reduce the size of one particular area of your body, but it is possible to reduce your overall fat by eating fewer calories and exercising more.

Many women find that, in spite of a consistent program of diet and exercise, they have areas of fat on their body (often the thighs, abdomen, or buttocks) that resist all efforts at reduction. Fatty deposits that stubbornly accumulate in one or more areas are often the result of a person's genetic makeup and the aging process. Liposuction and tummy tucks are surgical procedures that are performed to eliminate localized areas of fat on the body.

LIPOSUCTION

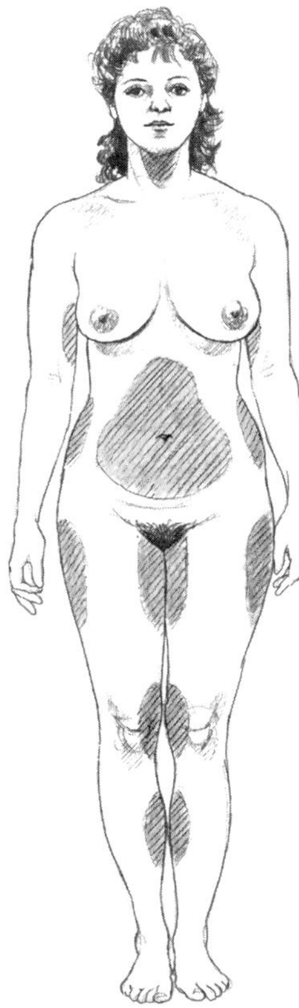

COMMON SITES FOR LIPOSUCTION
Liposuction is not a good solution for people who have excess fat over large areas of their body. It is most effective when performed on small areas of the body that are particularly resistant to fat reduction. Among the most common areas (shaded) for liposuction are the thighs, hips, abdomen, upper arms, neck, knees, calves, and ankles. The buttocks (not shown) are also a common site.

Liposuction ("lipos" is the Greek word for fat), also called suction-assisted lipectomy, is a procedure in which fatty deposits are suctioned out of specific areas of the body through a long, hollow tube attached to a vacuum device. Liposuction is the most frequently performed cosmetic surgical procedure in the US. Your age is not as important as the condition of your skin in determining whether liposuction might work for you. The procedure is most effective in people who have firm, resilient skin that will conform to the new, smaller contour. Liposuction will not eliminate dimpling of your skin (cellulite) or improve your skin's resiliency, but it can reduce the amount of underlying fat.

After you have liposuction, fat will not reappear in the treated areas unless you gain weight. For this reason, your doctor will recommend that you eat a low-fat diet and exercise regularly to increase your chances of keeping the fat off after you have liposuction.

Before surgery Make sure the doctor you choose has performed liposuction many times over a number of years; ask about his or her experience. During your initial consultation with your surgeon, he or she will evaluate the areas of your body in which fat accumulates and will explain the risks and limitations of the procedure in treating those areas. Ask your doctor about possible additional costs for any follow-up or touch-up procedures, which are sometimes necessary. Make sure you understand and carefully follow your doctor's instructions about what to do after the procedure to help ensure the best long-term results.

The procedure If the area on your body that is to be treated with liposuction is small, the procedure can be performed in your doctor's office. Liposuction to remove more extensive areas of fat may be done in an operating room in the hospital. Local anesthesia (see page 260) is often used unless a particularly large area is treated. An overnight stay in the hospital is seldom necessary. The procedure can take from 1 to 2½ hours.

Small, thin suction tubes are used to remove fat in the neck and face; wider tubes are used to remove fat on the abdomen, thighs, or buttocks. The surgeon makes a small incision and inserts the tube under your skin. (The number of incisions depends on the size of the area to be treated.) The surgeon manipulates the tube back and forth between layers of fat and muscle to dislodge the fatty tissue. A vacuum pump that is connected to the tube sucks out the dislodged fatty tissue and deposits it into a collecting bottle.

During the procedure, you will receive intravenous fluids to replace any fluids you may lose. You will not feel pain during the procedure, but you may feel vibrations and friction. When the suction procedure is complete, the surgeon removes the tube and closes the incisions with stitches that will dissolve on their own. The treated area will be covered with bandages.

After the procedure When the anesthesia wears off, you may feel some painful burning. Your doctor will prescribe pain relievers that you can take for the next several days if necessary. If you had liposuction on your lower body anywhere below the waist, you will need to wear an elastic girdle or elastic garments for 1 to 3 weeks. Wearing these garments helps the treated area heal smoothly and symmetrically and reduces the risk of skin irregularities.

Because liposuction naturally causes bruising and swelling, you will not notice an immediate improvement. The bruising will disappear in about 2 to 3 weeks and the swelling will subside in about 3 months. Your doctor will ask you to begin walking again as soon as you can after the procedure; activity helps reduce the accumulation of excess fluid and swelling. You can resume your usual activities as soon as you feel comfortable doing so, but wait about 2 to 3 weeks before engaging in strenuous exercise. You may bathe normally immediately after the surgery. If you have had liposuction on your lower body, having sex may be uncomfortable; wait about 2 weeks before resuming sexual activity.

Complications Complications from liposuction are extremely rare when the procedure is performed by a plastic surgeon who is trained and experienced in liposuction techniques. Your skin may appear rippled, which can occur from suctioning too close to the surface. If too much fat is removed, the skin may sag or appear loose. The two sides of your body may not match. Because swelling occurs almost immediately after the procedure begins, it is often difficult for the doctor to tell if the two sides match exactly. This problem, which can be corrected in another, later, procedure to restore symmetry, occurs in fewer than 10 percent of cases. The vast majority of women who have had liposuction are pleased with the results.

LIPOSUCTION
For liposuction on the buttocks, the surgeon makes a small incision (about 1/8 to 1/4 inch long) in the crease under each buttock, where it will not be visible. He or she then inserts a thin, hollow tube (right) through the incision and moves it back and forth to loosen and suction out the fat. The surgeon removes the tube and closes the incision with dissolvable stitches (far right).

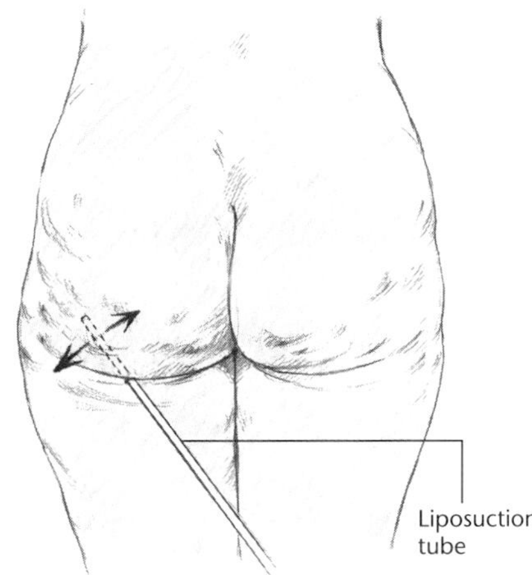

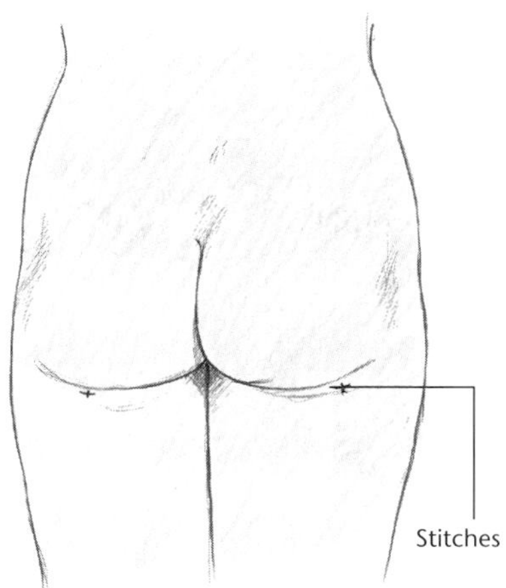

TUMMY TUCK

A tummy tuck (abdominoplasty) is a surgical procedure to remove excess skin and fat from the abdomen. The procedure may sound simple, but it is major surgery. A tummy tuck leaves a permanent scar and usually requires at least 2 weeks of recovery at home. The procedure is usually performed on women who are unhappy about excess skin or fat in their abdominal area that they have not been able to reduce with diet and exercise. The accumulation of excess skin in the lower abdomen often results from multiple pregnancies or a large weight loss. If you are considering having a tummy tuck, educate yourself about the surgery so you know what to expect.

The procedure A tummy tuck is usually performed in a hospital operating room and may require an overnight stay. A less extensive procedure, sometimes called a mini-tuck, often does not require an overnight stay. A tummy tuck is done using general anesthesia (see page 261) and takes about 2 to 2½ hours. A mini-tuck may require only local anesthesia (see page 260) to numb the abdominal area and a sedative to relax you; a mini-tuck takes about 1½ to 2 hours.

For a standard tummy tuck, the surgeon makes an incision across your abdomen from one hipbone to the other just above your pubic area. A short incision may seem more appealing, but the longer incision actually gives smoother results. Another incision is made around your navel so that it can be moved to a position at the center of your new waistline. The doctor may then perform liposuction (see page 704), in which he or she inserts a thin, hollow tube into the incision around your navel and vacuums out the excess fat. He or she will then free your skin (from the abdominal incision all the way up to your ribs) from the underlying tissues.

If the two major vertical muscles in your abdomen have weakened, the surgeon may tighten them by pulling them close together (in a line down the center of your abdomen) and stitching them in place. Your navel is then repositioned at your new waistline. The large, loosened flap of skin is stretched down to the lower edge of the incision and clamped in place. Most of the skin that previously extended from the navel to the lower incision is trimmed away. Drainage tubes may be inserted into your skin to remove excess fluid. Bandages and firm, elastic dressings similar to a girdle will be applied over your entire abdomen and around your buttocks to help hold the stitches together while your incisions heal. The dressings also help minimize fluid buildup and swelling.

In a mini-tuck, the navel does not have to be moved and only excess skin and fat from below the navel are removed. The horizontal abdominal incision is smaller than that in a regular tummy tuck. A small incision may be made near the navel to insert a liposuction tube to remove fat.

After surgery Recovery from a mini-tuck is usually faster than from a standard tummy tuck—about 2 days compared with 2 to 3 weeks. The drainage tubes will be removed after 1 day. Your abdomen will feel tight for 2 to 6 weeks and it may be 10 days before you can walk straightened up. However, it is important to walk as soon as possible (within 24 hours) after the surgery to avoid complications, such as blood clots in your legs. If needed, your doctor will prescribe medication to relieve pain. You will have substantial swelling in the treated area.

After you are released from the hospital, you will need to rest at home. Follow your doctor's instructions about rest, bathing, and other activities. You will feel tired for the first few weeks. Although you may be able to return to work after 2 weeks, many people require about 4 weeks to regain their usual strength. Avoid strenuous exercise or sexual activity for about 3 weeks to prevent your scars from widening from excessive pressure on them. Avoid lifting heavy objects for a month to avoid straining your stomach muscles.

Complications Serious complications from tummy tuck procedures are unusual. Rarely, a blood clot will form in the legs or groin that can be dangerous if it travels to the heart, brain, or lungs. Getting up and walking around within a day of the surgery increases the blood flow naturally and significantly reduces the risk of this potentially serious complication. Other complications include infection, heavy scarring, and fluid buildup. If you develop an infection, your doctor will prescribe antibiotics. A buildup of fluid under your skin may have to be drained with a needle.

Scars may be visible at first and, in some cases, may widen over time. It usually takes about a year for the scars to fade and flatten out. You can hide your scars with clothing. Most bathing suits will hide the long abdominal scar.

STANDARD TUMMY TUCK

For a standard tummy tuck, the surgeon makes an incision across your abdomen from one hipbone to the other just above your pubic area (right). He or she then separates the skin from the incision up to your ribs (shaded area) from the underlying tissues and stretches the loosened skin flap down to the lower edge of the incision. He or she then trims off the extra skin and closes the incision with stitches (far right). Your navel is stitched in place at your new waistline.

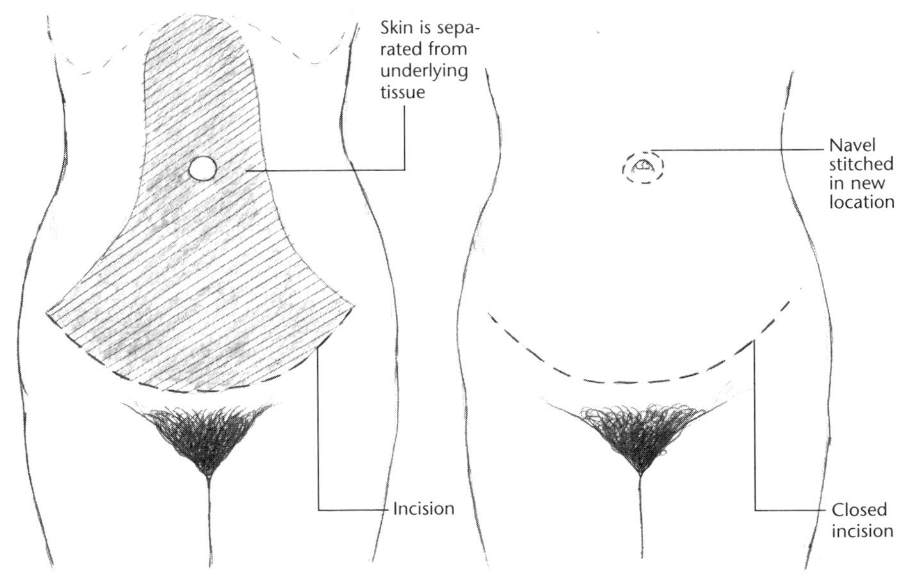

CHAPTER 29

Death and bereavement

Contents

Generally, you cannot anticipate exactly how or when you will die, but if you have a life-threatening chronic or terminal illness, you will need to evaluate your options and make important decisions. If your condition becomes irreversibly life threatening, have you expressed your wishes to a loved one about limitations on end-of-life medical care? How will you cope with the idea of your own death or that of a close family member? This chapter will give you practical information to help you take an active part in decisions about your well-being or that of a loved one.

If you have a serious illness, you will also have to decide who will provide the continuing help and care you will need. For information about the many alternatives for assisted living, see page 143.

End-of-life decisions

Like most people, you may find it difficult to think about your own death, or the death of people you love. But death is a natural part of our existence. You may find it worthwhile to take the time now to plan ahead and think about the many decisions you may be faced with when your health or that of a family member begins to fail. Learning about your options and expressing your feelings about how you want to die can help give you and your loved ones a sense of completeness about life and some control over these final days.

COPING WITH YOUR FEELINGS ABOUT DEATH

Each of us will face death differently. If you are diagnosed with a serious illness, you may want your doctor to inform you of all the details of your condition and your chances of survival, or you may feel overwhelmed by and anxious about such information and want to know very little. You may welcome death as a release from a long period of severe pain and emotional distress. You may fear death, as many people do. You may be afraid of being alone at the end of your life, or of being treated differently. You may not want to consider even the possibility of death.

A person who is dying needs opportunities to talk about his or her fears and concerns. A close friend, family member, doctor, or member of the clergy may be helpful, and may be able to open up the discussion of death in a family that is reluctant to talk about it.

When first told that they are dying, many people refuse to believe it. This stage of denial may gradually give way to anger, which is sometimes directed at the people who are closest—relatives and caregivers who are providing help and comfort. In trying to come to terms with the situation, a person may then enter a bargaining stage, in which he or she attempts to buy time, sometimes by promising in prayer to be a better person. Gradually, the person begins to acknowledge the reality of the situation. At this time, he or she is likely to experience severe depression or grief, and begin to lose interest in life in general. When the depression lifts, the final stage of acceptance can occur.

Not everyone goes through these stages in the same way. Some people skip a stage or experience several at the same time. Some people remain in a state of denial until the very end. But those who finally come to accept death usually have gone through some version of this process.

ADVANCE DIRECTIVES

Advance directives are documents that spell out your wishes regarding medical treatment in case you have a physically or mentally disabling illness or accident and cannot speak for yourself. The most common types of advance directives are living wills, durable powers of attorney for health care decisions, and single documents that combine a living will and durable power of attorney. As long as you can speak for yourself and are competent, you can continue to make your own decisions about medical treatments.

Medical technology can often prolong the life of a person who is terminally ill or who may have lapsed into a comatose or vegetative state in which his or her brain is no longer functioning. If you cannot express your wishes about end-of-life treatments and you have not previously indicated them in an advance directive, hospital and health care workers may make decisions for you about life-sustaining treatments that are inconsistent with your wishes.

A living will is designed to ensure that you receive the kind of medical treatment you want when you are dying. If you wish to be treated with a ventilator, surgery, or feeding tubes, you can give instructions for such care in your living will. Conversely, you can indicate in your living will that you do not want these treatments. A durable power of attorney for health care decisions gives a trusted person of your choosing—who is usually called your health care proxy—the authority to make decisions about your medical care if you are unable to make them yourself. He or she can be a family member, close friend, or other person you trust. The most important thing is for you and your proxy to understand each other and for you to trust him or her to act in accordance with your wishes and with good judgment on your behalf.

Many advance directive forms, especially living will forms, apply only when you become terminally ill or permanently unconscious. Make sure, by reading it carefully, that the document you use will take effect when you want it to.

Specify in your living will any requests you may have, such as your desire to die at home. Among the items you may want to include in your living will are statements about whether or not you want to receive the following treatments if you have a serious condition that is incurable and irreversible:

- **Cardiopulmonary resuscitation** When a person's heart stops beating, cardiopulmonary resuscitation (CPR), along with other medical treatments, is usually performed to try to reestablish a normal heartbeat. In many cases, a person who is terminally ill or has undergone a prolonged period of severe pain may decline such life-sustaining treatment. His or her doctor may then issue a "do-not-resuscitate" order, which prevents attempts at resuscitation if his or her heart should stop beating. You can make this order part of your living will.
- **Artificial breathing** When a person's lungs stop functioning, usually as a result of damage to the respiratory center of the brain from a stroke or head injury, emergency measures are often taken to

Urge loved ones to sign living wills and powers of attorney

Most people do not like to think about their own death, let alone talk about it. If someone close to you has not signed a living will and durable power of attorney for health care decisions, you will be doing the person a service by helping him or her begin the process. Here are some guidelines:

- The best time to create and sign an advance directive is long before a crisis arises. Bring up the subject sensitively with your relative or friend and then let a few days pass before you mention it again.
- If you meet resistance to the idea, back off for a few days but bring up the subject again later. Be persistent. Assure your loved one that as long as he or she is conscious and understands what is going on, he or she will have full control over all health care decisions.
- Give the person written information that describes what an advance directive does and why it can be useful.
- If your relative or friend objects to making a living will for religious reasons, consult a member of the clergy to find out if the particular religion has objections to signing advance directives. Most major religions do not prohibit the withdrawal of artificial measures to prolong the life of a person who is terminally ill beyond his or her body's natural ability to sustain itself, especially if the person is experiencing extreme physical pain or suffering.
- If your relative or friend is in the hospital or is in a home-care program (see page 143), a member of the clergy or a social worker is usually available to discuss the advantages of an advance directive and let family members know what the implications are for them.
- If your loved one is resistant to the idea of signing a document that calls for withholding specific treatments, discuss the option of specifying someone else to have durable power of attorney. A durable power-of-attorney directive gives a trusted relative or friend the authority to make medical and other decisions if, at some time in the future, the person is unable to do so.

reactivate the breathing process, usually by connecting the person to a mechanical breathing machine called a ventilator (also called a respirator).

■ **Artificial feeding** Some people who are seriously ill cannot eat or drink by mouth. In many cases, tubes are inserted through the person's nose into the stomach or directly into the stomach through a surgically created incision in the abdominal wall to provide nutrients and fluids to keep him or her alive.

■ **Medication** People with some terminal illnesses actually die of infections, such as pneumonia, caused by bacteria. Antibiotics may prevent you from dying of an infection but, if you have a terminal illness, you may choose not to have your life sustained with medication. If you have terminal cancer that has spread, you may choose to forego further treatment with chemotherapy, which can have severe, painful side effects. You may also request that you be given the maximum amount of pain-relief medication even if it might somewhat hasten your death because it can interfere with your breathing.

You can work with a lawyer to draw up a living will and durable power of attorney. You can also do this yourself by obtaining legal forms from a local hospital (ask for the department of social work) or a local or state medical society or bar association. An advance directive form that has been designed jointly by the American Medical Association, the American Bar Association, and the American Association of Retired Persons is also available. This form can be used in any state and applies to a broad range of circumstances. You can obtain a copy of this form by writing to the American Association of Retired Persons in Washington, DC. Make sure you have your signature witnessed by two responsible adults who are not relatives or beneficiaries of your estate. If your state requires it, have the documents notarized by a notary public.

In addition to preparing both of these documents, you should make your spouse, children, and other key family

One woman's story
Living wills

When my mother was 75, she had her first stroke. After that, she was unable to move her right arm and she couldn't walk very well. For the next 8 years, she experienced mini-strokes that caused dizziness and fainting. She became progressively weak, confused, and withdrawn.

When she could no longer live alone, she and I agreed it would be best for her to have around-the-clock care in a nursing home. She needed more attention and assistance than I could provide with a full-time job and two teenagers at home. Also, my mother did not want to burden her family.

Visits with my mother at the nursing home were sad and frustrating. She became more withdrawn and disabled, and it seemed she was waiting to die. We hoped the end would come painlessly and peacefully. One night, her heart stopped. Because she had not made out a living will with instructions to the contrary, the paramedics performed CPR and got her heart beating again.

When I saw her in the hospital the next morning, she had tubes down her throat and was unable to talk or function at all. She suffered in this condition for 3 months, getting progressively worse. Finally, her heart stopped again, and this time attempts to resuscitate her failed.

Over the years, I had raised the issue with my mother of preparing a living will, but she resisted so I let it go. After witnessing her prolonged misery, my husband and I have signed living wills and durable powers of attorney for health care decisions. We want to make sure we have some control over decisions that will be made at the end of our lives. We also want to spare our family the pain of sustaining our lives beyond the point of hope—and the pain of making a difficult decision.

"We want to make sure we have some control over decisions that will be made at the end of our lives."

members aware of your wishes. Tell them about your living will, durable power of attorney, or other advance directives. Give them copies of the documents or let them know where they can find the documents when necessary. Give your doctor copies and tell him or her the name of your health care proxy. Make sure you find out whether or not your doctor is willing to honor your requests; some doctors may not be. If not, you will need to look for another doctor. You should also give copies of your advance directives to your nursing home, hospital, or any other medical facility where you might have treatment.

ORGAN DONATION

The need for donated organs for transplants far exceeds the supply. The waiting lists of people who would benefit from receiving a transplanted organ are long. Many will die without one. Most families who have donated a loved one's organs find comfort in knowing that they and their loved one have given life or health to another person. If you want to donate your organs after your death, make your intentions clear to your relatives and sign a donor card. You can obtain information and applications from a local hospital, health care organizations such as the American Red Cross, or your local library. You can also indicate your wish to be an organ donor on your driver's license. Ask your secretary of state's office how to do so.

However, even if you have signed a donor card, all states require the permission of a close relative (spouse, adult child, or adult sibling) before your organs can be donated upon your death. For this reason it is especially important to make your wishes clear to your family.

Organ donation does not conflict with the beliefs of most religions or affect funeral practices, including an open casket. The organs are removed from the donor's body immediately after his or her death. In ideal circumstances, the organs are removed while the person (who has been medically certified brain-dead) is still connected to a heart-lung machine, which circulates blood and oxygen to the organs to keep them viable for transplantation. The organs are removed quickly, refrigerated, and transported immediately to a designated hospital, where they are transplanted into a waiting patient.

Living with loss

When someone you love dies, it is normal for you to feel sad and empty as you deal with the loss. Feelings of grief or bereavement are a universal human emotion and are necessary for the healing process. Most people go through a series of stages in their grief before they finally come to accept their loss.

STAGES OF GRIEF

Grief is the process of mourning the loss of a loved one. Although each person experiences grief in his or her own way, most people follow a common pattern. Some stages of the grieving process may overlap or be difficult to recognize but you are likely to go through some version of the following:

- **Numbness** When you experience the death of a loved one, you will probably feel numb at first. You may be unable to grasp the reality of the death and deny it. You may be so busy taking care of funeral arrangements and legal matters that you temporarily postpone dealing with your emotional needs. Many people feel alone, empty, and in shock at this time.
- **Guilt and anger** After the death of a loved one, many people question whether they did enough to ease the person's pain or try to prevent the death. They may also feel anger toward the people who are trying to help them, including doctors, nurses, family members, and friends.
- **Depression and loneliness** It is common to feel depression and loneliness after you experience a severe loss. After a time, intense emotions will begin to ease. You may feel tired, run-down, sad, and hopeless and have difficulty resuming normal activities. A sense of isolation may set in, as friends and family who were present immediately after the death

Helping the bereaved

Many people do not know what to say to a person who is grieving. They may avoid the person altogether. But the most helpful thing you can do for a grieving person is to be there to listen if he or she wants to talk. Don't feel that you have to do anything or give any advice to help the person get over the grief. Grieving is a gradual process that will occur naturally.

Try to avoid saying things—such as "It was God's will" or "It was meant to be"—that dismiss the pain the person is feeling. Keep yourself from sharing your own losses with the bereaved person; this is not helpful. The bereaved person may feel a need to describe over and over again in detail the last days of his or her loved one, the death itself, the funeral arrangements, or the service. Instead of trying to divert the person's attention, listen patiently and ask questions such as "Where were you when it happened?" or "What did you think of the funeral service?" to help him or her come to terms with the experience.

You should become concerned if the person expresses only negative feelings or seems depressed. If you think he or she may be having suicidal thoughts, ask "Are you feeling so bad that you are thinking about hurting yourself?" If the answer is "yes," get professional help for the person immediately by calling 911 or a crisis hotline at a local hospital. You may also encourage the grieving person to join a support group of other people who are experiencing bereavement. Ask your doctor to recommend one in your area.

may now be less available even though you still need reassurance and a sympathetic ear. This is a transitional stage during which you will gradually get back on your feet.

■ **Acceptance** Acceptance is the final stage of grief, when you begin to function normally again. You will still think about your loved one, but less often and with less pain. You will gradually be able to enjoy your friends again and participate in social activities. You may still experience some relapses of deep sadness. This is normal. You may be caught off guard by a sudden reminder of the person who died (such as discovering an old sweater in a drawer) or you may be reminded of the person during special times, such as holidays and birthdays. The length of the grieving process is different for every person. It can take many weeks, months, or even years for you to finally be able to reach full acceptance and closure.

The pattern of grieving can also vary, depending on an individual's situation. When death occurs after a prolonged terminal illness, the grieving process is sometimes delayed. In these circumstances, death may seem acceptable, even a relief, if the loved one was in severe pain. Later, especially when you return to a place or situation that has strong associations with your loved one, your feelings of grief may reemerge. You should use this as an opportunity to deal with those feelings, which will help you begin to heal.

Many people find it helpful to observe traditional or religious rituals that are associated with dying or to create their own private or family rituals. A funeral or memorial service is the customary, public acknowledgment of a person's death. A memorial service brings people together to share their grief and provide emotional support for each other. A short, simple service is often the least painful for the closest relatives and friends, who are most affected by the death. Some people prefer a more elaborate, longer service with calling hours, a formal funeral in a house of worship, and a burial service.

Many people gain a feeling of comfort by having a small, informal gathering of the people who were closest to the deceased. They share personal recollections of the person and may participate in a simple ritual, such as lighting a candle in his or her memory. Funerals can be expensive. You should not feel guilty about choosing a simple, less expensive service, particularly if your financial resources are already drained by the expense of a long illness.

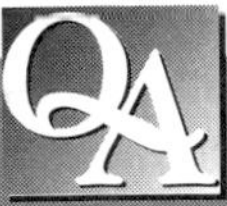

QUESTIONS WOMEN ASK
GRIEVING

Q I cared for my mother in my home until she died 6 months ago. I still feel sad often and can't seem to get over her death. My husband tells me it is time to get on with my life. Is something wrong with me?

A No. Your feelings are normal. Grief is different for everyone. Although some people recover from the death of a loved one in a matter of months, the process can often take a year or longer. If your feelings are affecting your ability to function and you think you may be depressed, see your doctor. Otherwise, try to resume your usual activities and take steps to rebuild your social life. A person with a strong social support system is better able to cope with the effects of a serious loss than a person who is socially isolated.

Q My husband has been ill with cancer for some time and the doctor now says that his condition is terminal. I feel unbearably sad and find myself crying almost every day. I'm worried that I will have trouble coping when he dies.

A Even though your husband is still living, you may already be going through the grieving process. You are preparing yourself for his death in a normal, natural way. People whose loved one experienced a prolonged illness often recover more quickly after the death than people who experience a sudden loss. Take time now to say the things to your husband that you would like him to know.

PHYSICAL EFFECTS OF GRIEF

Grief can have physical as well as emotional effects. Severe, prolonged grief can lead to depression (see page 594), which affects both the mind and body. Many people who are grieving experience the following symptoms:

- Difficulty sleeping; nightmares
- Stomach and intestinal upset; loss of appetite
- Fantasies and preoccupation with images of the deceased
- Headaches
- Tiredness and fatigue
- Aches and pains
- Tight feeling in the chest or throat
- Memory problems; inability to concentrate on ideas or tasks
- Heart flutters

These symptoms are a normal part of the grieving process. However, if any become particularly troublesome, affect your ability to function, or last longer than a few months, talk to your doctor. Your doctor can give you a complete physical examination and a psychiatric evaluation to rule out depression. If you are diagnosed with depression, your doctor may prescribe antidepressant medication for you to take for a short period or recommend that you talk with a qualified mental health professional, such as a psychiatrist.

The emotional stress of bereavement may lower your resistance to all types of illnesses. It is especially important at this time to pay close attention to your own health needs, which can help you cope better with your grief. Eat a nutritious, well-balanced diet (see page 44) and get plenty of exercise (see page 78). As soon as you are able, take daily walks by yourself or with a friend or engage in other forms of physical activity. Regular exercise is an excellent way to help relieve stress, boost your mood, and work out your emotions.

UNRESOLVED GRIEF

Grief can become a problem if it is not expressed or if it lasts an unusually long time without resolution. Some people deny or suppress their grief. After the death of a loved one, they are unable to express the sadness, anger, or other emotions they feel. They may be acting on the misconception that a courageous person endures pain silently—holds back the tears and continues to function in spite of the pain. Some people preoccupy themselves with funeral arrangements and other details that need to be taken care of after a death, which can postpone their emotional reaction to the loss.

Unexpressed grief can make it harder for you to ultimately accept the death of a loved one. You may isolate yourself from others, become indifferent, or refuse to talk about the deceased. You may work excessively or avoid social contact. In some people, unexpressed grief can lead to harmful behaviors such as abusing alcohol or other drugs. Over time, unexpressed grief can make it difficult for a person to develop a close relationship with or love another person.

Grief also becomes a problem when it is prolonged. Failure to reach the final stage of grieving—acceptance—can prevent you from going on with your life. Prolonged grief can cause unrelieved feelings of sadness, physical problems for which no medical cause can be found, inability to function normally, and social isolation. Some people begin to have the same physical symptoms as the person who died. Others may come to view their loved one and their relationship as different than they actually were. Unreconciled feelings may affect your own well-being and the nature of your relationships.

If you are unable to express your grief, or if it becomes prolonged, seek professional help. Talk to your doctor, who will be able to recommend a mental health professional, such as a psychiatrist. Most therapists are trained to help people cope with grief. A therapist can help you resolve feelings that may be interfering with your ability to acknowledge or accept the death of your loved one. The difficult part of this process is that, in order to resolve your feelings, you must experience them again. But it is important to go through each stage of the mourning process before you are finally able to accept the death.

MOVING ON

If you are grieving, the emotions you feel are a normal part of the process of bereavement. Talk about your feelings to a close friend, family member, member of the clergy, or a therapist who will listen to you objectively. Joining a support group of other people who are grieving can help make you feel less alone. Ask your doctor or the social services office of a local hospital for a support group in your area. For many people, talking with others who have moved beyond grief helps them come to terms with their own loss.

After the first weeks of grieving, try to rejoin the world. Return to your usual social activities, even if you don't feel like it yet; you can always leave a social situation. Get together with relatives who have also felt the loss of your loved one. By connecting with others, you can prevent your grief from becoming overwhelming or prolonged.

For many people who have lost a partner, recovery from grief can lead to new confidence and independence. For example, a woman who has depended on her husband to make all the financial decisions in the household may discover that she can competently manage her own affairs. A shy woman whose spouse was outgoing may become more extroverted.

A woman who has been married for a long time may feel that marriage is the only comfortable or acceptable state for her. After her spouse dies, she may feel she cannot live alone. If you are in this situation, talk with other women who live alone and enjoy it. Find out how they manage their social and financial lives.

If you have lost a partner, take time to think about what you want in life. Setting goals for the future is an important part of recovering from grief. Begin with short-term goals, such as making a date to go to a movie with a friend. When you are ready, set long-term goals such as finding a job or moving to a new home.

To recover fully from a severe loss is to successfully reach the stage of acceptance. Accepting the death of your loved one does not mean you are forgetting him or her or discarding your memories. Accepting the death can help relieve much of your pain and sorrow. How do you know when you have gotten through the grieving process? If you can think of your loved one without feeling pain, if you can incorporate the fact of his or her death into your life, if you can look forward to your future without your loved one and still retain your memories as a cherished part of your past, you are ready to move on.

CHAPTER 30

Sexual assault and family violence

Contents

Violence against women and children has reached epidemic proportions in the US. Most of this violence occurs in the home. Nearly one fourth of all women may be physically assaulted by a husband or boyfriend at some time in their life. Millions of children are abused each year; many die of their injuries. As the population ages, mistreatment and neglect of older Americans is a growing problem. Older people are most often abused by a family member, usually one of their adult children who is their primary caregiver. Family violence cuts across all racial, ethnic, religious, educational, and socioeconomic lines.

In response, doctors and other health care professionals, educators, and law enforcement officials are taking steps to help the victims of abuse and stop the pattern of violence. Doctors are learning how to recognize signs of physical, sexual, or emotional abuse in their patients—including children, women, and the elderly—and how to intervene on their behalf. Public education efforts are making people aware of the scope of the problem and what they can do to help the victims of abuse. Mental health experts are uncovering the stresses within a family that may lead to abuse and are developing intervention programs to help defuse those stresses. Organizations, such as local shelters for abused women, are available to provide safety, protection, and other lifesaving and support services to battered women and their children. Stronger laws are making it easier to prosecute offenders.

Sexual assault

Sexual assault is forced or manipulated nonconsensual sexual contact. The term nonconsensual means without mutual consent or agreement. Legally, the crime of sexual assault includes forced vaginal or anal intercourse, oral sex, or penetration with an object. These activities are usually referred to as rape. Sexual assault also includes involuntary sexual contact, such as forced touching and fondling.

Consensual sex occurs between two people who mutually agree to have sex and are both participating. A woman's consent to sex is legally defined as a clear "yes." The fact that she does not fight back, resist an attack, or try to escape does not indicate that she has consented. Rape is never the victim's fault. Rape can occur at any time, anywhere, to anyone—by a stranger or by a family member or acquaintance. Women are at much greater risk of being raped by a person they know—a present or former husband or boyfriend, a date, friend, neighbor, employer, or someone they have just met—than by a total stranger.

THE FACTS ABOUT RAPE

Rape is a crime of violence and aggression; it has nothing to do with sexual seduction or healthy, consensual sex. Consensual sex occurs between two people who mutually and freely agree to it. Rape occurs because an offender (usually a man) chooses to force sex on a victim (usually a woman) in order to feel powerful—to dominate and control. Rape is not the result of sudden, uncontrollable sexual urges stimulated by a woman's appearance or behavior.

A person who rapes is driven by a combination of anger and sexual urges that varies among individual offenders. He may use a weapon or his fists, verbal threats, drugs or alcohol, or physical isolation to overpower his victim. He may take advantage of a woman's smaller size, younger age or lack of experience, or impaired mental capacity (which can result from consumption of alcohol or other drugs, mental illness, developmental disability, or reduced level of consciousness).

Some rapists cause physical harm and are taking revenge on women in general. Others may want to control, punish, or humiliate a woman, or believe they are entitled to sex regardless of what she wants. These men rape when they are in a situation—often on a date—that they see as an opportunity to have sex, usually after they and their date have been drinking alcohol or using other drugs. These men often think they can get away with it and, even after the fact, do not view it as forced sex. Some rapists have fantasies that a woman that they force sex on will fall in love with them. Some rapists are angry at the world in general; others are simply sadistic, cruel people who become sexually aroused by their victim's fears.

Common misconceptions Common misconceptions about rape prevent most women from seeking help after they have been raped. Many think no one will believe them, especially if they were raped by an acquaintance. The legal system has not always been sympathetic to women who were raped; the victims often have been held at least partly responsible for the incident. It is a myth that women invite rape if they dress or act seductively. You have a right to dress or act however you want without having it be interpreted as an invitation for sex.

Being in a man's house, car, or dormitory room does not mean you have agreed to have sex with him. Even if you have previously consented to kissing and touching, you have the right to say "no," to stop at any time, and to have your wishes respected. Even if you have previously had consensual sex with a particular man, you have the right to later refuse to have sex with him. Some men believe that a woman who says "no" to sex really means "yes." It is illegal for a man to have sex with you without a clear indication of your consent. You do not owe sex as a payment to a man who takes you to dinner or a movie. Men do not physically need to have sex after becoming aroused any more than women do. They are able to control themselves; a rapist has chosen not to.

PREVENTING RAPE

You are much more likely to be raped by someone you know than by a stranger. In many cases, a woman has developed a trusting relationship with a person who later rapes her. But you can take measures to help you avoid being raped—by an acquaintance or by a stranger.

Preventing acquaintance rape Acquaintance rape is forced sexual contact with someone you know—such as a friend, neighbor, fellow student, or employer. One of the most important things you can do to decrease your risk of being raped by someone you know casually is to increase your sense of awareness. Be aware of the people around you, their behavior, and what they say. Watch for signs that they may be encroaching on your personal space. The concept of personal space is critical. Set your limits and don't allow your personal space to be invaded. Many women tend to be too polite to casual acquaintances and often hold back for fear of hurting their feelings. Here are some things you can do to reduce your risk of being raped by an acquaintance:

- Do not let people come too close to you physically or allow them to take you to secluded places or areas from which escape would be difficult.
- Tell a person to back off if he is standing too close to you or pretending to accidentally bump into you.
- Do not allow casual acquaintances into your home when you are alone, even if they have an innocent request, such as to use the bathroom.
- Do not get talked into driving a person home if you don't know him well, especially at night or to an area you are unfamiliar with.
- Take notice if a person appears to have been consuming alcohol or drugs.
- Do not use alcohol or other drugs in a way that may impair your judgment or your ability to evaluate and avoid a dangerous situation.
- Be wary of a neighbor who seems too knowledgeable about your activities. Try to avoid the person as much as possible.
- If the comments of a neighbor or coworker become too friendly, such as saying you look sexy or asking about your dating life, tell him firmly that he is overstepping his bounds. If he is a coworker, inform your supervisor. Avoid him as much as possible.

Preventing date rape Date rape is forced sexual contact with a person you are seeing socially. Date rape is most common among women between ages 16 and 24 and occurs frequently on college campuses. It often results from a lack of communication and understanding between men and women and differences in sexual expectations that they learned from their background and culture. At any age, a woman has the right to reject unwanted attention, to change her mind whenever she wants, and to say "no" and have it respected.

Recognizing a potential rapist

It is difficult to recognize a potential rapist. However, if you are dating or have a relationship with a person who has the following characteristics, discontinue the relationship as soon as you can. These are warning signs that this person may harm you and should be avoided:

- He tries to control you. For example, he may tell you who your friends can be or how you should dress.
- He has used physical violence—including grabbing or pushing—against you or others.
- He intimidates you. For example, he may be too familiar with you, sit too close, or touch you even when you ask him not to.
- He gets jealous for no reason.
- He abuses you emotionally. For example, he may insult you with belittling comments or ignore your opinion.
- He talks negatively about women in general.
- He drinks heavily or uses other drugs, or tries to get you intoxicated.
- He criticizes you for not wanting to drink, take other drugs, have sex, or go to an isolated place with him.
- He does not view you as an equal.

The following guidelines may help prevent you from becoming a victim of date rape:

- Establish clear limits in any relationship you have. In a romantic relationship, clearly express what you are willing to do sexually and what you are not willing to do.
- Remain in control. If you drink, do so only in moderation and do not take illegal drugs. Alcohol and other drugs can impair your judgment and your ability to defend yourself from an attack.
- Be aware that your nonverbal actions may send unintended messages; agreement to kiss and touch may be misinterpreted as an invitation to intercourse.
- Be aware that most attacks occur in isolated areas, such as parked cars, apartments, or dormitory rooms. Don't set yourself up for a potentially dangerous situation, especially with someone you don't know very well. Stay with a group of people if you are unsure.
- Pay attention to what is happening around you.
- Trust your instincts. If you feel afraid, get out of the situation quickly. Don't worry about being polite.
- If the person will not take "no" for an answer, shout, scream, fight back, or run away.

Preventing stranger rape Like acquaintance rape, rape by a stranger can occur at any time and any place to anyone. Although you cannot predict when or where a rape might occur, taking the following precautions in your daily life can help reduce your risk:

- Keep the lights on at all the entrances to your home.
- Always keep the doors and windows of your home locked.
- Do not hide your key under the doormat or in any other obvious place.
- If you move into a new house or apartment, change the locks.
- Have a chain or peephole on your door so you can identify all visitors before you open your door. If you do not know the person and are not expecting him, do not open the door. Ask delivery people to leave the item outside, and you can get it later.
- Keep curtains, blinds, and shades drawn at night. Do not get dressed or undressed in front of open windows.
- Before you get into your car, always glance into the back seat to make sure no one is there.
- If you arrive home and suspect someone has broken in, do not go in. Go to a nearby phone and call the police.
- List only your last name on the mailbox or door.
- In an elevator, stand near the buttons. If you are attacked, push as many buttons as you can, including the alarm. If there is a lone, suspicious-looking man in an elevator, do not get on alone.
- Have your keys ready as you approach your car; get in and lock the doors immediately.
- Park in well-lighted areas.
- If your car is disabled, stay inside the car with the windows and doors locked and flasher lights on. Wait for a uniformed police officer.
- If you spend a significant amount of time on the road or commuting, invest in a cellular phone so that you can call for help if you are ever stranded.
- On a bus or train, sit near the driver or conductor and stay awake.
- On the street, stay alert and watch for suspicious-looking people. Walk in a confident manner.
- Walk only in well-lighted areas.
- Do not walk through or near suspicious-looking groups of men; cross the street if necessary.

■ Carry a whistle around your neck or wrist and blow it if you are in danger.
■ Wear flat shoes and unrestrictive clothing when you are out in public so you can run if you need to escape from a threatening situation.
■ If you think you are being followed, head for a populated area.

IF YOU ARE ASSAULTED

It is impossible to know how you would react if you were sexually assaulted. Your actions would depend on the circumstances. Most experts agree that fighting back immediately and trying to run away from an attacker is usually a woman's best defense. However, whatever your response, you should never feel to blame for being sexually assaulted, even if you are unable to fight off your attacker.

Defending yourself Keep in mind that your attacker is motivated, at least in part, by the need to overpower, control, and humiliate you. Scream before the attack begins. If a suspicious-looking person comes toward you, quickly and aggressively shout, "Get away from me!" If you are forceful enough, the would-be attacker may be taken aback and decide to leave you alone.

Sometimes a loud noise, such as a whistle or other alarm, can surprise the attacker enough to make him back off. Seize this opportunity to run. Make a scene and try to attract attention. Get other people's attention by yelling "911!" "Fire!" or "Call the police!" If you choose to carry a weapon, such as a can of pepper spray, you must act quickly and decisively to use it. Make sure you are trained in how to use any weapon you carry. Be aware that your attacker may try to take it away and use it against you.

Physical resistance is usually more successful than verbal resistance alone or no resistance at all, especially if you act immediately. Women who fight hard early in the attack are more likely to escape. Scratch the assailant with your fingernails or keys, jab him hard in the eyes with your fingers, knee him in the groin, or bite his hand or any other part of his body that comes near your mouth. Use whatever is available—a pen, book, or umbrella—to fight back. If he throws you to the ground, kick back quickly and try to prevent him from getting on top of you. Grab a handful of dirt and throw it in his eyes.

If you cannot get away, try talking calmly with your attacker. Try not to show any emotion. Do not cry, plead, or moralize. These responses may be what the attacker wants and may increase his sense of power over you. Do not argue with an assailant or use obscenities, which may escalate the situation. Some women have dissuaded an attacker by telling him they are ill, pregnant, or have their period or a sexually transmitted disease.

If your assailant is armed with a lethal weapon, do everything you can to avoid being forced into a car. He is less likely to use the weapon against you in an open, public area. The vast majority of women who are forced into a car are raped, seriously injured, or killed. In cases of severe physical violence or the threat of death, a wiser strategy may be not to resist but to try to save your life. Giving in is not consenting to have sex; it may be the only way for you to survive the attack. Be alert to things that might help you

Self-defense training

Before you are in a position to have to fight off an attacker, consider taking a course in self-defense. Many community organizations—such as YWCAs, health clubs, rape crisis centers, and hospitals—offer courses or provide information about how to avoid becoming a victim of assault and how to protect yourself during an assault. In addition to teaching you how to recognize dangerous situations, self-defense classes can also help build your confidence, so that you look less vulnerable.

Once you learn self-defense techniques, it is important to practice them enough to be able to use them efficiently and effectively during an attack. You may get only one chance to inflict sufficient injury on an attacker to enable you to escape; being able to recognize that chance and acting immediately can save your life.

If you are raped
If you have been raped, get help immediately.
DO NOT change clothes
DO NOT bathe or shower
DO NOT brush your teeth

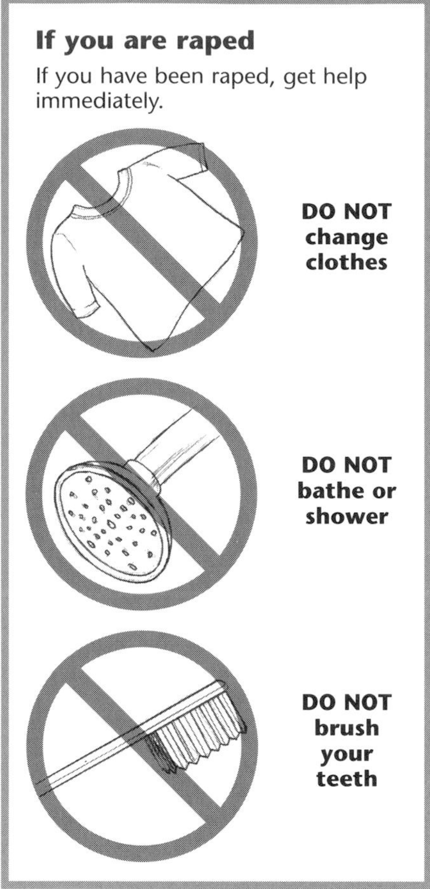

identify the man later. Note his height, hair color, eye color, scars or birthmarks, accent, and clothing.

Getting help after a sexual assault If you have been raped, get help immediately. Do not shower or bathe. Call the police or go to a hospital emergency room or a rape crisis center. Ask a person you trust to be with you during this time to help you and give you emotional support and reassurance.

Seeking medical treatment If you have been raped, seek medical treatment immediately, even if you do not think you have been injured seriously. If your gynecologist's office is near and open, go there. Otherwise, go to the emergency room of a local hospital or to a rape crisis center. The medical personnel in these facilities are usually very understanding and supportive of women in your situation. Many emergency rooms have volunteers who serve as advocates for rape victims. They are available to guide a woman who has been raped through the necessary medical and legal procedures and give her emotional support throughout the process and afterward. Rape crisis centers provide a variety of services, including counseling and help finding experienced legal assistance.

Do not change your clothes, take a shower, or brush your teeth. As much as you would like to bathe, it is important to wait until after the medical examination to avoid washing away evidence of the attack, such as semen from the attacker left in your vagina or on your clothing. This is extremely important evidence. DNA (genetic) analysis of semen, pubic hair, or other body particles can help confirm the identity of a rapist.

You may want to have a friend—or a female nurse or counselor—stay with you during the physical examination. The examination may include undressing while you stand on a white sheet or piece of paper so that any hair, dirt, leaves, or other debris can be collected as evidence. Your underwear and any torn or stained clothing should be kept as evidence. The doctor will scrape under your fingernails for material from the attacker's skin or clothing and comb your pubic hair for further evidence. Your body will be examined for traces of the attacker's sperm, hair, and skin cells, which will be removed and sent to the laboratory for genetic analysis.

After asking your permission, the doctor will perform a pelvic examination (see page 124). He or she will take samples of fluid from your vagina, rectum, and throat to test for semen and sexually transmitted diseases (STDs). He or she may prescribe medication that can prevent you from developing some STDs. However, you will still need to be tested 4 to 6 weeks after the assault because many STDs cannot be detected before then. Photographs will be taken of your injuries and kept with all of your medical records for use in legal proceedings against your assailant, if you decide to press charges. Make sure you get a copy of all your medical records to use as evidence in court.

The chance of becoming pregnant after a rape is small—1 in 100. Nevertheless, your doctor can prescribe medication that will eliminate that possibility completely, unless you were already pregnant before the attack. To be effective, this medication, called the morning-after pill (see page 317), must be taken within 72 hours of the rape. This preventive measure is another good reason not to delay reporting a rape.

Notifying the police Instead of going straight to an emergency room or rape crisis center, you can call the police immediately after the attack. The police usually will take you to a hospital or a rape crisis center.

You may choose not to report the crime to police. However, reporting it can be a positive step for you to take toward emotional healing. You can press charges against the offender, or you can report the crime without pressing charges. A report can at least give police evidence they may need in the future if the offender rapes another woman. Most rapists assault many women before they are convicted and punished. You may be saving another woman's life by reporting your own attack.

Emotional healing If you have been raped, you are dealing with many emotions, including a deep sense of invasion, loss, sadness, and anger. Some women who do not go through the healing process after a rape have symptoms many years later—including anxiety; nightmares; feelings of alienation, isolation, and vulnerability; mistrust of other people; sexual dysfunction; physical problems; and self-blame. In severe cases, women may experience posttraumatic stress disorder (see page 607), a mental disorder that may include recurring, vivid memories or nightmares of the traumatic event, easy startling, emotional numbness, depression (see page 594), or suicidal thoughts.

Although each woman responds in a unique way to being sexually assaulted, most women go through three general stages of emotional healing after a sexual assault. At first, they may feel shock, anger, fear, and numbness. They may withdraw from their usual social interactions and activities. Many women deny to themselves that the rape occurred. During this initial stage, they must decide whether or not to tell family members and friends and whether or not to report the incident to police.

For most women who have been raped, counseling can be helpful. Talking with an experienced doctor or rape counselor and discovering that your feelings are similar to those of other women who have been raped can be reassuring.

The second stage of healing after a sexual assault is outward adjustment. The woman resumes her usual activities, and may seem to be doing well. At this point, she may have pushed the memory of the rape aside but has not yet dealt with all of her feelings. The longer this phase goes on, the more difficult it will be for her to recover completely.

In the last stage of healing, the woman begins to resolve her feelings about the rape in her own mind. During this process, it is common for a woman to change her residence and phone number to avoid possible contact with her attacker (especially if he was an acquaintance). She may now be able to talk about the experience without becoming upset. Learning to face her anxieties and fears enables her to recover from the incident. If she has decided to prosecute the offender, she will need ongoing support from family, friends, and a counselor.

Family violence

When people think about violence, they often think of street crime, such as muggings or murders, which are physical attacks committed by strangers. But most violence is committed in the home by family members—usually by men against their partners. Family violence can also affect children and older family members.

DOMESTIC VIOLENCE

Domestic violence—also called battering, spouse abuse, or partner abuse—is the most common form of family violence and the most common cause of injuries to women that require medical attention. The abuse can take the form of physical, sexual, or emotional mistreatment. The violence usually recurs and

Could your partner be a batterer?

Early signs of domestic abuse can be subtle, progressing gradually from overly controlling behavior to threats and, ultimately, to violence. Initially, some women find their partner's controlling behavior flattering if they are not accustomed to a lot of attention. If you notice any of the following qualities in your partner, he is a potential batterer and you are at risk. It is important to recognize an abusive relationship and get out of it as quickly as possible, before it escalates.

- He imagines that other men are interested in you or that you are interested in other men. He may even be jealous of your relationships with family members or female friends.
- He abuses you verbally; he may frequently disparage you with insults, such as calling you stupid, fat, ugly, or lazy.
- He seems unusually concerned with your whereabouts, activities, and contacts with friends and family.
- He threatens to do something violent to you if you do something he doesn't like.
- When he is angry, he throws things; damages your possessions; or threatens to hurt you, your pets, or even your children.
- He uses force—such as pushing, shoving, or restraining you—during an argument.
- He blames you for his anger or violence.
- After a violent episode he promises it won't happen again, says he loves you, or buys you gifts, but repeats the behavior another day.

escalates over time. Battering occurs among people of all racial, ethnic, educational, and socioeconomic groups.

Recognizing abusive behavior A woman is a victim of abuse if her spouse or partner has harmed her physically, using physical force, or mentally, using threats or intimidation. Battering can include throwing objects, pushing, hitting, slapping, kicking, choking, beating, or attacking with a weapon, including dangerous household objects. Many batterers hit their partner in areas of the body that are usually covered by clothing so that bruises and scars will not be noticed.

In some cases, an abuser never actually hits his partner, but takes extreme measures to control her behavior—such as monitoring her phone calls and mail and limiting her contact with friends or family members. He may prevent his partner from getting a job; limit her access to medical care; or deprive her of money, food, clothing, or transportation. This type of emotional abuse can include actions such as destroying the woman's possessions or harming or killing her pets.

Men who abuse their partners are more likely to have witnessed or experienced abuse or violence themselves during their childhood. Many abusers have low self-esteem and a lack of confidence that surface as violent behavior at home. In many cases, a batterer appears to be a respectable member of the community who has a good job and provides well for his family. Episodes of violence are often triggered by the use of alcohol or other drugs that reduce inhibitions and suppress a person's ability to control his or her impulses.

Sexual abuse can be one of the most devastating forms of domestic violence and one that is difficult for women to discuss. Sexual abuse includes forcing a partner to perform sexual activities against her will; flaunting affairs outside the relationship; or preventing a woman from using birth control or protecting herself against sexually transmitted diseases, including HIV, the virus that causes AIDS.

If a friend is at risk of abuse Many women who are victims of abuse find it extremely difficult to talk about their situation.

They may stay in an abusive relationship for a variety of reasons. A woman who experienced physical or sexual abuse as a child, or witnessed domestic violence, may have a difficult time recognizing a relationship as abusive or taking steps to protect herself. Low self-esteem may make a woman believe she is to blame for the abuse.

She may still love her partner and want desperately for the relationship to work. She feels that, if she changes, things will improve. Some women, for religious or moral reasons, believe that families should stay together at all cost. Economic pressures, concerns about children, and a desire to protect an abuser make it difficult for many women to leave abusive relationships.

If you know that a friend or family member is being abused, approach her in a gentle, supportive way. Let her know that she is not to blame for the situation and that you are there for her if she needs you. Give her the telephone number of a domestic violence hotline. Do not encourage her to stay in the situation and try to make it work. Such attempts at reconciliation rarely work in violent relationships. However, you should not pressure her to leave if she does not feel ready; and do not make her ending of the relationship a condition of your friendship.

Look for the following signs if you suspect that a friend or family member may be in an abusive situation:

- Does she offer a variety of excuses (such as claiming to be accident-prone) for why she has frequent injuries, including black eyes, bruises, or broken bones? Does she avoid seeking medical treatment for her injuries? If she does go to the doctor for these injuries, does her partner always accompany her?
- Does her partner seem to exert an unusual amount of control over her activities, the family finances, the way she dresses, and her contact with friends and family?
- Does her partner seem overprotective, speaking for her and making decisions for her?
- Does her partner ridicule or insult her publicly?
- Have you noticed changes in her behavior or her children's behavior? Does she appear frightened, exhausted, or on edge? Do her children become upset easily?

Getting help For many battered women, leaving the relationship and breaking the cycle of violence is extremely difficult, especially if their abuser is excessively controlling. Many batterers threaten to kill their partner if she tries to leave. In many cases, a woman's leaving triggers an escalation of the violence if the abuser tracks her down.

The important first step in breaking the pattern of abuse is to ask for help from someone you trust, such as a friend or family member, your doctor, a nurse, social worker, or member of the clergy. You may find it difficult to publicly acknowledge the violence in your home because of feelings of shame, fear, and humiliation. But discussing your situation with another person makes it less threatening. It is important for you to

Effects of domestic violence on children

Children are profoundly influenced by any violence they witness at home. The majority of children whose mothers are battered are themselves hurt both physically and emotionally. The stress of domestic violence can disrupt a child's eating and sleeping patterns and cause physical problems, such as headaches or frequent abdominal pain. It can trigger regressive behaviors such as thumb sucking or bed-wetting, or make a child overly aggressive and difficult to control or unusually passive and withdrawn. A decline in school performance is common.

Children from violent homes often experience depression, anxiety, fear, and guilt. They may blame themselves for the violence or feel helpless to stop it. They may come to view violence as an effective way to resolve conflicts and problems. They are at increased risk of juvenile delinquency and abuse of alcohol and other drugs. If you are in an abusive situation and you have children, getting out of the situation is essential for the safety, health, and well-being of your children as well as yourself.

understand that the violence is not your fault and you have a right to be safe. Domestic violence is a crime, and other people can help you (and your children) get out of danger.

Most communities provide services to help women who are victims of domestic violence. Look for brochures, posters, or other materials that describe the services that are available in your community, or try the following:

- Look in the white or yellow pages of your phone book for a domestic violence shelter, women's shelter, shelter for battered or abused women, or domestic violence hotline. Keep the numbers handy (in a secret place) so you can use them immediately in an emergency.
- Call your community or county government information and referral office, mental health agency, or human services division and ask for the name, address, and phone number of the nearest program for battered women.
- Contact your state coalition or task force on domestic violence and request information.
- Call a local hospital emergency room and ask about programs that can help you.

Even if you have not decided to leave your abuser, you can call a battered women's shelter or hotline for advice and counseling. Shelters and hotlines are staffed by people who are very knowledgeable and concerned about your welfare and that of your children. Domestic violence counselors will not tell you what to do or make decisions for you, but they will give you information and support to help you make the best possible decisions for you and your family.

Counselors can help arrange for a place for you (and your children) to stay in case you need to leave home quickly. It might be the home of a friend or family member or a local shelter for battered women. In addition to providing you with a safe space, food, and clothing, a shelter will provide care for your children; work with the police and the criminal justice system; act as your advocate in obtaining services from other agencies and organizations; help you obtain emergency medical attention; assist you in finding permanent housing, job training, and employment; and inform you of support groups and counseling services for both you and your children. A shelter can also help you get an order of protection (see page 725), a written court order designed to protect you from further abuse.

Breaking the cycle of violence Ultimately, you will need to make some decisions about resolving your situation. You may decide to help your partner get treatment for his violent behavior and try to work things out. It is difficult but possible for some violent men to change. Individual psychotherapy (see page 194) with a qualified mental health professional, such as a psychiatrist, can be useful for both of you. Your partner will probably need therapy to help him understand the reasons for his behavior and to learn how to change it. You may need therapy to help you regain control of your life and build your self-esteem and confidence. Marriage or couples therapy is not recommended until after the violence has been absent from the relationship for a long time.

Although it may seem impossible to leave your abusive relationship, many women in your situation have done so and are leading happy, productive lives. You do not deserve to be abused or live in constant fear of being harmed. Learn to recognize the warning signs of a violent episode so that you can escape before it escalates. Have a plan for leaving home quickly (with your children) as soon as you notice signs of impending danger. Here are some steps you can take to develop a plan of action to escape from harm:

- Be prepared; know ahead of time where you will go. Make arrangements with a local shelter for battered women, a hotel, or a friend, neighbor, or family member. Explain that you are likely to show up unexpectedly.
- Pack a suitcase in advance and store it with a friend or neighbor in case you have to leave in a hurry. Include clothing and toilet articles for yourself and your children, an extra set of keys to the house and car, and some cash. Pack a special toy for each child.
- Keep the following items in an easy-to-locate but safe place (remember, you may not be coming back immediately, or you may decide to stay away permanently): medical prescriptions for you and your children and important documents such as birth certificates, social security cards, driver's license, the titles to your car and

house, and mortgage or rent receipts. Have cash available and a checkbook or extra checks and credit cards if possible.

■ If you are hurt, call 911, go to the emergency room immediately, or call your doctor once you are safe. When you see your doctor, tell him or her exactly how you were injured. Ask for a copy of the medical record to give to the police if you decide to press charges against your partner.

■ Call the police. Physical assault is a crime—even if you are living with or married to the abuser. Police forces in many communities have female officers who are specially trained to help women who have been abused. Most states have improved the legal options—including orders of protection—that are available to battered women.

Seeking medical treatment If you are a victim of domestic violence, talk to your doctor. Doctors can recognize the signs of physical abuse and they can help you. A doctor first will treat your immediate problem or injuries. He or she may recommend that you have testing and counseling for sexually transmitted diseases (see chapter 12), prescribe medication to help relieve depression or anxiety, or recommend counseling by a mental health professional (see page 194).

Together, you and your doctor will design a follow-up treatment and evaluation program. The success of this program depends on your taking an active role in making decisions and helping to develop the treatment plan. If your trauma is preventing you from getting the medical examinations and tests you need, discuss it with your doctor. Initially, you may feel more comfortable having a close friend or relative accompany you and stay with you during any medical procedures.

A doctor can reassure you and encourage you to seek further help when you feel you are ready and able to do so. Many doctors provide lists of local resources for victims of domestic violence, including counseling services, crisis intervention services, shelters, support groups of other victims of sexual assault, and legal groups.

Getting legal help Along with providing medical treatment, your doctor will also provide appropriate follow-up during any legal proceedings. If you acknowledge that you are a victim of battering, your doctor will ask whether or not you want the police to be notified. Depending on the laws in your state and the seriousness of your injuries, your doctor may be required to report the crime to the police. However, both your doctor and the police are required to ensure your safety. They will work with you to evaluate whether or not you are in immediate danger and in need of emergency shelter or other resources.

In many states, reporting a sexual crime assault does not mean that the victim will have to go to court, see the assailant again, or testify at a trial. In some states, the police will keep on file a record of the assailant's name, if it is known, and details of the crime. If he assaults the woman again and she chooses to press charges, these records may be helpful in the prosecution. Make sure you ask for a copy of the medical report in case you decide to press charges against your partner or seek an order of protection.

If you fear that your abuser may harm you or your children, hire a lawyer who has experience handling cases of battering. Ask for information about legal assistance from a shelter or domestic violence hotline. You may be able to get legal assistance at a relatively low cost by using a legal assistance foundation (look it up in your yellow pages under "attorneys"). Ask your lawyer to file an order of protection on your behalf, or you can seek an order of protection on your own.

An order of protection is a very important remedy for women who have been abused. It is a written court order, signed by a judge, that forbids or requires certain actions by an abusive family or household member. For example, an order of protection can prohibit a batterer from committing further abuse; prohibit him from entering your shared home for a period of time or from entering or remaining present at your school, place of employment, or other specified place when you are present; or require that he have counseling with a qualified mental health professional. The police are legally responsible for enforcing an order of protection.

Once you have an order of protection, which can last for up to 2 years (as determined by a judge), you should get several copies of the document and keep one with you at all times. If your abuser violates any condition of the order, call the police immediately. Show them a copy of the order (or they can check with police records). If the police find evidence that the order of protection was violated, they will arrest the abuser. The police will also assist you by providing transportation to a hospital, if necessary, or to a safe place such as the home of a relative or friend or a shelter.

CHILD ABUSE

Violence in the home frequently extends to children. Child abuse is a growing problem in the US. Child abuse includes neglect, physical abuse, emotional abuse, and sexual abuse. Girls are more likely to be sexually abused than boys. Child abuse occurs in all racial, ethnic, educational, and socioeconomic groups. The abuser is usually someone who provides care for the child—including a biological parent, adoptive parent, foster parent, grandparent, sibling, other relative, or a neighbor or friend.

Physical abuse and neglect Child abuse occurs most often in families that are under stress, which can result from problems such as loss of a job, financial difficulties, marital conflicts, abuse of alcohol or other drugs, or mental illness. Families that are socially isolated and lack strong support systems are also vulnerable to child abuse. Many adults who abuse their children were themselves abused as children. The psychological and physical effects of abuse on a child can be severe and long lasting. Abuse can affect the development of a child's brain, intellect, and personality, and can influence his or her behavior and emotions throughout his or her life.

Recognizing signs of abuse Many cases of child abuse go unnoticed and unreported. The only way to get help for a child who is a victim of abuse is to be aware of the signs of abuse, including the following:

- Repeated injuries with implausible explanations of the cause
- Injuries that leave scars that resemble cigarette burns or marks from an electrical cord, especially in areas of the body that are very sensitive, such as the genitals, nipples, and face
- Behavior problems—behavior that is either passive and withdrawn or hyperactive and aggressive
- Reticence or fear when asked about life at home
- Self-destructive, delinquent, or reckless behaviors, such as substance abuse, crime, or running away from home

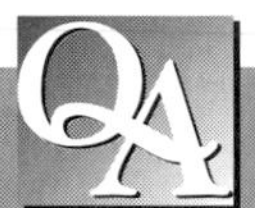

QUESTIONS WOMEN ASK
CHILD ABUSE

Q Is an abused child likely to become an abuser as an adult?

A It is possible, but the chances are small. Although the majority of child abusers were abused or neglected as children, most abused children do not grow up to be abusers themselves. Many come to recognize the destructiveness of such behavior and do not want to repeat the pattern. For many people who were abused as children, psychotherapy (see page 194) can help them resolve their feelings about their childhood.

Q How can I teach my children about sexual abuse without scaring them?

A Teach your children the difference between good, or OK, touching and bad touching. Friendly hugs or pats on the back are examples of OK touching. Bad touching includes feeling private parts (areas covered by a bathing suit) as well as touching (such as kissing or rubbing) anywhere on their body that makes them feel uncomfortable. Reinforce the idea with your children that their body is their private zone and that no one may touch them without their permission.

WARNING SIGNS
SEXUAL ABUSE

Be alert to the following signs of possible sexual abuse in your child:

- Bruising, redness, swelling, discharge, or other signs of injury in the rectal or genital area
- Regressive behavior, such as bed-wetting, thumb sucking, or excessive clinging
- Frequent nightmares or fearfulness
- An increase in hostile or aggressive behavior
- Withdrawal from friends, family, or school activities
- Provocative, promiscuous, or sexually precocious behavior

- Low self-esteem
- Learning problems and lack of motivation in school
- Neglected appearance
- No desire to make friends or invite them home
- Depression
- Suicide attempts

Getting help Any parent can make mistakes in judgment that may look like abuse to someone outside the family. If you are concerned that a child you know is a victim of abuse, do not directly confront the person you suspect of abuse. Contact one of the local service agencies that can provide help for the child and the family. These agencies—local child protective service agencies, welfare departments or social service agencies, public health authorities, or the police—will respect the legal and confidentiality rights of the family.

If you are abusing your child or you think you might be at risk of doing so, talk to your doctor, a member of the clergy, or a school counselor (if you are a teen mother), or join a support group of people in similar situations. Your community is likely to have many effective intervention and prevention programs, such as those described below, to help you learn positive parenting skills.

Preventing child abuse The causes of child abuse and neglect are complex and differ from family to family. Both children and parents need help. The most effective way to prevent or reduce child abuse is for at-risk children and families to participate in intervention and prevention programs that help them develop the skills for finding practical solutions to serious family problems. Many such programs are available in communities across the country to provide the information and support necessary to help strengthen family life and enhance the growth and development of children.

Some of these programs focus on health care; home health visitors go to a family's home to give parents and children emotional support, teach them about health, and provide prenatal care for at-risk pregnant women and their unborn children. Community-based programs provide services to troubled families such as self-help and support groups, child-care programs, and educational programs for latchkey children to help reduce their emotional and physical risks. These programs also work with parents to educate them about the far-reaching negative effects that child abuse and neglect can have on their children. Many employers are initiating programs to help employees cope with the challenges of parenthood. These employer efforts include flexible work schedules and benefits, parent education programs, parental leave policies, and employer-supported child-care facilities.

Many school-based programs help children develop positive coping skills to help them deal successfully with the challenges of childhood and adolescence. Such programs often include self-protection training to enable children to protect themselves from abuse and to seek appropriate help if they are abused. Classes in family living can give children and adolescents skills for coping with family problems in a positive way.

Children who are abused or who grow up in violent homes are more likely to see violence as an effective way to resolve problems. Many schools have counselors and social workers who work with abused children to try to prevent them from becoming abusers themselves. Counselors teach abused children that they are not responsible for the violence in their home (most abused children blame themselves) and encourage them to express their feelings in healthy, respectful ways.

Sexual abuse Physical contact, such as hugging, is an essential part of human development. Children need it to achieve healthy emotional and intellectual growth. All children have natural sexual responses. Boys have erections from infancy on and both boys and girls get pleasant feelings from touching their own genitals. Some children seek sexual contact with their peers at an early age, exploring each other's genitals or "playing doctor."

However, children do not seek out sexual contact with adults. If your child describes any sexual experience or genital contact with an adult or older child, you should be immediately concerned that he or she is a victim of sexual abuse. Sexual abuse can include fondling, undressing, looking at or photographing the child nude, or any other activity that gives the person in control sexual gratification.

A person who sexually abuses a child is usually a male member of the extended family—father, stepfather, brother, stepbrother, uncle, grandfather, or mother's boyfriend. In most cases, the abuser has had enough contact with the child to gain the child's trust and the trust of other family members, who are comfortable leaving the child alone with him.

A child sex abuser does not have to be an adult. A growing percentage of abusers are now under the age of 16. They may be going through puberty and becoming curious about sex and decide to experiment with a younger child who has been temporarily placed under their supervision. The victim is often a stepsister, half-sister, cousin, or neighbor for whom the sex abuser has volunteered to babysit.

Divorce and changing social customs have altered the traditional structure of the family. Increasing numbers of children grow up in households with minimal supervision because both parents work. They often live with older children whose relationship to them is not clearly defined. In these situations, the possibility of sexual abuse by an older child against a younger one is greater.

Preventing sexual abuse To reduce the risk that your children will be victims of sexual abuse, make sure they understand which parts of their body are private (the area covered by a bathing suit) and should not be touched by anyone except a doctor during a physical examination or (for very young children) by a parent or caregiver during washing or bathing. They need to know that unwanted touching by anyone, either within or outside the family, is unacceptable. Begin this education as early as possible.

Maintain an open, honest, and forgiving relationship with your children so they will feel free to tell you immediately of any improper sexual or physical contact from others. Let your children know they can tell you anything without having to worry about being blamed or punished for it or harmed by someone else. Sexual abusers frequently coerce children into secrecy by threatening to hurt them, the people they love, or their pets. If your child tells you about a possibly abusive situation, make sure you make it clear to the child that you believe him or her.

Getting help If you suspect your child may have been sexually abused, get help immediately. Call your pediatrician or contact the police, a social worker, or a school guidance counselor. Do not hesitate to contact local authorities. Most child abusers have abused many more than one child. Bringing a sex offender to justice may prevent the same thing from happening to other children.

Long-term consequences Child abuse can have serious, long-term consequences for a child. Children who were abused by their own parents are often the most severely affected later in life. Abuse by a parent usually begins earlier than abuse by someone else. The child usually has no one to turn to because the parent is the person who would normally be his or her major source of protection.

Many abused children develop a condition called posttraumatic stress disorder (see page 607). They experience symptoms such as irritability and sleep problems (including nightmares). They may have frequent flashbacks (vivid memories) of their experience and physical symptoms when they are exposed to reminders of it. Many people with posttraumatic stress disorder become emotionally numb; they may avoid showing their feelings or developing relationships with others. Many women who were sexually abused as children have difficulties developing healthy relationships with men.

Childhood sexual abuse can also have later adverse effects on a person's health.

Women who were sexually abused as children often begin smoking at a young age and are more likely to abuse alcohol and other drugs. They are at greater risk of obesity or eating disorders, such as anorexia (see page 114) or bulimia (see page 610). They are likely to begin having sex earlier in life and to have more sexual partners than other women, which puts them at increased risk of early pregnancy, sexually transmitted diseases (see chapter 12), pelvic inflammatory disease (PID; see page 232), infertility (see page 382), and cervical cancer (see page 250).

Many of these women put their health at further risk by not having annual pelvic examinations (see page 124) to test for sexually transmitted diseases and other reproductive disorders, and Pap smears (see page 127) to test for cervical cancer. If you were sexually abused as a child, it is essential to have these examinations regularly. Establish a relationship with a gynecologist or other doctor you trust and tell him or her about your past experience. Counseling may help you sort through your experiences and learn how to build trusting, healthy relationships in your adult life.

ELDER ABUSE

Each year, as many as 2 million older Americans may be victims of some form of long-term or temporary abuse or neglect, usually by a caregiver, such as an adult child or the child's spouse. Abuse of older people, called elder abuse, can involve physical abuse, verbal intimidation, exploitation (such as mishandling of financial resources or property), medical neglect (such as withholding necessary medications or treatment or devices such as false teeth, eyeglasses, hearing aids, or walkers), or physical neglect or abandonment. Elder abuse frequently goes unreported, but it affects people of all racial, ethnic, educational, and socioeconomic groups.

Most people who are victims of elder abuse live with the abuser because they are too frail or ill to live on their own. In some cases, the abuser is financially dependent on the person. For example, the older person may own the home they are living in together or pay most of the expenses. The majority of abused older people are women, although older men are also victims of abuse.

Recognizing elder abuse Elder abuse is difficult to detect because the victim is often confined to home and does not visit places, such as local senior centers, where other people might notice signs of abuse (such as bruises). Because many older people have frequent contact with their doctor, the medical profession has established guidelines to help doctors recognize, treat, and prevent abuse and neglect in their older patients. They can intervene by contacting local social service agencies, government services, or police or other authorities.

Even if a doctor recognizes a problem, in some cases, the person may not want the abuse to be reported to authorities. Their pride may be injured by public acknowledgment of their abuse; they may fear retaliation, isolation, or abandonment; they may be afraid of being moved to a nursing home; or they may have a sense of guilt or responsibility toward the abuser. A doctor can talk to the person, try to determine if he or she is willing to seek or accept help, and perhaps encourage the person to do so.

Be alert to the following warning signs of possible abuse in your older friends and relatives:

Signs of physical or emotional abuse or neglect:

- Unexplained burns, bruises, cuts, or scars
- Frequent falls
- Noticeable fear of caregiver
- Withdrawal; isolation
- Lack of responsiveness
- Agitation; anxiety
- Confusion; disorientation
- Depression
- Anger
- Poor hygiene
- Bedsores
- Unexplained weight loss or malnutrition
- Lethargy
- Changes in personality

Signs of financial exploitation:

- Mismanagement of person's assets
- Diversion of the person's income
- Withdrawal of funds against the person's will
- Withdrawal of funds without the person's permission

Getting help If you think a person you know is being abused or exploited, try to help him or her. Keep in touch with your friends and relatives who are dependent on caregivers. Ask how they are doing. If you sense that something is wrong, visit them. If you cannot reach them by phone, make an impromptu visit. If for some reason you are not allowed to see your friend or family member, ask about his or her condition and try to visit another day. Keep trying. If you have an elderly neighbor whom you have not seen in some time, ask a family member about his or her health. Ask to see the person on the spur of the moment or show up unexpectedly with the excuse of bringing him or her a small gift, such as a book or flowers.

If all attempts to see your friend or relative fail, or if, when you do see him or her, you suspect that something is wrong, consider reporting it to the local protective services agency. A local senior center or senior citizens agency can give you information about where to call for help. You should be able to provide the person's name and address, the nature of the suspected abuse, and the names of other people who may have knowledge of the situation. Tell the agency how best to contact the person you think is being abused. Your identity will be kept confidential.

Index

B

C

E

F

G

H

J

K

L

M

P

Q

R

U

V

W

X

Y

Z